Flexible Bronchoscopy
（4th Edition）

可弯曲支气管镜技术
（第4版）

主 编　〔美〕王国本（Ko-Pen Wang）
　　　　〔美〕阿图尔·C.梅塔（Atul C. Mehta）
　　　　〔美〕J.弗兰克斯·特纳, Jr.（J. Francis Turner, Jr.）

主 译　黄海东　董宇超　白　冲

上海科学普及出版社

著作权合同登记号：图字：09-2023-1125

图书在版编目（CIP）数据

可弯曲支气管镜技术：第 4 版 /（美）王国本（Ko-Pen Wang），（美）阿图尔·C. 梅塔（Atul C. Mehta），（美）J. 弗兰克斯·特纳，Jr.（J. Francis Turner, Jr.）主编；黄海东，董宇超，白冲主译 . -- 上海：上海科学普及出版社，2025.6. -- ISBN 978-7-5427-8819-1

I. R768.1

中国国家版本馆 CIP 数据核字第 2025YM1062 号

This edition first published 2020 © 2020 by John Wiley & Sons Ltd.
Edition History [3e, 2012]
　　All rights reserved. No part of this publication may be reproduced, stored in a retrieval system, or transmitted, in any form or by any means, electronic, mechanical, photocopying, recording or otherwise, except as permitted by law. Advice on how to obtain permission to reuse material from this title is available at http://www.wiley.com/go/permissions.
　　The right of Ko - Pen Wang, Atul C. Mehta, and J. Francis Turner, Jr. be identified as the authors of editorial work has been asserted in accordance with law.

责任编辑　李　蕾

可弯曲支气管镜技术（第 4 版）

（美）王国本（Ko-Pen Wang）（美）阿图尔·C. 梅塔（Atul C. Mehta）
（美）J. 弗兰克斯·特纳，Jr.（J. Francis Turner, Jr.）　主编
黄海东　董宇超　白　冲　主译
上海科学普及出版社出版发行
（上海中山北路 832 号　邮政编码 200070）
http://www.pspsh.com

各地新华书店经销　广东虎彩云印刷有限公司印刷
开本 787×1092　1/16　印张 25.75　字数 600 000
2025 年 6 月第 1 版　2025 年 6 月第 1 次印刷

ISBN 978-7-5427-8819-1　定价：168.00 元

译者名单

主 审

李 强 同济大学附属东方医院

主 译

黄海东 董宇超 白 冲

副主译

田 森 胥武剑 刘庆华

主译助理

张艺菲 方 晨

译 者（按姓氏拼音排序）

白 冲 海军军医大学第一附属医院
陈 慧 海军军医大学第一附属医院
陈来娟 浙江大学医学院附属第二医院
陈 婷 浙江大学医学院附属第二医院
陈 巍 上海交通大学医学院附属瑞金医院
陈 愉 广州医科大学附属第一医院
邓常文 同济大学附属东方医院
董宇超 海军军医大学第一附属医院
方 晨 海军军医大学第一附属医院
顾 晔 同济大学附属上海市肺科医院
官振标 海军军医大学第一附属医院
侯 刚 中日友好医院
黄海东 海军军医大学第一附属医院
黄 怡 海军军医大学第一附属医院
焦 洋 海军军医大学第一附属医院
柯明耀 厦门医学院附属第二医院

林　欢	海军军医大学第一附属医院
刘庆华	同济大学附属东方医院
马　静	山东大学附属儿童医院
秦　浩	海军军医大学第一附属医院
石　荟	海军军医大学第一附属医院
孙加源	上海市胸科医院／上海交通大学医学院附属胸科医院
田　森	联勤保障部队第906医院
王　俊	海军军医大学第一附属医院
王绮霞	广州医科大学附属第一医院
王　琴	海军军医大学第一附属医院
温梓键	广州医科大学附属第一医院
吴晓东	同济大学附属东方医院
夏　旸	浙江大学医学院附属第二医院
熊　叶	中国医学科学院阜外医院
胥武剑	同济大学附属东方医院
徐冬阳	上海市胸科医院／上海交通大学医学院附属胸科医院
徐　浩	浙江大学医学院附属第二医院
徐逸铧	广州医科大学附属第一医院
许　菲	应急总医院
杨宇光	海军军医大学第一附属医院
游振锭	广州医科大学附属第一医院
曾俊莉	厦门医学院附属第二医院
张　楠	应急总医院
张　伟	海军军医大学第一附属医院
张艺菲	海军军医大学第一附属医院
郑筱轩	上海交通大学医学院附属胸科医院
郑　宇	上海交通大学医学院附属仁济医院
钟长镐	广州医科大学附属第一医院
周国武	中日友好医院
周凌霄	浙江大学医学院附属第二医院
朱敏辉	海军军医大学第一附属医院
朱　莹	解放军总医院

编者名单

Jason Akulian, MD, MPH
Section of Interventional Pulmonology
Division of Pulmonary and Critical Care Medicine
University of North Carolina at Chapel Hill
Chapel Hill, NC, USA

Chong Bai, MD, PhD
Respiratory and Critical Care Medicine
Changhai Hospital
Second Military Hospital
Shanghai, China

Swati Baveja, MBBS
Division of Pulmonary and Critical Care Medicine
University of Tennessee Graduate School of Medicine
Knoxville, TN, USA

Heinrich D. Becker, MD
Formerly Department of Interdisiplinary Endoscopy
Thoraxclinic at Heidelberg University
Heidelberg, Germany

Ben Bevill, MD
Division of Pulmonary and Critical Care Medicine
University of Tennessee Graduate School of Medicine
Knoxville, TN, USA

Semra Bilaceroglu, MD
Izmir Dr Suat Seren Training and Research Hospital for Thoracic Medicine and Surgery
Health Sciences University
Izmir, Turkey

Martina Bonifazi, MD
Department of Biomedical Sciences and Public Health
Università Politecnica delle Marche, Ancona;
Pulmonary Diseases Unit
Department of Internal Medicine
Azienda Ospedaliero-Universitaria 'Ospedali Riuniti'
Ancona, Italy

Robert F. Browning Jr., MD, FACP, FCCP
Interventional Pulmonology
Walter Reed National Military Medical Center, Bethesda;
Uniformed Services University of Health Sciences
Bethesda, MD, USA

Eric R. Carlson, DMD, MD, FACS
Department of Oral and Maxillofacial Surgery
University of Tennessee Medical Center University of Tennessee Cancer Institute
Knoxville, TN, USA

Alexander Chen, MD
Division of Pulmonary and Critical Care
Washington University School of Medicine
St Louis, MO, USA

Ara A. Chrissian, MD
Pulmonary and Critical Care
Loma Linda University
Loma Linda, CA, USA

David Feller-Kopman, MD
Interventional Pulmonology
Division of Pulmonary and Critical Care Medicine
Johns Hopkins University School of Medicine
Baltimore, MD, USA

Erik E. Folch, MD, MSc
Division of Pulmonary and Critical Care Medicine
Massachusetts General Hospital
Boston, MA, USA

Stefano Gasparini, MD, FCCP
Department of Biomedical Sciences and Public Health
Universita Politecnica delle Marche
Ancona; and
Pulmonary Diseases Unit
Department of Internal Medicine
Azienda Ospedaliero-Universitaria 'spedali Riuniti'
Ancona, Italy

Thomas R. Gildea, MD, MS, FCCP
Department of Pulmonary
Allergy and Critical Care Medicine
Respiratory Institute
Cleveland Clinic
Cleveland, OH, USA

Sarah Hadique, MD
Department of Pulmonary and Critical Care Medicine
West Virginia University
Morgantown, WV, USA

Richard Helmers, MD
Mayo Clinic Health System
Eau Claire, WI, USA

Wolfgang Hohenforst-Schmidt, MD
Sana Clinic Group Franken
Department of Cardiology/Pulmonology/Intensive Care/Nephrology
"Hof" Clinics
University of Erlangen
Hof, Germany

Hai-dong Huang, MD
Shanghai Changhai Hospital
Shanghai, China

Yi Huang, MD
Shanghai Changhai Hospital
Shanghai, China

Takeo Inoue, MD
Division of Respiratory Medicine
Department of Internal Medicine
St Marianna University School of Medicine
Kawasaki, Japan

Takeshi Isobe, MD
Division of Medical Oncology and Respiratory Medicine
Department of Internal Medicine
Shimane University Hospital
Izumo, Japan

Prasoon Jain, MD, FCCP
Louis A. Johnson VA Medical Center
Clarksburg, WV, USA

Michael A. Jantz, MD
Division of Pulmonary, Critical Care, and Sleep Medicine
University of Florida
Gainesville, FL, USA

Mani S. Kavuru, MD
Division of Pulmonary and Critical Care Medicine
Jefferson Center for Critical Care
Thomas Jefferson University and Hospital
Philadelphia, PA, USA

Ming-yao Ke, MD
Department of the Respiratory Centre
Second Affiliated Hospital of XiaMen Medical College
Xiamen, Fujian, China

Danai Khemasuwan, MD, MBA
Tufts University School of Medicine and
St Elizabeth's Medical Center
Boston, MA, USA

Noriaki Kurimoto, MD
Division of Medical Oncology and Respiratory Medicine
Department of Internal Medicine
Shimane University Hospital
Izumo, Japan

Jonathan S. Kurman, MD
Division of Pulmonary and Critical Care
Department of Medicine
Medical College of Wisconsin
Milwaukee, WI, USA

Stephen C.T. Lam, MD, FCCP
Department of Integrative Oncology
British Columbia Cancer Agency
Vancouver, British Columbia;
Cancer Imaging Department and
Department of Medicine
University of British Columbia
Vancouver, British Columbia, Canada

Carlos Aravena Leon, MD
Department of Pulmonary
Allergy and Critical Care Medicine
Respiratory Institute
Cleveland Clinic
Cleveland, OH, USA;
Department of Respiratory Diseases
Faculty of Medicine
Pontificia Universidad Catolica de Chile
Santiago, Chile

Qiang Li, MD
Department of Respiratory and Critical Care Medicine
Shanghai East Hospital
Tongji University School of Medicine
Shanghai, China

Xicheng Liu, MD
Department of Interventional Pulmonology
Beijing Children's Hospital
Capital University of Medicine
Beijing, China

Jing Ma, MD
Department of Interventional Pulmonology
Qilu Children's Hospital of Shandong University
Jinan, China

Samir Makani, MD
Division of Pulmonary and Critical Care Medicine Henry Ford Hospital
Detroit, MI, USA

Sean McKay, MD
Interventional Pulmonology
Walter Reed National Military Medical Center
Uniformed Services University of Health Sciences
Bethesda, MD, USA

Atul C. Mehta, MD, FACP, FCCP
Professor of Medicine
Lerner College of Medicine
Buoncore Family Endowed Chair in Lung Transplantation
Department of Pulmonary Medicine
Respiratory Institute
Cleveland Clinic
Cleveland, OH, USA

Chen Meng, MD
Department of Interventional Pulmonology
Qilu Children's Hospital of Shandong University
Jinan, China

Teruomi Miyazawa, MD, PhD, FCCP
Division of Respiratory Medicine
Department of Internal Medicine
St Marianna University School of Medicine
Kawasaki, Japan

Blake A. Moore, MD
Section on Cardiothoracic Anesthesia
University of Tennessee Graduate School of Medicine
Knoxville, TN, USA

Septimiu D. Murgu, MD
Department of Medicine
Section of Pulmonary and Critical Care
University of Chicago
Chicago, IL, USA

Renelle Myers, MD, FRCPC
Department of Integrative Oncology
British Columbia Cancer Agency
Vancouver, British Columbia;
Department of Medicine
University of British Columbia
Vancouver, British Columbia, Canada

David E. Ost, MD, MPH, FACP
Division of Internal Medicine
Department of Pulmonary Medicine
MD Anderson Cancer Center
University of Texas
Houston, TX, USA

Luca Paoletti, MD
Division of Pulmonary and Critical Care Medicine
Medical University of South Carolina
Charleston, SC, USA

Nicholas J. Pastis Jr., MD, FCCP
Division of Pulmonary and Critical Care Medicine
Medical University of South Carolina
Charleston, SC, USA

Sunit R. Patel, MD
Medical Group
Trulock, CA, USA

Andrew Pattison, MD
Division of Thoracic Surgery
Toronto General Hospital
University Health Network
University of Toronto
Toronto, Ontario, Canada

Alexander S. Rabin, MD
Department of Pulmonary and Critical Care Medicine
Massachusetts General Hospital
Boston, MA, USA

Ali Sadoughi, MD
Division of Pulmonary and Critical Care
Albert Einstein College of Medicine/Montefiore Medical Center
New York, USA

Ala Eddin Sagar, MD
Banner MD Anderson Cancer Center
Phoenix, AZ, USA

Thomas Schlieve, DDS, MD
Division of Oral and Maxillofacial Surgery
University of Texas Southwestern Medical School
Parkland Memorial Hospital
Dallas, TX, USA

Michael J. Simoff, MD, FCCP
Division of Pulmonary and Critical Care Medicine Henry Ford Hospital
Detroit, MI, USA

J. Francis Turner, Jr., MD, FACP, FCCP, FCCM
Division of Pulmonary and Critical Care Medicine
University of Tennessee Graduate School of Medicine
Knoxville, TN;
National Supercomputing Institute
University of Nevada
Las Vegas, NV, USA

Ko-Pen Wang, MD
Division of Pulmonary and Critical Care Medicine
Johns Hopkins Bayview Medical Center
Johns Hopkins University School of Medicine
Baltimore, MD, USA

Wei Zhang, MD
Shanghai Changhai Hospital
Shanghai, China

Yang Xia, MD
Division of Pulmonary and Critical Care Medicine
Second Affiliated Hospital of Zhejiang University School of Medicine
Hangzhou, China

Kazuhiro Yasufuku, MD, PhD
Division of Thoracic Surgery
Toronto General Hospital
University Health Network
University of Toronto
Toronto, Ontario, Canada

Shunying Zhao, MD
Department of Interventional Pulmonology
Beijing Children's Hospital
Capital University of Medicine
Beijing, China

Guo-wu Zhou, MD, PhD
Respiratory and Critical Care Medicine
Changhai Hospital
Second Military Hospital
Shanghai;
Respiratory and Critical Care Medicine
China-Japan Friendship Hospital
Beijing, China

中文版序言一

欣闻由王国本教授、阿图尔·C.梅塔教授和J.弗兰克斯·特纳,Jr.教授共同主编的《可弯曲支气管镜技术》(第4版)中文版即将面世。应主译黄海东教授的邀请,欣然接受撰写此序的任务。

本书的三位主编均是中国介入呼吸病学界的老朋友,他们多次来过中国,尤其是王国本教授,在过去的30多年间,来华次数不下几十次。从最初的示教、帮扶,到后来的规范和引领,可以说以他们为代表的一大批国外专家,为中国可弯曲支气管镜技术的临床应用、普及以及介入呼吸病临床诊疗体系的建立做出了重要贡献。因此,我们可以说他们三位都是中国介入呼吸病学建设和发展的主要贡献者。同时,他们也是中国介入呼吸病学发展的见证者,亲眼目睹了中国介入呼吸病学从无到有、从小到大、由弱变强的发展历程。在此,我谨代表所有从事介入呼吸病学的同仁,向该书的三位主编及所有为中国介入呼吸病学发展给予过关心、支持和帮助的国际友人表示深深的感谢!

正如王国本教授在前言里所言,为了提升《可弯曲支气管镜技术》(第4版)的临床参考价值,主编们在第3版的基础上,增加了部分支气管镜技术用于处理临床常见病症的相关内容,极大地丰富了本书的内涵。同时,主编们还特意邀请了部分中国介入呼吸病学领域的专家参与本书英文版原著的撰写。通过这一合作,大家有机会深入了解国际同行的严谨治学态度,学习他们在临床技术创新方面的先进经验,同时也向世界展示了中国专家的临床经验和技术创新成果。这对于加深国际同行间的交流与合作,共同推动学科的发展具有重要意义。

回顾支气管镜的发展历程,从硬质支气管镜到可弯曲支气管镜,再到近年兴起的支气管镜机器人技术,每一次设备迭代和技术革新,都离不开一批又一批专业人士的大胆探索和不懈努力。正是这份对医学的热爱和对技术的精益求精,推动了介入呼吸病学的不断向前发展。

作为第一代中国介入呼吸病学界的一员,我欣喜地看到在众多同行的共同努力下,一个具有中国特色的经支气管、经皮、经血管以及经消化道的"大介入呼吸病学临床诊疗体系"理念已在呼吸学界深入人心,并在众多大型教学医院得以落地并实践。我们完全有理由相信,随着这一体系的建立,将为我国现代呼吸病学的高水平发展提供有力支撑。衷心期望中青年学者能从本书中吸取更多的知识养分,立足于当前介入呼吸病学的发展阶段,思考如何将前沿科学的新技术、新理念融入介入呼吸病学的发展中,为呼吸病患者的临床诊治提供重要支撑,同时也为未来我国介入呼吸病学的发展贡献力量。

衷心感谢英文版的三位主编以及所有作者为世界介入呼吸病学界奉献了这样一本宝贵且值得研读的专著。同时,也感谢国内为中文版翻译工作付出辛勤努力的译者和编辑人员。谢谢大家!

2024年12月17日于上海

中文版序言二

拿到《可弯曲支气管镜技术》(第 4 版)的翻译稿,王国本教授嘱我为该书作序,我诚惶诚恐。再次细读全文,追今抚昔,思绪万千。在认真梳理思路后,我归纳了以下三点体会。

首先,掌握支气管镜技术必须要有理论指导。支气管镜技术操作性非常强,是科学和艺术的完美结合。以往,我们多是通过"师傅带徒弟"的方式手把手地教和学。我从事介入支气管镜操作已有 30 多年的时间,先后师从刘忠令教授和王国本教授,基本上掌握了所有的操作技术。我个人体会最深的是,要真正全面地掌握这项技术,必须通过系统的理论学习,尤其要精读一两本经典专著。通过系统学习,我们才能对整个学科的各项技术和操作细节有所了解,做到融会贯通。而《可弯曲支气管镜技术》(第 4 版)汇聚了国际上许多专家的经验和智慧,也包括很多教训。通过学习研读该书,我们可以真正全面掌握支气管镜技术,也可以避免重蹈覆辙。

其次,对支气管镜技术必须与时俱进。我与该书的主编王国本、梅塔、特纳三位教授相识多年,王教授于我而言,更是亦师亦友。他每年奔波于中国、美国以及世界各地,传授支气管镜技术。最令我敬佩的是,王教授始终如一、孜孜以求地学习新技术和新方法,绝不墨守成规、故步自封。王教授曾对我说:"对于一项新技术,只有当你能够熟练掌握了这项技术,并成为这方面的顶级专家之时,你才有资格去评价这项技术。"我分别在 2008 年和 2019 年两次到美国霍普金斯医院,跟随王教授学习介入支气管镜技术,第一次学习 EBUS-TBNA 和激光技术,第二次学习肺外周导航技术。近几年,各项支气管镜技术都处于飞速发展的过程中,我们必须抱着认真的态度去学习。而《可弯曲支气管镜技术》(第 4 版)中有很多新的观念、新的知识,以及新的作者,他们不断地把自己的经验和成果介绍给我们,所以本书的内容远远超出了以往几版。

第三,在探索支气管镜技术的过程中,付出的努力一定会有收获。我和黄海东教授都曾是《可弯曲支气管镜技术》第 1 版、第 2 版的读者,后来成为了第 3 版的译者,到第 4 版时,我们和国内很多优秀的同道一起,已经加入到这本书的编写团队中,成为了作者。这个从读者到译者,再到作者的过程,其实也真正体现了我们这批从事支气管镜技术的同道对学问孜孜不倦的追求,而同道们所做出的贡献也为大家所认可。同时,我们也希望通过这本书,将我们所做的这些工作和收获能够播散出去,使更多的读者受益。所以,你今天可能是这本书的读者,但如果你能够在这个行业中默默耕耘、不断探索,未来你也可以成为这方面的专家、成为作者。非常欣喜的是,本书已有 11 位国内专家参与了撰写,近 50 名国内学者参与了翻译工作,他们都是呼吸介入诊疗方面的翘楚。尤其是黄海东教授、方晨大夫和张艺菲技师,在本书的撰写、翻译过程中倾注了大量的心血,使《可弯曲支气管镜技术》(第 4 版)能够顺利出版,在此一并表示感谢。

再次感谢所有热爱呼吸介入、从事呼吸介入的同道们。

2024 年 11 月

《可弯曲支气管镜技术》（第4版）序言

非常荣幸能为《可弯曲支气管镜技术》（第4版）作序，本书是众多呼吸内镜专家们共同努力的结晶。

采用支气管镜技术，我们可以获取肺部病原及病理组织，开展各种镜下介入治疗。这项技术不仅是一种重要的获取诊断和开展镜下治疗的方法，也是肺部疾病微创诊治技术的最佳选择。现代支气管镜技术诞生于100多年前，自1897年Gustav Killian医生使用硬质支气管镜开始，直至1964年Shigeto Ikeda教授设计和参与研发了可弯曲支气管镜后，支气管镜技术得以持续稳定地发展。自20世纪70年代开始，随着呼吸内镜领域的开拓者们对于支气管镜技术更深入的研究，我们实现了介入呼吸病亚专科的高速发展。

在本书中，我们邀请了全球呼吸内镜领域资深专家们介绍先进的支气管镜技术及进展，如Heinrich Becker、Teruomi Miyazawa、Kazuhiro Yasufuku教授等，他们分享了超声支气管镜相关技术以及器械的发展和使用，介绍了可弯曲支气管镜淋巴结穿刺技术和肺癌分期的经支气管穿刺针；本书也介绍了如François Dumon教授开创性的工作和气道硅酮支架相关内容。这些全球知名专家及其发明，在介入呼吸病领域都起着举足轻重的作用。本书还涵盖了支气管镜的基础技术，如内镜麻醉、硬质支气管镜技术和支气管镜肺活检技术，以及超声支气管镜技术、导航支气管镜技术等，对临床常用的治疗性支气管镜操作提出了规范化诊疗建议。例如，"热"消融技术（如激光、高频电凝、氩等离子体凝固术）和"冷"消融技术（如喷雾冷冻技术）。

随着支气管镜技术和介入呼吸病亚专科的日趋成熟，让支气管镜技术以更加高效、安全和经济的方式蓬勃发展是未来的发展方向之一。此外，考虑到许多原有成熟的内镜诊疗技术在良恶性疾病的诊断、分期方面仍然起着十分重要的作用，对于新技术的推广应用及其价值，我们仍需要进行非常严谨的科学论证。

我们非常荣幸可以通过支气管镜技术对罹患胸部疾病的患者们提供极大的帮助。我们也希望本书作者们所分享的支气管镜技术、智慧和热情，能够助力您在职业生涯中脱颖而出，并能更好地为患者提供最佳医疗照护。

阿图尔·C.梅塔

J.弗兰克斯·特纳,Jr.

《可弯曲支气管镜技术》（第4版）前言

自1964年池田茂人教授发明可弯曲支气管镜以来，历经60年，支气管镜技术已经实现了从光纤到机器人支气管镜的跨越式发展。相关诊疗技术的不断发展和迭代，使得可弯曲支气管镜技术为基础的介入呼吸病学迅速向系统化、专业化和亚专科方向推进。目前，介入呼吸病已成为呼吸与危重症医学的重要亚学科，而支气管镜技术也成为全球从事呼吸系统疾病各亚专科方向专业医师必须掌握的临床诊疗技术。鉴于此，我们再次以极大的热忱推出了《可弯曲支气管镜技术》（第4版）。

在章节编排上，我们改变了第3版的偏向诊断性和治疗性操作的技术介绍，在此基础上，第4版将围绕常见气道疾病（如良性气道狭窄、慢性气道疾病和气道瘘等）的支气管镜下诊治策略展开介绍。此外，我们增加了6个章节的内容，丰富了相关学科领域的介绍，旨在让不同阶段的支气管镜从业者都能从中获益。

经过30余年技术的全球化推广和普及，我们力求在第4版中展现更多的国际化特色，我们邀请了来自美国、中国、日本、加拿大、德国、意大利和土耳其等8个国家的共58名全球知名专家参与撰写。我们欣喜地见证了中国介入呼吸病学的快速发展和蓬勃态势，中国已经实现了支气管镜技术从追赶到赶超的转变。因此，我们高兴地邀请了来自中国的13名介入呼吸病专家共同完成本书部分章节的撰写，旨在让更多的中国支气管镜技术跃入全球视野，让更多的中国介入呼吸病专家融入国际介入呼吸病的大家庭。

在各项可弯曲支气管镜技术蓬勃发展之时，我们仍然建议同道们循着支气管镜发展的轨迹，回顾其被接受和发展的历程。因为只有深刻理解其历史和发展脉络，同时具备坚持不懈和永不言弃的执着信念，才能真正掌握和开拓支气管镜这一门科学和艺术。技术创新是介入呼吸病发展的动力源泉，但我们必须强调，技术创新是在原有技术基础上进一步优化和改进。本书介绍的一些具有里程碑意义的支气管镜技术，将潜移默化地增进同道们对可弯曲支气管镜技术的深入理解。

池田教授曾提出这样的哲学观点："吾必以吾之最佳精神力量和永不放弃之生活信念，竭尽吾之所能地工作，来服务大众。"同样在今天，我们仍然倡导医学的终极目标是为我们的患者提供优质的服务。

我们希望《可弯曲支气管镜技术》（第4版）能够帮助同道们更好地理解可弯曲支气管镜技术以及池田教授在追求支气管病学这一门科学和艺术过程中所展现的永不放弃的精神。

阿图尔·C.梅塔

J.弗兰克斯·特纳, Jr.

（黄海东 译）

目 录

第 1 章　可弯曲支气管镜发展简史 ··· 1

第 2 章　可弯曲支气管镜技术培训 ··· 18

第 3 章　气道实用解剖学 ·· 24

第 4 章　支气管镜室的感染控制及放射安全 ··· 30

第 5 章　可弯曲支气管镜诊断和治疗的麻醉管理 ··· 54

第 6 章　可弯曲支气管镜的适应证和禁忌证 ··· 68

第 7 章　径向探头超声技术在可弯曲支气管镜中的应用 ··· 87

第 8 章　凸阵扫描超声支气管镜在可弯曲支气管镜中的应用 ··· 94

第 9 章　光学成像技术在肺癌早期诊断中的应用 ··· 108

第 10 章　电磁导航支气管镜 ··· 117

第 11 章　虚拟支气管镜导航 ··· 131

第 12 章　间接喉镜 ··· 137

第 13 章　气道病变的支气管镜检查 ·· 150

第 14 章　支气管肺泡灌洗术 ··· 154

第 15 章　支气管镜肺活检术 ··· 174

第 16 章　经支气管针吸活检术获取细胞学和组织学标本 ··· 185

第 17 章　支气管肺癌的分期 ··· 211

第 18 章　介入肺脏病学的未来 ··· 221

第 19 章　可弯曲支气管镜下的激光、电凝、氩等离子体凝固术及冷冻治疗 ··················· 228

第 20 章　可弯曲支气管镜技术在支气管腔内近距离放射治疗、标记物定位、射频消融和微波消融中的应用 ·· 241

第 21 章　气道异物吸入与可弯曲支气管镜技术 ··· 268

第 22 章　支气管镜在咯血中的应用 ·· 279

第 23 章　气道支架 ··· 295

第 24 章　球囊扩张支气管成形术 ·· 319

第 25 章　硬质支气管镜技术 ··· 325

第 26 章	儿科可弯曲支气管镜	334
第 27 章	可弯曲支气管镜在重症监护室中的应用	345
第 28 章	支气管热成形术治疗哮喘	353
第 29 章	肺气肿的内镜下治疗	363
第 30 章	支气管胸膜瘘的内镜管理	373
第 31 章	良性气道狭窄和气管支气管软化症的临床诊疗	383
附录	本书配套视频资源汇总	397

第 1 章

可弯曲支气管镜发展简史

Heinrich D. Becker
Department of Interdisiplinary Endoscopy, Thoraxclinic at Heidelberg University,
Heidelberg, Germany

（译者：林 欢 黄海东 译者单位：海军军医大学第一附属医院）

支气管镜技术问世至今已有70余年的历史，可弯曲纤维支气管镜的问世标志着支气管镜技术翻开了新的篇章。未来支气管镜技术也将在可弯曲纤维支气管镜这一里程碑上取得进一步的发展。

（池田茂人[1]）

1.1 引言

大量著作介绍了支气管镜检查的历史。在这一章节中将给大家介绍从第一个可弯曲支气管镜原型机逐步发展至今的过程，以及从纤维支气管镜，到电子支气管镜，进而到超声支气管镜，和最新的机器人可弯曲支气管镜演变的关键步骤。辅助技术的引入进一步扩展了可弯曲支气管镜在临床诊断和治疗中应用的范围，目前可弯曲支气管镜已成为肺部医学中不可或缺的工具。下面笔者将阐述在不断变化的概念和技术环境中，有计划或偶然地寻找解决方案的驱动下，如何将新技术与现有技术融合，从而产生全新的概念和策略。这些例子包括早期和晚期肺癌、中央气道阻塞、孤立性肺结节（solitary pulmonary nodules，SPN）、肺实质疾病、肺气肿和哮喘。最后，本文将基于目前可弯曲支气管镜的发展现状展望可弯曲支气管镜的未来。

1.2 池田茂人与可弯曲支气管镜的发明

1897年，Gustav Killian使用硬质支气管镜观察气道，在随后的70年，硬质支气管镜一直是观察气道的标准设备。由于硬质支气管镜的操作相对复杂，需要特殊的技巧，还需要全身麻醉。因此，其应用主要局限于耳鼻喉科、胸外科和专科肺科中心。直到池田茂人在1967年引入可弯曲支气管镜之后，支气管镜技术才广泛传播到世界各地的医学中心。

池田茂人生于1925年（图1.1）。高中毕业后，自1944年起就读于庆应大学学习医学。然而，他因罹患特异性胸膜炎接受了外科胸廓成形术不得不休学一年。康复以后，他于1952年毕业。但同年，他在结核外科实习期间因罹患结核而再次进行肺切除术。自此，他开始潜心研究支气管解剖结构，包括支气管造影及动态成像技术。为了解决硬质支气管镜顶端的电灯泡照明效果欠佳的问题，1962年，他设计了一台带有"冷光"的镜子，将玻璃纤维束的一端连接到500 W的氙气光源上，另一端连接到透视镜上，这为观察图像和拍摄照片提供了足够的照明。

受限于解剖结构，当时的硬镜对两肺上叶支气管进行检查通常比较困难。因此，人们觉得很有必要发明一种可弯曲的支气管镜，它的灵感来自于1961年Basil Hirshowitz提出的纤维胃肠道镜的概念，临床中尚缺

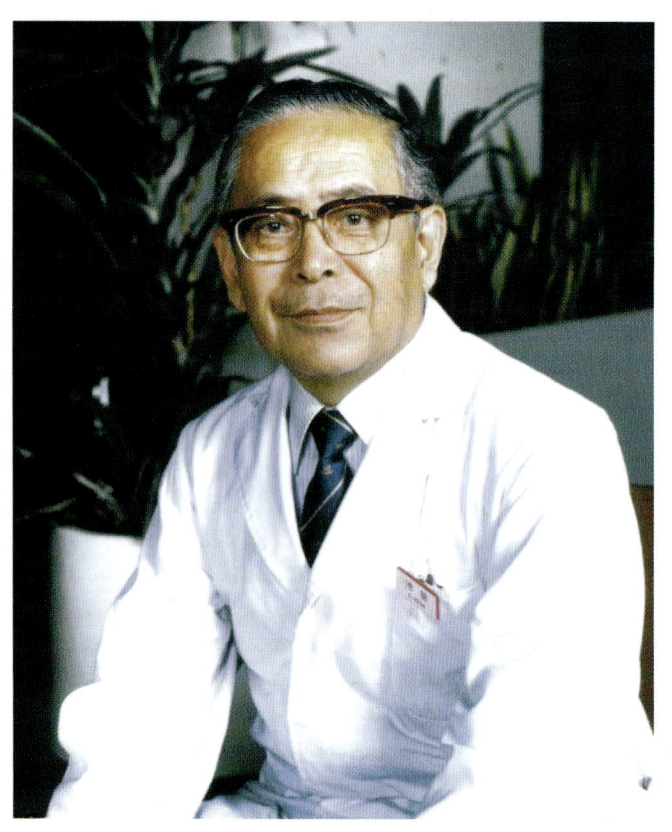

图 1.1 池田茂人（1925—2001 年）

乏一种灵活的支气管镜[2,3]。1962 年，町田公司和奥林巴斯光学公司在日本生产了第一台纤维胃镜。为了制造支气管镜原型机，池田茂人于 1964 年和町田公司、1965 年和奥林巴斯公司合作，对可弯曲支气管镜的光纤直径、数量、光导灵活度、先端部定长（<1 cm）、气管镜长度（1 m）、定焦（0.5~3 cm）、视角（80°）、顶端屈曲度（60°）等方面提出了具体要求。他还设计了一种特殊的半硬质的经口气管插管，拉直后应用于气管插管后使用硬质活检钳获取组织（图 1.2）。

1966 年，池田茂人在丹麦哥本哈根举行的第九届国际胸部疾病大会上展示第一个可弯曲支气管镜原型机时，引起了巨大的轰动并被《纽约时报》报道。后续他对原型机做了进一步的改进：增加了用于旋转和插入端弯曲的控制部分，用规则排列更细的玻璃纤维来改进成像，并且在插入端配备了透镜（图 1.3）。他在第 7 版设计模型中，增加了一个可以用于采样的工作通道，并将其整合到了支气管镜里。此时，池田茂人才认为这个版本的可弯曲纤维支气管镜可以商业化生产并在全球范围内推广使用了。

在接下来的几年里，可弯曲纤维支气管镜的临床应用经验越来越多，到 1980 年纤维支气管镜检查已经成为一种常规检查方法，并在全球范围内推广。1980 年，池田的团队在马赛访问了 Dumon 后，开始使用激光和光动力疗法（photodynamic therapy，PDT）对恶性肿瘤进行治疗。为了获得更好的图像分辨率，池田与朝日宾得公司一起引入了电荷耦合器件（charge-

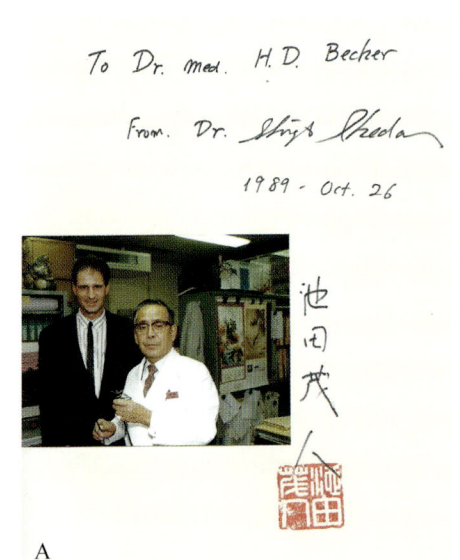
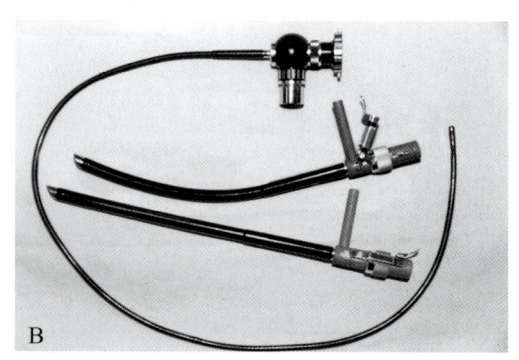

图 1.2 池田茂人与可弯曲支气管镜

A. 作者访问日本时，与池田茂人合影，池田茂人展示了首个支气管镜（他是左利手者，这就是光源连接线和可弯曲支气管镜吸引器设置向左延伸的原因，故支气管镜的控制部分和连接线部分易于左手操作）；B. 首个可弯曲支气管镜，设置有特殊的经口气管插管，气管插管可以在置入硬质活检钳时保持伸直状态。

coupled device，CCD）芯片技术，并开发了第一台电子内镜，这台电子内镜最终被万田-东芝和奥林巴斯公司生产出来。为了促进可弯曲纤维支气管镜检查技术的发展，池田茂人遍访世界各地，并于1978年成立了世界支气管病学协会（WAB），即现在的世界支气管和介入呼吸病学协会（WABIP），将各个国家和欧洲大陆的相关机构联合了起来。

为了表彰他的杰出成就，池田茂人获得了许多日本国内和国际奖项。1991年，他虽然因退休辞去了临床和学术任职，但仍对支气管镜技术的发展保持着浓厚的兴趣并与众多科学协会保持密切联系。晚年的池田茂人虽然因数次中风和心脏病发作而身体虚弱，但正如其毕生的座右铭"永不放弃"所形容的那样（图1.4），他直至2001年去世前仍坚持参加了所有的学术会议[1,4-8]。

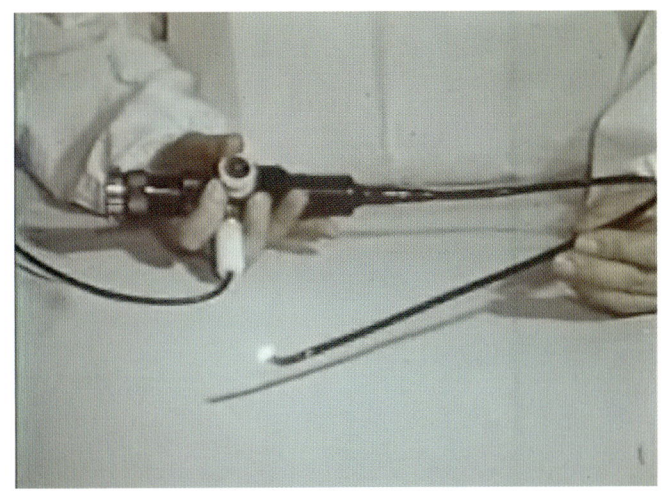

图1.3　首个可弯曲纤维支气管镜的影片截图

详见视频1.1。资料来源：白川方明提供。

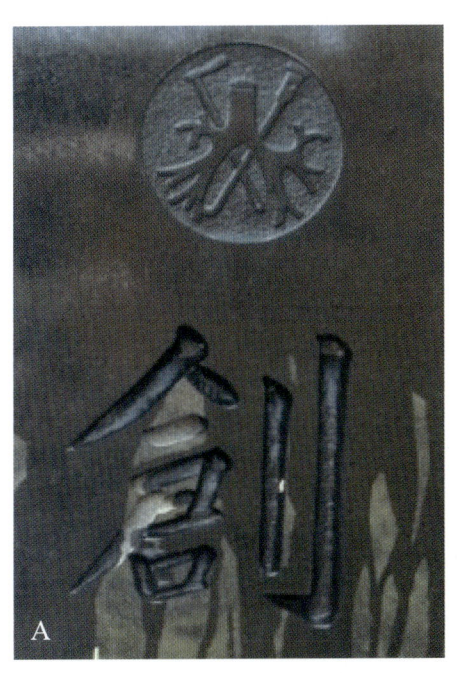
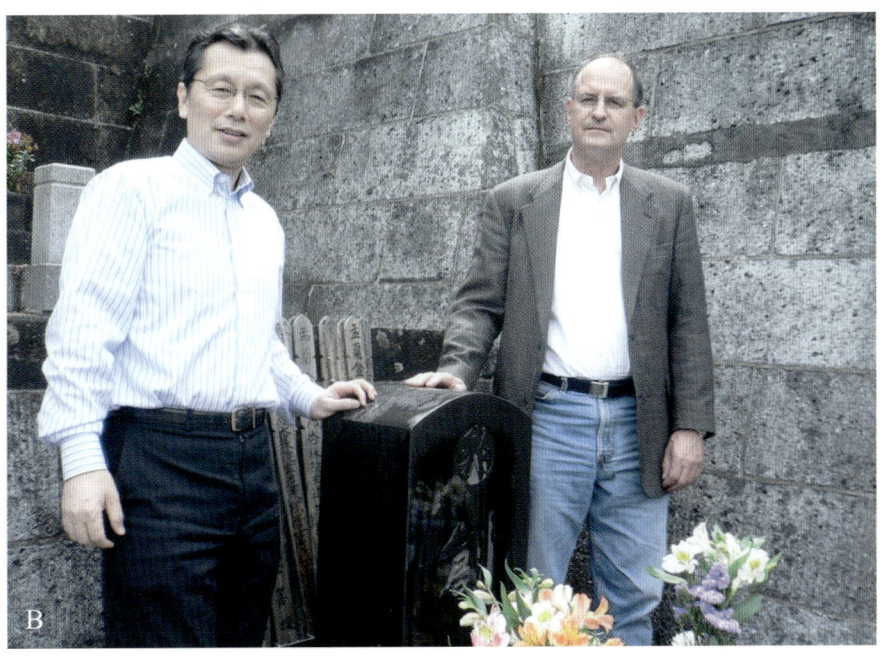

图1.4　池田茂人墓

A. 墓碑上印有WAB的会徽，会徽下方的铭文为"创造"；B. 本文作者（右）和宫泽泰美（左）在池田茂人墓前的合影。

视频1.1　具有弯曲和旋转功能的可弯曲支气管镜

1.3　可弯曲支气管镜的发展

起初，町田和奥林巴斯是仅有的两家可弯曲纤维支气管镜制造商，但很快日本、美国和欧洲的其他公司开始进入市场，如今已有约20家公司。由于奥林巴斯拥有最广泛的分销网络，它仍是主要的设备供应商。随着操作者使用纤维支气管镜经验的增加，同时其他学科，如麻醉科、儿科和重症医学科，也认识到这项新技术的重要价值，临床上使用支气管镜进行特殊诊治的需求也随之增加。

影像技术和治疗技术的进步推动了可弯曲支气管镜的发展。改良后的纤维支气管镜相继进入市场，市场上

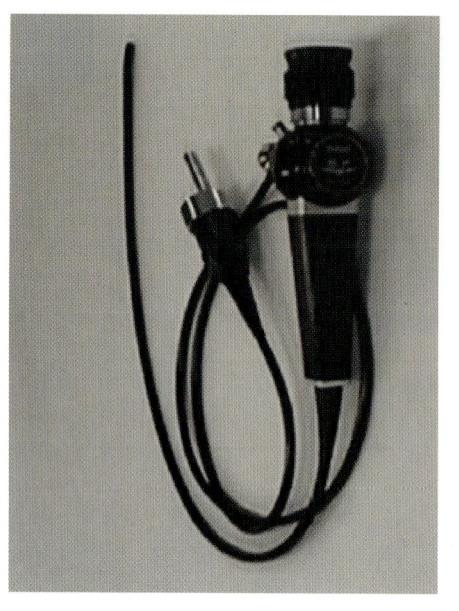
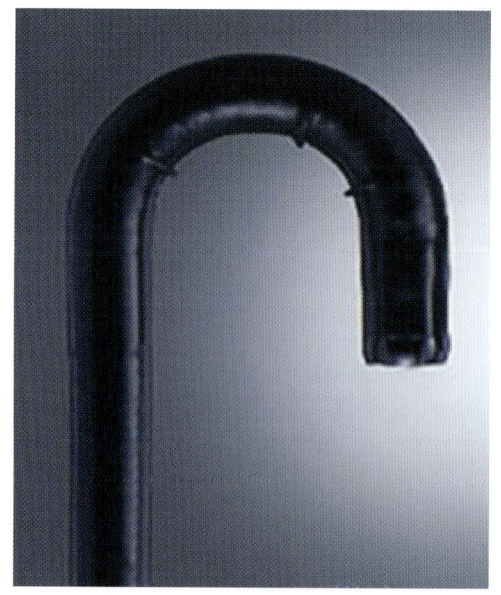
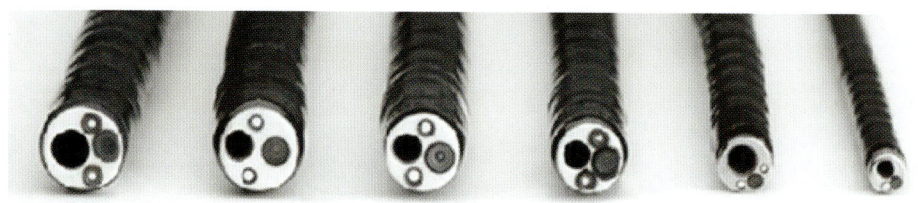

图 1.5 具有不同外径和活检通道的现代可弯曲支气管镜

已有外径从 2.2 mm 到 6 mm 不等的用于肺外周气道和儿科的可弯曲支气管镜（图 1.5）。最近，外径不到 1 mm 的小型支气管镜已经被制造出来，目前正处于动物实验研究阶段。如今，临床上有多种支气管镜可以选择，比如用于治疗性操作的工作通道直径为 3 mm 的支气管镜和针对肺外周病变的工作通道直径为 1.2 mm 的支气管镜。纤维光学技术的进步有利于医生更好地观察细微结构和记录影像。为了便于教学，操作者可使用安装有教学附件的支气管镜（教学内镜），而带有电池照明和交互式监视器的便携式光纤镜也适用于 ICU、睡眠实验室、病房和门诊部。

1987 年，宾得公司推出了电子支气管镜，其使用微型化的 CCD 芯片替代原有的光学纤维，CCD 被整合到可弯曲支气管镜插入端的末端[9]（图 1.6）。通过视频处理器，可以在监视器上观察动态图像，将其存储在胶片和数据库中并打印出来。同时，这些数据可以整合到报告中，并能在线发送给其他科室。CCD 最大的优势是可以根据颜色、轮廓增强、放大倍数和不同的光源优化影像资料，既可以直接整合到报告中，也可以在网上传递给其他部门对图像进行处理。得益于 CCD，现

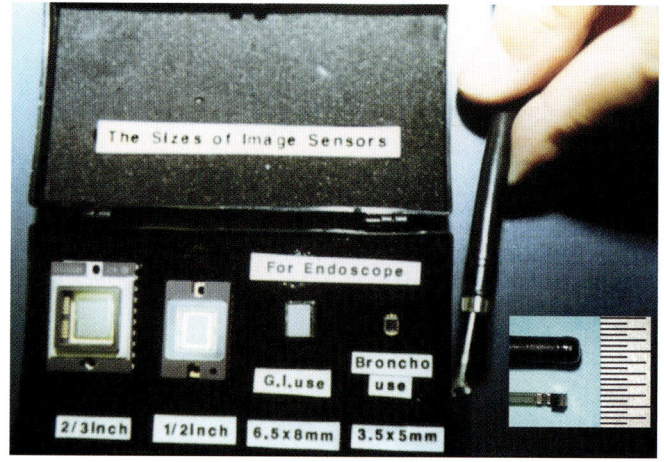

图 1.6 内窥镜 CCD 芯片

在的可视支气管镜可以连接高清电视（high definition television，HDTV），从而获得高分辨率的图像。在外径很小的可弯曲支气管镜中，CCD 被整合到可弯曲支气管镜的控制位置，进而通过纤维光镜技术把光纤图像传输到处理器，即 Hybird 镜。

1996 年，支气管腔内超声（endobronchial ultrsound，

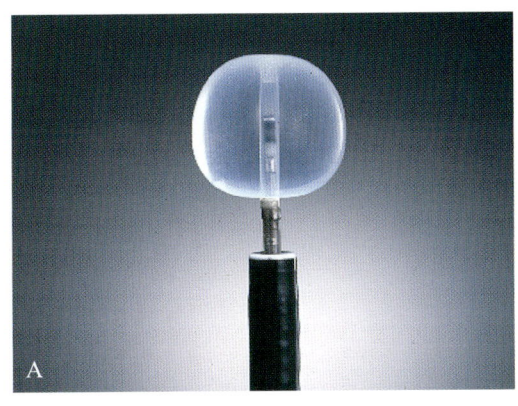 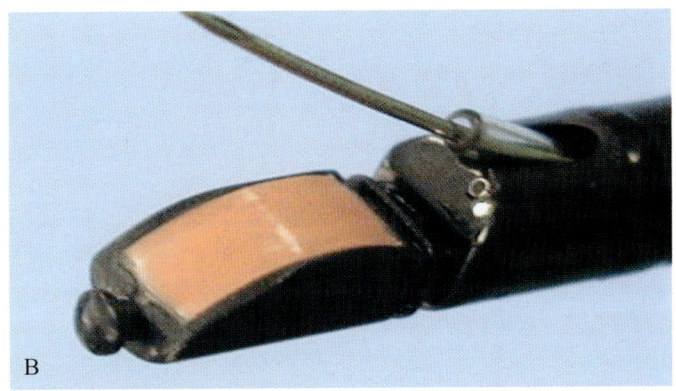

图 1.7　支气管腔内径向超声探头和超声支气管镜

A. 插入可弯曲支气管镜工作通道的径向微型腔内径向超声探头；B. 超声支气管镜（也被称为凸阵扫描超声支气管镜）。

EBUS）的引入扩大了支气管镜医师的视野，使可弯曲支气管镜的检查范围超出了气管管腔和内表面。1999年，微型腔内径向超声探头问世，该探头可以通过可弯曲支气管镜的工作通道插入支气管的远端[10]。随着操作者对实时经支气管镜针吸活检术（transbronchial needle aspiration，TBNA）的需求不断增加，2002年生产出第一台专用超声支气管镜[11]（图1.7）。如今，EBUS-TBNA已成为纵隔肿瘤分期的标准检查方式，支气管腔内径向超声也是肺外周病变的标准检查方式。"EBUS技术是几十年来最有用的肺部检查方法，适用于所有需要评估的胸廓内不明原因肿大淋巴结的患者"（Kevin L. Kovitz）。

可弯曲支气管镜最新的革命性突破是机器人支气管镜的引入。为了使支气管镜技术不依赖于操作者个体的操作技能并保持准确性，已开发出的机器人支气管镜具有更好的柔性和稳定性，可以通过遥控器将工具准确地送达肺外周病灶。2018年笔者的前同事Jose Rojas-Solano等发表了一篇关于首台机器人支气管镜临床应用的论文（Monarch®，Auris Surgical Robotics Inc.）[12]（图1.8）。除了Monarch®，另一个机器人平台是Intuitive Surgical, Inc.的Ion™系统。

消毒是可弯曲支气管镜常见的问题，因为细小的工作通道存在交叉感染风险[13]。由于很少有光学系统可以承受高压灭菌的过程，现已开发出一次性支气管镜[14]。复用型支气管镜的成本—效益已在ICU中进行了评估，尽管有许多不可预测的因素，但总体而言是利大于弊的。目前，从可弯曲支气管镜广泛的临床应用上看，一次性支气管镜的市场份额不太可能超过30%。对此，唯一切实可行的解决办法是严格遵守卫生指南对器械进行高水平消毒。

随着科技的进步，支气管镜技术已成为肺部医学

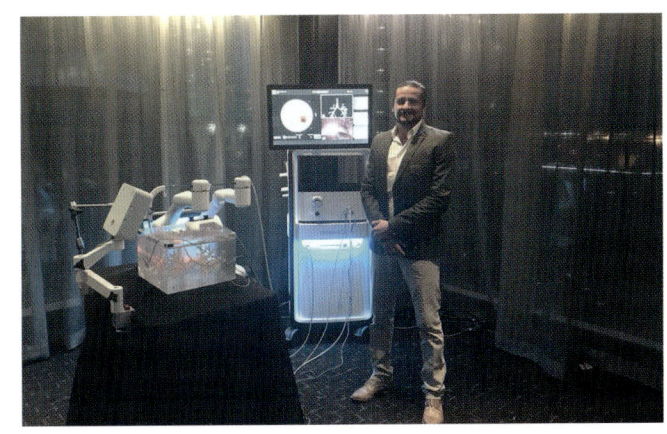

图 1.8　J. Rojas-Solano 和 Monarch 机器人支气管镜

的重要组成部分。驱动支气管镜市场发展的因素包括日益增多的需支气管镜微创操作诊治的肺部疾病、医疗报销份额的增加和科技的进步。2017年，支气管镜技术全球市场价值约为154亿美元，预计到2025年都将以每年8.3%的速度递增，对制造商而言，这些利好消息是对研究投入和创新投资的重要激励[15]。

1.4　可弯曲支气管镜技术的进一步发展

可弯曲支气管镜技术应用的简便性和可进一步拓展到达中央呼吸道以外的细支气管的快速发展，为引入新的光学、诊断和治疗技术提供了巨大的机遇[16]，在池田访问美国后，Anderson和Zavala医生首先开展了经支气管镜肺活检技术（transbronchial lung biopsy，TBLB）[17]。

1974年，Reynolds首次发表了有关支气管肺泡灌洗（bronchoalveolar lavage，BAL）的临床应用经验[18]。1978年，Cortese等证实了通过注射血卟啉衍生物（hematoporphyrin derivates，HPD）诱导的荧光技术可检测早期肺癌的潜在应用前景[19]。同年，Wang等开始通过可弯曲支气管镜对纵隔淋巴结进行TBNA分期，当时该项工作仅少数人采用硬质支气管镜进行操作[20]。此外，在治疗方面，Toty等首次在气道内应用了Nd:YAG激光[21]。1980年，Dumon等发表了气道内激光消融治疗气道狭窄相关的研究结果，这在当时很长一段时间内是应用最多的治疗性技术[22,23]。同时，Hayata等在HPD诱导荧光染色后应用光动力疗法治疗早期中央型肺癌[24]。1979年，Hilarss等使用放射性探针进行气道内近距离高剂量放射疗法治疗中央气道癌[25]。

随着电荷耦合器件电子成像技术的快速发展和小型化改进，1987年，池田与朝日宾得公司合作开发了第一台电子支气管镜。1990年，Dumon设计了首个用于呼吸道的气道硅酮支架[26]。由于可弯曲支气管镜下植入硅酮支架很困难且血管内金属支架被证明不适合呼吸道，Becker于1992年推出了Ultraflex® Nitinol®支架[27]。1991年，Lam等报道了无须注射HPD的自荧光支气管镜检查（autofluorescence bronchoscopy，AFB），该项技术可用于肺癌的早期检测[28]。1999年，径向EBUS技术的引入满足了对肺癌进行分期的需求[10]。此外，该技术还为纵隔和肺内的诊断开辟了广泛的应用领域。目前，专门为针吸活检术设计的EBUS正在广泛取代纵隔镜用于肺癌的分期[29]。肺癌的早期筛查进一步推动了对新的成像模式的需求，通过放大电子支气管镜和窄带成像技术（narrow band imaging，NBI）来分析细微的血管结构[30]。而目前正在开展研究的经支气管镜光学相干断层扫描（endoscopic optical coherence tomography，EOCT）可以提供比EBUS更高分辨率的支气管壁层结构信息[31]。

新的智能化的电磁导航技术（electromagnetic navigation，EMN）将大气道内可见病灶的诊断范围拓展到了肺外周病变[32,33]，它还支持通过插入近距离治疗导管对肺外周病变进行介入治疗[34]。有关通过射频消融破坏哮喘发作中引起气道收缩的平滑肌治疗支气管哮喘[35]和通过植入支气管内单向活瓣治疗肺气肿[36]的首批研究成果已经发表。

互联网的快速发展为学术交流、合作研究和教学互动提供了新的传播途径。2000年，在第12届世界支气管病和支气管食管病大会（WCB）期间，在德国海德堡和日本横滨之间进行了首次远程直播（图1.9）。

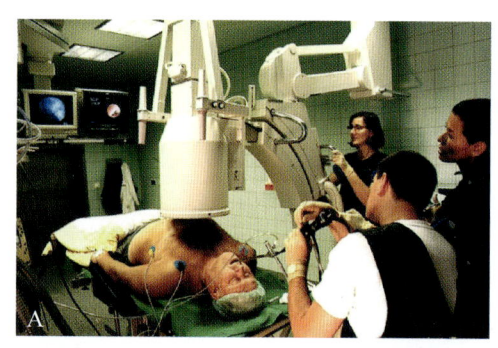
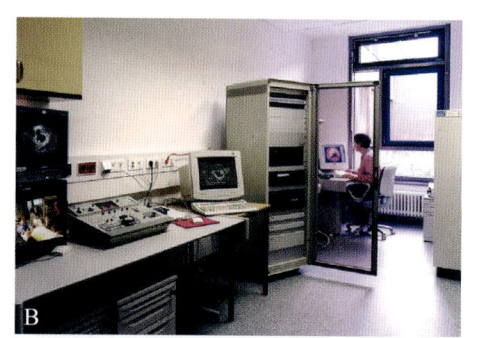
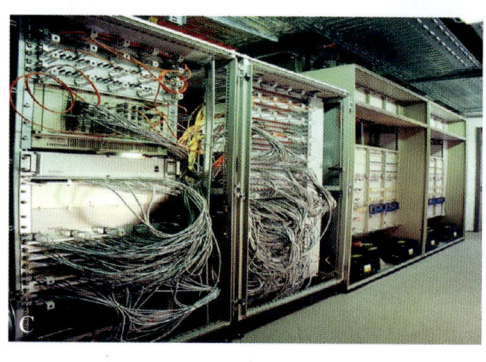
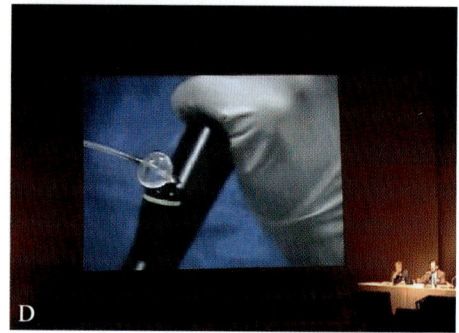

图1.9 第12届WCB期间EBUS操作直播

A. 德国内镜操作现场；B. 内镜室的电子通信中心；C. 电子通信传输的硬件设备（处理器）；D. 会议报告厅屏幕上直播的EBUS操作视频。

感兴趣的读者可以通过参考文献中获取更多的内容。

1.5 当前可弯曲支气管镜技术的概念和策略

在笔者的职业生涯中,大约有来自世界各地的600名医生至笔者中心学习了各种支气管镜操作。对年轻医生而言,除了掌握这项特殊技能外,更重要的是要认识到支气管镜技术是呼吸病学领域的一部分。这一章节重点介绍了基于介入肺脏病学的临床问题促使可弯曲支气管镜技术不断发展演化的历程。

1.5.1 中央气道早期肺癌的诊断和分期

在应用PDT治疗晚期肺癌时,笔者团队观察到,HPD激发的荧光使得不可见的小病变在支气管黏膜上变得可见,这对检测早期肺癌非常有用。也就是说,在痰细胞学阳性的患者中,那些在传统影像学上难以察觉的病变可能被治愈。进一步的研究表明,在特殊光源的照射下,支气管黏膜在没有被HPD激发的情况下也会发出荧光。基于这一发现,纤维镜和电子镜中已开发出了多种系统,用于检测早期癌症的自发荧光。

由于自荧光系统对恶性肿瘤的诊断特异性不佳,因此新近开发的技术增加了进一步分析的方法。例如,电子放大支气管镜可以更详细地分析上皮内和上皮下的结构,特别是病理血管,这是早期肺癌的特征。通过RGB成像和NBI,可以显著提高对特征性病变血管的可视化效果。EOCT技术可根据黏膜不同层次的反射,提供光学组织学图像,从而进一步提高分辨率,接近显微镜水平。最新的共聚焦显微内镜技术将光学分辨率提高到了细胞水平[37]。

预计这些方法的结合最终可能会取代活检标本的组织病理学检查。虽然早期病变能被有效的局部治疗(如PDT),但仍有相当数量的肿瘤患者只能得到部分缓解。根据定义,原位癌不侵犯黏膜固有层,早期肺癌不侵犯软骨及软骨之间的结缔组织层。这两者都无法用上述光学方法进行评估,尤其是后者。

20世纪90年代,笔者团队与奥林巴斯公司一起开发了20 MHz的专用径向EBUS探头,其高分辨率图像清楚地显示了支气管壁的全层结构。当使用EBUS技术分析自发荧光发现的所谓"早期癌症"时,有些病变已侵犯到支气管壁全层,甚至侵犯到邻近的组织和小淋巴结,而这些超微结构是计算机断层扫描(computed tomography,CT)无法诊断出来的[38]。在采用径向EBUS严格探查后,仅对局限性的肿瘤进行PDT治疗,所有患者均获得长期完全缓解[39]。事实证明,以往的所谓PDT疗法失败,并非真正意义上的失败,而是并未对这些病变进行正确的局部分期。这意味着,在决定镜下治疗之前,应该用上述方法来严格筛查所谓的早期病变。因此,在侵犯范围更为广泛的局部病变中,如果不考虑手术,支气管近距离放射治疗可能更为适合,因为其穿透深度更大(图1.10)。

1.5.2 晚期肺癌的诊断和分期

正确的肺癌分期是成功治疗的先决条件[40]。可弯曲支气管镜的使用拓展了气道内观察范围,使得段支气管和亚段支气管腔内可视化,这有助于评估癌症的腔内情况和胸部手术术前规划切除范围(图1.11)。此外,术前支气管镜检查对于排除其他支气管腔内转移也是必不可少的。由于支气管镜的视野仅限于管腔内和支气管壁的内表面,更深层的受累或对纵隔结构的侵犯只能通过间接的方式进行评估。如纵隔的影像学检查主要是依据水、空气、脂肪或钙的不同密度进行对比成像,临床工作中往往因密度接近或不存在典型的特征而导致影像学误诊。例如,一部分邻近纵隔的实体肿瘤,影像学认为该实体肿瘤侵犯到纵隔,但在手术中确认无纵隔侵犯。此外,基于影像学病灶大小诊断淋巴结转移的价值也有限。

以上就是笔者团队在1989年找到奥林巴斯公司,一起开发用于探查腔外淋巴结EBUS技术的原因。当时了解到奥林巴斯公司已经在开发针对淋巴结进行肿瘤分期的胃肠超声系统并取得了进展。故在接下来的10年里,鉴于呼吸道的特殊性,团队克服了重重困难,在开发出众多样机之后最终形成了两种支气管超声系统,即径向超声探头和超声支气管镜,现已广泛应用于临床。使用EBUS进行评估可以准确地区分肿瘤对呼吸道的压迫和对管壁的侵犯[41]。

明确纵隔淋巴结是否转移对支气管镜下分期非常重要。既往曾在硬质支气管镜检查中对纵隔肿块和肿大的淋巴结进行TBNA检查,但未被广泛应用。这种情况随着可弯曲支气管镜的应用发生了改变,操作者首先在CT上根据支气管位置(如隆突和支气管分支)定位肿大的淋巴结,即使是在角度较大的位置也可通过可弯曲支气管镜进行TBNA检查,使用专用的细胞针或组织针很容易穿过气道壁,而在以往采用硬质支

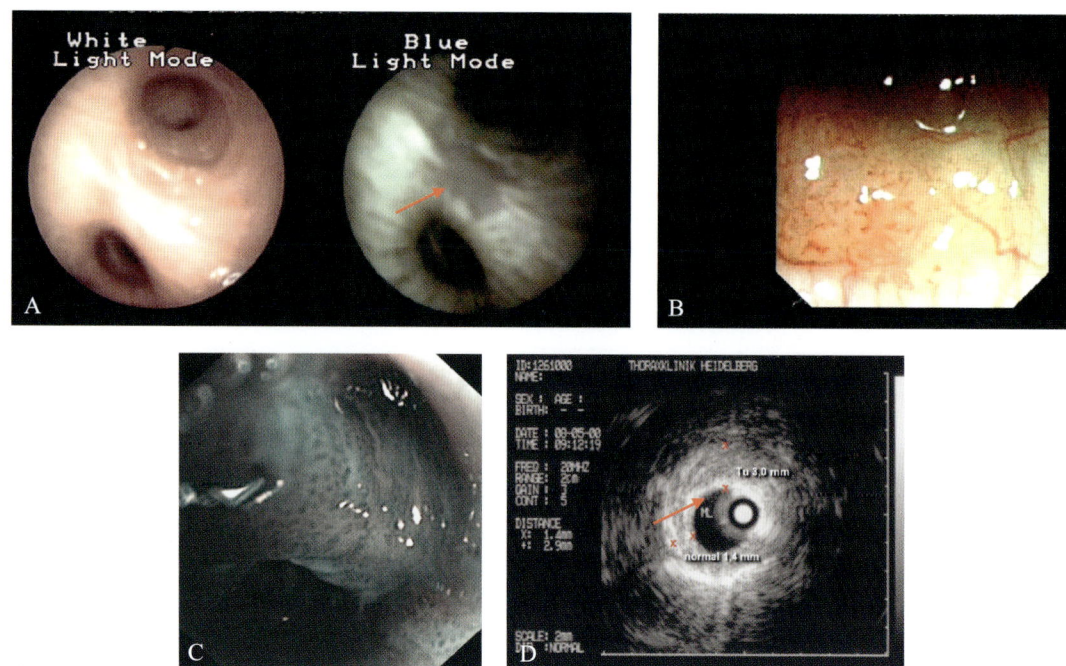

图 1.10　早期肺癌

A. 普通白光下病灶轻微变色而在自荧光模式下非常明显；B. 通过放大内镜可见到病理血管形成；C. 在 NBI 模式下更加明显；D. 采用径向 EBUS 探查，径向超声图像显示病变（上方）厚度（3 mm），而与左侧正常支气管管壁（1.4 mm）相比，病变仅限于支气管壁内，可通过支气管镜介入实施治疗。

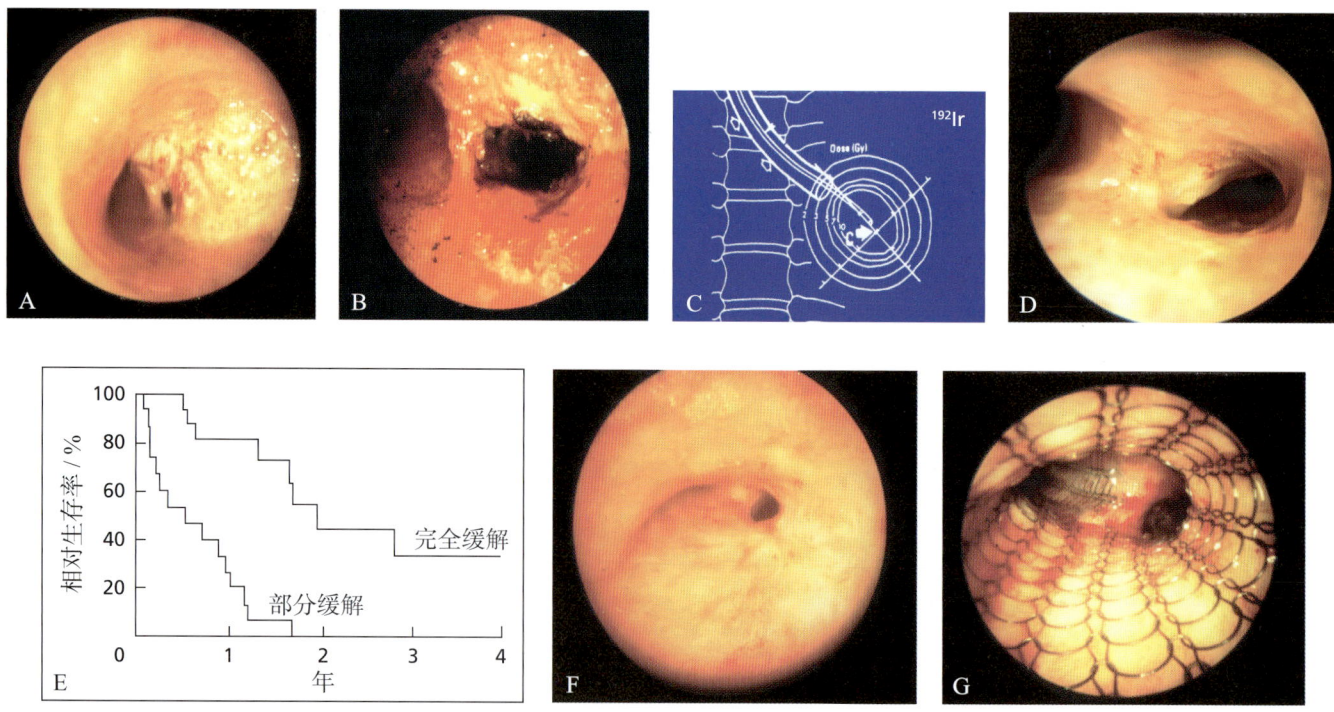

图 1.11　隆突鳞癌广泛侵犯累及器官

A. 隆突鳞癌广泛侵犯累及气管；B. Nd:YAG 激光治疗后；C. 后续实施铱-192 腔内近距离放疗的等剂量线；D. HDR 近距离放疗后 2 年，镜下隆突部所见；E. 近距离放疗后完全缓解与部分缓解患者的生存曲线；F. 完全缓解患者镜下所见气管隆突部位重度瘢痕狭窄（4 年后）；G. 球囊扩张再通后，置入 3 枚镍钛合金气道支架。

气管镜下硬针很难实施。这种方法非常安全，并发症少，效果非常理想，可弯曲支气管镜下的TBNA技术在一定程度上取代了纵隔镜检查，后者当时是进行分期的"金标准"。尽管如此，TBNA仍未广泛使用，主要原因可能是操作者担心因穿刺到较粗的纵隔内血管而导致大出血。

径向EBUS技术的应用使纵隔淋巴结的定位变得非常可靠，特别是在没有明确标志的气管旁区域。在气管旁区域EBUS引导下的TBNA的结果明显优于其他部位。然而，在专用的EBUS出现后，EBUS引导下的TBNA技术才被广泛使用。如今，EBUS引导下的TBNA已成为纵隔分期的推荐方式，从而取代了纵隔镜检查[42]。

1.5.3 中央气道肿瘤：从缓解到治愈

随着肺癌发病率的增加，中央气道阻塞是支气管镜操作的一个主要适应证。使用可弯曲支气管镜进行消融治疗，相比硬质支气管镜，除了一些坏死的易清理的组织碎片以外，大多并不成功。由于可弯曲支气管镜匹配的钳子、刮匙等工具尺寸较小，使得新生物体的机械清除变得十分繁琐。使用球囊扩张治疗外压性恶性气道狭窄则是例外[43]。但球囊扩张这种治疗方式效果短暂，对改善呼吸困难也不是很有效。

以下是几种可迅速解除气道阻塞的方法：1982年，Dumon采用Nd:YAG激光对肿瘤组织行热消融术，以快速解除中央气道阻塞。1980年，池田茂人去了马赛，参加了Dumon的专项技术学习班后立即将激光技术引入了日本。激光消融的优势是通过气化组织的方式进行非接触性消融，操作期间将最大功率设置在40 W以下，降低供氧至50%以下，并使用短波脉冲波模式，这是非常安全的。1997年，Homasson描述了高频电治疗术，高频电治疗的原理是利用电流的热效应对组织进行破坏，其瞬时效果与Nd:YAG激光相当。与激光相比，高频电具有类似的效果，成本却要低得多，故Sutedja等将其称为"穷人的激光"[44,45]。高频电消融的另一种方式是氩等离子体凝固术（argon plasma coagulation，APC）[46]，这是一种非接触的热消融术，电流作用于氩气，使电子与原子分离，同时产生的氩等离子体是电流传递的媒介。冷冻疗法与通过加热破坏组织的方法不同，其利用焦耳—汤姆孙效应，通过导管内液性气体迅速膨胀汽化来制冷。冷冻治疗包括通过快速拔出冷冻探头来移除粘连的冰冻组织（冻切术），也可致肿瘤细胞内冰晶形成诱导肿瘤细胞延迟性坏死（冻融术）[47]。

上述方法都能立即缓解症状。对于恶性肿瘤而言，除非有根治性的办法，否则复发后必须重复治疗。根据笔者团队的经验，激光切除恶性肿瘤的患者3年后的存活率约为20%。对于腔内治疗后不能通过手术或放射治疗治愈的患者，内镜下的长期管理方法有待进一步探索。

20世纪90年代初，人们采用腔内高剂量近距离放疗的方法使得气道内肿瘤获得了长期的局部控制，该方法的原理是在支气管腔内植入装有放射性铱-192粒子的导管，在放射源附近形成高剂量的辐射且以变化较大的梯度能量递减，以避免周围组织的损伤。笔者团队在激光治疗后采用高剂量率腔内照射治疗，当内镜下病灶达到完全缓解时，效果可持续很多年，甚至一些患者达到了治愈。故笔者团队认为可先应用2~3次外照射来缩小肿瘤体积，然后进行腔内近距离放疗，建议单次放射剂量为5 Gy，共计4次[48]。

在完全缓解的患者中，长期并发症主要是广泛气道内瘢痕形成导致重度中央气道狭窄复发，这些只能通过腔内介入治疗来解决。1989年，Dumon展示了通过硬质支气管镜放置专用的硅酮支架的方法，也有报道经可弯曲支气管镜置入的技术，但并未广泛使用。当时，将血管支架应用于呼吸道较为常见，但由不锈钢和钽制成的可膨胀和自膨胀的金属合金支架要么因内部支撑力过小而塌陷，要么因张力过大而易致气道壁穿孔。在经历了钽支架的失败后，笔者团队开发了Boston Scientific镍钛合金支架，后来被称为Ultraflex支架（图1.12）。在改进了置入方式和开发出覆膜金属支架后，它已成为易于可弯曲支气管镜置入的标准支架。笔者的一些患者是在20年前置入的该支架，其中最小的一个是在2岁的时候置入的。

除激光治疗外，光动力疗法同样可用于肺癌患者的治疗。具体而言，在注射HPD后，肿瘤组织内浓度明显高于周围正常组织。在适当时间用特定波长的激光照射肿瘤组织，激活HPD，产生氧自由基，特异性破坏肿瘤细胞及肿瘤新生血管。与激光切除相比，PDT治疗效果延迟，不建议在紧急情况下使用，但可作为一种腔内介入治疗后的非常有效的辅助手段，它也可以与近距离放射治疗联合使用，或者在放置非覆膜支架后应用，以治疗向腔内生长的肿瘤。

支气管镜下在瘤体内注射抗肿瘤药物，如乙醇、化疗药物或免疫刺激因子，对于不可手术的肺癌患者而言是一种很有前景的治疗方法。为了更好地控制局

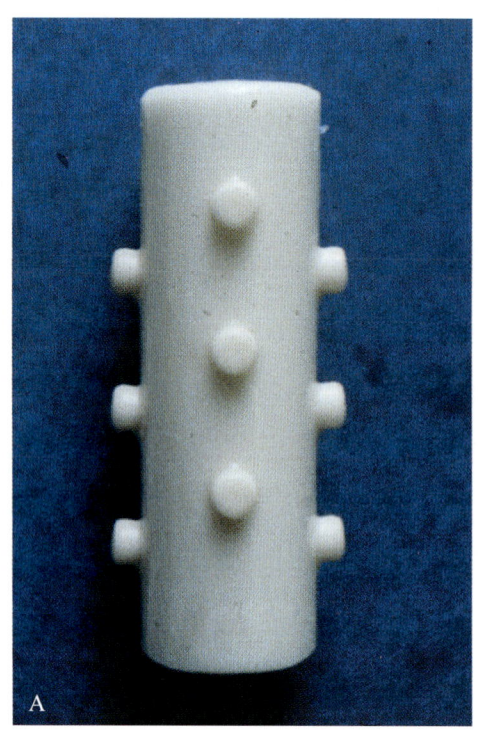 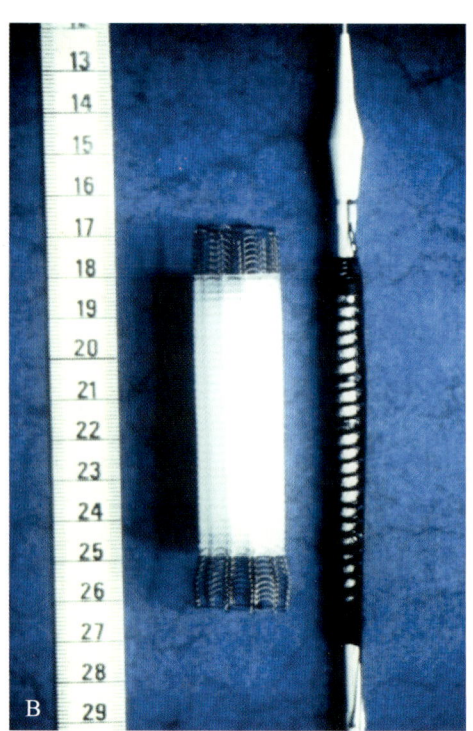

图 1.12 Dumon 硅酮气道支架（A）和镍钛合金覆膜气道支架（B）

部注射范围，EBUS 引导下经支气管细针注射（EBUS-guided transbronchial needle injection，EBUS-TBNI）可以精准测量肿瘤体积从而确定给药剂量，最大限度地减少与这些药物相关的全身毒性，还增加了药物的瘤内浓度。此外，该技术不仅可以直接观察到肿瘤中的药物注射情况，还可以最大限度地降低针头插入高度血管化区域的风险[49]。

1.5.4 周围型肺癌的诊断和治疗

近几十年来，中央型肺癌逐渐向周围型肺癌转变。与早期支气管癌一样，周围型肺癌被发现得越早，预后就越好。使用低剂量螺旋 CT 有利于肺癌筛查。经过长期随访，可以发现更多更小的病变，病死率可降低 20%[50]。但当外科常规切除 SPN 时，发现一半是不需要手术治疗的良性病变[51]。这就是在外科术前需明确病理的原因。获取组织病理学的方法包括灌洗、刷检、刮匙、针吸穿刺活检术和活检钳活检术。

诊断周围型肺癌的挑战在于找到通往周围病灶的路径。根据 X 线或 CT 定位，然后通过支气管镜到达病灶的成功率非常低。实时 X 线透视下经支气管活检的成功率更高[52]。但是，2 cm 以下的病变和磨玻璃样阴影的显影效果很差。有文献报道实时 CT 可视化下经支气管活检的成功率更高，但不同科室间的协调困难和辐射暴露阻碍了该技术的广泛应用[53]。径向 EBUS 的应用有助于确定 SPN 的确切位置和接近它的路径，当探头通过引导鞘管引入时，可以将引导鞘管置于适当的位置，并作为引入活检工具的"扩展的工作通道"，成功率更高[54]。但径向探头无法控制前进方向，且无法找到通往病灶的路径（尤其是肺上叶）。因此，笔者团队研究了一种类似于 GPS 电磁导航的 EMN 系统，以便将引导导管引入肺外周病变中。

患者的上半身被置于低强度电磁场中（充当"卫星"），传感器（GPS 中的板载计算机）可以通过患者 CT 扫描的叠加图像（路线图）在监视器上跟随，传感器安装在可转向导管的尖端，该导管可 360° 旋转并带有引导鞘管，带引导鞘管的导管通过导航技术到达肺外周病变后，取出带有传感器的导管，留置鞘管后再用径向 EBUS 确定病变内的实时位置。使用超细支气管镜可以观察支气管管腔内的情况，进而评估是使用活检钳钳夹腔内新生物，还是使用针吸活检管壁外病灶。另一种导航技术是将支气管镜沿着由虚拟支气管镜创建的路径导航下引入肺外周病变[55]。

导航技术显著提高了 SPN 的诊断率，并有希望成为这些病变的标准诊断方法。然而，就像所有的支气管镜介入操作一样，成功与否也取决于支气管镜操

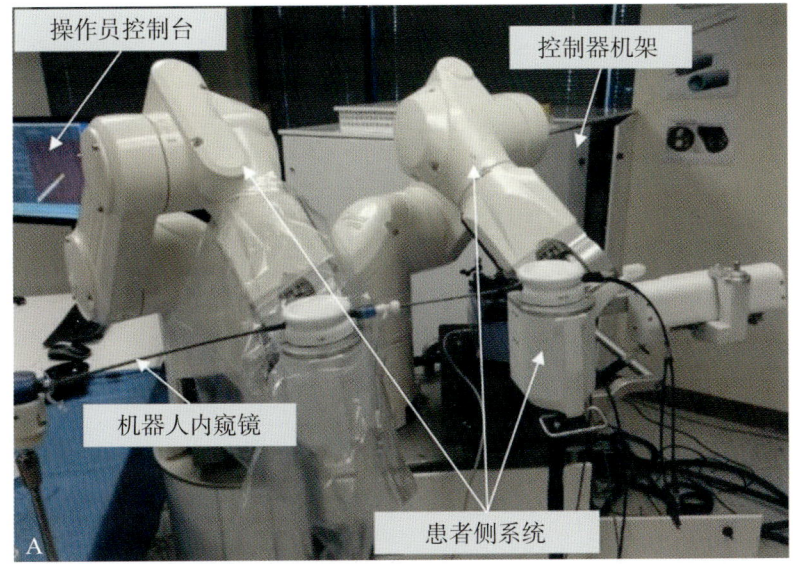
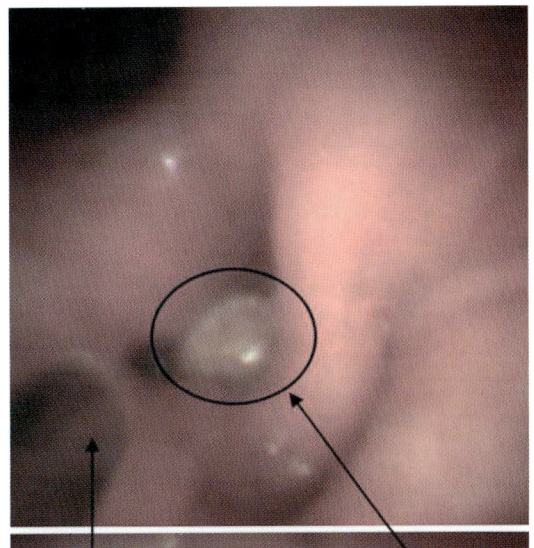
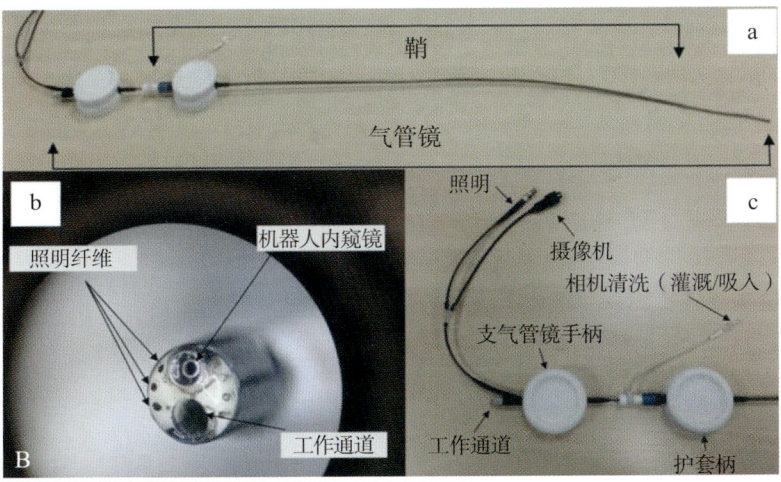
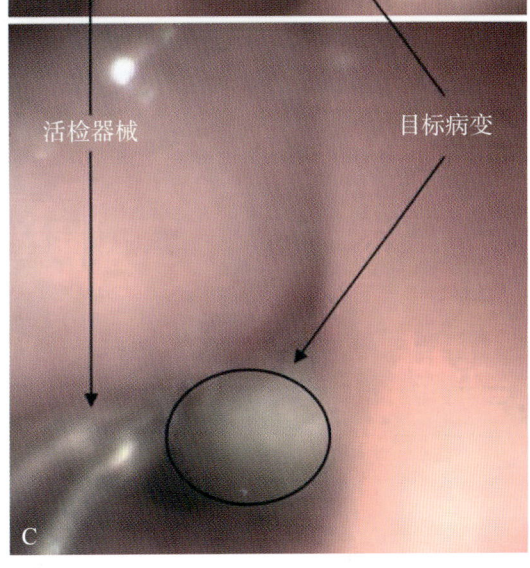

图 1.13　Monarch 机器人支气管镜系统

A. 近端控制系统和机器人内窥镜；B. 支气管镜；C. 肺周围病变的内镜下所见和活检。有关视频剪辑，请参阅 www.aurishealth.com/monarch-platform。

作者的个人技能。因此，研究者们开发了机器人支气管镜，用于解决目前支气管镜技术在肺外周病变活检中的局限性。笔者的前同事 Rojas-Solano 博士最近报道了首个商业化的机器人内窥镜（robotic endoscopy，RES）（Auris Surgical Robotics，San Carlos，CA），并展现出非常有希望的研究结果。

RES 由 1 个 3.2 mm 的电子支气管镜、1 个 1.2 mm 的工作通道和 1 个外鞘组成，它的 2 个机械臂可以连续地进行 4 个方向上转向，可以通过远程遥控、直接操作和视觉控制下实现 180°任意方向的偏转，并在近端设有冲洗和抽吸功能（图 1.13）。

有了可靠的 SPN 定位工具和径向 EBUS 稳定定位的延长工作通道，使不能手术的周围型肺癌在内镜下治疗成为可能。借鉴内镜治疗中央气道肿瘤的经验，采用近距离放射治疗肺外周病变，既可易于将放射剂量与原发肿瘤相匹配，也可控制剂量与转移性的支气管周淋巴管和肺门淋巴结相匹配。笔者团队首次开展了一项小型研究，大多数病例实现了长期完全缓解[56]（图 1.14）。其他正在计划中或目前正在研究的方法包括射频消融（radiofrequency ablation，RFA）、激光治疗、冷冻治疗、PDT 和蒸汽消融术。

1.5.5　实质性肺疾病

随着 CT 成像技术的发展，尽管许多间质性肺疾病呈现出不同的病原学形态特征，但常常需要组织形态学或微生物学的进一步确认。纤维支气管镜检查可通过灌

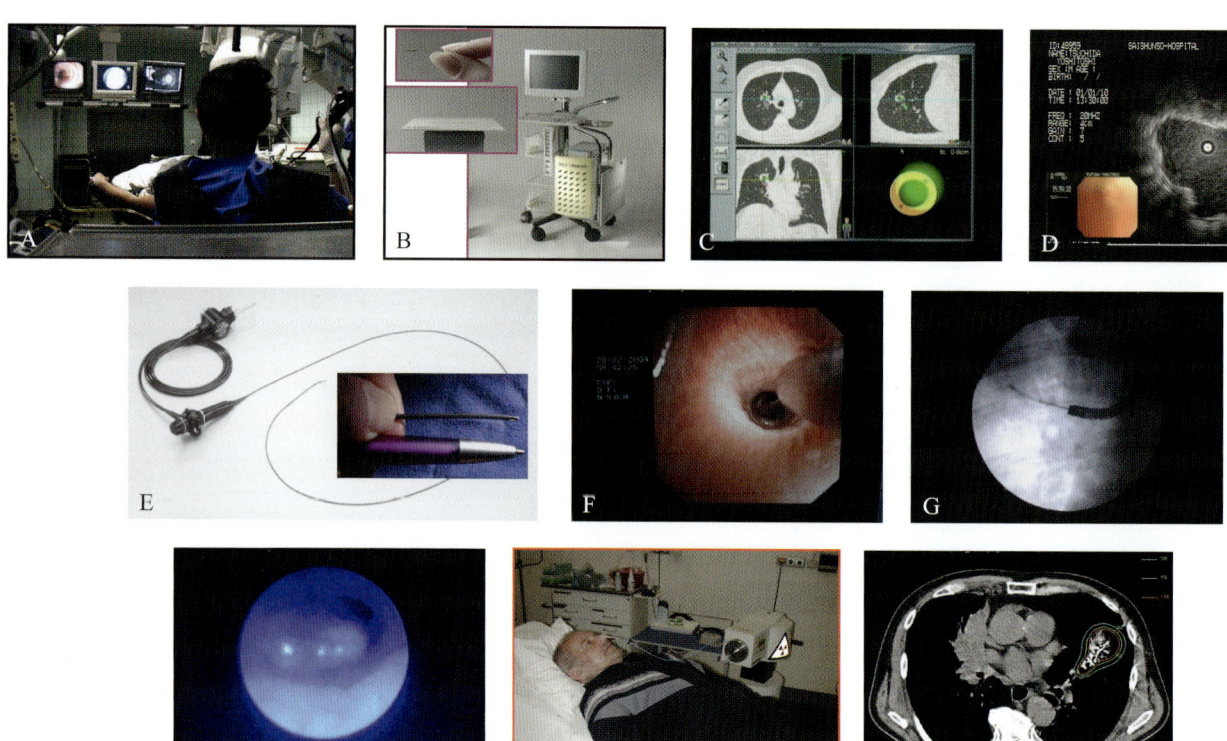

图 1.14 肺外周病变诊疗

A. 在内窥镜、X 线透视和 EBUS 三个监视器开展电磁导航操作；B. 电磁导航系统（EMN）由传感器、电磁板和计算机与控制监视器组成；C. 在螺旋三维 CT 指导下 EMN 传感器（绿色）进入目标病灶（黄色）；D. 通过引入径向 EBUS 探头确认病灶位置；E~G. 介绍了一种超细奥林巴斯支气管镜并将其引导到肺外周病变；H. 镜下所见病灶为突入管腔内时，使用活检钳活检是获取组织样本的最佳技术；I、J. 病理为不能手术的恶性病灶时，可通过相同的方式置入近距离放射治疗导管，并且可以根据等剂量线的计算进行经支气管近距离放疗（如 HDR 治疗）。

洗和刷检的方式采集标本。虽然细胞学阳性对诊断感染性肺部疾病和肺癌很有用，但这不足以诊断实质性肺疾病。

然而，正如有时观察到的特征性细胞一样，20 世纪 80 年代初，一种从支气管肺泡腔中注入大量液体以采集标本的方法——BAL 开始应用。最初，人们认为 BAL 是一种非出血性的活检方法。例如，通过 T 辅助细胞和 T 抑制细胞之间的关系来诊断结节病。但在进一步研究中，研究结果仍不明确。这些发现仅限于相对罕见的疾病，如嗜酸性肺炎或肺泡蛋白沉着症。只有在严重感染中，特别是在免疫功能低下的患者中才被广泛使用。在大多数情况下，需要取材肺组织以明确诊断。

在 Anderson 证明了可弯曲支气管镜下经活检钳夹肺组织术的安全性后，这种方法成为诊断肺部疾病和 SPN 的最新手段。由于取材标本小，从一个肺的不同部位采集几份标本检查可以减少抽样误差。笔者团队采用更大的活检钳，不通过活检通道和内镜一起退出的方法增加了阳性结果。如池田茂人在他的第一篇论文中所描述的那样，笔者团队通过气管内插管插入可弯曲支气管镜，并将钳子放在镜头尖端的前面。这样，从一个肺的每个节段最多采集一个标本，并发症发生率非常低，也提供了关于肺不同部位疾病的信息[57]。保证安全性的情况下采集更大的标本促进了冷冻探头的应用，通过这种探头可以以同样低的并发症发生率获得更大的组织碎片。此外，病理科医师更喜欢冻切的标本，因为它们的机械损伤比活检钳活检获取的组织要小得多[58]（图 1.15）。

1.5.6 肺功能障碍的治疗：肺气肿和哮喘

1996 年，Cooper 等发表了一篇关于严重肺气肿患者经双侧肺减容后取得较好治疗效果的论文[59]。在这些结果的基础上，国家肺气肿治疗试验（National Emphysema Treatment Trial，NETT）研究小组成立并开展了外科肺减容手术的前瞻性临床试验[60]。由于患者在外科肺减容术后死亡风险很高，使得人们对

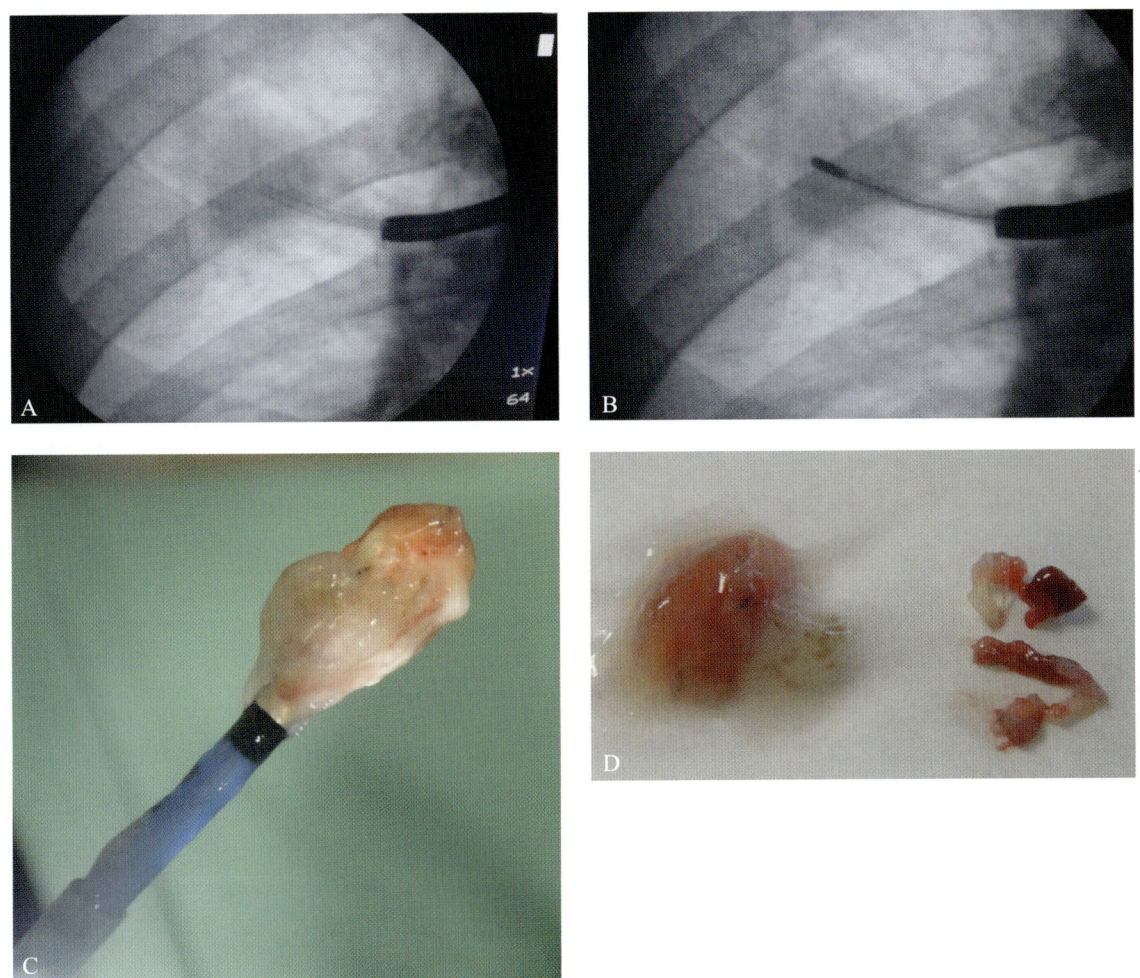

图 1.15 EMN 导航支气管镜肺外周病灶冷冻活检术

A. 导航下将引导鞘管留置于肺外周病灶内；B. 经引导鞘管置入冷冻探头；C. 实施肺外周病灶冷冻活检后取出的冷冻探头（黏附标本的冷冻探头、导管和支气管镜一起取出）；D. 冷冻探头冻切取得的标本和活检钳取材所获得的标本的大小比较。

预后乐观的情绪有所变化[61]。由于胸部手术后的结果不可逆转，因此人们开始研究可逆性内镜下肺减容术（endoscopic lung volume reduction，ELVR）。慢性阻塞性肺疾病（chronic obstructive pulmonary disease，COPD）患者的潜在市场是巨大的，多家公司开始开发不同的设备，如活瓣、线圈和蒸汽消融，用于 COPD 患者的肺减容。

在 3 个随机对照试验和几个非对照试验中对活瓣植入术进行了研究，结果表明，叶间通气量最小或没有侧支通气的患者能从活瓣植入术中获益。在以上叶肺气肿为主的患者中，肺叶体积可减少 56%~80%，同时肺功能显著改善约 20%。主要并发症是气胸，占 23%[62,63]。一项随机对照试验的结果显示，置入弹簧线圈患者的生活质量显著改善。对以上叶肺气肿为主的患者使用支气管镜热消融治疗，肺叶体积平均缩小

48%。其中活瓣可取出，是可逆的。线圈不容易取出，蒸汽减容是不可逆的。目前，仅限于有经验的中心可进行 ELVR 的治疗[64]。

通过支气管热成形术（bronchial thermoplasty，BT）治疗严重难治性哮喘的原理是通过减少呼吸道平滑肌来控制气道收缩，以减少重度哮喘发作。通过一个像篮子外形的射频探头，控制热量传递到气道壁，阻断平滑肌，但不会对其他结构造成持久的损害。经可行性研究证实了该方法的有效性、安全性以及更持久的效果后，研究人员进行了一项长期的多中心研究，数据表明，BT 是一种安全且有效的治疗方法。根据严重恶化和急诊就诊次数的减少情况来看，哮喘控制的改善可以维持很长时间。一个疗程的 BT 治疗包括 3 次支气管镜下治疗，效果可维持 5 年以上[65]。BT 已成为一些通过长效 β 激动剂和吸入皮质类固醇控制效

果欠佳的严重持续性哮喘患者的重要补充治疗手段。

1.6 可弯曲支气管镜的未来

我们可以通过将这些点点滴滴串在一起以回首过去。所以你必须相信，那些点点滴滴，会在你未来的生命里，以某种方式串联起来。

（史蒂夫·乔布斯[66]）

1.6.1 预测未来发展的因素

根据既往的经验和研究，可以预测可弯曲支气管镜技术未来的发展[67-69]。当然，准确预测未来是不可能的，但可以根据现有技术的改进，以及目前需要解决的问题来预测未来的发展方向。一些原本用于其他目的而发明的技术，后来被应用于支气管镜技术（如纤维支气管镜技术和EBUS）。有些是全新的技术，如芯片、计算机技术和机器人技术等，这些新技术可能是颠覆性的，甚至阻止其他技术的迭代。此外，还有一种纯属偶然的发现，如青霉素、聚合酶链式反应等，这是完全不可预测的。随着新技术的出现，所有这些因素都将以指数级速度增长。

此外，新技术的使用取决于客户的接受程度。根据笔者经验，这是让任何创新者都感到进退两难的最不可预测的因素。只有那些足够幸运、有耐心并获得足够支持的创新者，才有可能成功地创造出一项新技术。就径向EBUS技术而言，自1989年该技术首次亮相，历经公司投资、技术研发、医生接纳等多个阶段，最终于10年后成功进入市场化阶段。3年后，凸阵探头的EBUS技术问世，由于市场需求旺盛，几乎扼杀了径向EBUS技术（尤其在其用于肺周围病灶得到承认之前）。此外，振动响应成像（vibration response imaging，VRI）——一种使呼吸可见的电子听诊器新技术——尽管已获得FDA的批准，但由于从未被理解和接受，最终未能进入市场[70,71]。

1.6.2 成像

成像技术在分辨率、视野和穿透力等方面不断精进。因此，高倍率的EOTC、共聚焦显微内镜的细胞分析和体内免疫染色光学活检将成为现实。对于评估功能状态的新体内成像方法，如纤毛摆动、局部支气管和肺间质炎症、支气管平滑肌收缩、支气管和纵隔血流以及气管支气管气流等将为病理机制提供新的见解，并推动非侵入性局部治疗新技术的发展。

1.6.3 导航技术

机器人支气管镜通过遥控器作为人机界面进行导航。新的光学和触觉传感器将帮助指导内镜下操作。器械力反馈系统将被整合到"智能"工具中，如钳子、穿刺针、圈套器、网篮等。操作者不再通过他们的手来操纵这些器械，而是利用远程操纵器甚至监视器上的操纵杆遥控。就像使用机器人支气管镜一样。仪器直径变得越来越小，以至于传统的钢丝束技术不再适用。形状记忆合金（shape memory alloy，SMA）可实现更大的弯曲角度，其微型机械可用于气管镜尖端。真正的机器人将不再与人类交互，而是将根据计算机化的反馈数据独立执行诊断和治疗程序，人类只需在排除故障时进行干预。

1.6.4 介入治疗

由SMA制成的微型器械，如钳子、穿刺针和缝合装置，将使介入治疗发生革命性变化。新一代内镜可应用细胞毒剂或基因疗法、无线电波、微波和高强度聚集超声（high-intensity focused ultrasound，HIFU）穿刺注药法。生物技术被应用于移植物种植和生物可降解气道临时支架中。未来，还可能通过在3D打印支架上种植细胞或植入自体干细胞的生物假体来取代插管后狭窄的黏膜和软骨等受损结构。

1.6.5 电子通信

系统集成对于文档的完整和电子通信至关重要。这些不同种类的设备必须由系统整合在一起，以便实现连接、将图像转换为MPEG标准、在电子服务器上存储数据以及控制复杂的电子网络。数字通信系统不仅支持文档和数据存储，还具备介入诊疗操作规划、资源和人力合理管理以及结果跟踪的能力，从而涵盖全面质量管理的所有要素。目前，越来越多的医院通过互联网实现互连，而通过远程会诊系统将患者投送给远程专家的电子会诊将越来越少，外科医师与病理学家的直接联系也将减少，但有效降低了会诊时间和成本。将外科医师的手部运动转换为电信号，在虚拟模型上开展培训，通过力反馈系统可实现对所有的诊断性和治疗性操作"真实手感"的培训。目前，介入操作已经可以通过计算机控制台对仪器进行远程控制。借助高速网络，医院间，甚至跨大陆的远程医疗干预将成为可能（图1.16）。

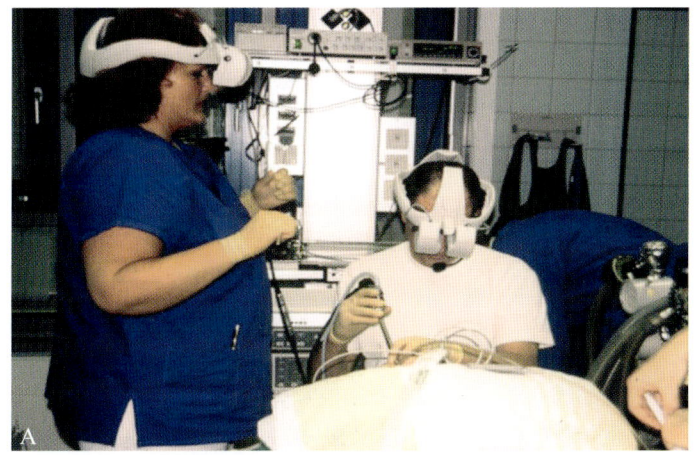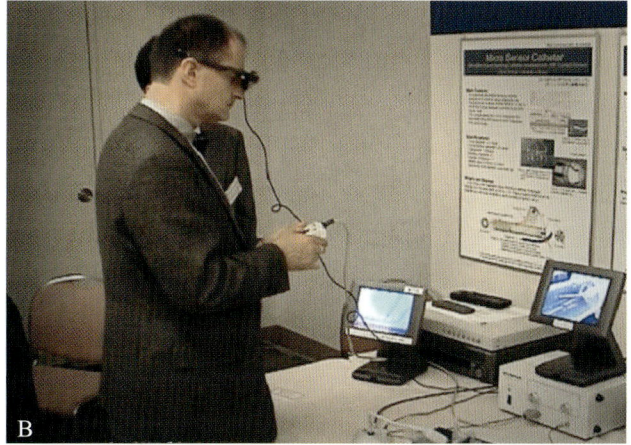
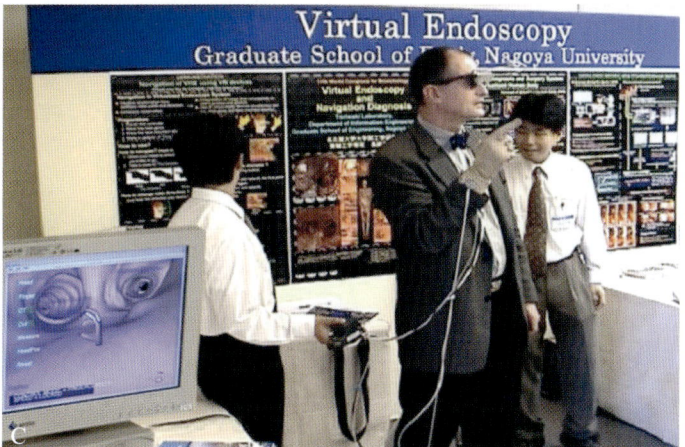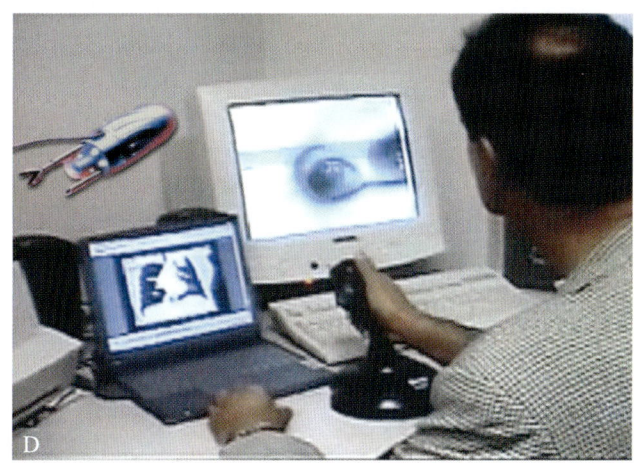

图 1.16 展望

A. 用于 3D 成像的配有两个监视器的头戴式装置；B. 使用轨迹球实施的远程导航系统；C. 电子手套式虚拟支气管镜导航系统；D. 操纵杆式远程虚拟胶囊内镜导航系统。

参考文献

1. Ikeda, S., Yanai, N., and Ishikawa, S. (1968). Flexible bronchofiberscope. *Keio J. Med.* 17 (1): 1–16.
2. Hirschowitz, B.I. (2000). Endoscopy – 40 years since fiber optics. *Dig. Surg.* 17 (2): 115–117.
3. Wilcox, C.M. (2014). Fiberoptic endoscopy: the singular transformative event of our time. *Dig. Dis. Sci.* 59: 2619–2622.
4. Ikeda, S. (1974). *Atlas of Flexible Bronchoscopy*. Tokyo: Igaku-Shoin.
5. Ikeda, S. (1982) Never give up. English edition. Studio Cockpit Tetsuya, Fukushima.
6. Miyazawa, T. (2000). History of the flexible bronchoscope. In: *Interventional Bronchoscopy*, vol. 30 (eds. C.T. Bolliger and P.N. Mathur), 16–21. Basel: Karger.
7. Shirakawa, T. (2007). History of bronchoscopy. Lecture in Slovenia, 5.10.2007.
8. Ohata, M. (1998). History and progress of bronchology in Japan. *J. Jpn. Soc. Respirat. Endosc.* 20 (6): 539–546.
9. Toshiaki, K., Koshiishi, H., Kawate, N. et al. (1994). The performance of prototype videobronchoscopes: the Pentax EB-TM1830 and EBTM1530. *J. Bronchology* 1: 160–167.
10. Becker, H.D. (1996). Endobronchial ultrasound: a new perspective in bronchology. *J. Ultraschall Med.* 17: 106–112.
11. Yasufuku, K., Sekine, Y., Chhajed, P.N. et al. (2003). Direct endobronchial ultrasound guided transbronchial needle aspiration of mediastinal lymph nodes using a new convex probe bronchoscope: a novel approach [abstract]. *Am. J. Respir. Crit. Care Med.* 167: A577.
12. Rojas-Solano, J., Ugalde-Gamboa, J., and Machuzak, M. (2018). Robotic bronchoscopy for diagnosis of suspected lung cancer, a feasibility study. *J. Bronchol. Intervent. Pulmonol.* 25 (3): 168–175.
13. Mehta, A. and Gildea, T. (2018). Burying our heads in the sand. *Chest* 154 (5): 1001–1003.
14. Terjesen, C.L., Kovaleva, J., and Ehlers, L. (2017). Early assessment of the likely cost effectiveness of single-use flexible video bronchoscopes. *PharmacoEconomics Open* 1 (2): 133–141.
15. No author. Bronchoscopes Market Size, Share, Industry Trends Report, 2018–2025. www.grandviewresearch.com/industry-analysis/bronchoscopes-market

16 Dionísio, J. (2012). Diagnostic flexible bronchoscopy and accessory techniques. *Rev. Port. Pneumol.* 18 (2): 99–106.

17 Andersen, H.A. and Fontana, R.S. (1972). Transbronchoscopic lung biopsy for diffuse pulmonary diseases: technique and results in 450 cases. *Chest* 62: 125–128.

18 Reynolds, H.J. and Newbau, H.H. (1974). Analysis of proteins and respiratory cells obtained from human lungs by bronchial lavage. *J. Lab. Clin. Med.* 84: 559–573.

19 Kinsey, J.H., Cortese, D.A., and Sanderson, D.R. (1978). Detection of hematoporphyrin fluorescence during fiberoptic bronchoscopy to localise bronchogenic carcinoma. *Mayo Clin. Proc.* 53: 594–599.

20 Wang, K.P., Terry, P., and Marsh, B. (1978). Bronchoscopic needle aspiration biopsy of paratracheal tumors. *Am. Rev. Respir. Dis.* 118: 17–21.

21 Toty, L., Personne, C., Colchen, A., and Vourc'h, G. (1981). Bronchoscopic management of tracheal lesions using the neodynium yttrium aluminium garnet laser. *Thorax* 36: 175–178.

22 Dumon, J.F., Reboud, E., Garbe, L. et al. (1982). Treatment of tracheobronchial lesions by laser photoresection. *Chest* 81: 278–284.

23 Dumon, J.F., Shapshay, S., Bourcereau, J. et al. (1984). Principles for safety in application of neodymium-YAG laser in bronchology. *Chest* 86 (2): 163–168.

24 Hayata, Y., Kato, H., Tanaka, C. et al. (1982). Hematoporphyrin derivative and laser photoradiation in the treatment of lung cancer. *Chest* 81: 269–277.

25 Speiser, B. and Spratling, L. (1993). Remote afterloading brachytherapy for the local control of endobronchial carcinoma. *Int. J. Radiat. Oncol. Biol. Phys.* 25: 579–587.

26 Dumon, J.F. (1990). A dedicated tracheobronchial stent. *Chest* 97: 328–332.

27 Becker, H.D., Wagner, B., Liermann, D. et al. (1995). Stenting of the central airways. In: *Medical Stents: State of the Art and Future Developments* (ed. D. Liermann), 249–255. Laval, Canada: Polyscience Publications, Inc.

28 Lam, S., Hung, J.Y., Kennedy, S.M. et al. (1992). Detection of dysplasia and carcinoma in situ by ratio Fluorometry 1-3. *Am. Rev. Respir. Dis.* 146: 1458–1461.

29 Yasufuku, K., Chiyo, M., Sekine, Y. et al. (2004). Real-time endobronchial ultrasound-guided transbronchial needle aspiration of mediastinal and hilar lymph nodes. *Chest* 126: 122–128.

30 Shibuya, K., Hoshino, H., Chiyo, M. et al. (2002). Subepithelial vascular patterns in bronchial dysplasias using a high magnification bronchovideoscope. *Thorax* 57: 902–907.

31 Laemmel, E., Genet, M., Le Goualher, G. et al. (2004). Fibered confocal fluorescence microscopy (CellviZio) facilitates extended imaging in the field of microcirculation: a comparison with intravital microscopy. *J. Vasc. Res.* 41: 400–411.

32 Schwarz, Y., Mehta, A.C., Ernst, A. et al. (2003). Electromagnetic navigation during flexible bronchoscopy. *Respiration* 70: 516–522.

33 Becker, H.D., Herth, F., Ernst, A., and Schwarz, Y. (2005). Bronchoscopic biopsy of peripheral lung lesions under electromagnetic guidance: a pilot study. *J. Bronchol. Interv. Pulmonol.* 12: 9.

34 Harms, W., Krempien, R., Grehn, C. et al. (2006). Electromagnetically navigated brachytherapy as a new treatment option for peripheral pulmonary tumors. *Strahlenther. Onkol.* 182: 108–111.

35 Cox, P.G., Miller, J., Mitzner, W., and Leffz, A.R. (2004). Radiofrequency ablation of airway smooth muscle for sustained treatment of asthma: preliminary investigations. *Eur. Respir. J.* 24: 659–663.

36 Toma, T.P., Hopkinson, N.S., Hillier, J. et al. (2003). Bronchoscopic volume reduction with valve implants in patients with severe emphysema. *Lancet* 361: 931–933.

37 Thiberville, L., Moreno-Swirc, S., Vercauteren, T. et al. (2007). In vivo imaging of the bronchial wall microstructure using fibered confocal fluorescence microscopy. *Am. J. Respir. Crit. Care Med.* 175: 22–31.

38 Lam, S. and Becker, H.D. Future diagnostic procedures. *Chest Surg. Clin. North Am.* 6 (2): 363–380.

39 Miyazu, Y., Miyazawa, T., Kurimoto, N. et al. (2002). Endobronchial ultrasonography in the assessment of centrally located early-stage lung cancer before photodynamic therapy. *Am. J. Respir. Crit. Care Med.* 165: 832–837.

40 Herth, F.J.F., Eberhardt, R., and Ernst, A. (2006). The future of bronchoscopy in diagnosing, staging and treatment of lung cancer. *Respiration* 73: 399–409.

41 Herth, F., Ernst, A., Schulz, M., and Becker, H.D. (2003). Endobronchial ultrasound reliably differentiates between airway infiltration and compression by tumor. *Chest* 123: 458–462.

42 Wahidi, M.M., .H.F., .Y.K. et al. (2016). Technical aspects of endobronchial ultrasound-guided transbronchial needle aspiration: CHEST guideline and expert panel report. *Chest* 149 (3): 816–835.

43 Hautmann, H., Gamarra, F., Pfeifer, K.J., and Huber, R.M. (2001). Fiberoptic bronchoscopic balloon dilatation in malignant tracheobronchial disease: indications and results. *Chest* 120 (1): 43–49.

44 Sutedja, G., van Kralingen, K., Schramel, F.M. et al. (1994). Fiberoptic bronchoscopic electrosurgery under local anaesthesia for rapid palliation in patients with central airway malignancies: a preliminary report. *Thorax* 49: 1243–1246.

45 Horinouchi, H., Miyazawa, T., and Takada, K. (2008). Safety study of endobronchial electrosurgery for tracheobronchial lesions: multicenter prospective study. *J. Bronchol.* 15: 228–232.

46 Morice, R.C., Ece, T., Ece, F. et al. (2001). Endobronchial argon plasma coagulation for treatment of hemoptysis and neoplastic airway obstruction. *Chest* 119: 781–787.

47 Schumann, C., Hetzel, M., Babiak, A.J. et al. (2010). Endobronchial tumor debulking with a flexible cryoprobe for immediate treatment of malignant stenosis. *J. Thorac. Cardiovasc. Surg.* 139: 997–1000.

48 Harms, W., Latz, D., Becker, H. et al. (1999). HDR-brachytherapy boost for residual tumour after external beam radiotherapy in patients with tracheal malignancies. *Radiother.*

Oncol. 52: 251–255.

49 Khan, F., Anker, C., Garrison, G., and Kinsey, C.M. (2015). Endobronchial ultrasound-guided transbronchial needle injection for local control of recurrent non-small cell lung cancer. *Ann. Am. Thorac. Soc.* 12 (1): 101–104.

50 National Lung Screening Trial Research Team (2011). Reduced lung-cancer mortality with low-dose computed tomographic screening. *N. Engl. J. Med.* 365 (5): 395–409.

51 Hoffmann, H. and Dienemann, H. (2000). Der pulmonale Rundherd: Prinzipien der Diagnostik. *Dtsch. Arztebl.* 97 (16): A-1065/B-907/C-822.

52 Chechani, V. (1996). Bronchoscopic diagnosis of solitary pulmonary nodules and lung masses in the absence of endobronchial abnormality. *Chest* 109 (3): 620–625.

53 Hautmann, H., Henke, O., and Bitterling, H. (2010). High diagnostic yield from transbronchial biopsy of solitary pulmonary nodules using low-dose CT-guidance. *Respirology* 15: 677–682.

54 Kurimoto, N., Miyazawa, T., and Okimasa, S. (2004). Endobronchial ultrasonography using a guide sheath increases the ability to diagnose peripheral pulmonary lesions endoscopically. *Chest* 126 (3): 959–965.

55 Asano, F., Eberhardt, R., and Herth, F.J. (2014). Virtual bronchoscopic navigation for peripheral pulmonary lesions. *Respiration* 88: 430–440.

56 Harms, W., Krempien, R., Grehn, C. et al. (2005). Electromagnetically navigated brachytherapy as a new treatment option for peripheral pulmonary tumors. *Strahlenther. Onkol.* 2: 108–111.

57 Becker, H.D., Shirakawa, T., Tanaka, F. et al. (1989). Transbronchial (transbronchoscopic) lung biopsy in the immunocompromised patient. *Eur. Respir. Mon.* 9: 193–208.

58 Babiak, A., Hetzel, J., Krishna, G. et al. (2009). Transbronchial cryobiopsy: a new tool for lung biopsies. *Respiration* 78: 203–208.

59 Cooper, J.D., Patterson, G.A., Sundaresan, R.S. et al. (1996). Results of 150 consecutive bilateral lung volume reduction procedures in patients with severe emphysema. *J. Thorac. Cardiovasc. Surg.* 112: 1319–1330.

60 National Emphysema Treatment Trial Research Group (1999). Rationale and design of the National Emphysema Treatment Trial (NETT): a prospective randomized trial of lung volume reduction surgery. *J. Thorac. Cardiovasc. Surg.* 118: 518–528.

61 National Emphysema Treatment Trial Research Group (2001). Patients at high risk of death after lung-volume reduction surgery. *N. Engl. J. Med.* 345: 1075–1083.

62 Sciurba, F.C., Ernst, A., Herth, F.J., and VENT Study Research Group (2010). A randomized study of endobronchial valves for advanced emphysema. *N. Engl. J. Med.* 363: 1233–1244.

63 Gasparini, S., Zuccatosta, L., Bonifazi, M., and Bolliger, C.T. (2012). Bronchoscopic treatment of emphysema: state of the art. *Respiration* 84 (3): 250–263.

64 Gompelmann, D., Eberhardt, R., and Herth, F. (2014). Endoscopic volume reduction in COPD – a critical review. *Dtsch. Arztebl. Int.* 111: 827–833.

65 Wechsler, M.E., Laviolette, M., Rubin, A. et al. (2013). Bronchial thermoplasty – long term safety and effectiveness in severe persistent asthma. *J. Allergy Clin. Immunol.* 132 (6): 1295–1302.

66 Panchabhai, T.S. and Mehta, A. (2015). Historical perspectives of bronchoscopy: connecting the dots. *Ann. Am. Thorac. Soc.* 12 (5): 631–641.

67 Becker, H.D. (1999). Heading into a virtual world, editorial. *J. Bronchol.* 6: 151–152.

68 Becker, H.D. (2001). Bronchoscopy. Year 2001 and beyond. *Clin. Chest Med.* 22 (2): 225–239.

69 Becker, H.D. (2006). Bronchoscopy and computer technology. In: *Thoracic Endoscopy: Advances in Interventional Pulmonology* (eds. M.J. Simoff and E.A. Sterman DH), 88–118. Malden, MA: Blackwell.

70 Becker, H.D., Slawik, M., Miyazawa, T. et al. (2009). Vibration response imaging as a new tool for interventional-bronchoscopy outcome assessment: a prospective pilot study. *Respiration* 77: 179–194.

71 Becker, H.D. (2009). Vibration response imaging – finally a real stethoscope. *Respiration* 77: 236–239.

第 2 章

可弯曲支气管镜技术培训

Jason Akulian[1] and David Feller-Kopman[2]

[1] Section of Interventional Pulmonology, Division of Pulmonary and Critical Care Medicine, University of North Carolina at Chapel Hill, Chapel Hill, NC, USA

[2] Interventional Pulmonology, Division of Pulmonary and Critical Care Medicine, Johns Hopkins University School of Medicine, Baltimore, MD, USA

（译者：焦　洋　董宇超　译者单位：海军军医大学第一附属医院）

2.1 池田茂人（1925—2001年）：可弯曲支气管镜之父

在1965年可弯曲支气管镜问世之前，支气管内评估与治疗是通过直视下的硬质支气管镜进行的。Gustav Killian 于 1876 年引入了硬质支气管镜，随后被耳鼻喉科医师采用，这使气管和中央气道得以可视化。硬质支气管镜的应用从简单的气道可视化发展到清除异物、诊断主动脉瘤和肿大淋巴结、去除白喉假膜和治疗肺结核[1,2]。这些发展体现了在气道疾病治疗上取得的重大进展，但必须承认的是，硬质支气管镜的刚性结构设计具有其固有的局限性，包括无法可视化上叶或中叶和双侧下叶的亚段[2]。1962年，日本国家癌症中心成立[3]。同年，池田茂人（图 2.1）领导的团队开发了用于食管镜和硬质支气管镜检查的玻璃纤维光导，取代了远端电灯泡，改善了支气管镜远端的照明。

在玻璃纤维光导开发后的 5 年里，两项重要的进展巩固了池田茂人作为"可弯曲支气管镜之父"的声誉。首先是池田茂人在东京新成立的国家癌症中心进行病例数据收集期间，描述了肺癌切除病例的气道分布情况，并注意到 48 例病例可被考虑是"早期肺癌"（切除的标本小于 3 cm）。他继续报告说，只有 20.8%（10/48）的病例可以通过硬质性支气管镜发现。池田茂人描述了可弯曲支气管镜的需求，即不仅可以看到上叶，还能够到达远端气道（Ⅱ~Ⅳ段）。在他看来，这种可弯曲支气管镜的使用可能会在气道腔内看到另外 62.4%（30/48）的病变[2]。池田茂人对这些问题的认识，以及他与町田公司合作开发玻璃纤维光导的经验，促使他在 1964 年春天萌生出生产可弯曲性支气管镜原型机的想法[4]。该原型机的规格包括但不限于小于 6 mm 的外径，15 μm 的图像和光导纤维，以及可弯曲的远端尖端（表 2.1）。1 年后，类似规格的设计被提交给了奥林巴斯光学公司。1966 年夏天，町田和奥林巴斯公司都提交了他们的原型机设计，随后在丹麦哥本哈根举行的第九届国际胸部疾病大会上展示。

可弯曲支气管镜的后续迭代包括但不限于增加工作通道、提高耐久性和远端尖端的可弯曲度。可弯曲支气管镜的另一个重要进展出现在 1987 年，宾得公司推出了一种在远端配有微型摄影机和在尖端配有微型电荷耦合器的支气管镜，取代了传统的纤维图像束传导，进而提高了图像分辨率[5]。奥林巴斯和东芝–町田公司也纷纷效仿，并很快推出了类似的产品。这种"视频支气管镜"代表了"现代"支气管镜中的第一代产品，自问世以来经历了迭代发展，包括各种尺寸的

表 2.1 可弯曲纤维支气管镜规格表（1964 年）

外径（mm）	<6
图像传导光纤（厚度和数量）	15 μm，>15 000
光导光纤（厚度和数量）	15~20 μm，>10 000
远端刚性部长度（mm）	<10
焦距（固定焦距，cm）	0.5~3.0
尖端屈曲角度	60°，距离远端尖端 30 mm
视野	80°
总长度（cm）	100

2.2 可弯曲支气管镜技术培训与教育

随着可弯曲支气管镜的不断发展，人们认识到需要对其进行专门的技术培训和教育。最初，教育集中在阐释支气管解剖学、疾病状态和支气管镜操作的教科书上[8-10]。1975 年，Zavala 发表了 1971—1974 年间对 600 例患者进行诊断性纤维支气管镜检查的数据[11]。Zavala 描述了其团队在支气管镜插入、移动和活检方面的技术。他还讨论了标本的处理，以及所使用设备的术后处理。在这项工作中，通过支气管镜活检建立了两种最常见的诊断：恶性和感染性疾病。最后，他试图量化每种技术的诊断率以及操作并发症。1974 年，Zavala 发表上述研究结果之前，美国胸科医师学会（ACCP）指派了一个代表胸外科医师、耳鼻喉科医师和内科医师的小组委员会来制定内窥镜检查方面的培训标准。1976 年发布的标准相当宽泛，代表了内窥镜检查的最低预期标准[12]。

1976 年，Zavala 开发了第一个支气管镜教学模型（图 2.2）。该模型采用成人气道插管模型作为上气道，用 Zavala 自制的气道替代声门下气道的远端。该模型可让学员进行支气管镜检查训练，同时避免了新手直接在患者上进行操作[13]。1978 年的一篇论文对支气管镜检查培训的现状提出了质疑，强调观察者需要识别特定的病理。此外，该论文还首次提出基本的操作技能需求，受训者实施支气管镜操作的例数应不低于 50 次[14]。1980 年，Dull 等发表的研究表明，接受 100~4 000 次支气管镜检查的指导医生，在支气管镜诊断的准确性上没有显著差异。他们认为，通过 100 次支气管镜操作足以熟练掌握该技术。

1982 年，ACCP 再次制定了技能水平和培训标准，这一次是专门针对纤维支气管镜检查推进的[16]。

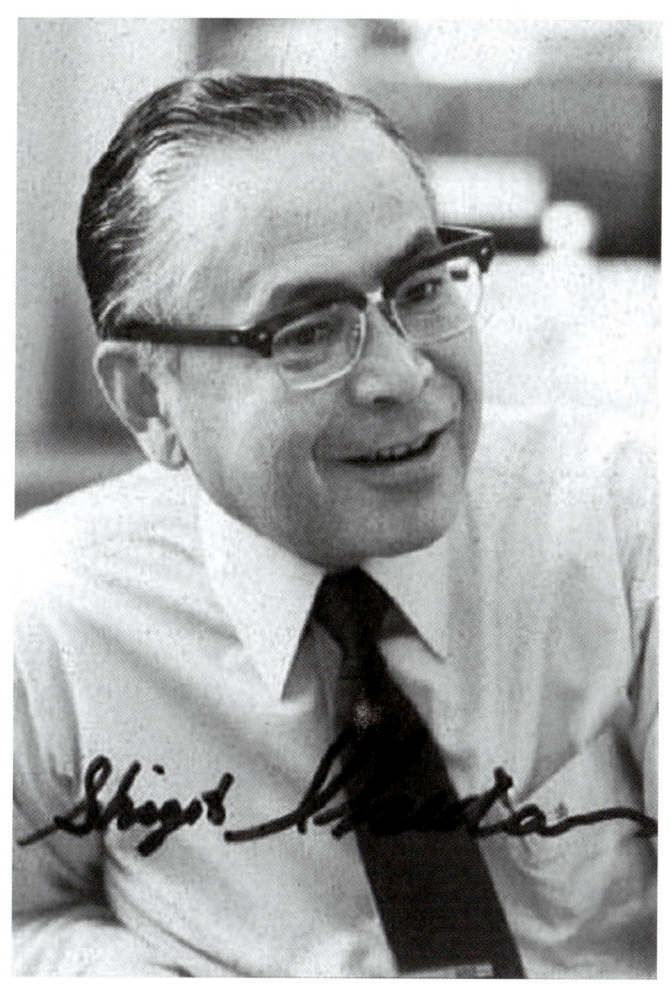

图 2.1　池田茂人

资料来源：经 Wolters Kluwer 健康公司许可复制。

气管镜或工作通道，以及各种成像方法和屈曲、旋转、自由度，并成为肺科和胸外科实践中必不可少的工具，其用途也进一步扩展到军事、执法和工业应用中，包括飞机发动机和公共供水系统的检查。

2004 年，随着可弯曲经支气管镜腔内超声（endobronchial ultrasonography，EBUS）[6,7]的引入，可弯曲视频支气管镜得以进一步发展。EBUS 将混合纤维视频支气管镜与超声探头相结合，可以对气道外的结构和常规支气管镜无法直视的结构进行实时评估和取样。在池田博士首次构想出可弯曲纤维支气管镜以来的 60 多年里，我们已见证了这项技术惊人的进步。我们现在不仅可以"看见"，还能进行活检、对肺门和纵隔淋巴结进行分期，以及研发出超薄支气管镜等众多的产品迭代。在可弯曲支气管镜的基础上，先进的技术如电磁导航支气管镜，甚至机器人支气管镜都在不断革新中。

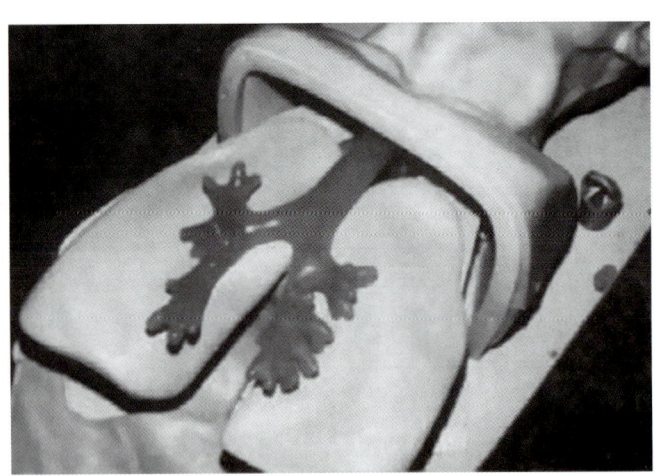

图 2.2 Zavala 肺模型
早期供医生进行支气管镜操作训练的肺模型。

指南推荐至少需要在监督下完成 50 次的诊断性支气管镜检查，并被分为认知和临床培训目标。尽管作者有专业知识背景，但并未提供任何数据支持该指导建议。1987 年，美国胸科学会（ATS）发布的指南遵循了 1982 年的 ACCP 指南，该指南针对纤维支气管镜的适应证和应用，而不是技能水平[17]。在接下来的 20 年里，大部分纤维支气管镜培训都集中在床旁或术中教学，秉承一日课程和"看一个，做一个，教一个"的原则。虽然这样的培训方式有效地培养出了许多能够熟练进行支气管镜检查的医生，但少有公开数据，基本的操作标准流程仍然缺乏。

从 20 世纪 90 年代开始，许多因素使人们对支气管镜检查培训的兴趣日益高涨。其中一个因素是，美国内科委员会要求在呼吸危重症监护认证的特定流程中证明相关操作的胜任能力，并声明无论 ACCP，还是 ATS 都未提供以数据为依据的"授予医院特权以进行与呼吸危重症亚专科相关的重要操作的综合指南"[18]。另外两个因素分别是引入了高保真支气管镜模拟器用于住院医师和呼吸内镜专科医师培训，以及介入肺病学（interventional pulmonology，IP）作为一个亚专科的发展。

2.3 可弯曲支气管镜技术培训的扩展工具

2000 年，Haponik 等对肺科专科医生开展了一项问卷调查，旨在了解一些有关支气管镜培训的情况。调查显示，支气管镜技术培训主要以导师的个人指导、讲座和病例讨论的形式为主，但很少采用肺模型和教学视频的形式。此外，作者指出，近 1/3 的受训者不熟悉经支气管镜插管技术，且很少进行治疗性的支气管镜操作，但值得注意的是，他们在使用支气管镜模型时都热情高涨。本研究没有对技能或培训质量进行评价[19]。随后，一系列验证和评估高保真支气管镜模型的研究相继发表。这些数据证实："专家级支气管镜操作者"、"中等级别支气管镜操作者"和"初学者"在手术时间、主观的技术评价和定量的支气管镜操作评分方面存在显著差异[20]。此外，通过高保真支气管镜模型训练还能够提高进入叶段数和减少碰撞次数，进而提高受训者的灵巧度和准确性[21]。在意识到模型在支气管镜培训中的重要性后，Domenico 等还提出了一个建立低保真支气管镜模型的方案，作为那些无法负担高保真支气管镜模型机构的替代选择[22]。

此后，很多研究将说教式教学和基于模型的培训相结合。从公开发表的数据可以看出，模型培训可以极大地提高操作技能，并有助于支气管镜培训的标准化[23,24]。

Wahidi 等发表了一项有关支气管镜技术培训的前瞻性、多中心的队列研究，研究对象是新入职的肺科专科医生，分成两组展开培训，第 1 组学员接受现行的多中心统一的支气管镜培训方案，第 2 组学员则接受模型培训以及在线支气管镜培训课程。两组学员均被要求完成一系列操作，并通过支气管镜技能评估量表（bronchoscopy skills and tasks assessment tool，BSTAT）进行评分。结果显示：所有学员在操作前 30 例支气管镜技能获得速度较快，而在操作 30~100 例时虽然支气管镜技能仍有不断提升，但速度变缓；值得注意的是，学员操作技能的提升并未在 50 例时达到最大值。此外，与第 1 组学员相比，除了 75 例的操作节点，第 2 组学员在其他所有例数的操作节点上的 BSTAT 评分均显著提高[25]。

2013 年，一项基于模型的支气管镜培训的荟萃分析表明，与未干预组相比，采用了支气管镜模型培训的学员在支气管镜技能水平和操作时间上有了显著提高；但与标准的教学组相比，相关指标并未发现有显著改善[26]。综上所述，基于模型的支气管镜培训至少对于支气管镜初学者来说是非常有益的。

2.4 介入肺脏病和支气管镜技术训练

介入肺脏病尽管已经存在一段时间了，但 2001 年在《新英格兰医学杂志》(The New England Journal of Medicine)上发表的关于该领域的综述，才真正意义上将其作为一个亚专科引入到医学和肺病领域[27]。在这篇综述中，Seijo 和 Sterman 详细介绍了介入肺脏病专科医生在临床实践中所使用到的各种操作技术。介入肺脏病相关研究项目的逐渐增加促使该领域愈发成熟。而随着介入肺脏病的发展，各种先进的诊断和治疗性支气管镜技术不断更新，专科医生开始意识到技能水平衡量和培训标准化的必要性。

2002 年和 2003 年，欧洲呼吸学会 (ERS)、ATS 和 ACCP 都发表了关于介入肺脏病实践的指南[28,29]。这些指南都经过深思熟虑，试图制定出支气管镜相关的操作规范，以及为获得支气管镜操作技能的最小操作数量提供指导。尽管做了最大努力，研究者也仅能依靠有限的研究数据来提出指导意见。ACCP 发表了一份专家小组报告，该报告使用了 PICO 问题构建表，以最大程度地了解各研究所报道的支气管镜培训的差异，并为建立培训标准提供指导。该小组发现，尽管可用的数据有限（每个 PICO 问题只有 3~11 项研究可评估），但各研究在培训方法上存在较大差异。同时，该报告还提出了 ERS、ATS 和 ACCP 关于支气管镜操作指南的汇总表，但需要强调的是，这些指南主要代表专家意见。

根据上述指南，无论在培训模型验证还是在常规支气管镜培训方法上都取得了积极的发展[23,24,30-34]。而随着 EBUS、导航支气管镜的引入和硬质支气管镜的重新引入，支气管镜领域继续不断发展。这些新技术体现了支气管镜在对肺癌患者和良性肺部疾病患者的微创诊断方面取得了巨大进步。而介入肺脏病的飞速发展也给操作技能评估、培训和实践模式转变带来了新的挑战。2012 年，Davoudi 等发表了一篇旨在评估支气管内超声技能和经验评估工具（EBUS-skills and tasks assessment tool，EBUS-STAT）的论文。EBUS-STAT 被用于评估 3 个机构的 24 名支气管镜操作者（根据技能水平分为 3 个等级——初级、中级和专家级）的技能水平，结果显示 EBUS-STAT 具有高度的测试者间可靠性，并可将经 EBUS 进行支气管针吸活检（transbronchial needle aspiration，TBNA）操作者的技能水平从初级到专家级进行分类[35]。2013 年，Feller-Kopman 等在一个大型学术医疗中心评估了 EBUS 的引入对传统 TBNA（conventional TBNA，cTBNA）培训的影响。研究发现，与 cTBNA 相比，EBUS 的实施与患者数量的显著增加和诊断率的显著提高密切相关。此外，与 EBUS 相比，肺科专科医生进行 cTBNA 操作的数量、诊断率和准确性都显著下降[36]。

2016 年，Mahmood 等开发了一种评估硬质支气管镜技术和能力的工具（RIGID-TASC）。RIGID-TASC 作为一种客观、能力导向的评估工具，可以评价基础的硬质支气管镜操作技能，包括硬镜下插管和导航技术。该研究纳入了来自美国两个不同学术医疗中心的共 30 名专科医生（初级、中级和专家级医生各 10 名）并评估了他们操作硬质支气管镜的情况。研究显示，RIGID-TASC 具有高度的测试者间可靠性，且不同级别的医生之间的 RIGID-TASC 评分存在显著差异[37]。

支气管镜技术的评估工具，如 BSTAT、EBUS-STAT 和 RIGID-TASC，是最近开发的，用以量化评估进行基础和进阶的支气管镜操作医生的技能水平。虽然上述评估工具所采用的方法具有一定的局限性，但它们为改进支气管镜实践和标准化支气管镜操作提供了数据支持。在支气管镜技能评估系统中，仍然缺乏对周围型病变导航的支气管镜评估工具，目前只有有限的仿真模型数据可用[38,39]。由于先进的支气管镜检查技术在实践中的应用愈发普遍，因此迫切需要与该技术培训、操作技能获取、设备维护等方面相关的数据。在最近的一项评估使用 EBUS-TNBA 进行适当的肺癌纵隔分期的研究中，操作例数的不同导致专科医生在进行适当的纵隔分期方面存在显著差异[40]。这些数据表明，掌握一项技能，不仅需要充分练习，还需要在规定的时间内进行特定数量的练习，同时也需要正确且规范化的操作流程。随着支气管镜技术的不断革新，这些复杂的问题将变得越来越具有挑战性。因此，需要进一步的研究来解决这些问题。

2.5 结论

我们目前站在一个巨人——池田博士的肩膀上。如果没有他的远见和开发可弯曲纤维支气管镜的动力，我们评估气道和肺部疾病的能力可能仍然受到严重的限制。虽然池田博士从未设想过外周支气管镜、EBUS 或现代硬质支气管镜的发展，但他以患者为中心的技术应用、教育和指导的核心价值观，将继续推动着我们今天的实践。最后，我们一定要牢记，只有不忘初心，才能继续砥砺前行。

参考文献

1 Shirakawa, T. and Becker, H.D. (2002). The dawn of bronchoscopy – the biography of Ino Kubo, the Japanese pioneer of bronchoscopy. *Journal of Bronchoscopy* 9: 59–64.

2 Ikeda, S., Yanai, N., and Ishikawa, S. (1968). Flexible bronchofiberscope. *Keio Journal of Medicine* 17 (1): 1–16.

3 Shirakawa, T. (2003). The history of bronchoscopy in Japan – the keynote lecture at 12th WCB & WCBE. *Journal of Bronchology* 10: 223–230.

4 Ikeda, S., Tsuboi, E., Ono, R., and Ishikawa, S. (1971). Flexible bronchofiberscope. *Japanese Journal of Clinical Oncology* 1 (1): 55–65.

5 Miyazawa, T. (2000). History of the flexible bronchoscope. In: *Interventional Bronchoscopy* (eds. C.T. Bolliger and P.N. Mathur), 16–21. Basel: Karger.

6 Yasufuku, K., Chiyo, M., Sekine, Y. et al. (2004). Real-time endobronchial ultrasound-guided transbronchial needle aspiration of mediastinal and hilar lymph nodes. *Chest* 126 (1): 122–128. https://doi.org/10.1378/chest.126.1.122.

7 Yasufuku, K., Chhajed, P.N., Sekine, Y. et al. (2004). Endobronchial ultrasound using a new convex probe: a preliminary study on surgically resected specimens. *Oncology Reports* 11 (2): 293–296.

8 Ikeda, S. (1974). *Atlas of Flexible Bronchofiberscopy*. Tokyo: Igaku Shoin Ltd.

9 Stradling, P. (1973). *Diagnostic Bronchoscopy*. London: Churchill Livingstone.

10 Sackner, M.A. (1975). Bronchofiberscopy. *American Review of Respiratory Disease* 111 (1): 62–88. https://doi.org/10.1164/arrd.1975.111.1.62.

11 Zavala, D.C. (1975). Diagnostic fiberoptic bronchoscopy: techniques and results of biopsy in 600 patients. *Chest* 68 (1): 12–19.

12 American College of Chest Physicians (1976). Standards for training in endoscopy. Statement of the Committee on Bronchoesophagology, American College of Chest Physicians. *Chest* 69 (5): 665–666.

13 King, E.G., Sproule, B.J., and Yamamoto, I. (1976). A teaching model for bronchoscopy. *Chest* 70 (1): 72–73.

14 Faber, L.P. (1978). Bronchoscopy training. *Chest* 73 (5 Suppl): 776–778.

15 Dull, W.L. (1980). Flexible fiberoptic bronchoscopy: an analysis of proficiency. *Chest* 77 (1): 65–67.

16 American College of Chest Physicians (1982). Guidelines for competency and training in fiberoptic bronchoscopy. Section on Bronchoscopy, American College of Chest Physicians. *Chest* 81 (6): 739.

17 American Thoracic Society (1987). Position paper on guidelines for fiberoptic bronchoscopy in adults. *American Review of Respiratory Disease* 136 (4): 1066. https://doi.org/10.1164/ajrccm/136.4.1066.

18 Hansen-Flaschen, J. (1995). Pulmonary and critical care procedures: under the spotlight. *American Journal of Respiratory and Critical Care Medicine* 151 (2 Pt 1): 275–277. https://doi.org/10.1164/ajrccm.151.2.7842177.

19 Haponik, E.F., Russell, G.B., Beamis, J.F. Jr. et al. (2000). Bronchoscopy training: current fellows' experiences and some concerns for the future. *Chest* 118 (3): 625–630.

20 Ost, D., DeRosiers, A., Britt, E.J. et al. (2001). Assessment of a bronchoscopy simulator. *American Journal of Respiratory and Critical Care Medicine* 164 (12): 2248–2255. https://doi.org/10.1164/ajrccm.164.12.2102087.

21 Colt, H.G., Crawford, S.W., and Galbraith, O. 3rd (2001). Virtual reality bronchoscopy simulation: a revolution in procedural training. *Chest* 120 (4): 1333–1339.

22 Di Domenico, S., Simonassi, C., and Chessa, L. (2007). Inexpensive anatomical trainer for bronchoscopy. *Interactive Cardiovascular and Thoracic Surgery* 6 (4): 567–569. https://doi.org/10.1510/icvts.2007.153601.

23 Crawford, S.W. and Colt, H.G. (2004). Virtual reality and written assessments are of potential value to determine knowledge and skill in flexible bronchoscopy. *Respiration* 71 (3): 269–275. https://doi.org/10.1159/000077425.

24 Davoudi, M., Osann, K., and Colt, H.G. (2008). Validation of two instruments to assess technical bronchoscopic skill using virtual reality simulation. *Respiration* 76 (1): 92–101. https://doi.org/10.1159/000126493.

25 Wahidi, M.M., Silvestri, G.A., Coakley, R.D. et al. (2010). A prospective multicenter study of competency metrics and educational interventions in the learning of bronchoscopy among new pulmonary fellows. *Chest* 137 (5): 1040–1049. https://doi.org/10.1378/chest.09-1234.

26 Kennedy, C.C., Maldonado, F., and Cook, D.A. (2013). Simulation-based bronchoscopy training: systematic review and meta-analysis. *Chest* 144 (1): 183–192. https://doi.org/10.1378/chest.12-1786.

27 Seijo, L.M. and Sterman, D.H. (2001). Interventional pulmonology. *New England Journal of Medicine* 344 (10): 740–749. https://doi.org/10.1056/NEJM200103083441007.

28 Bolliger, C.T., Mathur, P.N., Beamis, J.F. et al. (2002). ERS/ATS statement on interventional pulmonology. European Respiratory Society/American Thoracic Society. *European Respiratory Journal* 19 (2): 356–373.

29 Ernst, A., Silvestri, G.A., and Johnstone, D. (2003). Interventional pulmonary procedures: guidelines from the American College of Chest Physicians. *Chest* 123 (5): 1693–1717.

30 Davoudi, M., Quadrelli, S., Osann, K., and Colt, H.G. (2008). A competency-based test of bronchoscopic knowledge using the Essential Bronchoscopist: an initial concept study. *Respirology* 13 (5): 736–743. https://doi.org/10.1111/j.1440-1843.2008.01320.x.

31 Davoudi, M. and Colt, H.G. (2009). Bronchoscopy simulation: a brief review. *Advances in Health Sciences Education: Theory and Practice* 14 (2): 287–296. https://doi.org/10.1007/s10459-007-9095-x.

32 Quadrelli, S., Davoudi, M., Galindez, F., and Colt, H.G. (2009). Reliability of a 25-item low-stakes multiple-choice assessment of bronchoscopic knowledge. *Chest* 135 (2): 315–321. https://doi.org/10.1378/chest.08-0867.

33 Goldberg, R., Colt, H.G., Davoudi, M., and Cherrison, L. (2009). Realistic and affordable lo-fidelity model for learning bronchoscopic transbronchial needle aspiration. *Surgical Endoscopy* 23 (9): 2047–2052. https://doi.org/10.1007/s00464-008-9951-7.

34 Chen, J.S., Hsu, H.H., Lai, I.R. et al. (2006). Validation of a computer-based bronchoscopy simulator developed in Taiwan. *Journal of the Formosan Medical Association* 105 (7): 569–576. https://doi.org/10.1016/S0929-6646(09)60152-2.

35 Davoudi, M., Colt, H.G., Osann, K.E. et al. (2012). Endobronchial ultrasound skills and tasks assessment tool: assessing the validity evidence for a test of endobronchial ultrasound-guided transbronchial needle aspiration operator skill. *American Journal of Respiratory and Critical Care Medicine* 186 (8): 773–779. https://doi.org/10.1164/rccm.201111-1968OC.

36 Feller-Kopman, D.J., Brigham, E., Lechtzin, N. et al. (2013). Training perspective: the impact of starting an endobronchial ultrasound program at a major academic center on fellows training of transbronchial needle aspiration. *Annals of the American Thoracic Society* 10 (2): 127–130. https://doi.org/10.1513/AnnalsATS.201208-052OC.

37 Mahmood, K., Wahidi, M.M., Osann, K.E. et al. (2016). Development of a tool to assess basic competency in the performance of rigid bronchoscopy. *Annals of the American Thoracic Society* 13 (4): 502–511. https://doi.org/10.1513/AnnalsATS.201509-593OC.

38 Chen, A., Machuzak, M., Edell, E., and Silvestri, G.A. (2016). Peripheral bronchoscopy training using a human cadaveric model and simulated tumor targets. *Journal of Bronchology and Interventional Pulmonology* 23 (1): 83–86. https://doi.org/10.1097/LBR.0000000000000200.

39 Asano, F., Eberhardt, R., and Herth, F.J. (2014). Virtual bronchoscopic navigation for peripheral pulmonary lesions. *Respiration* 88 (5): 430–440. https://doi.org/10.1159/000367900.

40 Miller, R.J., Mudambi, L., Vial, M.R. et al. (2017). Evaluation of appropriate mediastinal staging among endobronchial ultrasound bronchoscopists. Annals of the *American Thoracic Society* 14 (7): 1162–1168. https://doi.org/10.1513/AnnalsATS.201606-487OC.

第 3 章

气道实用解剖学

Mani S. Kavuru[1], Atul C. Mehta[2], and J. Francis Turner, Jr.[3,4]

[1] Division of Pulmonary and Critical Care Medicine, Jefferson Center for Critical Care, Thomas Jefferson University and Hospital, Philadelphia, PA, USA

[2] Lerner College of Medicine, Buoncore Family Endowed Chair in Lung Transplantation, Department of Pulmonary Medicine, Respiratory Institute, Cleveland Clinic, Cleveland, OH, USA

[3] Division of Pulmonary and Critical Care Medicine, University of Tennessee Graduate School of Medicine, Knoxville, TN, USA

[4] National Supercomputing Institute, University of Nevada, Las Vegas, NV, USA

（译者：方 晨 张艺菲 译者单位：海军军医大学第一附属医院）

3.1 咽和喉

可弯曲支气管镜检查通常是经口或经鼻进入气管。因此，熟悉口和鼻的正常解剖和病理对于支气管镜顺利进入气管是非常重要的。当然，对于咯血和喘息的患者行支气管镜检查时需要对其上呼吸道进行仔细评估。鼻自外向内依次分为鼻孔、鼻腔和鼻咽。鼻腔被鼻中隔平均分为左右两侧，每侧鼻腔又被3个鼻甲（贝壳状的骨性结构）分开，鼻腔下方以硬腭为界将鼻腔与口腔分开。鼻旁窦开口于鼻甲下部的鼻道。鼻黏膜的血液供应来自Kisselbach丛，其通过上颌动脉和面动脉的分支在鼻腔前内侧壁汇合形成，这是鼻出血的常见部位[1]。

咽部长12~15 cm，包括下咽部和喉，连接鼻腔（鼻咽）和口腔（口咽），延伸到环状软骨[1]。咽部的肌肉包括环咽肌在内，主要起到近端食管括约肌的作用，以防食管反流。腺样体（又称咽扁桃体）位于鼻咽后壁。口咽侧壁以扁桃体柱为界，上壁以软腭为界，前壁和下壁以舌为界，后壁以C2、C3脊椎为界。口咽腔不是骨性结构，很容易受到损伤。喉咽位于会厌和环状软骨下缘之间。

喉部长5~7 cm，位于C4、C5、C6水平，是一个由软骨、韧带和肌肉组成的复杂器官[1]。通过内镜可以观察到会厌前端，杓状会厌皱襞两侧以及旁边的鼻窦梨状隐窝。声门是由上方的前庭襞（假声带）、下方的声襞（真声带）和后方的杓状软骨构成[2]。在吸气过程中，声带远离中线，声门裂呈三角形。在呼气过程中，声带内收，声门裂仅为一个非常小的开口。男性声带内收的最大距离为19 mm，女性为12 mm。与儿童不同，成人的声门裂是喉部最狭窄的部分[2]。

3.2 气管支气管树

正常成人气管起始于环状软骨下缘，延伸10~14 cm，直到T5水平分为左主支气管和右主支气管。以胸骨上切迹为界，上1/3的气管位于胸腔外，下2/3的气管位于胸腔内。气管直径平均为2.5 cm，其前壁由18~24个缺口向后的C形软骨组成，其后壁缺口由膜部肌肉组织组成。在正常成年人中，由于气道壁结构的支撑作用，气管的直径在整个呼吸周期中能够维持稳定。而对于阻塞性气道疾病患者或老年人，由于气管膜部向前塌陷，在其咳嗽或呼气过程中，气管的动态顺应性有所降低[3]。

正常情况下，主动脉弓压迫气管的左侧将其推向右侧。成人气管宽深比范围为0.6~3.0。气管隆突通常很锐利，可以在呼吸周期中移动[4]。右主支气管与气管纵轴的延长线夹角为25°~30°，管腔直径约为16 mm，分叉前的平均长度为2 cm。右上叶开口直径平均为10 mm，远端分支分为尖段、后段和前段支气管[5]。继分出右上叶后，右主支气管延伸为右中间段支气管。

右中间段前壁继续延伸，成为右中叶支气管，其亚段分为内段和外段。由于位置靠前，异物通常会从气管落入右中间段支气管进而进入右中叶支气管。右下叶支气管为右中间段支气管后壁的延续，进而演变成5段，且位置多变[6]。右下叶背段通常在右中叶的反方向位置从右中间段分出。接下来，右下叶内侧基底段从内壁分出形成亚段后进一步细分。随后，右下叶从上到下依次分为前、外侧和后基底段3个亚段结构（A-L-P）。

左主支气管与气管纵轴呈45°角，比右主支气管更窄、更长，平均长度为5 cm。左主支气管远端分为左上、下叶支气管。左上叶支气管分为舌叶（由上舌段和下舌段组成）和固有上叶（由尖后段和前段组成）。左下叶支气管首先分出后位的左下叶背段分支，随后延伸为左下叶基底段，进一步分为前内段、外侧段和后基底段，左下叶基底段的变异也多见[6,7]。

3.3 气道、淋巴和血管之间的关系

全面了解支气管正常解剖结构、常见的先天性变异以及紧邻气道外部的正常结构均十分重要[8]，掌握这些知识有助于提高支气管镜相关诊疗操作水平，包括经支气管针吸活检术（transbronchial needle aspiration，TBNA）、激光治疗术、支气管腔内放射治疗。掌握这些解剖知识有助于识别淋巴结或腔外占位性病变，在疾病诊断或分期中非常重要[9,10]，也有助于避免因疏忽误入某些与气道相邻的血供丰富区域。

食管位于气管后方、紧贴气管膜部。主动脉弓位于气管远端1/3的左前方，此处气管壁可见动脉搏动，应避免在此区域进行有创操作[8]。上腔静脉和奇静脉位于气管远端1/3的右前方。主动脉弓和无名动脉位于气管正前方平隆崎水平。右肺动脉紧贴右主支气管前壁及右上叶支气管开口。右中叶和下叶支气管与周围血管相对位置变异度较大。主动脉弓和左肺动脉的解剖位置与左主支气管和左肺上叶支气管的解剖位置毗邻。

淋巴结与气道关系密切。气管旁淋巴结位于气管两侧，右气管旁淋巴结位于气管下段倒数第1~2个软骨环的右后外侧（图3.1）。隆崎下淋巴结通常位于气管隆

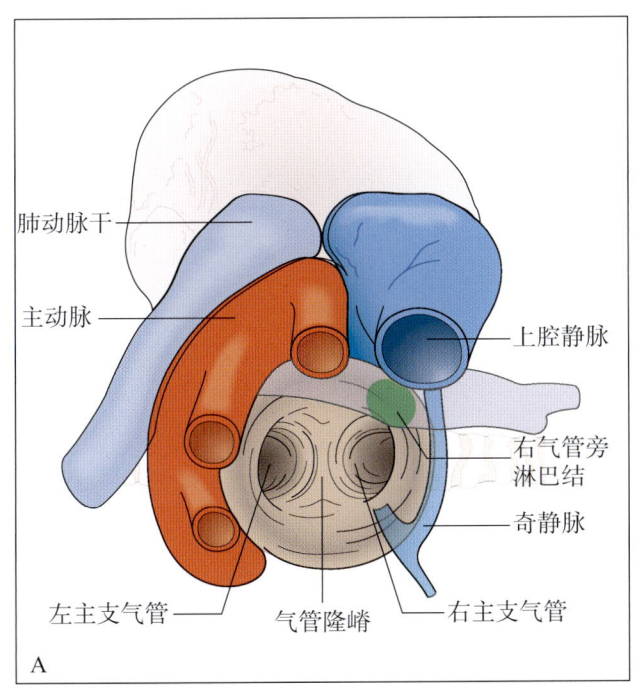
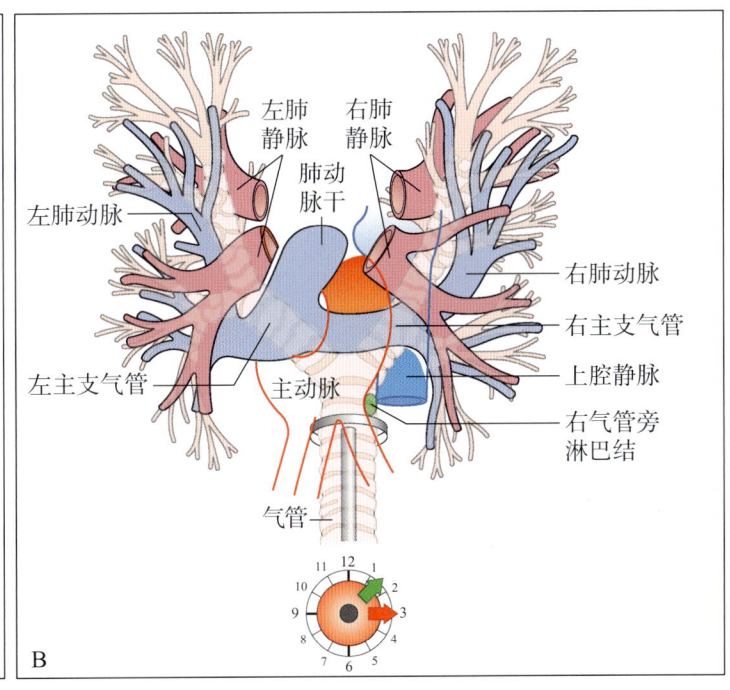

图3.1 气管远端的正常解剖关系

A. 与邻近血管和淋巴结叠加后气管远端的镜下所见，右气管旁淋巴结位于1点钟和2点钟方向之间，奇静脉位于3点钟方向；B. 支气管镜钟面视图，1点钟和2点钟方向之间是右气管旁淋巴结TBNA的穿刺位置，3点钟方向TBNA穿刺不安全（奇静脉）。

嵴下方内侧，可以通过在隆嵴两侧任意一方从外向内进针 3~5 mm 取样（图 3.2），而非直接穿刺隆嵴，避免穿刺到软骨。肺门淋巴结可以通过穿刺左右两侧小隆嵴获取，右侧位于平右上叶开口层面，左侧位于平左上叶开口层面（图 3.3）。由于右上叶支气管前壁紧贴右肺动脉，该区域需慎行 TBNA 和其他类似操作（图 3.4、图 3.5）。

左气管旁淋巴结位于左主支气管开口近气管下段（图 3.6），这组淋巴结较难穿刺取样，但可以通过先将穿刺针挂在气管下段平隆嵴左侧壁，然后将气管镜和穿刺针整体下送，从而使穿刺针从侧面进入气管进行抽吸取样。图 3.7 显示了左肺上叶支气管和左肺动脉之间的联系。图 3.8 显示了左肺门淋巴结的位置。

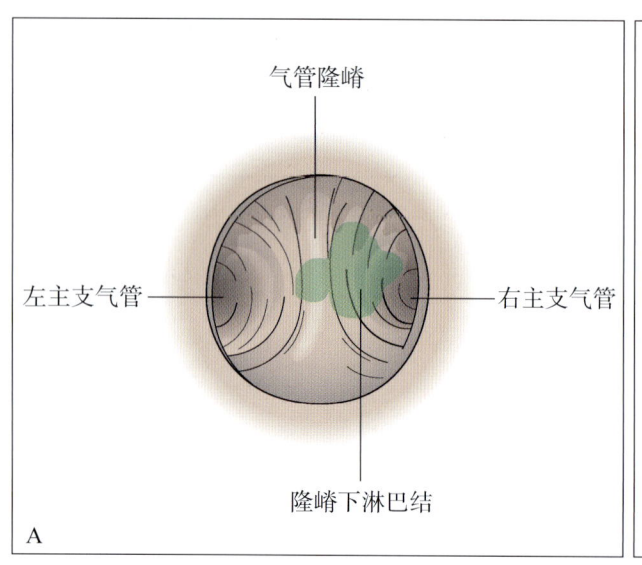
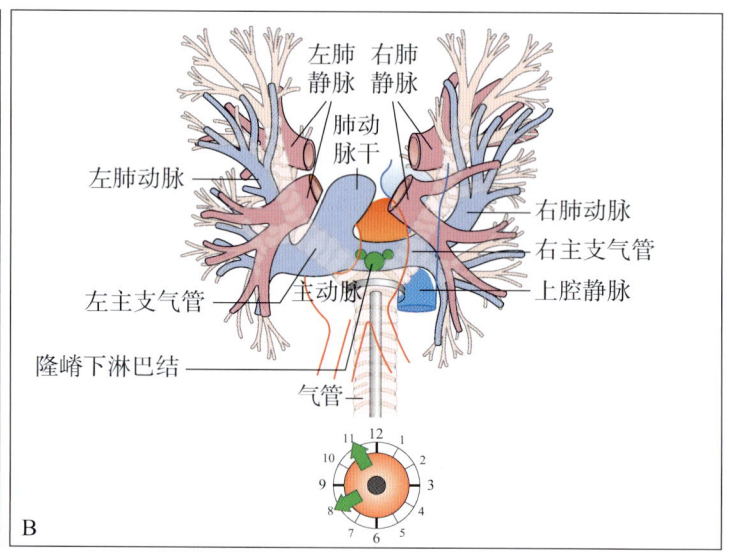

图 3.2　气管隆嵴的正常解剖关系
A. 与周围淋巴结叠加后气管隆嵴的镜下所见；B. 右主支气管开口处支气管镜钟面视图，8~11 点钟方向之间是隆嵴下淋巴结 TBNA 穿刺位置。

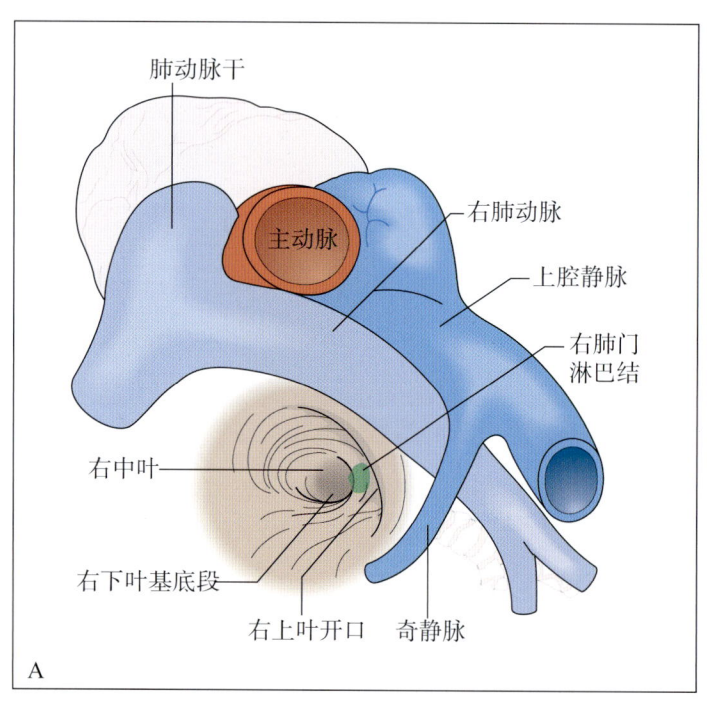
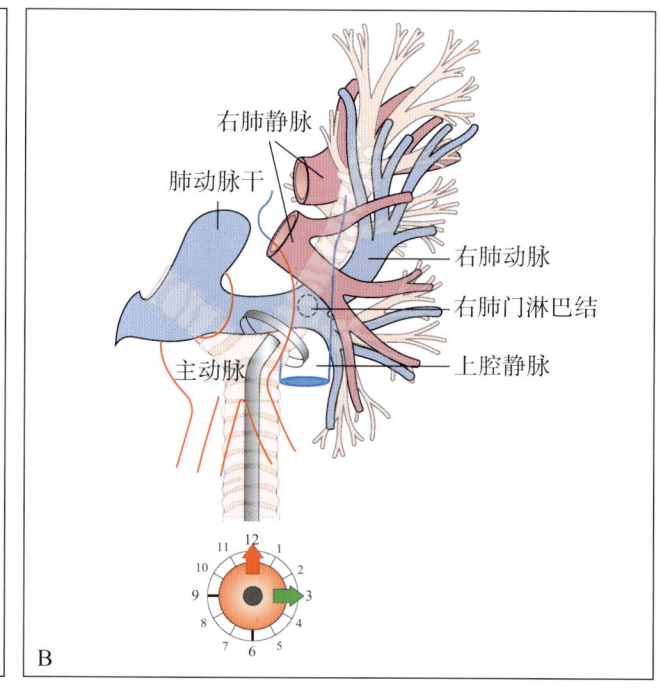

图 3.3　右中间段支气管层面的正常解剖关系
A. 与血管和淋巴结叠加后右中间段支气管镜下所见；B. 支气管镜钟面视图，3 点钟方向是 TBNA 右肺门淋巴结穿刺位点。12 点钟方向 TBNA 穿刺不安全（右肺动脉）。

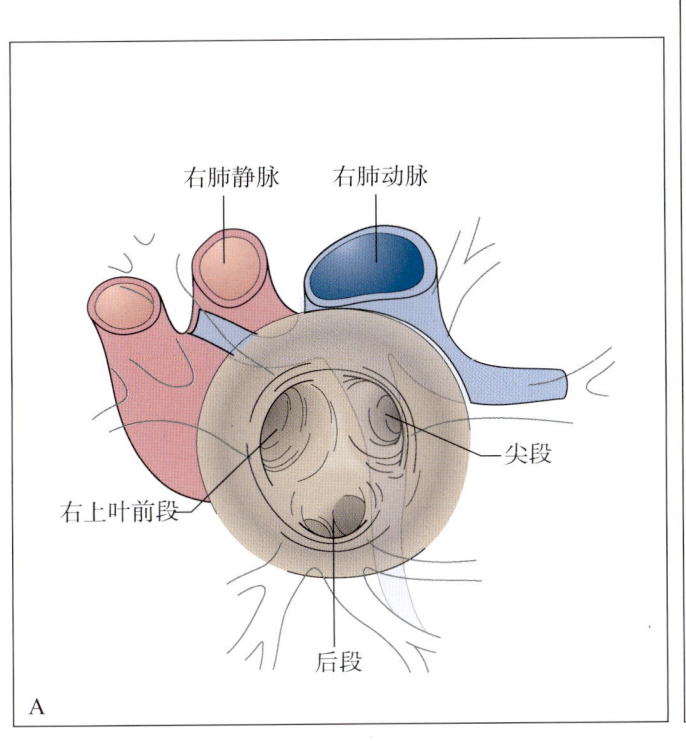 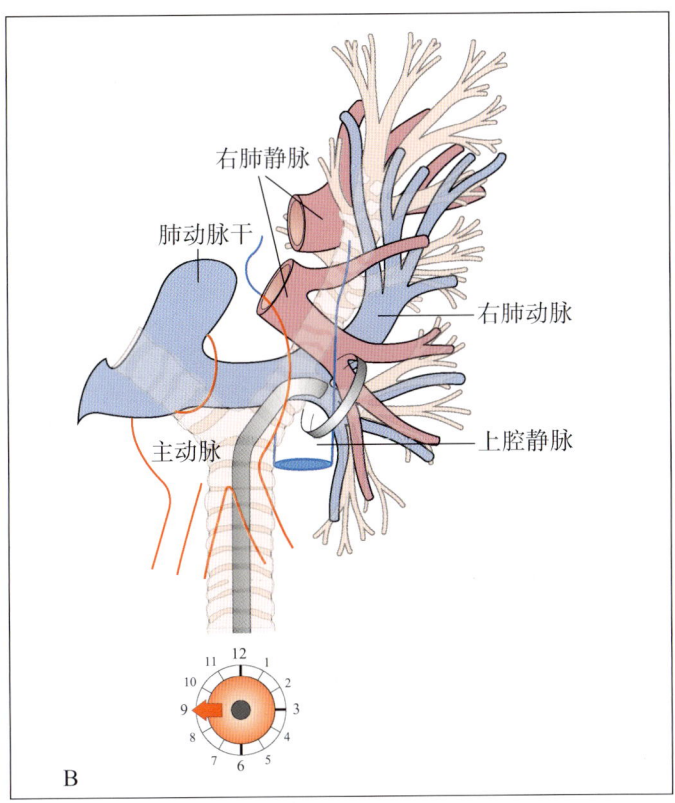

图 3.4 右肺上叶的正常解剖关系

A. 与周围血管和淋巴结叠加后右上叶支气管开口的镜下所见；B. 支气管镜钟面视图，9 点钟方向是右肺动脉所在位置。

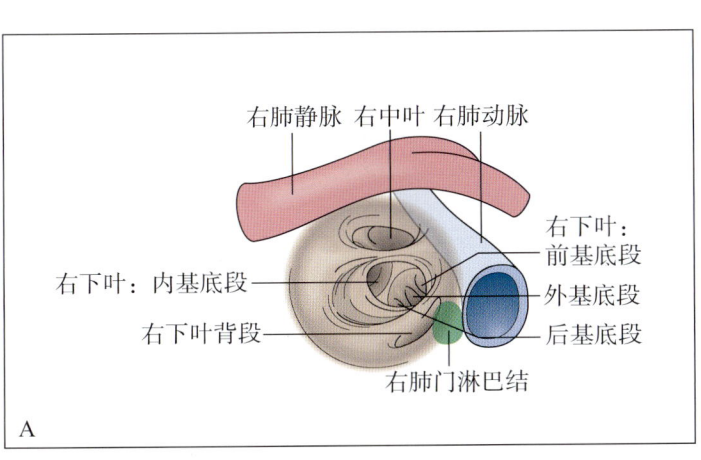 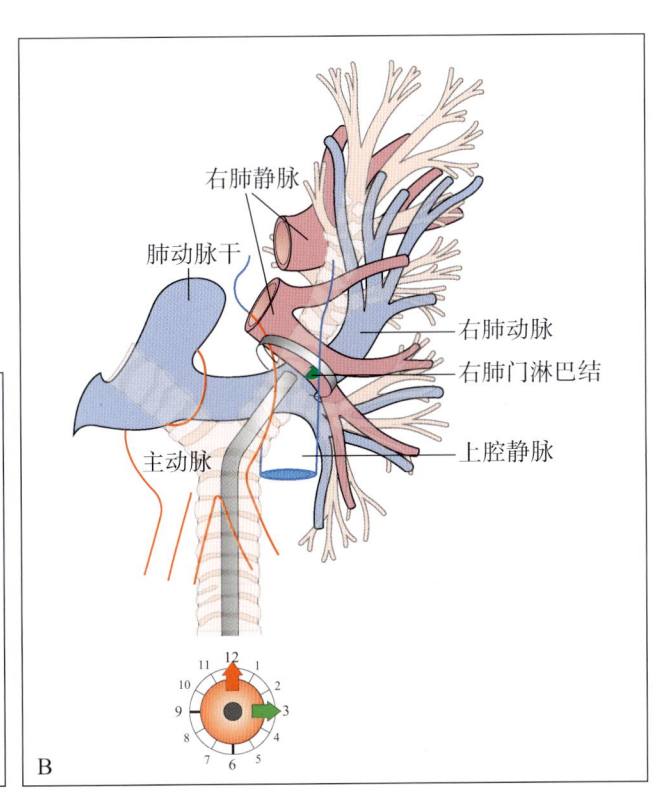

图 3.5 右中间段支气管远端正常解剖关系

A. 右中间段支气管镜下所见，右肺门淋巴结位于 3 点钟位置；B. 支气管镜钟面视图，3 点钟方向是 TBNA 右肺门淋巴结穿刺位点。12 点钟方向 TBNA 穿刺不安全（右肺静脉）。需注意右中叶支气管和周围血管结构之间的关系。

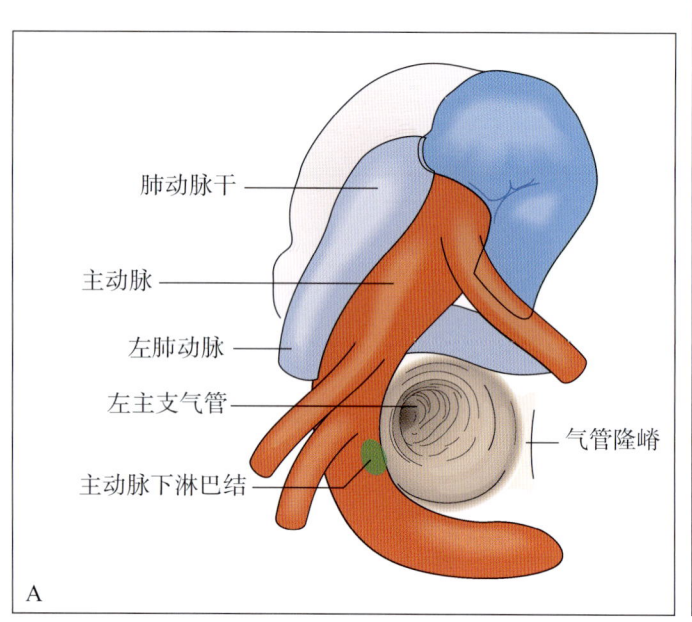
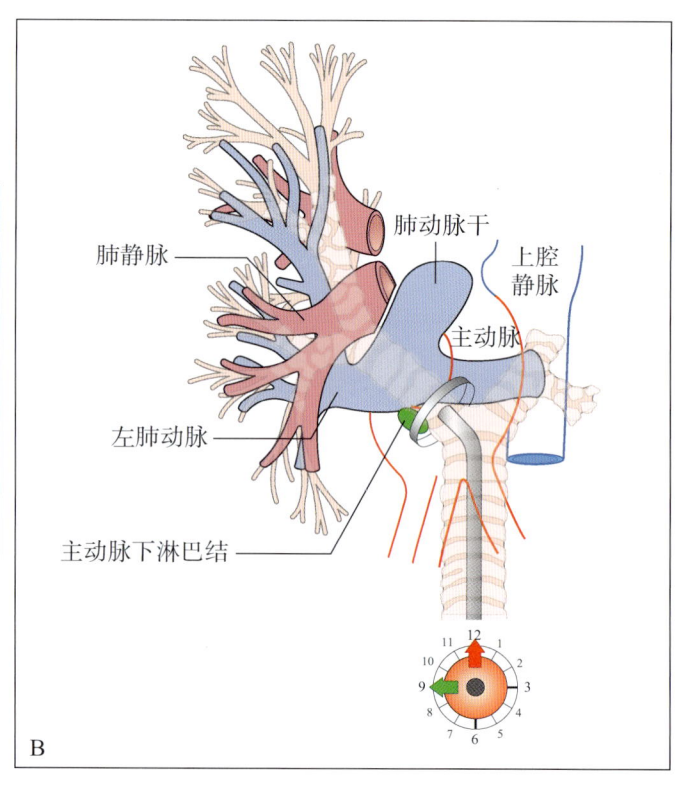

图 3.6　左主支气管开口层面的正常解剖关系

A. 左主支气管的镜下所见，血管和主动脉下淋巴结均位于 9 点钟方向；B. 支气管镜钟面视图，9 点钟方向是主动脉下淋巴结 TBNA 的穿刺位点，12 点钟方向 TBNA 不安全（左肺动脉）。

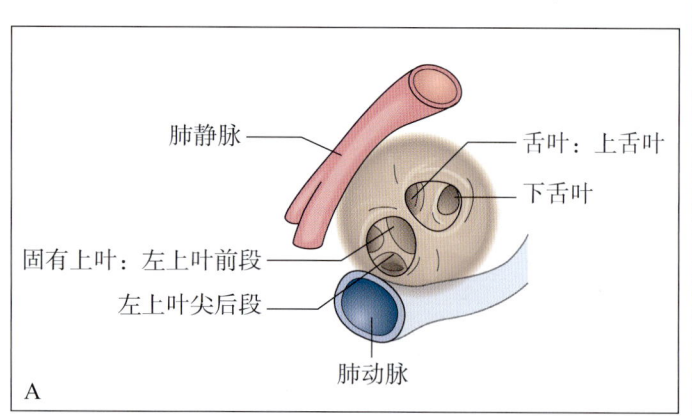
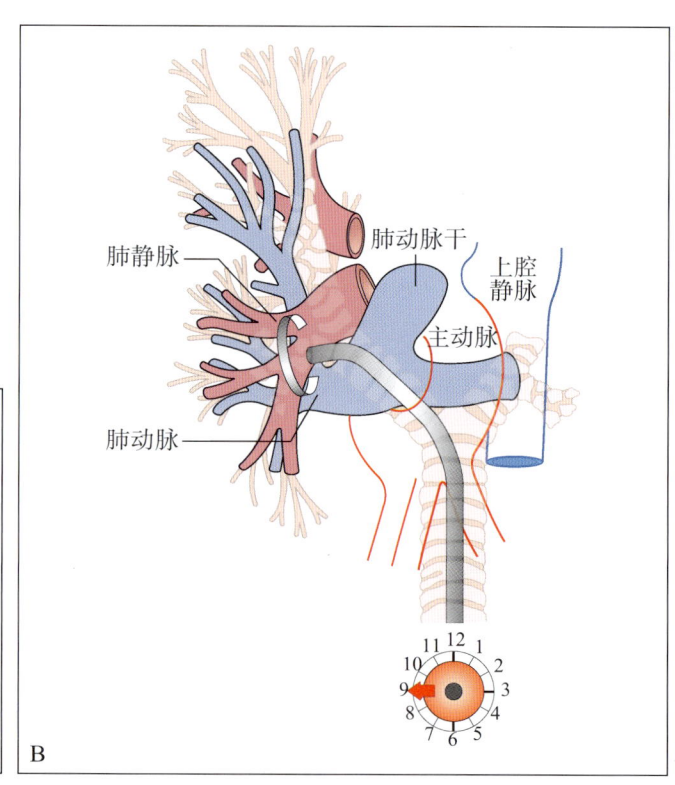

图 3.7　左肺上叶开口的正常解剖关系

A. 与支气管周围血管叠加后左肺上叶支气管镜下所见；B. 支气管镜钟面视图，9 点钟方向是左肺门淋巴结 TBNA 穿刺位点。

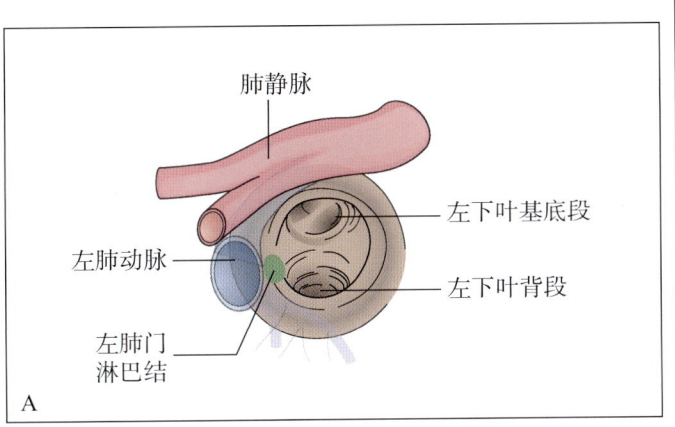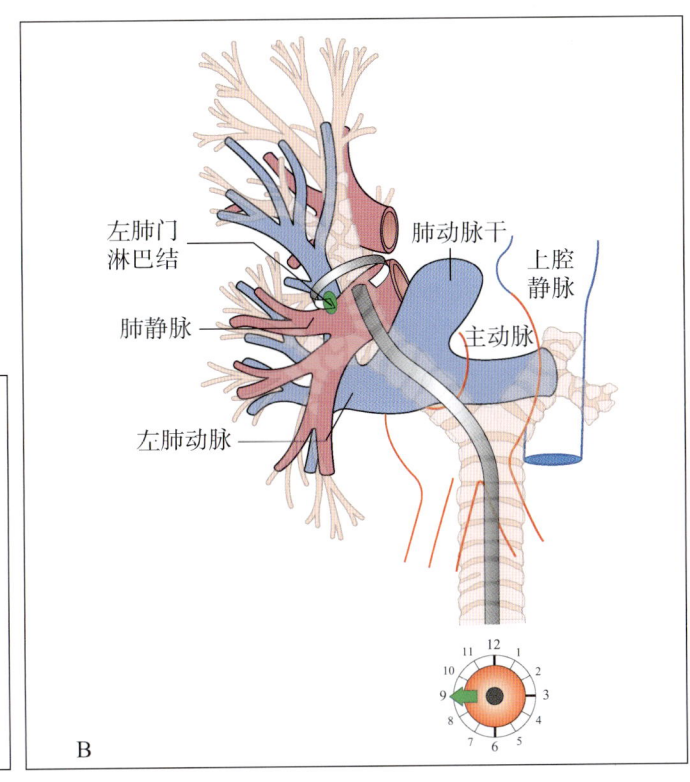

图 3.8 左下叶的正常解剖关系

A. 左主支气管远端支气管镜下所见，左肺门淋巴结位于 9 点钟位置和血管重叠；B. 支气管镜钟面视图，9 点钟方向是左肺门淋巴结 TBNA 穿刺位点。

参考文献

1. Ovassapian, A. (ed.) (1990). Anatomy of the airway. In: Fiberoptic Airway Endoscopy in Anesthesia and Critical Care, 15–25. New York: Raven Press.
2. Peter, L.G. and Sasaki, C.T. (1991). Laryngeal anatomy and physiology. In: Clinics in Chest Medicine: Airway Management in the Critically Ill Patient (ed. J.E. Heffuer), 415–423. Philadelphia: W.B. Saunders.
3. Stradling, P. (1981). Diagnostic Bronchoscopy, 4e, 34–59. Edinburgh: Churchill Livingstone.
4. Ikeda, S. (1974). Atlas of Flexible Bronchofiberscopy. Baltimore: University Park Press.
5. Zavala, D.C. (1978). Flexible Fiberoptic Bronchoscopy: A Training Handbook. Iowa City: Iowa University Press.
6. Boyden, E.A. (1955). Developmental anomalies of the lung. *Am. J. Surg.* 89: 78–89.
7. Mehta, A.C., Ahmad, M., Golish, J.A., and Buonocore, E. (1983). Congenital anomalies of the lung in the adult. *Cleve. Clin. Q.* 50: 401–416.
8. Durnon, J.F. and Merlc, B. (1983). Handbook of Endobronchial Laser Surgery, 7–22. Marseilles: Salvator Hospital Publication.
9. Mehta, A.C., Kavuru, M.S., Meeker, D.P. et al. (1989). Transbronchial needle aspiration for histology specimens. *Chest* 96: 1228–1232.
10. Mountain, C.F. (1997). Revisions in international system for staging lung cancer. *Chest* 111: 1710–1717.

第 4 章

支气管镜室的感染控制及放射安全

Prasoon Jain[1], Sarah Hadique[2], and Atul C. Mehta[3]

[1] Louis A Johnson VA Medical Center, Clarksburg, WV, USA

[2] Department of Pulmonary and Critical Care Medicine, West Virginia University, Morgantown, WV, USA

[3] Lerner College of Medicine, Buoncore Family Endowed Chair in Lung Transplantation, Department of Pulmonary Medicine, Respiratory Institute, Cleveland Clinic, Cleveland, OH, USA

(译者：王 琴[1] 陈 慧[1] 邓常文[2] 译者单位：[1] 海军军医大学第一附属医院 [2] 同济大学附属东方医院)

4.1 感染控制

对支气管镜进行规范化的清洗和消毒至关重要，该过程中的任何一环出现问题都将威胁到患者的健康。本章将讨论支气管镜操作相关的感染控制问题，围绕支气管镜的相关感染问题，阐述目前采用的支气管镜清洗和消毒指南，并就如何尽可能降低支气管镜操作中感染传播的风险进行讨论。

4.1.1 感染的传播

支气管镜可导致感染传播，目前已成为一个严重威胁患者安全的问题并引起了足够的重视[1,2]。临床上支气管镜检查相关的感染被分为真感染和伪感染[3,4]。真感染是指患者在支气管镜检查过程中由于微生物的传播而出现了新的疾病。大部分真感染是由高致病性的微生物引起的。随着对高龄、多种基础疾病、肿瘤、器官移植和其他免疫抑制状态等高危患者行支气管镜检查的例次增多，发生真感染的潜在风险也在增加。这些患者更容易感染耐药的病原体。支气管镜清洗和消毒不彻底可将这些耐药微生物传播给其他易感患者，进而引发交叉感染，产生严重的安全隐患。

伪感染是指行支气管镜检查后抽样分离出微生物但没有出现任何感染的临床证据。大部分伪感染是由于清洗和消毒不彻底，即便患者没有出现临床症状，伪感染仍然会对患者产生间接的伤害[5,6]，包括延误诊断而导致严重的后果。例如，有研究报道由于支气管镜取样后分离出抗酸杆菌而漏诊了早期肺癌，而且由于错误的诊断使患者接受了不必要的抗生素或抗结核药物的治疗，这些药物的使用又会发生相关的不良反应。这不仅增加了患者个人的费用，同时增加了调查费用，因为对感染暴发进行流行病学调查花费巨大。支气管镜设备相关的伪感染提示支气管镜清洗和消毒不彻底，因此需立即停用内镜室的所有支气管镜，直至查明原因并进行正确的整改。如果未采取适当措施，所有行支气管镜检查的患者检查后都存在并发感染的风险。

4.1.2 支气管镜感染相关问题

通过支气管镜传播感染并不常见，这可能是不够重视或疏于报告所致。常规的微生物学研究大多不从支气管镜检查中取样，并且大部分行支气管镜检查的研究中心缺少前瞻性监督系统。因此，很难获取准确的评估数据。有关支气管镜传播感染的报道多源自于回顾性病例分析。Culver 等在 2003 年发表的一篇详尽的文献综述中，报道了 953 例患者行可弯曲支气管镜检查后发生了伪感染或真感染[7]。这些患者绝大多数都是伪感染，仅 3%~4% 的患者为真感染。全球每年进行的支气管镜检查数以万计,虽然支气管镜检查相关感染发生率相对较低,但我们绝不能因此掉以轻心。每一次支气管镜检查后出现的感染,都可能严重威胁患者的健康。有报道称支气管镜检查相关的感染已导致数例患者的死亡[1,2]。

4.1.3 病原学微生物

大部分不同种类的细菌和真菌都可能引起支气管镜相关感染的暴发(表 4.1)。铜绿假单胞菌和黏质沙雷菌是发生真感染和伪感染最常见的病原体。嗜麦芽窄食单胞菌也可引起多种伪感染[8]。最近关于耐碳青霉烯类鲍曼不动杆菌和肺炎克雷伯菌通过支气管镜传播的报道引发了广泛关注[9,10]。环境因素导致的分枝杆菌感染也可引起大规模的伪暴发[11],其中,龟分枝杆菌和戈登分枝杆菌最为常见[12-19]。环境中分枝杆菌引起的真感染极其罕见[20]。结核病的传播是一个关注的热点,所幸仅有少数病例是通过支气管镜检查导致了结核分枝杆菌感染[21-26]。

文献中报道的大部分真菌暴发是由于环境中存在的真菌(如深红酵母菌)引起的伪感染[27-29]。人类免疫缺陷病毒(human immunodeficiency virus,HIV)感染的患者行支气管镜检查后支气管镜中可分离出 HIV-RNA[30]。然而,严格的清洗和消毒对于消灭病毒是非常有效的,目前没有发现行支气管镜检查可传播 HIV 的证据。同样,关于行支气管镜检查导致乙型肝炎或丙型肝炎病毒传播的病例,未见相关报道。

表 4.1 引起支气管镜检查相关感染的病原体

细菌
铜绿假单胞菌[a]
黏质沙雷菌[a]
肺炎克雷伯菌
嗜肺军团菌
类鼻疽伯克霍尔德菌[a]
变形杆菌
芽孢杆菌
嗜中温甲基杆菌
摩氏摩根菌
阴沟肠杆菌
嗜麦芽窄食单胞菌

分枝杆菌
结核分枝杆菌[a]
龟分枝杆菌[a]
鸟-胞内分枝杆菌
蟾分枝杆菌

(续表)

偶发分枝杆菌
戈登分枝杆菌
分枝杆菌脓肿亚种

真菌
深红酵母菌
短梗霉属
皮炎芽生酵母菌
皮肤丝孢酵母菌
青霉属
芽枝霉属
瓶梗孢子菌属

[a] 导致支气管镜检查相关感染暴发的病原微生物。

4.1.4 超声支气管镜感染相关问题

随着超声支气管镜(endobronchial ultrasound,EBUS)的普及,对感染并发症的担忧也随之增加[31]。EBUS 的设计较标准支气管镜更为复杂,目前关于其清洗和消毒有效性的数据有限。EBUS 的清洗和消毒应予以足够的重视,因为多篇报道称患者在 EBUS 检查后出现了纵隔脓肿、化脓性心包感染和脓毒血症[32-35],这些均是严重且危及生命的感染。根据日本的一项全国性调查,14例(0.19%)接受 EBUS 检查的患者发生了感染性并发症,包括纵隔炎($n=7$)、肺炎($n=4$)、心包炎($n=1$)、囊肿感染($n=1$)和脓毒血症($n=1$)[36]。此外,还有研究报道了患者在 EBUS 检查后出现了 A 族链球菌导致的脓毒血症和死亡[37]。

目前尚不清楚这些感染性并发症是由上呼吸道分泌物污染内镜所致,还是支气管镜清洗和消毒不彻底所致。尽管前者可能性更大,但新出现的证据使人们开始关注 EBUS 清洗和消毒的规范性。例如,最近有报道称在使用 EBUS 后出现了阴沟肠杆菌的伪传播[38]。即使在严格遵守清洗和消毒规范的情况下,仍多次分离培养出阴沟肠杆菌。因此,研究者对设备制造厂商关于内镜的质量控制评估提出了质疑。此外,最近的一项多中心前瞻性研究评估了真实世界中支气管镜清洗和消毒的效果,结果显示,高水平消毒后,6根超声支气管镜中仍有 4 根存在有机残留物和微生物生长[39]。综上所述,今后迫切需要更多的研究来解决与 EBUS 感染相关的问题。

4.1.5 感染控制相关术语

近年来,支气管镜相关感染已对患者健康造成严重威胁。因此,所有医护人员都肩负着尽最大努力减少支气管镜操作中感染传播风险的重任。为实现这一目标，掌握相关知识是必备的先决条件。首先，所有医护人员都必须掌握感染控制的基本概念，如灭菌、消毒（包括高水平、中等水平、低水平）。不同等级消毒水平的定义及常用方法见表4.2。

Spaulding根据感染传播的风险将医疗器械分为高度危险、中度危险、低度危险器3类（表4.3）[40,41]。根据分类，支气管镜归为中度危险器械，因此至少应进行高水平消毒。相比之下，由于经支气管镜针吸活检术（transbronchial needle aspiration，TBNA）或支气管镜下肺活检会导致黏膜损伤，支气管镜操作辅助器械被归类为高度危险器械。因此，对辅助器械推荐的最低消毒级别为灭菌。

近些年来，对清洗和消毒失败的原因和机制的研究不断深入。采用分子生物技术诊断和观察感染暴发也取得了令人振奋的进展。同时，近年来多项研究评估了生物膜在内镜操作相关感染中所起的重要作用。此外，还出现了各种新方法以快速判断支气管镜清洗和消毒是否达到规定标准。这些技术的广泛应用，为减少支气管镜操作中感染传播的风险带来了巨大希望。

表4.2 消毒的等级、常用药剂及应用

等级	定义	常用药剂	支气管镜操作中的应用
灭菌	消除所有微生物，包括细菌芽孢	蒸汽、环氧乙烷	重复使用的活检钳、清洁刷、雾化器
高水平消毒	消除所有微生物，减少但不能消除所有的细菌芽孢；理论上，高水平消毒可以使分枝杆菌细菌负荷降低6 log	2%戊二醛、1%过氧乙酸、0.55%邻苯二甲醛	支气管镜
中等水平消毒	消除活体细菌、分枝杆菌，以及大部分真菌、病毒，不包括细菌芽孢	葡萄糖酸氯己定、氯二甲苯酚、载碘化合物	非FDA证明的高度危险或中度危险的器械；皮肤抑菌液和清洁低度危险器械如支气管镜台车、有肉眼血迹的侧栏
低水平消毒	消除活体细菌、部分真菌、病毒但不包括分枝杆菌和细菌芽孢	季铵盐化合物（如苯紫氯胺）	用于没有肉眼血迹的低度危险器械

FDA，美国食品药品监督管理局。

表4.3 医疗设备的Spaulding分类

设备	定义	用于支气管镜检查的物品	推荐的清洗方法
高度危险	进入无菌组织或血管	活检钳、经支气管穿刺针	灭菌
中度危险	接触无菌黏膜但不穿透无菌组织	支气管镜	高水平消毒
低度危险	不接触患者或仅接触完整的皮肤	听诊器、血压计、支气管镜操作台车	一般预防和中至低水平的消毒

4.1.6 生物膜的作用

生物膜在医疗器械与假体的继发感染中起着重要的作用[42]。很多支气管镜操作相关感染的暴发可以追溯到支气管镜全自动内镜清洗消毒机（automated endoscopic reprocessors，AER）中的生物膜。生物膜是指病原微生物菌落被多糖基质和蛋白包绕（图4.1和4.2）。包被生物膜的病原体呈现了不同于浮游微生物的生理学特性。包被生物膜的细菌之间紧密结合并黏附于表面，形成微菌落。微菌落中的单个细胞间相互影响，具有高度协同的作用。这种特性被称为群体感应，生物膜是作为一个整体形成和存活的。细胞外基质允许水的自由循环并可作为细菌的营养储备。

与独立生存的微生物相比，生物膜的毒力并非更强，而是比较适宜定植细菌存活。生物膜一旦形成，很难通过常规的抗生素和消毒剂清除。高度耐药细菌生物膜发生的几种机制参见表4.4[43]。生物膜含有大量的细胞外聚合物，这些胞外基质能够起到屏障作用，阻碍抗

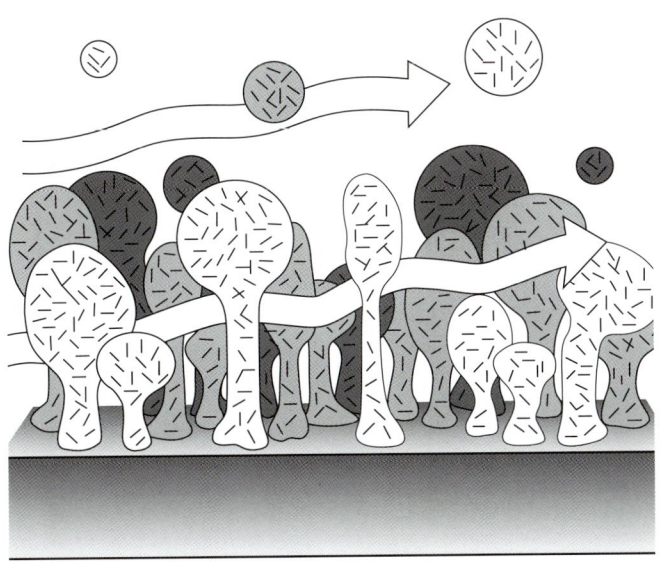

图 4.1 生物膜

微生物附着于实性表面形成生物膜，由菌落和细胞外基质组成，生物膜表面液体流动提供营养并排出代谢废物。（资料来源：Reproduced with permission from Wang et al. Flexible Bronchoscopy, 2003; Blackwell Publishing Ltd.）

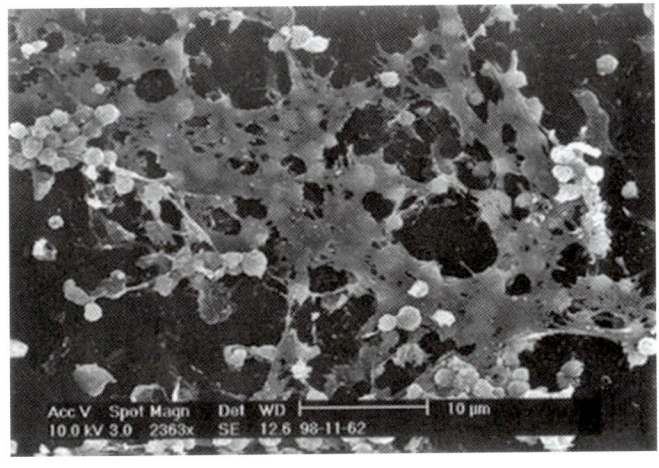

图 4.2 生物膜的电镜图片

资料来源：Courtesy of Drs Rodney Dolan and Janice Carr, Centers for Disease Control, Atalant, GA.

生素的渗透，从而使微生物对抗生素产生耐药。有趣的是，在粗糙表面形成细菌生物膜的病原体对消毒剂的耐药性更强。这也可以解释内镜操作中工作通道损坏导致了生物膜更容易形成。目前的证据表明，工作通道的细微损伤和正常的磨损、裂缝也可能促进生物膜的形成。

多项报道都认为支气管镜生物膜的形成与真感染、伪感染相关。例如，行支气管镜操作后铜绿假单胞菌、黏质沙雷菌感染的暴发追溯起源是由于活检口的螺纹与活检口盖帽上形成了生物膜[1,2]。生物膜也可在支气管镜管腔内出现。Pajkos 等检查了 13 根支气管镜的管腔，通过电镜扫描发现了生物膜和细菌。所有测试样品都检测出了生物沉积物。在 13 根支气管镜中，5 根支气管镜的吸引或活检孔道发现了生物膜。细菌的微菌落与管道的表面缺陷有关，但部分也存在于肉眼未见损坏的通道中[44]。

从设计上看，支气管镜很容易出现生物膜。该装置结构比较复杂，支气管镜的工作通道细长，每一次操作都可能被细菌和病原体污染。尽管可以通过"管道镜"直视观察支气管镜工作通道内的情况，但在每次支气管镜检查后都明确最初的清洗是否彻底或形成的生物膜是否处于早期阶段显然不切实际。消毒前进行彻底的机械性清洗仍然是预防生物膜形成最有效的手段。然而，几种常用清洗支气管镜的清洗剂对于清除已形成的生物膜效果不佳[45]。因此，寻找有效的清洗剂仍需更进一步的研究[46]。

AER 也可能形成生物膜。Alvarado 等报道，AER 清洗剂存储容器、接水的软管和气孔中形成了厚重的生物膜，使支气管镜出现了铜绿假单胞菌污染[47]。使用由制造厂商制定的 AER 消毒标准仍未能解决问题。另有报道，Fraser 等从 14 例患者使用的内镜和支气管冲洗液中分离出龟分枝杆菌[15]，并且发现污染源是 AER 使用的冲洗用水，尝试对 AER 进行消毒却没有解决问题，可能是机器内部有生物膜。生物膜一旦形成，使用 AER 很难灭菌，很多情况下，只能更换整套设备来解决这个问题[48]。

表 4.4 生物膜的耐药机制

细胞外聚合物
弥散屏障
中和抗生素
细菌生长速度缓慢
营养的储存
细胞表面分子促使抗生素的钝化
膜转运系统发生改变
产生过氧化氢酶
存留对抗生素高耐药的细胞
质粒介导的耐药

4.1.7 支气管镜的清洗和消毒

如上所述，可弯曲支气管镜设计上的几个特征增加了设备病原体污染和定植的风险。可弯曲支气管镜的工作通道细长、有一定的角度、表面粗糙,所有这些问题都可促进生物膜的形成,并增加支气管镜腔内清洗的难度。由于这些设备大多对热比较敏感,不能使用蒸汽消毒。

严格按照支气管镜清洗和消毒规范执行可有效减少支气管镜相关感染传播的风险。当工作人员不执行既定的指南,不按照规定的方法和准则清洗和消毒医疗设备时,常会出现问题。其中有些问题是人为因素,另外一部分则是由于缺乏相关的知识和培训。

支气管镜清洗和消毒的推荐方法详见表4.5。让支气管镜检查涉及的所有人员掌握目前使用的清洗和消毒指南非常有必要[49-51]。在下文,我们将简要讨论支气管镜清洗和消毒步骤的基本理论依据,并介绍不严格执行推荐指南导致的支气管镜检查相关感染的传播。

表4.5 可弯曲支气管镜清洗和消毒的步骤

步骤	主要目的	流程	注释
机械性清洗	预防有机物干结在支气管镜内外表面	1) 使用浸泡清洁剂的纱布或海绵擦拭插入部外表面 2) 通过工作通道抽吸清洁剂溶液 3) 通过工作通道抽吸生理盐水 4) 分拆吸引接口和活检附件,丢弃一次性用品	
测漏试验	检测工作通道或外鞘是否有破损 支气管镜测漏试验阳性不能保证充分消毒	1) 使用测漏装置对设备加压 2) 将设备完全浸入水中 3) 观察有无气泡溢出 4) 轻柔地弯曲和伸直弯曲部检测小的气泡溢出	1) 不能使用损坏的支气管镜 2) 回收支气管镜至厂商处维修 3) 将送修支气管镜标记为可能被污染的医疗设备
清洁剂清洗	进一步减少有机物和预防生物膜的形成	1) 含酶清洁剂和水浸泡支气管镜5 min 2) 使用含酶清洁剂清洗和擦拭支气管镜的外表面 3) 使用消毒刷清洁工作通道和所有的接口 4) 反复流水冲洗工作通道,清除管腔内疏松物 5) 用水冲洗支气管镜外表面和管腔,清除残留的清洗剂	1) 彻底清洗可以减少3.5~4 log级别的细菌负荷 2) 既可以使用一次性清洁刷也可使用机械清洗和灭菌的刷子
高水平消毒	尽可能清除残留的病原微生物	1) 可手动或自动进行(使用AER) 2) 如果严格执行操作流程,两种方法同样有效 3) 环氧乙烷消毒效果最好,但需严格按照要求操作,并且清洗消毒过程较长。此外,对于减少经支气管镜传播感染而言,进一步消毒并没有更好的效果	1) 确认支气管镜适合于该型号的AER 2) 核实支气管镜工作通道和AER管道已正确连接。如果不按规范操作可能导致工作通道未完全暴露在消毒剂中 3) 严格执行厂商推荐的高水平消毒流程 4) 根据厂商的推荐使用AER
最后冲洗和干燥	1) 清除工作通道和外表面残留的消毒液 2) 储存过程中工作通道潮湿会加重支气管镜的微生物再污染	1) 使用无菌或过滤水冲洗工作通道和外表面 2) 使用70%乙醇或干燥空气灌注工作通道以干燥设备	1) 最后冲洗不能使用自来水 2) AER冲洗水的质量需要监测 3) 不能重复使用冲洗水 4) 最初清洗和最后冲洗不能使用同一水槽
储存	不正确地储存设备也可导致潜在病原体的再污染	1) 储存于通风良好的橱柜 2) 推荐使用干燥剂保持橱柜干燥 3) 设备需悬挂储存 4) 储存过程中不能连接任何一次性或可拆卸物品	5) 不能储存在最初的转运箱内

AER,全自动内镜清洗消毒机。

4.1.8 清洗

首先，对支气管镜进行彻底的人工清洗可以减少生物污染、感染的暴发以及预防支气管镜内生物膜的形成。上气道分泌物导致的器械污染在支气管镜操作中不可避免。一次常规检查后，支气管镜可以检测到细菌的数量为 6.4×10^4 CFU/mL[52]。大部分分离出的常见病原体是链球菌和口腔内其他共生菌。有毒力的病原体污染支气管镜多发生于行支气管镜操作时本身存在高风险的患者，如有肺部浸润的器官移植受体与 HIV 感染患者。

机械性清洗支气管镜的目的在于清除支气管镜表面附着的炎性分泌物和有机物。支气管镜检查后立即进行彻底的机械性清洗可减少 3.5~4 log 的细菌负荷[53]。清洗不彻底导致工作通道内有机物残留会显著降低消毒剂的有效性。此外，机械性清洗不彻底也可促进生物膜形成，导致后续的感染。

目前的指南特别强调在进行高水平消毒前要彻底手动清洗支气管镜（表 4.5）。清洗过程属于劳动密集型工作，清洗操作时间至少 15 min。因此不难理解国外有综述报道实施推荐的清洗指南依从性很差。例如，厂商推荐清洗过程中内镜必须在含酶清洗剂中充分浸泡 5 min，但这一条通常被忽视[54]。而新型的全自动内镜清洗消毒机可在高水平消毒前进行自动清洗，逐渐可替代人工手动洗刷，标准流程操作也可减少人为的错误。美国食品药品监督管理局（FDA）已批准此类"清洗—消毒一体机"在临床实践中的应用。研究表明，全自动清洗消毒机和手动清洗对人工污染的支气管镜同样有效[55]。

正确清洗支气管镜，需将所有可拆部分拆下来，如活检孔和吸引活塞阀。所有一次性物品使用后均应丢弃。由于可重复使用的支气管镜吸引活塞阀清洗和消毒不彻底可导致感染暴发，目前，ACCP 指南推荐使用一次性支气管镜吸引活塞阀[1,2,23,56]。

测漏试验是支气管镜清洗和消毒过程中必不可少的一环。测漏试验可以检测出支气管镜工作通道内有无损坏，而其他方法则很难发现。支气管镜腔内损坏可促进生物膜形成，一旦发生，无法保证相关设备能达到高水平消毒标准。几次感染暴发都是由于工作通道损坏没有进行测漏试验。其中最严重的情况是，损坏的支气管镜感染了结核分枝杆菌并传播，进而使几例患者感染了结核[21]。在这个报道中，已确诊的结核患者使用过的支气管镜工作通道有个洞，导致没有充分消毒。因为并非每次支气管镜操作后都常规进行测漏试验，所以没有及时发现支气管镜的损坏。

清洗支气管镜的含酶清洗剂应一次性使用。同样，清洗支气管镜的冲洗用水也不能再用于冲洗其他支气管镜。

4.1.8.1 高水平消毒

支气管镜是中度危险器械，每次操作结束后需要进行高水平消毒。需要将整根支气管镜完全浸泡在已批准使用的消毒剂中。只要进行充足的预清洗，并按指南推荐的操作流程进行，整个消毒过程是非常有效的。FDA 已批准了用于高水平消毒内镜的几种化学消毒剂，其中 2% 戊二醛、过氧乙酸和邻苯二甲醛最为常用。这些化学消毒剂的优缺点和副作用见表 4.6，其他文献也有相关报道[57,58]。

尽管 FDA 指南过于严格，但 ACCP 专家委员会表示为达到支气管镜高水平消毒的标准，仍应按照推荐的方法充分预清洗后，20℃ 下将气管镜置于 2% 戊二醛溶液中浸泡 20 min[51]。该指南是基于几项验证的研究结果所提出的。多学会指南也支持 FDA 关于进行高水平消毒时可弯曲胃肠镜所需的浸泡时间和温度的建议[59]。高水平消毒可通过手工方法或 AER 完成（图 4.3）。只要严格按照流程操作，两种方法均可使内镜达到高水平消毒的标准[60]。二者的优缺点详见表 4.7。

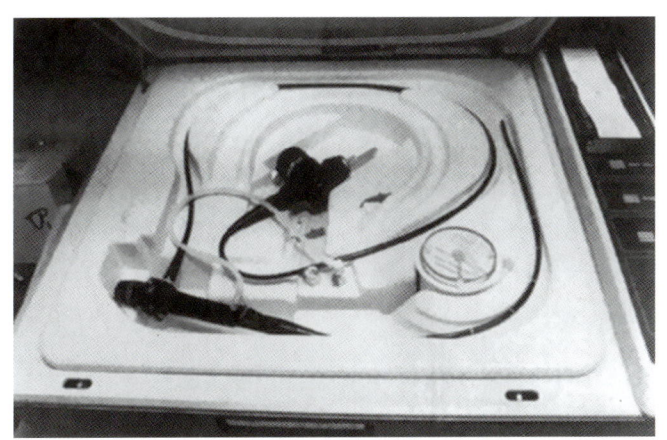

图 4.3　**全自动内镜洗消机**
置入支气管镜的 Steris 系统全自动内镜洗消机（Steris Corp, Mentor, OH），可用于自动化学灭菌。

通过手工方法进行高水平消毒最主要担心的问题是洗镜人员对戊二醛的职业暴露存在的健康风险。鉴于此，越来越多的支气管镜检查机构采用 AER 对内镜进行高水平消毒。不管采用哪种方法消毒，要确保支气管镜所有部件（包括内部工作通道）都灌满消毒剂，并保证充足的接触时间。采用手工方法消毒时，需要使用注射器将消毒剂注满工作通道。使用 AER 时，需要注意支气管镜的部件与厂商提供的模具、连接孔道配套。如不配套则不能保证消毒液灌注整根支气管镜，可能达不到高水平消毒的标准[61]。

被污染 AER 已导致了数次支气管镜操作相关的感染暴发，包括非结核分枝杆菌、铜绿假单胞菌和其他几种微生物的真感染和伪感染[11,48,62]。如上所述，生物膜形成是导致部分病例反复感染的原因，一旦出现，便很难通过常规的消毒方法清除。AER 需根据厂商推荐的方法定期维护，从而保证其正常使用。嵌入的滤水器需定期更换。如没有定期更换，可引起龟分枝杆菌的伪暴发[62]。

表 4.6　用于支气管镜高水平消毒的常用药物

药物	优点	缺点	副作用	注释
2% 戊二醛	1) 便宜 2) 易获得 3) 丰富的经验 4) 对支气管镜无损伤	1) 副作用多 2) 需要维持 pH 值在 7.5~8.5 之间 3) 由于自发聚合和损失游离醛基，保质期限制为 14 天 4) 清洗不彻底可能黏附血液及有机物在镜表面 5) 因重复使用而被稀释 6) 最终冲洗不彻底遗留黏膜及炎性成分在工作通道 7) 分枝杆菌、真菌的生长、子囊孢子影响消毒效果	1) 刺鼻的气味 2) 刺激呼吸道 3) 导致职业性哮喘 4) 刺激皮肤及眼睛 5) 接触性皮炎	1) 干扰微生物 DNA、RNA 和蛋白质合成 2) 每天监测 pH 值和浓度，并做好记录 3) 20-2-20 规则：暴露至少 20 min，浓度 2%，温度为 20℃ 4) 镜表面及内部充分接触药物 5) 尽量减少操作者与消毒药物的接触 6) 环境戊二醛浓度应<0.05 mg/m³ 7) 操作间充分通风 8) 每小时 7~15 次空气交换 9) 使用管道式排气罩或无管道吸烟罩减少暴露
过氧乙酸	1) 无毒环境友好型产品 2) 良好的杀菌活性 3) 易于清除工作通道的有机材料 4) 不会在镜表面黏附血液及有机物	1) 较贵 2) 可能造成严重皮肤及眼睛损伤	1) 通常情况下没有特别的副作用 2) 挥发气体可刺激鼻、喉咙及肺	1) 可用于自动清洗系统如 Steris 1 2) 充分浸泡时间为 30~45 min 3) 一次性使用避免了常规浓度的监测
邻苯二甲醛	1) 快速高水平消毒 2) pH 值为 3~9，极其稳定 3) 不会在镜表面黏附血液及有机物 4) 无刺激性气味	1) 较昂贵 2) 慢杀芽孢作用	1) 接触时对眼睛刺激	1) 在美国不常用

DNA，脱氧核糖核酸；RNA，核糖核酸。

表 4.7　手动方法和全自动内镜清洗消毒机进行高水平消毒的优点和缺点

	手动方法	全自动内镜清洗消毒机
优点	1) 成本低 2) 复杂性低 3) 没有机械故障风险	1) 省时 2) 确保标准的清洗浓度及合适的接触时间 3) 对操作者的健康危害较低 4) 较少的人为错误
缺点	1) 耗时 2) 蒸汽、化学试剂对操作者产生健康风险 3) 需要每天监测戊二醛浓度 4) 人为因素导致洗消时间不充分 5) 溶剂使用次数多于推荐次数	1) 启动费用较高 2) 较人工方法操作更为复杂 3) 机械故障风险 4) 不恰当的连接可能 5) 洗涤剂罐污染的可能性 6) 水和水过滤器污染 7) 污染后昂贵的修理和置换费用

4.1.9 冲洗、干燥和储存

完成高水平消毒后,还需要冲洗支气管镜外表面和工作通道,以去除残留的消毒剂。理论上,最好使用灭菌水冲洗,但实践中也可使用过滤水,但不能使用未经过滤的自来水冲洗,因为会存在被非结核分枝杆菌和其他致病菌污染的风险。冲洗用水质量不过关导致了几次感染的暴发。因此,一些作者建议用于冲洗内镜的冲洗用水应常规行微生物采样[63-65],但由于费用和资源利用的问题,常规检测冲洗用水仍存在争议。此外需要注意的是,冲洗用水不得重复使用。

工作通道潮湿的环境易促进细菌和真菌生长。因此,用水冲洗后,插入管和工作通道需彻底干燥[66]。最近的一项研究在三家医院通过肉眼观察和其他方法检测内镜上的液体和污染情况[67],结果显示在近一半(49%)的内镜中检测到液体,22%的内镜中检测到升高的三磷酸腺苷水平,71%的内镜中检测到微生物生长。潴留的液体与三磷酸腺苷水平显著升高相关。此外,还发现两家医院在洗消和干燥上未符合相关标准。

使工作通道干燥最好是先用70%的乙醇冲洗,然后注入压缩的医用级高效空气过滤器(HEPA)过滤的空气持续至少10 min。乙醇除了有干燥作用,还可以抑制病原微生物生长。最近的一项研究表明,使用70%的乙醇冲洗工作通道可将潜在致病微生物的污染风险从4.1%降低至0.6%[68]。

合适的储存方法对预防支气管镜再污染也很重要。彻底干燥后,将支气管镜垂直悬挂在较干燥的柜子中,并使用干燥剂降低相对湿度[69,70]。

支气管镜吸引和活检部位在储存前不需要组装好。有文献报道,清洗后立即更换吸引活检阀门,这些部位的积水可使支气管镜出现深红酵母菌污染[27]。清洗消毒后的支气管镜不能储存在转运箱中,也不要将支气管镜盘绕,这些均可能增加支气管镜操作后感染暴发的风险[71]。

4.1.10 配件的清洗和消毒

从感染控制角度来看,支气管镜检查中使用的大部分配件如活检钳等都是高度危险医疗器械。临床实践中最好使用预先灭菌的一次性活检钳。可重复使用的活检钳在每次使用后都需要使用清洗剂彻底清洗。活检钳的头端设计比较复杂,钳身呈螺旋形,限制了手工清洗的有效性。为了避免发生这种情况,建议使用效果更好的医用超声清洗器清洗污染的活检钳[72]。

彻底清洗后,应根据制造厂商推荐的高压蒸汽灭菌对活检钳进行灭菌。环氧乙烷灭菌同样有效,也可以采用。所有出现故障的活检钳都应被丢弃,因为此类活检钳可能损坏内部孔道,从而导致患者发生支气管镜操作相关的铜绿假单胞菌感染[73]。此外,严禁对一次性用品(如活检钳、TBNA针或三通开关等)进行消毒灭菌后重复使用[74]。

雾化器使用一次后,雾化器管和储液罐常被微生物污染[75]。有报道,一组行支气管镜检查的患者在局部麻醉时,因共用一台雾化器而感染了结核[24]。我们建议使用一次性雾化器。如果是可重复使用的雾化器,应在每次使用后进行彻底清洗和蒸汽灭菌。雾化器堵塞的喷嘴很难清洗,应丢弃。

清洗刷使用一次会受到严重污染,可引起支气管镜操作相关的感染[28]。一次性的清洗刷价格低廉,推荐用于清洗支气管镜的内部孔道。非一次性的清洗刷每次使用后需用清洗剂彻底清洗,然后进行高水平消毒或灭菌。

4.1.11 预防感染暴发

表4.8总结了支气管镜检查过程中的污染源。

感染暴发的主要原因是由于没有执行标准的清洗消毒方案。国外的综述和邮寄问卷调查结果都表明,许多机构在支气管镜清洗和消毒方面都存在严重问题。例如,有调查者对马萨诸塞州18家医院的光导纤维内镜的清洗和消毒进行现场调查,结果发现各医院内和各医院间清洗和消毒操作存在很大差异[76]。调查者发现了几个问题,如消毒剂的使用时间短、内部孔道消毒不彻底、最后使用自来水冲洗内镜、活检钳灭菌不足等。有趣的是,几个例子中,对已知感染了HIV、肝炎病毒或结核的患者行内镜检查后,内镜清洗消毒的方法与未感染的患者所使用的内镜清洗消毒方法不同。与从事内镜清洗消毒的工作人员进行交谈发现,对高水平消毒的管理制度缺乏了解是导致实际操作与规范操作之间存在差距的重要原因。

同样对北卡罗来纳107家医院进行的调查也发现了几个问题[77]。该项研究中,44%的医院内镜在消毒剂中浸泡的时间少于10 min,55%的医院最后冲洗使用自来水。对英国159个开展支气管镜检查的医院进行的一项大规模问卷调查表明,遵守清洗消毒规范方面存在突出问题[78]。这项研究中,35%的医院行支气管镜检查后消毒支气管镜的时间少于推荐的最短消毒时间,更让人担忧的是,34%的医院行急诊支气管镜

表 4.8 支气管镜检查污染的来源

清洗不充分
　手工清洗不充分
　腔内孔道有生物膜
　腔内孔道的损坏
　未做测漏试验
　吸引活阀松动
　工作通道接口

高水平消毒不彻底
　消毒剂类型选择不当
　消毒剂的浓度不合适
　消毒剂污染
　与清洗消毒机的接口不匹配
　内部孔道消毒剂不够
　清洗消毒机机械故障

清洗消毒机的污染
　生物膜的形成
　冲洗槽
　管路
　过滤器

高水平消毒后的污染
　终末冲洗使用自来水
　过滤水污染
　重复使用蒸馏水冲洗
　支气管镜未行干燥处理
　存储前把吸引和活检头装配在支气管镜上
　把支气管镜盘绕放置

仪器配件的污染
　清洗刷
　活检钳
　重复使用三通开关
　重复使用未灭菌的雾化器
　局麻液污染

检查前未进行消毒，43%的单位最后冲洗未使用无菌水或过滤水。该项研究提出了一个尖锐的问题，当内镜清洗消毒人员不上班时，急诊支气管镜检查后谁负责支气管镜的清洗和消毒？显然，所有的医院在周末、非正常工作时间都需要安排训练有素、操作熟练的内镜清洗消毒人员。

来自北美的另一项调查进一步反映了支气管镜清洗消毒过程中护工的熟练程度和基础知识存在严重问题[79]。这项调查中，65%的调查对象，包括55%的支气管镜室的主任，都不了解已发布的支气管镜清洗消毒的指南。接近40%的调查对象不了解清洗消毒的方法，35%的调查对象不知道他们科室使用的是哪种消毒剂，接近50%的操作者没有记录每个患者使用哪根支气管镜，30%的调查对象在清洗消毒支气管镜后例行定期的支气管镜培养以检测支气管镜有无持续的污染，只有1/3的调查对象记录了支气管镜操作后细菌培养的结果。大部分地区的清洗消毒人员都缺乏具体的清洗消毒步骤相关知识。

所有这些研究都反映出支气管镜从业人员缺乏清洗、消毒知识和相关培训。这些研究也提出，对所有支气管镜室从事支气管镜清洗和消毒的人员进行教育的重要性。

例行的环境采样可以警示并预防支气管镜检查相关感染的暴发[5,61]。然而，并没有研究特别调查定期支气管镜培养或环境采样在预防支气管镜检查相关的感染暴发中的作用。实施该项目花费巨大，因此并不推荐将常规环境微生物的监控（包括对高水平消毒后支气管镜最终冲洗用水进行的微生物监测）用于预防支气管镜检查相关感染的暴发。相反，强烈推荐对支气管镜检查分离出的菌种施行监管机制。当一些不常见或意外分离出来的病原微生物（如结核病支原体、环境分枝杆菌等）比率出现异常时，应成立调查组审查清洗消毒过程并进行流行病学调查。例如，有研究报道1例患者在胸外科手术后不久，意外发现铜绿假单胞菌肺部感染，随之进行流行病学调查[80]。结果显示使用污染的支气管镜就是感染的源头。

4.1.12　质量保证

目前指南并不建议监测可弯曲支气管镜清洗消毒的效果。传统的微生物监测培养十分耗时。因此，对清洗消毒后的支气管镜进行微生物学培养仅作为感染暴发调查的一部分。在过去10年间，不断涌现出各种新兴技术，可快速且准确地评估清洗消毒的有效性[81]。

目前已探索出多种方法来检测内镜手动清洗后残留的微生物负荷和有机物。可用试纸检测用无菌水冲洗工作通道后所得液体中残留的糖类、蛋白质和血红蛋白[82]，结果在90 s内便可获得。手动清洗后无明显有机残留物的基准为糖类$<1.2\ \mu g/cm^3$、蛋白质$<6.4\ \mu g/cm^3$和血红蛋白$<2.2\ \mu g/cm^3$[83]。此外，还开发了用于快速检测内镜表面或工作通道内三磷酸腺苷含量的技术。三磷酸腺苷与荧光素和荧光素酶反应产生生物发光，可用光度计检测，并以相对光单位（relative light units，RLU）表示。手动清洗或高水平消毒后内镜中存在生物发光表明存在残留有机物和

微生物负荷[84]。检测品可采用冲洗法或毛刷冲洗法获得。整个检测在 5 min 内便可完成。对于有效的手动清洗和高水平消毒，制定的基准分别为 <200 RLU 和 <40 RLU[85,86]。用于微生物检测的三磷酸腺苷技术已得到验证，目前已经有几种市售版本可用于临床实践。

上述生物分子检测结果表明，内镜手动清洗后，在表面和内部孔道中经常可检测到残留有机物。有研究报道，在手动清洗后无任何肉眼可见残留物的情况下，82% 的胃肠道内镜至少有一次快速指示剂测试呈阳性[87]。

也有技术可直接检查工作通道是否存在其他方法无法检测到的损坏。如上所述，工作通道内部的损坏可促进生物膜的形成，从而增加交叉感染的风险。而使用超细管道镜可直接检查内部孔道[88]。

这些新兴技术为评估内镜清洗消毒的有效性提供了强有力的支持。这些快速检测工具可提供有关手动清洗有效性的即时反馈。然而，需要进行前瞻性研究来评估这些检测在支气管镜常规操作中的成本效益和临床价值。

4.1.13 暴发调查

在支气管镜操作过程中因违反感染控制原则而导致的感染传播，对患者、支气管镜室工作人员乃至整个科室都将带来严重的影响。一旦怀疑感染暴发流行，就需要采取多项综合措施。根据当时情况的严重性，支气管镜室主任或负责人需立即停用内镜室的设备，整体进行清查直至查明原因并进行正确的整改。忽视或故意回避问题只会使事情变得更糟。

4.1.13.1 调查组

支气管镜操作引起的感染暴发需要成立调查组彻底清查。调查组成员包括支气管镜室主任或负责人、感染控制专家、感染科医师、从事微生物和分子检测技术的实验人员、流行病学专家、生物医学工程人员、支气管镜操作助手。早期将支气管镜、AER、消毒剂厂商的代表纳入调查组中，在很多情况下也非常有用。

4.1.13.2 资料收集

调查开始需要仔细回顾感染暴发期间所有的操作。为追溯每位患者的资料，行支气管镜检查的所有设备都需要详细记录患者姓名和病历号、支气管镜操作医师、每次操作所使用的支气管镜的编号或其他的唯一识别码[49,51]。每次支气管镜操作的助手信息也需要记录。没有这些信息就无法进行流行病学调查。这些信息同时也包括支气管镜检查的适应证、临床和影像学表现、支气管镜检查步骤、支气管镜下微生物标本鉴定结果以及其他微生物检测结果，如痰和血培养。对感染暴发期间所有行支气管镜检查的患者结果进行统计学分析，与患者进行电话联系，并进行临床评估以及相应的影像学和实验室检查。感染暴发期间支气管镜相关的微生物检测结果需要与前几个月的结果进行对比，以确定感染率是否增加。通过这些数据，调查组要尝试确定感染和一些常见的确定变量之间的关系。例如，同一根支气管镜、同一天做的操作等。

下一个重要的步骤是需要彻底地回顾该机构前几个月设备的清洗消毒过程。专家组需要彻底调查所有违反清洗消毒制度会导致污染的行为（表 4.8）。暴发流行中可能不止一个污染环节[89]。每一位负责清洗消毒的员工都需要面谈。清洗消毒仪器配件都要进行记录。任何仅限一次性使用的配件被重复使用也需要进行记录。AER 的日常维护记录、戊二醛浓度日常监测结果、滤水器的更换等也要进行调查。任何与设备制造商推荐的使用方法不一致的操作都要记录。

4.1.13.3 环境采样

从环境、支气管镜、支气管镜的配件中采样对于感染暴发的流行病学调查至关重要。需要从清洁瓶、消毒剂、洗涤盆、AER 的容器、自来水、用于终末消毒的过滤水、支气管镜、清洗刷、多剂量给药瓶、雾化器、重复使用的支气管镜配件中取样培养。支气管镜中取样培养需要顺行和逆行取样。顺行取样培养是将 50 mL 无菌的生理盐水从活检孔道注入取标本。逆行取样培养是将一半容量的无菌生理盐水通过内镜吸入吸引瓶中收集标本。

使用棉签擦拭法对工作通道的外表面和远端部分进行采样。具体而言，用经无菌去离子水润湿的无菌棉签从工作通道中获取标本，用于微生物培养。"冲—刷—冲"的方法是从工作通道中获取标本的首选技术。具体而言，首先需要用无菌水冲洗工作通道，然后使用无菌刷子刷洗，之后用无菌水再次冲洗工作通道。应将标本送至具有微生物培养资质的实验室进行检测。此外，活检孔道和吸引口使用棉签蘸取标本后送检也可以。

4.1.13.4 分子技术

一种病原体分离出的比例过高时常提示感染暴发。

分离出的病原体有相似的表型特征。例如，生物型、血清型或有独特的细菌耐药性，能早期预警支气管镜检查的院内感染。表型分析在早期确定流行情况中非常重要，但其区分能力较差，限制了在进一步流行病学调查中的应用。环境中和支气管镜中分离的病原体表型类似可能是巧合。调查支气管镜操作相关的感染暴发，用分子技术鉴定不同来源取样之间的关联性准确度更高。近期大部分研究调查支气管镜检查相关感染暴发都是采用基因型分析来确认感染的源头。最常用的基因分型方法是脉冲场凝胶电泳法（pulsed-field gel electrophoresis，PFGE）[90]。另一个常用的技术是聚合酶链式反应（polymerase chain reaction，PCR）[62,91]。

4.1.13.5 改进措施

改进措施取决于感染暴发的根本原因。无论根本原因如何，教育和监督都是改进措施的重要组成部分。流行病学调查并不是以完成改进措施而告终。更重要的是，适当的调整后继续监测采样培养结果和监督清洗消毒方法数周至数月。

4.1.13.6 注意事项

所有支气管镜检查相关的感染暴发必须上报至感染控制部门，如当地和州立健康部门、疾病控制中心、FDA，也应通报支气管镜、AER、消毒剂的生产厂商。患者和参与支气管镜检查的全体人员在感染暴发期间都可能暴露于感染，也应被告知相关信息。

4.1.14 支气管镜操作人员的感染风险

支气管镜操作会引起患者咳嗽。研究表明，在支气管镜操作后，可在周围空气中检测到多种细菌[92]。支气管镜操作过程中产生的气溶胶可能会将严重的呼吸道病毒传播给支气管镜操作人员，如结核、水痘、麻疹和其他呼吸道病毒。幸运的是，除1例腺病毒感染的病例报道外[93]，支气管镜操作期间由于职业暴露导致的活动性呼吸道感染目前尚未报道。

尽管如此，医务人员暴露于结核中进行支气管镜检查很可能发生感染，这个问题应该引起重视，并且有一些间接的证据支持。例如，采用结核菌素试验的方法判断结核的暴露情况，结果发现肺科医师的阳性率比感染科医师要高[94]。考虑这种差异产生的原因为：从事支气管镜操作的肺科医师的结核分枝杆菌的暴露风险更高。另一个间接的证据显示，支气管镜操作和气管插管与透析病房的结核暴发有关[95]。在低收入地区，结核病的传播是一个非常值得关注的问题，因为在这些地区，接受支气管镜操作的患者中存在较高比例的结核感染[96]。内镜医师在行支气管镜操作过程中可以采取一些预防措施以减少结核播散的风险。首先，对疑似结核的患者应尽量避免行支气管镜检查。拟行支气管镜操作前至少3次痰抗酸杆菌检查阴性。特殊情况下可以检查消化道和尿标本的抗酸杆菌。如不能明确诊断，对患者行支气管镜操作时，需要权衡工作人员受感染的风险。如该项操作无法避免，可以采取一些防范措施来减少传播风险，提高操作的安全性。支气管镜操作在负压房间内进行，空气被排出室外或再循环前通过HEPA过滤器过滤（图4.4）。在操作过程中尽可能为患者戴上面罩。局部麻醉充分，并使用镇咳药物，尽可能减少操作过程中患者的咳嗽。所有支气管镜室工作人员佩戴空气净化器口罩可以有效地减少结核的传播[97]。如果没有这些设备，至少也应该使用N95口罩作为替代。使用普通的外科口罩不起作用。

针刺损伤是支气管镜操作中另一个可能传播感染的原因。有报道称，操作者在使用皮下注射针挑取活检钳钳取的标本时不慎被针刺伤，感染了乙肝病毒[98]。

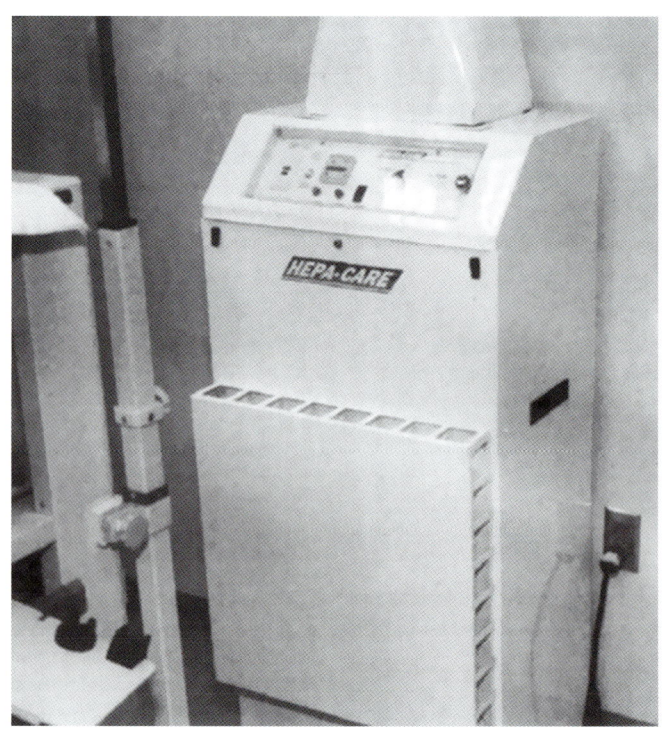

图4.4 HEPA-Care 高效空气过滤器
HEPA-Care 空气过滤器可循环室内空气至少14次/h。

这种做法应严格禁止。

在 CO_2 激光和电凝治疗皮肤损害的烟雾中已发现人乳头状瘤病毒 DNA[99]。提示支气管镜下治疗人乳头状瘤病毒的感染也要注意职业防护。目前尚无患者将人乳头状瘤病毒传染给医务人员的相关报道。尽管如此，所有参与支气管镜操作的医务人员均应采取呼吸道防护措施，如戴呼吸面具。贴合度很好的外科口罩对于保护操作者并减少吸入人乳头状瘤病毒的暴露风险十分有效。使用排烟设备对减少术者的暴露也有帮助。同样需要注意传播 HIV 感染的潜在风险。到目前为止，还没有发现支气管镜操作人员因为支气管镜操作的相关暴露发生 HIV 血清抗体转阳的报道。

严格执行综合预防措施是预防感染从患者传播给术者最好的方法。所有从事支气管镜操作的医务人员都要全身防护，包括隔离衣、手套、口罩和防护眼镜[49-51]。同样的防护措施也适用于完成支气管镜操作后从事清洗、消毒的工作人员。不过，调查显示支气管镜操作过程中推荐使用的综合防护措施在实际操作中依从性很差[78]。

4.1.15 特殊情况的清洗和消毒

4.1.15.1 分枝杆菌病

给怀疑结核感染的患者行支气管镜操作后，采用标准的清洗消毒方法消毒支气管镜也是有效的[100,101]。只要严格遵守清洗和消毒指南，则无须特殊的预防措施[49,51]。

4.1.15.2 病毒性疾病

如上所述，AIDS 患者行支气管镜检查后支气管镜上一定会污染 HIV[30]。目前清洗消毒的方法对于清除所有 HIV 的痕迹是非常有效的。一项实验性研究证实，使用戊二醛溶液浸泡污染的支气管镜 2 min 就可以清除所有的 HIV 痕迹[102]。目前没有由于污染或清洗消毒不彻底发生患者之间传播 HIV 的报道。同样，支气管镜检查后没有乙型肝炎和丙型肝炎传播的情况。胃肠镜文献中的研究表明，目前清洗消毒内镜的方法都可以消除乙型肝炎或丙型肝炎病毒[103]。然而，清洗前需要充分的机械预清洗才能清除工作通道内的肝炎病毒。肠息肉摘除术后预清洗不充分与丙型肝炎的传播有关[104]。

4.1.15.3 其他病原体

炭疽的孢子对高水平消毒是耐药的。孢子主要在土壤和死亡组织中产生，在血液和活体组织中无法存活。因此，一般不需要担心患者间通过支气管镜传播炭疽。所以，对怀疑或确诊炭疽的患者行支气管镜检查后，对支气管镜进行高水平消毒即可[7]。

而对怀疑或确诊克-雅脑病（Creutzfeldt-Jakob disease，CJD）的患者行支气管镜操作则比较麻烦。根据专家建议，疑似或确诊 CJD 的病例行支气管镜检查后，支气管镜的清洗和消毒不需要特殊的预防措施[7,105]。相反，欧洲胃肠内镜学会（ESGE）却建议尽可能避免对这些患者行支气管镜操作，如不可避免，最好使用快到使用期限的内镜[106]。CJD 患者使用的内镜要销毁或隔离，以后仅用于确诊为 CJD 的患者。这一观点缺少文献支持，对疑似 CJD 患者使用支气管镜进行操作，医师可以选择遵循同样的指南。最近一次性支气管镜已上市，但其作用仍仅限于检查气道和获取呼吸道分泌物。

4.1.16 结论

尽管严格遵守清洗和消毒指南，但抽查的内镜中仍可检测到活菌[107]。而未严格遵守清洗和消毒指南则会使上述情况变得更糟。这是一个威胁到患者生命健康的问题，因此需要引起足够的重视。围绕超声支气管镜感染相关的问题也需要持续关注。快速指示剂检测为评估手动清洗的有效性提供了强有力的工具，但仍需进一步的研究来明确其在常规临床实践中的价值。同时，必须尽一切努力严格遵守推荐的清洗和消毒指南。必须强调的是，目前对支气管镜进行清洗消毒的方法并非在所有情况下都有效。因此，需要进行研究以开发更有效的支气管镜清洗和消毒方法。

4.2 放射安全

在支气管镜检查过程中，X 线透视的使用可能会使患者和操作人员遭受过量的辐射暴露，但该问题尚未受到足够的重视。本节将讨论支气管镜操作期间辐射暴露对患者和医护人员造成的潜在健康威胁，并提供实用的指南以减少暴露风险。

4.2.1 背景

X 线透视是非放射科专业人员辐射暴露的主要来源。支气管镜操作者在很多诊断性和治疗性支气管镜操作中常使用 X 线透视（表 4.9），在这些操作中，患者和操作者都会不可避免地暴露在电离辐射下[108]。辐射暴露存在威胁健康的潜在风险，其中人们最为担心的是低剂量的辐射暴露可能会致癌。因此，在支气管镜操作过程中应尽可能地减少放射剂量，为了实现这一目标，我们需要充分了解辐射防护的基本原则。

表4.9 使用X线透视的常用操作

经支气管镜活检
支气管腔内径向超声引导下活检
导航支气管镜
肺外周病灶的细胞刷检
肺外周病灶经支气管镜针吸活检
定位不透X线的异物
近距离放疗
气道支架置入
术后排除气胸

尽管长期低剂量的辐射暴露令人担忧，但一次诊断性和治疗性内镜操作所接受的辐射剂量几乎不会出现任何不良反应。因为没有急性的不良反应，医务人员通常会低估辐射带来的危害，且经常忽视放射卫生规范。更糟糕的是，有医务人员在放射科以外的场所使用诊断性的放射检查，这其中的大部分医务人员从未接受放射物理学或辐射防护规范的正式培训。本节将对放射术语和诊断性的放射检查可能带来的相关风险展开讨论。

4.2.2 放射医学术语

放射医学术语比较复杂。操作医师和医务人员对一些放射医学术语并不了解。本节将简要介绍放射医学常用的术语。如需要更进一步了解相关知识，读者可参考该领域详细的综述[109,110]。

X线是电离辐射的一种类型，包含了高能量的光子。X线照射至人体，一些光子可穿透组织，另一些光子向不同方向反射。这些光子的一部分被组织吸收，一部分光子可透过机体。透过组织的这部分光子就传递了诊断的信息。

用于描述辐射源发出的X线的亮度或强度的一个量化指标就是照射量，用X线在单位体积空气内产生的电离作用来衡量。照射量是以空气为标准定义的，它计量了直接到达底片或影像增强器的射线的量。照射量本身并不能衡量辐射给患者带来的健康风险，因为很多其他的因素也会影响组织吸收的辐射量。在国际单位制系统中，照射量单位为库伦每千克（C/kg），传统单位是伦琴（R）。1 R=2.58×10^{-4} C/kg。另一个用于计量X线辐射强度的参数是比释动能，代表了每单位体积释放的动能。比释动能计量了从X线光子到媒介带电粒子传递的能量的多少，媒介可以是空气或其他物质，如人体组织。比释动能的单位是戈瑞（Gy）。1 Gy 相当于在每千克媒介内，X线向带电粒子传递1焦耳（J）能量。

照射量和比释动能计量的是X线的强度。因为组织只吸收了一小部分入射X线，这些方法没有计量射线的吸收剂量。吸收剂量是指单位质量的组织接受电离辐射的能量。吸收剂量的国际制单位是Gy。1 Gy=1 J/kg。吸收剂量的传统单位是辐射吸收剂量或拉德（rad）。1 Gy=100 rad。另一个与透视相关的重要参数是吸收剂量率，即每单位时间内组织吸收的辐射剂量，单位为Gy/min。

组织损伤的程度不仅取决于辐射量，还取决于导致损伤的射线的生物学效应的类型和组织对射线损伤的易感性。一些射线更容易损伤组织。例如，对于给定的吸收剂量，中子较X线对组织的损伤更严重。等效剂量是对一种射线的潜在组织损伤能力进行加权后的衡量。等效剂量的国际制单位是西弗（Sv）。等效剂量的旧制单位是雷姆（rem）。1 Sv=100 rem。不同类型射线潜在损伤能力的定义为辐射权重因子（W_r）。等效剂量的计算公式如下：

等效剂量（Sv）= 吸收剂量（Gy）× W_r

国际放射防护委员会（ICRP）最近修订了不同射线的W_r值[111]。X线的辐射权重因子等于1；所以其以Sv为单位的等效剂量等同于以Gy为单位的吸收剂量。

医务人员在放射检查过程中，身体的不同部位接受的射线剂量不同，身体的不同部位对放射损伤作用的易感性也不同。不同组织对放射损伤的易感性用组织权重因子（W_t）衡量。为衡量剂量和每个器官对辐射损伤的易感性，引入有效剂量（ED）的概念以评估身体对放射的总体风险。ED是各组织辐射敏感性加权后的等效剂量之和：

有效剂量（Sv）= $\Sigma_T D_T W_t$

其中，D_T是每个器官的等效剂量，W_t是组织权重因子。

ED是衡量患者和因职业暴露于射线中的医务人员的辐射风险的最佳指标。其衡量了辐射暴露对人体的总体风险。使用 ED 定义辐射剂量的辐射防护指南仅限于公众和专业人员的辐射暴露。ED 的国际制单位是 Sv，ED 的旧制单位是 rem，1 Sv=100 rem。

4.2.2.1 放射检查的健康风险

众所周知，辐射会带来生物学风险[112]。辐射的直接损害主要是由于其可导致组织发生电离。电离作用是原子或分子增减电荷的过程中产生了带正电或负电的离子。水分子是人体细胞受到射线照射后产生电离作用最初的靶位。电离反应产生的羟自由基破坏了DNA 单链或双链的连续性。单链 DNA 被破坏后很快就会修复，但双链 DNA 被破坏后很难修复。DNA 修复不彻底可引起点突变和其他不同的染色体异常。这些遗传物质的变化与后期诱导肿瘤的发生相关。染色体 DNA 的严重损坏会导致细胞死亡。

辐射对人体的危害分为两种：确定性效应和随机性效应（表 4.10）。确定性效应发生的基本机制是辐射诱导的细胞死亡。随机性效应与剂量阈值相关。组织损伤的程度与辐射剂量有关。低于剂量阈值时，组织的损伤没有临床表现。超过阈值后，组织损伤的严重程度与辐射剂量成正比。通常在 1~2 Gy 之间的大辐射剂量才会引起确定性效应。行介入操作时间较长时的皮肤暴露，如进行难度较大的血管成形术和血管支架置入术，可达到这样的剂量[113]。而在支气管镜检查中使用 X 线透视引起辐射确定性效应的可能性不大。

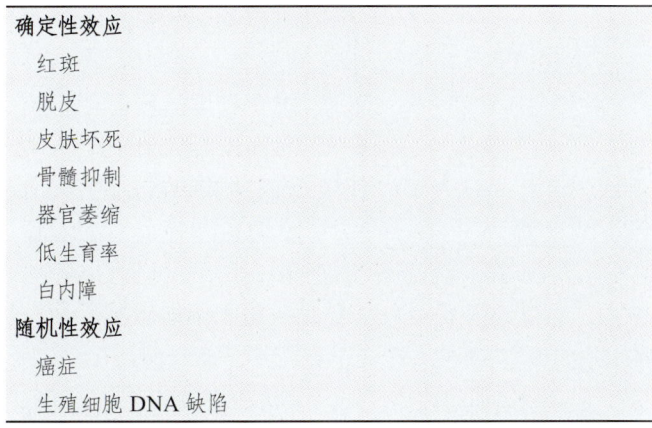

表 4.10 辐射对人体健康的危害

确定性效应
红斑
脱皮
皮肤坏死
骨髓抑制
器官萎缩
低生育率
白内障
随机性效应
癌症
生殖细胞 DNA 缺陷

DNA，脱氧核糖核酸。

随机性效应中，受到的辐射剂量越大，不良事件出现的概率越高，但不良反应的强度却不会随之增加。随机性效应的典型例子是辐射暴露导致癌症的发生。高辐射剂量的致癌性容易理解，但低剂量的辐射暴露与致癌风险之间的相关性仍存在较大争议[114]。预测低水平的辐射暴露致癌的风险很大一部分也是通过一些接受高剂量辐射暴露的实验性研究推断出来的[115]，或源自于对核辐射存活者长期的随访观察[116]。据估计，在接受诊断性放射检查的患者中，仅有 1% 发生白血病，不到 1% 发生乳腺癌[117]。目前有明确的证据表明，长时间暴露于超过 50 mSv 的辐射剂量会增加个体罹患癌症的风险[118]。

由于疾病的严重性，医护人员应重视职业辐射暴露可能带来的致癌风险。因此，大部分专家，包括电离辐射生物学效应委员会在 1990 年的报告（BEIR V）在该问题上都持保守态度，建议只要接触到辐射，辐射诱导的癌症发生的风险便可采用线性剂量-反应曲线进行预测[119]。这样可以最大限度地限制职业辐射暴露到尽可能低的水平。

4.2.2.2 限制辐射暴露

人的一生所接触的放射线中，天然放射源占 85%，其余 15% 才是人造辐射[111]，后者大部分来自于诊断性或介入性放射操作。正确使用放射学检查方法给患者带来的健康益处是毫无争议的，真正的挑战是在不损害健康的前提下尽量减少辐射暴露。关于这点需要注意的是，不同的放射操作或同样的操作由不同的术者完成时带来的辐射剂量差异很大。但有一点是明确的，即在不影响操作质量的情况下尽可能减少辐射剂量，这将有助于降低操作者的辐射暴露。

近年来，医务人员过度的辐射暴露已受到越来越多的关注[120]。很多研究发现，放射介入科医师[121]、介入心血管医师[122]、骨科医师[123]、泌尿科医师[124]、麻醉医师[125]和其他专科的内科医师的辐射暴露都在可接受的最高上限以下。这些数据极大程度上消除了医务人员对其在工作环境安全性上的顾虑。同样，这些证据也出现在支气管镜介入医师及团队的相关研究中。一项研究对在透视引导下对 45 个周围型肺结节和肿块进行活检期间患者和操作者受到的平均辐射剂量进行了评估[126]。结果显示，平均透视时间为（96±55）s。患者的 ED 中位数是（0.49±0.37）mSv，范围是 0.16~1.3 mSv。据估计，支气管镜医师和助手的 ED 分别为 0.4 μSv 和 0.2 μSv。虽然这些结果是可靠的，但仍需要更多的研究进一步验证，并关注其他介入操作相关的辐射暴露，如气道支架置入术。

许多国内、国际科学委员会和监管机构正在努力制订辐射暴露高风险人员的辐射暴露限值。除了收集和分析相关辐射数据外，这些组织机构还制订了职业暴露的安全辐射剂量值上限。ICRP 推荐，5 年以上的职业暴露中，每年平均的 ED 不能超过 20 mSv，并且任何一年的 ED 都不能超过 50 mSv[111,127]。各器官的辐射剂量值上限见表 4.11。

表 4.11 职业性辐射暴露的剂量限值

有效剂量上限	5 年平均剂量 20 mSv/年，其中任何 1 年不超过 50 mSv
各器官有效剂量上限	
晶状体	5 年平均剂量 20 mSv/年，其中任何 1 年不超过 50 mSv
皮肤	500 mSv
手部和足部	500 mSv

4.2.3 患者的辐射暴露

有关医务人员辐射暴露的风险问题已经讨论得很充分，但减少患者辐射暴露的重要性还没有得到科学界的足够重视。这几年情况正在逐渐改善，专家开始关注这一问题：由于过度使用放射诊疗技术给患者带来了过量的辐射暴露[128,129]。考虑到放射诊断的净效益，目前还没有监管机构设定患者接受放射诊疗过程中辐射剂量限值。ICRP 和这个领域的其他专家建议医师在放射诊断时应遵循正当性、最优化的原则[127,130]。所有医务人员包括支气管镜介入医师都应遵循这样的原则。

正当性原则是指在进行放射检查前需仔细分析风险-获益。当获益明显超过风险时，进行放射检查才被认为是合适的。医师准备行放射性操作一定要有明确的理由。此外，在选择诊断方法时，辐射剂量是一个重要的考虑因素。例如，有条件进行支气管腔内超声引导下 TBNA 时，就不应该选择 CT 透视引导的 TBNA[131]。

研究表明，实时 CT 引导下进行支气管镜检查和周围小结节活检，该操作与患者和操作人员接受更多的辐射剂量显著相关[132]。当可以使用导航支气管镜和支气管腔内超声时，CT 的使用便违反了正当性原则[133]。定期进行外部审查是确定这些操作必要性的重要方法。

最优化原则是指在不影响检查效果的前提下选择辐射剂量最小的检查方法、影像技术和设备。这一原则也被称为"合理可行尽量低原则（ALARA）"[134]。其中的一些要素包括高标准的质量保证、审查制度和有计划地更换落后的或未达标的设备。再次强调，诊断方法的选择同样很重要。

例如，肺外周病变的新型诊断技术的应用降低了患者和操作者的辐射剂量。在日本的一项研究中，使用常规技术对肺外周病变患者进行活检时，透视时间为（7.06±3.27）min，而使用支气管腔内超声技术时，透视时间缩短至（4.08±3.99）min[135]。

又如，在同一个部门中比较不同术者进行同一操作时的透视时间。此类信息是很容易获得的。这样，可以对那些进行特定操作时，使用透视时间明显比其同事长的操作者及时进行教育和辅导。研究表明，对操作者的个体化辐射剂量反馈可以提高其辐射剂量意识，并改变其使用透视的习惯[136]。

因为 X 线透视是患者辐射暴露的主要来源，所以所有操作者都应了解透视技术和设备操作原理。这有助于在不影响检查效果的前提下，降低患者和医务人员的辐射剂量。

4.2.3.1 透视

透视用于实时显示体内器官的图像。透视系统的主要组成为一个 X 线球管和一个图像增强装置（将获得图像传递给视频摄像单元）（图 4.5）。在覆盖有铅和钢制成的防护层的真空玻璃管中，阴极电子被加速后撞击阳极，当电子束被金属钨阻挡时，便会产生 X 线。初始 X 射线束从外壳射线口中释放出来。当初始射线照射到人体时，一部分被组织完全吸收，一部分被组织部分吸收、改变方向并作为散射辐射释放出来，其余射线穿过身体被影像增强器接收。组织的类型和密度决定了这些不同作用的程度。从初始射线穿过患者进入影像增强器的那部分射线即携带着诊断信息。影像增强器将摄像头捕获的 X 线转换为可视的图像，显示在监视器上。

在一个经典的 C 形臂透视系统中，X 线球管在床下方，影像增强器在患者上方。这被称为床下系统，其明显优于床上系统。在床上系统中，X 线源位于患者上方，影像增强器在床下方，这使患者和医务人员的辐射剂量明显增高[137]。对患者产生辐射损伤的主要是那部分被组织吸收的射线。现代透视系统可以降低这部分对成像质量无明显作用的射线。散射辐射是那部分改变了方向，从患者的各个方向释放出来的射线。散射辐射是危害室内医护人员的主要原因。有几种方法可以有效减少医护人员使用透视时的辐射暴露[138,139]。

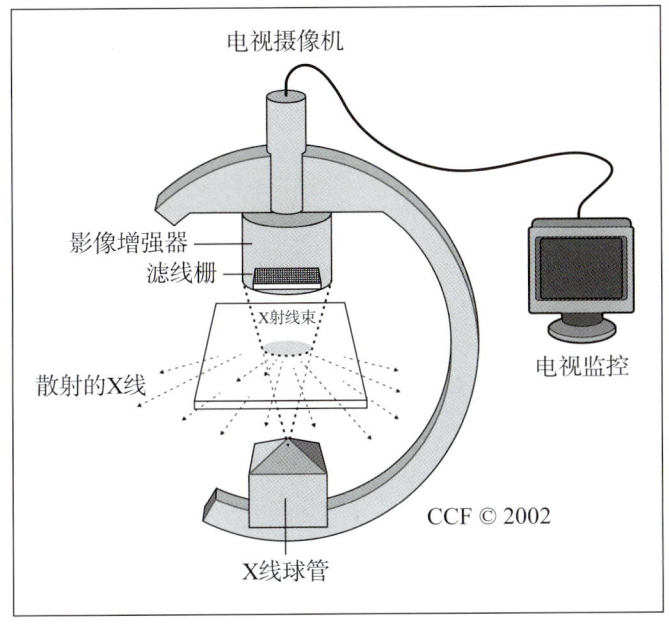

图 4.5 C 形臂透视设备的基本部件

4.2.3.1.1 X 线的特性

玻璃球管内的电子流被称为球管电流,以毫安(mA)表示。X 线的强度与球管电流成正比。增加管内电流时,X 线强度增加。增加管内电流可改善成像质量,但会增加患者及其附近人员的辐射暴露。在包含支气管镜检查在内的大部分介入操作中,不需要使用高毫安球管电流来获得高质量的图像。即在透视检查中,应该尽可能减小球管电流的毫安数。用于常规透视系统的经典球管电流范围是 1~5 mA。

初始 X 线的能量取决于球管电压,以千伏峰值(kVp)表示。电压影响 X 线的硬度和穿透力。高千伏峰值可增加 X 线穿透力,使低球管电流情况下也能进行透视操作。高电压(kVp)、低电流(mA)的 X 线较低电压、高电流的 X 线对患者的辐射剂量更小。对于超重和体型较大的患者来说,使用高千伏峰值和低毫安的 X 线尤其重要,因为他们在透视时更需使用穿透能力强的 X 线。

透视的电压范围为 60~125 kVp。目标是尽可能保持较高的千伏峰值。使用高千伏峰值的主要缺点是降低了图像的对比度,但对大部分支气管镜操作来说,这不是主要的问题。大部分现代透视系统有自动剂量率控制(automatic dose rate control,ADRC)和自动亮度控制(automatic brightness control,ABC)功能,这可以通过预定义调节毫安和千伏峰值来实现。许多系统的 ADRC 有低、中、高剂量率设定。高剂量率提供了高质量图像,但也增加了辐射剂量。低 ADRC 设定将患者的辐射剂量降到最低,但图像会出现雪花点。对于一般的检查,低剂量率设定适用于大多数病例,因此值得推荐。比较旧的透视设备需要手动调节毫安和千伏峰值。支气管镜医师使用这些设备时需要学会如何调节,以最小的毫安和最高的千伏峰值使图像达到可接受的质量。而还在使用老式透视设备的工作者应考虑将其升级至新一代系统。

4.2.3.1.2 滤过器

透视球管产生的 X 线能量各不相同。初始产生的低能量 X 线穿过人体时会被组织大部分吸收,不产生图像但会影响图像的对比度。大部分透视系统装备有一个金属片或金属箔,其遮盖住 X 线球管的射线口,过滤初始射线中的低能量 X 线。从初始射线中去除低能量 X 线,降低了患者的辐射剂量。还能使高电流、低电压 X 线不会产生放射剂量和干扰图像对比度。滤过器有不同的类型。操作者应该知道自己使用的透视系统中这个特性。

4.2.3.1.3 准直器

在现代透视系统中,初始射线的范围和形状是可以调节的,以尽量减少辐射场的范围。这是通过准直器完成的。准直器是位于 X 线球管窗口前方的一种 X 线准直装置。操作者通过控制面板调节准直器的边界,使照射野的面积尽可能小。这不仅减少了患者的辐射剂量,还降低了影响图像级别的散射辐射,提高成像质量。同时,初始射线通过准直器严格准直后,室内的散射辐射和医务人员的暴露也随暴露组织的减少而降低。

4.2.3.1.4 放射源到皮肤的距离

当 X 线源到目标的距离增加时,X 线强度急剧下降。通过增加 X 线源到患者的距离,可以明显降低皮肤的辐射剂量,减少可能的皮肤辐射损伤。增加距离后,图像质量会轻度受损,但不会明显影响支气管镜操作。对于增加距离会使散射的 X 线增加,人们也有所顾虑。但通过适当的准直,室内的散射射线不会明显改变。国际指南规定射线口到皮肤的最小距离为 30 cm。移动式 C 形臂 X 线机在 X 线球管顶部配有隔离锥以保证这个距离。

4.2.3.1.5 影像增强器到皮肤的距离

影像增强器要尽量靠近患者。这一简单的保护措施明显降低了患者和操作者的辐射剂量。大部分 C 形臂机 X 线源和影像增强器之间的距离（source to image distance，SID）是固定的。在这些系统中，当影像增强器靠近患者时，X 线源会自动远离患者，这样就减少了患者皮肤的辐射剂量。减少这个距离也会降低操作者的辐射剂量，因为影像增强器吸收了大部分患者反射的 X 线，从而为操作者提供了辐射屏蔽。

4.2.3.2　滤线栅

滤线栅是一种位于影像增强器前方的平板装置，用于屏蔽影响图像的射线，但允许成像射线通过。因此，滤线栅改善了图像对比度，但也会增加患者和操作者的辐射剂量。大多数情况下，去除滤线栅将使患者和操作者的辐射剂量降低 1/3~1/2，且不会明显影响成像质量。当影像增强器不能靠近患者时，去除滤线栅特别有效。在一些系统中，滤线栅是可以通过面板控制的自动系统进行伸缩的；而在另一些系统中滤线栅只能手动去除。在大部分透视下的支气管镜操作中，滤线栅是可以去除的。

4.2.3.2.1　射线持续时间

操作者在使用透视时，只能在观察监视器上图像的同时进行手控内镜操作。所以操作者需要同时控制透视的开启。在大部分设备中，射线束启动是由控制面板上的按钮或脚踏板来控制的。只有按下按钮或踏板时，才会有射线。支气管镜操作中，操作者通常在操作中使用脚踏板控制透视设备。在大部分系统中，有两个并列的踏板：一个控制正常剂量透视，另一个控制高剂量透视。在操作中，支气管镜医师应该只使用正常剂量而不是高剂量的透视踏板。支气管镜医师应该学习如何使透视时间降到最低。这会大大减少对患者和医务人员的总辐射暴露。

4.2.3.2.2　最终图像的保存

在大部分现代透视系统中，图像可以数字化冻结。这是非常有用的功能，可以让操作者回顾图像并进行下一步的操作，从而避免额外的辐射暴露。这一功能可显著减少支气管镜操作过程中患者的辐射暴露。我们发现这一功能在支气管镜教学时也是非常有用的。

4.2.3.2.3　脉冲式透视

现代透视系统中另一个可以降低辐射剂量的创新点为脉冲式透视[140]。与产生持续 X 线的传统透视不同，脉冲透视的 X 线是短促爆发式产生的。在经典的脉冲透视系统中，以每秒 15 幅的速度获得图像，而传统透视是每秒 30 幅。这减少了患者 25%~30% 的辐射剂量。还可以进一步减少每秒的图像数，但这会导致运动器官成像的不稳定。

4.2.3.2.4　图像放大

现代透视系统的创新点还有图像放大。更大的图像改善操作中的可视性，但会增加辐射剂量。图像放大可以是几何放大或电子放大。几何放大是通过改变患者相对 X 线或影像增强器的位置来实现的。通过增加患者与影像增强器之间的距离或减小患者与 X 线球管间的距离，都能使图像放大。如前所述，两种方法患者的辐射剂量都会增加。几何放大的另一个缺点是降低图像的空间分辨率。

在许多现代透视系统中都有电子放大功能。操作者可以在控制面板的多个电子放大选项中选择一个。一般来说，电子放大增加的辐射剂量较几何放大更小。总之，在介入操作过程中要慎重使用放大功能。

4.2.3.3　降低支气管镜操作中的辐射暴露

多种方法可以将透视引导下介入操作中的辐射暴露降至最低[141]。因为散射辐射是医务人员主要的辐射源，所以控制患者的辐射暴露自然能降低医务人员的辐射暴露。在这些措施中，关键是要开展对使用透视系统和放射卫生学实践知识的教育。对正确使用透视进行全面的教育，可以明显降低患者和医务人员的辐射暴露[142]。教育和培训可以减少透视的不规范使用，提高对安全指南的依从性。例如，一项研究发现，全面的培训项目将经支气管活检的平均透视暴露时间从 121.5 s 降低至 41.7 s，同时并未影响诊断率和并发症发生率[143]。表 4.12 总结了降低患者和医务人员在支气管镜检查过程中的辐射暴露的措施。

表 4.12　降低支气管镜操作中辐射暴露的措施

一般措施
对所有可能接触辐射的医务人员进行防辐射教育
避免不必要的操作
尽量缩短透视时间
尽量远离患者
避免直接暴露在射线中
全程穿戴铅衣
穿戴甲状腺防护装置
正确校验和维护透视系统
具体措施
使用尽可能低的球管电流（mA）
使用尽可能高的电压（kVp）

(续表)

使用低或中档自动剂量率控制设置
使 X 线源尽量远离患者
使影像增强器尽量靠近患者
使用滤过器
正确使用准直器
移除滤线栅
控制射线持续时间
使用影像冻结
使用脉冲式透视
避免图像放大

4.2.3.3.1 避免不必要的操作

所有需要透视引导的支气管镜操作都要有明确的适应证。为避免辐射暴露要尽量选择更为安全的方法。

4.2.3.3.2 保持距离

根据平方反比定律,辐射剂量与距离的平方成反比[144]。对于医务人员来说,辐射暴露主要来源于散射辐射。如果与患者的距离增加 1 倍,医务人员能将其辐射暴露降至原来的 1/4。这对主要术者来说是不现实的,但其他未直接参与操作的医务人员可以在透视时保持尽量远的距离。术者应尽可能将他们的手避开主射线。

4.2.3.3.3 正确使用透视系统

如上所述,正确使用透视系统可以成倍降低患者和医务人员的辐射暴露(表 4.12)。所有支气管镜工作人员必须熟悉现有透视系统的操作界面,并进行辐射防护相关的培训。

4.2.3.3.4 限制透视时间

透视的过程随病例复杂程度和支气管镜医师经验的不同而有所差异。从我们的经验来看,肺科专科住院医师在其培训的早期阶段,会在经支气管活检时倾向于过度使用透视。带教医师需要反复强调操作中控制透视使用时间的必要性。

4.2.3.3.5 穿戴防护设备

穿戴铅衣是支气管镜操作中减少辐射暴露最有效的方法。铅衣的防护值用铅当量表示,单位是毫米(mm)。标准铅衣的铅当量厚度约 0.5 mm,可以屏蔽操作者至少 90% 的散射辐射。这种铅衣一般都较重,当穿的时间较长时,会感觉疲劳和背痛。一些医务人员发现较薄的 0.25 mm 铅衣更舒适,但其吸收射线的能力不如标准的 0.5 mm 铅衣[145]。妊娠期间要穿特殊铅衣以进一步降低腹部和盆腔的辐射。

标准铅衣不保护甲状腺。因为甲状腺癌的发生与既往辐射暴露明确相关。因此,避免颈部过多辐射暴露非常重要。最好的方法就是佩戴甲状腺防护围脖,防护围脖不昂贵,佩戴也较舒适。甲状腺围脖至少将甲状腺的辐射暴露降低 20 倍[146]。然而,医务人员在检查操作中常常未佩戴甲状腺防护围脖,对这种行为应强力谴责。

眼部的过量辐射暴露会导致更早出现视力障碍,如白内障等,一些医师在透视时常规佩戴眼防护装置。普通眼镜也有一些保护作用,但最佳的防护装置是 0.6 mm 铅眼镜,其可以将眼的辐射暴露降低 6~8 倍[147]。然而,铅眼镜都比较重,长时间佩戴会很不舒适。而且铅眼镜的视觉质量较差,且易碎,破碎后会损伤眼睛。临床实践中,支气管镜操作中是否佩戴眼防护装置很大程度上取决于个人选择。可移动铅玻璃挡板通常用于放射科,目前尚未在支气管镜操作中使用。

铅衣、甲状腺防护围脖等所有个人防护装置,应该在每个使用透视的支气管镜中心都有备用。支气管镜医师有责任确认,每个进入支气管镜操作间的医务人员都已佩戴了合适的防护装置。卫生组织认证联合委员会(JCAHO)要求卫生机构每年在透视下测试铅衣有无缺损,并仔细记录测试结果。

4.2.3.4 监测辐射暴露

所有与透视相关的医务人员都必须监测其职业辐射暴露情况。目前有多种可用的监测方法。一般来说,可将个人监测分为主动监测和被动监测。被动监测包括胶片剂量计、热释光剂量计(thermoluminescent dosimeters,TLD)和光致发光(optically stimulated luminescence,OSL)剂量计[148]。这些设备可以记录操作者的累计辐射剂量,通常以月为单位进行计算。对于支气管镜医师而言,这些仪器是如何监测辐射并不重要,重要的是,医务人员在所有环节都应该严格遵守规范,并每月提交监测设备进行分析。

多种电子剂量计也可用于个人辐射监测[149]。其中大部分配有报警装置,只要辐射暴露超过了预先设置的限值,警报器便会鸣叫报警。电子剂量计可以立即读出数据,方便统计每个人每天的辐射暴露剂量。如果要求更准确地监测辐射暴露,比如妊娠的医务人员或操作需要较长时间,电子剂量监测器可联合胶片剂量计或 TLD 进行监测。

目前建议在铅衣胸部水平佩戴辐射监测仪[112]。但是,还没有任何一种个人用的剂量计可准确评估全身辐射剂量[150]。佩戴于铅衣外颈部的监测仪可以估测头部、晶状体和甲状腺的辐射暴露，但会将 ED 值高估 5~20 倍。相反，佩戴在铅衣下腰部水平的监测仪，提供了更准确的估测 ED 值，但会低估头、颈和手部的辐射剂量。因此，一些作者建议使用 2 个监测器。但这不常用，除非用于妊娠的员工。

个人辐射剂量的详细记录是十分必要的。因为一些医务人员不重视辐射风险，依从性的问题只是被偶然发现。在这一问题上是不能松懈的，否则会使对医务人员和机构辐射安全负责的人员面临法律风险。

当发现个人的辐射剂量超过正常值上限时，或在某月医务人员的辐射剂量异常增加时，需进行彻底调查。正确的调查方法包括仔细审查个人工作量、设备工作状态、透视使用的时间、个人防护设备使用的依从性以及个人辐射安全事件。在未仔细查明过度辐射暴露的原因之前让个人暂时离职是不可取的。实践中，每个支气管镜室都需要遵循标准流程调查辐射暴露意外增加的原因，类似于放射科所采取的方案。此时，强烈推荐放射科专家介入调查。

4.2.3.5 未来方向

近年来，由于偶然发现或胸部 CT 筛查时发现的肺部小结节越来越多，对组织活检提出了更高的要求。传统的支气管镜的诊断率较低，主要问题是操作者无法实时确认活检仪器是否到达了目标位置。为了解决该问题，在支气管镜检查中使用锥形束 CT 引起了人们的兴趣。锥形束 CT 通常在支气管镜室或复合手术室中使用，只需将 CT 数据与实时 X 线透视数据相结合，便可确定活检仪器和目标的相对位置[151]。一项针对 33 个偶发肺结节的初步研究显示，在支气管镜检查中使用锥形束 CT 后，总诊断率和恶性病变诊断率分别为 70% 和 82%[152]。

由于锥形束 CT 涉及辐射问题，因此需要明确将锥形束 CT 常规用于肺外周病变的诊断中，会对患者增加多少辐射剂量。有研究表明，持续 20 min 的透视和锥形束 CT 检查，其辐射剂量为 0.98~1.5 mSv[153]。这个辐射剂量是安全的，且不会对患者造成严重伤害。锥形束 CT 也被用于电磁导航支气管镜（electromagnetic navigation bronchoscopy，ENB）检查中。最近的一个报道显示，在 ENB 检查中，透视的平均辐射剂量是 1.5 mSv，每进行一次锥形束 CT，增加的辐射剂量为 2.0 mSv[154]。同样，另一项研究结果显示，在 7 例使用锥形束 CT 和经支气管通路工具的肺外周病变患者中，平均有效辐射剂量为 4.3 mSv[155]。

基于上述证据，对患者或操作者造成的辐射暴露可能不会阻碍锥形束 CT 在支气管镜检查中的应用。尽管如此，在将其纳入常规临床实践之前，仍需要大量的研究对锥形束 CT 和现有的诊断技术如支气管腔内超声等在诊断率上的比较。

4.3 结论

尽管临床实践中经常使用透视的医师的职业辐射暴露在可接受范围内，但仍需严格执行各项预防及防护措施，以尽量减少职业辐射暴露。对此，引入一位合格的放射专科医师无论对透视设备的初始化准备，还是定期校正和对透视设备的质量控制评估，都是非常有用的。此外，放射专科医师也应当参与到个人辐射暴露监测、过度辐射暴露原因调查，以及对医护人员的教育培训中。现在，应该对那些没有经过正式培训就经常使用透视的支气管镜医师加强辐射相关的教育和培训，且建议对所有在支气管镜室工作的医护人员都开展放射诊断学原理、健康风险和辐射防护等方面的规范化培训。最后，必须尽一切努力降低患者的辐射暴露风险。

参考文献

1 Srinivasan, A., Wolfenden, L.L., Song, X. et al. (2003). An outbreak of *Pseudomonas aeruginosa* infections associated with flexible bronchoscopes. *N. Engl. J. Med.* 348: 221–227.

2 Kirschke, D.L., Jones, T.F., Craig, A.S. et al. (2003). Outbreak of *Pseudomonas aeruginosa* and *Seratia marcescens* associated with a manufacturing defect in bronchoscopes. *N. Engl. J. Med.* 348: 214–220.

3 Mehta, A.C. and Minai, O.A. (1999). Infection control in the bronchoscopy suite: a review. *Clin. Chest Med.* 20: 19–32.

4 Prakash, U.B.S. (1993). Does the bronchoscope propagate infection? *Chest* 104: 552–559.

5 Harvey, J. and Yates, M. (1996). Do you clean or contaminate your bronchoscope? *Respir. Med.* 90: 63–67.

6 Mughal, M.M., Minai, O.A., Culver, D.A., and Mehta, A.C. (2004). Reprocessing the bronchoscope: the challenges. *Semin. Respir. Crit. Care Med.* 25: 443–449.

7 Culver, D.A., Gordon, S.M., and Mehta, A.C. (2003). Infection control in the bronchoscopy suite. *Am. J. Respir. Crit. Care Med.* 167: 1050–1056.

8 Botana-Rial, M., Leiro-Fernández, V., Núñez-Delgado, M. et al. (2016). A pseudo-outbreak of pseudomonas putida and *Stenotrophomonas maltophilia* in bronchoscopy unit. *Respiration* 92: 274–278.

9 Xia, Y., Lu, C., Zhao, J. et al. (2012). A bronchofiberscopy associated outbreak of multidrug resistant *Acinetobacter baumannii* in an intensive care unit in Beijing, China. *BMC Infect. Dis.* 12: 335–344.

10 Zweigner, J., Gastmeier, P., and Kola, A. (2014). A carbapenem-resistant *Klebsiella pneumoniae* outbreak following bronchoscopy. *Am. J. Infect. Control* 42: 935–940.

11 Gubler, J.G., Salfinger, M., and von Graevenitz, A. (1992). Pseudoepidemic of nontuberculous mycobacteria due to a contaminated bronchoscope cleaning machine. *Chest* 101: 1245–1249.

12 Brown, N.M., Hellyar, E.A., Harvey, J.E. et al. (1993). Mycobacterial contamination of fibreoptic bronchoscopes. *Thorax*: 1283–1285.

13 Nye, K., Chadha, D.K., Hodgkin, P. et al. (1990). *Mycobacterium chelonae* isolation from broncho-alveolar lavage fluid and its practical implications. *J. Hosp. Infect.* 16: 257–261.

14 Centers for Disease Control and Prevention (1991). Nosocomial infection and pseudoinfection from contaminated endoscopes and bronchoscopes – Wisconsin and Missouri. *MMWR Morb. Mortal. Wkly. Rep.* 40: 675–678.

15 Fraser, V.J., Jones, M., Murray, P.R. et al. (1992). Contamination of flexible fiberoptic bronchoscopes with *Mycobacterium chelonae* linked to an automated bronchoscope disinfection machine. *Am. Rev. Respir. Dis.* 145: 853–855.

16 Campagnaro, R.L., Teichtahl, H., and Dwyer, B.A. (1994). Pseudoepidemic of *Mycobacterium chelonae*: contamination of a bronchoscope and autocleaner. *Aust. NZ J. Med.* 24: 693–695.

17 Wang, H.C., Liaw, Y.S., Yang, P.C. et al. (1995). A pseudoepidemic of *Mycobacterium chelonae* infection caused by contamination of a fiberoptic bronchoscope suction channel. *Eur. Respir. J.* 8: 1259–1262.

18 Cox, R., deBorja, K., and Bach, M.C. (1997). A pseudo-outbreak of *Mycobacterium chelonae* infections related to bronchoscopy. *Infect. Control Hosp. Epidemiol.* 18: 136–137.

19 Scorzolini, L., Mengoni, F., Mastroianni, C.M. et al. (2016). Pseudo-outbreak of Mycobacterium gordonae in a teaching hospital: importance of strictly following decontamination procedures and emerging issues concerning sterilization. *New Microbiol.* 39: 25–34.

20 Wallace, R.J., Brown, B.A., and Griffith, D.E. (1998). Nosocomial outbreaks/pseudo-outbreaks caused by nontuberculous mycobacteria. *Annu. Rev. Microbiol.* 52: 453–490.

21 Ramsey, A.H., Oemig, T.V., Davis, J.P. et al. (2002). An outbreak of bronchoscopy-related *Mycobacterium tuberculosis* infections due to lack of bronchoscope leak testing. *Chest* 121: 976–981.

22 Pappas, S.A., Schaff, D.M., DiCostanzo, M.B. et al. (1983). Contamination of flexible fiberoptic bronchoscopes [letter]. *Am. Rev. Respir. Dis.* 127: 391–392.

23 Wheeler, P.W., Lancaster, D., and Kaiser, A.B. (1989). Bronchopulmonary cross-colonization and infection related to mycobacterial contamination of suction valves of bronchoscopes. *J. Infect. Dis.* 159: 954–958.

24 Southwick, K.L., Hoffmann, K., Ferree, K. et al. (2001). Cluster of tuberculosis cases in North Carolina: possible association with atomizer reuse. *Am. J. Infect. Control* 29: 1–6.

25 Agerton, T., Valway, S., Gore, B. et al. (1997). Transmission of a highly drug-resistant strain (strain W1) of *Mycobacterium tuberculosis*. *JAMA* 278: 1073–1077.

26 Michele, T.M., Cronin, W.A., Graham, N.M.H. et al. (1997). Transmission of *Mycobacterium tuberculosis* by a fiberoptic bronchoscope. *JAMA* 278: 1093–1095.

27 Whitlock, W.L., Dietrich, R.A., Steimke, E.H. et al. (1992). *Rhodotorula rubra* contamination in fiberoptic bronchoscopy. *Chest* 102: 1516–1519.

28 Hoffmann, K.K., Weber, D.J., and Rutala, W.A. (1989). Pseudoepidemic of *Rhodotorula rubra* in patients undergoing fiberoptic bronchoscopy. *Infect. Control Hosp. Epidemiol.* 10: 511–514.

29 Hagan, M.E., Klotz, S.A., Bartholomew, W. et al. (1995). A pseudoepidemic of *Rhodotorula rubra*: a marker for microbial contamination of the bronchoscope. *Infect. Control Hosp. Epidemiol.* 16: 727–728.

30 Hanson, P.J., Gor, D., Clarke, J.R. et al. (1991). Recovery of the human immunodeficiency virus from fibreoptic bronchoscopes. *Thorax* 46: 410–412.

31 Vaidya, P.J., Munavvar, M., Leuppi, J.D. et al. (2017). Endobronchial ultrasound guided transbronchial needle aspiration: safe as it sounds. *Respirology* 22: 1093–1101.

32 Lee, H.Y., Kim, J., Jo, Y.S., and Park, Y.S. (2015). Bacterial pericarditis as a fatal complication after endobronchial ultrasound-guided transbronchial needle aspiration. *Eur. J. Cardiothorac. Surg.* 48: 630–632.

33 McGovern Murphy, F., Grondin-Beaudoin, B., Poulin, Y. et al. (2015). Mediastinal abscess following endobronchial ultrasound transbronchial needle aspiration in a patient with sarcoidosis. *J. Bronchology Interv. Pulmonol.* 22: 370–372.

34 Matsuoka, K., Ito, A., Murata, Y. et al. (2015). Severe mediastinitis and pericarditis after transbronchial needle aspiration. *Ann. Thorac. Surg.* 100: 1881–1883.

35 Voldby, N., Folkersen, B.H., and Rasmussen, T.R. (2017). Mediastinitis: a serious complication of endobronchial ultrasound-guided transbronchial needle aspiration. *J. Bronchology Interv. Pulmonol.* 24: 75–79.

36 Asano, F., Aoe, M., Ohsaki, Y. et al. (2013). Complications associated with endobronchial ultrasound-guided transbronchial needle aspiration: a nationwide survey by the Japan Society for Respiratory Endoscopy. *Respir. Res.* 14: 50.

37 Navani, N., Brown, J.M., Nankivell, M. et al. (2012). Suitability of endobronchial ultrasound-guided transbronchial needle aspiration specimens for subtyping and genotyping of non-small cell lung cancer: a multicenter study of 774 patients. *Am. J. Respir. Crit. Care Med.* 185: 1316–1322.

38 Dickson, A., Kondal, P., Hilken, L. et al. (2018). Possible pseudotransmission of *Enterobacter cloacae* associated with an endobronchial ultrasound scope. *Am. J. Infect. Control* 46 (11): 1296–1298.

39 Ofstead, C.L., Quick, M.R., Wetzler, H.P. et al. (2018). Effectiveness of reprocessing for flexible bronchoscopes and endobronchial ultrasound bronchoscopes. *Chest* 154: 1024–

1034. https://doi.org/10.1016/j.chest.2018.04.045.

40 Rutala, W.A. and Weber, D.J. (1999). Disinfection of endoscope: review of new chemical sterilents used for high-level disinfection. *Infect. Control Hosp. Epidemiol.* 20: 69–76.

41 Spaulding, E.H. (1958). Chemical disinfection in the operating room. *Mil. Med.* 123: 437–443.

42 Talsma, S.S. (2007). Biofilms on medical devices. *Home Healthc. Nurse* 25: 589–594.

43 Stewart, P.S. and Costorton, J.W. (2001). Antibiotic resistance of bacteria in biofilms. *Lancet* 358: 135–138.

44 Pajkos, A., Vickery, K., and Cossart, Y. (2004). Is biofilm accumulation on endoscope tubing a contributor to the failure of cleaning and decontamination? *J. Hosp. Infect.* 58: 224–229.

45 Vickery, K., Pajkos, A., and Cossart, Y. (2004). Removal of biofilm from endoscopes: evaluation of detergent efficiency. *Am. J. Infect. Control* 32: 170–176.

46 Marion, K., Freney, J., James, G. et al. (2006). Using an efficient biofilm detaching agent: an essential step for the improvement of endoscope reprocessing protocols. *J. Hosp. Infect.* 64: 136–142.

47 Alvarado, C.J., Stolz, S.M., and Maki, D.G. (1991). Nosocomial infections from contaminated endoscopes: a flawed automated endoscope washer. An investigation using molecular epidemiology. *Am. J. Med.* 91 (3B): 272S–280S.

48 Kressel, A.B. and Kidd, F. (2001). Pseudo-outbreak of *Mycobacterium chelonae* and *Methylobacterium mesophilicum* caused by contamination of an automated endoscopy washer. *Infect. Control Hosp. Epidemiol.* 22: 414–418.

49 Alvarado, C.J. and Reichelderfer, M. (2000). APIC guideline for infection prevention and control in flexible endoscopy. *Am. J. Infect. Control* 28: 138–155.

50 Honeybourne, D., Babb, J., Bowie, P. et al. (2001). British Thoracic Society guidelines on diagnostic flexible bronchoscopy. *Thorax* 56: I1–I21.

51 Mehta, A.C., Prakash, U.B.S., Garland, R. et al. (2005). American College of Chest Physicians and American Association of Bronchology consensus statement. *Chest* 128: 1742–1755.

52 Alfa, M.J. and Sitter, D.L. (1994). In-hospital evaluation of orthophthalaldehyde as a high level disinfectant for flexible endoscopes. *J. Hosp. Infect.* 26: 15–26.

53 Hanson, P.J.V., Chadwick, M.V., Gaya, H. et al. (1992). A study of gluterladehyde disinfection of fiberoptic bronchoscope experimentally contaminated with *Mycobacterium tuberculosis*. *J. Hosp. Infect.* 22: 137–142.

54 Alfa, M.J., Olson, N., DeGagne, P., and Jackson, M. (2002). A survey of reprocessing methods, residual viable bioburden, and soil levels in patient-ready endoscopic retrograde choliangiopancreatography duodenoscopes used in Canadian centers. *Infect. Control Hosp. Epidemiol.* 23: 198–206.

55 Alfa, M.J., Olson, N., and DeGagne, P. (2006). Automated washing with the Reliance Endoscope Processing System and its equivalence to optimal manual cleaning. *Am. J. Infect. Control* 34: 561–570.

56 Cêtre, J.C., Nicolle, M.C., Salord, H. et al. (2005). Outbreaks of contaminated broncho-alveolar lavage related to intrinsically defective bronchoscopes. *J. Hosp. Infect.* 61: 39–45.

57 Wendt, C. and Kampf, B. (2008). Evidence-based spectrum of antimicrobial activity for disinfection of bronchoscopes. *J. Hosp. Infect.* 70 (suppl 1): 60–68.

58 Rutala, W.A. and Weber, D.J. (2004). Disinfection and sterilization in health care facilities: what clinicians need to know. *Clin. Infect. Dis.* 39: 702–709.

59 Petersen, B.T., Cohen, J., Hambrick, D.R. III et al. (2017). Multi-society guideline for reprocessing flexible gastrointestinal endoscopes: 2016 update. *Gastrointest. Endosc.* 85: 282–294.

60 Fraser, V.J., Zuckerman, G., Clouse, R.E. et al. (1993). A prospective randomized trial comparing manual and automated endoscope disinfection methods. *Infect. Control Hosp. Epidemiol.* 14: 383–393.

61 Sorin, M., Segal-Maurer, S., Mariano, N. et al. (2001). Nosocomial transmission of imipenem-resistant *Pseudomonas aeruginosa* following bronchoscopy associated with improper connection to the Steris System 1 processor. *Infect. Control Hosp. Epidemiol.* 22: 409–413.

62 Chroneou, A., Zimmerman, S.K., Cook, S. et al. (2008). Molecular typing of *Mycobacterium chelonae* isolates from a pseudo-outbreak involving an automated bronchoscope washer. *Infect. Control Hosp. Epidemiol.* 29: 1088–1090.

63 Muscarella, L.F. (2002). Application of environmental sampling to flexible endoscope reprocessing: the importance of monitoring the rinse water. *Infect. Control Hosp. Epidemiol.* 23: 285–289.

64 Muscarella, L.F. (2004). The importance of bronchoscope reprocessing guidelines: raising the standard of care. *Chest* 126: 1001–1002.

65 Pang, J., Perry, P., Ross, A., and Forbes, G.M. (2002). Bacteria-free rinse water for endoscope disinfection. *Gastrointest. Endosc.* 56: 402–406.

66 Muscarella, L.F. (2006). Inconsistencies in endoscope-reprocessing and infection control guidelines: the importance of endoscope drying. *Am. J. Gastroenterol.* 101: 2147–2147.

67 Ofstead, C.L., Heymann, O.L., Quick, M.R. et al. (2018). Residual moisture and waterborne pathogens inside flexible endoscopes: evidence from a multisite study of endoscope drying effectiveness. *Am. J. Infect. Control* 46: 689–696.

68 Gavalda, L., Olmo, A.R., Hernandez, R. et al. (2015). Microbiological monitoring of flexible bronchoscopes after high-level disinfection and flushing channels with alcohol: results and cost. *Respir. Med.* 109: 1079–1085.

69 Pineau, L., Villard, E., Duc, D.L., and Marchetti, B. (2008). Endoscope drying/storage cabinet: interest and efficacy. *J. Hosp. Infect.* 68: 59–65.

70 Kovaleva, J. (2017). Endoscope drying and its pitfalls. *J. Hosp. Infect.* 97: 319–328.

71 Vandenbroucke-Grauls, C.M., Baars, A.C., Visser, M.R. et al. (1993). An outbreak of Serratia marcescens traced to a contaminated bronchoscope. *J. Hosp. Infect.* 23: 263–270.

72 Kruse, A. and Rey, J.-F. (2000). Guidelines on cleaning and disinfection in GI endoscopy. *Endoscopy* 32: 77–83.

73 Corne, P., Godreuil, S., Jean-Pierre, H. et al. (2005). Unusual implication of biopsy forceps in outbreaks of *Pseudomonas*

74 Wilson, S.J., Everts, R.J., Kirkland, K.B., and Sexton, D.J. (2000). A pseudo-outbreak of Aureobasidium species lower respiratory tract infections caused by reuse of single-use stopcocks during bronchoscopy. *Infect. Control Hosp. Epidemiol.* 21: 470–472.

75 Spraggs, P.D., Hanekom, W.H., Mochloulis, G. et al. (1994). The assessment of risk of cross-contamination with a multi-use nasal atomizer. *J. Hosp. Infect.* 28: 315–321.

76 Reynolds, C.D., Rhinehart, E., Dreyer, P., and Goldmann, D.A. (1992). Variability in reprocessing policies and procedures for flexible fiberoptic endoscopes in Massachusetts hospitals. *Am. J. Infect. Control* 20: 283–290.

77 Rutala, W.A., Clontz, E.P., Weber, D.J., and Hoffmann, K.K. (1991). Disinfection practices for endoscopes and other semicritical items. *Infect. Control Hosp. Epidemiol.* 12: 282–288.

78 Honeybourne, D. and Neumann, C.S. (1997). An audit of bronchoscopy practice in the United Kingdom: a survey of adherence to national guidelines. *Thorax* 52: 709–713.

79 Srinivasan, A., Wolfenden, L.L., Song, X. et al. (2004). Bronchoscope reprocessing and infection prevention and control: bronchoscopy-specific guidelines are needed. *Chest* 125: 307–314.

80 Shimono, N., Takuma, T., Tsuchimochi, N. et al. (2008). An outbreak of *Pseudomonas aeruginosa* infections following thoracic surgeries occurring via the contamination of bronchoscopes and an automatic endoscope reprocessor. *J. Infect. Chemother.* 14: 418–423.

81 American Society for Gastrointestinal Endoscopy (ASGE) Technology Committee (2014). Technologies for monitoring the quality of endoscope reprocessing. *Gastrointest. Endosc.* 80: 369–373.

82 Alfa, M.J., Olson, N., DeGagne, P., and Simner, P.J. (2012). Development and validation of rapid use scope test strips to determine the efficacy of manual cleaning for flexible endoscope channels. *Am. J. Infect. Control* 40: 860–865.

83 Alfa, M.J., Sepehri, S., Olson, N. et al. (2012). Establishing a clinically relevant bioburden benchmark: a quality indicator for adequate reprocessing and storage of flexible gastrointestinal endoscopes. *Am. J. Infect. Control* 40: 233–236.

84 Alfa, M.J., Fatima, I., and Olson, N. (2013). Validation of adenosine triphosphate to audit manual cleaning of flexible endoscope channels. *Am. J. Infect. Control* 41: 245–248.

85 Alfa, M.J., Fatima, I., and Olson, N. (2013). The adenosine triphosphate test is a rapid and reliable audit tool to assess manual cleaning adequacy of flexible endoscope channels. *Am. J. Infect. Control* 41: 249–253.

86 Alfa, M.J., Olson, N., and Murray, B.L. (2014). Comparison of clinically relevant benchmarks and channel sampling methods used to assess manual cleaning compliance for flexible gastrointestinal endoscopes. *Am. J. Infect. Control* 42: e1–e5.

87 Visrodia, K.H., Ofstead, C.L., Yellin, H.L. et al. (2014). The use of rapid indicators for the detection of organic residues on clinically used gastrointestinal endoscopes with and without visually apparent debris. *Infect. Control Hosp. Epidemiol.* 35: 987–994.

88 Ofstead, C.L., Wetzler, H.P., Eiland, J.E. et al. (2016). Assessing residual contamination and damage inside flexible endoscopes over time. *Am. J. Infect. Control* 44: 1675–1677.

89 Silva, C.V., Magalhães, V.D., Pereira, C.R. et al. (2003). Pseudo-outbreak of *Pseudomonas aeruginosa* and *Serratia marcescens* related to bronchoscopes. *Infect. Control Hosp. Epidemiol.* 24: 195–197.

90 Singh, A., Goering, R.V., Simjee, S. et al. (2006). Application of molecular techniques to the study of hospital infection. *Clin. Microbiol. Rev.* 19: 512–530.

91 Bou, R., Aguilar, A., Perpiñán, J. et al. (2006). Nosocomial outbreak of *Pseudomonas aeruginosa* infections related to a flexible bronchoscope. *J. Hosp. Infect.* 64: 129–135.

92 Marchand, G., Duchaaine, C., Lavoie, J. et al. (2016). Bacteria emitted in ambient air during bronchoscopy – a risk to health care workers? *Am. J. Infect. Control* 44: 1634–1638.

93 Morice, A. (1989). Hazard to bronchoscopists. (Letter). *Lancet* 1: 448.

94 Malasky, C., Jordan, T., Potulski, F., and Reichman, L.B. (1990). Occupational tuberculous infections among pulmonary physicians in training. *Am. Rev. Respir. Dis.* 142: 505–507.

95 Jereb, J.A., Burwen, D.R., and Dooley, S.W. (1993). Nosocomial outbreak of tuberculosis in a renal transplant unit: application of a new technique for restriction fragment length polymorphism analysis of *Mycobacterium tuberculosis* isolates. *J. Infect. Dis.* 168: 1219–1224.

96 Saeed, D.K., Shakoor, S., Irfan, S., and Hasan, R. (2016). Mycobacterial contamination of bronchoscopes: challenges and possible solutions in low resource settings. *Int. J. Mycobacteriol.* 5: 408–411.

97 Fennelly, K.P. (1997). Personal respiratory protection against *Mycobacterium tuberculosis*. *Clin. Chest Med.* 18: 1–17.

98 Birnie, G.G., Quigley, E.M., Clements, G.B. et al. (1983). Endoscopic transmission of hepatitis B virus. *Gut* 24: 171–174.

99 Sawchuk, W.S., Weber, P.J., Lowy, D.R., and Dzubow, L.M. (1989). Infectious papillomavirus in the vapor of warts treated with carbon dioxide laser or electrocoagulation: detection and protection. *J. Am. Acad. Dermatol.* 21: 41–49.

100 Hanson, P.J.V., Chadwick, M.V., Gaya, H., and Collins, J.V. (1992). A study of glutaraldehyde insinfection of fiberoptic bronchoscopes experimentally contaminated with *Mycobacterium tuberculosis*. *J. Hosp. Infect.* 22: 137–142.

101 Seballos, R.L., Walsh, A.L., and Mehta, A.C. (1995). Clinical evaluation of a liquid chemical sterilization system for the flexible bronchoscopes. *J. Bronchol.* 2: 192–199.

102 Hanson, P.J., Gor, D., Jeffries, D.J., and Collins, J.V. (1990). Elimination of high titer HIV from fibreoptic endoscopes. *Gut* 31: 657–659.

103 American Association for Gastrointestinal Endoscopy (2008). Infection control during GI endoscopy. *Gastrointest. Endosc.* 67: 781–790.

104 Bronowicki, J.P., Venard, V., Botté, C. et al. (1997). Patient-to-patient transmission of hepatitis C virus during colonoscopy. *N. Engl. J. Med.* 337: 237–240.

105 Rutala, W.A. and Weber, D.J. (2001). Creutzfeldt-Jakob disease: recommendations for disinfection and sterilization. *Clin. Infect. Dis.* 32: 1348–1356.

106 Axon, A.T., Beilenhoff, U., Brumble, M.G. et al. (2001). Variant Creutzfeldt-Jacob disease (vCJD) and gastrointestinal endoscopy. *Endoscopy* 33: 1070–1080.

107 Ofstead, C.L., Wetzler, H.P., Doyle, E.M. et al. (2015). Persistent contamination on colonoscopies and gastroscopes detected by biological cultures and rapid indicators despite reprocessing performed in accordance with guidelines. *Am. J. Infect. Control* 43: 794–801.

108 Jain, P., Fleming, P., and Mehta, A.C. (1999). Radiation safety for the health care workers in bronchoscopy suite. *Clin. Chest Med.* 20: 33–38.

109 Harrison, J.D. and Streffer, C. (2007). The ICRP protection quantities, equivalent, and effective dose: their basis and application. *Radiat. Prot. Dosim.* 127: 12–18.

110 Huda, W. (1997). Radiation dosimetry in diagnostic radiology. *Am. J. Roentgenol.* 169: 1487–1488.

111 Wrixon, A.D. (2008). New recommendations from the international commission on radiological protection – a review. *Phys. Med. Biol.* 53: 41–60.

112 Dewar, C. (2013). Occupational radiation safety. *Radiol. Technol.* 84: 467–484.

113 Mettler, F.A., Koenig, T.R., Wagner, L.K., and Kelsey, C.A. (2002). Radiation injuries after fluoroscopic procedures. *Semin. Ultrasound CT MR* 23: 428–442.

114 Wall, B.F., Kendall, G.M., A, E. et al. (2006). What are the risks from medical x-rays and other low dose radiation? *Br. J. Radiol.* 79: 285–294.

115 Cohen, B.L. (1980). The cancer risk from low-level radiation. *Health Phys.* 39: 659–678.

116 Shimizu, Y., Schull, W.J., and Kato, H. (1990). Cancer risk among atomic bomb survivors: the RERF life span study. *JAMA* 264: 601–604.

117 Evans, J.S., Wennberg, J.E., and McNeil, B.J. (1986). The influence of diagnostic radiography on the incidence of breast cancer and leukemia. *N. Engl. J. Med.* 315: 810–815.

118 Brenner, D.J., Doll, R., Goodhead, D.T. et al. (2003). Cancer risk attributable to low dose ionizing radiation: assessing what we really know. *Proc. Natl. Acad. Sci.* 100: 13761–13766.

119 Committee on the Biological Effects of Ionizing Radiation (BEIR V) (1990). *Health Effects of Exposure to Low Levels of Ionizing Radiation. National Academy of Science*. Washington (DC): National Research Council.

120 Valentin, J. (2000). Avoidance of radiation injuries from medical interventional procedures. *Ann. ICRP* 30: 7–67.

121 Niklason, L.T., Marx, M.V., and Chan, H.P. (1993). Interventional radiologists: occupational radiation doses and risks. *Radiology* 187: 729–733.

122 Johnson, L.W., Moore, R.J., and Balter, S. (1992). Review of radiation safety in the cardiac catheterization laboratory. *Catheter. Cardiovasc. Diagn.* 25: 186–194.

123 Goldstone, K.E., Wright, I.H., and Cohen, B. (1993). Radiation exposure to the hands of orthopedic surgeons during procedures under fluoroscopic control. *Br. J. Radiol.* 66: 899–901.

124 Giblin, J.G., Rubenstein, J., Taylor, A., and Pahira, J. (1996). Radiation risk to the urologist during endourologic procedures, and a new shield that reduces exposure. *Urology* 48: 624–627.

125 McGowan, C., Heaton, B., and Stephenson, R.N. (1996). Occupational x-ray exposure of anesthetists. *Br. J. Anaesth.* 76: 868–869.

126 Steinfort, D.L., Einsiedel, P., and Irving, L.B. (2010). Radiation dose to patients and clinicians during fluoroscopically-guided biopsy of peripheral pulmonary lesions. *Respir. Care* 55: 1469–1474.

127 Wrixon, A.D. (2008). New ICRP recommendations. *J. Radiol. Prot.* 28: 161–168.

128 Dendy, P.P. (2008). Radiation risks in interventional radiology. *Br. J. Radiol.* 81: 1–7.

129 Rehani, M.M. and Ortiz-Lopez, P. (2006). Radiation effects in fluoroscopically guided cardiac interventions – keeping them under control. *Int. J. Cardiol.* 109: 147–151.

130 Wall, B.F. (2004). Radiation protection dosimetry for diagnostic radiology patients. *Radiat. Prot. Dosim.* 109: 409–419.

131 Ost, D., Shah, R., Anasco, E. et al. (2008). A randomized trial of CT fluoroscopic-guided bronchoscopy vs conventional bronchoscopy in patients with suspected lung cancer. *Chest* 134: 507–513.

132 Tsushimaa, K., Sonea, S., Hanaokaa, T. et al. (2006). Comparison of bronchoscopic diagnosis for peripheral pulmonary nodule under fluoroscopic guidance with CT guidance. *Respir. Med.* 100: 737–745.

133 Yoshikawa, M., Sukoh, N., Yamazaki, K. et al. (2007). Diagnostic value of endobronchial ultrasonography with a guide sheath for peripheral pulmonary lesions without X-ray fluoroscopy. *Chest* 131: 1788–1793.

134 National Council on Radiation Protection and Measurement (1990). Implementation of the principle of as low as reasonably achievable (ALARA) for medical and dental personnel. NCRP Report No. 107. Bethesda: NCRP.

135 Fujita, Y., Seki, N., Kurimoto, N. et al. (2011). Introduction of endobronchial ultrasonography (EBUS) in bronchoscopy clearly reduces fluoroscopy time: comparison of 147 cases in groups before and after EBUS introduction. *Jpn. J. Clin. Oncol.* 41: 1177–1181.

136 Sailer, A.M., Vergoossen, L., and Paulis, L. (2017). Personalized feedback on staff dose in fluoroscopy-guided interventions: a new era in radiation dose monitoring. *Cardiovasc. Intervent. Radiol.* 40: 1756–1762.

137 Faulknar, K. and Moores, B.M. (1982). An assessment of the radiation dose received by staff using fluoroscopic equipment. *Br. J. Radiol.* 55: 272–276.

138 Mahesh, M. (2001). Fluoroscopy: patient radiation exposure issues. *Radiographics* 21: 1033–1045.

139 Chaffins, J. (2008). Radiation protection and procedures in OR. *Radiol. Technol.* 79: 415–428.

140 Herman-Schulman, M. (2006). Can fluoroscopic radiation

dose be substantially reduced. *Radiology* 238: 1–2.

141 Norris, T.G. (2002). Radiation safety in fluoroscopy. *Radiol. Technol.* 73: 911–933.

142 Lakkireddy, D., Nadzam, G., Verma, A. et al. (2009). Impact of a comprehensive safety program on radiation exposure during catheter ablation of atrial fibrillation: a prospective study. *J. Interv. Card. Electrophysiol.* 24: 105–112.

143 Ernst, A., Smith, L., Gryniuk, L. et al. (2004). A simple teaching intervention significantly decreases radiation exposure during transbronchial biopsy. *J. Bronchol.* 11: 109–111.

144 Brateman, L. (1999). Radiation safety considerations for diagnostic radiology personnel. *Radiographics* 19: 1037–1055.

145 Hubbert, T.E., Vucich, J.J., and Armstrong, M.R. (1993). Light weight aprons for protection against scattered radiation during fluoroscopy. *Am. J. Roentgenol.* 161: 1079–1083.

146 Tse, V., Lising, J., Khadra, M. et al. (1999). Radiation exposure during fluoroscopy: should we be protecting our thyroids? *Aust. N. Z. J. Surg.* 69: 847–848.

147 Richman, A.H., Chan, B., and Katz, M. (1976). Effectiveness of leaded glasses in reducing radiation exposure. *Radiology* 121: 357–359.

148 Yukihara, E.G. and McKeever, S.W. (2008). Optically stimulated luminescence (OSL) dosimetry in medicine. *Phys. Med. Biol.* 53: R351–R379.

149 Luszig-Bhadra, M. and Perle, S. (2006). Electronic personal dosimeters will replace passive dosimeters in the near future. *Radiat. Prot. Dosim.* 123: 546–553.

150 Al-Shakhrah, A. and Abu-Kaled, Y.S. (2000). Estimation of effective radiation dose for physicians and staff members in contrast angiocardiography. *Heart Lung* 29: 417–423.

151 Schroeder, C., Chung, J.M., Mitchell, A.B. et al. (2018). Using the hybrid operating room in thoracic surgery: a paradigm shift. *Innovations* 13: 372–377. https://doi.org/10.1097/IMI.0000000000000531.

152 Hohenforst-Schmidt, W., Zarogoulidis, P., Vogl, T. et al. (2014). Cone beam computer tomography (CBCT) in interventional chest medicine – high feasibility for endobronchial real-time navigation. *J. Cancer* 5: 231–241.

153 Hohenforst-Schmidt, W., Banckwitz, R., Zarogoulidis, P. et al. (2014). Radiation exposure of patients by cone beam CT during endobronchial navigation – a phantom study. *J. Cancer* 5: 192–202.

154 Pritchett, M.A., Schampaert, S., de Groot, J.A.H. et al. (2018). Cone-beam cCT with augmented fluoroscopy combined with electromagnetic navigation bronchoscopy for biopsy of pulmonary nodules. *J. Bronchology. Interv. Pulmonol.* 25: 274–282. https://doi.org/10.1097/LBR.0000000000000536.

155 Bowling, M.R., Brown, C., and Anciano, C.J. (2017). Feasibility and safety of the transbronchial access tool for peripheral pulmonary nodule and mass. *Ann. Thorac. Surg.* 104: 443–449.

第 5 章

可弯曲支气管镜诊断和治疗的麻醉管理

Blake A. Moore[1], J. Francis Turner, Jr.[2,3], and Ko-Pen Wang[4]

[1] Section on Cardiothoracic Anesthesia,
University of Tennessee Graduate School of Medicine, Knoxville, TN, USA
[2] Division of Pulmonary and Critical Care Medicine,
University of Tennessee Graduate School of Medicine, Knoxville, TN, USA
[3] National Supercomputing Institute, University of Nevada, Las Vegas, NV, USA
[4] Division of Pulmonary and Critical Care Medicine, Johns Hopkins Bayview Medical Center,
Johns Hopkins University School of Medicine, Baltimore, MD, USA

（译者：杨宇光　译者单位：海军军医大学第一附属医院）

5.1　引言

支气管镜诊疗的临床应用日益广泛，这项技术需要支气管镜操作医师和麻醉医师之间协作和沟通，以确保其安全性和舒适度。对于两个专业医疗领域而言，在共同解剖区域进行最佳干预或诊疗至关重要。鉴于在美国每年进行超过50万例次的支气管镜诊疗服务，麻醉医师和支气管镜医师都需要熟悉这些操作、麻醉技术和相关风险[1]。当存在重大并发症的潜在风险时，应在麻醉给药之前根据患者的风险级别来讨论制定相应计划。此外，也应优先考虑患者的身心舒适。随着介入操作的日益复杂，根据患者合并症和临床情况，应对患者进行抗焦虑干预，以提供最佳的医护服务条件。患者的不适可导致不必要的体动，这可能延长内镜诊疗时间或增加受伤和产生并发症的风险，极端情况下可能会产生严重后果。随着病例数量不断增加，操作变得更加复杂，选择合适的麻醉团队和麻醉技术（如深度镇静或全身麻醉）可提升这项医疗服务的安全和效率。

本章将概述各种气管镜操作的围术期评估和管理，包括每种操作的复杂性和相关风险状况。

5.2　麻醉前评估

美国麻醉医师协会（American Society of Anesthesiologists，ASA）麻醉前评估实践标准包括以下5个方面：现病史、既往史、体格检查（如心脏、肺部、气道等）、术前检查和必要的会诊。时间安排取决于外科手术以及疾病严重程度[2]。根据ASA评估标准应包括既往麻醉史和用药史。此外，麻醉医师应当根据需要给予适当的术前药物。评估后，麻醉医师应和患者签署知情同意书，并根据ASA PS评分系统对每一位患者进行评分[3,4]。

术前评估有助于风险评估和制订相应的诊疗计划。ASA状态分级如表5.1所示，从Ⅰ级到Ⅵ级全面评估患者的并发症和风险。若数字评分后加"E"，则认定为紧急手术。脑死亡捐献患者ASA评级为Ⅵ级。对于更新的最新版本的评级系统提供了一些适合特定ASA PS评分的标准。

表 5.1 美国麻醉医师学会（ASA）身体状况分级评价系统[4]

分级	定义	示例，但不限于
I	健康患者	健康，不吸烟，无或极少饮酒
II	轻度全身性疾病患者	仅有轻度疾病且功能无实质性限制。例如（但不限于），当前吸烟者，社交饮酒者，孕妇，肥胖（30<BMI<40），控制良好的糖尿病或高血压，轻度肺部疾病
III	重度全身性疾病患者	有实质性功能限制；1 个或多个中度到重度疾病。例如（但不限于），糖尿病或高血压控制不良，慢性阻塞性肺病，病态肥胖（BMI≥40），活动性肝炎，酒精依赖或滥用，植入起搏器，中度降低的射血分数，定期进行血液透析的 ESRD，校正年龄<60 周的早产儿，心肌梗死、脑血管意外、短暂性脑缺血发作或冠心病/支架置入史（>3 个月）
IV	威胁生命的重度全身性疾病患者	例如（但不限于），近期（<3 个月）发生的心肌梗死、脑血管意外、短暂性脑缺血发作或冠心病/支架置入，持续的心肌缺血或严重瓣膜功能障碍，严重降低的射血分数，败血症，DIC，ARD 或不定期接受透析的 ESRD
V	病情濒临死亡，手术前预计无法生存的患者	例如（但不限于），腹部/胸部动脉瘤破裂，重大创伤，颅内出血伴有占位效应，心脏病理学或多器官/系统功能紊乱情况下的缺血性肠病变
VI	宣告脑死亡并且器官用于捐献的患者	

添加"E"表示紧急手术。紧急情况是指当延误治疗时会导致患者生命或身体部位受到威胁显著增加。ARD，急性呼吸道疾病；BMI，体重指数；DIC，弥散性血管内凝血；ESRD，终末期肾病。

可弯曲支气管镜的评估和干预，主要是针对心血管系统和肺部的病史和症状，评估操作过程的刺激对心肺功能的影响，以及正压通气和药物引起的潜在生理变化。气道操作对自主神经系统的强烈刺激，引起交感神经兴奋，儿茶酚胺释放增加，随后心输出量增加和心动过速，造成需氧量增多[5]。通气和氧合的改变导致缺氧，甚至一些氧储备有限的患者在呼吸暂停期就可能产生严重的缺氧。

5.2.1 心肺评估

有呼吸系统症状的患者，如喘鸣、进行性呼吸困难、声音嘶哑、运动耐量下降或喘息等，可以通过简要的病史和体格检查快速评估，从而了解肺部疾病的严重和紧急程度。与肺部疾病相关的重要病史要素包括吸烟史和戒烟时间、阻塞性睡眠呼吸暂停和持续气道正压通气（continuous positive airway pressure，CPAP）的耐受性，哮喘发作史包括目前的治疗药物、插管史。慢性阻塞性肺病（chronic obstructive pulmonary disease，COPD）和氧气依赖程度。对于哮喘患者来说，需重点评估患者的用药方案和哮喘的严重程度，并且评估目前治疗方案对患者症状控制的稳定性情况。对于阻塞性睡眠呼吸暂停患者，存在多种分型，觉醒阈值是影响患者对镇静药物耐受性的重要因素。具有较高觉醒阈值的患者（即根据患者发生皮层觉醒时会厌负压值确定）会在多导睡眠图中观察到觉醒的发生，其可能对镇静药物更敏感[6]。

应当对患者进行心脏病史询问，其中以下因素很重要：心力衰竭伴左心室射血分数降低、严重冠状动脉疾病、过去 6 个月到 1 年内的心肌梗死、心脏支架或手术史、因缺血性或出血性中风而导致的脑血管疾病，或者严重的外周动脉疾病。在经皮冠状动脉介入术后，对于冠脉非覆膜金属支架术后，可弯曲支气管镜应该延迟 30 天；对于药物洗脱支架植入术后，可弯曲支气管镜应该延迟 6 个月；对于药物洗脱支架植入术后，当延迟风险高于血栓形成或缺血事件的风险时，可弯曲支气管镜操作应该延迟 3 个月[7]。严重的心脏瓣膜疾病，尤其是主动脉或二尖瓣狭窄，应该根据手术的复杂性和预计的麻醉深度来考虑有创动脉监测。

可弯曲支气管镜操作患者预防性使用抗生素取决于具体的操作和患者情况。2007 年，美国心脏协会（AHA）指南建议高风险患者和组织活检或气道黏膜出现切口后预防性使用抗生素[8]。预防性抗生素应用于 4 种特定的高危心脏疾病：人工心脏瓣膜、感染性心膜炎病史、心脏移植患者和明确有先天性心脏病患者[9]。支气管镜检查期间菌血症的发生与心内膜炎感染相关。Matveychuk 等进行了一项前瞻性研究，评估了经支气管镜进行氩等离子电凝治疗后菌血症的发生率，结果显示严重的临床感染十分罕见，菌血症的发生率仅为 2.3%，总体菌血症的发生率在 0~6%之间[10]。随着支气管内超声引导下的针吸活检的出现，一项关于可能感染并发症的前瞻性研究表明，在行超声引导下经支气管针吸活检（endobronchial ultrasound-guided transbronchial needle aspiration, EBUS-TBNA）的患者中,菌血症的发生率为7%,这一结果与常规支气管镜检查的结果相当[11]。随着支气管镜检查变得越来越复杂,我们建议谨慎并仔细评估风险因素。Janszky等最近的研究结果显示,在一些"侵入性非牙科诊疗操作"中感染性心内膜炎的风险增加[12]。

心血管症状包括心绞痛、呼吸困难、跛行,或体格检查中出现如颈静脉压升高、外周水肿或肺部啰音的迹象,都是重点记录的内容。失代偿性心力衰竭或急性肺部感染患者通常需要在术前进行优化治疗,除非需要紧急手术的患者。

5.2.2 气道检查

麻醉医师使用多种指标来预测面罩通气和插管的困难程度。为了通过直接观察声门来更好地管理患者的气道,喉镜医生会要求患者口腔、咽部和喉部的轴线保持一致。嗅位是使喉镜医生的视线与声门开口一致的最佳位置。此外,还有一些标准作为插管困难的预测因素进行评分。

Mallampati分级是对咽喉部可视化的评估,按照图5.1中的示例,分为Ⅰ~Ⅳ级。甲状腺舌距或舌骨下距用来评估下颌前突的程度,这可能会增加喉镜检查的难度。它以手指的宽度为单位,从1到4个手指不等进行测量。口腔张开度,也以手指宽度来测量,用来估计在喉镜检查时是否能够看到声门。Mallampati评级为Ⅲ级或Ⅳ级,通常认为喉镜检查困难程度较高。

气道评估中还包括颈椎活动度,因为颈椎活动度的受限会使轴线的对齐更加具有挑战性。就面罩通气而言,所有这些解剖特征都可能对成功的气道管理提出挑战,而在多次尝试喉镜检查失败后,面罩通气可能会变得更加困难。还应考虑其他特征包括颈围、体重指数（BMI）>30 kg/m^2、年龄>55岁、颈部放疗史、大舌头或气道内肿物。

5.2.3 纵隔疾病

前纵隔肿块可能带来重大挑战和显著风险,必须在手术前根据其大小和位置加以确认。一旦患者麻醉并进行正压通气,生理上可能会有显著变化。此外,患者为了进行手术而处于仰卧位,也会导致通气和循环方面出现明显的生理学变化。

在病史和体格检查中有一个重要特征可用于判断纵隔病变是否会影响操作安全性,即患者是否能在仰卧位时不出现明显的呼吸困难。如果前纵隔肿块足够大,以至于在仰卧位时压迫气管或心脏结构,维持自主呼吸可能是必要的,以防止气道堵塞或心输出量下降。一些学者认为,在大型前纵隔肿块患者中,可以通过正压通气来观察气道,这对正压通气时患者气管塌陷的假设提出了挑战[14]。此外,心包积液可能是相关恶性肿瘤的症状之一,包括纵隔肿瘤,极端情况下,甚至可能表现为心包填塞[15,16]。

如果存在较大的前纵隔肿块,了解患者在仰卧位时最舒适的体位可能很有帮助:他们是否能够仰卧入睡,还是必须采取侧卧或俯卧位才能舒适地呼吸?在这些患者中,自主呼吸的丧失和体位的改变可

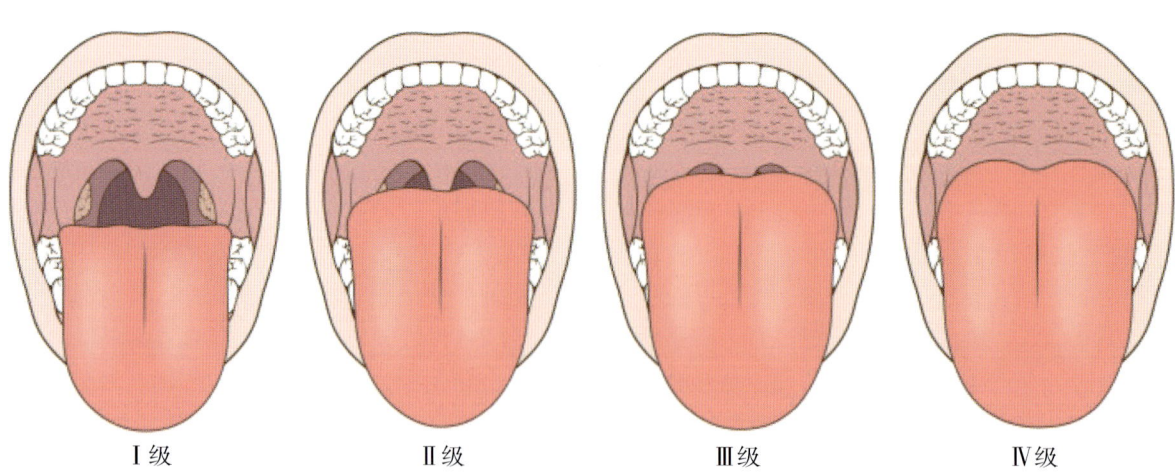

Ⅰ级　　　　Ⅱ级　　　　Ⅲ级　　　　Ⅳ级

图5.1　Mallampati分级

来源：Samsoon and Young[13]。

能会影响胸腔内的解剖关系，从而对患者产生毁灭性的后果。此外，对血管结构的压迫可能导致患者右心室充盈减少，在严重情况下可引起心输出量下降，需要进行抢救。尽管不常见，但在评估接受支气管镜检查患者的风险时，应将未诊断的心包压塞或未预料到的前纵隔肿物（可能会压迫血管结构或影响气管通畅）纳入风险评估范畴。严重的症状、混合性阻塞性/限制性肺疾病和气管横截面积小于正常水平50%的情况，是纵隔受累及患者围手术期并发症相关的预测因素[17]。

5.2.4 中央气道阻塞性病变

流量-容积曲线有助于明确气道阻塞的病变。肺功能测试（pulmonary function testing，PFT）可以显示阻塞类型，其特征是FEV_1/FVC比值降低。通过肺活量描绘流量-容积曲线，可以深入了解患者的限制性或阻塞性肺疾病，或者帮助明确中央气道病变。根据流量-容积曲线的描绘特征，可将中央气道阻塞性病变分为两种类型。可变性胸内阻塞表现出流量-容积曲线的呼气相扁平化。这些病变呈现生理学纯粹的特点是，当患者自发呼吸时，肺部病变将在气道周围塌陷，将阻塞性病变引向中央气道并减弱呼气段。可变性胸外阻塞则表现出流量-容积曲线的吸气相变钝，因为自主呼吸时气管内压力小于大气压。

尽管这些典型的流量-容积曲线的描绘显示阻塞性类型的多样性，但应将它们视为理想的呈现方式，临床表现可能有所不同。例如，所有类型的中央气道阻塞可能表现为吸气流量减小，但当吸气流量平台减小的比例大于呼气流量减小，或者出现单独的吸气流量

减弱时，就可以明确诊断为可变性胸外阻塞[18]。胸腔内外的固定性病变都会表现出吸气和呼气曲线的变平。气道阻塞性病变预期的流量-容积曲线见图5.2。

5.3 监测与设备

5.3.1 ASA麻醉效应对意识和心肺生理的连续性

麻醉药物的使用会导致生理学变化，这些变化在大脑皮质功能上呈现为从清醒和警觉到无反应和失去意识的连续变化，同时还会伴随着与用药剂量相关的心脏和呼吸功能的变化。ASA已经明确划分了这个连续的镇静深度，以指导医务人员了解关于意识程度、可唤醒性以及气道通畅性、呼吸功能和心血管变化相关的预期生理变化。

这一专家共识也指导从业者，关于何时需要合格的麻醉医师参与，独立管理气道和生理方面的副作用或并发症。

ASA认为，实施中度镇静和镇痛（以前称为"有意识的镇静"）的麻醉医师应具备相应的知识和技能，以逆转无意中引起的过度镇静效应，并提供抢救措施来纠正呼吸过缓/呼吸暂停、低血压以及过度镇静，以使患者恢复到预期的镇静状态。ASA将中度镇静/镇痛定义为在保持气道通畅和自主呼吸的同时，通常不会对心血管功能产生影响，同时保持对轻微触碰或口头指令有明确的或有意识的反应[19]。ASA共识声明中概述了镇静的连续性和已接受的定义（表5.2）。有

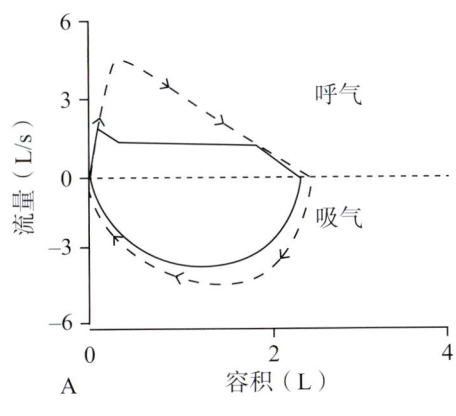 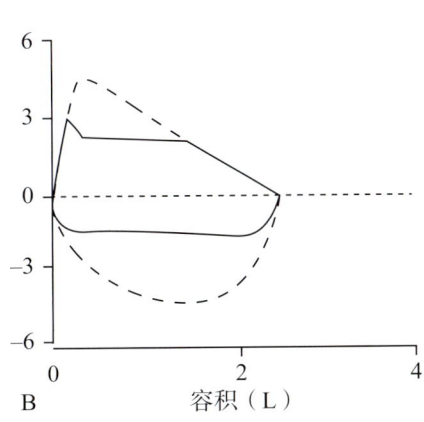 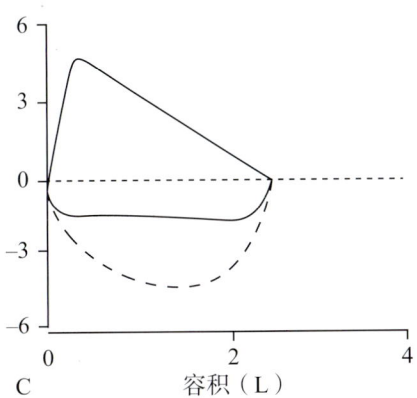

图5.2 流量-容积曲线

A. 可变胸内阻塞；B. 固定胸内或胸外阻塞；C. 可变胸外阻塞。来源：Williamson[18]。

意识的反应并不是指对疼痛刺激的反射性回避。存在心血管功能受损的患者，中度镇静下镇静剂可能会影响心脏生理，包括全身血管阻力（systemic vascular resistance，SVR）、心脏收缩能力或心率。在极端情况下，如存在明显的心包积液、心力衰竭或瓣膜疾病等，即使轻度到中度的镇静也可能导致心血管生理变化。应始终考虑与心肺患者相关的重要合并症，以安全提供任何程度的镇静。

表 5.2　ASA 持续镇静深度：全身麻醉的定义和镇静/镇痛水平[a]

	轻度镇静/抗焦虑	中度镇静/镇痛（"意识镇静"）	深度镇静/镇痛	全身麻醉
意识反应	对语言刺激反应正常	对语言或触觉刺激有反应[b]	反复的疼痛刺激后有反应[b]	即使受到疼痛刺激也无法唤醒
气道	无影响	无须干预	可能需要干预	经常需要干预
自发通气	无影响	充足	可能不足	频繁不足
心血管功能	无影响	可以维持	可以维持	可能受损

[a] 监测下的麻醉护理（MAC）不是一种持续的镇静。准确地说，它是"一种特殊的麻醉服务，要求麻醉医师参与对正在接受诊疗性操作的患者的护理"。
[b] 戒断过程中的疼痛刺激反射不被认为是有目的的反应。
来源：ASA 专家共识。

5.3.2　ASA 的麻醉监测标准

ASA 提出了两项关于使用麻醉药物患者的监测标准。第一项标准规定，接受监测麻醉（monitored anesthesia care，MAC）、全身麻醉或局部麻醉的所有患者都应由合格的麻醉医师进行监护。第二个标准概述了在不同镇静深度下进行手术的患者监护中应包括的生理参数。为了持续评估氧合情况，接受麻醉的患者，无论是中度镇静、MAC 还是全身麻醉，都应通过可视的脉搏血氧饱和度读数进行监测，对患者的评估应由团队中受过适当培训的成员独自负责。对于中度镇静，除非手术或患者情况不允许外，通气状况均应通过呼吸末二氧化碳监测进行监护。为了监测心脏功能，所有麻醉都要求进行连续心电图监测，并每 5 min 至少进行一次血压监测[20]。当进行全身麻醉手术时，将有更多的监测要求，这超出了本章讨论的范围。

5.4　常用于支气管镜检查的麻醉药物

支气管镜检查的麻醉药物选择需考虑多方面因素，包括患者的个体特征、支气管镜医师的技术、麻醉医师的经验，以及设备可用性和既往使用特定药物的病史。在药物短缺和供应链存在问题的时代，因地制宜对于提供一致和高质量的镇静镇痛至关重要。本章的目的不是详细描述现代麻醉实践的四大目标：遗忘、镇痛、自主神经控制和肌松。相反，本章应作为一个指南为团队提供安全和可预测效应的药物来满足患者需求并及时完成支气管镜检查。在涉及技术方面时，它并不意味着要成为麻醉管理的明确指南，而是展示如何使用和组合各种药物来为患者提供舒适和安全的麻醉。这里介绍的都是常用药物，但绝不是支气管镜操作可能用到的所有药物的详尽清单。省略的常见药物要么不适合手术时机，要么在本书概述的手术中不常用。

刺激声门上结构，如进行喉镜检查、插管，或使用硬质支气管镜、可弯曲支气管镜，会引起强烈的交感神经反射，导致儿茶酚胺释放增加，从而引起高血压和心动过速。这种反应与口咽内所受刺激的程度直接相关[21]。在进行气道干预期间出现这种生理反应需要麻醉处理和气道控制。

通过采用复合麻醉的方法来减轻这种反应，对于确保支气管镜检查的安全和成功至关重要，尤其对于心肺生理储备有限的患者。通常情况下，可通过局部麻醉或有针对性的局麻药物对气道进行麻醉，并结合阿片类药物（如静脉注射芬太尼 1~3 μg/kg 或瑞芬太尼 0.5~1.5 μg/kg）进行镇痛，或使用艾司洛尔（1~1.5 mg/kg）来对抗心动过速，从而减轻气道刺激引起的生理反应。对于出现高血压的情况，可以根据需要使用硝酸甘油静脉滴注（10~200 μg/min）。在为接受支气管镜操作的患者提供全面医护服务时，一个重要的原则是能够迅速进行调整和控制。因此，通常情况下，快速起效的药物优于起效时间长的药物。综上，本章将重点介绍常见的、易调节的和短效的药物。

5.4.1 丙泊酚

丙泊酚是一种镇静催眠药,主要作用于γ-氨基丁酸(gamma-aminobutyric acid,GABA)受体亚型A,会导致可预测的催眠、遗忘、心肌抑制以及体循环阻力降低。随着剂量的增加,其呼吸抑制作用逐渐显现,最终导致呼吸停止。丙泊酚是最常用的麻醉诱导药物,在输注时还具有止吐作用。通常以 1~2 mg/kg 的剂量作为单次静脉注射,或以 10~150 μg/(kg·min)的剂量进行静脉滴注。丙泊酚具有可预测的代谢特点,经过肝脏清除后,很快通过肾脏排泄。然而,长时间(数天)输注丙泊酚可能导致高甘油三酯血症和肝功能异常。此外,丙泊酚是以脂溶性乳剂的形式包装,在静脉注射时可引起患者不适。磷丙泊酚二钠作为一种水溶性丙泊酚前药,注射时不会引起疼痛,但由于成本和可用性原因,其使用并不广泛。

5.4.2 右美托咪定

右美托咪定与降压药可乐定属于同一类,是 α_2 肾上腺素能受体激动剂,具有抑制交感神经和镇静作用。在重症监护室或操作性镇静中,如支气管镜操作中,右美托咪定得到广泛应用。右美托咪定可与其他药物以及局麻药联合使用,用于清醒下纤维支气管镜插管的镇静。右美托咪定还可用于缓解酒精戒断症状。虽然它不是一种遗忘剂,但可以增强镇静作用同时保持呼吸驱动力。右美托咪定可引起心动过缓和低血压反应。通常在静脉注射 0.25~1 μg/kg 后,以 0.2~1.2 μg/(kg·h)的速度维持注射,即可开始支气管镜检查。在使用挥发性麻醉药的情况下,右美托咪定可降低最小肺泡浓度(minimum alveolar concentration,MAC),从而减少挥发性麻醉剂的使用。

5.4.3 氯胺酮

氯胺酮作为苯环己哌啶的衍生物,是常用的静脉全身麻醉药物。氯胺酮能提供可靠的镇痛和遗忘效果,被称为分离性麻醉药,与其他麻醉药物所产生的无反应特征不同,患者可以与外界互动,但对自己所处环境没有意识。尽管它有多个作用位点,但主要作用机制是对 N-甲基-D-天门冬氨酸(N-methyl-d-aspartate,NMDA)受体的非竞争性拮抗。单独使用氯胺酮不会导致呼吸抑制,但与其他常用药物联合使用时可能出现呼吸暂停。此外,氯胺酮具有抗胆碱能和肾上腺素能效应,可用于扩张支气管,缓解支气管痉挛症状。

心血管系统方面,氯胺酮可引起交感神经反应,导致血压升高、心输出量和心肌氧耗增加。此外,氯胺酮还可引起视觉和听觉幻觉,以及兴奋、恐惧或愉快感,使其成为潜在的滥用药物。在临床环境中,这些症状可能表现为激动或谵妄。通过使用苯二氮䓬类药物进行预处理可以减轻这种风险,如给予咪达唑仑 1~2 mg。氯胺酮有多种给药途径,包括口服、肌内、静脉、直肠和鼻内给药。作为镇痛增强剂,静脉注射 0.25~0.5 mg/kg 的剂量通常有效,预计 1~2 h 内恢复。若作为插管诱导剂量,通常在 1.0~1.5 mg/kg 的给药浓度范围内进行静脉注射。

5.4.4 咪达唑仑

咪达唑仑是一种短效苯二氮䓬类药物,具有抗焦虑、镇静和致顺行性遗忘效应、抗癫痫作用,是围术期预处理的理想药物。它可以口服、静脉注射、肌内注射或鼻内给药。对于小儿患者,咪达唑仑有助于配合静脉置管和适应与家人的分离。苯二氮䓬类药物在围手术期起到的镇静作用是通过促进中枢神经系统中 GABA 与 $GABA_A$ 受体的结合实现的。成年患者的静脉剂量通常为 0.5~5 mg。咪达唑仑可导致显著的血管舒张,其作用可通过与其他药物(如阿片类药物)的联合使用而增强。由于中枢神经系统的快速重新分布和肝脏代谢,咪达唑仑作用时间较短。氟马西尼(Romazicon®)是苯二氮䓬类药物过量的竞争性拮抗剂和解毒剂,可迅速逆转苯二氮䓬类药物的效应,包括咪达唑仑的作用。咪达唑仑具有相对较短的半衰期,因此在其清除后应监测患者是否出现再次麻醉。在长期使用苯二氮䓬类药物的情况下,可能使患者更容易发生癫痫,因此在易感人群中应慎用。

5.4.5 芬太尼和纳洛酮

芬太尼是一种常用的、强效且持续时间较短的静脉注射阿片类药物,作用起效较快,用于围手术期镇痛以及减轻喉镜检查的刺激。芬太尼广泛用于诊疗操作的镇静或镇痛。其使用剂量为 1~2 μg/kg,更高剂量会导致可预测的呼吸减慢和呼吸暂停。呼吸抑制是由于对二氧化碳浓度反应性的改变而引起的。单次给药时,芬太尼会迅速被肝脏清除,但在持续输注或多次给予情况下,其效应可能会延长。

纳洛酮是一种阿片类拮抗剂,对所有阿片受体产生拮抗作用。纳洛酮作为 μ 受体拮抗剂,可以逆转与阿片类药物过量相关的镇静和呼吸抑制作用。类似于氟马西尼，纳洛酮的拮抗效应持续时间相对较短，因此对使用纳洛酮的患者需要进行持续监测，必要时可能需要重新给药。通过每隔几分钟以 40~80 μg 的较低剂量静脉给予纳洛酮时，其逆转效应并不显著，如果患者情况稳定但怀疑有阿片类药物过量时，应优先考虑该剂量，而不是使用 400 μg 以上的大剂量。

5.4.6 瑞芬太尼

瑞芬太尼（Ultiva®）是一种与芬太尼等效的阿片类药物，但其代谢特性独特，主要由血浆酯酶代谢，半衰期较短，时量相关半衰期不依赖于输注时间，即使在长时间输注时也无蓄积风险。瑞芬太尼并不适合用作镇痛药，因为它代谢迅速，即使短期输注也可能导致疼痛高度敏感，因此几乎不考虑用作围术期镇痛。但它可以抑制交感自主神经和控制血流动力学变化，并通过降低 MAC 来减少其他药物的使用量。痛觉过敏的机制似乎是通过 NMDA 受体的激活来介导的[22,23]。在全凭静脉麻醉（total intravenous anesthesia，TIVA）中，瑞芬太尼与丙泊酚联合可以作为一种选择，特别是在需要考虑苏醒时间和控制血流动力学的情况下（在气道操作中需要减轻交感兴奋）。

对于接受支气管镜检查的患者，即使存在神经生理缺陷，也可不需要使用肌松药，作为均衡麻醉的一部分，瑞芬太尼可以通过允许逐步调整剂量和可预测的代谢来帮助实现麻醉目标。通常以 0.05~0.20 μg/（kg·min）的剂量输注使用。患者会出现可预测的剂量相关性低平均动脉压（mean arterial pressures，MAP），如果出现低血压，应考虑调整瑞芬太尼的输注剂量或给予去氧肾上腺素输注（50~200 μg/min）。

5.4.7 挥发性麻醉药物

异氟醚、七氟醚和氟烷是复合麻醉中的主要遗忘剂，用于需要或希望使用吸入麻醉药物的情况。尽管本章不涵盖挥发性麻醉药物的详尽讨论，但它们具有复杂的作用机制，已证实能够通过增强 $GABA_A$ 受体的作用以及抑制 NMDA 谷氨酸亚型受体来改变神经传递。这些神经化学效应的综合作用导致抑制性突触通信的增加和兴奋性突触通信的减少。在现代医学中，它们主要产生遗忘效应，尽管剂量不同也会导致意识丧失和对刺激无反应的状态。

MAC 提供了标准化的吸入麻醉剂量，其测量单位是使患者对外科刺激无体动所需浓度来确定。1.0 MAC 定义为挥发性麻醉药物的 ED50，即 50% 的受试者对手术刺激无反应所需要的药物浓度。MAC 会随年龄增长和联合使用其他镇静药物和镇痛药物（如阿片类药物）而降低。在 MAC 为 0.3~0.5 的水平时，患者可能会出现意识，称术中知晓。紧急使用兴奋剂（如可卡因或安非他命）会增加 MAC，而长期使用阿片类药物和苯二氮䓬类药物也会增加 MAC。

挥发性麻醉剂几乎完全在密闭和废气回收系统中使用。在大多数手术操作中这是可以实现的，但通常需要控制气道。因此，密闭通气系统能够充分发挥挥发性麻醉剂在支气管镜操作中的效果，并可监测药物浓度及 MAC，同时避免室内的大气污染。当使用喉罩或气管插管全麻行纤维支气管镜操作时，通常会使用挥发性麻醉剂。相反，硬质支气管镜操作因存在挥发性麻醉剂泄漏风险，可能不适合使用挥发性麻醉剂。

5.4.8 局部麻醉药物

可以使用各种局部麻醉药来安全地进行鼻咽、咽喉和喉部的局部麻醉或有针对性的神经阻滞。局部麻醉药物分为氨基酯和氨基酰胺两类，其中酰胺类麻醉药（如利多卡因、罗哌卡因和布比卡因）极少引起变态反应。氨基酯麻醉剂代谢为对氨基苯甲酸（p-aminobenzoic acid，PABA）酯类化合物，因此更容易引起变态反应[24]。局部麻醉药物通过阻断电压门控钠通道，从而减少在刺激时感觉神经元的去极化，进而产生麻醉效果。

在使用这些药物时，必须考虑局部麻醉药全身毒性反应（local anesthetic systemic toxicity，LAST），临床医生应遵循指南中每种局部麻醉药的剂量。中枢神经系统症状可能包括口周麻木、耳鸣或言语不清，这可能会进一步发展为癫痫。局部麻醉药血浆水平过高会产生心血管毒性，最初可能表现为低血压，并逐渐发展为心电图改变，包括 QRS 波段的延长，最终导致心功能衰竭。在某些情况下，可能需要进行心肺转流术，直到局部麻醉药的血浆浓度下降到安全水平为止。

英脱利匹特是一种 20% 浓度的脂质乳剂，用于局麻药物过量的情况，当出现毒性症状时，首先给予 1.5 mL/kg 的初始剂量（快速注射）。然后以 0.25 mL/（kg·min）的速度持续输注。脂质乳剂用于提取结合血浆中的游离局麻药。有关脂质乳剂在 LAST 的使用指南，以及由美国区域阻滞麻醉学会（ASRA）提供的高级心脏生命支持（ACLS）复苏措施的修改，包括将肾上腺素剂量减少到 1 μg/kg。

利多卡因作用时间相对较短，且安全性较高，是用于气道操作局部麻醉的首选药物。它可以通过靶向神经阻滞直接应用，或者以雾化溶液吸入的形式给予。雾化利多卡因的疗效尚不清楚，其起效时间较长，但已有成功的应用案例[25]。美国胸科医师学会（ACCP）和英国胸科学会都支持在可弯曲支气管镜操作中使用利多卡因[26,27]。

其他局部麻醉药物（如苯佐卡因和替卡因）也可考虑用于可弯曲支气管镜操作，但由于可能引起高铁血红蛋白症的风险，临床实践中很少使用。4%浓度可卡因局部应用是另一种替代治疗方法，但由于其具有成瘾性和不良心血管效应，ACCP也不建议使用。然而，可卡因具有明显的血管收缩作用。如果采用鼻腔途径进行气道管理，其血管收缩作用可能是有益的。必须注意的是，可卡因会被全身吸收，可能产生不良反应，如高血压和室性心律失常[28]，因此应谨慎使用，特别是在存在严重心血管疾病的患者中最好避免使用。可卡因通常适用于内窥镜鼻窦手术，是一种可接受的鼻部局部麻醉药，可减少鼻孔黏膜出血。氯普洛卡因等酯类局部麻醉药已经成功应用于临床，通常作为腰麻或硬膜外麻醉的短效药物[29]。由于其半衰期较短，在使用上有一定限制。

5.5 清醒插管或可弯曲支气管镜操作的气道局部麻醉技术

ASA已经制定了关于困难气道管理的指南（图5.3）。对于无法进行通气或插管的患者而言，这种情况可能会危及生命。在伴有严重肺部疾病或纵隔病变的患者中，介入肺科医师和麻醉医师应该了解困难气道的预测因素，以及纵隔病变引起的严重心肺功能障碍的体征和症状。同样，两个团队都应熟悉ASA处理困难气道的流程，以便在手术前制订相应计划。

在支配气道的特定部位适当使用局部麻醉药是成功实施纤维光学引导插管的有效方法，也适用于支气管镜检查操作。气道由以下颅神经支配：三叉神经（V）、舌咽神经（IX）和迷走神经（X）。对于清醒状态下的插管，三叉神经通常没有影响，因为经常采用口腔入路（除非有其他禁忌）。对于鼻腔途径，在鼻孔内使用局部麻醉药效果显著。迷走神经的喉内支是迷走神经的一个分支，它穿过甲状舌软膜，可在甲状软骨近端进行双侧注射。通过将手指放在甲状切迹上，使用23号针在甲状舌软膜上的两侧行2%利多卡因3 mL浅表注射。在这一平面上，局部麻醉药应能轻松注入而几乎没有阻力。在超过扁桃体前柱之后，需要使用麻醉剂来减轻咳嗽和呕吐反射。

舌咽神经为舌部的后1/3、咽喉和会厌提供感觉支配。它可以通过颞骨突（经颞骨突途径）的水平，或更常用的通过口腔内在扁桃体后柱处进行局部麻醉药注射。对于插管或支气管镜检查，在双侧扁桃体后柱的黏膜下注射2%利多卡因2 mL，可提供足够的麻醉来抑制舌咽神经的感觉和反射刺激。可以将舌头向对侧移位，使用Miller 2号喉镜片有助于直视扁桃体后柱。使用足够长的细针头，以便在后口咽部轻松注射。

最后，气管内注射局部麻醉药可以使气管（声带以下的迷走神经支配区域）局部麻醉，可以使用4%利多卡因以5 mL、10 mL注射器或21号针进行迅速注射。使用21号针头穿过环状甲状膜，同时不断抽吸，直到空气返回注射器中，然后进行快速注射。大多数情况下，通过适当的镇静，该过程可以迅速完成，而且患者通常不会感到明显的不适。如果存在颈部肿块或解剖结构变异，那么这可能不是一种理想的气道麻醉方法。

5.6 肌肉松弛药物

常用的肌肉松弛药物包括罗库溴铵、维库溴铵和西沙库溴铵。在过去，通常使用5~15 μg/kg的格隆溴铵和25~75 μg/kg的新斯的明来拮抗肌松残余。新斯的明是一种乙酰胆碱酯酶抑制剂，同时也会导致心动过缓。格隆溴铵是一种抗胆碱药，用于对抗新斯的明引起的心动过缓。舒更葡萄糖钠通过不可逆地与残余肌肉松弛药物结合，然后以原型通过尿液排出，使肌肉松弛的逆转发生革命性的转变。不建议在晚期肾脏疾病患者中使用，但可以通过透析清除。氨基甾类的罗库溴铵和维库溴铵是唯一可以通过舒更葡萄糖钠进行逆转的神经肌肉松弛药，使用剂量根据残余的神经肌肉松弛程度分别为1 mg/kg、2 mg/kg或16 mg/kg。在给予逆转神经肌肉松弛药时，应始终使用"四个成串刺激"模式来监测肌松情况。对神经肌肉松弛的深入讨论超出了本章的范围。

琥珀胆碱是一种去极化肌肉松弛药，以1.5 mg/kg的剂量（根据总体重计算）可以在30~45 s内迅速提供插管条件。它通过去极化神经肌肉连接处的运动

1. 评估基本管理问题的可能性和临床影响：
   - 患者合作或同意方面存在困难
   - 面罩通气困难
   - 喉上气道置入困难
   - 喉镜检查困难
   - 插管困难
   - 建立外科气道困难
2. 在困难气道管理过程中，积极寻求提供补充氧的机会。
3. 考虑基本管理选择的相对优点和可行性：
   - 清醒插管与全麻诱导后插管
   - 非侵入性技术与侵入性技术作为插管的初始方法
   - 视频辅助喉镜作为插管的初始方法
   - 保留自主通气与破坏自主通气
4. 制定主要和备选策略。

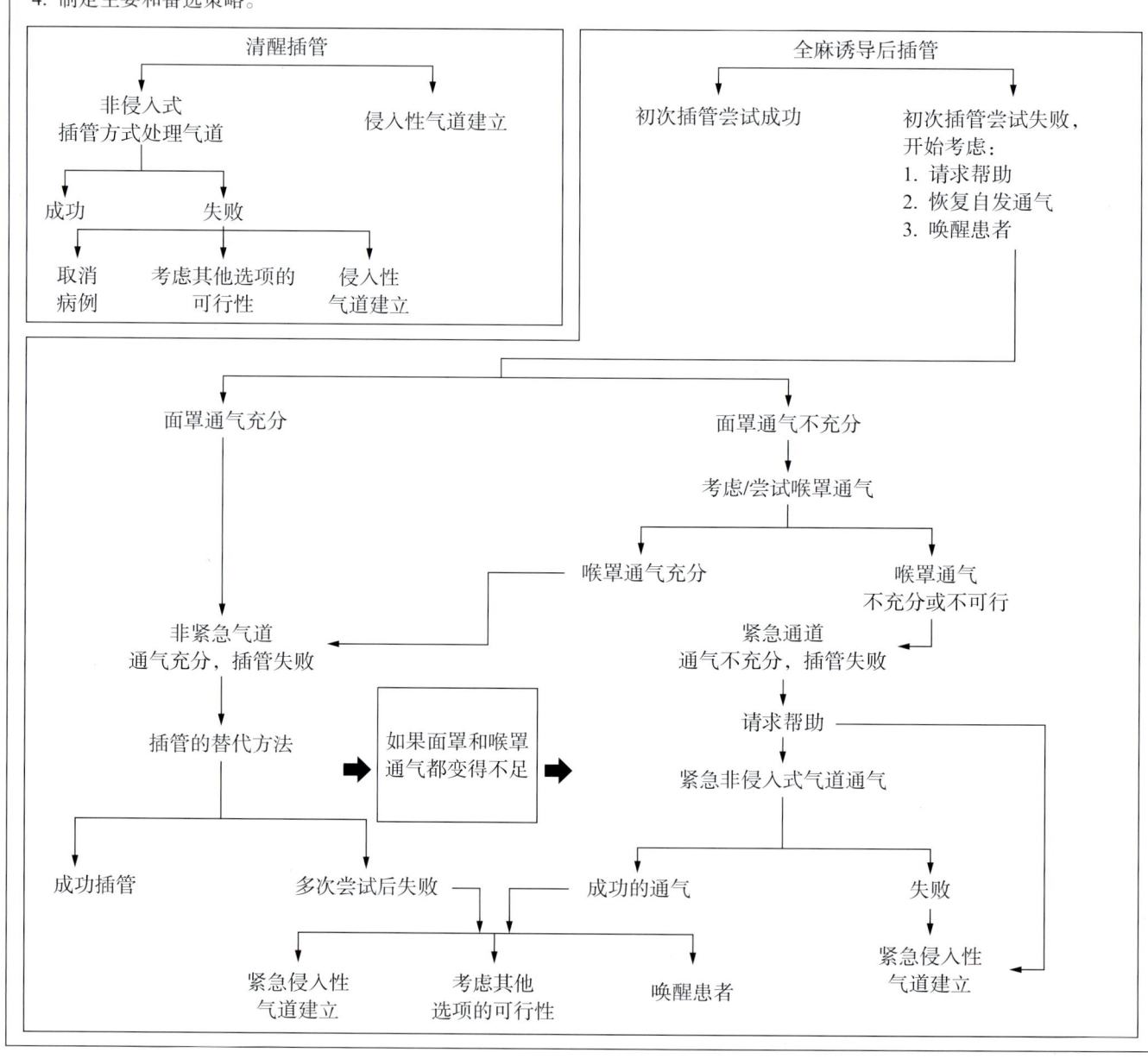

图 5.3　ASA 困难气道处理流程

来源：Apfelbaum 等[13]。

神经元，导致全身骨骼肌松弛瘫痪，有效防止喉痉挛或患者体动。琥珀胆碱并无镇痛或镇静效应，其主要用途仅仅是使声带麻痹，以便在正常情况下进行插管。在输注时，可以使用神经刺激仪的4个成串刺激模式来进行滴定，以维持诸如支气管镜检查等操作所需的肌松状态。琥珀胆碱应避免在血钾升高或存在恶性高热风险的患者中使用。对于假性胆碱酯酶缺乏症的患者，使用琥珀胆碱可能导致其作用时间明显延长，甚至可能需要机械通气，这取决于患者的遗传基因特征。要进行深入讨论，请参阅《米勒麻醉学》第8版相关章节[31]。

在历史上，琥珀胆碱输注曾被用于复合麻醉，尽管在某种程度上来说有点过时，但在没有禁忌证的患者中使用仍被认为是安全的。在诱导阶段，可以选择使用琥珀胆碱的插管剂量或不使用，随后以40~100 μg/（kg·min）的速度开始持续输注，同时连续监测Ⅰ期阻滞（即每次肌颤搐幅度相等，但在4个成串刺激监测下整体减弱）。在某个时刻，具体时间因个体差异而异，可能会出现Ⅱ期阻滞（4个成串刺激反应递减），这是一种类似非去极化肌松药物反应，具体取决于手术的持续时间[32]。不管是Ⅰ期还是Ⅱ期阻滞，只要患者没有假性胆碱酯酶缺乏，解除阻滞都应该是自发的，即使持续时间较长。在全身麻醉下进行神经肌肉阻滞时，使用脑电图监测（如 BIS 监测、脑电双频指数）有助于确保患者对因药物引起的麻痹状态以及对进行的操作事件没有记忆。对于 MAC 的效用，目前并不认为其比传统的麻醉深度监测更优越。

5.7 不同支气管镜操作的镇静管理

对于可弯曲支气管镜操作，通常可以通过适度的镇静和局部麻醉或神经阻滞来实现抗焦虑、镇痛、抑制交感反应。或者，这类操作也可以在全身麻醉下进行。在全身麻醉下，可以使用气管插管或喉罩，患者将在手术期间失去意识。在这些情况下，由于回路是封闭的，通常可以使用挥发性麻醉药物，这些药物几乎不会散发到手术室内。如果需要辅助气管插管，可以使用琥珀胆碱或罗库溴铵等肌肉松弛药物。非去极化肌肉松弛药物用于维持肌肉松弛状态。肌松效果必须通过舒更葡糖或抗胆碱酯酶抑制剂新斯的明（25~75 μg/kg）联合抗胆碱能药物格隆溴铵（5~15 μg/kg）来逆转。这些药物的作用可以通过在不同部位的神经进行电刺激来监测，如尺神经、面神经或胫后神经。需要注意的是，对常用的全身麻醉药物进行详尽讨论超出了本章的范围，但静吸复合麻醉基本原则适用于中度镇静或全身麻醉。

5.8 气道管理

5.8.1 喉罩

喉罩（Laryngeal mask airway，LMA）于1983年问世，作为一种声门上的通气装置，广泛用于多种日间手术。自1989年首次在可弯曲支气管镜检查中使用以来，LMA一直安全地应用于各类可弯曲支气管镜操作。在第二代产品中，LMA已经发展成为一种多功能工具，能够根据患者需求提供多种选择。在 ASA 的困难气道处理流程中，LMA 因其在无法插管/无法通气的情况下的独特价值而备受推崇。LMA 可确保患者不会因气道未得到有效保障而面临气道受损和死亡的风险。LMA 提供从小儿到成人的各种类型尺寸，儿科患者尺寸的选择是基于年龄或体重，而成年患者则基于体重。

最初的 LMA 是可重复使用的设备，带有充气套囊，可获得密封气道并提供正压通气。随后，它发展成具有高级功能的产品，包括可变的密封压力阈值和用于胃减压和减小吸入风险的通道。例如，可重复使用的 LMA ProSeal™ 或 LMA Supreme™。先进的第二代设备 LMA Protector™ 配备了减压胃通道和连续套囊压力指示器，由硅胶制成，比 PVC 材质的型号更好地适应咽喉部位。LMA FasTrach™ 具有插管功能，并配备了一个手柄，可用于调整位置以优化通气。Intersurgical 的 i-gel® LMA 也采用硅胶材质咽喉密封和胃减压通道，成人3~5号尺寸可进行可弯曲支气管镜操作或插管。具有特殊解剖结构或合并其他疾病（如习惯性呕吐反流、咽喉部感染等）的患者可能不适合使用任何 LMA 通气，在这种情况下，应当使用气管插管进行可弯曲支气管镜操作。

5.8.2 经硬质支气管镜喷射通气

使用 Sanders 手动喷射通气装置（图5.4），麻醉医师可以通过连接到硬质支气管镜侧口的装置，来为未经气道保护的患者进行通气。这是硬支气管镜检查中一种常见和广泛使用的通气方法。在正常情况下，麻醉医师会手动进行通气，频率控制在每分钟10~14

次，直至观察到胸廓起伏。这种方法利用了文丘里效应，即在开放的气道中，高压喷射气流能够吸引周围空气进入，实现气体交换，可媲美带充气套囊的气管内插管获得的大气流[34]。喷射通气会导致更高的平均气道压力，能够改善如间质性肺病患者的肺不张区域的氧合，这也是使用高频通气来治疗急性呼吸窘迫综合征（acute respiratory distress syndrome，ARDS）的基本原理。但在肺动脉高压患者中，这种通气方法可

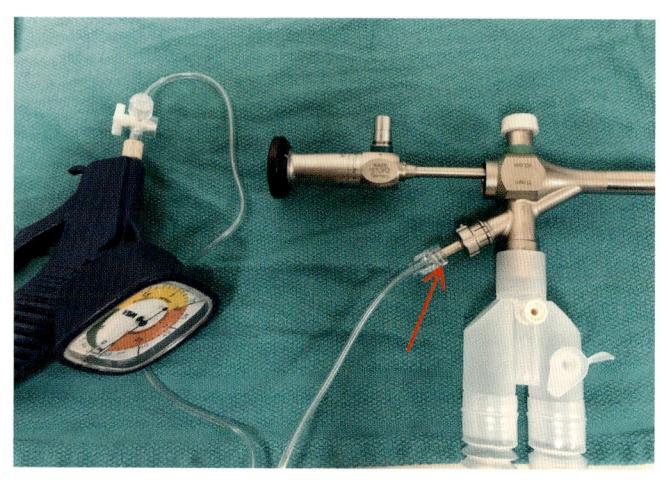

图 5.4　手动喷射通气装置
红色箭头显示了正压通气管路与硬质支气管镜的连接，在硬质支气管镜检查期间进行手动喷射通气。

能是有害的，因为气道压力的增加将通过增加肺血管阻力进一步减少肺血流[35]。

5.9　专题

5.9.1　中度镇静："WANG 氏法"

在西方国家，全身麻醉和 MAC 的使用在内窥镜检查中大幅增加；然而，作者（JFT，KPW）注意到，在美国许多地区以及其他国家，仍然以仅使用局部麻醉或局部麻醉加轻度镇静为标准。甚至在一些需要较大直径支气管镜操作中，如 EBUS-TBNA，已被发现无论是在中度镇静还是深度镇静下进行，其诊断效果和安全性都相当。对于任何在中度镇静下进行的麻醉操作，我们建议遵循 ASA 的最新准则（2018 年）[36]。

回顾这些最新的指南，我们强烈赞同"以小剂量递增或通过输注的方式给予静脉镇静/镇痛药物，以逐渐调整到所需的终点"。因此，我们将在以下章节中详细介绍中度镇静的实际操作方法，这是由 Ko-Pen Wang 医师传授的"我如何操作"的实际操作方法。

在患者经过本章概述的适当评估和准备后，使用局部麻醉联合逐渐增加的静脉药物进行麻醉。首先，给予患者 0.5 mg 的咪达唑仑和 25 μg 的芬太尼静脉注射。当患者更加安静时，分别在每个鼻孔中缓慢注入 2~3 mL 1% 利多卡因。在此期间，每 3 min 记录一次生命体征，如果患者有失控的咳嗽或不适，可以额外给予相同剂量的芬太尼和咪达唑仑。在鼻腔给予利多卡因溶液后，使用长棉签（Q-tip）涂抹利多卡因凝胶进一步麻醉每个鼻孔。这不仅可以利用利多卡因的局部镇痛作用，还可以帮助操作者评估每个鼻孔的通畅程度，以及确定哪个鼻孔最容易通过可弯曲支气管镜。

完成上述步骤后，此时患者可能已经静脉注射了 1.0 mg 的咪达唑仑和 50 μg 的芬太尼，可弯曲支气管镜可通过鼻腔直至声带水平。这种方法允许更全面地观察口咽部气道和声带，包括它们的功能状态，相对于 LMA 或气管插管的视野更优。声带清晰可见后，直接在声带之间喷洒利多卡因。通常 1.5 mL 的利多卡因喷洒量已足够，并且效果立竿见影。然后，支气管镜进一步进入会厌下区域，向下到达主支气管分叉处。在这里，再喷洒 1.5 mL 1% 利多卡因，然后在右主干支气管和左主干支气管重复相似的操作。咪达唑仑和芬太尼的总量因患者和具体操作而异，但通常不会超过 2.0 mg 咪达唑仑 +100 μg 芬太尼。

这些建议仅作为两位作者在支气管镜检查中使用中度镇静实践的一般指南，需要根据患者、操作和团队成员进行个别调整，不应被视为绝对的标准。

5.9.2　硬质支气管镜

对于硬镜操作而言，通常需要使用全身麻醉，操作过程中无论是否用到气管插管，均需确保患者的舒适和安全。在插入硬质支气管镜时，患者的体动可能会导致气管或其他纵隔结构的严重损伤。通常情况下，不建议在没有气管插管或 LMA（用于可弯曲支气管镜检查）的情况下使用挥发性麻醉剂，因为这将导致手术室内出现不受控制的挥发性麻醉药物污染，并且无法可靠地测量 MAC。是否需要使用肌肉松弛药物可能因情况而异。在这些情况下，TIVA 通过与多种药物联合使用以实现复合麻醉。有些医疗机构仅使用丙泊酚作为持续输注的药物。也可以使用丙泊酚和瑞芬太尼输注的组合。当需要神经肌肉松弛时，可以使用罗库溴铵或维库溴铵来维持无体动。

5.10 紧急情况

5.10.1 气道内医源性出血

支气管镜操作中医源性出血的发生率很低，取决于定义、患者群体和所进行的操作，发生率为 0.26%~5%[37]。近端气道出血最常见的原因是恶性病变，而远端气道出血的原因更为多样[38]。

尽管医源性出血罕见，但可能会导致灾难性后果。因此，应在手术前制订相应计划，特别是如果风险较大。在气管插管的患者中，可能需要在紧急情况下将气管插管推进至气管隆突以下，以进行单肺通气和隔离。鉴于右主支气管的角度，气管插管很可能会进入右肺。处理气道出血的基本原则包括确保气道通畅、维持通气和循环，以及确保获得足够的静脉通路进行复苏。如果凝血功能障碍导致出血，那么可能需要尝试逆转。如果需要外科手术来控制出血，那么死亡率高达 25%[38]。

除了肺科医师可以使用的止血气囊导管外，支气管内封堵器是广泛用于胸科手术的气道工具，通常与双腔气管插管（endotracheal tubes，ETT）一起使用，也可用于介入性呼吸病操作。其功能是在胸科手术期间隔离手术肺脏，不进行通气。虽然双腔气管插管不太可能用于可弯曲支气管镜操作，因可弯曲支气管镜无法通过双腔气管插管，但支气管内封堵器在紧急情况下有潜在用途。作者认为，支气管内封堵器应该提供肺部隔离作用，以便在出现大出血时进行暂时控制或将出血隔离至一侧肺。此外，根据出血部位，支气管内封堵器还可以在出血部位进行止血。支气管内封堵器可以放置在气管插管的外部，易于可弯曲支气管镜下控制出血[39]（图 5.5）。在某些情况下，硬质支气管镜可能更适合用于去除大块凝血物或经支气管镜冷冻肺活检等介入操作。

实际上，如果出现严重的气道出血，由于血液遮挡了气道，可能很难通过可弯曲支气管镜来隔离肺部。Rusch® EZ-Blocker™ 是最适合的隔离工具之一，它具有叉状双气囊设计，使双气囊的分叉部位位于气管隆突处。其他支气管内封堵器包括 Fuji Uniblocker™ 或 Arndt Endobronchial Blocker™。熟悉这些产品非常重要，以便在紧急情况下可以使用这些工具。肺科医师还应熟悉用于处理这些情况的替代性封堵工具。

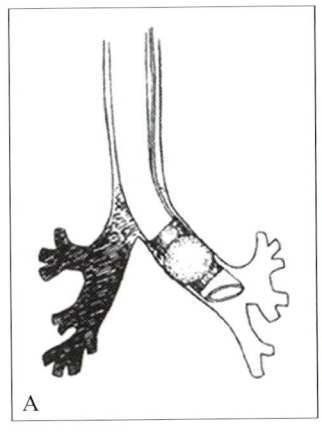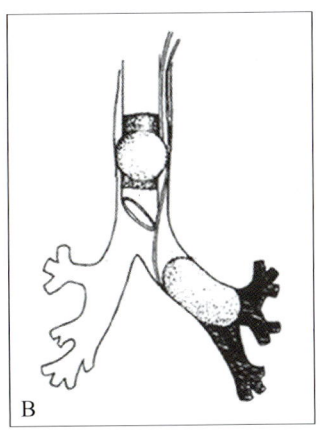

图 5.5 支气管内封堵器

A. 在右侧支气管出血过程中，放置在左主支气管中的双腔气管插管提供肺部隔离作用；B. 在左侧支气管出血过程中，放置在左主支气管的支气管内封堵器膨胀，进而起到隔离左肺的作用，同时放置在气管中的双腔气管插管可对右肺进行通气。资料来源：经 Gourin 和 Garzon 许可复制[40]。

5.10.2 喉痉挛

喉痉挛如果未能正确识别和治疗可能危及生命。合并心脏和肺部疾病或肥胖等相关患者在介入呼吸病操作中经常出现这种情况，由于呼吸和氧合的能力受到限制，氧饱和度可能会下降更快。喉痉挛的处理可以首选面罩正压通气来缓解。如果无效，给予丙泊酚可能会受益[41]。如果喉痉挛得不到缓解，可能有必要迅速使用琥珀酰胆碱或非去极化肌肉松弛药。

5.10.3 气道着火

气道着火很大程度上取决正在进行的介入操作。气道着火直接威胁到患者的安全，为了避免其发生，需要医务人员熟悉相关操作的基本知识。如果在介入过程中使用热消融设备"烧"，如激光、电凝或射频消融，那么就可能引起气道着火。着火的发生，必须具备 3 个因素：燃料、氧化气体和火源。其中，燃料是患者的组织，氧化剂是氧气或笑气，而火源则是电凝或激光。为预防气道着火，需要在实施介入操作前评估潜在的风险，热消融时需保持吸入氧浓度（FiO_2）低于 30%。此外，还应避免使用笑气。如果不能耐受 $FiO_2<30\%$ 的条件可能会使患者无法进行相关的诊疗操作。麻醉回路中，较高的气体流速将迅速降低或增加吸入和呼出的氧气浓度，以避免气道着火和长时间低氧血症。尽管降低了氧浓度，但在使用热消融设备前，必须将呼出的氧浓度降低到安全水平[42]。

如果发生气道着火，应立即清除气道中可能充当燃料的任何物质。此外，铺巾、纱布、海绵或其他易燃材料，均需移除以避免组织损伤。同时应切断氧气供应，以去除氧化剂。避免进一步损害，应向气道内注射生理盐水以冷却组织。在扑灭火源后，需及时进行气道管理和评估患者[43,44]。

5.11 结论

随着医疗技术水平不断发展，重症患者的症状得到改善，并发症发生率降低，进而生活质量得以显著提高。随着患者对操作安全性和有效性以及舒适度上的需求不断增加，医护人员在进行介入操作时的挑战随之增加。对此，本文提供了一个框架，用于建立高质量、安全且高效的医护服务，强调了以团队合作为中心的方式，并在术前预测并发症的风险，从而最大限度地减少不良反应的发生。毫无疑问，随着现代医疗的不断进步、治疗方法的不断更新，相关理念也在不断发展。本文提出了以团队沟通为中心、基于患者风险预测罕见严重并发症，以及对共享气道的理解，这些知识将有助于最大限度地减少对患者的危害，并让医师在遇到这些具有挑战性的患者时能够从容面对。

感谢田纳西大学研究生医学院麻醉科主任、教授 Robert M. Craft 博士协助并审阅了本手稿。

参考文献

1 Mehta, A.C., Prakash, U.B., Garland, R. et al. (2005). American College of Chest Physicians and American Association for bronchoscopy consensus statement: prevention of flexible bronchoscopy-associated infection. *Chest* 128: 1742–1755.

2 Apfelbaum, J.L., Connis, R.T., Nickinovich, D.G. et al. (2012). American Society of Anesthesiologists Task Force on Preanesthesia evaluation: practice advisory for preanesthesia evaluation. *Anesthesiology* 116 (3): 522–538.

3 American Society of Anesthesiologists (2015). *Committee on Practice Standards: Basic Standards of Preanesthesia Care*. Schaumburg: American Society of Anesthesiologists.

4 American Society of Anesthesiologists (2014). *ASA Physical Status Classification System*. Schaumburg: American Society of Anesthesiologists.

5 Russell, W.J., Morris, R.G., Frewin, D.B., and Drew, S.E. (1981). Changes in plasma catecholamine concentrations during endotracheal intubation. *Br. J. Anaesth.* 53 (8): 837–839.

6 Subramani, Y., Singh, M., Wong, J. et al. (2017). Understanding the phenotypes of obstructive sleep apnea: applications in anesthesia, surgery, and perioperative medicine. *Anesth. Analg.* 124 (1): 179–191.

7 Levine, G.N., Bates, E.R., Bittl, J.A. et al. (2016). 2016 ACC/AHA Guideline Focused Update on Duration of Dual Antiplatelet Therapy in Patients with Coronary Artery Disease: A Report of the American College of Cardiology/American Heart Association Task Force on Clinical Practice Guidelines: An Update of the 2011 ACCF/AHA/SCAI Guideline for Percutaneous Coronary Intervention, 2011 ACCF/AHA Guideline for Coronary Artery Bypass Graft Surgery, 2012 ACC/AHA/ACP/AATS/PCNA/SCAI/STS Guideline for the Diagnosis and Management of Patients with Stable Ischemic Heart Disease, 2013 ACCF/AHA Guideline for the Management of ST-Elevation Myocardial Infarction, 2014 AHA/ACC Guideline for the Management of Patients with Non-ST-Elevation Acute Coronary Syndromes, and 2014 ACC/AHA Guideline on Perioperative Cardiovascular Evaluation and Management of Patients Undergoing Noncardiac Surgery. *Circulation* 134 (10): e123–e155.

8 Wilson, W., Taubert, K.A., and Gewitz, M. (2007). Prevention of infective endocarditis: guidelines from the American Heart Association. *Circulation* 116: 1736–1754.

9 Neves, S.E. (2016). Anesthesia for patients with peripheral vascular disease and cardiac dysfunction. *Anesthesiol. Clin.* 34 (4): 775–795.

10 Matveychuk, A., Guber, A., Talker, O., and Shitrit, D. (2014). Incidence of bacteremia following bronchoscopy with argon plasma coagulation: a prospective study. *Lung* 192: 615–618.

11 Steinfort, D.P., Johnson, D.F., and Irving, L.B. (2010). Incidence of bacteremia following endobronchial ultrasound-guided transbronchial needle aspiration. *Eur. Respir. J.* 36: 28–32.

12 Janszky, I., Gémes, K., Ahnve, S. et al. (2018). Invasive procedures associated with the development of infective endocarditis. *J. Am. Coll. Cardiol.* 71: 2744–2752.

13 Samsoon, G.L.T. and Young, J.R.B. (1987). Difficult tracheal intubation: a retrospective study. *Anaesthesia* 42: 487–490.

14 Hartigan, P.M., Ng, J.M., and Gill, R.R. (2018). Anesthesia in a patient with a large mediastinal mass. *N. Engl. J. Med.* 379 (6): 587–588.

15 Ben-Horin, S., Bank, I., Guetta, V., and Livneh, A. (2006). Large symptomatic pericardial effusion as the presentation of unrecognized cancer: a study in 173 consecutive patients undergoing pericardiocentesis. *Medicine* 85 (1): 49–53.

16 Azarbal, A. and LeWinter, M.M. (2017). Pericardial effusion. *Cardiol. Clin.* 35 (4): 515–524.

17 Blank, R.S. and de Souza, D.G. (2011). Anesthetic management of patients with an anterior mediastinal mass: continuing professional development. *Can. J. Anesth.* 58 (9): 853–867.

18 Williamson, J.P., Phillips, M.J., Hillman, D.R., and Eastwood, P.R. (2010). Managing obstruction of the central airways. *Intern. Med. J.* 40: 399–410.

19 ASA Expert Consensus (2014). Continuum of Depth of Sedation: Definition of General Anesthesia and Levels of Sedation/Analgesia. Approved by the ASA House of Delegates October 13, 1999. Revised October 10, 2014.

20 ASA Committee of Standards and Practice Parameters (2015). *Standards for Basic Anesthetic Monitoring*. Schaumburg: ASA, American Society of Anesthesiologists.

21 McCoy, E.P., Mirakhur, R.K., and McCloskey, B.V. (1995). A comparison of the stress response to laryngoscopy. *Anaesthesia* 50: 943–946.

22 Angst, M.S., Koppert, W., Pahl, I. et al. (2003). Short-term infusion of the mu-opioid agonist remifentanil in humans causes hyperalgesia during withdrawal. *Pain* 106 (1–2): 49–57.

23 Wang, Z., Yuan, Y., Xie, K. et al. (2016). PICK1 regulates the expression and trafficking of AMPA receptors in remifentanil-induced hyperalgesia. *Anesth. Analg.* 123 (3): 771–781.

24 Eggleston, S.T. and Lush, L.W. (1996). Understanding allergic reactions to local anesthetics. *Ann. Pharmacother.* 30 (7–8): 851–857.

25 McCambridge, A.J., Boesch, R.P., and Mullon, J.J. (2018). Sedation in bronchoscopy: a review. *Clin. Chest Med.* 39 (1): 65–77.

26 Wahidi, M.M., Jain, P., Jantz, M. et al. (2011). American College of Chest Physicians consensus statement on the use of topical anesthesia, analgesia, and sedation during flexible bronchoscopy in adult patients. *Chest* 140 (5): 1342–1350.

27 Du Rand, I.A., Blaikley, J., Booton, R. et al. (2013). British Thoracic Society guideline for diagnostic flexible bronchoscopy in adults. *Thorax* 68 (Suppl 1): i1–i44.

28 Liao, B.S., Hilsinger, R.L. Jr., Rasgon, B.M. et al. (1999). A preliminary study of cocaine absorption from the nasal mucosa. *Laryngoscope* 109 (1): 98–102.

29 Hensley, M. and Singer, B.H. (2018). Alternative topical anesthesia for bronchoscopy in a case of severe lidocaine allergy. *Respir. Med. Case Rep.* 23: 90–92.

30 Apfelbaum, J.L., Hagberg, C.A., Caplan, R.A. et al. (2013). Practice guidelines for management of the difficult airway: an updated report by the American Society of Anesthesiologists Task Force on Management of the Difficult Airway. *Anesthesiology* 118 (2): 251–270.

31 Viby-Morgensen, J. and Claudius, C. (2015). Neuromuscular monitoring. In: *Miller's Anesthesia* (ed. R.D. Miller), 1604–1621. St Louis: Elsevier.

32 Delisle, S., Lebrun, M., and Bevan, D.R. (1982). Plasma cholinesterase activity and tachyphylaxis during prolonged succinylcholine infusion. *Anesth. Analg.* 61 (11): 941–944.

33 Alon, D., Pertzov, B., Gershman, E. et al. (2017). The safety of laryngeal mask airway-assisted bronchoscopy versus standard nasal bronchoscopy. *Respiration* 93 (4): 279–284.

34 Pathak, V., Welsby, I., Mahmood, K. et al. (2014). Ventilation and anesthetic approaches for rigid bronchoscopy. *Ann. Am. Thorac. Soc.* 11 (4): 628–634.

35 Goudra, B.G., Singh, P.M., Borle, A. et al. (2015). Anesthesia for advanced bronchoscopic procedures: state-of-the-art review. *Lung* 193 (4): 453–465.

36 Apfelbaum, J.L., Gross, J.B., Connis, R.T. et al. (2018). Practice guidelines for moderate procedural sedation and analgesia 2018. *Anesthesiology* 128 (3): 437–479.

37 Bernasconi, M., Koegelenberg, C.F.N., Koutsokera, A. et al. (2017). Iatrogenic bleeding during flexible bronchoscopy: risk factors, prophylactic measures, and management. *ERJ Open Res.* 3 (2): 00084–02016.

38 Yendamuri, S. (2015). Massive airway hemorrhage. *Thorac. Surg. Clin.* 25: 255–260.

39 Templeton, T.W., Morris, B.N., Goenaga-Diaz, E.J. et al. (2017). A prospective comparison of intraluminal and extraluminal placement of the 9-french arndt bronchial blocker in adult thoracic surgery patients. *J. Cardiothorac. Vasc. Anesth.* 31 (4): 1335–1340.

40 Gourin, A. and Garzon, A. (1975). Control of hemorrhage in emergency pulmonary resection for massive hemoptysis. *Chest* 68: 120–121.

41 Nawfal, M. (2002). Propofol for relief of extubation laryngospasm. *Anaesthesia* 57 (10): 1036.

42 Remz, M., Luria, I., Gravenstein, M. et al. (2013). Prevention of airway fires: do not overlook the expired oxygen concentration. *Anesth. Analg.* 117 (5): 1172–1176.

43 Fire Safety Video: Prevention and Management of Operating Room Fires. (2010). www.apsf.org/resources_video.php.

44 Apfelbaum, J.L., Caplan, R.A., Barker, S.J. et al. (2013). Practice advisory for the prevention and management of operating room fires: an updated report by the American Society of Anesthesiologists task force on operating room fires. *Anesthesiology* 118: 271–290.

第 6 章

可弯曲支气管镜的适应证和禁忌证

Robert F. Browning Jr.[1], J. Francis Turner, Jr.[2,3], and Ko-Pen Wang[4]

[1] Interventional Pulmonology, Walter Reed National Military Medical Center;
Uniformed Services University of Health Sciences, Bethesda, MD, USA

[2] Division of Pulmonary and Critical Care Medicine,
University of Tennessee Graduate School of Medicine, Knoxville, TN, USA

[3] National Supercomputing Institute, University of Nevada, Las Vegas, NV, USA

[4] Division of Pulmonary and Critical Care Medicine, Johns Hopkins Bayview Medical Center,
Johns Hopkins University School of Medicine, Baltimore, MD, USA

（译者：熊　叶　译者单位：中国医学科学院阜外医院）

6.1 引言

自1897年Killian引入支气管镜以来，其作用与地位与日俱增，随着不断与其他新技术发展融合，支气管镜逐渐形成了一门独立的医学应用技术[1]。硬质支气管镜最初用于气管及近端支气管的检查，同时可去除气道异物[2]。1964年，Shigeto Ikeda发明了享誉全球的可弯曲支气管镜的原型机。随着町田和奥林巴斯公司制造原型机不断取得成功，第7代支气管镜样机在1966年问世并首次应用于临床[3,4]。在池田教授不断指导和技术改良下，支气管镜技术较Killian时代取得了巨大进步。这些新手段能让支气管镜医师更加清晰地观察肺上叶及下叶远端支气管。新型支气管镜易于被患者接受，且无须全身麻醉，同时还可作为门诊患者的常规诊疗措施。

随着可弯曲支气管镜下操作技术的发展，气道内病变组织可在内镜下进行活检取样[5,6]。王氏穿刺针甚至能够在气管支气管树可视状态下进行管壁外病变的细胞学和组织学穿刺活检[7,8]。

随着诊断性可弯曲支气管镜技术的广泛应用，我们必须牢记医学教父之一的希波克拉底（公元前460—公元前370年），他曾建议将芦苇秆插入气道以缓解患者的窒息状况。而内镜技术的核心是对患者呼吸系统疾病进行积极治疗，因此可弯曲支气管镜在治疗中的应用得以飞速发展。本章旨在阐述目前在可弯曲支气管镜实际应用中的适应证和禁忌证，适应证和禁忌证来源于患者的症状、体征和影像学资料，也是支气管镜医师在患者就诊时得到的第一手资料（表6.1）。

6.2 咳嗽

咳嗽是评价患者存在肺部基础疾病的重要症状。尽管因咳嗽而应用支气管镜的高频率和低收益率被认为这是一项过度检查，然而，我们仍建议对存在以下表现的患者进行直接的肺部评估检查[9,10]。

无免疫缺陷且胸部X线检查正常的患者，其急性咳嗽通常变化快，可不考虑支气管镜检查。然而，对于CD4计数低（<200/mm³）的免疫缺陷患者而

表 6.1 诊断性支气管镜的适应证

恶性肿瘤
  支气管肺癌的诊断
  支气管肺癌的分期
  治疗和/或首次纵隔镜检查后的再分期
  痰细胞学异常
  恶性肿瘤治疗后的随访复查
  头颈部恶性肿瘤患者的评估
  食管恶性肿瘤患者的评估
  转移癌
  纵隔肿块

感染
  复发或难治性肺炎
  免疫功能不全患者的肺内渗出性病变
  空洞样病变

不明原因的肺不张

间质性肺病

咯血

不明原因的慢性咳嗽

局限性哮鸣音

喘鸣

异物吸入

胸部外伤
  挫裂伤或穿透伤
  化学性损伤
  热损伤

不明原因的胸腔积液

肺移植患者术后评估

气管插管
  确认气管插管位置
  评估气管插管相关损伤
  确认经气管氧气导管的位置

气管、支气管狭窄

声音嘶哑或声带麻痹

上腔静脉综合征

瘘管
  支气管胸膜瘘
  气管-支气管食管瘘
  气管-支气管主动脉瘘

难治性气胸

气管、支气管、细支气管或残端吻合术后评估

支气管造影

言,即使其胸片正常,若无法进行诱导痰检查,仍需考虑施行支气管镜检查[11]。对于症状持续3~8周和8周以上的亚急性和慢性咳嗽[12],应根据患者的年龄、家族史、危险因素以及伴随症状进行评估,判断咳嗽是否为严重疾病的先兆。对于亚急性和慢性咳嗽的免疫缺陷患者,在针对常见病因如上气道咳嗽综合征、哮喘、非哮喘性嗜酸性粒细胞性肺炎、胃食管反流病(gastroesophageal reflux disease,GERD)给予经验性治疗后,可进行支气管镜检查,用于评估一些罕见病因[12]。即使是免疫功能正常的患者,其慢性咳嗽仍可能作为某些严重疾病的早期表现。21%~87%的支气管肺癌患者初始症状为慢性咳嗽,而70%~90%的患者在整个病程中均有该症状[13]。使用支气管镜对经验性治疗无效后的阵发性夜间呼吸困难(paroxysmal nocturnal dyspneal,PND)、哮喘和GERD患者进行评估,能成功明确大部分原因未明的慢性咳嗽的病因[14]。

因此,我们建议对于胸片提示肺内局灶性病变、咯血、局限性哮鸣音的急性咳嗽患者,或需明确诊断的免疫缺陷的急性咳嗽患者,应早期进行支气管镜检查。而对于慢性咳嗽或咳嗽加重且特征改变、戒烟后无改善以及需要明确病因的患者,我们建议进行痰细胞学检查和支气管镜检查[14,15]。

6.3 哮鸣音

虽然哮鸣音在哮喘患者中多见,但其鉴别诊断仍复杂多变且十分广泛。非哮喘患者出现哮鸣音或存在哮鸣音的患者应用支气管扩张剂疗效不佳时,需要进行全面的检查(包括能够直视上下气道的支气管镜检查),以评估哮鸣音产生的原因。有时"并非所有哮鸣音都是哮喘"仍然是个难题。此类情况下的鉴别诊断包括异物、气管畸形、由肿块引起的外源性或内源性阻塞、血管畸形或气管支气管狭窄性病变,或发生在声带水平的声带功能障碍(vocal cord dysfunction,VCD)和声带矛盾运动(paradoxical vocal fold motion,PVFM)[16-20]。

胸片检查和流量-容积肺功能检查可以为鉴别诊断提供线索[21]。然而,如果诊断仍不明确,可借助纤维支气管镜(fiberoptic bronchoscopy,FOB)直视化气道,寻找气道阻塞性病变。出现局限性哮鸣音的阻塞性病变可在胸片上提示局部肺透亮度增加,需要使用支气管镜进行相关评估检查。此外,支气管镜也是清除病灶的重要治疗工具。

6.4 喘鸣

喘鸣是一个提示上气道阻塞乃至危及生命的重要征象，需要尽快明确病因。导致喘鸣的病因繁多，可根据发病年龄将其归类[22]。在婴幼儿和儿童中，鉴别诊断包括会厌炎、喉炎、喉畸形、喉乳头状瘤、喉气管裂、会厌下血管瘤、肺动脉吊带、无名动脉异常和气管异物[23,24]。而在成人患者中，需考虑以下诊断：急性双侧声带麻痹、快速进展的气管病变、纵隔或食管病变引起的外源性气道压迫、风湿性疾病引起的环杓关节异常、韦格纳肉芽肿、感染或急性喉头水肿[23,25]。影像学检查应同时包括颈部和胸部。颈部软组织X线检查或CT可协助诊断会厌炎或咽后脓肿。正确的可视化上气道检查能明确诊断，部分情况下尚能给予治疗，如解除阻塞性病变或去除气道异物。在实施内镜术之前，内镜医师应确保有设备和专业人员在紧急情况下行气管插管或气管切开术。

6.5 声音嘶哑和声带麻痹

许多声音嘶哑或声带麻痹的患者往往首诊五官科医师而不是胸科医师。导致声带麻痹的病因有很多，由于病变可能位于胸部，因此很有必要就诊胸科医师[26]。Terris等回顾了20年来有关声带麻痹病因的文献，发现36%的病因是新生物[27]，其中55%是肺癌。当患者病史、体格检查和影像学检查均无法明确诊断时，应进行支气管镜检查，它能使20%的患者明确诊断[27]。由于左侧喉返神经在胸腔内行走，因此可被左侧肺门病变所累及，该部位病变可经支气管针吸活检确诊。而右侧喉返神经仅在病变扩展至右侧颈部时才会被累及。

6.6 吸入性损伤

吸入性损伤可由吸入蒸汽或高温空气、浓烟、毒性气体造成，可以导致毁灭性的损伤，当患者同时存在皮肤烧伤和吸入性损伤时，死亡率可达30%~90%[28]。仅仅依据临床标准，如面部或口咽部烧伤、碳质痰液产生、哮鸣音、声音嘶哑或鼻毛烧焦，很容易造成大部分患者的误诊[29,30]。

热损伤可表现为喘鸣，同时伴有声音嘶哑和吞咽困难。面部烧伤、口咽部水肿或碳质痰液都是热损伤或浓烟吸入的警示症状，提示患者必须采取气道评估措施。早期的放射检查对于气道黏膜损伤的诊断十分困难且敏感性差。有报道提示10例烧伤患者使用CT仿真气管镜可明确诊断吸入性损伤，但其作用是否等同或优于支气管镜尚未可知[31]。支气管镜可作为明确气道黏膜炎症和水肿的早期评估手段之一。急性浓烟吸入损伤的患者，应尽快进行纤维支气管镜检查，以快速明确喉部区域的早期炎症、溃疡或肿胀[32]。患者可能需要同时进行气管插管，使用纤维支气管镜可方便插管[33]。纤维支气管镜还能协同组织学诊断，帮助判断疾病预后[34,35]。急性损伤可引起严重的气道水肿、红斑和黏膜塌陷。亚急性损伤能造成黏膜坏死和出血性气管支气管炎，而慢性损伤可导致瘢痕形成和气道狭窄、肺不张以及肉芽组织形成。损伤慢性期行支气管镜活检可提示闭塞性毛细支气管炎性改变[23]。因此，使用支气管镜能评估气道损伤情况，及时做出早期诊断并根据诊断结果迅速采取治疗措施，包括应用糖皮质激素、湿化空气、抗生素和解除气道阻塞。

碳氧血红蛋白暴露于毒性物质、燃烧后产生的氨气、氮气、二氧化硫和氯气均可引起气道损伤[36]。由工业事故和战争造成的化学泄漏亦是引起肺损伤的潜在危险因素。Freitag等报道了他们对21例在20世纪80年代两伊战争时期吸入芥子毒气（二氯二乙硫醚）及其他吸入毒气引发肺损伤的伊朗士兵的诊疗经验[37]。在气道损伤急性期，使用支气管镜评估其受损程度并去除气道内的烧焦和坏死物。这些患者分泌了大量的浓稠痰液，在虚弱状态下无法自行咳出。后期形成的气道狭窄和肉芽组织需要支气管镜进行积极的治疗[37]。

6.7 咯血

咯血是肺部疾病的常见症状，可表现为痰中少量带血，也可表现为每日100~600 mL的大咯血[38]。其最常见的病因包括支气管炎、肺不张和肺癌，咯血也是支气管镜检查的第二大常见适应证[39-41]。消化道出血、咽部出血、鼻腔出血和肺内出血的鉴别非常重要[42]。对于持续性出血、出血速度快或量大、存在恶性病变可能的情况下均应使用可弯曲支气管镜检查。

应仔细查找出血原因。若应用得当，支气管镜可在 75%~93% 的病例中成功定位到出血部位[43]。细支气管镜能对远端支气管树进行彻底检查[44]。如果初始检查无法明确诊断，很有必要在出现咯血后复查支气管镜。虽然早期（48 h 内）支气管镜检查较晚期诊断率更高，但具体的检查时机对患者总体处理是否有影响尚无定论[45-47]。

通常 CT 检查是诊断出血的第一步。如果扫描图像上存在局部异常，CT 能快速确定病变部位。但如果 CT 扫描提示弥漫性出血，那就不能区分该出血是病灶出血后蔓延导致还是弥漫性肺泡出血（diffuse alveolar hemorrhage，DAH）。尽管缺乏正式研究予以佐证，但我们认为了解咯血的原因和部位对于患者后续处理至关重要。因此，我们建议早期使用支气管镜进行评估检查。在大咯血的情况下，硬质支气管镜和可弯曲气管镜的作用一直存在争议，但并没有对二者进行过头对头的比较研究。一般来说，大咯血最大的威胁是血液凝结致严重气道阻塞。硬质支气管镜吸引能力强，镜下能使用较大的器械工具，可有效控制气道通气，并可直接对出血部位进行填塞。而使用带气囊的气管插管给患者提供了最有效的气道通气控制，可弯曲支气管镜为小气道提供了更大的可视性[48]，同时还可应用肾上腺素、凝血酶、Fogarty 球囊和其他的支气管内阻滞器进行止血[49,50]。

此外，一些新型设备，如氩等离子体凝固术（argon plasma coagulation，APC），也被用以控制咯血，如果出血部位在大气道内，还可同时治疗恶性气道阻塞[51]。最后，对咯血的处理还依赖于支气管镜医师所接受的培训、器械工具的适用程度和出血量。

6.8 上腔静脉综合征

纵隔病变可影响静脉回流，造成上腔静脉综合征。此时可使用支气管镜行经气管或支气管针吸活检该部位肿块或肿大的淋巴结。取样时，应明确该部位大血管的解剖学定位。此外，在对上腔静脉综合征患者进行评估时，应在进行任何侵入性操作前排除血管异常。抗生素治疗期间出现上腔静脉综合征主要与恶性病变相关[52]，但也不能排除良性疾病。因此，在给予此类患者治疗之前，必须有明确的病理诊断。支气管镜活检能确诊 60%~70% 的病例[53,54]，这对于有巨大纵隔肿块的患者至关重要，因其可避免不必要的全麻开胸手术及相关脱机拔管困难[55]。

6.9 纵隔肿块

对于纵隔肿块的评估，支气管镜的使用能让患者避免有创的纵隔镜手术。传统和超声引导经支气管针吸活检都能取得并诊断纵隔肿块[8,56]。由于该操作能安全地在门诊开展，诊疗费用亦随之下降。可弯曲支气管镜对麻醉医师同样重要，其能协助麻醉医师对因前纵隔肿块而气道受压的患者行局麻下气管插管[57]。先前的指南提示对于纵隔肿块患者需术前行直立和卧位流量–容积肺功能检查，现已被证实对危险分层和手术规划并无帮助[58]。

6.10 间质性肺病

表现为间质性肺病的疾病种类繁多[59]。同样，支气管镜在这些疾病的评估中也发挥着不同的作用。支气管肺泡灌洗（bronchoalveolar lavage，BAL）可用于研究特发性肺间质纤维化（interstitial pulmonary fibrosis，IPF）中引发炎症反应的细胞类型和数目，并能够排除其他可能的诊断[60]。

支气管镜下行 BAL 和活检能诊断的疾病包括结节病、癌性淋巴管炎、嗜酸性粒细胞性肺炎和肺泡蛋白沉着症。当 BAL 发现肺部存在非典型物质或细胞时，其临床诊断倾向于组织细胞增多症、肺泡蛋白沉着症、石棉肺和铍肺等[61-64]。此外，所发现的不同炎症细胞计数亦有助于缩小纤维化间质性肺炎的鉴别诊断范围，但并不能诊断 IPF。结节病、铍肺、过敏性肺炎、结核以及真菌感染中辅助 T 细胞/抑制 T 细胞比例会发生变化[65]。在特发性肺纤维化、胶原性血管病、肺沉着病和闭塞性毛细支气管肺炎中可发现中性粒细胞水平增高[66]。在慢性嗜酸性粒细胞肺炎和 Churg-Strauss 综合征中可发现嗜酸性粒细胞水平增高[67,68]。富含脂质的巨噬细胞提示患者有胺碘酮接触史，而含铁血黄素巨噬细胞提示出血综合征。

在诊断间质性肺疾病时，应考虑经支气管肺活检，尤其是对手术肺活检有禁忌证的患者。然而，由于经支气管肺活检获得的组织块相对较小，往往不能明确诊断，只能协助鉴别诊断，因此手术肺活检仍是诊断的"金标准"[69,70]。最近，有文献支持经支气管镜冷冻肺活检来诊断间质性肺疾病，但由于数据有限，且气胸和出血的发生率较高，该技术尚未成为间质性肺疾病的一线诊断方法[71]。

6.11 感染

肺炎对于胸科医师而言是一种常见疾病，通常是经验性或根据痰培养结果给予抗感染药物。社区获得性肺炎的影像学转归取决于患者的年龄及其是否合并基础性肺病。总体而言，73%的患者可在6周内完全缓解[72]。而当肺炎反复发作或未吸收缓解时，则有必要行支气管镜检查[73]。Feinsilver等分析了35例未吸收缓解的肺炎患者，阐述了可弯曲支气管镜在其中的作用[74]。对于社区获得性肺炎以外的特殊类型的肺炎患者，可弯曲支气管镜的确诊率为85.7%（12/14）。在23例未行支气管镜检查的患者中，有21例诊断为社区获得性肺炎，提示非支气管镜检查具有高阴性预测值。当患者存在炎性渗出30天以上、多叶而非单叶或局灶渗出，年龄小于55岁时，支气管镜有助于一些特定疾病的诊断[74]。而年龄大于55岁或存在免疫系统缺陷（如慢性阻塞性肺病、酗酒和糖尿病等）的患者肺炎转归较慢[74]。因此，在此类患者中应推迟进行支气管镜检查。

免疫抑制患者易罹患多种病原体相关的机会性肺炎。Huang等回顾性地评估了支气管镜在诱导痰无法确诊的患者中的作用。研究表明50.5%的气管镜检查能够获得明确诊断，其中64%的病例得以早期诊断或确诊为肺结核[75]。支气管镜下BAL能安全、快速地获取下呼吸道标本。在获得性免疫缺陷患者中，主要感染病原体是卡氏肺孢子菌，同时行BAL和经支气管活检，其敏感性可达100%[76]。在一项针对100例免疫缺陷患者的研究中，Martin等确诊33%的患者存在机会性感染，从而避免了开胸肺活检[77]。通过涂片、染色和单克隆抗体检测方法，能快速筛查肺泡灌洗液中的病原体。如果初步结果为阴性，则有必要在数小时内行开胸肺活检。因此，即便BAL阴性也不会耽误开胸肺活检术来明确病因。

纤维支气管镜检查对于伴有发热和肺内浸润渗出、疑似肺炎的危重患者的评估是一种重要的补充手段[78]。通过纤维支气管镜BAL是获取下呼吸道标本的常用方法，能直接观察气道状况并及时清除残留分泌物。对于重症癌症患者，尤其对于那些中性粒细胞减少的患者，有必要行经支气管镜BAL和经支气管肺活检以明确诊断[79,80]。对凝血功能障碍或血小板减少的正压通气患者，BAL检查更为安全[81]。

空洞样肺内病变的诊断对胸科医师来说是一项巨大挑战。虽然多数情况下由感染所致，但恶性肿瘤的发生率也可达7.6%~17%[82]。因此，支气管镜检查对于出现肺内空洞样病变的患者是否存在恶性肿瘤非常必要。除了评估空洞病变的良恶性，支气管镜还能收集到标本进行病原体检查。另有报道提示，通过经支气管置入引流导管能成功地进行肺部脓肿引流[83]。

6.12 肺不张

在放射学检查异常的患者中，最常使用支气管镜确诊肺不张[84]。顽固性肺不张可提示存在支气管内病变导致阻塞后肺实变，这种情况下应做内镜检查进行评估和治疗。Su等报道的54例行支气管镜检查的肺不张患者中，35例（65%）发现支气管内肿物，8例（15%）存在支气管黏膜异常，4例（7%）发现气道管腔缩小、受压或狭窄[84]。

纤维支气管镜亦能治疗肺叶萎陷或肺不张的重症患者。Hasegawa等指出，27%的急诊支气管镜检查是为了治疗肺不张和黏液阻塞患者[85]。存在神经肌肉基础疾病的患者，如脊髓损伤或吉兰-巴雷综合征，通过支气管镜去除气道内残留的分泌物后能得到显著改善[86]。因此，推荐对于那些胸部物理治疗无效的大面积肺不张患者或危及生命的全肺不张患者进行支气管镜检查。

6.13 胸腔积液

胸腔积液通常使用胸腔穿刺、闭式胸膜活检、内科胸腔镜或视频辅助胸腔镜术（video-assisted thoracoscopic surgery，VATS）进行诊断[87]。最近广泛使用的胸腔镜下胸膜活检成为支气管镜检查的替代方法。与Abram活检针相比，半硬质胸腔镜（Olympus™ LTF）的敏感性更高（81%比62%），胸膜视野更佳，有助于查找出引起复杂胸腔积液的病因[88]。大部分原因未明的胸腔积液，其恶性来源可能性高[89,90]，尤其对于那些咳嗽、咯血或合并肺不张的患者，应进行支气管镜检查。此外，支气管镜检查还可用于评估可能导致肺不张和胸腔积液的支气管内阻塞。

6.14 胸部创伤

胸部常受到各种各样的创伤。物理性创伤分为肺挫裂伤或穿透伤。对于胸部重大创伤（肺挫裂伤和穿透伤）的进行支气管镜检查，能进一步评估气道的损伤情况[91,92]。Hara 和 Prakash 进行的一项回顾性研究报道，在进行支气管镜检查的 53 例胸部外伤患者中，有 28 例（53%）可明确诊断[93]。此外，由于忽视了高位气道损伤而导致了部分患者死亡，因此有学者建议所有的胸部创伤患者均应行支气管镜检查[94-97]。

在胸部创伤患者中行可弯曲支气管镜检查能同时发挥诊断和治疗的双重作用。特别是对于颈部严重损伤的患者，可弯曲支气管镜检查能直接观察气道和声带情况，同时还能进行插管。在对多发伤患者进行评估时，如出现颈椎或胸骨骨折、纵隔气肿和持续性胸腔闭式引流管漏气等情况常提示存在严重的气道损伤可能，因此必须考虑行可弯曲支气管镜检查。

支气管镜除了对创伤患者进行早期评估，还能诊断和处理创伤后并发症，包括误吸和黏液阻塞。

6.15 肺移植

随着肺移植患者术后生存率的提高，患者的术后管理对胸科医师也是一项严峻的考验。肺移植患者更易发生支气管吻合瘘、排异反应、感染和闭塞性毛细支气管炎等相关并发症。支气管镜对于评估和处理气道并发症以及鉴别排异反应或感染非常重要[97-99]。虽然外科技术的发展降低了吻合口瘘发生的风险，但在持续胸导管漏气患者中仍须使用支气管镜检查吻合口情况。肺移植患者还可并发缝合部位肉芽组织增生而阻塞气道。支气管镜检查能避免此类现象的发生并进行相应的治疗（如气道支架植入或缝合部位肉芽组织激光切除）[100]。

肺移植患者的排异反应和感染的临床表现和影像学表现非常相似。由于两者的治疗方法截然不同，因此必须通过经支气管活检将二者区分开[97-99,101]。闭塞性细支气管炎，表现为新发或进展的气道阻塞或限制性通气功能障碍，显著影响肺移植患者的长期生存。然而，其仍需通过经支气管活检获取组织标本以明确诊断[102]。

6.16 支气管造影

支气管镜和CT检查问世之前，广泛使用支气管造影来明确气道解剖结构。如今，三维重建CT和虚拟气管镜（virtual bronchoscopy, VB）已经取代了支气管造影。然而，实时气道内支气管造影仍然有助于定位局灶性空洞和病变。Ono 等应用此项技术，通过可弯曲支气管镜在选择性支气管造影术下对肺外周病变进行定位[103]。

6.17 肺结节

肺外周病变无法通过支气管镜直接观察。结节部位、大小和使用的诊断技术会显著影响肺外周病变的诊断率。直径<2 cm的病变的诊断率为30%，而直径>4 cm的病变可达80%[104-108]。随着先进的影像学和导航技术的应用，直径<2 cm的肺外周病变的诊断率可高达74%[109]。病变与肺门的距离也对诊断率有显著影响，肺外周1/3的病变诊断率明显低于中央型病变[110]。直觉上，这一观点似乎合理，尽管一些经验丰富的支气管镜医师认为，结节与气道的距离、角度和支气管镜到达病变所需转弯次数是能否成功检出的决定性因素。

活检和诊断工具常常难以触及位于上叶尖段和下叶背段的病灶。肺外周病变合并气胸的风险高，尤其在使用超声探头检测时。通常，径向超声探头、电磁导航支气管镜（electromagnetic navigation bronchoscopy, ENB）探头、引导鞘管和经支气管穿刺针往往难以在气道内进行大幅转向。双平面或C形臂X线透视机引导下经支气管活检曾作为肺外周病变的标准活检方式，但是经过近十年的发展，支气管腔内超声、CT透视、CT引导、VB、ENB或以上技术联合应用在临床实践和研究中变得越来越普遍，并且较单纯使用X线透视有更高的诊断率[109,110]。

活检工具也可能对诊断率有显著影响。目前，多种工具可用于活检，包括活检钳、毛刷、穿刺针、带针刷和刮匙。如果要使用细胞学毛刷对肺外周病变采样，则应在经支气管活检前进行，可防止毛刷上附带血液而影响检测结果[105]。相较于标准经支气管钳活检，TBNA对肺外周病变的诊断率更高[111,112]。而在活检钳、灌洗和刷检基础上联合应用 TBNA 能将诊断率从 48% 提高到 69%[111]。

6.18 肺部肿块与纵隔占位

肺癌是美国死亡率最高的恶性疾病。最近一项对北美支气管镜医师调查研究显示，因其发病率高，胸部影像提示的肺部肿块成为支气管镜检查中最常见的适应证[9]。

支气管镜医师认为，肿块可分为中央型和周围型[113]。中央型肿块及其对中央气道的影响，如外压性阻塞，通常可以通过支气管镜直接观察到。支气管内病变可以很容易通过活检钳进行取样。一般认为，需要进行 3~4 次活检才能满足病理学检查要求[114,115]。活检钳活检对于中央型病变的诊断率为 55%~85%，具体取决于病变的细胞学类型[113]。此外，灌洗液和细胞刷检标本也可用于中央型病变的细胞学分析。细胞刷检的诊断率可达 62%~78%[116]。TBNA 更常用于黏膜下病变或气管外压性病变，也推荐应用于坏死或出血性病变。适当快速的标本准备可提高 TBNA 的诊断率。TBNA 最重要的作用在于肺癌分期，如下文所述，它可对肺门或纵隔淋巴结行针吸活检[117]。

Shure 和 Fedullo 通过联合 TBNA 和灌洗、活检和刷检能将中央型病变的诊断率提高至 97%[118]。Dasgupta 等对 55 例黏膜下或管腔外病变患者进行前瞻性研究，比较单独 TBNA 或联合传统灌洗、刷检和活检钳活检的阳性率，结果显示后者的诊断率达 96%，而单独使用 TBNA 也达到 95.6%[119]。纤维支气管镜能够直视气道，然而仅能在 3.5% 的肺癌患者中发现支气管内恶性病灶[46]。

Wang 等开展了一项前瞻性研究，评估了 329 例中央型和周围型病变患者使用 TBNA 或经胸壁针吸穿刺（transthoracic needle aspiration，TTNA）的诊断情况[120]。TBNA 的总诊断率为 68.1%，其中，纵隔病变阳性诊断率为 89.3%，肺外周病变且无纵隔异常的诊断率为 45.6%。TTNA 对于纵隔病变的诊断率为 83.3%，肺部病变的诊断率为 66.7%。该研究证实对胸部中央型病变患者，TBNA 优于 TTNA。对于无纵隔或肺门累及的患者，还是应首选 TBNA，因为其能在进行有效诊断的同时，通过可视化中央气道从而排除其他病变，且并发症发生率较 TTNA 更低。

在痰液中找到可疑或恶性细胞的患者需行诊断性支气管镜检查，目前已不推荐使用痰细胞学检查作为肺癌筛查方法。但由于其无创、价廉的优点，仍不失为肺部疾病的一种检查手段[121]。是否对痰检阳性但胸片正常的患者行支气管镜检查尚不明确[122]，对此，可先从口腔、咽部、喉部进行逐步排查，若结果为阴性，再行支气管镜检查。若未发现大气道内病变，则应检查各个段及亚段支气管，同时在各个部位收集细胞学标本。

Lam 等对 82 例有石棉或石油接触史的患者行自荧光支气管镜检查（autofluorescence bronchoscopy，AFB），结果提示：对于中重度不典型增生和原位癌，普通白光支气管镜（white light bronchoscopy，WLB）和 AFB 的敏感性分别为 52% 和 86%；特异性分别为 81% 和 79%[123]。Nakhosteen 和 Khanavkar 的研究显示，AFB 诊断不典型增生和原位癌的敏感性是 WLB 的 2.6 倍[124]。

然而，在加拿大，当应用 AFB 于肺癌高危人群筛查时，并未显示出明显的优势，并因此基本停止了 AFB 在肺癌筛查中的应用[125]。在有条件实施该技术的医学中心，AFB 通常用于确定病灶边缘和选择活检部位。

可弯曲支气管镜和 TBNA 的联合应用除了诊断支气管肺癌之外，还能对疾病进行诊断分期。通过额外的成像引导技术，如在支气管腔内超声（endobronchial ultrasound，EBUS）、CT、X 线透视、VB 和 ENB 引导下行 TBNA，可提高诊断率。据报道，凸阵探头（convex probe，CP）或径向探头 EBUS 可将 TBNA 的敏感性、特异性和准确性分别提高至 95%、100% 和 97%[56]。

使用支气管镜对肺癌治疗后患者疗效的评估和再分期尤为重要。影像学检查（如 CT、PET）常规用于支气管肺癌患者的随访复查。需要强调的是，任何复发或肿瘤生长的影像学证据都需要通过组织学或细胞学评估来证实。早期曾接受纵隔镜或纵隔手术的患者，常常需要对治疗期间或治疗后的纵隔异常病变或进展进行诊断。由于复查纵隔镜在技术层面上难以实现，特别是在纵隔放疗之后，因此常使用 TBNA 作为最佳的纵隔病变分期方法。

由于食管与气道毗邻，食管癌常累及气道，其侵犯程度直接影响手术指征。在对 525 例行支气管镜的食管癌患者进行的回顾性研究中，Choi 等发现 91 例（17.3%）累及气道，另 87 例（16.6%）直接侵犯至呼吸道黏膜[126,127]。尽管有明确的手术指征，但对于气道正常或单纯性外压而无明显侵犯的患者，通过支气管镜检查进行评估仍存在一定缺陷。7% 的"正常"患者和

20%的"外压"患者在术中被发现病灶侵犯到呼吸道。

转移性肿瘤常累及肺脏,因此行支气管镜检查非常重要。Argyros 和 Torrington 在一项针对111例转移性肿瘤的报告中指出,44例(39.6%)患者的支气管镜检查结果存在异常[128]。而出现咳嗽、咯血、胸痛以及局限性哮鸣音或干啰音的患者更可能在支气管镜检查中发现异常[128,129]。此外,如果胸片提示肺不张,则支气管镜下也很容易发现病变[128,129]。恶性肿瘤转移至气道内多见于肾细胞癌、腺癌、黑色素瘤、肉瘤、卡波西肉瘤和淋巴瘤[128]。

6.19 支气管镜治疗

如前所述,希波克拉底最早使用内镜是为了缓解病痛。该作用在1897年得以扩展,Gustav Killian 报道在检查气管支气管树时取出了一枚气道骨性异物,即著名的"鸡骨头"[1]。

在21世纪,我们使用支气管镜亦是为了解除病痛。可弯曲支气管镜的引进大大扩展了支气管镜在临床操作中的作用。表6.2列举了支气管镜在治疗方面的应用。

通常情况下,支气管镜可同时发挥诊断和治疗作用。可弯曲支气管镜的治疗作用将在后面的章节中详细阐述,下文中仅做简要说明。

表6.2 支气管镜治疗的适应证

肺部清洗
异物取出术
解除气道内梗阻
恶性肿瘤
近距离放疗
激光治疗
冷冻治疗
高频电刀/氩等离子凝固
光动力治疗
非恶性肿瘤
支架置入
支气管肺泡灌洗
囊肿抽吸
纵隔囊肿
支气管源性囊肿
脓肿引流

(续表)

肺不张
瘤内注射治疗
胸部创伤
支气管镜下支气管胸膜瘘(BPF)封堵术
严重哮喘患者支气管热成形术
无侧支通气肺气肿患者支气管内活瓣植入术
保持气道通畅(填塞止血)
科研指征
经支气管镜肺减容术(BLVR)

6.19.1 异物取出

最初支气管镜的使用即为了去除吸入的异物[1]。支气管镜在这方面一直发挥着重要作用,使患者避免接受创伤较大的外科手术。青少年和成年患者能提供可靠的异物吸入史,然而,对于幼童和部分成人可能无法提供明确的误吸史。Pasaoglu等报道,822例儿童中仅有48%能明确地说出误吸史[130]。不透射线的物体在胸片上显示为肺内阴影,但可穿透射线的物体常表现为正常胸片或局部透亮度增高、浸润或肺不张[130]。我们传统上首选硬质支气管镜,因其异物取出成功率可达85%[131]。然而,可弯曲支气管镜也能达到类似效果,且并发症发生率和死亡率更低[132,133]。培训新手肺科医师使用硬质支气管镜往往经验不足,导致异物的取出更多地依赖于可弯曲支气管镜,其探查外周病变更有优势,也适用于颈椎不稳或使用机械通气的患者。多种夹取异物工具适用于可弯曲支气管镜,如异物网篮、三爪异物钳、支气管球囊和冷冻探针,均可成功取出异物。如果异物吸入时间较长,则会被增生的肉芽组织包绕,此时,应在镜下仔细清除肉芽组织并找到异物。

6.19.2 肺部廓清

肺部清洗可能是最常用的支气管镜治疗方式,适用于由各种原因引起的咳嗽机制受损或气道灼伤导致的支气管内膜塌陷[134]。通常需要有大口径工作通道的支气管镜去除分泌物。术中应时刻警惕防止因清除分泌物和黏液而发生医源性感染。

6.19.3 高频电刀和氩等离子体凝固术(APC)

支气管镜除了作为激光和放疗导管的传送工具,它还能传送电力进行电灼消融治疗。由电流产生的热能发挥作用,其应用模式可呈接触式或非接触式。传统的接触式电刀已在外科手术中应用数十年，通过多种辅助器械在可弯曲支气管镜介导下实施。

近期新兴的另一项可弯曲支气管镜下治疗方法是APC，通过电离氩产生电流作用于病灶，这是一种非接触式技术，多用于支气管腔内凝血和腔内质脆易出血病变或肿瘤病变的处理[135]。

与激光相比，高频电刀对支气管黏膜表面作用更强，价格更低且手术时间更短[136]。尽管电刀、激光、电灼和APC降低了穿透气管壁的风险，但它们仍可能引起气道内燃烧。因此，在使用热治疗时，吸氧浓度必须低于 0.4 FiO$_2$。高频电刀或APC治疗前应将气道内可燃物质（如气管内套管、硅酮支架、覆膜支架等）取出，以免发生气道内燃烧。由于APC是通过喷射氩离子气体携带的电流作用于腔内病变，因此有报道称在APC治疗过程中会发生气体栓塞和气管壁穿孔[137,138]。动物实验表明，气体流速水平与气体栓塞发生密切相关，但仍需进一步研究明确最佳的气体流速，将风险降至最低[138]。

6.19.4　冷冻治疗

尽管支气管镜冷冻治疗早在20世纪70年代就已问世[139]，但其应用十分受限。与激光治疗和近距离放疗相比，冷冻治疗存在较大争议。支持者认为其比较安全，因为不存在气管壁穿透和支气管内燃烧的风险，对术中吸氧流量没有限制，不会对操作者的眼睛造成损害，费用也相对较低[140,141]。此外，软骨、结缔组织和纤维组织可耐受冷冻治疗，而黏膜、肉芽组织和肿瘤组织则较为敏感，因此它能选择性破坏异常组织[142]。反对者则认为冷冻治疗常需要多次行支气管镜才能去除组织坏死物，大大延长了治疗后所预期的气道充分开放的时间[143]。

Mathura等报道了22例经可弯曲支气管镜介导下行冷冻治疗的患者[144]。其中，20例存在支气管恶性病变导致腔内阻塞，2例肺移植患者术后出现气道狭窄。所有治疗在患者镇静状态下于气管镜室内实施。18例患者的腔内恶性病变被完全去除，其中2例出现支气管痉挛，但后续处理相对容易。研究亦提示冷冻治疗对于无法手术的气管腔内肿瘤十分有效，包括早期使用冷冻探针即可帮助气道再通[145]。正如我们在上述异物去除部分中提到的，可弯曲冷冻探针也可用于去除腔内大血块或黏液栓。

液氮喷射是一种较新的冷冻治疗方式，可通过柔性导管在支气管镜下对组织进行非接触式冷冻治疗，其温度远低于以前的冷冻治疗设备[146]。经支气管镜喷射冷冻治疗（spray cryotherapy，SCT）可用于多种良性和恶性气道疾病。SCT的主要限制因素在于对液氮挥发产生的氮气的管理[147]。为了安全地从肺部排出多余氮气，术中需要使用适当尺寸的气管导管，并在喷射过程中将气管插管与呼吸机断开，使用放气阀排气[148]。定量SCT是目前最新的技术进展，该技术正在实验性地应用于慢性支气管炎的治疗，并显示出初步的安全性和良好的组织特异性[149]。更大规模的定量SCT研究正在进行中。

6.19.5　激光治疗

内镜下行激光治疗的适应证和禁忌证取决于阻塞病灶的解剖学特点和临床症状[150]（表 6.3）。

表 6.3　激光治疗的禁忌证

解剖禁忌
无腔内病变的外压性阻塞
病变侵犯大血管（如肺动脉）边缘，有窦道形成可能
病变侵犯食管边缘，有窦道形成可能
病变侵犯纵隔边缘，有窦道形成可能
临床禁忌
即将行外科手术患者
预后差，无法缓解症状
不能耐受镇静或全身麻醉
凝血功能障碍
完全阻塞超过4周

来源：Turner 和 Wang[150]。

激光治疗应用于阻塞性病变，能迅速恢复气道通畅，从而保证远端肺组织的通气和阻塞性肺炎的引流。激光的止血作用能缓解气道内出血性肿瘤患者的症状。有报道提示，激光治疗可改善79%~92%患者的气道通畅情况[151-154]。激光治疗仅适用于管腔内的可见病变，而不适用于管腔外的巨大肿瘤。这些管腔外肿瘤可行辅助放疗，通过外照射放疗或在支气管镜介导下行近距离放疗。气道再通后可置入气道支架以防再次阻塞。由于腔内病灶易复发，因此需多次行激光治疗。激光治疗的并发症包括低氧血症、出血、邻近结构穿孔和支气管内燃烧[144,154]。

激光疗法可用于一些少见的良性气道阻塞性病

变,效果较为显著。气道内的良性肿瘤(如支气管错构瘤)使用激光治疗可以避免创伤更大的外科手术[151,152,155]。其他可使用激光治疗的良性气道阻塞性病变包括主气管肉芽肿(如瘢痕性肉芽肿)、气管狭窄(如气管插管后损伤)、气管淀粉样变、梅毒树胶肿、骨化性气管支气管病[151,152,156]和支气管胸膜瘘(bronchopleural fistula,BPF)封堵[157,158]。

6.19.6 光动力疗法

光动力疗法(photodynamic therapy,PDT)需要注射血卟啉衍生物作为光敏剂,在支气管镜介导下,激光可活化血卟啉衍生物继而导致组织坏死。近十多年来,PDT用于姑息治疗无法手术的气道内肿瘤。最近,多项研究提示,单独或联合外照射放疗能够成功治愈一部分患者[159-165]。另外,PDT在控制气管乳头状瘤方面也有显著疗效[166]。治疗相关并发症包括暴露于光线导致的皮肤晒伤、咯血和坏死组织脱落阻塞气道。考虑到费用和患者对光线敏感的问题,PDT仅在少数中心开展。

6.19.7 近距离放疗

良恶性肿瘤或其他良性病变导致的气道阻塞常需要紧急处理,而支气管镜则充当了这样一种能够介导局部治疗的特殊媒介。体积较大的气道内恶性肿瘤可根据肿瘤特点和以往治疗方案采用多种处理方式。腔内可见的肿瘤仅是冰山一角,黏膜下和肺实质肿瘤负荷更大,因此胸壁外照射是首选的治疗方式。然而,当危及到邻近组织而无法行胸壁外照射时,可选用近距离放疗。Paradelo等在支气管镜介导下对阻塞气道的恶性肿瘤内植入放射性粒子,结果提示34例患者中有30例(88%)症状明显改善。此外,24例患者中有22例(92%)影像学显示改善或稳定[167]。近距离放疗的并发症包括坏死性空洞、瘘管形成和出血[168]。近期有不少无法手术的恶性肿瘤患者经植入放射性粒子成功治疗的病例,它作为近距离放疗的另一种形式,可更精确地传送照射剂量,也可减少并发症的发生率[169]。

6.19.8 支气管肺泡灌洗术(BAL)

众所周知,BAL具备诊断作用,特别在肺部感染性病变或弥漫性病变中广泛使用,同时也能在支气管镜介导下发挥治疗作用。对于肺泡蛋白沉着症患者,BAL能同时进行诊断和治疗。通过分析灌洗液能明确诊断,并避免了开胸肺活检。治疗上,灌洗能直接去除肺泡内沉积的磷脂[170,171]。约2/3的患者需要行肺泡灌洗,将近50%的患者仅需要单次治疗,剩余患者则需要多次灌洗[172]。BAL禁忌证相对较少,包括FEV_1<1 L、哮喘伴中度气道阻塞、难以纠正的高碳酸血症和低氧血症、严重心律失常、血流动力学不稳定或存在出血倾向[173]。

6.19.9 囊肿抽吸

支气管源性囊肿的诊断和治疗都十分困难,尤其是对那些其他方面健康且无症状的患者,通常在病理确诊后或囊肿压迫邻近结构时需行外科手术。然而,也有报道提示通过经支气管针吸即可明确诊断,同时可行囊肿减压治疗[174,175]。

6.19.10 肺脓肿引流

肺脓肿常用抗生素和适当引流治疗,后者包括胸部物理方法和体位引流。上述引流方法无效可考虑外科介入[176,177]。而使用支气管镜不仅能够取得病原学培养标本,还能有效引流空洞[178]。在少部分患者中通过支气管镜放置引流管获得了良好的效果[83]。患者在清醒状态下放置导管的舒适性和误吸风险是该技术广泛应用的主要障碍。在对肺脓肿进行支气管镜评估时,必须注意避免脓液溢出到其他气道。

6.19.11 支架置入

上述所提及的解除气道阻塞的方法中,大多数仅适用于腔内病变。在气道外源性受压或气道软骨环缺失时,置入气道支架能保证气道通畅。另外,支架还应用于肺袖状切除术后或肺移植术后气道狭窄的患者[179,180]。可弯曲支气管镜或硬质支气管镜介导下均可实施支架置入术[181,182],相关讨论在本书的后续章节中会详细阐述。

6.19.12 球囊扩张

长期以来,一直使用硬质支气管镜对良恶性病变导致的气道狭窄和中央气道梗阻进行扩张[183,184]。可弯曲支气管镜也被证实可进行有效的球囊扩张。Hautmann等报道了78例共接受了126次扩张术的气管支气管恶性疾病患者[185]。球囊扩张的适应证包括有症状的气管支气管狭窄(如呼吸困难、喘鸣等)、复发性肺炎、肺不张、分泌物潴留或肺脓肿。2例肺脓肿患者均已好转,此外,肺不张、肺炎和呼吸困难的改善率分别为62%、92%和37%。并发症包括1例因肺动脉破裂导致的危及生命的咯血以及无须特殊处理的少量出血。

可弯曲支气管镜介导下行球囊扩张和激光治疗可成功治疗良性喉-气管狭窄（laryngotracheostenosis，LTS）患者，避免了气管手术，而且对于大多数患者而言仅需单次治疗[186]。球囊扩张术在评估气道可膨胀金属支架置入中也发挥重要的作用[187]。扩张常用器械包括标准型可弯曲支气管镜、8~16F的球囊导管和2.5~4.0 cm长的球囊[188]。

6.19.13 瘘

瘘是气道及其周围结构之间形成的通道。支气管胸膜瘘是最常见的瘘，通常发生于手术后。支气管胸膜瘘也常见于肺结核、肺炎、肺气肿和肺脓肿患者[189,190]。位于气道近端的瘘管可以直接观察到，而在可弯曲支气管镜介导下检查位于远端的瘘管是非常困难的。此时应系统地对各个段及亚段支气管进行球囊充气检查。如果球囊充气后气体泄漏减少，则能确认瘘管所在亚段[189,191]。一旦确认瘘管位置，可通过支气管镜用多种组织封堵器或活瓣封堵瘘口[192-195]。

气管食管瘘可以是先天性的，而更多的是与成人气道消化道肿瘤及其治疗不当有关。其常见的症状是咳嗽，尤其在进行吞咽动作或卧位时可诱发，通过支气管镜能发现83%的气管食管瘘[196]。支气管镜除了能诊断气管食管瘘，还能联合食管镜行术前评估检查、制订手术方案。

主动脉支气管瘘少见但常危及生命。梅毒、动脉粥样硬化动脉瘤以及结核浸润至主动脉壁患者均可能发生主动脉支气管瘘，常用的处理方法是主动脉修复手术[197]。主动脉造影往往不能显示瘘管。Graeber等报道只有1/5的主动脉造影有阳性发现[197]。支气管镜能诊断50%的病例（14例中有7例确诊）[198]。支气管镜医师必须知晓主动脉支气管瘘患者行支气管镜的固有风险。触碰瘘管或其上附着的血块可能引起大出血[197]。因此，必须立即隔离出血的一侧肺，同时行修复手术。

6.19.14 气管插管

我们常规使用喉镜在直视会厌下进行正确的气管插管。然而，在插管困难的情况下，可择优选择可弯曲支气管镜。固定或不稳定的颈椎状况、颞下颌关节僵直和巨大口咽部肿瘤患者可在可弯曲支气管镜引导下行气管插管[199]。此外，在难以直视声门的情况下，也需立即使用可弯曲支气管镜，以确认气管内插管的正确位置。虽然床旁胸片也能确认气管插管位置，但在X线纵隔穿透较弱的肥胖患者和无法立即实施X线胸片的危重症患者中，使用支气管镜确认更佳。有些医师亦使用支气管镜确认小儿患者气管插管位置以减少胸部X线的放射性损伤[200]。

气管插管和气管切开是医源性气道损伤的潜在原因。气管插管过程中对声带的直接损伤可导致声门前隙瘢痕形成[201]。气管插管对所接触的气管壁的压力不同可导致缺血性溃疡形成[202]。通常情况下这些损伤能快速愈合。然而，损伤迁延时，则导致环杓关节僵直和声门后隙瘢痕形成[203,204]。气管插管固定气囊的过度充气会导致气管周围缺血坏死，造成气管软骨环支撑结构丧失和气管软化或在修复过程中形成纤维化狭窄[205]。气管插管气囊对气管壁的压力可能会损伤喉返神经，造成声带麻痹[202]。虽然气管切开能避免声门及声门下损伤，但切开孔的肉芽增生、瘢痕形成和收缩会造成患者气道狭窄[202]。支气管镜和喉镜能对此类损伤情况行全面的解剖学评估检查并制订正确的治疗方法。

可弯曲支气管镜和硬质支气管镜都能用于检查气管近端至狭窄部位。然而，在明显狭窄情况下，气管远端的检查往往无法使用可弯曲支气管镜。这种情况下，需借助于硬质支气管镜，在机械通气作用下进行全面的气道检查。支气管镜医师应当知晓任何针对严重气道狭窄的处理措施都可引起分泌物增加、出血或水肿，继而导致气道完全阻塞。因此，应立即准备行扩张术。

支气管镜可用于评估经气管供氧导管的适当长度和位置。接受经气管氧疗的患者可能会因导管反折穿过声带，或导管过长刺激隆突、损伤支气管。虽然这些情况可通过胸部X线片进行评估，但有时也需要使用支气管镜直接观察。经气管供氧导管的刺激可能导致气管瘘口肉芽组织形成，需要进行支气管镜检查和治疗。经气管供氧导管还导致大块黏液栓形成，同样需要利用支气管镜评估与清除[206]。

6.19.15 基因治疗

可弯曲支气管镜也被用于将基因治疗载体输送到气管支气管树。利用支气管镜向支气管黏膜、肺泡输送基因治疗载体以及靶向血管内皮细胞的临床试验，正在进行中[207-210]。

6.19.16 支气管热成形术

近期有许多针对难治性哮喘的研究，对支气管壁进行射频消融以破坏哮喘发作中引起气道收缩的平滑肌[211]。最早的哮喘干预研究（asthma intervention research，AIR）试验和危重哮喘试验研究结果显示，6～12个月内哮喘患者的控制情况有所改善，但危重哮喘患者组的术后并发症和住院率较对照组明显增加[211,212]。AIR2试验5年延长试验显示，AIR试验的效果在5年内仍能持续[213]。最近，PAS2［FDA批准的评估支气管热成形术（bronchial thermoplasty，BT）治疗严重持续性哮喘患者的临床研究］的结果显示，接受BT治疗的重症哮喘患者的急性加重、急诊就诊和住院次数均显著减少[214]。研究结果都支持将BT作为一种辅助手段，用于治疗特定的重症哮喘患者。

6.19.17 支气管镜肺减容术

目前开展的多种支气管镜肺减容术（bronchoscopic lung volume reduction，BLVR）都希望达到2003年全国肺气肿治疗研究（NETT）中的治疗效果[215]。这些BLVR具体可分为以下3类：支气管内活瓣、气道旁路系统和生物重塑。在过度充气和肺气肿的支气管内植入支气管内活瓣能使肺远端的气体和分泌物流出，但气体无法进入，由此可减小该部位的肺组织容积或使其完全萎陷[216,217]。气道旁路系统通过应用射频球囊导管从中央气道至过度充气部位的肺组织之间建立旁路气道，使气体进入大的气道从而减小肺容积[218]。第三项主要技术是生物重塑——支气管镜进入肺内目标区域，在镜下注入生物胶，促使过度充气的肺组织萎陷[219]。

目前，支气管内活瓣是FDA唯一批准使用的BLVR技术[220,221]。其他技术都还在进一步评估研究中，早期研究的初步结果提示在不久的将来，它们将在支气管镜治疗肺气肿中发挥重要作用。

6.20 禁忌证

支气管镜操作从一开始就被证实是一种安全的检查方法[222,223]。

虽然总体上来说它是一项安全的操作，但出现以下情况，支气管镜相关并发症的风险会相对升高（表6.4），尤其对于恶性心律失常、严重难治性低氧血症或

表6.4 支气管镜操作的禁忌证

绝对禁忌证
- 术中氧供不足
- 硬质支气管镜
- 颈部不稳定
- 严重颈椎强直
- 颞下颌关节活动受限

相对禁忌证
- 恶性心律失常
- 心功能不稳定
- 难治性低氧血症
- 出血倾向或严重血小板减低症（如果需要活检）

发生并发症的高危因素
- 患者无法配合
- 近期或不稳定型心绞痛
- 不稳定型哮喘
- 中度或重度低氧血症
- 高碳酸血症
- 尿毒症
- 血小板减少症
- 肺动脉高压
- 肺脓肿
- 免疫抑制
- 上腔静脉阻塞
- 虚弱、高龄或营养不良
- 近期服用氯吡格雷

有严重出血倾向（如果需要活检）的患者而言[224,225]。

多项研究评估了合并冠脉疾病患者行气管镜检查的安全性。Matot等研究了患者在镇静状态下行纤维支气管镜检查发生心肌缺血的发病率。在29例年龄≥50岁的进行择期支气管检查的患者中[226]，心率明显升高，其中17%的患者出现心肌缺血。心电图提示ST段改变的5例患者中，只有1例曾有心肌梗死和心绞痛病史。随后，Dunagan等对心肌梗死10天后行支气管镜检查的患者进行随访，结果并没有发现胸痛或缺血事件的发生，主要并发症也没有显著增加[227]。这些相关研究的结果提示，对存在潜在冠脉疾病的患者而言，支气管镜检查仍是一项非常安全的操作，但对于存在心源性危险因素的患者，在实施支气管镜检查前应仔细审查相关禁忌证[228-233]。

出血倾向评估的重要性取决于实施支气管镜检查时的具体操作。气道检查和BAL通常均可安全实施。为了减少鼻腔出血，首选经口而非经鼻置入支气管镜。如果需行活检或镜下切除，应及时纠正凝血障碍。未

纠正的血小板减少症（低于 50 000/dL）或尿毒症期的血小板功能障碍被认为是支气管镜的相对禁忌证[223]。非直视下使用剪切或撕裂法进行大块组织活检，如经支气管活检，存在较高的风险。由于靠近大血管，气道近端活检也存在大量出血的风险。在这种存在出血高危因素情况下，如果用 TBNA 替代经支气管活检，可减少出血风险[202]。然而，必要时仍可在低血小板计数条件下行经支气管活检，也曾有过成功案例的报道。对服用血小板抑制剂——氯吡格雷的患者，经支气管活检后出血明显增加，因此建议患者在活检前停用该药物[234]。需要强调的是，这并非绝对禁忌证，但如果时间允许，仍建议在术前 5~7 天停用氯吡格雷，能明显降低出血风险。

对于基础肺功能差的患者，应考虑到操作过程中活检或器械造成气胸的风险。而对于部分患者而言，可能为相对禁忌证，因此建议使用 X 线透视直接观察器械在体内的情况，以免器械过于接近胸膜。气胸的发生率因医院、支气管镜医师、器械类型、活检操作以及引导活检的成像方法的不同而变化。总之，支气管镜引起医源性气胸的发生率较低，即便在重症慢阻肺患者并发气胸时，致死率也相对较低[235,236]。

参考文献

1. Nakhosten, J. (1994). History of bronchoscopy: removal of tracheobronchial foreign body, Gustav Killian. *J. Bronchol.* 1: 76.
2. Jackson, C. (1928). Bronchoscopy; past, present and future. *N. Engl. J. Med.* 199: 759–763.
3. Ikeda, S., Yawai, N., and Ishikawa, S. (1968). Flexible bronchofiberscope. *Keio J. Med.* 17 (1): 133.
4. Miyazawa, T. (2000). History of the flexible bronchoscopy. In: Interventional Bronchoscopy, vol. 30 (eds. C.T. Bollger and P.N. Mathur), 16–21. Basel: Karger.
5. Popavich, J., Kvale, P.A., and Ikanhornit, L. (1982). Diagnostic accuracy of multiple biopsies from flexible fiberoptic bronchoscopy. A comparison of central vs. peripheral carcinoma. *Am. Rev. Respir. Dis.* 125: 521–523.
6. Chur, D. and Asterita, R.W. (1983). Carcinoma presenting as endobronchial mass. Optimum number of biopsies specimens for diagnosis. *Chest* 83: 865–867.
7. Wang, K.P., Terry, P.B., and Marsh, B. (1978). Bronchoscopic needle aspiration, biopsy of paratracheal tumors. *Respir. Dis.* 118: 17–21.
8. Wang, K.P., Marsh, B., Summer, D.R. et al. (1981). Transbronchial needle aspiration for diagnosis for lung cancer. *Chest* 80: 48–50.
9. Prakash, U.B.S. and Stubbs, S.E. (1991). Bronchoscopy in North America: the ACCP survey. *Chest* 100: 1660–1675.
10. Poe, R.H., Israel, R.H., Utell, M.J., and Hall, W.J. (1982). Chronic cough: bronchoscopy or pulmonary function testing? *Am. Rev. Respir. Dis.* 126: 160–162.
11. Rosen, M.J. (1996). Overview of pulmonary complications. *Clin. Chest Med.* 17 (4): 621–631.
12. Pratter, M.R., Brightling, C.E., Boulet, L.P., and Irwin, R.S. (2006). An empiric integrative approach to the management of cough. *Chest* 129: 222–231S.
13. Hyde, L. and Hyde, C.I. (1974). Clinical manifestations of lung cancer. *Chest* 65: 299–306.
14. Decalmer, S., Woodcock, A., Greaves, M. et al. (2007). Airway abnormalities at flexible bronchoscopy in patients with chronic cough. *Eur. Respir. J.* 30: 1138–1142.
15. Kennedy, T.C., McWilliams, A., Edell, E. et al. (2007). Bronchial intraepithelial neoplasia/early central airways lung cancer: ACCP evidence-based clinical practice guidelines (2nd edition). *Chest* 132: 221S–233S.
16. Aslan, A.T., Kiper, N., Dogru, D. et al. (2005). Diagnostic value of flexible bronchoscopy in children with persistent and recurrent wheezing. *Allergy Asthma Proc.* 26: 483–486.
17. Schellhase, D.E., Fawcett, D.D., Schutze, G.E. et al. (1998). Clinical utility of flexible bronchoscopy and bronchoalveolar lavage in young children with recurrent wheezing. *J. Pediatr.* 132 (2): 312–318.
18. Wood, R.E. (2001). The emerging role of flexible bronchoscopy in pediatrics. *Clin. Chest Med.* 22 (2): 311–317.
19. Mehra, P.K. and Woessner, K.M. (2005). Dyspnea, wheezing, and airways obstruction: is it asthma? *Allergy Asthma Proc.* 26: 319–322.
20. Forrest, L.A., Husein, T., and Husein, O. (2012). Paradoxical vocal cord motion: classification and treatment. *Laryngoscope* 122 (4): 844–853.
21. Kryger, M., Bode, F., Antic, R., and Anthonisen, N. (1976). Diagnosis of obstruction of the upper and central airways. *Am. J. Med.* 61: 85–93.
22. O'Hollaren, M.T. and Everts, E.C. (1991). Evaluating the patient with stridor. *Ann. Allergy* 67: 301–305.
23. Prakash, U.B.S. (1993). Bronchoscopy. In: Pulmonary and Critical Care Medicine, vol. (5) (ed. R.C. Bone), 1–18. St Louis: Mosby-Yearbook.
24. Mancuso, R.F. (1996). Pediatric otolaryngology. Stridor in neonates. *Pediatr. Clin. North Am.* 43 (6): 1339–1355.
25. Langford, C.A. and van Waes, C. (1997). Life-threatening complications of autoimmune disease. *Rheum. Dis. Clin. North Am.* 23 (2): 345–363.
26. Parnell, F.W. and Brandenburg, J.H. (1970). Vocal cord paralysis: a review of 100 cases. *Laryngoscope* 80: 1036–1045.
27. Terris, D.J., Arnstein, D.P., and Nguyen, H.H. (1992). Contemporary evaluation of unilateral vocal cord paralysis. *Otolaryngol. Head Neck Surg.* 107: 84–90.
28. Mlcak, R.P., Suman, O.E., and Herndon, D.N. (2007). Respiratory management of inhalation injury. *Burns* 33: 2–13.
29. Hunt, J.L., Agee, R.N., and Pruitt, B.A. (1975). Fiberoptic bronchoscopy in acute inhalation injury. *J. Trauma* 15: 641.
30. Moylan, J.A. (1980). Smoke inhalation and burn injury. *Surg. Clin. North Am.* 60: 1533–1540.
31. Gore, M.A., Joshi, A.R., Nagarajan, G. et al. (2004). Virtual

bronchoscopy for diagnosis of inhalation injury in burnt patients. *Burns* 30: 165–168.

32 Marek, K., Piotr, W., Stanislaw, S. et al. (2007). Fibreoptic bronchoscopy in routine clinical practice in confirming the diagnosis and treatment of inhalation burns. *Burns* 33: 554–560.

33 Raoof, S., Mehrishi, S., and Prakash, U.B.S. (2001). Role of bronchoscopy in modern medical intensive care unit. *Clin. Chest Med.* 22 (2): 241–261.

34 Masanes, M.J., Legendre, C., Lioret, N. et al. (1994). Fiberoptic bronchoscopy for the early diagnosis of subglottal inhalation injury. *J. Trauma* 36: 59–67.

35 Endorf, F.W. and Gamelli, R.L. (2007). Inhalation injury, pulmonary perturbations, and fluid resuscitation. *J. Burn Care Res.* 28: 80–83.

36 Moylan, J.A., Adib, K., and Birnbaum, M. (1975). Fiberoptic bronchoscopy following thermal injury. *Surg. Gynecol. Obstet.* 140: 541–543.

37 Freitag, L., Firusian, N., Stamatis, G., and Greschuchuna, D. (1991). Bronchoscopy: the role of bronchoscopy in pulmonary complications due to mustard gas inhalation. *Chest* 100: 1436–1441.

38 Thompson, A.B., Teschler, H., and Rennard, S.I. (1992). Pathogenesis, evaluation, and therapy for massive hemoptysis. *Clin. Chest Med.* 13: 69.

39 Johnston, H. and Reisz, G. (1989). Changing spectrum of hemoptysis. Underlying causes in 148 patients undergoing diagnostic flexible fiberoptic bronchoscopy. *Arch. Intern. Med.* 149: 1666.

40 Santiago, S., Tobias, J., and Williams, A.J. (1991). A reappraisal of the causes of hemoptysis. *Arch. Intern. Med.* 151: 2449.

41 Hirshberg, B., Biran, I., Glazer, M., and Kramer, M.R. (1997). Hemoptysis: etiology, evaluation, and outcome in a tertiary referral hospital. *Chest* 112: 440.

42 Lyons, H.A. (1976). Differential diagnosis of hemoptysis and its treatment. *Basics Respir. Dis.* 5: 26–30.

43 Smiddy, J.F. and Elliot, R.C. (1973). The evaluation of hemoptysis with fiberoptic bronchoscopy. *Chest* 92: 77–82.

44 Prakash, U.B.S. (1985). The use of the pediatric fiberoptic bronchoscope in adults. *Am. Rev. Respir. Dis.* 132: 715–717.

45 Pursel, S.E. and Lindskog, G.E. (1961). Hemoptysis: a clinical evaluation of 105 patients examined consecutively on a thoracic surgical service. *Am. Rev. Respir. Dis.* 84: 329–336.

46 Gong, H. Jr. and Salvatierra, C. (1981). Clinical efficacy of early and delayed fiberoptic bronchoscopy in patients with hemoptysis. *Am. Rev. Respir. Dis.* 124: 221–225.

47 Stoller, J.K. (1992). Diagnosis and management of massive hemoptysis: a review. *Respir. Care* 37 (6): 564–581.

48 Jean-Baptiste, E. (2000). Clinical assessment and management of massive hemoptysis. *Crit. Care Med.* 28 (5): 1642–1646.

49 Freitag, L. (1993). Development of a new balloon catheter for management of hemoptysis with bronchofiberscopes. *Chest* 103: 593.

50 Saw, E., Gottlieb, L., Yokoyama, T. et al. (1976). Flexible fiberoptic bronchoscopy and endobronchial tamponade in the management of massive hemoptysis. *Chest* 70: 589–591.

51 Morice, R.C., Ece, T., Ece, F. et al. (2001). Endobronchial argon plasma coagulation for the treatment of hemoptysis and neoplastic airway obstruction. *Chest* 119 (3): 781–787.

52 Abner, A. (1993). Approach to the patient who presents with superior vena cava obstruction. *Chest* 103: 394S–397S.

53 Armstrong, B.A., Perez, C.A., Simpson, J.R. et al. (1987). Role of irradiation in the management of superior vena cava syndrome. *Int. J. Radiat. Oncol. Biol. Phys.* 13: 531–539.

54 Chen, J.C., Bongard, F., and Klein, S.R. (1990). A contemporary perspective on superior vena cava syndrome. *Am. J. Surg.* 160: 207–211.

55 Ferrari, L.R. and Bedford, R.F. (1990). General anesthesia prior to treatment of anterior mediastinal masses in pediatric cancer patients. *Anesthesiology* 72: 991–995.

56 Yasufuku, K., Chiyo, M., Sekine, Y. et al. (2004). Real-time endobronchial ultrasound-guided transbronchial needle aspiration of mediastinal and hilar lymph nodes. *Chest* 126: 122–128.

57 Ovassapian, A. (2001). The flexible bronchoscope: a tool of anesthesiologists. *Clin. Chest Med.* 22 (2): 281–299.

58 Hnatiuk, O.W., Corcoran, P.C., and Sierra, A. (2001). Spirometry in surgery for anterior mediastinal masses. *Chest* 120: 1152–1156.

59 Depaso, W.J. and Winterbauer, R.H. (1991). Interstitial lung disease. *Dis. Mon.* 37: 61–133.

60 Meyer, K.C., Raghu, G., Baughman, R.P. et al. (2012). An official American Thoracic Society clinical practice guideline: the clinical utility of bronchoalveolar lavage cellular analysis in interstitial lung disease. *Am. J. Respir. Crit. Care Med.* 185: 1004.

61 Chollet, S., Soler, P., Dournovo, P. et al. (1984). The diagnosis of pulmonary histiocytosis X by immunodetection of Langerhan's cell in BALF. *Am. J. Pathol.* 115: 225–232.

62 Martin, R.J., Coalsen, J.J., Rogers, R.M. et al. (1980). Pulmonary alveolar proteinosis: the diagnosis by segmental lavage. *Am. Rev. Respir. Dis.* 121: 819–825.

63 Helmers, R.A. and Hunninghake, G.W. (1989). Broncho-alveolar lavage in the non-immunocompromised patient. *Chest* 96: 1184–1190.

64 Rossman, M.D., Kern, J.A., Elias, J.A. et al. (1988). Proliferative response of bronchoalveolar lymphocytes to beryllium, a test for chronic beryllium disease. *Ann. Intern. Med.* 108: 687–693.

65 Hunninghake, G.W. and Crystal, R.G. (1981). Pulmonary sarcoidosis: a disorder mediated by excess helper T-lymphocyte activity at sites of disease activity. *N. Engl. J. Med.* 305: 429–434.

66 Hunninghake, G.W., Kawanami, O., Ferrans, V.J. et al. (1981). Characterization of inflammatory and immune effector cells in the lung parenchyma of patients with interstitial lung disease. *Am. Rev. Respir. Dis.* 123: 407.

67 Aguayo, S.M., Niccole, S.A., Martin, R.J. et al. (1989). Is BAL eosinophilia clinically useful in the differential diagnosis of unexplained pulmonary infiltrates? *Am. Rev. Respir. Dis.* 139: 385. Abstract.

68 Pesci, A., Bertorelli, G., Manganelli, P. et al. (1988).

Bronchoalveolar lavage in chronic eosinophilic pneumonia: analysis of six cases in comparison with other interstitial lung diseases. *Respiration* 54: 16–22.

69 Bradley, B., Branley, H.M., Egan, J.J. et al. (2008). Interstitial lung disease guideline: the British Thoracic Society in collaboration with the Thoracic Society of Australia and New Zealand and the Irish Thoracic Society. *Thorax* 63 (Suppl 5): v1.

70 Raghu, G., Collard, H.R., Egan, J.J. et al. (2011). An official ATS/ERS/JRS/ALAT statement: idiopathic pulmonary fibrosis: evidence-based guidelines for diagnosis and management. *Am. J. Respir. Crit. Care Med.* 183: 788.

71 Johannson, K.A., Marcoux, V.S., Ronksley, P.E., and Ryerson, C.J. (2016). Diagnostic yield and complications of transbronchial lung cryobiopsy for interstitial lung disease. A systematic review and metaanalysis. *Ann. Am. Thorac. Soc.* 13: 1828.

72 Mittle, R.L. Jr., Schwab, R.J., Duchin, J.S. et al. (1994). Radiographic resolution of community acquired pneumonia. *Am. J. Respir. Crit. Care Med.* 149: 630–635.

73 Kuru, T. and Lynch, J.P. 3rd. (1999). Nonresolving or slowly resolving pneumonia. *Clin. Chest Med.* 20: 623–651.

74 Feinsilver, S.H., Fein, A.M., Niederman, M.S. et al. (1990). Utility of fiberoptic bronchoscopy in nonresolving pneumonia. *Chest* 98: 1322–1326.

75 Huang, L., Hecht, F.M., Stansell, J.D. et al. (1995). Suspected pneumocystis carinii pneumonia with a negative induced sputum examination. Is bronchoscopy useful? *Am. J. Respir. Crit. Care Med.* 151: 1866–1871.

76 Gal, A.A., Klatt, E.C., Koss, M.N. et al. (1987). The effectiveness of bronchoscopy in the diagnosis of *Pneumocystis carinii* and cytomegalovirus pulmonary infections in acquired immunodeficiency syndrome. *Arch. Pathol. Lab. Med.* 111: 238–241.

77 Martin, W.J. II, Smith, T.F., Sanderson, D.R. et al. (1987). Role of bronchoalveolar lavage in the assessment of opportunistic pulmonary infections: utility and complications. *Mayo Clin. Proc.* 62: 549–557.

78 Liebler, J.M. and Markin, C.J. (2000). Fiberoptic bronchoscopy for diagnosis and treatment. *Crit. Care Med.* 16 (1): 83–100.

79 White, P. (2001). Evaluation of pulmonary infiltrates in critically ill patients with cancer and marrow transplant. *Crit. Care Clin.* 17 (3): 647–670.

80 Jain, P., Sandur, S., Meli, Y. et al. (2004). Role of flexible bronchoscopy in immunocompromised patients with lung infiltrates. *Chest* 125: 712–722.

81 Peikert, T., Rana, S., and Edell, E.S. (2005). Safety, diagnostic yield, and therapeutic implications of flexible bronchoscopy in patients with febrile neutropenia and pulmonary infiltrates. *Mayo Clin. Proc.* 80: 1414–1420.

82 Sosenko, A. and Glassroth, J. (1985). Fiberoptic bronchoscopy in the evaluation of lung abscesses. *Chest* 87: 489–494.

83 Herth, F., Ernst, A., and Becker, H.D. (2005). Endoscopic drainage of lung abscesses: technique and outcome. *Chest* 127: 1378–1381.

84 Su, W.J., Lee, P.Y., and Perng, R.P. (1993). Chest roentgenographic guidelines in the selection of patients for fiberoptic bronchoscopy. *Chest* 103: 1198–1201.

85 Hasegawa, S., Terada, Y., Murakawa, M. et al. (1998). Emergency bronchoscopy. *J. Bronchol.* 44: 284–287.

86 Jolliet, P. and Chevrolet, J.C. (1992). Bronchoscopy in the intensive care unit. *Intensive Care Med.* 18: 160–169.

87 Frank, W. (2004). Current diagnostic approach to pleural effusion. *Pneumologie* 58: 777–790.

88 Lee, P., Hsu, A., Lo, C. et al. (2007). Prospective evaluation of flex-rigid pleuroscopy for indeterminate pleural effusion: accuracy, safety and outcome. *Respirology* 12: 881–886.

89 Gunnels, J.J. (1978). Perplexing pleural effusion. *Chest* 74: 390–393.

90 Chang, S.C. and Perng, R.P. (1989). The role of fiberoptic bronchoscopy in evaluating the causes of pleural effusions. *Arch. Intern. Med.* 149: 855–857.

91 Balci, A.E., Eren, N., Eren, S. et al. (2002). Surgical treatment of post-traumatic tracheobronchial injuries: 14-year experience. *Eur. J. Cardiothorac. Surg.* 22: 984–989.

92 Eckert, M.J., Clagett, C., Martin, M. et al. (2006). Bronchoscopy in the blast injury patient. *Arch. Surg.* 141: 806–809; discussion 810–801.

93 Hara, K.S. and Prakash, U.B.S. (1989). Fiberoptic bronchoscopy in the evaluation of acute chest and upper airway trauma. *Chest* 96: 627–630.

94 Baumgartner, F., Seppard, B., de Virgilio, C. et al. (1990). Tracheal and main bronchial disruptions after blunt chest trauma. *Ann. Thorac. Surg.* 50: 569–574.

95 Payne, W.S. and DeRemee, R.A. (1971). Injuries of the trachea and major bronchi. *Postgrad. Med.* 49: 152–158.

96 Travis, S.P.L. and Layer, G.T. (1983). Traumatic transection of the thoracic trachea. *Ann. R. Coll. Surg. Engl.* 65: 240–241.

97 Lehto, J.T., Koskinen, P.K., Anttila, V.J. et al. (2005). Bronchoscopy in the diagnosis and surveillance of respiratory infections in lung and heart-lung transplant recipients. *Transpl. Int.* 18: 562–571.

98 Glanville, A.R. (2006). The role of bronchoscopic surveillance monitoring in the care of lung transplant recipients. *Semin. Respir. Crit. Care Med.* 27: 480–491.

99 Greene, C.L., Reemtsen, B., Polimenakos, A. et al. (2008). Role of clinically indicated transbronchial lung biopsies in the management of pediatric post-lung transplant patients. *Ann. Thorac. Surg.* 86: 198–203.

100 Seballos, R.J., Mehta, A.C., McCarthy, P.M., and Kirby, T.J. (1993). The management of airway complications following lung transplantation [abstract]. *Am. Rev. Respir. Dis.* 147: A602.

101 Sibley, R.K., Berry, G.J., Tazelaar, H.D. et al. (1993). The role of transbronchial biopsies in the management of lung transplant recipients. *J. Heart Lung Transplant.* 12: 308–324.

102 Paradis, I., Yousem, S., and Griffith, B. (1993). Airway obstruction and bronchiolitis obliterans after lung transplantation. *Clin. Chest Med.* 14: 751–763.

103 Ono, R., Loke, J., and Ikeda, S. (1981). Bronchofiberscopy with curette biopsy bronchography in the evaluation of peripheral lung lesions. *Chest* 79: 162–166.

104 Cortese, D.A. and McDougall, J.C. (1979). Biopsy and brushing of peripheral lung cancer with fluoroscopic

guidance. *Chest* 75: 141–145.
105 Radke, J.R., Conway, W.A., Eyler, W.R. et al. (1979). Diagnostic accuracy in peripheral lung lesions. *Chest* 76: 176–179.
106 Zavala, D.C. (1975). Diagnostic fiberoptic bronchoscopy: techniques and results of biopsy in 600 patients. *Chest* 68: 12–19.
107 Stringfield, J.T., Markowitz, D.J., Bentz, R.R. et al. (1977). The effect of tumor size and location on diagnosis by fiberoptic bronchoscopy. *Chest* 72: 474–476.
108 Wallace, J.M. and Deutsch, A.L. (1982). Flexible fiberoptic bronchoscopy and percutaneous needle lung aspiration for evaluating the solitary pulmonary nodule. *Chest* 81: 665–671.
109 Asano, F., Eberhardt, R., and Herth, F.J. (2014). Virtual bronchoscopic navigation for peripheral pulmonary lesions. *Respiration* 88: 430.
110 Mondoni, M., Sotgiu, G., Bonifazi, M. et al. (2016). Transbronchial needle aspiration in peripheral pulmonary lesions: a systematic review and meta-analysis. *Eur. Respir. J.* 48: 196.
111 Shure, D. and Fedullo, P.F. (1983). Transbronchial needle aspiration of peripheral masses. *Am. Rev. Respir. Dis.* 128: 1090–1092.
112 Wang, K.P., Haponik, E.F., Britt, E.J.B. et al. (1984). Transbronchial needle aspiration of peripheral pulmonary nodules. *Chest* 86: 819–823.
113 Mori, K., Yanase, N., Kaneko, M. et al. (1989). Diagnosis of peripheral lung cancer in cases of tumors 2 cm or less in size. *Chest* 95: 304–308.
114 Popovich, J. Jr., Kvale, P.A., Eichenhorn, M.S. et al. (1982). Diagnostic accuracy of multiple biopsies from flexible fiberoptic bronchoscopy: a comparison of central versus peripheral carcinoma. *Am. Rev. Respir. Dis.* 125: 521–523.
115 Shure, D. and Astarita, R.W. (1983). Bronchoscopic carcinoma presenting as an endobronchial mass: optimal number of biopsy specimens for diagnosis. *Chest* 83: 865–867.
116 Buccheri, G., Barberis, P., and Delfino, M.S. (1991). Diagnostic, morphologic and histopathologic correlates in bronchogenic carcinoma: a review of 1,045 bronchoscopic examinations. *Chest* 99: 809–814.
117 Wang, K.P., Gupta, P.K., Haponik, E.F. et al. (1984). Flexible transbronchial needle aspiration: technical considered. *Ann. Otol. Rhinol. Laryngol.* 93: 233–236.
118 Shure D, F.P.F. (1985). Transbronchial needle aspiration in the diagnosis of submucosal and peribronchial bronchogenic carcinoma. *Chest* 88 (1): 49–51.
119 Dasgupta, A., Jain, P., Minai, O.A. et al. (1999). Utility of transbronchial needle aspiration in the diagnosis of endobronchial lesions. *Chest* 115 (5): 1237–1241.
120 Wang, K.P., Gonullu, U., and Baker, R. (1994). Transbronchial needle aspiraiton versus transthoracic needle aspiration in the diagnosis of pulmonary lesions. *J. Bronchol.* 1: 199–204.
121 Raab, S.S., Hornberger, J., and Raffin, T. (1997). The importance of sputum cytology in the diagnosis of lung cancer a cost-effective analysis. *Chest* 112 (4): 937–945.
122 Martini, N. and Melamed, M.R. (1980). Occult carcinomas of the lung. *Ann. Thorac. Surg.* 30: 215–223.
123 Lam, S., Hung, J., Kennedy, S.M. et al. (1992). Detection of dysplasia and carcinoma in situ by ration fluorometry. *Am. Rev. Respir. Dis.* 146: 1458–1461.
124 Nakhosteen, J.A. and Khanavkar, B. (1999). Autofluorescence bronchoscopy: the laser imaging fluorescence endoscope. In: Interventional Bronchoscopy (eds. C.T. Bolliger and P.N. Mathur), 236–242. Basel: Karger.
125 Tremblay, A. Low prevalence of high-grade lesions detected with autofluorescence bronchoscopy in the setting of lung cancer screening in the pan-Canadian lung cancer screening study. *Chest* 150 (5): 1015–1022.
126 Choi, T.K., Siu, K.F., Lam, K.H., and Wong, J. (1984). Bronchoscopy and carcinoma of the esophagus I: findings of bronchoscopy in carcinoma of the esophagus. *Am. J. Surg.* 147: 757–759.
127 Choi, T.K., Siu, K.F., Lam, K.H., and Wong, J. (1984). Bronchoscopy and carcinoma of the esophagus II: carcinoma of the esophagus with tracheobronchial involvement. *Am. J. Surg.* 147: 760–762.
128 Argyros, G.J. and Torrington, K.G. (1994). Fiberoptic bronchoscopy in the evaluation of carcinoma metastatic to the lung. *Chest* 105: 454–457.
129 Poe, R.H., Ortiz, C., Isreal, R.H. et al. (1985). Sensitivity, specificity, and predictive values of bronchoscopy in neoplasm metastatic to lung. *Chest* 88: 84–88.
130 Pasoglu, I., Dogan, R., Demircin, M. et al. (1991). Bronchoscopic removal of foreign bodies in children: retrospective analysis of 822 cases. *Thorac. Cardiovasc. Surg.* 39: 95–98.
131 Weissberg, D. and Schwartz, I. (1987). Foreign bodies in the tracheobronchial tree. *Chest* 91: 730–773.
132 Cunanan, O.S. (1978). The flexible fiberoptic bronchoscope in foreign body removal: experience in 300 cases. *Chest* 73: 725–726.
133 Lan, R.S., Lee, C.H., Chaing, Y.C., and Wang, W.J. (1989). Use of fiberoptic bronchoscopy to retrieve bronchial foreign bodies in adults. *Am. Rev. Respir. Dis.* 140: 1734–1737.
134 Cha, S.I., Kim, C.H., Lee, J.H. et al. (2007). Isolated smoke inhalation injuries: acute respiratory dysfunction, clinical outcomes, and short-term evolution of pulmonary functions with the effects of steroids. *Burns* 33: 200–208.
135 Reichle, G. (2000). Argon plasma coagulation in bronchology: a new method – alternative or complimentary? *Pneumologie* 54 (11): 508–516.
136 Gerasin, V.A. and Shafrovsky, B.B. (1988). Endobronchial electrosurgery. *Chest* 93: 270–274.
137 Reddy, C., Majid, A., Michaud, G. et al. (2008). Gas embolism following bronchoscopic argon plasma coagulation: a case series. *Chest* 134: 1066–1069.
138 Feller-Kopman, D., Lukanich, J.M., Shapira, G. et al. (2008). Gas flow during bronchoscopic ablation therapy causes gas emboli to the heart: a comparative animal study. *Chest* 133:

139 Carpenter, R.J., Neel, H.B., and Sanderson, D.R. (1977). Cryosurgery of bronchopulmonary structures. *Chest* 72: 279–284.

140 Marasso, A., Gallo, E., Massaglia, G.M. et al. (1993). Cryosurgery in bronchoscopic treatment of tracheobronchial stenosis: indications, limits, personal experience. *Chest* 103: 472–474.

141 Walsh, D.A., Maiwand, M.O., Nath, A.R. et al. (1990). Bronchoscopic cryotherapy for advanced bronchial carcinoma. *Thorax* 45: 509–513.

142 Gage, A.A. and Baust, J.G. (2007). Cryosurgery for tumors. *J. Am. Coll. Surg.* 205: 342–356.

143 George, P.J.M. and Rudd, R.M. (1991). Bronchoscopic cryotherapy for advanced bronchial carcinoma. *Thorax* 46: 150.

144 Mathur, P.N., Wolf, K.M., Busk, M.F. et al. (1996). Fiberoptic bronchoscopiccryotherapy in the management of tracheobronchial obstruction. *Chest* 110 (3): 718–723.

145 Hetzel, M., Hetzel, J., Schumann, C. et al. (2004). Cryorecanalization: a new approach for the immediate management of acute airway obstruction. *J. Thorac. Cardiovasc. Surg.* 127: 1427–1431.

146 Browning, R., Parrish, S., Sarkar, S., and Turner, J.F. Jr. (2013). First report of a novel liquid nitrogen adjustable flow spray cryotherapy (SCT) device in the bronchoscopic treatment of disease of the central tracheo-bronchial airways. *J. Thorac. Dis.* 5 (3): E103–E106.

147 O'Connor, J.P., Hanley, B.M., Mulcahey, T.I. et al. (2017). N2 gas egress from patients' airways during LN2 spray cryotherapy. *Med. Eng. Phys.* 44: 63–72.

148 Browning, R., Turner, J.F. Jr., and Parrish, S. (2015). Spray cryotherapy (SCT): institutional evolution of techniques and clinical practice from early experience in the treatment of malignant airway disease. *J. Thorac. Dis.* 7 (Suppl 4): S405–S414.

149 Slebos, D.J., Breen, D., Coad, J. et al. (2017). Safety and histological effect of liquid nitrogen metered spray cryotherapy in the lung. *Am. J. Respir. Crit. Care Med.* 196 (10): 1351–1352.

150 Turner, J.F. and Wang, K.P. (1999). Endobronchial laser therapy. *Clin. Chest Med.* 20 (1): 107–122.

151 Brutinel, W.M., Cortese, D.A., McDougall, J.C. et al. (1987). A two-year experience with the neodymium-YAG laser in endobronchial obstruction. *Chest* 91: 159–165.

152 Cavaliere, S., Foccoli, P., and Farina, P.L. (1988). Nd:YAG laser bronchoscopy: a five-year experience with 1,396 applications in 1,000 patients. *Chest* 94: 15–21.

153 Unger, M. (1984). Bronchoscopic utilization of the Nd:YAG laser for obstructing lesions of the trachea and bronchi. *Surg. Clin. NorthAm.* 64: 931–938.

154 Unger, M. (1992). Lasers and their role in pulmonary medicine: present and future. In: Update: Pulmonary Diseases and Disorders (ed. A.P. Fishman), 419–432. New York: McGraw Hill.

155 Wang, K.P. and Turner, J.F. (1196). Nd:YAG resection of hamartoma. *J. Bronchol.* 3: 112–115.

156 Mehta, A.C. (1988). Laser applications in respiratory care. In: Current Respiratory Care (eds. R.M. Kacmarek and J.K. Stoller), 100–106. Toronto: Mosby-Year Book.

157 Wang, K.P. and Turner, J.F. (1995). Closure of bronchopleural fistula with Nd-YAG laser. *AJRCCM* 151: A847.

158 Wang, K.P., Schaeffer, L., Heitmiller, R. et al. (1993). Nd:YAG laser closure of a bronchopleural fistula. *Monaldi Arch. Chest Dis.* 48: 301–303.

159 Abramson, A.L., Shikowitz, M.J., Mullooly, V.M. et al. (1992). Clinical effects of photodynamic therapy on recurrent laryngeal papillomas. *Ann. Otol. Head Neck Surg.* 118: 25–29.

160 Patel, S.R., DeBoer, G., and Mehta, A.C. (1993). Role of photodynamic therapy in juvenile laryngotracheobronchial papillomatosis [abstract]. *Chest* 161S: 104.

161 Imamura, S., Kusunoki, Y., Takifuji, N. et al. (1994). Photodynamic therapy and/or external beam radiation therapy for roentgenological occult lung cancer. *Cancer* 73: 1608–1614.

162 Balchum, O. and Doiron, D.R. (1985). Photoradiation therapy of endobronchial lung cancer. *Clin. Chest Med.* 6: 255–275.

163 McCaughan, J.S. (1987). Overview of experience with photodynamic therapy for malignancies in 192 patients. *Photochem. Photobiol.* 46: 903–909.

164 Freitag, L., Ernst, A., Thomas, M. et al. (2004). Sequential photodynamic therapy (PDT) and high dose brachytherapy for endobronchial tumour control in patients with limited bronchogenic carcinoma. *Thorax* 59: 790–793.

165 Moghissi, K., Dixon, K., Thorpe, J.A. et al. (2007). Photodynamic therapy (PDT) in early central lung cancer: a treatment option for patients ineligible for surgical resection. *Thorax* 62: 391–395.

166 Dweik, R.A., Patel, S.R., and Mehta, A.C. (1994). Tracheal papillomatosis. *J. Bronchol.* 1: 226.

167 Paradelo, J.C., Waxman, M.J., Throne, B.J. et al. (1992). Endobronchial irradiation with 192Ir in the treatment of malignant endobronchial obstruction. *Chest* 102: 1072–1074.

168 Khanavkar, B., Stern, P., Alberti, W., and Nakhosteen, J.A. (1991). Complications associated with brachytherapy alone or with laser in lung cancer. *Chest* 99: 1062–1065.

169 Lee, W., Daly, B.D., DiPetrillo, T.A. et al. (2003). Limited resection for non-small cell lung cancer: observed local control with implantation of I-125 brachytherapy seeds. *Ann. Thorac. Surg.* 75: 237–242; discussion 242–233.

170 Goldstein, R.A., Rohatgi, P.K., Bergofsky, E.H., and Block, E.R. (1990). Clinical role of bronchoalveolar lavage in adults with pulmonary disease. *Am. Rev. Respir. Dis.* 142: 481–486.

171 Prakash, U.B.S., Barham, S., Carpenter, H.A. et al. (1987). Pulmonary alveolar phospholipoproteinosis: experience with 34 cases and a review. *Mayo Clin. Proc.* 62: 499–518.

172 Murray, M.J., DeRuyter, M.L., and Harrison, B.A. (1998). "How I do it" bilateral lung washings for pulmonary alveolar proteinosis. *J. Bronchol.* 5: 324–326.

173 Colt, H.G. (1995). "How I do it" bronchoalveolar lavage. *J.*

Bronchol. 2: 154–156.

174 Schwartz, D.B., Beals, T.F., Wimbish, K.J., and Hammersley, J.R. (1985). Transbronchial fine needle aspiration of bronchogenic cysts. *Chest* 88: 573–575.

175 Schwartz, A.R., Fishman, E.K., and Wang, K.P. (1986). Diagnosis and treatment of a bronchogenic cyst using transbronchial needle aspiration. *Thorax* 41: 326–327.

176 Delarue, N.C., Pearson, F.G., Nelems, J.M., and Cooper, J.D. (1980). Lung abscess: surgical implications. *Can. J. Surg.* 23: 297–302.

177 Estrera, A.S., Platt, M.R., Mills, L.J., and Shaw, R.R. (1980). Primary lung abscess. *J. Thorac. Cardiovasc. Surg.* 79: 275–282.

178 Connors, J.P., Roper, C.L., and Ferguson, T.B. (1975). Transbronchial catheterization of pulmonary abscesses. *Ann. Thorac. Surg.* 19: 254.

179 Colt, H.G., Janssen, J.P., Dumon, J.F., and Noirclerc, M.J. (1992). Endoscopic management of bronchial stenosis after double lung transplantation. *Chest* 102: 10–16.

180 Tsang, V. and Goldstraw, P. (1989). Endobronchial stenting for anastomotic stenosis after sleeve resection. *Ann. Thorac. Surg.* 48: 568–571.

181 Dumon, J.F. (1990). A dedicated tracheobronchial stent. *Chest* 97: 328–332.

182 deCastro, F.R., Lopez, L., Varela, A. et al. (1991). Tracheobronchial stents and fiberoptic bronchoscopy [letter]. *Chest* 99: 792.

183 Turner, J.F., Ernst, A., and Becker, H.D. (2000). "How I do it" rigid bronchoscopy. *J. Bronchol.* 7: 171–176.

184 Ayers, M.L. and Beamis, J.F. (2001). Rigid bronchoscopy in the twenty-first century. *Clin. Chest Med.* 22 (2): 355–364.

185 Hautmann, H., Gamarra, F., and Pfeifer, K.J. (2001). Fiberoptic bronchoscopic balloon dilatation in malignant tracheobronchial disease. *Chest* 120 (1): 43–49.

186 Andrews, B.T., Graham, S.M., Ross, A.F. et al. (2007). Technique, utility, and safety of awake tracheoplasty using combined laser and balloon dilation. *Laryngoscope* 117: 2159–2162.

187 Susanto, I., Peters, J.I., Levine, S.M. et al. (1998). Lung transplantation. Use of balloon-expandable metallic stents in the management of bronchial stenosis and bronchomalacia after lung transplantation. *Chest* 114 (5): 1330–1335.

188 Sheski, F.D. and Mathur, P.N. (1998). "How I do it" balloon bronchoplast using the flexible bronchoscope. *J. Bronchol.* 5: 242–246.

189 Baumann, M.H. and Sahn, S.A. (1990). Medical management and therapy of bronchopleural fistulas in the mechanically ventilated patient. *Chest* 97: 721–728.

190 Steiger, Z. and Wilson, R.F. (1984). Management of bronchopleural fistulas. *Surgery* 158: 267–271.

191 Regal, G., Sturm, A., Neumann, C. et al. (1989). Occlusion of bronchopleural fistula after lung injury: a new treatment by bronchoscopy. *J. Trauma* 29: 223–226.

192 Shah, A.M., Singhal, P., Chhajed, P.N. et al. (2004). Bronchoscopic closure of bronchopleural fistula using gelfoam. *J. Assoc. Physicians India* 52: 508–509.

193 Snell, G.I., Holsworth, L., Fowler, S. et al. (2005). Occlusion of a broncho-cutaneous fistula with endobronchial one-way valves. *Ann. Thorac. Surg.* 80: 1930–1932.

194 Ferguson, J.S., Sprenger, K., and van Natta, T. (2006). Closure of a bronchopleural fistula using bronchoscopic placement of an endobronchial valve designed for the treatment of emphysema. *Chest* 129: 479–481.

195 Travaline, J.M., McKenna, R.J. Jr., de Giacomo, T. et al. (2009). Treatment of persistent pulmonary air leaks using endobronchial valves. *Chest* 136: 355–360.

196 Campion, J.P., Bourdelat, D., and Launois, B. (1983). Surgical treatment of malignant esophagotracheal fistulas. *Am. J. Surg.* 148: 641–646.

197 Graeber, G.M., Farrell, B.G., Neville, J.F. Jr., and Parker, F.B. Jr. (1980). Successful diagnosis and management of fistulas between the aorta and the tracheobronchial tree. *Ann. Thorac. Surg.* 29: 555–561.

198 Ishizaki, Y., Tada, Y., Takagi, A. et al. (1990). Aortobronchial fistula after an aortic operation. *Ann. Thorac. Surg.* 50: 975–977.

199 Edens, E.T. and Sia, R.L. (1981). Flexible fiberoptic endoscopy in difficult intubations. *Ann. Otolaryngol.* 90: 307–309.

200 Dietrich, K.A., Strauss, R.H., Cabalka, A.K. et al. (1988). Use of flexible fiberoptic endoscopy for determination of endotracheal tube position in the pediatric patient. *Crit. Care Med.* 16: 884–887.

201 Streitz, J.M. and Shapshay, S.M. (1991). Airway injury after tracheotomy and endotracheal intubation. *Surg. Clin. North Am.* 71: 1211–1231.

202 Bishop, M.J. (1989). Mechanisms of laryngotracheal injury following prolonged tracheal intubation. *Chest* 96: 185–186.

203 Colice, G.L., Stukel, T.A., and Dain, B. (1989). Laryngeal complications of prolonged intubation. *Chest* 96: 877–884.

204 Whited, R.E. (1984). A prospective study of laryngotracheal sequelae on long term intubation. *Laryngoscope* 94: 376–377.

205 Kastanos, N., Estopa Miro, R., Marin Perez, A. et al. (1983). Laryngotracheal injury due to endotracheal intubation: incidence, evolution, and predisposing factors. A prospective long-term study. *Crit. Care Med.* 11: 362–367.

206 Rai, N.S., Mehta, A.C., Meeker, D.P., and Stoller, J.K. (1994). Transtracheal oxygen therapy – does practice make perfect? *J. Bronchol.* 1: 205–212.

207 Orkin, S.H., Motulsky, A.G. (1996). Report and recommendations of the panel to assess the NIH investment in research on gene therapy. NIH, Bethesda, MD.

208 Mastrangeli, A., Harvey, B.G., and Crystal, R.G. (1997). Gene therapy for lung disease. In: *The Lung: Scientific Foundation*, 2e (eds. R.G. Crystal, J.B. West, E.R. Wibel, et al.), 2795. Philadelphia: Lippincott-Raven.

209 Rochlitz, C.F. (2000). Gene therapy for lung cancer. In: *Interventional Bronchoscopy*, vol. 30 (eds. C.T. Bolliger and P.N. Mathur), 280–289. Basel: Karger.

210 Kruklitis, R.J. and Sterman, D.H. (2004). Endobronchial gene therapy. *Semin. Respir. Crit. Care Med.* 25: 433–442.

211 Cox, G., Thomson, N.C., Rubin, A.S. et al. (2007). Asthma control during the year after bronchial thermoplasty. *N. Engl.*

212 Pavord, I.D., Cox, G., Thomson, N.C. et al. (2007). Safety and efficacy of bronchial thermoplasty in symptomatic, severe asthma. *Am. J. Respir. Crit. Care Med.* 176: 1185–1191.

213 Thomson, N.C., Rubin, A.S., Niven, R.M. et al. (2011). Long-term (5 year) safety of bronchial thermoplasty: Asthma Intervention Research (AIR) trial. *BMC Pulm. Med.* 11: 8.

214 Chupp, G., Laviolette, M., Cohn, L. et al. (2017). Long-term outcomes of bronchial thermoplasty in subjects with severe asthma: a comparison of 3-year follow-up results from two prospective multicentre studies. *Eur. Respir. J.* 50.

215 Fishman, A., Martinez, F., Naunheim, K. et al. (2003). A randomized trial comparing lung-volume-reduction surgery with medical therapy for severe emphysema. *N. Engl. J. Med.* 348: 2059–2073.

216 Strange, C., Herth, F.J., Kovitz, K.L. et al. (2007). Design of the Endobronchial Valve for Emphysema Palliation Trial (VENT): a non-surgical method of lung volume reduction. *BMC Pulm. Med.* 7: 10.

217 Wood, D.E., McKenna, R.J. Jr., Yusen, R.D. et al. (2007). A multicenter trial of an intrabronchial valve for treatment of severe emphysema. *J. Thorac. Cardiovasc. Surg.* 133: 65–73.

218 Choong, C.K., Cardoso, P.F., Sybrecht, G.W. et al. (2009). Airway bypass treatment of severe homogeneous emphysema: taking advantage of collateral ventilation. *Thorac. Surg. Clin.* 19: 239–245.

219 Reilly, J., Washko, G., Pinto-Plata, V. et al. (2007). Biological lung volume reduction: a new bronchoscopic therapy for advanced emphysema. *Chest* 131: 1108–1113.

220 Ingenito, E.P., Wood, D.E., and Utz, J.P. (2008). Bronchoscopic lung volume reduction in severe emphysema. *Proc. Am. Thorac. Soc.* 5: 454–460.

221 Criner, G.J., Sue, R., Wright, S. et al. (2018). A multicenter RCT of Zephyr® endobronchial valve treatment in heterogeneous emphysema (LIBERATE). *Am. J. Respir. Crit. Care Med.* 198: 1151–1164.

222 Pereira, W. Jr., Kovnat, D.M., and Snider, G.L. (1978). A prospective cooperative study of complications following flexible fiberoptic bronchoscopy. *Chest* 73: 813–816.

223 Suratt, P.M., Smiddy, J.F., and Gruber, B. (1976). Deaths and complications associated with fiberoptic bronchoscopy. *Chest* 69: 747–751.

224 Burgher, L.W., Jones, F.L., Patterson, J.R., and Selecky, P.A. (1987). Guidelines for fiberoptic bronchoscopy in adults. *Am. Rev. Respir. Dis.* 136: 1066.

225 Katz, A.S., Michelson, E.L., Stawicki, J., and Holford, F.D. (1981). Cardiac arrhythmias: frequency during fiberoptic bronchoscopy and correlation with hypoxemia. *Arch. Intern. Med.* 141: 603–606.

226 Matot, I., Kramer, M.R., Glantz, L. et al. (1997). Myocardial ischemia in sedated patients undergoing fiberoptic bronchoscopy. *Chest* 112 (6): 1454–1458.

227 Dunagan, D.P., Burke, H.L., and Aquino, S.L. (1998). Fiberoptic bronchoscopy in coronary care unit patients. *Chest* 114 (6): 1660–1667.

228 Kvale, P.A. (1996). Is it really safe to perform bronchsocpy after a recent myocardial infarction? *Chest* 110 (3): 592.

229 Liebler, J.M. (2000). Fiberoptic bronchoscopy for diagnosis and treatment. *Crit. Care Clin.* 16 (1): 83–100.

230 Dweik, R.A., Mehta, A.C., Meeker, D.P., and Arroliga, A.C. (1996). Analysis of the safety of bronchoscopy after recent acute myocardial infarction. *Chest* 110 (3): 825–828.

231 Matot, I., Drenger, B., Glantz, L. et al. (1999). Coronary spasm during outpatient fiberoptic laser bronchsocpy. *Chest* 115 (6): 1744–1746.

232 Bein, T. and Pfeifer, M. (1997). Fiberoptic bronchoscopy after recent acute myocarcial infarciton: stress for the heart? *Chest* 112 (1): 295–296.

233 Prakash, U.B.S. and Stubbs, S.E. (1991). The bronchoscopy survey: some reflections. *Chest* 100: 1660–1667.

234 Ernst, A., Eberhardt, R., Wahidi, M. et al. (2006). Effect of routine clopidogrel use on bleeding complications after transbronchial biopsy in humans. *Chest* 129: 734–737.

235 Sun, S.W., Zabaneh, R.N., and Carrey, Z. (2003). Incidence of pneumothorax after fiberoptic bronchoscopy (FOB) in community-based hospital; are routine post-procedure chest roentgenograms necessary? *Chest* 124 (4): 145.

236 Hattotuwa, K., Gamble, E.A., O'Shaughnessy, T. et al. (2002). Safety of bronchoscopy, biopsy, and BAL in research patients with COPD. *Chest* 122: 1909–1912.

第 7 章

径向探头超声技术在可弯曲支气管镜中的应用

Noriaki Kurimoto[1], Takeshi Isobe[1], Takeo Inoue[2], and Teruomi Miyazawa[2]

[1] Division of Medical Oncology and Respiratory Medicine,
Department of Internal Medicine, Shimane University Hospital, Izumo, Japan
[2] Division of Respiratory Medicine, Department of Internal Medicine,
St Marianna University School of Medicine, Kawasaki, Japan

（译者：侯 刚 译者单位：中日友好医院）

7.1 引言

支气管镜检查期间使用的径向超声探头，通过旋转发射超声波并获得返回波的图像，产生支气管和周围结构的短轴图像。当从侧面观察径向超声探头时，探头的表面是凹形的，因此在距离探头 5~10 mm 处有一个超声聚焦区域。与其他区域相比，聚焦区域的超声图像具有较高的图像质量，这对评估疾病的性质具有重要意义。径向超声小探头的频率通常为 20 MHz，同样也有用于消化道的 30 MHz 超声探头。由于 20 MHz 探头具有较高的频率，因此探头的分辨率也较高；但其观察区域仅在探头周围半径的 1 cm 范围内，穿透距离较短。由于径向超声探头使用时周围存在介质，如果长时间使用，探头表面会产生气泡。被气泡覆盖的超声探头暂时无法获取超声图像，而通过摆动移除探头表面的气泡，则可以继续获得超声图像。

自 1994 年以来，笔者团队已经使用径向超声探头进行经支气管镜肺外周病变的诊断。径向支气管腔内超声检查（endobronchial ultrasonography，EBUS）对肺外周病变诊断的最大优势是能够实时详细地识别病变的位置。这意味着操作者可以观察探头是否位于病变内、邻近病变或远离病变。笔者团队正在研究如何利用肺外周病变的内部结构进行定性诊断。Ⅰ型——内部回声均匀，多提示良性病变；Ⅱ型——较多高回声小点，高度怀疑腺癌；Ⅲ型——内部回声异质性，多提示恶性病变。通过径向 EBUS 确定病变位置后，将引导鞘（guide sheath, GS）放置在该位置，然后进行活检。

在本章中，详细介绍了在笔者医院进行 EBUS-GS 操作的具体步骤，希望对医师在临床实践中实施 EBUS-GS 有所帮助。

7.2 EBUS-GS 的操作步骤

7.2.1 支气管镜检查前的准备

首先，需要考虑患者是否需进行支气管镜检查。根据笔者的经验，如果 1~2 mm 的薄层胸部 CT 显示支气管在肺部病变内部或旁边，那么使用 EBUS-GS 对肺外周病变具有可观的诊断率，并且并发症较少。其次，需要考虑患者的一般状况是否可以耐受支气管镜检查。

此外，与临床主管医生沟通患者是否应该停用抗凝/抗血小板药物，如果需要停用，则应进一步明确是否需要肝素化。

手术前应准备好支气管镜、超声探头等设备,并联系进行支气管镜检查的支气管镜医师和助手。

在对肺外周病变进行支气管镜检查前,应通过 CT 或虚拟支气管镜导航(virtual bronchoscopic navigation,VBN)确认病灶周围支气管的分布。当病灶中存在多条支气管路径时,应对最适合活检的支气管路径进行排序。分析 CT 解剖结构时,应在纸上绘制出手绘支气管导航图(图 7.1)。

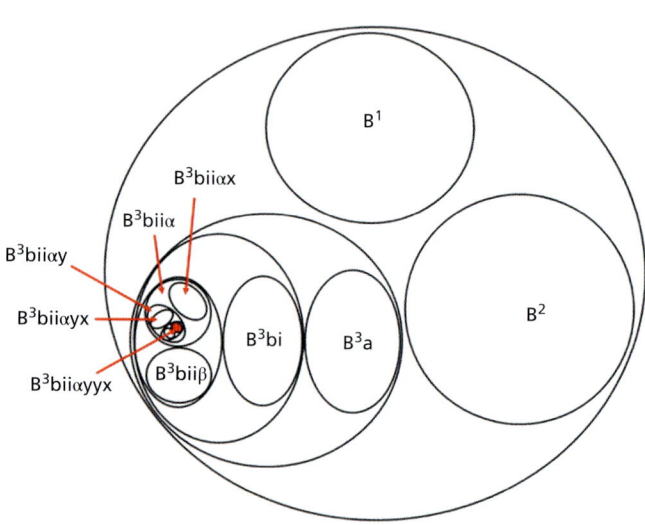

图 7.1　支气管分支手绘导航图
在对右侧 B^3b 支气管进行检查时,CT 解剖显示支气管($B^3bii\alpha yyx$)与病变相连。

7.2.2　在支气管镜检查室的准备工作

需要向参加支气管镜检查的护士、影像学技师、医生等介绍此次支气管镜检查的目的、注意事项、并发症等(快速信息传递:在笔者医院约 3 min)。

在进行支气管镜检查前,打开 GS 套件并准备 GS、刷子和活检钳。刷子和活检钳均应在 GS 中各自插入一个止动器,使刷子外鞘的尖端正好位于 GS 尖端,活检钳打开的钳杯应尽可能靠近 GS 尖端,并调整制动器的位置,使活检杯下端的铰链刚好从 GS 中出来。将超声探头固定在 GS 的近端,使二者成为一体(需要注意的是,在此固定状态下集成的超声探头和 GS 称为超声探头/GS)。

将超声探头连接到探头驱动单元时,请在超声主机关闭的情况下连接。连接后,按激活按钮激活超声机。如果连接成功,显示器上会显示 20 MHz 的频率。当在支气管镜检查之前解除 EBUS 图像的冻结并执行径向扫描时,探头周围出现多个圆形回波,这些回波是探头外壁的反射。如果看不到这多个圆形回波,则超声波探头表面的介质中存在气泡的可能性很高。此时,应将探头对着探头尖端用力摇晃或旋转探头,使气泡从表面移动到探头近端。设置超声波机时应记住的要点:① 将方向(超声波图像的观察方向)设为反向(从探头前方朝向探头前端获取图像);② 设为 I(图像);③ 保持增益和对比度恒定;④ 将超声波检查调整控制设为 0。

7.2.3　咽/喉麻醉前注意事项

1)首先,请患者说出自己的姓名和出生日期,或说出姓名并用腕带确认身份证。
2)确认利多卡因过敏史。
3)确认既往病史、停用药物等。
4)测量患者生命体征、SpO_2 等。

7.2.4　咽/喉麻醉

将 10 mL 2% 利多卡因倒入杰克逊喷雾器中。将喷雾器的喷嘴尖端慢慢地放入咽部,然后在患者吸气的同时向咽部和喉部喷射约 4 次,休息 20~30 s。随后,喷嘴的尖端指向声门。同样,当患者吸气时,在咽部和喉部喷 4 次。然后,等待 20~30 s 并重复上述过程,直至使用完约 10 mL 2% 利多卡因。注意事项包括:① 测量患者的生命体征、SpO_2 等;② 由于患者可能走路不稳,助手应紧靠患者以防摔倒。

7.2.5　进入支气管镜检查室

1)请患者说出自己的姓名和出生日期,或请患者说出姓名并用腕带确认身份证。
2)当患者处于仰卧位时,其头部应尽可能靠近支气管镜医师。
3)调整床的高度,使患者的鼻子和嘴与支气管镜医师髂前上棘的高度大致相同。
4)注射镇静剂前,握住口器。

7.2.6　支气管镜的插入

内窥镜制造商强调使用 A5 的对比度用于白色光和 B8 的对比度用于窄带成像(narrow-band imaging,NBI),这提供了最佳的支气管镜图像。

握住支气管镜手柄的下部。上/下杆可以通过拇指末端指骨的中心部分抓握并进行操作，这样可以在手掌中留有较大空间。

在拿起支气管镜的同时，操作者用右手的拇指、示指和中指抓住距尖端约 5 cm 的区域，并将其引导到口腔中。此后，操作者将内窥镜放入和取出，同时将右手的小拇指抵在患者的脸颊。内窥镜应从右嘴角和咽部稍微向右通过（以便右手操作者将小拇指固定在右脸颊上，使其从右嘴角通过右侧）。

从支气管镜的工作通道注入 1 mL 1% 盐酸利多卡因 2 次以遍布声带。当进入气管时，将 1 mL 1% 盐酸利多卡因在气管的上 1/3 处喷洒 1~2 次。从无病变的一侧支气管开始观察。例如，如果右侧有病变，则从左侧支气管开始观察。在左主支气管注射 1 mL 1% 盐酸利多卡因 1 次。继续向左上叶支气管和左下叶支气管注射 1 mL 1% 盐酸利多卡因各 1 次。然后，观察 B^{1+2} 至 B^{10} 的支气管。在观察过程中，记录静止图像，以便可以按照 B^{1+2} 到 B^{10} 的数字顺序看到亚段支气管。

内窥镜不断沿支气管管腔中心移动。然后，将内窥镜尖端朝向下一个分支的分叉（间嵴）推进，转向目标支气管，到达分叉（间嵴）前方。如果存在盲点，稍微拉回支气管镜观察。在拍摄静态图像时，如果操作者尝试在构图时将支气管分叉部分置于屏幕的一角拍摄，则在支气管镜检查结束后回顾支气管镜结果时很容易确认具体部位。

当有明显的支气管镜检查异常时，拍摄 3 种图像：远距离视图、中距离视图和近距离视图。在远距离视图中，观察周围支气管上皮的情况（检查是否存在肥大、萎缩等）并掌握病变的全貌。在中距离视图中，用白色光和 NBI 观察，并评估血管分布是否均匀，排列是否均匀。在近距离视图中，用白色光和 NBI 观察，并评估血管是否有扩张、弯曲或口径变化。

通过向每个肺叶支气管注射 1 mL 1% 盐酸利多卡因 1 次来观察患侧。之后，从 B^1 至 B^{10} 开始观察支气管。

7.2.7 肺外周病变的处理方法

当观察右侧和左侧支气管完成后，返回到病变的叶支气管之前，需根据手绘导航或 VBN 的结果进行下一步操作。助手会旋转手绘导航图（位于支气管镜监视器图像旁边）或 VBN 图像（放置在更接近支气管镜监视器的位置，如果它与支气管镜镜下结果显示在同一监视器上则更好）。助手会在手绘导航图或 VBN 图像上指向下一个要观察的支气管。

一般来说，操作员并不是看手绘导航图或 VBN 图像，而是观看显示支气管镜检查的显示器。

从叶支气管的入口开始，应在一个角落拍摄带有支气管分叉的静止图像，并逐级向外周推进。在观察支气管镜检查结果时，支气管镜医师将镜头尖端推向支气管分叉处，并在接触到支气管间嵴之前改变其方向，以便进一步进入目标支气管。在推动支气管管腔的同时，逐渐推进内窥镜至外周，当越过支气管间嵴时，应贴近并沿着位于支气管间嵴对面的支气管壁，使其越过支气管间嵴。

将支气管镜紧密嵌合在支气管，并通过内镜工作通道注入 1 mL 生理盐水冲洗。将总计 5~10 mL 生理盐水注入支气管，称为生理盐水注射技术。当整个外周病变为纯磨玻璃样阴影（ground glass opacity, GGO）或部分实性病变伴小实性部分时，不应进行这种盐水注射技术。因为当进行盐水注射疗法时，正常肺也出现高回声小点，此时不能区分 GGO 和正常肺。

操作者将内窥镜推向外周，助手用左手从工作通道的对侧抓住支气管镜，用右手将探头/GS 从工作通道插入支气管。

7.2.8 插入探头/GS

当探头/GS 插入工作通道时，可以将工作通道内的生理盐水推入支气管，并且可以在插入探头/GS 的同时清楚地观察支气管腔。由于支气管镜工作通道的尖端出口位于 3 点钟位置，如果支气管镜尖端位于狭窄的支气管内，则探头/GS 可能从支气管间嵴进入右侧分支。如果发生这种情况，操作者可能会看到一种现象，即支气管壁从监视器的 3 点钟位置略微突出。此时，应旋转并弯曲内窥镜尖端，使其面向 9 点钟方向，将探头/GS 拉回内窥镜末端并再次插入，如果仍然无法进入，则轻轻拉动内窥镜本身，然后旋转并弯曲内窥镜尖端，以便您可以将探头/GS 再次插入目标支气管。

将透视图像旋转 180° 并进行调整，使透视视图的底部为患者的头侧，透视视图的顶部为患者的尾侧，透视视图的右侧为患者的右侧。通过这种旋转，操作者可以感觉到内窥镜尖端的移动与控制上/下操作杆的手指的移动相关联。

根据手绘导航图和 VBN 图像，估算从内窥镜尖端到病变的距离并插入探头/GS。如果存在插入阻力，则在该位置停止并检查透视图像上的探头/GS 位置。

通过感觉将探头/GS 插入病变后，利用透视检查放置部位，之后解除冻结状态并进行扫描。原则上，使用透视的时间应当尽可能缩短,并且通过使用放射防护用具尽可能地减少辐射暴露。

7.2.9 EBUS 图像的评估

当 EBUS 可以显示病变时,将探头从病变的远端边缘移动到近端边缘,同时扫描整个病变。观察整个病变的内部结构,并评估内部回声的均匀性、血管的开口、高回声小点以及高回声弧线样改变。EBUS 对肺外周病变的分型有助于良/恶性的鉴别:如良性病变中肺炎与机化性肺炎的鉴别、恶性病变中高分化腺癌与低分化腺癌的鉴别等。

当内部回声均匀时归类为Ⅰ型,内部回声不均匀时归类为Ⅲ型,而病变中可见高回声小点时则归类为Ⅱ型。其中,Ⅰ型(内部回声均匀)可进一步分为:Ⅰa型(怀疑肺炎等)——病灶内可以见到自由舒缩的血管;Ⅰb型(怀疑机化性肺炎)——病灶内没有血管。Ⅲ型(内部回声不均匀)可进一步分为:Ⅲa型(包括多种恶性肿瘤)——伴有高回声短线的非均质性图像;Ⅲb型(低分化腺癌)——不伴有高回声短线的非均质性图像。Ⅱ型(病变中可见高回声小点)可进一步分为:Ⅱa型——不伴有血管显像(病灶中有含气的肺泡结构,阻碍了血管的显像);Ⅱb型——伴有血管显像(随着癌细胞密度增加,病变中残留气体减少,超声穿透更深)。纯 GGO 仅在探头附近具有高回声小点,被归类为Ⅱa型。

在类型分类中,我们关注的要点是病变内部回声的一致性以及病变内是否存在血管。关于内部回声的一致性,我们观察病变中散斑的对齐程度。当散斑分布均匀(即同心圆结构)时,超声波可以深入穿透,即使在距离探头超过 1 cm 的区域,图像通常也很亮。

当散斑分布不均匀(即无同心圆结构)时,超声图像的衰减较强,以至于距离探头约 1 cm 的区域变得较暗。病变内可见血管显像的类型为Ⅰa 和Ⅱb,推测为软组织病变(图 7.2)。

需要注意的是,具有疑似坏死表现的病变被分类为Ⅲa 型,即病变内部为无回声区域(将探头从远端缩回至近端,无回声区域的不连续表明它不是血管),这种情况下高度怀疑鳞癌。在段支气管以外的支气管区域,处于病灶内的探头周围出现的高回声环被怀疑是由肿瘤引起的支气管壁扩张。我们认为源自支气管的病变将支气管壁推向外侧,这种征象提示鳞癌或小细胞癌。

7.2.10 探头/GS 位置的调整

当引导探头/GS 进入病变内部时,将 GS 留在原位,并将刷子和活检钳插入 GS,以进行刷检和活检。即使探头/GS 被引导至病变处,EBUS 图像也无法被检测到(不可见),此时可以引导探头/GS 至远离病灶的支气管处。再次核对手绘导航或 VBN 图像,明确进入的支气管是否正确。如果第一个路径是错误的,重新尝试沿着正确的路线引导探头/GS 至靶病灶处。

当操作者可以通过透视设备识别病变位置时,旋转 X 线 C 臂,使病变位置距离探头/GS 尖端最远,或改变患者的体位(抬高右背部等)。如果通过观察透视图像发现病变位置距离探头/GS 尖端最远,则使用支气管镜的上/下角度杆弯曲支气管镜尖端以抵近病变。当操作者在保持支气管镜角度的同时撤回探头/GS 并重新插入时,如果存在通向病变的支气管,则可能会到达病变。如果透视设备上无法识别病变位置,那么可以在支气管镜检查前在 CT 定位图像上添加一个指向病变位置的箭头。在完成手绘导航或 VBN 后,将

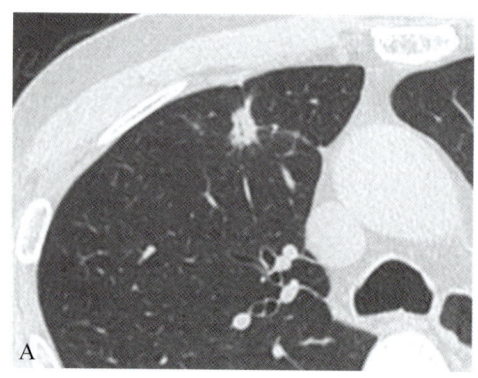
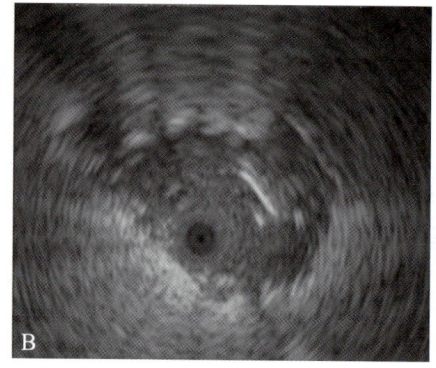
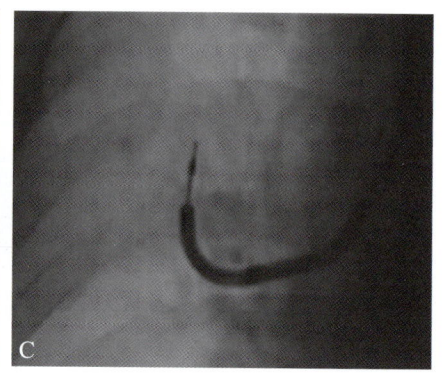

图 7.2 代表性案例

A. 该病变位于右肺 S^3b;B. EBUS 图像分为Ⅱ型和Ⅱb 型,Ⅱ型病变中发现高回声小点,Ⅱb 型病变中伴有血管显像(随着癌细胞密度增加,病变中残留气体减少,超声穿透更深);C. 显示探头/GS 位置的透视图像,X 线透视上未清楚显示病变。

探头/GS 的尖端引导至病变中的支气管，如果病灶在 EBUS 图像上可见并位于箭头周围时，则进行刷检和活检。如果病灶在 EBUS 图像上不可见，则在 CT 定位图像上的箭头区域进行刷检和活检。

当探头/GS 被引导至病变处，并且探头邻近 EBUS 图像上的病变边缘时，将需要进行 3 种操作。第 1 种操作是使用上/下角度杆弯曲支气管镜尖端，观察探头是否接近 EBUS 图像上的病变。例如，当应用向上角度时，探头接近 EBUS 图像上的病变。然后，尝试拉回并插入探头/GS，在抵近病灶的过程中保持内窥镜弯曲。如果支气管朝向病变分叉，则有可能将探头/GS 插入病变内（在超声导引下）。

在第 2 种操作中，当探头未接近病变时，通过使用上/下角度杆弯曲支气管镜尖端，探头在 EBUS 图像中沿病变边缘的切线方向移动。即使在支气管镜绕自身轴顺时针或逆时针旋转的情况下应用上/下角度变换，探头也会在 EBUS 图像上沿病变的切线方向移动。在某些病例中使用该操作方法可使探头接近 EBUS 图像上的病变。尝试拉回并插入探头/GS，在保持内窥镜弯曲的同时去抵近病灶。如果支气管超向病变分叉，则有可能将探头/GS 插入病变内（在超声导引下旋转支气管镜）。

如果在执行上述两个步骤后仍无法改变情况，需要第 3 种操作。将探头/GS 引导到病变附近的支气管位置，并使用上/下角度或旋转支气管镜使探头尖端更靠近病变。如果它靠近病变，用活检钳以定位活检组织，将 GS 的尖端留在该位置（精确活检）。当支气管壁和病变之间存在血管时，不要活检。在精确活检中，应轻轻推动活检钳以穿过支气管壁进行活检。因此，存在活检钳的尖端从病变移位并滑动到周边的可能性，鉴于此，需要在透视图像上仔细观察镊子尖端的移动。

7.2.11　将 GS 尖端保持在准确位置

执行上述程序并将 GS 放置到位。届时有一些具体问题需要注意。在 EBUS-GS 活检钳中，活检钳杯在远离 GS 尖端约 4 mm 的位置打开，并对该部位进行活检。因此，操作者需要将 GS 尖端放置在病变内近侧或病变近端。此外，GS 可由于呼吸而在支气管中移动。当 GS 尖端越过病变而到达更外周时，则无法获得病变的标本。

为了明确 GS 与病变之间的位置关系，将探头缓慢拉入 GS 并仔细观察 EBUS 图像。当探头的换能器完全在 GS 内时，EBUS 图像突然变暗，并且当探头稍

微离开 GS 时，它突然变亮。因此，当 EBUS 图像突然变暗时，将其设置为 EBUS 图像上的病变内近侧或病变近端附近，GS 的尖端位置变得更靠近病变内近侧或病变近端（图 7.3）。

7.2.12　刷检和活检技巧

对于刷检和活检，在三个点需要进行固定，包括：支气管镜医师在工作通道管口周围的 GS 上方抓握活检钳；第一助手将探头鞘管外的固定锁卡锁至活检口塞的凹槽里；第二助手在口腔或鼻腔出口附近握住支气管镜，以使活检钳不会在质地硬的病灶表面打滑。助手推动毛刷，在感受病变硬度的同时决定毛刷的远端位置。助手使毛刷在病灶远端和病灶中央之间刷检（避免从病灶远端刷到病灶周围）。

对于活检，将活检钳放入 GS 后，助手打开活检钳，外科医师在 GS 上方抓住活检钳，用闭合的钳杯抵住病变，然后打开钳杯。由于病变较硬，通常很难打开病变内的钳杯，但当操作者在打开活检钳时反复戳动活检钳，钳杯通常会打开。在确认以上 3 点固定后，支气管镜医师将打开的钳杯轻轻抵住病灶，第一助手慢慢闭合钳杯 3~5 s 以咬住组织。随后，第一助手用左手（右手为关闭活检钳的手）在略靠近 GS 出口的部位握住透明鞘管。抓住 GS 的出口并用右手拉动活检钳，透明鞘管可能变得像风箱一样，并且难以传递拉回活检钳的力。

刷检 5 次和活检 5 次交替进行，但如果刷检时出血过多，活检次数会相应减少。我们将 GS 留在活检部位附近止血约 2 min，然后将其撤回。出血很少时继续，然后将支气管镜楔入目标支气管。在确认止血后，我们连接收集支气管灌洗液的容器。

7.3　EBUS 在肺外周病变中的应用进展

Hürter 等[1]首次报道了径向 EBUS 在肺外周病变中的应用。笔者团队在 1994 年报道了径向 EBUS 在消化系统中的应用，他们将直径为 2.5 mm 的超声探头（UM-3R，奥林巴斯）插入到工作通道为 2.8 mm 的支气管镜中。尽管探头具有 2.5 mm 的直径，但其尖端是圆形的，因此它可以被引导至胸膜下直径为 1 mm 的支气管。尽管人们普遍认为肺因其含有大量的空气而不适合使用超声波，但对于含气较少的肺外周病变，

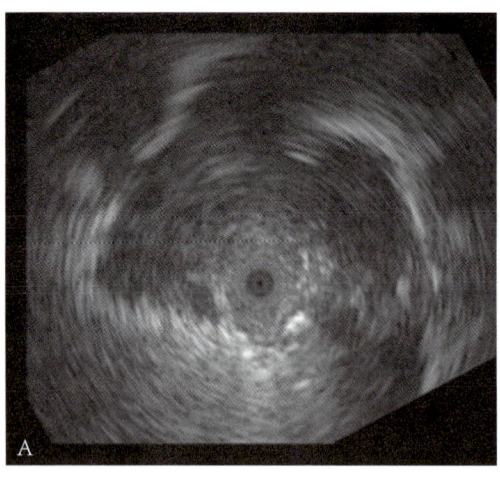 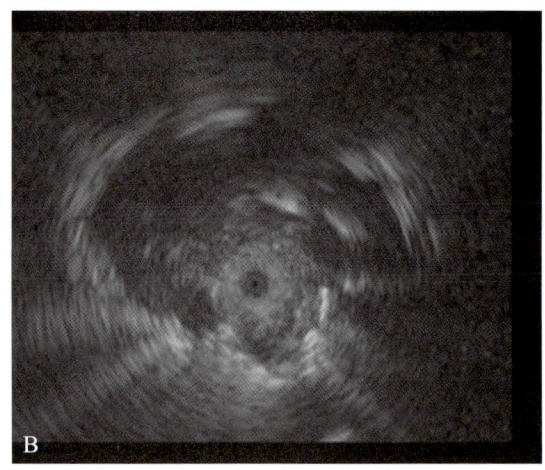

图 7.3 确认 GS 的位置

为了明确 GS 与病变之间的位置关系,将探头缓慢拉入 GS 并仔细观察 EBUS 图像。A. 当探头的换能器完全位于 GS 内时,EBUS 图像突然变暗;B. 当探头稍微离开 GS 时,它突然变亮。

通过超声波可以清楚地显示,并且以难以显示的肺作为背景,肺外周病变很容易被识别。

此外,超声波为 20 MHz,频率较高,能详细描绘病变的内部结构。我们将术前 EBUS 图像与手术标本进行对比,发现 EBUS 可以识别肺外周病变的血管、支气管、坏死、钙化、出血等[2]。此外,根据肺外周病变 EBUS 图像内部回声的均匀性、是否存在血管显像以及是否存在高回声小点和弧线样改变进行声像类型的分类。

在将径向超声探头插入肺外周病变获得 EBUS 图像后,需要移除探头并插入刷子和活检钳。当然,如果操作者拔出探头,病变有时会有大量出血,我们再插入活检刷和活检钳就很困难。因此,将鞘管套在超声探头上,并将其重新引导至病变处。1996 年,笔者团队开始仅将鞘管放置在病变中,随后插入刷子和活检钳。起初鞘管内插入 2.5 mm 探头,需要直径为 2.8 mm 的工作通道的支气管镜。他们报告使用此 GS 的 EBUS-GS 对肺外周病变的诊断率为 77%。另外,探头位于病变内的"内"状态下的诊断率约为探头与病变接触的"邻近"状态下的诊断率的 2 倍[3]。之后,其他机构也相继报告了 EBUS-GS 诊断率,并通过荟萃分析评估了 EBUS-GS 的有效性[4]。

此后,对影响 EBUS-GS 诊断率的因素也不断被报道,如"CT 支气管征"(CT 图像上支气管进入病变)[5]、"within"(探头位于病变内)[3]、活检次数[6]等,据报道,当进行 5~6 次活检时,诊断率达到阈值。随着 CT 的普及,以 GGO 为主的病变逐渐增多,关于其在 EBUS 图像上的表现也有讨论[7,8]。笔者团队认为,GGO 病变可能在 EBUS 图像上观察到高回声小点,这认为是残留在肺泡中的空气的反射引起的。

在其他国家和地区,应用径向 EBUS 检查肺外周病变在 2013 年 ACCP 指南[9]中已成为 Ic 级别推荐,并且正在逐渐推广应用,特别是在澳大利亚、泰国和中国台湾地区。

7.4 未来展望

如何诊断肺外周病变是目前关注的问题。由于支气管镜可以尽可能地插入外周支气管,因此这有利于选择支气管并插入探头/GS。在支气管镜操作中,抽吸痰和血液是必要的,因此支气管镜的工作通道的直径必须足够大。在笔者团队的临床经验中,当工作通道直径为 1.2 mm 时,很难抽吸,而工作通道直径 2 mm 时就可以充分进行抽吸,最佳直径可能接近 2 mm,即 1.2~2.0 mm。

最近,在日本,已经可以使用外径为 3 mm、工作通道直径为 1.7 mm 的支气管镜。Oki 等报道称,3 mm 的支气管镜联合径向超声探头而不使用 GS 的诊断率优于应用 4 mm 支气管镜联合 EBUS-GS 的诊断率。然而,对于这种仅使用超声探头而不使用 GS 的 3 mm 内窥镜,很难确认活检钳是否在对同一病变部位进行活检。此外,由于支气管镜的尖端是柔性的,其形状可能在活检后发生改变,并且可能难以将活检钳再放入同一支气管中。因此，需要更多关于该技术的研究报告来评估其有效性。

此外，目前应用的 EBUS-GS 技术，无法在刷检和活检期间实时进行 EBUS 操作。在不久的将来，如果凸阵扫描超声支气管镜的直径能够进一步缩小，那么在肺外周进行 EBUS-TBNA 将成为可能，并且能够实现"实时"活检。

参考文献

1. Hürter, T. and Hanrath, P. (1990). Endobronchial sonography in the diagnosis of pulmonary and mediastinal tumors. *Dtsch. Med. Wochenschr.* 115 (50): 1899–1905.
2. Kurimoto, N., Murayama, M., Yoshioka, S., and Nishisaka, T. (2002). Analysis of the internal structure of peripheral pulmonary lesions using endobronchial ultrasonography. *Chest* 122: 1887–1894.
3. Kurimoto, N., Miyazawa, T., Okimasa, S. et al. (2004). Endobronchial ultrasonography using a guide sheath increases the ability to diagnose peripheral pulmonary lesions endoscopically. *Chest* 126: 959–965.
4. Steinfort, D., Khor, Y., Manser, R. et al. (2011 Apr). Radial probe endobronchial ultrasound for the diagnosis of peripheral lung cancer: systematic review and meta-analysis. *Eur. Respir. J.* 37 (4): 902–910.
5. Minezawa, T., Okamura, T., Yatsuya, H. et al. (2015). Bronchus sign on thin-section computed tomography is a powerful predictive factor for successful transbronchial biopsy using endobronchial ultrasound with a guide sheath for small peripheral lung lesions: a retrospective observational study. *BMC Med. Imaging* 15: 21.
6. Yamada, N., Yamazaki, K., Kurimoto, N. et al. (2007). Factors related to diagnostic yield of transbronchial biopsy using endobronchial ultrasonography with a guide sheath in small peripheral pulmonary lesions. *Chest* 132 (2): 603–608.
7. Nakai, T., Matsumoto, Y., Suzuk, F. et al. (2017). Predictive factors for a successful diagnostic bronchoscopy of ground-glass nodules. *Ann. Thorac. Med.* 12 (3): 171–176.
8. Ikezawa, Y., Shinagawa, N., Sukoh, N. et al. (2017). Usefulness of endobronchial ultrasonography with a guide sheath and virtual bronchoscopic navigation for ground-glass opacity lesions. *Ann. Thorac. Surg.* 103 (2): 470–475.
9. Detterbeck, F.C., Lewis, S.Z., Diekemper, R. et al. (2013). Executive summary: diagnosis and management of lung cancer, 3rd ed: American College of Chest Physicians evidence-based clinical practice guidelines. *Chest* 143 (5 suppl): 7S–37S.

第 8 章

凸阵扫描超声支气管镜在可弯曲支气管镜中的应用

Andrew Pattison and Kazuhiro Yasufuku
Division of Thoracic Surgery, Toronto General Hospital, University Health Network,
University of Toronto, Toronto, Ontario, Canada
（译者：郑筱轩　译者单位：上海交通大学医学院附属胸科医院）

8.1 凸阵扫描超声支气管镜

8.1.1 发展史

约15年前，凸阵扫描超声支气管镜（convex-probe endobronchial ultrasonography，CP-EBUS）在多种临床实践中开始应用。最成熟和公认的临床应用就是支气管内超声引导下经支气管针吸活检（endobronchial ultrasound-guided transbronchial needle aspiration，EBUS-TBNA），特别是在侵袭性肺癌的纵隔分期中。CP-EBUS和EBUS-TBNA是由先前开创的多种其他支气管镜和内镜技术演变而来的[1]。

1949年，Schiepatti首次对纵隔淋巴结进行了TBNA术[2]。整个过程是使用硬质支气管镜通过隆突完成的。随着可弯曲支气管镜的广泛应用，促使开发了可通过可弯曲支气管镜工作通道使用的经支气管穿刺针[3]。Ko-Pen Wang团队于1978年首次发表了关于纵隔肿瘤的经可弯曲支气管镜TBNA获取诊断的报道[4]。5名气管旁恶性肿块患者中有3名获得了足够的组织且没有发生并发症。这项技术通常被称为常规TBNA（conventional TBNA，cTBNA），已发展应用于纵隔、肺门淋巴结或其他中央型病变的良恶性疾病诊断中。使用大规格型号的针头（18G）时，尽管诊断准确率较低，但可以获得组织学标本[5]。事实上，不同文献中关于cTBNA的诊断准确性差异很大（14%~100%），其准确性的预测因素包括淋巴结大小、位置是否存在异常以及是否由经验丰富的支气管镜医师使用组织活检针[6]。

20世纪80年代末，超声内镜检查术（endoscopic ultrasonography，EUS）首次被报道通过使用胃镜评估食管癌。特别是，EUS在肿瘤和淋巴结分期的精准度比计算机断层扫描（computed tomography，CT）成像更高[7,8]。随后，该技术被应用于对疑似恶性纵隔肿块进行细针抽吸（fine needle aspiration，FNA），并显示具有良好的诊断准确性和安全性[9]。支气管腔内超声最早是在20世纪90年代初被开发的，使用径向探头来观察和评估中央和外周病变[10,11]。使用20 MHz换能器、专用球囊和经支气管腔内径向超声（radial probe EBUS，RP-EBUS）可提供由黏膜、软骨和外膜组成的支气管壁三维视图。这使得对气管、支气管壁和气道内肿瘤侵袭的评估比CT成像更准确[12,13]。RP-EBUS也被证明能够识别其他中央和纵隔结构，包括淋巴结和血管系统。随后开发的20 MHz微型径向探头可用于肺外周实质病变的探查和活检[14]。

尽管RP-EBUS在评估肿瘤侵袭和诊断肺外周病变方面具有显著优势，但仍存在一些技术局限性。首先，360°径向探头无法准确地评估纵隔和肺门结构及其空间相关性。更重要的是，RP-EBUS 不能实时引导活检，因此必须在前期超声评估的基础上进行盲检[15]。将 RP-EBUS 与 cTBNA 联合使用的局限性促使了 CP-EBUS 和 EBUS-TBNA 技术的发展和进步。

随着 cTBNA 和 RP-EBUS 的引入，诊断性支气管镜检查取得了进一步发展，但它们各自的局限性促使 CP-EBUS 进一步发展为允许对 TBNA 操作进行实时超声引导。

CP-EBUS 支气管镜最初由日本东京奥林巴斯公司与 Yasufuku 团队共同开发，在可弯曲支气管镜尖端集成了频率为 7.5 MHz 的线性弯曲矩阵换能器。凸阵探头平行于支气管镜的插入方向进行扫描，图像由专用超声处理器处理。支气管镜外径为 6.7 mm，尖端外径为 6.9 mm，工作通道为 2.0 mm，其观察方向有 35° 前倾。超声图像是通过将探头直接贴紧气道壁而获得的，同时需要在探头外连接专用的水囊。可使用一根 22 G 的穿刺针通过工作通道，并以 20° 的角度出针。这种操作比其他技术采集的纵隔和肺门淋巴结标本更多。具体而言，EBUS-TBNA 可对气管旁淋巴结站（2R、2L、3、4R、4L 组）、隆突下（7 组）和肺门淋巴结站（10、11 和 12 组）的淋巴结进行检查。通常无法探及的淋巴结包括主动脉旁（5 组）、主动脉–肺动脉窗（6 组）、食管旁（8 组）和肺韧带（9 组）。

2004 年，Yasufuku 等报道了 EBUS-TBNA 在已知或疑似恶性纵隔和/或肺门淋巴结患者中的首次临床应用[16]，这是基于对手术切除标本进行的初步试验[17]。这项初步临床研究表明，EBUS-TBNA 在区分纵隔和肺门淋巴结良恶性方面具有非常高的敏感性（95.7%）、特异性（100%）和诊断准确性（97.1%）。随后的一项前瞻性研究证明了 EBUS-TBNA 在侵袭性肺癌分期中的作用，在预测淋巴结分期方面同样具有较高的诊断准确性（96.3%）[18]。因此，EBUS-TBNA 的使用可以让患者避免更具创伤性的诊断操作，如纵隔镜检查、胸腔镜检查和 CT 引导下的经皮穿刺活检。

自从早期证明 EBUS-TBNA 的可行性和诊断准确性以来，现在已有大量文献描述了该技术在纵隔和肺门病理微创评估中的各种临床应用价值。

8.1.2 超声仪器

目前，市场上有 3 种不同厂商的 CP-EBUS。奥林巴斯公司生产了第一台 CP-EBUS，随后是宾得医疗公司和富士胶片公司（图 8.1、表 8.1）。3 家不同公司的 CP-

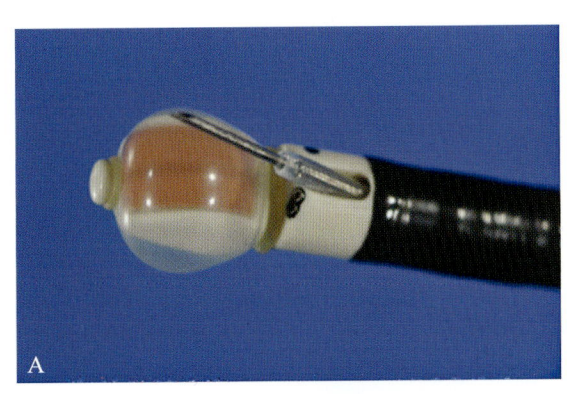
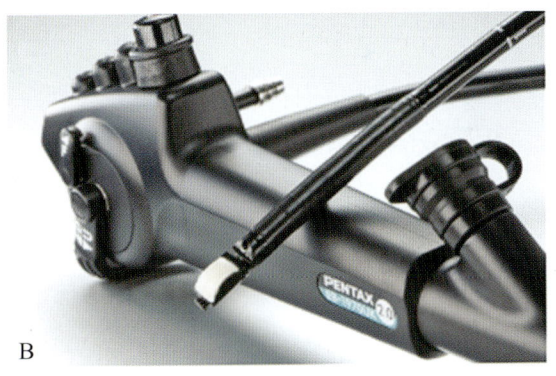
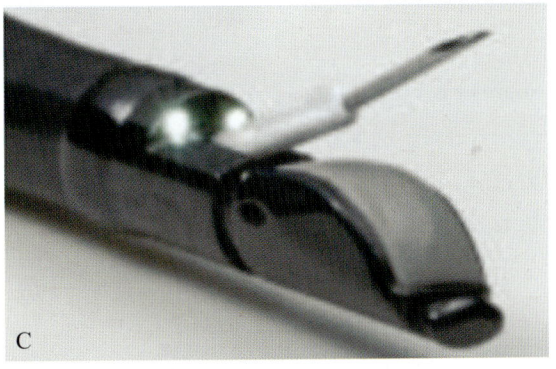

图 8.1 3 种不同类型的凸阵扫描超声支气管

A. 奥林巴斯；B. 宾得；C. 富士胶片。

EBUS 基本结构非常相似。凸阵扫描探头连接在配有工作通道的可弯曲支气管镜的尖端。通过工作通道，连接专用 EBUS-TBNA 针，用于支气管周围病变的采样（表 8.2）。3 种 CP-EBUS 之间的详细差异如表 8.1 所示。

表 8.1 凸阵扫描超声支气管镜

基本信息	奥林巴斯（BF-UC180F）	宾得（EB1970UK）	富士胶片（EB530US）
视频类型	集成	彩色电荷耦合器	超小型电荷耦合器
外径	6.9 mm（尖端）	6.3 mm	6.7 mm（尖端）
内镜角度	前倾 35°	前倾 45°	前倾 10°
视角	80°	80°	120°
弯曲范围	向上 120° 向下 90°	向上 120° 向下 90°	向上 130° 向下 90°
工作通道	2.2 mm	2.0 mm	2.0 mm

表 8.2 EBUS-TBNA 穿刺针

奥林巴斯	波士顿科学	库克医疗
Vizishot-21G，22G	Expect 22G，25G	EchoTip ProCore 22G，25G
Vizishot 2-21G，22G	Acquire 22G，25G	
Vizishot Flex-19G		

8.1.3 EBUS-TBNA

8.1.3.1 操作场所

EBUS-TBNA 可以在类似于传统支气管镜检查的操作场所中进行。包括内镜检查室、专用的呼吸内镜诊疗中心或手术室。

8.1.3.2 麻醉

除了应用于口咽、声带和气道的局部麻醉（同可弯曲支气管镜检查中的常规麻醉一致）外，CP-EBUS 还可以根据临床需要在全身麻醉、清醒镇静下进行，或者在某些情况下可不使用镇静剂。镇静的选择应基于操作的优化，以最安全、最有效的方式提供诊断，同时考虑患者的舒适度。医疗保健利用率也是一个值得考虑的因素。

选择麻醉方式的研究证据是有限的。由于 EBUS-TBNA 操作时间较长，限制了在常规可弯曲支气管镜检查中评估麻醉方法的研究的可行性。两项评估 EBUS-TBNA 在不同镇静水平下诊断准确性的研究结果存在冲突。一项多中心回顾性研究比较了深度镇静（静脉注射丙泊酚加喉罩通气管或气管插管）与中度镇静（静脉滴注芬太尼和咪唑安定，不加人工气道）[19]，结果显示深度镇静的诊断率（79.8%）高于中度镇静（66.4%）。深度镇静也缩短了手术时间，同时能够通过增加针吸活检次数以此获得更多的淋巴结样本。相反，一项前瞻性随机对照研究也评估了深度和中度镇静，但在诊断效果、患者耐受性和并发症发生率方面没有差异；然而，中度镇静的手术时间更短。其他研究也评估了患者在进行 EBUS-TBNA 时对深度和中度镇静的舒适度和耐受性，没有观察到显著差异[20,21]。

由于这些研究的结果相互矛盾，目前尚没有足够的证据推荐对 EBUS-TBNA 使用中度或深度镇静。在做出麻醉决定时应考虑多种因素。在经验丰富、操作流程高效和迅速的中心，可考虑中度镇静；但当操作人员经验不足且手术持续时间较长时，可考虑深度镇静。使用气管插管可能会限制对上叶支气管附近的病灶取样，因此喉罩（最小 4 号）应该是深度镇静时优先的选择。如果需要气管插管，则应选择最小的 8 号气管插管，以适应 CP-EBUS 支气管镜的尺寸，同时保证足够的通气。

8.1.3.3 操作流程

在进行 CP-EBUS 和 EBUS-TBNA 之前，建议先通过可弯曲支气管镜对声带和气道进行局部麻醉，并充分评估支气管内是否存在异常。然后，EBUS-TBNA 可以按照以下步骤进行（图 8.2）。

1）水囊连接：为了获得最佳的超声图像，应使用专用的乳胶水囊装载在 CP-EBUS 尖端并在操作过程中保持充盈状态。将一个装有 20 mL 生理盐水的注射器通过延长管和三通阀连接到水囊。随后使用专用水囊钳将水囊安装到超声探头的尖端。保持水囊充盈以防止漏气。只需 0.3~0.5 mL 生理盐水即可使水囊充分膨胀。若患者对乳胶过敏，则不应使用水囊。

2）插入支气管镜：尽管鼻腔进镜是可行的，通常是充分麻醉后通过口腔进镜。操作者必须注意 EBUS 支气管镜的前倾角度与白光气管镜是不同的。因此，EBUS 支气管镜应该在进入气管前保持观察声门的前半部分的同时完成插入。

3）淋巴结和纵隔结构检查：当进入气管后，水囊保持充盈并进行调整以获得最佳超声视图。使用双屏幕视图用于同时显示内窥镜图像和 EBUS 图像。超声镜尖端轻轻弯曲，贴在气道壁上。然后根据国际肺癌

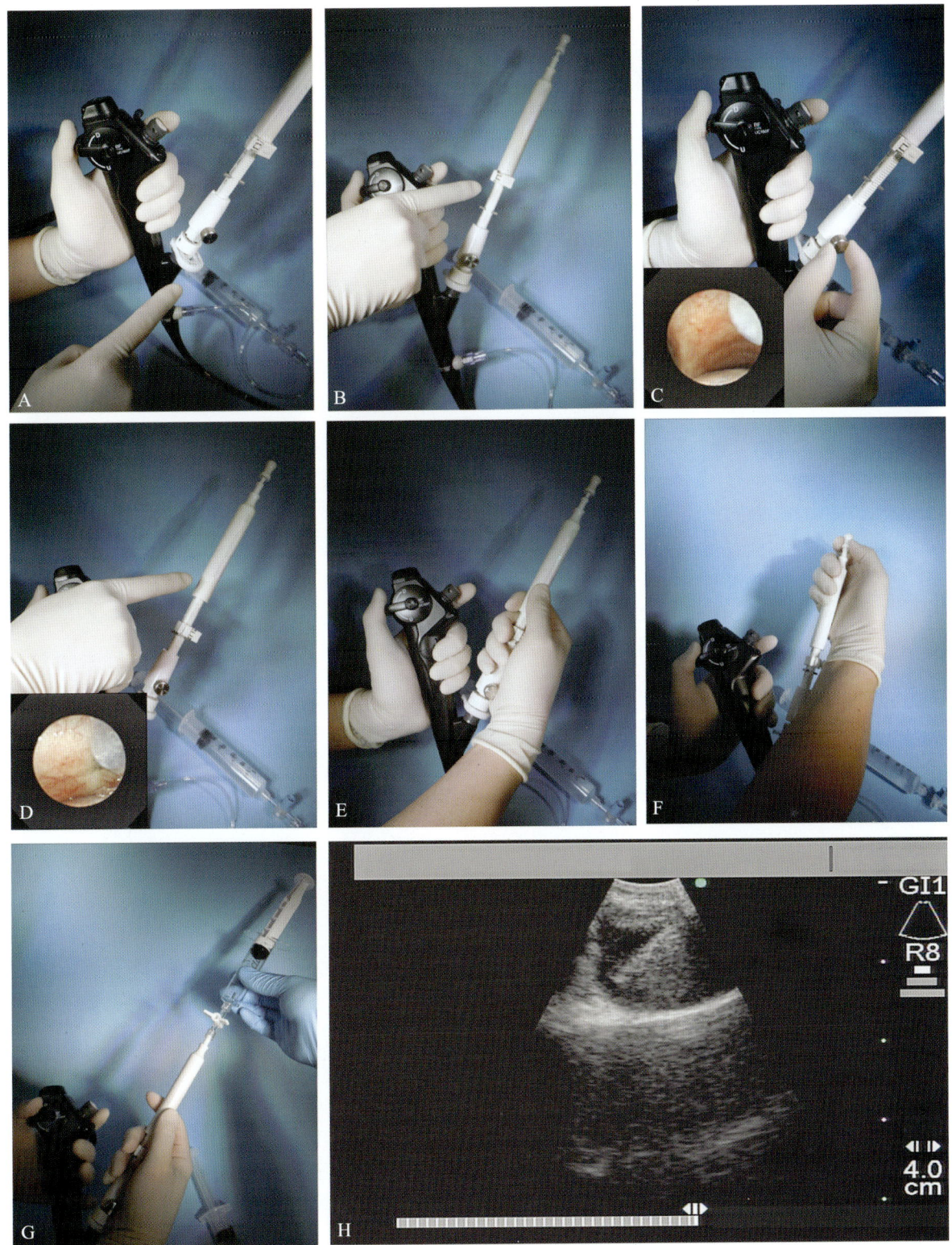

图 8.2　EBUS-TBNA 操作穿刺成功的重要步骤

A. 在识别目标淋巴结后，插入专用穿刺针并固定在通道适配器活检阀上，应确保针头已缩回鞘内；B. 目视检查穿刺针，以确保穿刺针滑块完全缩回，并且调节穿刺调节器旋钮进行锁定穿刺针，以防止针头滑出；C. 当在内窥镜图像上观察到鞘管出来时，松开鞘管调节器旋钮，并将其调整到适当长度；D. 将支气管镜尖端与针鞘推进到目标点，并将可弯曲支气管镜的尖端向上弯曲，使针头插入软骨间隙；E. 在 EBUS 上确认图像的同时，将针头插入淋巴结；F. 在超声波图像上确认穿刺针插入淋巴结后，使用针芯清除任何可能堵塞针尖的碎片；G. 将 Vaclok 注射器连接到穿刺针上，以获得持续负压抽吸；H. 当穿刺针在淋巴结内移动时，保持穿刺针始终在超声图像上可见。

研究协会(IASLC)淋巴结图谱对淋巴结进行系统的评估[22]。通过支气管内标志物和超声下血管标志的联合来辅助识别淋巴结(图 8.3)。可使用多普勒模式用于区分血管结构和淋巴结。

4)装载穿刺针：当目标淋巴结识别后，准备并装好穿刺针。准备穿刺针包括确认鞘管完全拉起并锁定。穿刺针必须处于鞘内的锁定位置。针芯也应该在适当的位置并稍微拉出。然后将穿刺针插入工作通道并固定在支气管镜上。

5)调整穿刺针鞘管末端：使用调节旋钮推进鞘管，确保鞘管尖端在内窥镜图像的角落中可见。

6)识别目标淋巴结：通过弯曲 EBUS 支气管镜的尖端来重新识别目标淋巴结。注意：当穿刺针在工作通道中时，支气管镜的尖端会变得稍硬一些。

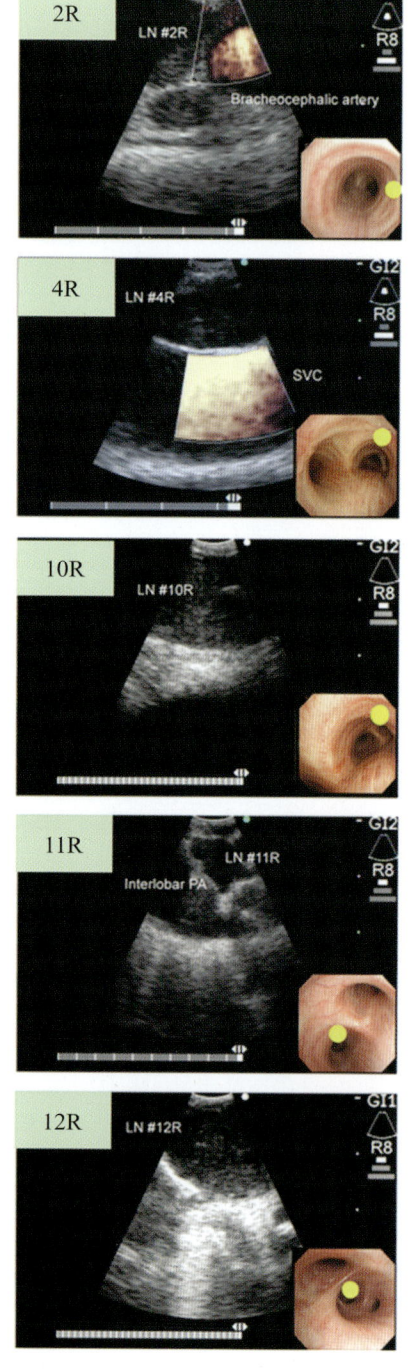
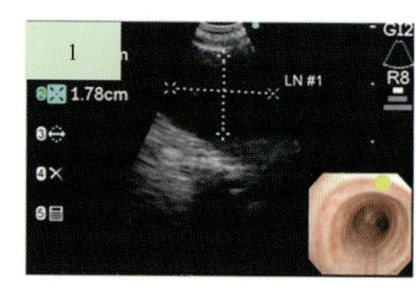
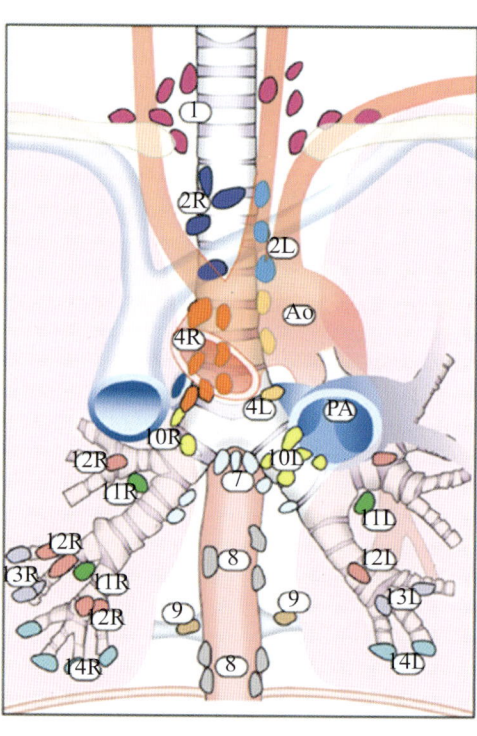
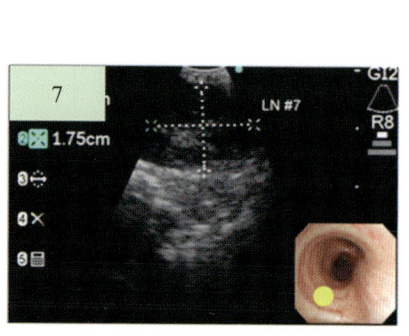
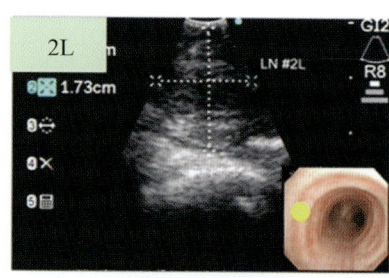
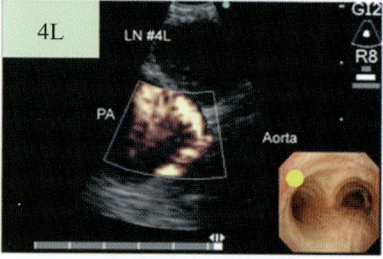
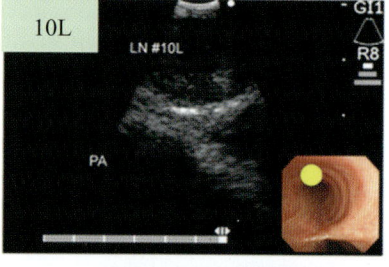
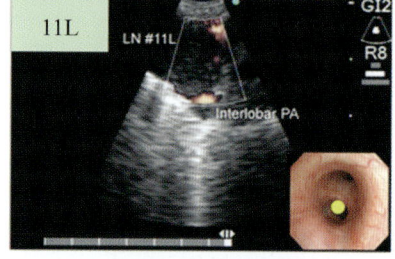

图 8.3 EBUS-TBNA 淋巴结定位图

7）针吸活检：当看到淋巴结，应将鞘管末端定位于软骨环之间。然后将穿刺针锁旋松并设置为所需深度。然后推进穿刺，同时一名助手将支气管镜固定在患者的口中。当穿刺针头插入气道壁，助手可以轻轻推一下支气管镜以帮助穿透气道壁。如果遇到软骨环有阻力时，穿刺针的位置应该在内窥镜图像的引导下重新调整。当穿刺针进入淋巴结后，拔出针芯，接负压抽吸注射器，穿刺针在淋巴中前后移动5~15次，然后取下注射器而穿刺针保持在淋巴结内。随后将针拉回鞘内并锁定。最后从支气管镜中取出穿刺针，并处理标本。

8.1.3.4 标本的处理流程和充分性评估

EBUS-TBNA标本的处理对于提高诊断率非常重要。当有条件进行快速现场评估（rapid on-site evaluation，ROSE）时，可用穿刺针针芯将几滴标本推到载玻片上直接涂抹。这些玻片可被快速染色，包括无需固定风干的Romanowsky染色（如Diff Quik）或利用乙醇固定的快速巴氏法[23]。然后让细胞学专家现场对这些涂片进行判读，确定样本的充分性和初步诊断。而剩余的标本存放在充满生理盐水的锥形容器中，用于细胞块的制备。当没有条件进行ROSE时，应将全部标本放置在一个装满防腐剂（细胞块制备的溶液，如Cytolyt®）的圆锥形容器中。

标本是否充分并没有公认的统一标准。一些标准采用描述淋巴细胞或淋巴组织的存在，而另一些则使用定量指标，如每个高倍视野中淋巴细胞的数量[24]。如果标本足够诊断肿瘤或肉芽肿性炎症，即使在没有淋巴细胞或淋巴组织的情况下通常也会认为标本是充分的。

8.1.3.5 注意事项

8.1.3.5.1 快速现场评估（ROSE）

经常与包括CP-EBUS在内的许多TBNA操作结合使用。ROSE已被证实可以减少穿刺的次数和额外操作的需求[25,26]。当然，诊断率似乎不受ROSE的影响[25-27]。尽管如此，ROSE能通过最少的针吸活检次数获取足够的诊断组织，特别是在一些EBUS-TBNA诊断率低的病例中，如疑似淋巴瘤患者。ROSE也有助于获取足够的恶性细胞数量用于分子和其他辅助细胞检测中。

8.1.3.5.2 穿刺针尺寸

多种TBNA穿刺针可适配CP-EBUS。穿刺针的直径和材质存在差异。此外，穿刺针的功效也因制造商的不同而有所差异。穿刺针包括19G、21G、22G和25G四种类型。如何选择合适的穿刺针已经在多项研究中进行了评估。Nakajima等报道了使用21G和22G针对于诊断率没有显著差异[28]。使用21G针组织学结构会保存得更好，但血液污染会更多。其他研究也报道了类似的结果，其中包括唯一的一项随机对照研究[29,30]。因此，穿刺针的选择应以个体情况而定，并受潜在的病理诊断和血液污染风险的影响。ROSE的实时细胞学反馈在判定标本充分性时也非常有用，必要时可更换穿刺针尺寸以获得足够的标本。

8.1.3.5.3 负压吸引

在EBUS-TBNA操作中使用负压吸引是一个有争议的话题。支持者认为负压吸引可以增加细胞的数量，而反对者则认为负压吸引会增加标本的组织损伤和血液污染的风险。事实上，只有一项研究对此进行了充分评估[31]。结果显示，无论淋巴结大小如何，标本的充分性或诊断率没有显著差异。在临床实践中，通常会首先使用负压吸引。如果有严重的血液污染，操作者应考虑在接下来的淋巴结穿刺中不使用负压吸引[32]。相反，如果最初没有使用负压吸引，且获取的标本经ROSE或肉眼评估效果欠佳，应考虑增加负压吸引。此外，还应使用带彩色多普勒的EBUS以评估目标淋巴结的血管分布，其可能会影响负压吸引的使用。

8.1.3.5.4 针吸活检次数

穿刺一针的定义是每次通过TBNA针穿过气道壁，对目标淋巴结或病变进行采样，然后再对标本进行移除和处理。所需的针吸活检次数取决于ROSE和抽吸标本的肉眼评估。当有条件使用ROSE时，诊断标本充分性的实时反馈可以提供帮助。因此，ROSE可以评价穿刺标本的质量，相比之下穿刺次数已经不那么重要了。在没有条件使用ROSE的情况下，通过肉眼评价可能有助于确定针吸活检次数，但这种评估非常主观。

一项研究评估了肺腺癌纵隔淋巴结转移的最佳针吸活检次数，结果显示，经过3次穿刺后，达到了最高的诊断率和最大的标本充分性。但由于该研究没有使用ROSE，上述结果还需进一步评估。随着最近分子检测技术的兴起，可能需要进行更多次的针吸活检以获取足够的标本。一项研究对此进行了探索，结果表明，在联合ROSE时，针吸活检4次可获取足够的标本用于分子检测[33]。每次针吸活检的移动次数通常为5~15次[32]。移动次数越多可能获得更多标本，但也可能导致血液污染程度更高。ROSE 对操作者调整穿刺针数上也很用。

8.1.4 临床应用

8.1.4.1 肺癌分期

尽管肺癌的发病率有所下降，但目前仍是全球癌症死亡的主要原因，特别对于男性患者[34]。目前肺癌分期是根据 IASLC 第 8 版 TNM 分期制定的[35]。在初次诊断的肺癌患者中进行准确分期是必不可少的，这对患者预后和全程管理有重要影响。有创和无创方法都可用于肺癌的分期，以评估局部和远处的转移情况。

无创方法主要包括 CT、氟脱氧葡萄糖-正电子发射型计算机体层成像（fluorodeoxyglucose positron emission tomography，FDG-PET）、磁共振成像（magnetic resonance imaging，MRI）和放射性核素骨显像等影像学检查。尽管这些方法在肺癌分期中发挥一定的作用，并且经常被使用，但都存在一定局限性，特别是 CT 和 FDG-PET 在鉴别纵隔淋巴结转移的准确性方面。CT 在预测淋巴结转移方面的敏感性和特异性相对较低，分别为 61% 和 79%[36]。而 PET 的敏感性和特异性相对较高，分别为 85% 和 90%，但值得注意的是：① PET 上高达 25% 的 FDG-avid 淋巴结为假阳性；②在正常淋巴结大小的评估中，约 20% 的非 FDG-avid 淋巴结是假阴性[37]。

由于 CT 和 FDG-PET 在预测淋巴结转移中的特异性较低，当淋巴结分期影响肺癌分期或治疗决策时，应对肿大或 FDG-avid 淋巴结进行有创性取样[37,38]。此外，对于潜在可手术患者进行有创纵隔分期的情况包括：①中央型肿瘤（病灶位于胸腔中内 1/3）；②肿大或 FDG-avid 的 N_1 淋巴结；③肿瘤直径 >3 cm 的（即临床分期ⅡA 及以上）[37]。

研究表明，与 CT 和 FDG-PET 对比，EBUS-TBNA 对肺癌纵隔分期的诊断准确性更高[39]。CT、PET 和 EBUS-TBNA 对纵隔和肺门淋巴结正确分期的敏感性分别为 76.9%、80.0% 和 92.3%，特异性分别为 55.3%、70.1% 和 100%，诊断准确率分别为 60.8%、72.5% 和 98.0%。

在有创纵隔分期中，EBUS-TBNA 已被证明在肺癌纵隔分期中与 CT 和 FDG-PET 相比，具有更高的诊断准确性[39]。在一项研究中，CT、PET 和 EBUS-TBNA 用于正确诊断纵隔肺门淋巴结分期的敏感性分别为 76.9%、80.0% 和 92.3%，特异性分别为 55.3%、70.1% 和 100%，诊断准确率分别为 60.8%、72.5% 和 98.0%。

CP-EBUS 在肺癌分期中的局限性是无法探及 8 组和 9 组淋巴结，不过这两组淋巴结可以通过 EUS 探及。联合使用 EBUS-TBNA 和 EUS-FNA 时的诊断率比单独使用一种方法诊断率更高[38,40,41]。此外，也可以通过插入食管的 CP-EBUS 支气管镜（通常称为 EUS-B-FNA）进行 EUS 分期[42]。尽管支气管镜和消化内镜联合应用的方法使得敏感性和阴性预测值（negative predictive value，NPV）都有提升，但这种提升并不显著，且所需的操作技能不同，因此在临床实践中很少实施。

除了潜在的可手术肺癌患者，EBUS-TBNA 对于不可手术的且正考虑其他替代疗法［如外照射放疗（external beam radiation therapy，EBRT）、立体定向放疗（stereotactic body radiotherapy，SBRT）、射频消融（radiofrequency ablation，RFA）和微波消融（microwave ablation，MWA）治疗］的患者也有作用。EBUS-TBNA 能准确识别纵隔和肺门淋巴结转移，而淋巴结转移将限制上述治疗方法的疗效[43,44]。相反，由于无创的影像分期如 PET 的特异性较低，EBUS-TBNA 可用于排除可疑 N_1 和 N_2 淋巴结转移的拟行 SBRT 的患者[45]。EBUS-TBNA 对于接受根治性放疗的肺癌患者也发挥重要作用。通过系统地对纵隔和肺门淋巴结取样，EBUS-TBNA 在确定淋巴结的受累范围方面相较无创的影像分期（如 PET）准确率更高[46]。

8.1.4.2 肺癌的诊断

除了分期，EBUS-TBNA 在肺癌的诊断中也扮演着重要角色。对于临床Ⅳ期的患者，建议采用最容易且最安全的活检方法。然而，对于Ⅰ~Ⅲ期患者，活检需要兼顾诊断和分期信息而变得更加复杂，因为这将直接影响到后续的治疗管理。在开发 CP-EBUS 之前，这种患者通常需要进行诊断性操作，如 CT 引导的经皮穿刺活检或支气管镜活检，然后如果需要进行有创纵隔分期的话，通常需要纵隔镜检查。而随着 CP-EBUS 的问世，诊断和分期都可以通过这一技术实现[47]。

在一项评估疑似Ⅰ~ⅢA 期肺癌患者的研究中，与传统诊断分期方法相比，使用 EBUS-TBNA 作为初步诊断方法显示缩短了治疗决策时间，减少侵入性手术的次数[48]。除此之外，这种有效的诊断方法还具有更高的成本效益。因此，在疑似肺癌临床Ⅰ~Ⅲ期纵隔和/或肺门淋巴结肿大患者中，或 PET 成像上 FDG-avid

淋巴结的患者中，应考虑 EBUS-TBNA 作为首选的诊断方法，以同时进行诊断和纵隔分期。

尽管大多数文献都围绕着 EBUS-TBNA 在非小细胞肺癌中的应用，但该方法在诊断其他原发性肺部恶性肿瘤疾病中也有一定作用。这包括经常发生纵隔或肺门淋巴结受累的小细胞肺癌[49]。在这种情况下，据研究显示，EBUS-TBNA 的总体诊断率达到 97%[50]。

有纵隔或肺门淋巴结受累或可通过 CP-EBUS 进行探查及评估的恶性间皮瘤也可以通过 EBUS-TBNA 进行诊断[51]。EBUS-TBNA 在恶性胸膜间皮瘤侵袭性纵隔分期中可能发挥一定作用，特别是对于一些在考虑进行积极治疗的患者，如胸膜切除术后半侧胸廓放疗，需要准确的病理分期以确定治疗方案[52]。

8.1.4.3 肺部肿块的直视下活检

实质性肺部肿块的诊断取样可以通过多种支气管镜检查方法实现，包括直视下的支气管内活检、荧光镜引导下经支气管活检、RP-EBUS、导航支气管镜检查，以及新的机器人支气管镜。如前所述，大多数方法的不足是缺乏 CP-EBUS 提供的实时可视化。CP-EBUS 的一个常被忽视的用途是使用 EBUS-TBNA 对近端肺部肿块进行直视下活检。虽然 6.9 mm 的支气管镜尖端限制了其进入亚段支气管，但它通常能够插入下叶支气管。在下叶，也可以进入基底段支气管。当肺部肿瘤位于这些位置，可以使用 EBUS-TBNA 直接对肿瘤进行取样[53]。对于靠近气管上叶的肿瘤也是如此。

8.1.4.4 转移性恶性肿瘤的诊断

有胸外恶性肿瘤病史的患者存在纵隔和/或肺门淋巴结肿大是一种常见的临床情况。尽管临床怀疑这些患者的淋巴结转移的概率可能很高，但在大多数情况下，需要通过病理明确诊断来指导治疗决策。EBUS-TBNA 是一种微创的诊断选择，可以提供相应的证据，以明确淋巴结转移的存在或排除转移的存在。这已在多篇文献中得到证实，包括一项多中心研究，该研究表明 EBUS-TBNA 具有较高的敏感性（87%）和诊断准确率（88%）[54]。因此，对于有纵隔和/或肺门淋巴结肿大和胸外恶性肿瘤病史的患者，特别是如果没有更好的方法可以提供相同的诊断和分期信息时，EBUS-TBNA 应被视为首选的诊断方法。

8.1.4.5 EBUS-TBNA 与纵隔镜检查比较

纵隔淋巴结分期也可以采用其他有创方法，包括 cTBNA 和纵隔镜检查。实时 EBUS-TBNA 已被证实在纵隔淋巴结分期中比"盲"cTBNA 具有更高的诊断准确性，尤其是 CT 或 FDG-PET 成像显示没有明显肿大的纵隔疾病[55,56]。在 EBUS-TBNA 问世之前，纵隔镜检查是肺癌侵袭性纵隔分期的"金标准"和最广泛使用的方法。

纵隔镜检查是指一系列主要用于肺癌侵袭性纵隔淋巴结分期的外科学方法。其中包括颈纵隔镜检查（传统和视频辅助）、左前纵隔镜和颈纵隔扩大镜。随后，开发了经颈扩大纵隔淋巴结切除术（transcervical extended mediastinal lymphadenectomy, TEMLA）和视频辅助纵隔淋巴结清扫术（video-assisted mediastinal lymphadenectomy, VAMLA），作为解剖和完全切除纵隔淋巴结的一种手段，而不仅仅为纵隔镜检查的淋巴结基础活检方式[57]。颈纵隔镜检查能够进入并采样上气管旁（2R 和 2L）、下气管旁（4R 和 4L）、前隆突下（7 组）和肺门（10R 和 10L）淋巴结。无法通过颈纵隔镜检查的纵隔淋巴结包括主动脉肺动脉窗（5 组）、主动脉旁（6 组）、后隆突下（7 组）、食管旁（8 组）和肺韧带（9 组）淋巴结。对于叶间（11R、11L）和肺叶（12R 和 12L）淋巴结，可通过 EBUS-TBNA 进行检查，但纵隔镜则无法获取。左前纵隔镜可检查主动脉肺动脉窗（5 组）和主动脉旁（6 组）淋巴结。

在肺癌的纵隔分期中，纵隔镜检查的作用和准确性已被明确并有足够的文献报道[58]。一项大型荟萃分析显示，传统的颈纵隔镜检查对于肺癌纵隔分期的敏感性为 78%，而视频辅助颈纵隔镜检查的敏感性为 89%，NPV 为 92%[38]。这些研究中的假阴性率在大多数情况下可归因于某些淋巴结无法从传统的颈椎入路进入。纵隔镜检查的并发症发生率为 2%，其中死亡率仅为 0.08%[38]。

Ernst 等首次将 EBUS-TBNA 与纵隔镜在肺癌分期中的效果进行直接比较，并以手术切除后的手术淋巴结标本作为"金标准"[59]。在最初的研究中，EBUS-TBNA 对淋巴结的诊断率高于纵隔镜检查（91% 比 78%），但两种技术在正确诊断病理分期方面的准确性没有显著性差异（93% 比 82%）。与纵隔镜检查相比，EBUS-TBNA 对第 7 组淋巴结具有更高的诊断率，其影响了每个淋巴结的总体诊断准确性的差异。在另一项研究中也报道了相似的结果[60]。Yasufuku 等的研究表明，在纵隔镜检查后再进行 EBUS-TBNA 时二者的敏感性、NPV 和诊断准确率分别为79%、90%、93%和81%、91%、93%，差异并无统计学意义。与EBUS-TBNA组未出现并发症相比，接受纵隔镜检查的患者中有2.6%出现并发症。随后的荟萃分析再次表明，EBUS-TBNA和纵隔镜检查在敏感性和诊断准确性上没有显著差异；然而，纵隔镜检查的假阴性结果更少，但并发症更多[61]。

综上，与纵隔镜检查相比，EBUS-TBNA具有相似的诊断准确性、更低的并发症发生率和更低的成本。因此，目前的指南建议EBUS-TBNA是疑似或已确诊肺癌的初始侵袭性纵隔分期的首选方法[38,58,62]。而纵隔镜检查应保留用于高度怀疑转移性淋巴结但初始EBUS-TBNA结果为阴性的病例[38,62,63]。

8.1.4.6 超声特征

CP-EBUS的一个常被忽视的用途是评估受检结构的超声特征。这包括淋巴结的大小、形状、边界、异质性、血管分布、中央窦门结构的存在和凝固性坏死的存在[32]。与恶性淋巴结相关的超声影像特征包括：① 圆形；② 边界清晰；③ 不均匀回声；④ 凝固性坏死[64]。当这4个特征都不存在时，良性病因的可能性非常高。淋巴结大小也可以预测是否存在转移性病变，尽管目前的研究证据相互矛盾[64-66]。

彩色多普勒超声观察到的淋巴结的血管模式也与恶性肿瘤有关，混合型或周边血流信号在预测转移性淋巴结方面具有高灵敏度和中等特异性[67]。相反，淋巴窦门中央血流信号与良性淋巴结有关[68]。除了淋巴结形态和血管模式的超声评估，EBUS弹性成像和灰度纹理分析也被证实能够以相对较高的准确性预测良恶性淋巴结[69,70]。CP-EBUS的影像特征在结节病的评估中也很有用。圆形、边缘清晰、回声均匀、淋巴结分隔和存在生发中心结构的淋巴结超声特征可预测结节病[71,72]。

虽然这些超声特征有助于预测恶性或良性淋巴结，但这些方法的预测价值不足以被视为诊断，因此仍建议通过经支气管穿刺进行确认。

8.1.4.7 EBUS-TBNA标本用于辅助检测

肺癌靶向治疗的发展对用于分子学检测的标本提出了更高的要求。通过EBUS-TBNA获取的标本已被证明可在90%以上的病例中进行免疫组织化学染色（immunohistochemistry staining，IHC）、分子和细胞遗传学检测（包括EGFR和KRAS突变以及ALK和ROS-1重排）[23,33,73]。PD-L1 IHC先前主要通过组织学标本进行检测，而目前，大多数病例可通过EBUS-TBNA获取的细胞学标本实现，并且与手术切除的标本有很强的相关性[74-77]。检测结果通常受到染色细胞块载玻片中有效的肿瘤细胞数量的限制，准确评估通常需要＞100个。

通过二代测序进行快速多重遗传分析是一种新型的、有前途的识别细胞信号通路突变的技术。该方法也可借助于EBUS-TBNA福尔马林固定石蜡包埋标本进行检测。最近的一项研究表明，EBUS-TBNA可为大约2/3的患者提供足够的DNA用于二代测序检测，这些患者已鉴定出46种潜在的体细胞突变[78]。

8.1.4.8 淋巴瘤

孤立性纵隔淋巴结肿大是淋巴瘤的常见临床表现。切除性淋巴结活检或组织（空心）针淋巴结活检仍然是非霍奇金淋巴瘤（non-Hodgkin lymphoma，NHL）和霍奇金淋巴瘤（Hodgkin lymphoma，HL）的推荐诊断技术[79,80]。尽管有这些指南推荐，但细针抽吸细胞学（fine needle aspirate cytology，FNAC）技术经常被用作初始的诊断方法，因为其风险较低，并且在临床实践中可能更容易操作[81]。在淋巴瘤的诊断中，细胞学和组织学标本之间可能存在不一致，这一点存在重大争议[82]。继EBUS-TBNA在原发性肺癌的诊断和分期中的作用被明确后，其在淋巴瘤中的价值也被多项研究评估。Kennedy等在2010年进行的一项初步研究表明，EBUS-TBNA对淋巴瘤的诊断具有较高的敏感性（90.9%）和NPV（92.9%）[83]。随后的研究显示EBUS-TBNA的诊断准确性各不相同，敏感性和NPV分别为38%~90%和83%~96%[84-90]。

这些结果的差异似乎与HL的低诊断准确性有关。这种低敏感性可能与HL诊断中鉴定Reed-Sternberg细胞和评估淋巴结形态的重要性有关。研究还表明，在部分淋巴结受累、淋巴结纤维化或反应性炎症细胞水平高的HL病例中，FNA敏感性降低[91]。与复发病例相比，新诊断淋巴瘤的准确性似乎更低。ROSE有助于确保获取足够的组织标本用于辅助检测，包括流式细胞术和IHC，从而提高细胞学评估的敏感性[89,91]。开发更粗的19号TBNA针（与21G和22G相比）也可能有助于获得更多的"核心"淋巴结标本，但还需要进一步的研究来确定EBUS-TBNA诊断淋巴瘤的潜在益处[92]。

因此，对于疑似淋巴瘤伴纵隔淋巴结肿大的患者，EBUS-TBNA可作为一种安全、微创的诊断方法。在检查结果呈阴性的情况下，且临床上仍高度怀疑淋巴瘤时，应考虑进行诊断性淋巴结切除性活检，如纵隔镜检查。

8.1.4.9 结节病

结节病是一种基于临床和放射学特征的诊断，通常有病理学结果支持。这些发现包括在1个或多个器官中存在非癌性上皮样细胞肉芽肿，同时也排除了其他潜在病[93]。传统上，经支气管肺活检术（transbronchial lung biopsy，TBLB）的组织学评估是最常用的诊断肺结节病的方法。然而，这种方法的诊断率在不同研究中差异较大，而且并发症发生率也较高，主要包括气胸和/或肺出血。在纵隔淋巴结肿大是唯一临床表现的情况下，纵隔镜检查已用于组织学确诊，但如前所述，其并发症发生率虽然较低但症状明显，并且无法进入结节病常见的叶间或叶淋巴结。

EBUS-TBNA已被证实可用于疑似结节病患者的病理评估[94]。在Ⅰ~Ⅱ期疾病患者中，与TBLB（37%~53%）相比，该方法提供了更高的诊断率（80%~90%）[95,96]。在Ⅰ期疾病的诊断准确性方面，EBUS-TBNA（84%~97%）优于TBLB（31%~38%）。与EBUS-TBNA相比，EBUS-TBNA与TBLB联合使用可进一步提高诊断准确性[97]。

因此，建议将EBUS-TBNA作为疑似结节病Ⅰ~Ⅱ期患者的首选诊断方法。此外，还可以联合TBLB以提高诊断准确性，但这需要与该技术观察到的增加的并发症发生率进行权衡。

8.1.4.10 肺结核

淋巴结炎是肺结核最常见的肺外表现。对于孤立性胸内淋巴结炎的患者，包括支气管镜检查和痰培养在内的传统诊断方法的诊断敏感性较低[98]。相比之下，EBUS-TBNA具有较高的诊断准确性，早期研究表明其敏感性为94%。在这项研究中，阳性诊断包括一致的病理结果，如干酪化肉芽肿或微生物学检查结果。微生物学阳性仅在53%的病例中得到证实（17%的抗酸杆菌涂片阳性，47%的结核分枝杆菌培养阳性）。随后对8项研究进行的荟萃分析再次表明，总体敏感性为87%（范围74%~95%）[99]。因此，EBUS-TBNA可作为诊断纵隔或肺门受累的疑似结核淋巴结炎的初步检查方法。然而，在一些结核病流行地区，CP-EBUS的低可用性可能会限制这一点，因此仍可以使用其他诊断技术。

8.1.4.11 并发症

EBUS-TBNA的并发症发生率通常较低。在一项包括7 000多例患者的大型队列研究中，总体并发症发生率为1.23%[100]。并发症包括出血（0.68%）、感染（0.19%）和气胸（0.03%），死亡率为0.01%。

8.2 CP-EBUS的发展方向

当前CP-EBUS支气管镜的局限性是相对较大的外径和较小的弯曲角度，这限制了其进入远端气道。目前正在开发的是一种细凸阵扫描探头超声支气管镜（thin convex-probe EBUS，TCP-EBUS），旨在到达更远端气道和目标病灶。它具有更细的尖端直径（5.9 mm）、更大的弯曲角度（向上170°）和视角（20°）。与目前的Olympus CP-EBUS相比，猪和尸体模型实验都显示出TCP具有更大的覆盖范围和更大的内窥镜视野角度[101,102]。因此，这些益处可以实现对更远端的目标直接实时采样。例如，以前用CP-EBUS无法到达的外周N_1淋巴结。这在早期肺癌的治疗中具有重要的临床意义。在考虑亚肺叶切除、SBRT和其他局部治疗的情况下，N_1淋巴结的状态在治疗计划中起到至关重要的作用。

TCP-EBUS的另一个潜在作用是改善对肺外周病变的探查和活检。目前可用于定位和采样肺外周病变的支气管镜检查方法包括RP-EBUS、导航支气管镜检查以及最新的机器人支气管镜检查。这些方法的局限性在于缺乏CP-EBUS提供的实时组织采样。TCP-EBUS可以实现对肺外周病变的实时采样，这可能对提高诊断率有所帮助。

目前，CP-EBUS在临床上可用于多种肺部疾病的诊断和肺癌淋巴结分期。然而，通过CP-EBUS进行治疗也是可能的，并且在未来几年内可能呈持续增长的趋势。

8.3 结论

凸阵扫描支气管镜技术已在临床应用超过15年，这项技术已经彻底改变了支气管镜下诊断的格局，堪称自可弯曲支气管镜问世以来，介入呼吸病领域最具影响力并改变临床实践的技术。EBUS-TBNA的使用已经显著减少了纵隔镜的使用，并在许多中心取代纵隔镜检查和其他侵入性诊断操作。CP-EBUS 在肺癌、淋巴瘤、转移性恶性肿瘤以及结节病和结核病等许多良性疾病的诊断和分期中具有明确的作用。通过在许多临床情况下提供准确和安全的诊断评估，CP-EBUS 成为肺科医师和胸外科医师的一项基本技能，尤其是对于在肺癌领域工作的医务人员。在当前微创诊断和治疗的时代，CP-EBUS 的潜在应用还有很多，发展前景不可限量。

参考文献

1 Mehta, A. and Panchabhai, T. (2015). Historical perspectives of bronchoscopy. Connecting the dots. *Ann. Am. Thorac. Soc.* 12: 631–641.

2 Schieppati, E. (1958). Mediastinal lymph node puncture through the tracheal carina. *Surg. Gynecol. Obstet.* 107: 243–246.

3 Oho, K., Kato, H., Ogawa, I. et al. (1979). A new needle for transfiberoptic bronchoscopic use. *Chest* 76: 492.

4 Wang, K.P., Terry, P., and Marsh, B. (1978). Bronchoscopic needle aspiration biopsy of paratracheal tumors. *Am. Rev. Respir. Dis.* 118: 17–21.

5 Mehta, A.C., Kavuru, M.S., Meeker, D.P. et al. (1989). Transbronchial needle aspiration for histology specimens. *Chest* 96 (6): 1228–1232.

6 Bonifazi, M., Zuccatosta, L., Trisolini, R. et al. (2013). Transbronchial needle aspiration: a systematic review on predictors of a successful aspirate. *Respiration* 86: 123–134.

7 Tio, T.L., Cohen, P., Coene, P.P. et al. (1989). Endosonography and computed tomography of esophageal carcinoma. *Gastroenterology* 96: 1478–1486.

8 Ziegler, K., Sanft, C., Zimmer, T. et al. (1993). Comparison of computed tomography, endosonography, and intraoperative assessment in TN staging of gastric carcinoma. *Gut* 34: 604–610.

9 Pederson, B.H., Vilman, P., Folke, K. et al. (1996). Endoscopic ultrasonography and real-time guided fine-needle aspiration biopsy of solid lesions of the mediastinum suspected of malignancy. *Chest* 110: 539–544.

10 Hurter, T. and Hanrath, P. (1992). Endobronchial sonography: feasibility and preliminary results. *Thorax* 47: 565–567.

11 Becker, H.D. (1996). Endobronchial ultrasound, a new perspective in bronchology. *Ultraschall. Med.* 17: 106–112.

12 Kurimoto, N., Murayama, M., Yoshioka, S. et al. (1999). Assessment of usefulness of endobronchial ultrasonography in determination of depth of tracheobronchial tumor invasion. *Chest* 115: 1500–1506.

13 Herth, F., Ernst, A., Schulz, M. et al. (2003). Endobronchial ultrasound reliably differentiates between airway infiltration and compression by tumor. *Chest* 123: 458–462.

14 Herth, F.J.F. and Becker, H.D. (2002). Endobronchial ultrasound-guided transbronchial lung biopsy in solitary pulmonary nodules and peripheral lesions. *Eur. Respir. J.* 20: 972–974.

15 Herth, F.J., Becker, H.D., and Ernst, A. (2003). Ultrasound-guided transbronchial needle aspiration: an experience in 242 patients. *Chest* 123: 604–607.

16 Yasufuku, K., Chiyo, M., Sekine, Y. et al. (2004). Real-time endobronchial ultrasound-guided transbronchial needle aspiration of mediastinal and hilar lymph nodes. *Chest* 126: 122–128.

17 Yasufuku, K., Chhajed, P.N., Sekine, Y. et al. (2004). Endobronchial ultrasound using a new convex probe: a preliminary study on surgically resected specimens. *Oncol. Rep.* 11: 293–296.

18 Yasufuku, K., Chiyo, M., Koh, E. et al. (2005). Endobronchial ultrasound guided transbronchial needle aspiration for staging of lung cancer. *Lung Cancer* 50: 347–354.

19 Yarmus, L.B., Akulian, J.A., Gilbert, C. et al. (2013). Comparison of moderate versus deep sedation for endobronchial ultrasound transbronchial needle aspiration. *Ann. Am. Thorac. Soc.* 10 (2): 121–126.

20 Dal, T., Sazak, H., Tunç, M. et al. (2014). A comparison of ketamine-midazolam and ketamine-propofol combinations used for sedation in the endobronchial ultrasound-guided transbronchial needle aspiration: a prospective, single-blind, randomized study. *J. Thorac. Dis.* 6 (6): 742–751.

21 Churton, J., Edwards, T., Fielding, D. et al. (2015). Comparison of comfort scores comparing bronchoscopy with conscious sedation or anaesthetist controlled sedation; a randomised prospective trial. *Eur. Respir. J.* 46 (suppl 59): PA322.

22 Rusch, V.W., Asamura, H., Watanabe, H. et al. (2009). The IASLC lung cancer staging project: a proposal for a new international lymph node map in the forthcoming seventh edition of the TNM classification for lung cancer. *J. Thorac. Oncol.* 4: 569–577.

23 Jain, D., Allen, T.C., Aisner, D.L. et al. (2018). Rapid on-site evaluation of endobronchial ultrasound-guided transbronchial needle aspirations for the diagnosis of lung cancer: a perspective from members of the pulmonary pathology society. *Arch. Pathol. Lab. Med.* 142 (2): 253–262.

24 VanderLaan, P.A., Wang, H.H., Majid, A. et al. (2014). Endobronchial ultrasound-guided transbronchial needle aspiration (EBUS-TBNA): an overview and update for the cytopathologist. *Cancer (Cancer Cytopathol.)* 122: 561–576.

25 Oki, M., Saka, H., Kitagawa, C. et al. (2013). Rapid on-site cytologic evaluation during endobronchial ultrasound-guided transbronchial needle aspiration for diagnosing lung cancer: a randomized study. *Respiration* 85 (6): 486–492.

26 Murakami, Y., Oki, M., Saka, H. et al. (2014). Endobronchial ultrasoundguided transbronchial needle aspiration in the diagnosis of small cell lung cancer. *Respir. Invest.* 52 (3): 173–178.

27 Griffin, A.C., Schwartz, L.E., and Baloch, Z.W. (2011). Utility of on-site evaluation of endobronchial ultrasound-guided transbronchial needle aspiration specimens. *Cytojournal* 8: 20.

28 Nakajima, T., Yasufuku, K., Takahashi, R. et al. (2011). Comparison of 21-gauge and 22-gauge aspiration needle during endobronchial ultrasound-guided transbronchial needle aspiration. *Respirology* 16: 90–94.

29 Yarmus, L.B., Akulian, J., Lechtzin, N. et al. (2013). Comparison of 21-gauge and 22-gauge aspiration needle in endobronchial ultrasound-guided transbronchial needle aspiration: results of the American College of Chest Physicians Quality Improvement Registry, Education, and Evaluation Registry. *Chest* 143 (4): 1036–1043.

30 Oki, M., Saka, H., Kitagawa, C. et al. (2011). Randomized study of 21-gauge versus 22-gauge endobronchial ultrasound-guided transbronchial needle aspiration needles for sampling histology specimens. *J. Bronchol. Interv. Pulmonol.* 18 (4): 306–310.

31 Casal, R.F., Staerkel, G.A., Ost, D. et al. (2012). Randomized clinical trial of endobronchial ultrasound needle biopsy with and without aspiration. *Chest* 142 (3): 568–573.

32 Wahidi, M.M., Herth, F., Yasufuku, K. et al. (2016). Technical aspects of endobronchial ultrasound-guided transbronchial needle aspiration. CHEST guideline and expert panel report. *Chest* 149 (3): 816–835.

33 Yarmus, L., Akulian, J., Gilbert, C. et al. (2013). Optimizing endobronchial ultrasound for molecular analysis. How many passes are needed? *Ann. Am. Thorac. Soc.* 10 (6): 636–643.

34 Siegel, R.L., Miller, K.D., and Jemal, A. (2017). Cancer statistics 2017. *CA Cancer J. Clin.* 67: 7–30.

35 Amin, M.B., Edge, S.B., Greene, F.L. et al. (2017). *Cancer Staging Manual*, 8e. Chicago: Springer.

36 Gould, M.K., Kuschner, W.G., and Rydzak, C.E. (2003). Test performance of positron emission tomography and computed tomography for mediastinal staging in patients with non-small-cell lung cancer a meta-analysis. *Ann. Intern. Med.* 39: 879–892.

37 Darling, G.E., Dickie, A.J., Malthaner, R.A. et al. (2011). Invasive mediastinal staging of non-small-cell cancer: a clinical practice guideline. *Curr. Oncol.* 18 (6): e304–e310.

38 Silvestri, G.A., Gonzales, A.V., and Jantz, M.A. (2013). Methods for staging non-small cell lung cancer. Diagnosis and management of lung cancer, 3rd ed: American College of Chest Physicians, evidence-based clinical practice guidelines. *Chest* 143 (5 (Suppl)): e211S–e250S.

39 Yasufuku, K., Nakajima, T., Motoori, K. et al. (2006). Comparison of endobronchial ultrasound, positron emission tomography, and CT for lymph node staging of lung cancer. *Chest* 130: 710–718.

40 Zang, R., Yink, K., Shi, L. et al. (2013). Combined endobronchial and endoscopic ultrasound-guided fine needle aspiration for mediastinal lymph node staging of lung cancer: a meta-analysis. *Eur. J. Cancer* 49: 1860–1867.

41 Korevaar, D.A., Crombag, L.M., Cohen, J.F. et al. (2016). Added value of combined endobronchial and oesophageal endosonography for mediastinal nodal staging in lung cancer: a systematic review and meta-analysis. *Lancet Respir. Med.* 4: 960–968.

42 Herth, F., Krasnik, M., Kahn, N. et al. (2010). Combined endoscopic-endobronchial ultrasound-guided fine-needle aspiration of mediastinal lymph nodes through a single bronchoscope in 150 patients with suspected lung cancer. *Chest* 138: 790–794.

43 Nakajima, T., Yasufuku, K., Nakajima, M. et al. (2010). Endobronchial ultrasound-guided transbronchial needle aspiration for lymph node staging in patients with non-small cell lung cancer in nonoperable patients pursuing radiotherapy as a primary treatment. *J. Thorac. Oncol.* 5: 606–611.

44 Yasufuku, K., Nakajima, T., Waddell, T. et al. (2013). Endobronchial ultrasound-guided transbronchial needle aspiration for differentiating N0 versus N1 lung cancer. *Ann. Thorac. Surg.* 96: 1756–1760.

45 Hashimoto, K., Daddi, N., Giuliani, M. et al. (2018). The role of endobronchial ultrasound-guided transbronchial needle aspiration in stereotactic body radiation therapy for non-small cell lung cancer. *Lung Cancer* 123: 1–6.

46 Steinfort, D.P., Siva, S., Leong, T.L. et al. (2016). Systematic endobronchial ultrasound-guided mediastinal staging versus positron emission tomography for comprehensive mediastinal staging in NSCLC before radical radiotherapy of non-small cell lung cancer. A pilot study. *Medicine* 95: 1–7.

47 Fielding, D. and Windsor, M. (2009). Endobronchial ultrasound convex-probe transbronchial needle aspiration as the first diagnostic test in patients with pulmonary masses and associated hilar or mediastinal nodes. *Intern. Med. J.* 39 (7): 435–440.

48 Navani, N., Nankivell, M., and Lawrence, D.R. (2015). Lung cancer diagnosis and staging with endobronchial ultrasound-guided transbronchial needle aspiration compared with conventional approaches: an open-label, pragmatic, randomised controlled trial. *Lancet Respir. Med.* 3: 282–289.

49 Wang, Z., Li, M., Huang, Y. et al. (2018). Clinical and radiological characteristics of central pulmonary adenocarcinoma: a comparison with central squamous cell carcinoma and small cell lung cancer and the impact on treatment response. *Oncol. Targets Ther.* 11: 2509–2517.

50 Murakami, Y., Oki, M., Saka, H. et al. (2014). Endobronchial ultrasound-guided transbronchial needle aspiration in the diagnosis of small cell lung cancer. *Respir. Invest.* 52: 173–178.

51 Ghigna, M.R., Crutu, A., Florea, V. et al. (2016). The role of endobronchial ultrasound-guided fine needle aspiration in the diagnosis of pleural mesothelioma. *Cytopathology* 27: 284–288.

52 De Perrot, M., Feld, R., Leighl, N. et al. (2016). Accelerated hemithoracic radiation followed by extrapleural pneumonectomy for malignant pleural mesothelioma. *J. Thorac. Cardiovasc. Surg.* 151: 468–475.

53 Yasufuku, K., Nakajima, T., Chiyo, M. et al. (2007). Endobronchial ultrasonography. Current status and future directions. *J. Thorac. Oncol.* 2: 970–979.

54 Navani, N., Nankivell, M., Woolhouse, I. et al. (2011). Endobronchial ultrasound-guided transbronchial needle aspiration for the diagnosis of intrathoracic lymphadenopathy in patients with extrathoracic malignancy: a multicenter study. *J. Thorac. Oncol.* 6 (9): 1505–1509.

55 Wallace, M.B., Pascual, J.M.S., and Raimondo, M. (2008). Minimally invasive endoscopic staging of suspected lung

56 Medford, A. (2014). Endobronchial ultrasound-guided versus conventional transbronchial needle aspiration: time to re-evaluate the relationship? *J. Thorac. Dis.* 6 (5): 411–415.

57 Kuzdzat, J., Szlubowski, A., Grochowski, Z. et al. (2005). Current evidence on transcervical mediastinal lymph node dissection. *Eur. J. Cardiothorac. Surg.* 27: 384–390.

58 Czarnecka-Kujawa, K. andYasufuku, K. (2017). The role of endobronchial ultrasound versus mediastinoscopy for non-small cell lung cancer. *J. Thorac. Dis.* 9 (Suppl 2): S83–S97.

59 Ernst, A., Anantham, D., Eberhardt, R. et al. (2008). Diagnosis of mediastinal adenopathy – real-time endobronchial ultrasound guided needle aspiration versus mediastinoscopy. *J. Thorac. Oncol.* 3: 577–582.

60 Um, S.W., Kim, H.K., Jung, S.H. et al. (2015). Endobronchial ultrasound versus mediastinoscopy for mediastinal nodal staging of non-small-cell lung cancer. *J. Thorac. Oncol.* 10: 331–337.

61 Ge, X., Guan, W., Han, F. et al. (2015). Comparison of endobronchial ultrasound-guided fine needle aspiration and video-assisted mediastinoscopy for mediastinal staging of lung cancer. *Lung* 193: 757–766.

62 De Leyn, P., Dooms, C., Kuzdzal, J. et al. (2014). Preoperative mediastinal lymph node staging for non-small cell lung cancer: 2014 update of the 2007 ESTS guidelines. *Transl. Lung Cancer Res.* 3: 225–233.

63 Czarnecka-Kujawa, K., Rochau, U., Siebert, U. et al. (2017). Cost-effectiveness of mediastinal lymph node staging in non-small cell lung cancer. *J. Thorac. Cardiovasc. Surg.* 153 (6): 1567–1568.

64 Fujiwara, T., Yasufuku, K., Nakajima, T. et al. (2010). The utility of sonographic features during endobronchial ultrasound-guided transbronchial needle aspiration for lymph node staging in patients with lung cancer: a standard endobronchial ultrasound image classification system. *Chest* 138 (3): 641–647.

65 Garcia-Olivé, I., Monsó, E., Andreo, F. et al. (2009). Sensitivity of linear endobronchial ultrasonography and guided transbronchial needle aspiration for the identification of nodal metastasis in lung cancer staging. *Ultrasound Med. Biol.* 35 (8): 1271–1277.

66 Memoli, J.S., El-Bayoumi, E., Pastis, N.J. et al. (2011). Using endobronchial ultrasound features to predict lymph node metastasis in patients with lung cancer. *Chest* 140 (6): 1550–1556.

67 Nakajima, T., Anayama, T., Shingyoji, M. et al. (2012). Vascular image patterns of lymph nodes for the prediction of metastatic disease during EBUS-TBNA for mediastinal staging of lung cancer. *J. Thorac. Oncol.* 7 (6): 1009–1014.

68 Satterwhite, L.G., Berkowitz, D.M., Parks, C.S., and Bechara, R.I. (2011). Central intranodal vessels to predict cytology during endobronchial ultrasound transbronchial needle aspiration. *J. Bronchol. Interv. Pulmonol.* 18 (4): 322–328.

69 Izumo, T., Sasada, S., Chavez, C. et al. (2014). Endobronchial ultrasound elastography in the diagnosis of mediastinal and hilar lymph nodes. *Jpn. J. Clin. Oncol.* 44 (10): 956–962.

70 Nguyen, P., Bashirzadeh, F., Hundloe, J. et al. (2012). Optical differentiation between malignant and benign lymphadenopathy by grey scale texture analysis of endobronchial ultrasound convex probe images. *Chest* 141: 709–715.

71 Imai, N., Imaizumi, K., Ando, M. et al. (2013). Echoic features of lymph nodes with sarcoidosis determined by endobronchial ultrasound. *Intern. Med.* 52 (13): 1473–1478.

72 Fielding, D., Bashirzadeh, F., and Nguyen, P. (2010). Review of the role of EBUS-TBNA for the pulmonologist, including lung cancer staging. *Thorac. Cancer* 1: 44–52.

73 Casadio, C., Guarize, J., Donghi, S. et al. (2015). Molecular testing for targeted therapy in advanced non-small cell lung cancer: suitability of endobronchial ultrasound transbronchial needle aspiration. *Am. J. Clin. Pathol.* 144: 629–634.

74 Biswas, A., Leon, M.E., Drew, P. et al. (2018). Clinical performance of endobronchial ultrasound-guided transbronchial needle aspiration for assessing programmed death ligand-1 expression in nonsmall cell lung cancer. *Diagn. Cytopathol.* 46 (5): 378–383.

75 Perotta, F., Adizie, B., Maqsood, U. et al. (2017). S100 utility of endobronchial ultrasound-guided transbronchial needle aspiration for pd-l1 testing in patients with nsclc. *Thorax* 72: A60–A61.

76 Lee, J.M., Heymann, J.J., Pagan, C. et al. (2017). Feasibility of Pd-L1 expression testing in non-small cell lung cancer from EBUS-TBNA samples. *Am. J. Respir. Crit. Care Med.* 195: A2883.

77 Sakata, K., Midthun, D., Mullon, J. et al. (2017). Comparison of PD-L1 immunohistochemical staining between EBUS-TBNA and resected non-small cell lung cancer specimens. *J. Thorac. Oncol.* 12 (Suppl 2): S2001–S2002.

78 Fielding, D., Dalley, A.J., Bashirzadeh, F. et al. (2017). Next-generation sequencing of endobronchial ultrasound transbronchial needle aspiration specimens in lung cancer. *Am. J. Respir. Crit. Care Med.* 196: 388–391.

79 Tilly, H., Gomes da Silva, M., Vitolo, U. et al. (2015). Diffuse large B-cell lymphoma (DLBCL): ESMO clinical practice guidelines for diagnosis, treatment and follow-up. *Ann. Oncol.* 26 (Suppl5): v116–v125.

80 Eichenauer, D.A., Aleman, B., Andre, M. et al. (2018). Hodgkin lymphoma: ESMO clinical practice guidelines for diagnosis, treatment and follow-up. *Ann. Oncol.* 29 (Suppl 4): iv1–iv11.

81 Frederiksen, J.K., Sharma, M., Casulo, C. et al. (2015). Systematic review of the effectiveness of fine-needle aspiration and/or core needle biopsy for subclassifying lymphoma. *Arch. Pathol. Lab. Med.* 139: 245–251.

82 Das, D.K., Francis, I.M., Sharma, P.N. et al. (2009). Hodgkin's lymphoma: diagnostic difficulties in fine-needle aspiration cytology. *Diagn. Cytopathol.* 37: 564–573.

83 Kennedy, M.P., Jimenez, C.A., Bruzzi, J.F. et al. (2008). Endobronchial ultrasound-guided transbronchial needle aspiration in the diagnosis of lymphoma. *Thorax* 63: 360–365.

84 Erer, O.F., Erol, S., Anar, C. et al. (2017). Diagnostic yield of EBUS-TBNA for lymphoma and review of the literature. *Endosc. Ultrasound* 6: 317–322.

85 Steinfort, D.P., Conron, M., Tsui, A. et al. (2010). Endobronchial ultrasoundguided transbronchial needle aspiration for the evaluation of suspected lymphoma. *J. Thorac. Oncol.* 5: 804–809.

86 Marshall, C.B., Jacob, B., Patel, S. et al. (2011). The utility of endobronchial ultrasound-guided transbronchial needle aspiration biopsy in the diagnosis of mediastinal lymphoproliferative disorders. *Cancer Cytopathol.* 119: 118–126.

87 Iqbal, S., DePew, Z.S., Kurtin, P.J. et al. (2012). Endobronchial ultrasound and lymphoproliferative disorders: a retrospective study. *Ann. Thorac. Surg.* 94: 1830–1834.

88 Moonim, M.T., Bren, R., Fields, P.A. et al. (2013). Diagnosis and subtyping of de novo and relapsed mediastinal lymphomas by endobronchial ultrasound needle aspiration. *Am. J. Respir. Crit. Care Med.* 188: 1216–1223.

89 Ko, H.M., da Cunha Santos, G., Darling, G. et al. (2013). Diagnosis and subclassification of lymphomas and non-neoplastic lesions involving mediastinal lymph nodes using endobronchial ultrasound-guided transbronchial needle aspiration. *Diagn. Cytopathol.* 41: 1023–1030.

90 Senturk, A., Babaoglu, E., Kilic, H. et al. (2014). Endobronchial ultrasound-guided transbronchial needle aspiration in the diagnosis of lymphoma. *Asian Pac. J. Cancer Prev.* 15: 4169–4173.

91 Chhieng, D.C., Cangiarella, J.F., Symmans, W.F. et al. (2001). Fine-needle aspiration cytology of Hodgkin disease: a study of 89 cases with emphasis on false-negative cases. *Cancer* 93: 52–59.

92 Kinoshita, T., Ujiie, H., Schwock, J. et al. (2018). Clinical evaluation of the utility of a flexible 19-gauge EBUS-TBNA needle. *J. Thorac. Dis.* 10 (4): 2388–2396.

93 Iannuzzi, M.C., Rybicki, B.A., and Teirstein, A.S. (2007). Sarcoidosis. *N. Engl. J. Med.* 357: 2153–2165.

94 Nakajima, T., Yasufuku, K., Kurosu, K. et al. (2009). The role of EBUS-TBNA for the diagnosis of sarcoidosis – comparisons with other bronchoscopic diagnostic modalities. *Respir. Med.* 103: 1796–1800.

95 Oki, M., Saka, H., Kitagawa, C. et al. (2012). Prospective study of endobronchial ultrasound-guided transbronchial needle aspiration of lymph nodes versus transbronchial lung biopsy of lung tissue for diagnosis of sarcoidosis. *J. Thorac. Cardiovasc. Surg.* 143: 1324–1329.

96 Von Barthled, M.B., Dekkers, O.M., Szlubowski, A. et al. (2013). Endosonography vs conventional bronchoscopy for the diagnosis of sarcoidosis The GRANULOMA randomized clinical trial. *JAMA* 309: 2457–2464.

97 Gupta, D., Dadhwal, D.S., Agarwal, R. et al. (2014). Endobronchial ultrasound-guided transbronchial needle aspiration vs conventional transbronchial needle aspiration in the diagnosis of sarcoidosis. *Chest* 146: 547–556.

98 Codecasa, L.R., Besozzi, G., de Cristofaro, L. et al. (1998). Epidemiological and clinical patterns of intrathoracic lymph node tuberculosis in 60 human immunodeficiency virus-negative adult patients. *Monaldi Arch. Chest Dis.* 53 (3): 277–280.

99 Ye, W., Zhang, R., Xu, X. et al. (2015). Diagnostic efficacy and safety of endobronchial ultrasound-guided transbronchial needle aspiration in intrathoracic tuberculosis: a meta-analysis. *J. Ultrasound Med.* 34: 1645–1650.

100 Asano, F., Aoe, M., and Ohsaki, Y. (2013). Complications associated with endobronchial ultrasound-guided transbronchial needle aspiration: a nationwide survey by the Japan Society for Respiratory Endoscopy. *Respir. Res.* 14: 50.

101 Wada, H., Hirohashi, K., Nakajima, T. et al. (2015). Assessment of the new thin convex probe endobronchial ultrasound bronchoscope and the dedicated aspiration needle: a preliminary study in the porcine lung. *J. Bronchol. Interv. Pulmonol.* 22: 20–27.

102 Callahan, S.P., Tanner, N.T., Chen, A. et al. (2017). Comparison of the thin convex probe endobronchial ultrasound bronchoscope to standard endobronchial ultrasound and flexible bronchoscope – a cadaveric study. *US Respir. Pulmon. Dis.* 2 (1): 33–36.

第 9 章

光学成像技术在肺癌早期诊断中的应用

Renelle Myers[1,2] and Stephen C.T. Lam[1,2]

[1] Department of Integrative Oncology, British Columbia Cancer Agency, Vancouver, British Columbia, Canada

[2] Cancer Imaging Department and Department of Medicine, University of British Columbia, Vancouver, British Columbia, Canada

（译者：孙加源　徐冬阳　译者单位：上海市胸科医院/上海交通大学医学院附属胸科医院）

9.1 引言

目前肺癌仍然是全球范围内致死率最高的癌症[1]。尽管肺癌的诊疗技术已取得重大进展，但其5年生存率仍不足18%。这主要是由于大部分患者在确诊时就已是肺癌晚期[2]。通过低剂量CT（low-dose computed tomography，LDCT）进行肺癌筛查有助于实现肺癌的早发现、早诊断，可将死亡率降低20%[3,4]。与晚期肺癌的低生存率相比，IA期非小细胞肺癌的5年生存率可超过80%。而通过普通光（白光）支气管镜检查（white light bronchoscopy，WLB）难以诊断早期肺癌，这也成了内镜医师们所面临的一大挑战。在WLB下往往难以识别黏膜光泽丧失、黏膜不规则、纵向皱褶或环形皱褶消失以及隆突增宽等细微的气道黏膜变化（表9.1）[5]。通过LDCT筛查发现的肺癌病灶大多＜20 mm（表9.2）[4,6-9]。利用支气管镜对这些多位于外周的小结节进行活检的平均诊断率仅为55%，而CT引导下经胸壁穿刺活检的诊断率可达66%~81%（表9.3）[3,4]。

尽管支气管镜技术已取得了许多进展，如高分辨率的白光支气管镜、可进一步进入远端支气管且具备可插入活检工具的工作通道的细支气管镜（外径为3 mm）、更大的旋转角度以及支气管腔内超声，但对于肺外周的小病灶，进行定位及活检仍然很困难。Ost等[10]利用AQuIRE数据库统计分析了不同的经支气管活检方法对＜2 cm的肺外周病变的诊断率。该研究纳入了来自美国15个中心的22名支气管镜医师的数据，结果显示，尽管使用径向支气管腔内超声和电磁导航支气管镜技术，但诊断率仍只有38.5%~57%。这表明，随着肺癌的主要类型发生转变（从多位于中央的鳞状细胞癌和小细胞肺癌转变为多位于外周的腺癌），早期肺癌的诊断也面临着新的挑战。因此，对新技术的需求不仅在于能引导工具到达病灶，还要能安全地获取足够多的活检标本以进行辅助检查。本章将重点介绍光学成像技术在诊断中央型肺癌与周围型肺癌中的应用。

表9.1　早期肺癌的镜下表现[5]

原位癌	黏膜下浸润	支气管周围侵犯
失去光泽	纵向皱褶消失	血管充血
黏膜不规则	环形皱褶消失	外源性压迫
黏膜肥厚	支气管软骨不明显	管腔狭窄
黏膜苍白	肿胀	
黏膜红肿	黏膜皱褶不明显	
结节样或息肉样病变		

表 9.2　低剂量 CT 扫描筛查出的肺癌大小[4,6-9]

尺寸	基线 CT			复查扫描		
(mm)	NLST	NELSON	PanCan	NLST	NELSON	PanCan
≤10	20%	30%	47%	45%	33%	62%
11~20	41%	53%	32%	31%	49%	25%
21~30	22%	14%	16%	15%	14%	8%
>30	17%	3%	5%	9%	4%	4%

NLST，美国国家肺癌筛查试验；NELSON，荷兰-比利时肺癌筛查试验；PanCan，泛加拿大早期肺癌检测研究。

表 9.3　支气管镜检查、CT 引导下经胸壁肺活检与手术切除对筛查发现的肺癌的诊断率[3,4]

方法	NLST		PanCan	
	占比	诊断率	占比	诊断率
支气管镜检查	34%	55.8%	20%	55.6%
CT 引导下经胸壁肺活检	19%	66.5%	38%	81.1%
手术	47%	73.9%[a]	42%	77.6%[a]

[a] 部分恶性。NLST，美国国家肺癌筛查试验；PanCan，泛加拿大早期肺癌检测研究。

9.2　光子成像原理

光子成像是基于光照射支气管表面时光与组织的相互作用。光由于光能分子振动状态改变，可以被支气管表面反射（镜面反射）、吸收，诱导自体荧光，也可以在支气管组织表面反向散射为入射光相同波长的光（弹性散射），或产生一个不同波长的散射（非弹性或拉曼散射）[11]。无论是 WLB、自发荧光支气管镜检查、使用光敏剂的光诊断、窄带成像、光学相干断层扫描（optical coherence tomography，OCT）还是拉曼光谱，图像都是基于光与组织相互作用的原理生成的。

9.3　自荧光支气管镜检查

白光支气管镜检查使用宽谱可见光（400~700 nm）来照亮支气管组织。其成像取决于穿透支气管组织、被组织吸收的光量与被组织散射、镜面反射的光量之间的差异。光还可以激发内源性荧光基团，使组织发出荧光。大多数内源性荧光基团参与了细胞代谢过程或与组织基质相关。最重要的荧光基团是结构蛋白，诸如胶原蛋白、弹性蛋白和参与细胞代谢的基团，如还原型烟酰胺腺嘌呤二核苷酸（NADH）与黄素。荧光基团还包括芳香族氨基酸、各种卟啉和脂质色素。在白光照射下，内源性荧光基团的自发荧光由于太弱而不可见。然而当支气管表面被紫光或蓝光（380~460 nm）照射，并由滤光片去除反射的紫光或蓝光时，即使没有图像增强剂也可以观察到自发荧光。正常的支气管组织呈绿色的强荧光（480~520 nm）。当支气管上皮由不典型增生转变为癌时，绿色和红色荧光都逐渐减弱，但后者减弱的比例相对较小。因此，异常组织的自发荧光表现为暗色、棕红色甚至红色。绿色荧光的减少主要是由于基质胶原交联的断裂、细胞代谢活性增加导致 NADH 和黄素腺嘌呤二核苷酸（FAD）辅酶的变化，以及新生血管内血红蛋白吸收较多蓝紫色光。肿瘤或坏死组织内细菌产物中较高的内源性卟啉也会增加红色荧光。区别肿瘤与正常组织的强度与对比度最佳的激发光波长为 405 nm[12-14]。正是基于这一原理开发了自荧光支气管镜（autofluorescence bronchoscope，AFB）设备，用以检查浸润前和早期浸润性支气管肺癌[15-18]。

为了突出正常组织和恶性组织的对比，通常将滤光光源或激光在反射后生成的少量蓝光或红光与自发荧光图像相结合，从而使正常组织呈绿色，而异常组织呈红色、紫色或棕红色[18-23]（表 9.4）。一些商用设

表 9.4　自荧光支气管镜设备[18-23]

设备	支气管镜	激发光 /nm	荧光 /nm	反射光 /nm	图像构成	异常病变
Onco-LIFE	光纤	395~445	500~720	675~720	绿色荧光，红色反光	绿色背景上的红/棕红色区域
SAFE-3000	视频内镜	408	430~700	408	绿/红色荧光，蓝色反光	蓝绿背景上的紫色区域
AFB	视频内镜	395~445	460~490	550, 610	绿色荧光，绿/红色反光	绿色背景上的洋红/紫色区域
DAFE	光纤	390~470	500~590	650~680	绿色荧光，红色反光	绿色背景上的红色区域
D-light	光纤	380~460	≥480	380~460	绿/红色荧光，蓝色反光	蓝绿背景上的紫色区域
ClearVu Elite	光纤	400~450	470~700	720~800	绿色荧光，红色反光	绿色背景上的红/棕红色区域

Onco-LIFE/Pin-point（Novadq，里士满，加拿大）；SAFE-3000（宾得-豪雅，东京，日本）；AFB（奥林巴斯，东京，日本）；DAFE（沃尔夫，克尼特林根，德国）；D-Light（史托斯，图林根，德国）；ClearVu Elite（Perceptronix 医疗公司，温哥华，加拿大）。

备允许同时显示白光和自发荧光图像，使气道检查更加方便和快捷。

目前已有的3项荟萃分析和多个多中心临床研究表明，在检测癌前病变方面，AFB或WLB+AFB较单独使用WLB具有更高的敏感性[24-26]。Sun等[24]发表了截至目前最大规模的荟萃分析，其纳入了21项研究，涉及3 266名患者。研究结果显示，在检查上皮内瘤变和浸润性癌方面，联用AFB与WLB相比单用WLB在每个病变基础上的相对敏感度分别为2.04（95% CI：1.72~2.42）和1.15（95% CI：1.05~1.26），而在每个病变基础上的相对特异性为0.65（95% CI：0.59~0.73）。AFB和WLB在检查浸润前病变（重度不典型增生和原位癌）方面优于单独使用WLB，但对于经验丰富的支气管镜医师来说，在检查浸润性癌症方面并没有显著优势[25]。较低的特异性主要是由炎症、感染和创伤导致的假阳性结果造成的。可以通过在AFB检查过程中尽量避免对支气管黏膜进行强力的吸引或接触来最小化假阳性表现的产生。具备AFB检查能力需要额外的训练，美国胸科医师协会的指南指出，在监督下完成20例检查操作才能达到AFB检查的基本能力[27]。

在开发出自荧光支气管镜检查技术之前，人们常使用光敏剂（如光卟啉®）进行光诊断。这些药物会被优先保留在肿瘤组织内，从而增强早期肺癌与邻近正常组织的对比，并引导光动力疗法（photodynamic therapy，PDT）[28]。由于该方法成本高且会引起皮肤长时间光敏，因此未能得到广泛应用。近来，随着LDCT筛查的落实，早期肺癌的检出率也随之提高，光诊断和PDT作为一种微创治疗手段，因可用于因心肺功能差或多发性肺癌而无法进行手术治疗的患者中而重新引发了人们的关注。新型光敏剂具有较短的皮肤光敏性持续时间，并且通过在正常组织中"关闭"其活性，在肿瘤细胞中"开启"其活性，从而最大限度地减少副作用[29-33]。利用外径为1 mm的超薄复合光纤镜，可实现沿外周支气管到达目标病灶，并在实时可视化与激光照射下进行PDT[34]。

9.4 窄带成像

窄带成像（narrow-band imaging，NBI）利用光学滤光器产生两种带宽的窄谱光生成图像，两种窄谱光分别为：会被浅表毛细血管中血红蛋白所吸收的390~445 nm蓝光，以及会被更深的黏膜下血管所吸收的530~550 nm绿光[35]。血管生成是恶性病变的特征之一，作为一种图像增强技术，NBI可以针对性地增强对支气管内微血管的成像[35,36]。浅表血管呈斑点状、迂曲或截断表现被认为是恶性病变与气道浸润的特征[35-37]。

有两项荟萃分析比较了AFB、AFB联合WLB与NBI诊断肺癌的敏感性和特异性。Iftikhar和Musani[38]分析了8项研究中632例接受NBI检查的患者数据，以及4项研究中413例同时接受NBI与AFB检查的患者数据。结果显示，NBI的合并敏感性和特异性分别为0.80（95% CI：0.77~0.83）和0.84（95% CI：0.81~0.86）。联合应用AFB与NBI的合并敏感性和特异性分别为0.86（95% CI：0.82~0.89）和0.75（95% CI：0.71~0.79），表明联合使用AFB和NBI并未显著提高诊断性能。作者推断NBI可能比AFB具有更高的敏感性和特异性。然而该荟萃分析所纳入研究的患者数量偏少，仅有22~136例不等。

另一项由Zhang等在2016年发表的更大规模的荟萃分析对WLB、AFB和NBI进行了比较[26]。作者共回顾了53项符合条件的研究（39项WLB、39项AFB、17项AFB和WLB，以及6项NBI）。其中，只有12项研究通过病理学评估了对高级别病变的诊断性能，包括诊断为中度不典型增生至浸润性癌症的2 880例患者和8 830例活检标本。该研究分析得出结论：单用AFB与联用AFB、WLB的表现接近，但均优于WLB。WLB的敏感性、特异性、诊断优势比（DOR）和曲线下面积（AUC）分别为51%（95% CI：34%~68%）、86%（95% CI：73%~84%）、6%（95% CI：3%~13%）和77%（95% CI：73%~81%）。而当使用AFB或联用AFB与WLB时则分别为93%（95% CI：77%~98%）和86%（95% CI：75%~97%），52%（95% CI：37%~67%）和71%（95% CI：56%~87%）。在其中一项研究中，NBI的敏感性为100%，特异性为43%。

AFB与NBI检查浸润前或早期浸润病灶的敏感性高于WLB，但特异性较低。观察者之间对血管分型的判断上存有显著差异可能是低特异性的原因。要充分实现NBI等新型图像增强内镜技术的临床效益，还需要基于图像帮助识别活检区域并进行能力评估的程序支持[39]。

检测浸润前病变的意义在于，它是一项重要的预测病变恶性风险的指标，不仅可以提示浸润前病变是否会发展为恶性肿瘤，还可以作为肺部其他部位出现恶性肿瘤的标志。van Boerdonk等进行的研究表明，在确诊存在浸润前病变的患者中，10年内有34%的患者通过 CT 与 AFB 联合进行的双峰监测诊断为肺癌，包括支气管内肿瘤和肺实质肿瘤[40]。

Tremblay 等研究了利用 AFB 在高危吸烟者中检测 LDCT 筛查不易发现的早期中央型肺癌。作为泛加拿大肺癌早期检测研究的一部分，该多中心试验在 6 年内对来自 7 个中心的 1 300 名具有≥2% 肺癌风险的参与者进行了 AFB 和 LDCT 扫描筛查[41]。其中，5.3% 的参与者被筛查出存在不典型增生、原位癌或浸润性癌。其中 CT 难以发现的隐匿性癌症占 0.15%（95% CI：0%~0.6%），仅有 1 例典型类癌和 1 例原位癌病灶是由 AFB 单独检出的。吸烟时长和 FEV_1% 预计值是发现不典型增生或原位癌的独立危险因素。该研究得出结论，随着肺癌的类型从鳞状细胞癌向常规支气管镜（外径 5.9 mm）不能到达的周围性腺癌转变，在 LDCT 扫描的基础上增加 AFB 所能检出的隐匿性癌症减少（0.15%），不足以支持将其纳入肺癌筛查计划。

在真实世界中，即使采用先进的支气管镜检查方法，如导航支气管镜检查和径向超声检查，对肺外周病变的诊断率也不到 60%[10,42]。对于肺外周病变，尤其是直径≤20 mm 的早期肺癌，我们需要更好的方法来实现内镜下的诊断。

9.5　光学相干断层扫描（OCT）

OCT 是一种可以提供接近组织学分辨率的成像方法，能够显示组织表面或以下的细胞和细胞外结构[43-47]。OCT 与超声原理相似，但 OCT 使用的是近红外光而不是声波。利用光学干涉测量技术可以根据被组织反向散射或反射的光生成一维的组织轮廓图。

被组织反向散射或反射的光使用光学干涉测量技术产生一维的组织轮廓图。通过在组织表面进行光束扫描，可以生成相应的二维图像或三维立体图像。在支气管镜检查中，通过向工作通道插入光纤探头至目标病灶来获得图像。该探头可用于气管直至末端细支气管的成像。根据成像条件的不同，OCT 的轴向和横向分辨率为 5~30 μm，成像深度为 2~3 mm。这种分辨率和成像深度适用于检查中央或外周气道的上皮改变。与超声波不同，光不需要液体耦合介质。用于 OCT 的弱近红外光源对患者也不会造成相关风险。

时域 OCT 利用低相干成像原理，通过参考臂的移动制造光程差与相对应深度的光发生干涉从而获得组织的深度信息，实现横向扫描是利用参考臂的水平移动或旋转[45,46]。频域 OCT 是在时域 OCT 的基础上发展改进，使用光谱仪代替参考臂的机械扫描结构，收集到的干涉图样通过测量谱密度函数并进行傅里叶变换从而获得组织的深度信息。谱密度函数可以通过干涉仪测量，包括宽带光源和光谱仪或是波长扫描光源和平方律检波器。研究显示，频域 OCT 检测的灵敏度相较时域 OCT 提高了几个数量级[47-51]。在切除的肺标本中，OCT 检查的结果与组织病理学结果密切相关[52-55]。软骨由于具有较低的散射特性，在 OCT 图像中通常表现为较暗的信号区。手术切除前根据 OCT 测量的平均管腔直径、管腔内面积、气道壁面积和气道壁厚度百分比，与切除标本中直至第 9 级支气管的组织学检查结果显著相关[56]。

OCT 成像的最新进展是自荧光联合 OCT（autofluorescence OCT，AF-OCT）[57,58]。AF-OCT 在中央气道中利用的光学原理与 AFB 相同。该技术克服了自荧光支气管镜的局限性，其成像探头比可弯曲支气管镜小得多，可以进入在支气管镜视野之外的外周小气道（图 9.1）。AF-OCT 可以快速地对气道结构进行扫描，相对多普勒 OCT 等其他检查方法更不易产生运动伪影[59]（图 9.2）。

临床研究表明，OCT 可被用于鉴别浸润性癌与原位癌或不典型增生[55,59]。一到两层细胞位于高度分散的基底膜和黏膜下层之上是正常组织或增生的特征。随着上皮组织从正常/增生变为化生、不同程度的不典型增生和原位癌，上皮层的厚度也不断增加。原位癌的基底膜仍然完整，但当癌症浸润后基底膜则变得不连续或消失[59]。鳞状细胞癌相比腺癌[57,60-62]或 CT 不可见中央型支气管肺癌具有不同的 OCT 特征。尽管 NBI 的一些特征（如血管迂曲）可提示存在黏膜下肿瘤浸润，通过 WLB、AFB 或 NBI 通常很难区分原位癌和浸润性癌[35]。准确判断肿瘤的浸润深度有助于更好地指导治疗。目前尚无研究对 OCT 与经支气管镜腔内超声（endobronchial ultrasound，EBUS）在确定肿瘤浸润支气管壁深度方面的准确性进行比较[63]。然而，中央型鳞状细胞肺癌患病率的显著下降使得这类研究难以开展。

OCT 是一种很有前途的指导诊断肺外周病变的方法。正常肺实质可以通过代表肺泡结构的蜂窝状信号空洞的存在来识别，而肺结节则表现为肺泡结构被实体组织所取代[58,64]。此外，呈附壁样生长模式的腺癌可以通过增厚的肺泡壁来识别（图 9.3）[63]。在完成 OCT 结果解读培训后，临床医生可以顺利地通过 OCT

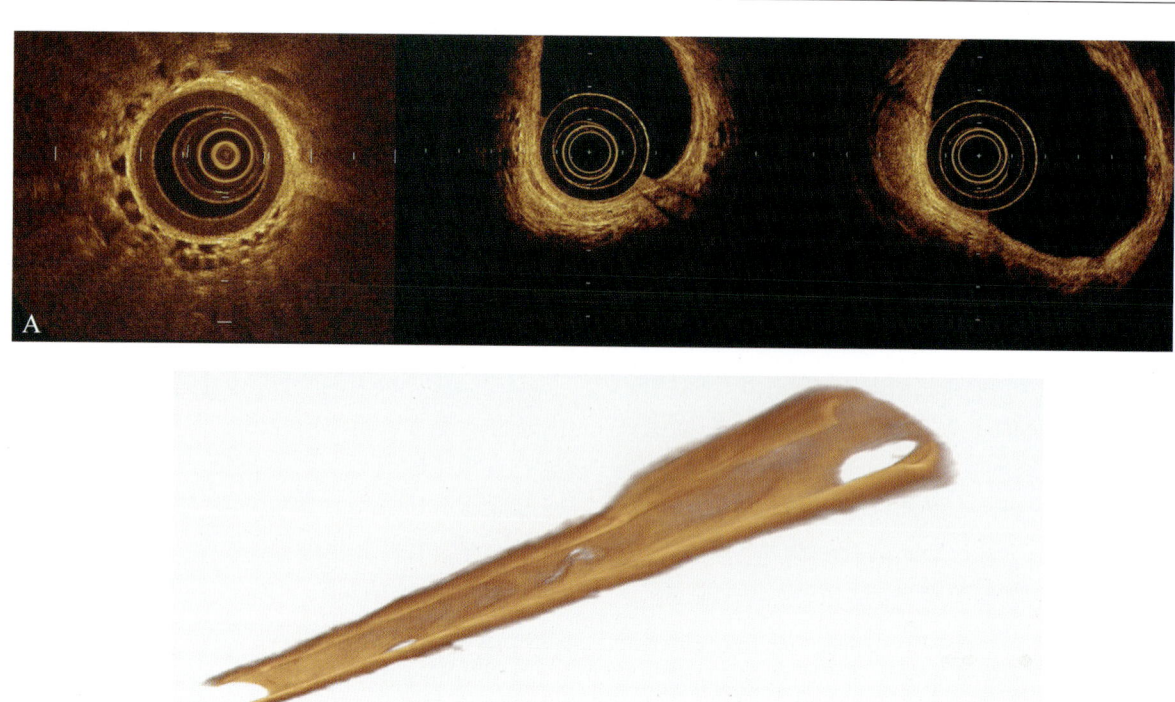

图 9.1　末端细支气管 OCT 图像

A. 正常末端细支气管与其邻近肺泡的 OCT 图像；B. 更近端气道的 3D 渲染图。

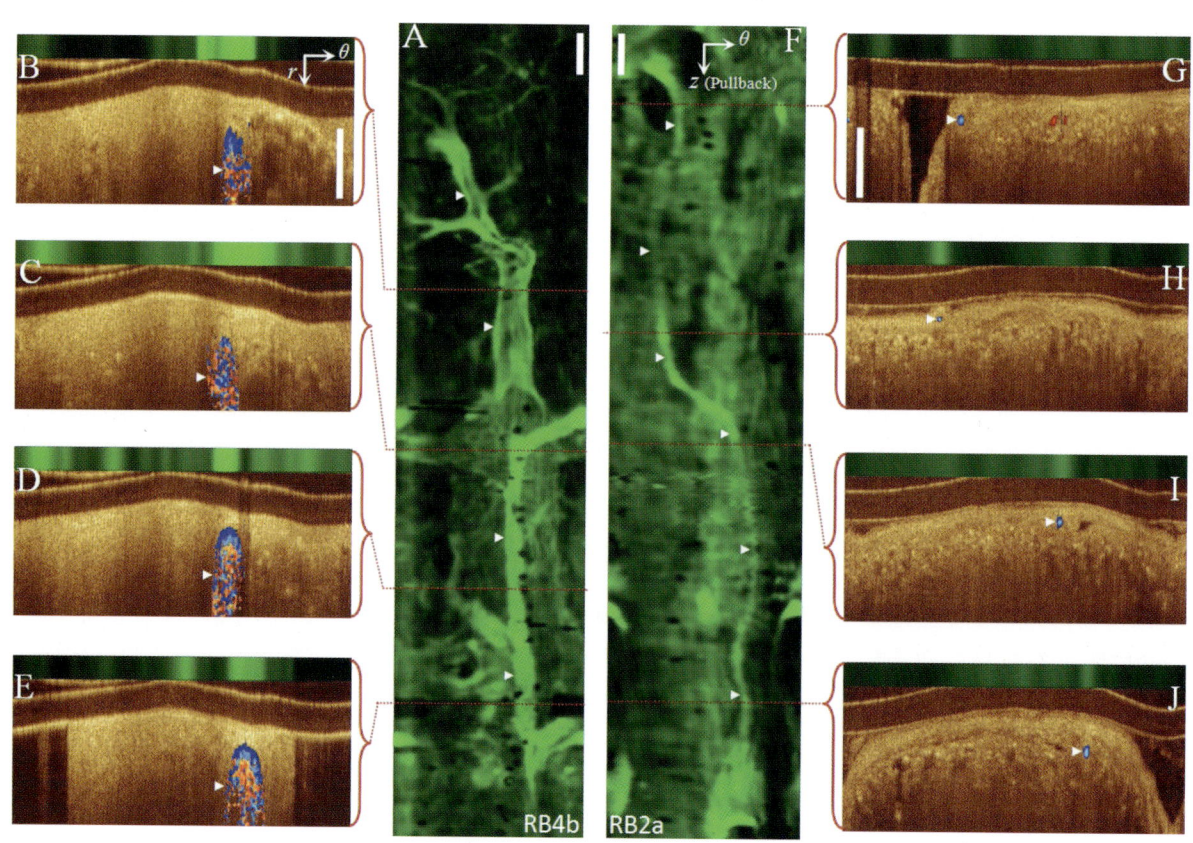

图 9.2　AF-OCT 图像

AF-OCT（A、F）与其相应的多普勒 OCT（B~E、G~J）显示血管大小。

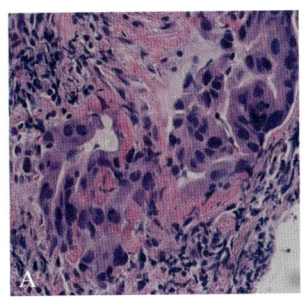 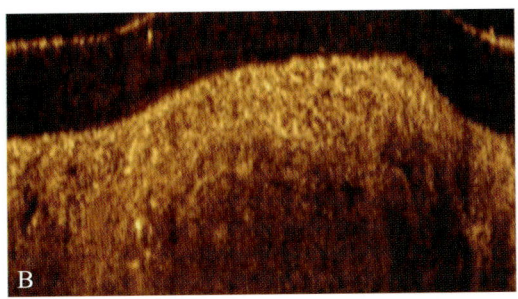 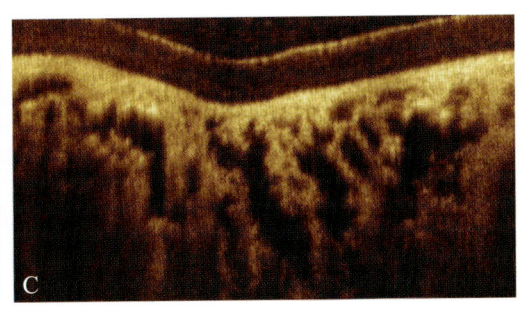

图9.3 腺癌

A. 腺癌的病理图像；B. 具有实性成分腺癌的OCT图像；C. 具有附壁样成分腺癌的OCT图像。

诊断常见的原发性肺癌（如腺癌、鳞状细胞癌、低分化癌），并达到平均82.6%（73.7%~94.7%）的诊断准确率[62]。虽然OCT在诊断肺癌中无法替代组织病理学的作用，但它可能有助于在活检前确认病变组织的性质。OCT探头直径较小，可以被直接插入活检针/导管内以实时指导活检。因此，无须将成像探头从引导鞘管中取出后再重新插入活检钳或针头，从而避免了在此过程中可能出现的移位或误入其他气道[65,66]。通过OCT或AF-OCT定位异常病变以指导活检的临床实用性还需要相关随机临床试验的进一步证实。其他技术方法，如共聚焦显微内镜等用以诊断肺外周病变的相关研究目前也在进行中。OCT或AF-OCT可以在不使用造影剂的情况下快速成像几厘米内的气道组织，而共聚焦显微内镜是一种点监测方法，并且需要使用造影剂[67]。

除了OCT之外，还有一些新兴技术可引导对肺外周病变进行精确活检，如0.8 mm的微型广角多光谱内镜成像系统，该系统可以进行反射与荧光成像[68]，且分辨率优于单独的反射成像[69]。

9.6 激光拉曼光谱

激光拉曼光谱（laser raman spectroscopy，LRS）是一种对组织进行低功率激光照射并收集其散射光来进行光谱分析的技术。这项技术的强大之处在于它可以无损地获取光谱，并且可以轻松地区分来自不同分子组成的标本产生的光散射[70,71]。拉曼效应是一种非弹性光散射过程，入射光子中有很小一部分会发生散射，同时频率也会发生相应的变化。入射与散射频率之间的差异取决于参与相互作用的分子的振动模式。拉曼光谱是通过绘制散射光子的强度作为频移的函数来描绘的。拉曼光谱可以捕获特定分子种类的特征性"指纹"，因此可以潜在地用于识别恶性组织。联合使用LRS、AFB与WLB在识别肺癌方面表现出了更高的特异性。一项探索性研究表明，LRS可能有助于减少活检取样的次数。不过，LRS目前仍只是一项实验性技术，尚待未来对其进行更深入的研究工作。

9.7 结论

AFB与NBI等光学成像方式在检测中央气道内早期肺癌方面表现出了卓越的敏感性，但使用这些技术需要进行额外的训练。随着肺癌的高发部位从中央气道转移到了超出标准支气管镜范围的肺外周，联合使用OCT与AF-OCT等成像方式也有助于气管镜医师在活检前评估病变，从而提高诊断率，减少不必要的活检，并指导后续内镜下的治疗。

参考文献

1 Fitzmaurice, C., Dicker, D., Pain, A. et al. (2015). The global burden of cancer 2013. *JAMA Oncol.* 1 (4): 505–527.

2 Coleman, M.P., Forman, D., Bryant, H. et al. (2011). Cancer survival in Australia, Canada, Denmark, Norway, Sweden, and the UK, 1995–2007 (the International Cancer Benchmarking Partnership): an analysis of population-based cancer registry data. *Lancet* 377 (9760): 127–138.

3 National Lung Screening Trial Research Team (2011). Reduced lung-cancer mortality with low-dose computed tomographic screening. *N. Engl. J. Med.* 365: 395–409.

4 Tammemagi, M.C., Schmidt, H., Martel, S. et al. (2017). Participant selection for lung cancer screening by risk modelling (the Pan-Canadian Early Detection of Lung Cancer [PanCan] study): a single-arm, prospective study. *Lancet Oncol.* 18: 1523–1531.

5 Hayata, Y. (1982). *Lung Cancer Diagnosis*. Tokyo: Igaku-Shoin.

6 Church, T.R., Black, W.C., Aberle, D.R. et al. (2013). Results

of initial low-dose computed tomographic screening for lung cancer. *N. Engl. J. Med.* 368 (21): 1980–1991.

7 McWilliams, A., Tammemagi, M.C., Mayo, J.R. et al. (2013). Probability of cancer in pulmonary nodules detected on first screening CT. *N. Engl. J. Med.* 369 (10): 910–919.

8 Aberle, D.R., DeMello, S., Berg, C.D. et al. (2013). Results of the two incidence screenings in the National Lung Screening Trial. *N. Engl. J. Med.* 369 (10): 920–931.

9 Horeweg, N., Rosmalen, J., Marjolein, A. et al. (2014). Lung cancer probability in patients with CT-detected pulmonary nodules: a prespecified analysis of data from the NELSON trial of low-dose CT screening. *Lancet Oncol.* 15: 1332–1341.

10 Ost, D.E., Ernst, A., Lei, X. et al. (2016). Diagnostic yield and complications of bronchoscopy for peripheral lung lesions. Results of the AQuIRE registry. *Am. J. Respir. Crit. Care Med.* 193 (1): 68–77.

11 Wagnieres, G., McWilliams, A., and Lam, S. (2003). Lung cancer imaging with fluorescence endoscopy. In: *Handbook of Biomedical Fluorescence* (eds. M. Mycek and B. Pogue), 361–396. New York: Marcel Dekker.

12 Hung, J., Lam, S., LeRiche, J.C. et al. (1991). Autofluorescence of normal and malignant bronchial tissue. *Lasers Surg. Med.* 11 (2): 99–105.

13 Zellweger, M., Grosjean, P., Goujon, D. et al. (2001). In vivo autofluorescence spectroscopy of human bronchial tissue to optimize the detection and imaging of early cancers. *J. Biomed. Opt.* 6 (1): 41–51.

14 Lam, S. (2005). The role of autofluorescence bronchoscopy in diagnosis of early lung cancer. In: *IASLC Textbook of Prevention and Early Detection of Lung Cancer* (eds. F.R. Hirsch, P.A. Bunn Jr., H. Kato and J.L. Mulshine), 160–172. Abingdon: Taylor and Francis.

15 Palcic, B., Lam, S., Hung, J. et al. (1991). Detection and localization of early lung cancer by imaging techniques. *Chest* 99 (3): 742–743.

16 Lam, S., MacAulay, C., Hung, J. et al. (1993). Detection of dysplasia and carcinoma in situ with a lung imaging fluorescence endoscope device. *J. Thorac. Cardiovasc. Surg.* 105 (6): 1035–1040.

17 Lam, S., Kennedy, T., Unger, M. et al. (1998). Localization of bronchial intraepithelial neoplastic lesions by fluorescence bronchoscopy. *Chest* 113 (3): 696–702.

18 Edell, E., Lam, S., Pass, H. et al. (2009). Detection and localization of intraepithelial neoplasia and invasive carcinoma using fluorescence-reflectance bronchoscopy: an international, multicenter clinical trial. *J. Thorac. Oncol.* 4 (1): 49–54.

19 Chiyo, M., Shibuya, K., Hoshino, H. et al. (2005). Effective detection of bronchial preinvasive lesions by a new autofluorescence imaging bronchovideoscope system. *Lung Cancer* 48 (3): 307–313.

20 Häussinger, K., Stanzel, F., Huber, R.M. et al. (1999). Autofluorescence detection of bronchial tumors with the D-Light/AF. *Diagn. Ther. Endosc.* 5 (2): 105–112.

21 Goujon, D., Zellweger, M., Radu, A. et al. (2003). In vivo autofluorescence imaging of early cancers in the human tracheobronchial tree with a spectrally optimized system. *J. Biomed. Opt.* 8 (1): 17–25.

22 Tercelj, M., Zeng, H., Petek, M. et al. (2005). Acquisition of fluorescence and reflectance spectra during routine bronchoscopy examinations using the ClearVu Elite device: pilot study. *Lung Cancer* 50: 35–42.

23 Ikeda, N., Honda, H., Hayashi, A. et al. (2005). Early detection of bronchial lesions using newly developed videoendoscopy-based autofluorescence bronchoscopy. *Lung Cancer* 52 (1): 21–27.

24 Sun, J., Garfield, D.H., Lam, B. et al. (2011). The value of autofluorescence bronchoscopy combined with white light bronchoscopy compared with white light alone in the diagnosis of intraepithelial neoplasia and invasive lung cancer: a meta-analysis. *J. Thorac. Oncol.* 6: 1336–1344.

25 Chen, W., Gao, X., Tian, Q. et al. (2011). A comparison of autofluorescence bronchoscopy and white light bronchoscopy in detection of lung cancer and preneoplastic lesions: a meta-analysis. *Lung Cancer* 73: 183–188.

26 Jianrong, Z., Jieye, W., Yujing, Y. et al. (2016). White light, autofluorescence and narrow band imaging bronchoscopy for diagnosing airway pre-cancerous and early cancer lesions: a systematic review and meta-analysis. *J. Thorac. Dis.* 8 (11): 3205–3216.

27 Ernst, A., Silvestri, G.A., and Johnstone, D. (2003). Interventional pulmonary procedures: guidelines from the American College of Chest Physicians. *Chest* 123 (5): 1693–1717.

28 Doiron, D.R., Profio, E., Vincent, R.G., and Dougherty, T.J. (1979 Jul). Fluorescence bronchoscopy for detection of lung cancer. *Chest* 76 (1): 27–32.

29 Usuda, J., Tsutsui, H., Honda, H. et al. (2007 Dec). Photodynamic therapy for lung cancers based on novel photodynamic diagnosis using talaporfin sodium (NPe6) and autofluorescence bronchoscopy. *Lung Cancer* 58 (3): 317–323.

30 Ohtani, K., Usuda, J., Ogawa, E. et al. (2017). Skin fluorescence following photodynamic therapy with NPe6 photosensitizer. *Photodiagn. Photodyn. Ther.* 20: 210–214.

31 Jin, C.S., Wada, H., Anayama, T. et al. (2016). An integrated nanotechnology-enabled transbronchial image-guided intervention strategy for peripheral lung cancer. *Cancer Res.* 76 (19): 5870–5880.

32 Kato, T., Jin, C., Ujiie, H. et al. (2017). Nanoparticle targeted folate-receptor 1 enhanced photodynamic therapy for lung cancer. *Lung Cancer* 113: 59–68.

33 Luby, B., Charron, D.M., MacLaughlin, C.M., and Zheng, G. (2016). Activatable fluorescence: from small molecule to nanoparticle. *Adv. Drug Deliv. Rev.* (16): 30242–30243.

34 Kasuya, K., Oka, K., Soya, R. et al. (2017). Photodynamic therapy for biliary tract organ via a novel ultrasmall composite optical fiberscope. *Exp. Ther. Med.* 14 (5): 4344–4348.

35 Shibuya, K., Nakajima, T., Fujiwara, T. et al. (2010). Narrow band imaging with high-resolution bronchovideoscopy: a new approach for visualizing angiogenesis in squamous cell carcinoma of the lung. *Lung Cancer* 69: 194–202.

36 Herth, F., Eberhardt, R., Anantham, D. et al. (2009). Narrow-band imaging bronchoscopy increases the specificity of

bronchoscopic early lung cancer detection. *J. Thorac. Oncol.* 4: 1060–1065.

37 Andolfi, M., Potenza, R., Capozzi, R. et al. (2016). The role of bronchoscopy in the diagnosis of early stage lung cancer: a review. *J. Thorac. Dis.* 8 (11): 3329–3337.

38 Iftikhar, I.H. and Musani, A.I. (2015). Narrow-band imaging bronchoscopy in the detection of premalignant airway lesions: a meta-analysis for diagnostic test accuracy. *Ther. Adv. Respir. Dis.* 9: 207–216.

39 Dumas, C., Fielding, D., Coles, T. et al. (2016). Development of a novel image-based program to teach narrow-band imaging. *Ther. Adv. Respir. Dis.* 10 (4): 300–309.

40 van Boerdonk, R.A., Smesseim, I., Heideman, D.A. et al. (2015). Close surveillance with long-term follow-up of subjects with preinvasive endobronchial lesions. *Am. J. Respir. Crit. Care Med.* 192 (12): 1483–1489.

41 Tremblay, A., Taghizadeh, N., McWilliams, A.M. et al. (2016). Low prevalence of high grade lesions detected with autofluorescence bronchoscopy in the setting of lung cancer screening in the Pan-Canadian lung cancer screening study. *Chest* 150 (5): 1015–1022.

42 Ali, M.S., Trick, W., Mba, B.I. et al. (2017). Radial endobronchial ultrasound for the diagnosis of peripheral pulmonary lesions: a systematic review and meta-analysis. *Respirology* 22 (3): 443–453.

43 Huang, D., Swanson, E.A., Lin, C.P. et al. (1991). Optical coherence tomography. *Science* 254 (5035): 1178–1181.

44 Tearney, G.J., Brezinski, M.E., Boppart, S.A. et al. (1996). Images in cardiovascular medicine. Catheter-based optical imaging of a human coronary artery. *Circulation* 94 (11): 3013.

45 Fujimoto, J.G., Brezinski, M.E., Tearney, G.J. et al. (1995). Optical biopsy and imaging using optical coherence tomography. *Nat. Med.* 1 (9): 970–972.

46 Tearney, G.J., Brezinski, M.E., Bouma, B.E. et al. (1997). In vivo endoscopic optical biopsy with optical coherence tomography. *Science* 276 (5321): 2037–2039.

47 Choma, M., Sarunic, M., Yang, C. et al. (2003). Sensitivity advantage of swept source and Fourier domain optical coherence tomography. *Opt. Express* 11 (18): 2183–2189.

48 de Boer, J.F., Cense, B., Park, B.H. et al. (2003). Improved signal-to-noise ratio in spectral-domain compared with time-domain optical coherence tomography. *Opt. Lett.* 28 (21): 2067–2069.

49 Leitgeb, R., Hitzenberger, C., and Fercher, A. (2003). Performance of fourier domain vs. time domain optical coherence tomography. *Opt. Express* 11 (8): 889–894.

50 Wojtkowski, M., Bajraszewski, T., Targowski, P. et al. (2003). Real-time in vivo imaging by high-speed spectral optical coherence tomography. *Opt. Lett.* 28 (19): 1745–1747.

51 Yun, S.H., Tearney, G.J., de Boer, J.F. et al. (2003). High-speed optical frequency-domain imaging. *Opt. Express* 11 (22): 2953–2963.

52 Hariri, L.P., Applegate, M.B., Mino-Kenudson, M. et al. (2013). Optical frequency domain imaging of ex vivo pulmonary resection specimens: obtaining one to one image to histopathology correlation. *J. Vis. Exp.* 71: ii.

53 Ohtani, K., Lee, A.M., and Lam, S. (2012). Frontiers in bronchoscopic imaging. *Respirology* 17 (2): 261–269.

54 Pahlevaninezhad, H., Lee, A.M., Lam, S. et al. (2014). Coregistered autofluorescence-optical coherence tomography imaging of human lung sections. *J. Biomed. Opt.* 19 (3): 36022.

55 Tsuboi, M., Hayashi, A., Ikeda, N. et al. (2005). Optical coherence tomography in the diagnosis of bronchial lesions. *Lung Cancer* 49 (3): 387–394.

56 Chen, Y., Ding, M., Guan, W.J. et al. (2015). Validation of human small airway measurements using endobronchial optical coherence tomography. *Respir. Med.* 109 (11): 1446–1453.

57 Pahlevaninezhad, H., Lee, A.M.D., Shaipanich, T. et al. (2014). A high-efficiency fiber-based imaging system for co-registered autofluorescence and optical coherence tomography. *Biomed. Opt. Express* 5 (9): 2978–2987.

58 Pahlevaninezhad, H., Lee, A.M., Hohert, G. et al. (2016). Endoscopic high-resolution autofluorescence imaging and OCT of pulmonary vascular networks. *Opt. Lett.* 41 (14): 3209–3212.

59 Lam, S., Standish, B., Baldwin, C. et al. (2008). In vivo optical coherence tomography imaging of preinvasive bronchial lesions. *Clin. Cancer Res.* 14 (7): 2006–2011.

60 Hariri, L.P., Applegate, M.B., Mino-Kenudson, M. et al. (2013). Volumetric optical frequency domain imaging of pulmonary pathology with precise correlation to histopathology. *Chest* 143 (1): 64–74.

61 Hariri, L.P., Villiger, M., Applegate, M.B. et al. (2013). Seeing beyond the bronchoscope to increase the diagnostic yield of bronchoscopic biopsy. *Am. J. Respir. Crit. Care Med.* 187 (2): 125–129.

62 Hariri, L.P., Mino-Kenudson, M., Lanuti, M. et al. (2015). Diagnosing lung carcinomas with optical coherence tomography. *Ann. Am. Thorac. Soc.* 12 (2): 193–201.

63 Herth, F., Ernst, A., Schulz, M. et al. (2003). Endobronchial ultrasound reliably differentiates between airway infiltration and compression by tumor. *Chest* 123 (2): 458–462.

64 Hariri, L.P., Mino-Kenudson, M., Applegate, M.B. et al. (2013). Toward the guidance of transbronchial biopsy: identifying pulmonary nodules with optical coherence tomography. *Chest* 144 (4): 1261–1268.

65 Tan, K.M., Shishkov, M., Chee, A. et al. (2012). Flexible transbronchial optical frequency domain imaging smart needle for biopsy guidance. *Biomed. Opt. Express* 3 (8): 1947–1954.

66 Gora, M.J., Suter, M.J., Tearney, G.J., and Li, X. (2017). Endoscopic optical coherence tomography: technologies and clinical applications [Invited]. *Biomed. Opt. Express* 8 (5): 2405–2444.

67 Thiberville, L. and Salaün, M. (2010). Bronchoscopic advances: on the way to the cells. *Respiration* 79 (6): 441–449.

68 Tate, T.H., Keenan, M., Black, J. et al. (2017). Ultraminiature optical design for multispectral fluorescence imaging endoscopes. *J. Biomed.* 22 (3): 036013.

69 Godbout, K., Martel, S., Simon, M. et al. (2016). Evaluation of pulmonary nodules using the spyglass direct visualization system combined with radial endobronchial ultrasound: a clinical feasibility study. *Open Respir. Med. J.* 10: 79–85.

70 McGregor, H.C., Short, M.A., McWilliams, A. et al. (2016). Real-time endoscopic Raman spectroscopy for in vivo early lung cancer detection. *J. Biophotonics* 10 (1): 98–110.

71 Short, M., Lam, S., McWilliams, A. et al. (2011 Jul). Using laser Raman spectroscopy to reduce false positives of autofluorescence bronchoscopies: a pilot study. *J. Thorac. Oncol.* 6 (7): 1206–1214.

第 10 章

电磁导航支气管镜

Carlos Aravena Leon[1,2] and Thomas R. Gildea[1]
[1] Department of Pulmonary, Allergy and Critical Care Medicine,
Respiratory Institute, Cleveland Clinic, Cleveland, OH, USA
[2] Department of Respiratory Diseases, Faculty of Medicine,
Pontificia Universidad Católica de Chile, Santiago, Chile
（译者：钟长镐　游振锭　译者单位：广州医科大学附属第一医院）

10.1 引言

自 1990 年以来，在美国，肺癌已成为导致死亡、残疾（伤残调整生命年）和早死所致生命损失年的主要原因之一。尽管在减轻肺癌疾病负担方面已取得重大进展，但截至 2016 年，肺癌仍然是伤残调整生命年和早死所致生命损失年的第二大原因，也是总体死亡率较高的主要原因之一[1]。此外，肺癌也是恶性肿瘤死亡的主要原因。2015 年，因肺癌死亡的人数为 153 722 人。此外，2018 年预计肺癌仍将是第二常见的癌症类型，预估新发病例数为 234 030 例[2]。

低剂量计算机体层成像（low-dose computed tomography，LDCT）筛查能有效地降低肺癌死亡率[3]。LDCT 能在 20% 的筛查人群中识别出单发或多发肺结节，其中约 1% 确诊为肺癌[4]。数据显示，每年约有 120 万人发现肺部有新发结节，其中超过 6.3 万人在后续 2 年的随访中被确诊为肺癌[5]。

在 LDCT 筛查或胸部影像学筛查中偶然发现的可疑肺结节患者，需要及时并有效地进行初步评估，判断可疑肺结节是否为肺癌[6]。然而，新发肺结节的增多也容易导致大量假阳性的出现，这就需要进行仔细的风险效益分析才能得出确切诊断[7]。临床医生将根据患者的肺癌风险评估、肺结节影像特征和合并症情况等来综合决定诊断的方法[8]。

对于呼吸专科医师而言，肺外周病变（peripheral pulmonary lesion，PPL）的诊断具有挑战性。传统支气管镜检查对 PPL 的检出率较低[9]。在小于 2 cm 且位于肺外 1/3 的结节中，检出率低至 14%[10]。2003 年，美国胸科医师学会（ACCP）建议不要对 PPL 患者进行经支气管活检[11-12]。而 2013 年的指南推荐，如果设备及专业知识许可（IC 级），建议使用电磁导航引导取样[13]。相关的诊断技术及证据也在不断更新。

10.2 发展史

20 世纪 90 年代，计算机技术的进步推动了虚拟现实的发展，尤其是在构建气管-支气管树中[14]。一种基于微型电磁传感器和低功率磁场发生器的方法可以进行实时的体内定位和导航，逐步成为支气管镜检查的辅助手段[14-16]。一篇关于电磁导航支气管镜（electromagnetic navigation bronchoscopy，ENB）的综述回顾了该技术的演变发展历史[17]（图 10.1）。

21 世纪初，随着胸部 CT 筛查的增加，外周病变与中央病变占比出现变化，加之传统支气管镜检查对 PPL 的低检出率，加快了 ENB 的发展，并试图通过该技术的应用取代一些高成本或有并发症风险的活检方法，如经胸壁针吸活检，电视辅助胸腔镜或诊断性开

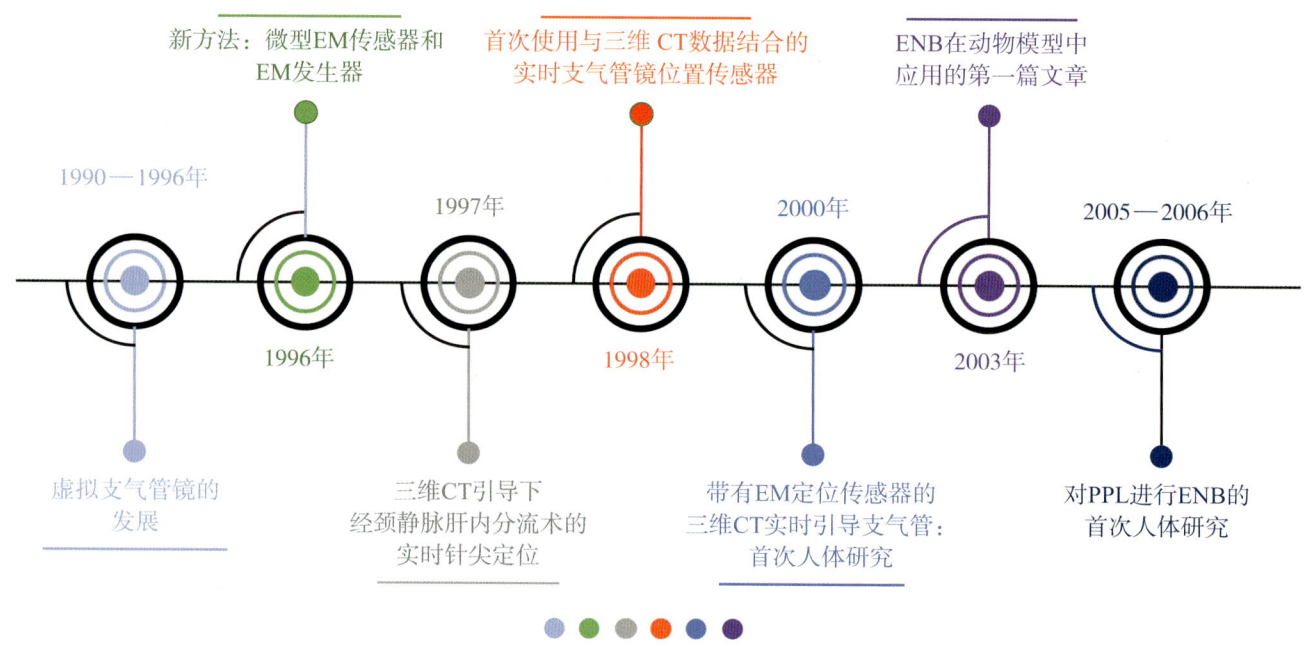

图 10.1　ENB 的发展历史时间轴

胸手术等[11,18-20]。

2003 年，Swartz 等发表了第一篇关于在动物模型中进行电磁导航引导可弯曲支气管镜检查的文章[19]。随后，Becker 等和 Schwarz 等首次在人体中开展 ENB 相关研究，针对 PPL 进行活检取样[20,21]。Gildea 等在一项前瞻性研究中评估了 ENB 在纵隔淋巴结病变中的应用价值[22]。

10.3　技术组成

电磁导航系统整合了几项关键技术，为操作者提供了术前支气管树规划模型和地图、实时定位和导航，以及用于置入专用器械的引导鞘管。在过去 15 年中，这些技术从各个层面均得到提升，也有许多同类竞品已进入市场，尽管呈现方式不同，但每种技术都促进了导航平台的发展。

目前最常用的 ENB 系统是 SuperDimension™（美国明尼苏达州明尼阿波利斯市，美敦力公司）。它主要由四部分构成[19,20,22]。

（1）磁导航电磁板

尺寸为 47 cm×56 cm×1 cm。它能发射低频电磁波，放置于支气管镜诊床头端，用于在患者躯干周边产生磁场（图 10.2）。

（2）附带传感器的定位探头

在最初版本中，探头内芯可通过控制杆和旋钮从近端实施主动调控。当前版本是被动式的，通过前端

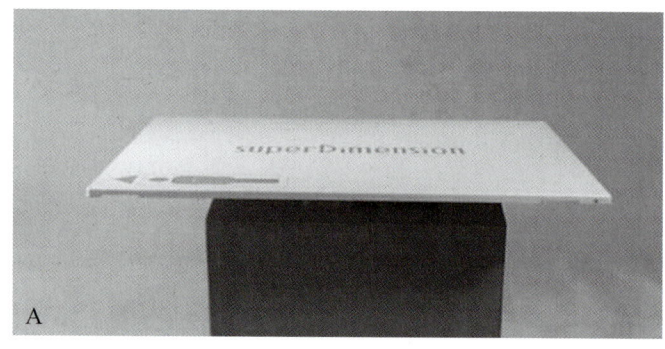
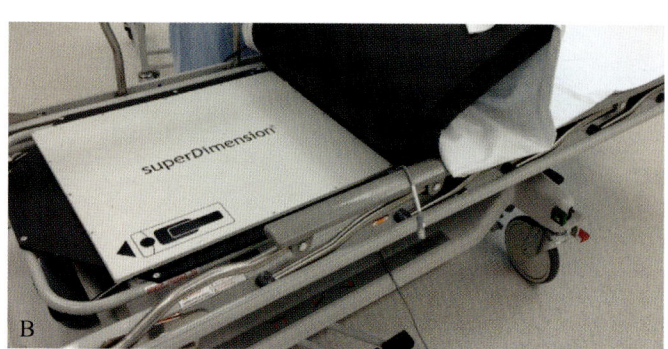

图 10.2　磁导航电磁板

A. 电磁板；B. 放置在支气管镜检查床头端下方的电磁板。

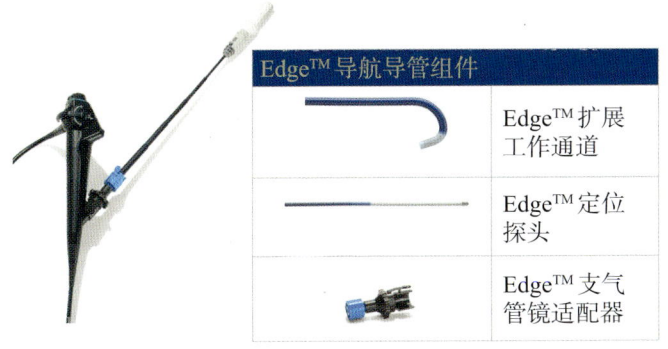

图 10.3　定位探头（当前版本）

预弯的定位导管实现各种角度的引导（图 10.3）。

（3）柔性导管

柔性导管作为延伸的工作通道（extended working channel，EWC），长 130 cm，直径 1.9 mm。定位探头（locatable guide，LG）被放置其中，当导航系统引导抵达靶点时，EWC 即被留置固定在靶点处，为支气管镜活检工具提供通道。当前版本中，导管长 106.95 cm，外径 2.68 mm，内径 2.08 mm，具备不同的预弯角度（如 45°、90°、180°、190° 等），以协助进入一些角度过大的气道拐角（图 10.4）。

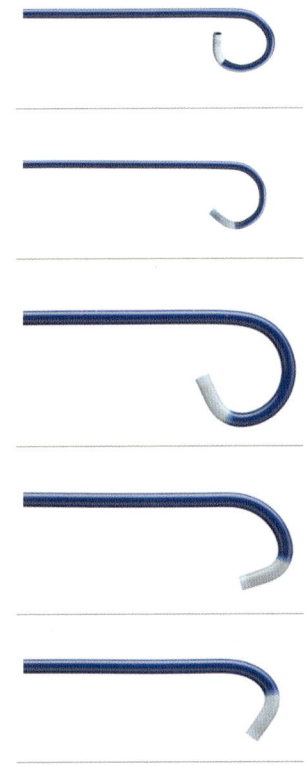

图 10.4　延长的工作通道导管

当前版本的所有角度类型。

（4）导航规划软件及硬件

软件系统可对高分辨螺旋 CT 的医学数字成像和通信（digital imaging and communication in medicine，DICOM）格式数据进行气道三维重建，构建虚拟支气管图像。构建的图像包括表示传感器探头位置的图形信息以及预先识别的解剖标志和目标病变的位置。路径最初是由内镜操作者规划，但随着计算机技术的发展，现在许多步骤都已实现自动化。关键是操作人员要学会使用三维重建后的气道模型来规划手术路径（图 10.5）。这个过程包括以下四个不同的阶段：

1）规划：即影像采集和绘图。在 ENB 软件中下载胸部高分辨螺旋 CT 扫描数据，通过多平面数字信息来重建支气管树的轴向、冠状和矢状位图以及虚拟图像。支气管镜医师利用这些信息规划通往目标病变的路径。虽然该系统现在仅用作备份系统，但系统会提示用户在 5 个标准解剖标志中进行选择，这些标志将有助于对齐虚拟支气管镜和电磁图，以便在需要时手动配准（图 10.5）。

2）注册及支气管内测绘：即支气管镜定位与配准。当患者躺在检查床上时，将 3 个传感器放置在被检查者的胸部，用以模拟和补偿患者的呼吸运动和在床上的位置移动。然后将支气管镜置入气管，沿支气管镜工作通道将已预置入 LG 的 EWC 送入气管中。LG 的传感器探头设置数百个配准点，这些配准点与建立的 3D 虚拟支气管图像中的注册点一一叠加校正。在操作过程中，为了提高模型的准确性，控制 LG 要以均匀的深度和平衡的方式探查肺部（图 10.6）。

3）导航：当配准完成后，远端装有传感器的支气管镜在通向肺部病变的气道中前进。LG 和 EWC 由电磁导航监视器引导，该监视器上会显示代表传感器探头、解剖标志和目标病变位置的图形信息。为了尽可能靠近病灶，需要 LG 末端到目标病变在正确的平面上并保持直线（图 10.7）。

4）活检：可通过透视来确认活检部位（推荐但非必需）[23]。把 EWC 固定在工作通道端口上，然后把 LG 从 EWC 上取出；EWC 中插入径向支气管腔内超声探头或其他仪器来进一步确认病变位置。在收回径向探头后，插入支气管镜工具以活检采集样本。

10.4　实施

在 2005 年，Becker 等发表了首个初步研究报告，

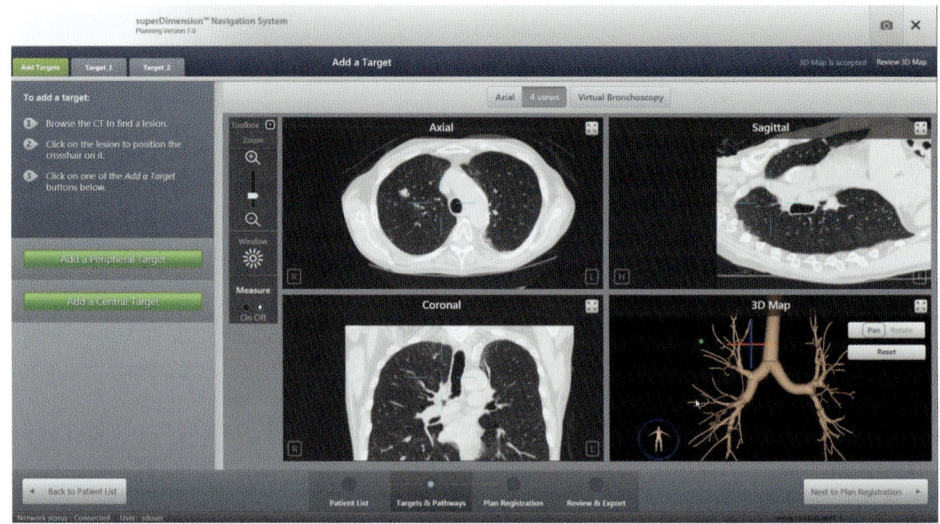

图 10.5　EMN 系统规划软件

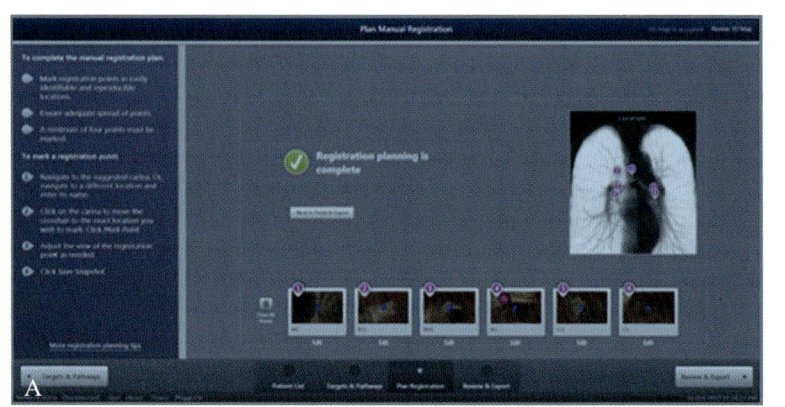 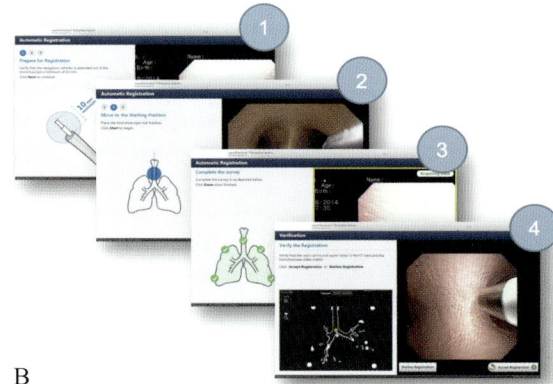

图 10.6　注册（A）和支气管镜定位与配准（B）界面

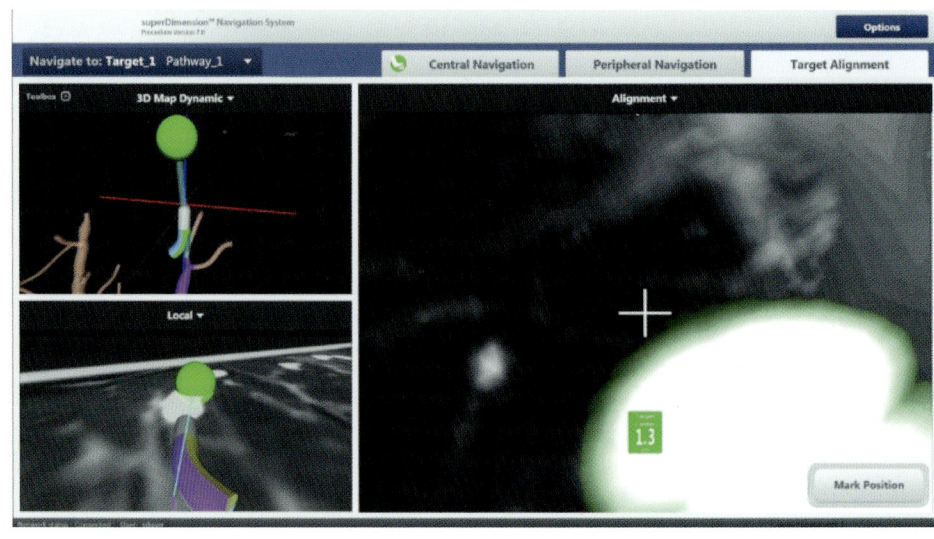

图 10.7　术中导航界面

对30个PPL患者进行电磁导航下支气管镜活检,诊断率达69%。病变大小为12~106 mm(平均39.8 mm),病灶距离胸膜的平均距离为1.9 mm(范围0~41 mm,标准差10.3 mm)。与传统支气管镜检查相比,ENB的手术时间增加了7.3 min[20]。在2006年,Schwarz等进行了一项研究,该研究纳入了13名内镜下未发现病变的患者,病变大小为15~50 mm(平均33.5 mm),诊断率为69%[21]。之后,Gildea等在克利夫兰临床医学中心进行了一项更大规模的前瞻性单中心研究。该研究共纳入了60名受试者。肺外周病变平均大小为22.8 mm(±12.6 mm),导航平均时间为7 min(±6 min),诊断率为74%[22]。除此以外,该研究还评估了ENB在纵隔淋巴结中的应用价值[22]。多项研究表明,ENB在不同条件下也能展现出类似的诊断性能[18-49](图10.8、表10.1)。

与ENB和径向支气管腔内超声(radial-probe endobronchial ultrasound,REBUS)有关的唯一一项随机化、前瞻性试验是相关研究中的例外,Eberhardt等报道,ENB与REBUS技术结合的诊断率为88%[46]。但该诊断率从未被其他研究复现,即使研究是由该团队进行的。

2012年,一篇纳入了39项经支气管镜诊断肺外周结节相关研究的meta分析报道,合并的诊断率为70%(范围为46%~86.2%,具有明显差异)[52]。2013年,ACCP肺癌指南报道,在14项研究中,对932例患者使用ENB协助诊断,其中在前瞻性试验中诊断率为68%,在回顾性试验中诊断率为74%[13]。2015年发表的一项纳入了15篇使用ENB诊断PPL相关研究的meta分析发现,合并的敏感性、特异性、阳性似然比和阴性似然比分别为82%、100%、19.36和0.2。由于患者选择了不同的活检技术,敏感性和阴性似然比具有显著异质性[53]。有趣的是,另一项meta分析报道导航

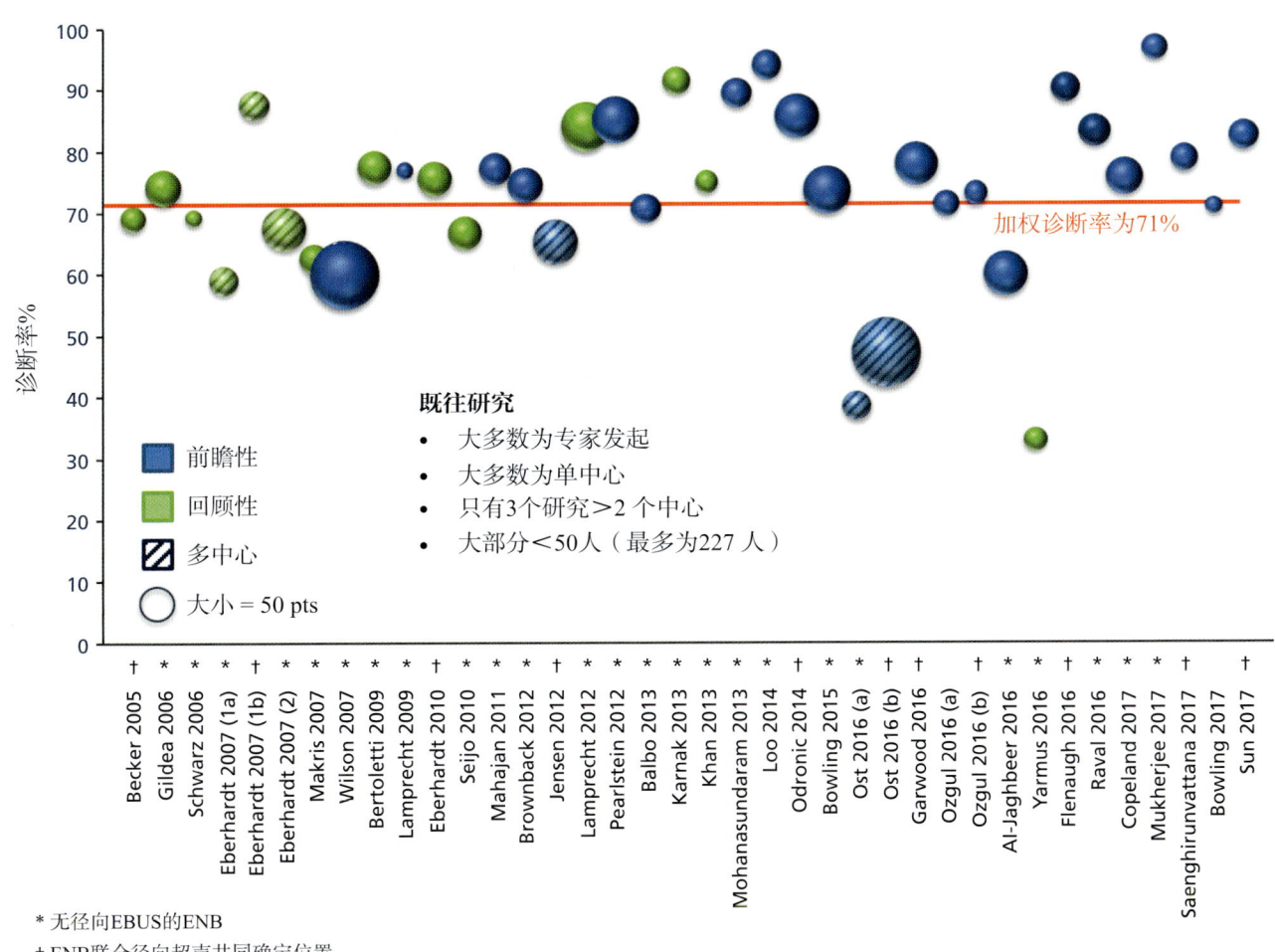

* 无径向EBUS的ENB
† ENB联合径向超声共同确定位置

图10.8 已发表ENB研究的诊断率

来源:允许转载自ENB对周围性肺部病变的诊断率:前瞻性、多中心NAVIGATE研究1年的结果。图片版权归Medtronic所有。

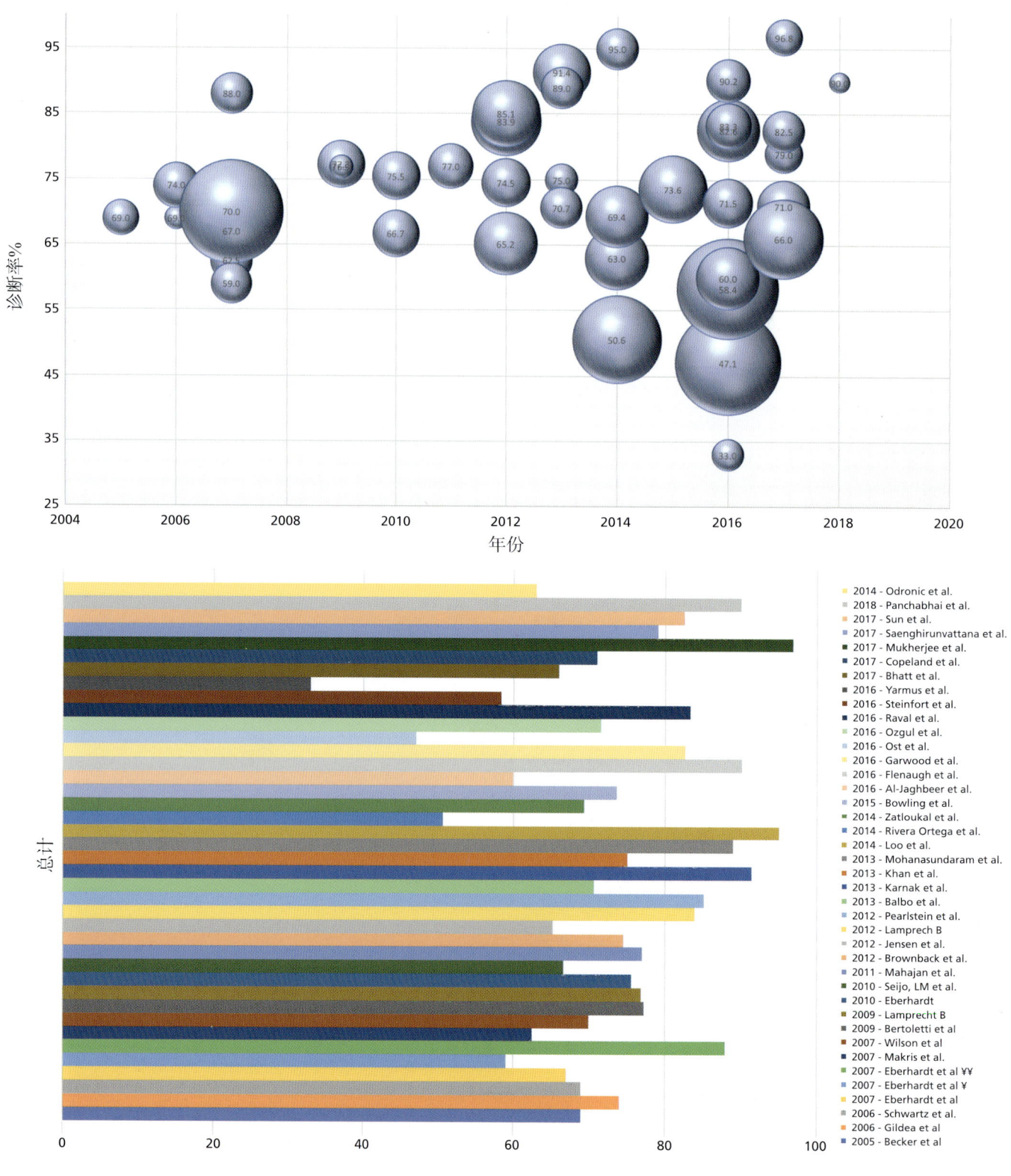

图 10.8 已发表 ENB 研究的诊断率（续）

成功率为 97.4%，但合并诊断率较低，仅为 64.9%[54]。

AQuIRE（ACCP 质量改进登记、评估和教育）登记处对接受支气管镜检查及经支气管活检的 PPL 患者进行了一项多中心研究。共 312 名患者接受了诊断性支气管镜检查。2016 年发表的结果显示，单独使用 ENB 的诊断率较低，仅为 38.5%，当 ENB 与 REBUS

表 10.1 ENB 相关研究的总结

研究	研究设计	SD/Veran	技术	活检	样本量	病变平均大小 (mm)	诊断率 (%)	并发症	其他评论
Becker 等[20]	回顾性	SD	RB/FB/Fluoro/EBUS	活检钳/细胞刷	30	24	69	1例气胸（插入胸管）(3.3%)	
Schwartz 等[21]	前瞻性	SD	FB/Fluoro	活检钳/TBNA/细胞刷	13	33.5±11	69	3例轻度出血，无气胸	
Gildea 等[22]	前瞻性	SD	FB/Fluoro	冲洗/细胞刷/TBNA	49	22.8	74	2例气胸（均插入胸管）(3.4%)	
Makris 等[23]	前瞻性	SD	FB	仅活检钳	40	23.5	62.5	3例气胸（1例插入胸管）(7.5%)，1例II型呼吸衰竭	(77例 AFTRE<4)
Eberhardt 等[46]	回顾性	SD	FB	活检钳/TBNA/细胞刷/冲洗	89	24±8	67	2例气胸（无插入胸管）(2.2%)	
Eberhardt 等[46]	前瞻性	SD	FB ENB	活检钳	39	28±8	59	2 (5%)	
Eberhardt 等[47]	前瞻性	SD	FB ENB REBUS	活检钳	40	24±5	88	3 (8%)	
Wilson 等[48]	回顾性	SD	FB/Fluoro/ROSE	活检钳/TBNA	248	21±14	70	3例气胸（无插入胸管，3例中度出血）(1.2%)	
Bertoletti 等[49]	前瞻性	SD	仅 ENB	活检钳	53	31.2±14.4	77.3	2例气胸（1例插入胸管）(4%)	
Lamprecht 等[50]	回顾性	SD	RB/FB/ROSE	活检钳/TBNA/细胞刷	13	30±12	76.9	无气胸 (0)	
Eberhardt (2010年)[24]	前瞻性	SD	RB/REBUS	SC/TBBX	54	23.3	75.5	1例气胸 (1.9%)	ENB 对 CT 支气管征阳性患者的诊断率为 79%
Seijo 等	前瞻性	SD	FB/ROSE	TBNA/活检钳	51	N/A	66.7	无气胸 (0)	
Mahajan 等[25]	回顾性	SD	FB/Fluoro	活检钳/细胞刷/BAL	48	20±13	77	5例气胸（2例插入胸管）(10%)	
Lamprech 等[26]	前瞻性	SD	RB/FB/ROSE	活检钳/TBNA	112	27.1	83.9	2例气胸（无插入胸管）(1.8%)	
Pearlstein 等[27]	回顾性	SD	FB/ROSE	活检钳/细胞刷	104	32.6±22.2	85.1	6例气胸（6例插入胸管）(5.8%)	胸外科医师
Brownback 等[28]	回顾性	SD	FB/Fluoro/ROSE	活检钳/TBNA/冲洗	55	30	74.5	无气胸，2例I型呼吸衰竭	56.4%的患者 CT 支气管征呈阳性
Jensen 等[29]	前瞻性	SD	FB	活检钳/细胞刷	92	26.1±14.2	65.2	3例气胸，1例出血	
Karnak 等[30]	前瞻性	SD	FB/ROSE	活检钳/TBNA	76	23	91.4	3例气胸 (3.9%)	
Khan 等[39]	前瞻性	SD	FB/Fluoro	N/A	24	N/A	75	无气胸 (0)	所有 PPL 患者均植入心脏设备
Mohanasundaram 等 (2013年)	回顾性	SD	FB/ROSE	活检钳/细胞刷	41	30.1±2.1	89	6例气胸 (13%)	
Balbo (2013年)	回顾性	SD	FB/Fluoro/ROSE	活检钳/TBNA/细胞刷	40	23.5±4.9	70.7	无气胸	ENB+Fluoro+ROSE 在 Bronch+ROSE 后进行；78% 的患者 CT 支气管征呈阳性
Odronic 等[40]	回顾性	SD	FB/Fluoro/ROSE	TBNA/活检钳/细胞刷	91	27（范围7~71）	63	5例气胸 (5.3%)	敏感性 63%，特异性 100%
Loo 等[31]	回顾性	SD	FB/ROSE	活检钳/TBNA/细胞刷	40	26（范围3~80）	95	无气胸 (0)	

(续表)

研究	研究设计	SD/Veran	技术	活检	样本量	病变平均大小（mm）	诊断率（%）	并发症	其他评论
Ortega 等[90]	前瞻性	N/A	FB/?	活检钳/TBNA	180	23.7	50.6	9例气胸（5%）	
Zatloukal 等[91]	前瞻性	SD	FB/?	活检钳/TBNA/细胞刷	89	23.1±10.2	69.4	无气胸	
Bowling 等[32]	回顾性	SD	FB/Fluoro/ROSE	活检钳/针刷/TBNA/BAL	107	N/A	73.6	3例气胸（1例需插入胸管），1例呼吸衰竭，1例心动过缓	
Ost 等[55]	前瞻性	SD(252) Veran(4)	REBUS	活检钳/TBNA/细胞刷/BAL	256	N/A	47.1	整项研究（n=581）中，10例气胸	
Garwood 等[41]	回顾性	N/A	N/A	N/A	90	N/A	82.6	6例气胸（5例需插入胸管）（6.7%）	敏感性和阴性预测值分别为90.0%和88.6%
Steinfort 等[33]	前瞻性	SD	REBUS/VB/ENB/Fluoro/ROSE	活检钳/细胞刷/冲洗	236	19.1	58.4	N/A	序贯多模态支气管镜检查（REBUS未能成功定位和ROSE未能成功诊断的57例患者接受ENB检查）
AlJaghbeer 等[92]	回顾性	SD	FB/REBUS/Fluoro/ROSE	不适用	92	26	60	气胸（6%）	
Ozgul 等[34]	回顾性	SD	FB/REBUS	活检钳/细胞刷/BAL	56	21.1±5.3	71.5	1例气胸（1.7%）	
Copeland 等[43]	回顾性	SD	FB/Fluoro	活检钳/细胞刷/BAL	64	23±9	71	?	
Mukherjee 和 Chacey[35]	回顾性	SD	FB/Fluoro/ROSE	活检钳/TBNA/细胞刷/BAL	31	18（范围4~40）	96.8	2例气胸（1例插入胸管）（6.5%）	
Bhatt 等[36]	回顾性	SD	N/A	N/A	146	22.0±9.0	66	6例气胸（4例插入胸管或入院）（4%），2例症状性出血	2个队列（TTNA vs ENB）
Saenghirunvattana 等[44]	回顾性	不适用	FB/REBUS	活检钳/TBNA/细胞刷	33	N/A	79	无气胸（0）	
Sun 等[45]	前瞻性	SD	FB/REBUS/Fluoro	活检钳/细胞刷/BAL	40	21.1±5.3	82.5	无气胸（0）	
Panchabhai 等[93]	回顾性	SD	FB/REBUS/Fluoro/ROSE	活检钳/TBNA/TNB/BAL	10	20.5（范围14~30）	90	无气胸	
Yarmus 等[42]	前瞻性	Veran	FB CEBUS ETTNA	活检钳/TBNA/细胞刷/BAL	24	20.3（范围12~29）	33	23例ETTNA患者中，5例气胸（2例插入胸管）24%	仅ETTNA的诊断率为83%，ENB+ETTNA的诊断率为87%，CEBUS+ENB+ETTNA的诊断率为92%
Raval 等[37]	回顾性	Veran	N/A	活检钳/细胞刷	48	19.3±10.7	83.3	1例气胸（2%）	
Flenaugh 等[38]	回顾性	Veran	FB/REBUS	活检钳/TBNA/细胞刷	44	22.1±9.8	90.2	无气胸	1例通过SPiN Perc完成经皮入路

ENB，电磁导航支气管镜；SD，SuperDimension™；Veran，Veran Spin™；FB，可弯曲支气管镜；Fluoro，荧光；ROSE，快速现场评估；TBNA，支气管针吸活检；PTX，气胸；BAL，支气管肺泡灌洗术；REBUS，径向支气管腔内超声；RB，硬质支气管镜；TBBX，经支气管活检；SC，导管抽吸；ETTNA，电磁引导经胸穿刺针吸术；CEBUS，凸阵扫描经支气管超声检查。

联合使用时诊断率为47.1%，这表明ENB和REBUS在既定研究环境或规模化的专科中心以外应用时表现不如过往报道[55]。

也有学者评估了有无X线透视辅助的ENB对PPL的诊断率和并发症发生率。Makris等进行了一项前瞻性研究，该研究共纳入了40例不适合手术或CT引导下经胸壁针吸活检（transthoracic needle aspiration，TTNA）的患者，在无透视辅助下通过ENB对小直径的PPL[病变直径为（23.5±1.5）mm，至胸膜的平均距离为（14.9±2）mm]进行诊断，总体诊断率为62.5%。发生了3例气胸，其中1例需要插管[23]。同样，Eberhardt等评估了无透视辅助下ENB在PPL患者中的应用价值，证实了单独使用ENB并不会影响诊断率或增加气胸风险[47]。

诊断率还与PPL的大小有关。Bowling等在一项回顾性研究中发现，超过3 cm的PPL诊断率更高[32]。此外，在一项针对51名受试者的前瞻性研究中，Seijo等在单因素变量分析中发现，结节大小会显著影响ENB的诊断率[24]。Wang等在一项共纳入22篇研究的meta分析中评估了PPL患者进行ENB检查的诊断率，病变≤20 mm的629例患者的加权诊断率为60.9%，病变≥20 mm的767名患者的加权诊断率为82.5%（相差19.6%，$P<0.001$）[52]。

平均基准点目标配准误差（AFTRE）分数（由软件计算，表示患者实际传感器探头尖端与其预期位置之间的差异半径）也可能与诊断率有关。Makris等发现，当CT-人体误差≤4 mm时，诊断率明显更高。其中，结节的位置也被认为是降低诊断率的一个因素。具体来说，通过肺下叶的导航可能会受到横膈膜运动的影响。Eberhardt等发现，当单独进行ENB（无REBUS）时，肺下叶结节的诊断率明显降低。当REBUS与ENB联合使用时，诊断率与结节肺叶分布无关[46]。

CT支气管征对PPL患者的诊断具有预测价值。在一项针对51名受试者的前瞻性单中心研究中，Seijo等发现，胸部CT支气管征的发现能将ENB的诊断率从31%提高至79%[24]。最近的一项meta分析显示，与CT支气管征阴性相比，CT支气管征阳性的PPL患者ENB的诊断率更高，成功诊断的比值为3.4[56]。

ENB是一种虚拟成像引导技术，当与可以进行实时图像定位的REBUS联合应用时，可以提高PPL的诊断率。Eberhardt等证实了ENB-REBUS在提高PPL诊断率中的作用。他们进行了一项前瞻性随机对照试验，共纳入118例患者，结果显示ENB-REBUS联合使用使诊断率从69%（仅REBUS）和59%（仅ENB）增加到88%（ENB-REBUS）。两组间气胸发生率无统计学差异[46]。

McLemore等对42例患者进行了相关研究，也发现了类似的结果：REBUS联合ENB的诊断率为90%，共避免了32例手术活检，仅出现1例气胸[57]。有趣的是，Eberhardt等进行了一项前瞻性研究，共纳入54例患者，结果显示使用REBUS确认ENB定位的病灶时，PPL的诊断率为93%，而未使用REBUS确认病灶时诊断率仅为48%[51]。

已有多项研究评估了在常规支气管检查中不同的活检工具对PPL的诊断效能。在第1版ACCP肺癌指南中发表且在第2版和第3版进行更新的系统性研究显示，PPL的总体诊断敏感性为78%（范围36%~88%）。其中，经支气管活检的敏感性最高（57%），其次是经支气管刷检（54%）和支气管肺泡灌洗（bronchoalveolar lavage，BAL）/冲洗（43%）。但多篇文献报道经支气管针吸活检的敏感性为65%[9,13]。

既往研究证实，将TBNA与其他活检工具联合使用可提高PPL的诊断率[9,58-64]。同样，在AQuIRE研究中，通过多因素分析发现，使用TBNA能提高PPL的诊断率。奇怪的是，尽管有越来越多的证据表明TBNA是有效的，但该技术在PPL的诊断中的使用率仅有16%[55]。

可以将上述结果推广到ENB引导的支气管镜活检中。然而，尚不完全清楚不同活检工具在ENB中的作用。在一项回顾性研究中，91例患者接受了ENB检查。对于恶性肿瘤的诊断，TBNA的敏感性为63%。但当TBNA、经支气管镜肺活检术（transbronchial lung biopsy，TBLB）和支气管刷检联合使用时，TBNA的敏感性提高至83%[40]。

在前瞻性研究中评估了导管抽吸的采样方法，该项研究显示，在接受ENB检查的PPL患者中，采用导管抽吸的诊断率高于传统的活检钳活检[51]。在其他未使用ENB的研究中也得出了类似的结论[65,66]。此外，与经支气管活检相比，导管抽吸效果更好，但二者联合使用的效果优于任一技术单独使用[67]。

快速现场评估（rapid on-site evaluation，ROSE）有助于快速诊断[48]。一项小型回顾性研究将ROSE与ENB获得的组织病理学结果进行了比较，发现敏感性为84.6%，特异性为100%[50]。但ROSE在提高ENB诊断率的作用尚不明确。

Makris等注意到操作者技术和学习曲线对PPL的影响。操作者A对前7例PPL和后7例PPL的诊断率均为 42.8%，操作者 B 对前 13 例 PPL 的诊断率为 76%，而对后 13 例 PPL 的诊断率下降至 62%[23]。

10.5 并发症

近几年，越来越多的证据表明，ENB 是一种安全的方法，发生呼吸衰竭、大出血或气胸等并发症的风险较低（表 10.1）。一项关于 SuperDimension 导航系统的前瞻性多中心研究（NAVIGATE）的早期研究结果（前 1 000 名受试者）表明，ENB 的不良事件发生率较低，其中，气胸发生率为 4.9%，至少需要一次干预的气胸发生率为 3.2%。ENB 相关的支气管肺出血和呼吸衰竭发生率分别为 1.0% 和 0.6%[68]。此外，慢性阻塞性肺疾病或肺功能下降患者在 ENB 术后的并发症发生率没有增加[69]。

最近一项研究比较了 ENB 与 CT 引导下的 TTNA 在 PPL 中的诊断率和并发症发生率。这项回顾性研究通过倾向性匹配的方法来调整选择偏倚，结果表明，CT 引导下的 TTNA 比 ENB 的诊断率更高。这个研究是存在固有偏倚的，即许多患者拒绝使用 TTNA 作为标准检查方法，而进行 ENB 检查，反之亦然[36]。

ENB 的另一个版本是 Veran Spin™ 导航支气管镜系统，该系统使用实时程序扫描来控制呼吸门控，以解决活检时的呼吸运动问题。该系统具有 ENB 构成的基本元件，不同的是，该系统在 CT 检查前使用 vPad™（带有电磁传感器的贴纸）贴在患者胸壁，减少了注册的环节，这样有助于指导导航并对患者呼吸运动进行监测。Veran Spin™ 导入了患者吸气和呼气的 CT 扫描数据，可自动计算结节的移动并进行跟踪，以提高导航的准确性。与 SuperDimension 系统相比，该系统的导管设计也具有显著的优势，在活检过程中导航始终保持开启状态。此外，可以在磁导航支气管镜检查为阴性后，进行磁导航引导的 TTNA[17,38,70]（图 10.9）。多项报道表明，当使用该系统时，对 CT 支气管征阴性的 PPL 的诊断率为 77%，

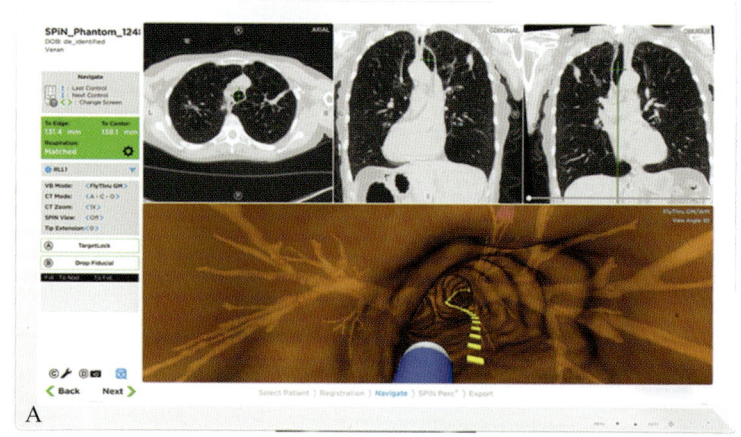

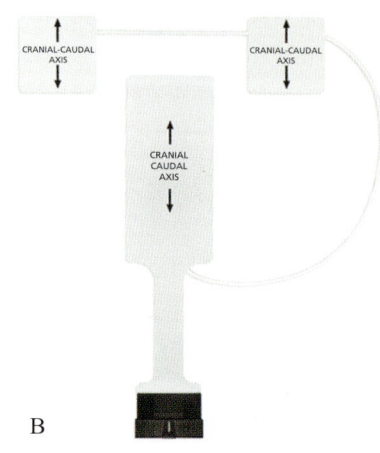

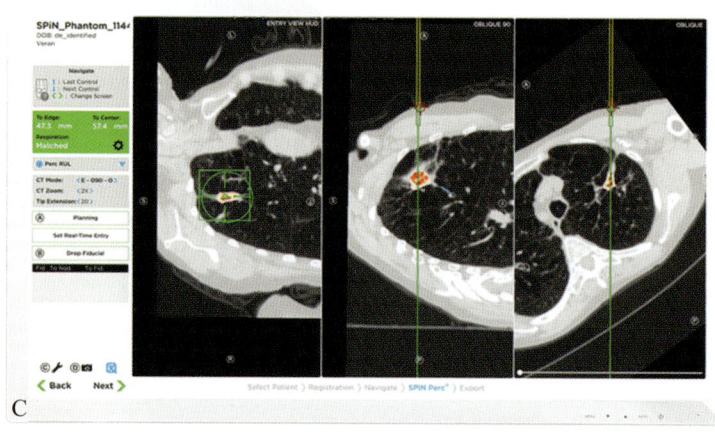

图 10.9　Veran Spin™ 导航支气管镜系统

A. Veran Spin™ 导航支气管镜系统界面；B. 带有电磁传感器的贴纸；C. Veran Spin™ 经胸廓针吸活检界面。

当 ENB 和 ENB-TTNA 联合使用时，诊断率高达 87%，气胸发生率分别为 21%，其中 8% 的气胸需要引流[37,38,42,71-75]。

10.6 治疗应用

ENB 已成为辅助其他治疗技术的有效手段。已有报道指出，ENB 能安全地植入基准标记物以帮助进行定向化疗和手术切除[76-79]。标记物可送达需行楔形切除的病变区域[76]。此外，它能准确定位需定向放疗的肿瘤位置，与气胸发生率高达 64% 的 CT 引导下经胸壁穿刺放置标记物相比，其气胸发生率更低[70-86]。ENB 根据治疗的需要可以放置一个或数个标记物。已有学者研究了最佳的基准标记物，研究发现，相比于双波段标记物和金属标记物，线圈标记物具有更高的保留率，差异具有统计学意义[79,81]（图 10.10）。

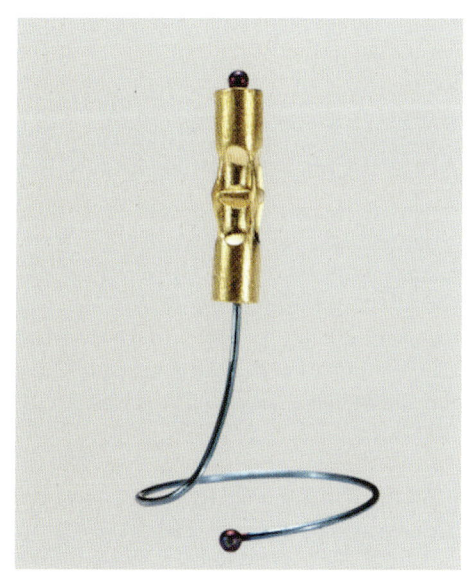

图 10.10　基准定位标记装置

同样，对于无法手术的患者，特别是不能进行定向放疗的患者，有研究报道可使用 ENB 引导的近距离放射导管进行高剂量短距离放疗（在肿瘤内进行放疗）[87,88]。此外，经肺表面放置胸膜染料标记物或基准标记物的技术已被用于视频辅助胸腔镜手术（video-assisted thoracoscopic surgery，VATS）。目前，一项使用 ENB 和锥体束 CT 引导的微波消融导管的研究正在进行中。

10.7 结论

电磁导航支气管镜技术是一个包含多种技术的平台，可以提高操作者对患者 CT 影像的解读能力，方便操作者通过留置的操作导管对目标病变进行活检。目前关于电磁导航支气管镜技术的文献很多，但缺乏直接对比研究。因此，该技术的价值并未被广泛接受。此外，大多数发表的数据都来自使用单中心研究，进行荟萃分析可能没有价值。AQuIRE 研究和 NAVIGATE 研究数据有很大差异。因此，关于操作技术、患者选择和与操作相关的其他方面仍然存在许多问题，但该技术是安全的。目前关于最佳的麻醉方式、合适的活检工具以及 REBUS、透视和锥形束 CT 等辅助成像技术的应用等相关研究仍在不断进行。因此，ENB 技术在临床实践中的最佳使用方法仍需进一步探讨。

参考文献

1 Mokdad, A.H., Ballestros, K., Echko, M. et al.(2018). The state of US health, 1990–2016. *JAMA* 319: 1444.

2 Siegel, R.L., Miller, K.D., and Jemal, A.(2018). Cancer statistics, 2018. *CA Cancer J. Clin.* 68: 7–30.

3 National Lung Screening Trial Research Team (2011). Reduced lung-cancer mortality with low-dose computed tomographic screening. *N. Engl. J. Med.* 365: 395–409.

4 Bach, P.B., Mirkin,J.N., Oliver, T.K. et al.(2012). Benefits and harms of CT screening for lung cancer. *JAMA* 307: 2418.

5 Gould, M.K., Tang,T., Liu, I.L.A. et al.(2015). Recent trends in the identification of incidental pulmonary nodules. *Am. J. Respir. Crit. Care Med.* 192: 1208–1214.

6 Almeida, F.A., Uzbeck, M., and Ost, D.(2010). Initial evaluation of the nonsmall cell lung cancer patient: diagnosis and staging. *Curr. Opin. Pulm. Med.* 16: 307–314.

7 MacMahon, H., Naidich, D.P., Goo, J.M. et al. (2017). Guidelines for management of incidental pulmonary nodules detected on CT images: from the Fleischner Society 2017. *Radiology* 284: 228–243.

8 Ost, D.E., JimYeung, S.-C., Tanoue, L.T., and Gould, M.K.(2013). Clinical and organizational factors in the initial evaluation of patients with lung cancer. *Chest* 143: e121S-e141S.

9 Schreiber, G. and McCrory, D.C. (2003). Performance characteristics of different modalities for diagnosis of suspected lung cancer: summary of published evidence. *Chest* 123: 115S–128S.

10 Baaklini,W.A., Reinoso, M.A., Gorin, A.B. et al. (2000). Diagnostic yield of fiberoptic bronchoscopy in evaluating solitary pulmonary nodules. *Chest* 117: 1049–1054.

11 Stoller, J.K., Ahmad, M., and Rice, T.W. (1988). Solitary

pulmonary nodule. *Cleve. Clin. J. Med.* 55: 68–74.

12 Rivera, M.P., Detterbeck, F., Mehta, A.C., and Franklin, W.A. (2003). Diagnosis of lung cancer. *Chest* 123: 119S–123S.

13 Rivera, M.P., Mehta, A.C., and Wahidi, M.M. (2013). Establishing the diagnosis of lung cancer: diagnosis and management of lung cancer, 3rd ed: American college of chest physicians evidence-based clinical practice guidelines. *Chest* 143: e142S–e165S.

14 Vining, D.J., Liu, K., Choplin, R.H., and Haponik, E.F. (1996). Virtual bronchoscopy: relationships of virtual reality endobronchial simulations to actual bronchoscopic findings. *Chest* 109: 549–553.

15 Ben-Haim, S.A., Osadchy, D., Schuster, I. et al. (1996). Nonfluoroscopic, in vivo navigation and mapping technology. *Nat. Med.* 2: 1393–1395.

16 Solomon, S.B., White, P., Acker, D.E. et al. (1998). Real-time bronchoscope tip localization enables three-dimensional CT image guidance for transbronchial needle aspiration in swine. *Chest* 114: 1405–1410.

17 Mehta, A.C., Hood, K.L., Schwarz, Y., and Solomon, S.B. (2018). The evolutional history of electromagnetic navigation bronchoscopy: state of the art. *Chest* 154 (4): 935–947.

18 Baaklini, W.A., Reinoso, M.A., Gorin, A.B. et al. (2000). Diagnostic yield of fiberoptic bronchoscopy in evaluating solitary pulmonary nodules. *Chest* 117: 1049–1054.

19 Schwarz, Y., Mehta, A.C., Ernst, A. et al. (2003). Electromagnetic navigation during flexible bronchoscopy. *Respiration* 70: 516–522.

20 Becker, H.D., Herth, F., Ernst, A., and Schwarz, Y. (2005). Bronchoscopic biopsy of peripheral lung lesions under electromagnetic guidance: a pilot study. *J. Bronchol.* 12: 9–13.

21 Schwarz, Y., Greif, J., Becker, H.D. et al. (2006). Real-time electromagnetic navigation bronchoscopy to peripheral lung lesion using overlaid CT images: the first human study. *Chest* 129: 988–994.

22 Gildea, T.R., Mazzone, P.J., Karnak, D. et al. (2006). Electromagnetic navigation diagnostic bronchoscopy: a prospective study. *Am. J. Respir. Crit. Care Med.* 174: 982–989.

23 Makris, D., Scherpereel, A., Leroy, S. et al. (2007). Electromagnetic navigation diagnostic bronchoscopy for small peripheral lung lesions. *Eur. Respir. J.* 29: 1187–1192.

24 Seijo, L.M., de Torres, J.P., Lozano, M.D. et al. (2010). Diagnostic yield of electromagnetic navigation bronchoscopy is highly dependent on the presence of a bronchus sign on CT imaging: results from a prospective study. *Chest* 138: 1316–1321.

25 Mahajan, A.K., Patel, S., Hogarth, D.K., and Wightman, R. (2011). Electromagnetic navigational bronchoscopy an effective and safe approach to diagnose peripheral lung lesions unreachable by conventional bronchoscopy in high-risk patients. *J. Bronchol. Interv. Pulmonol.* 18: 133–137.

26 Lamprecht, B., Porsch, P., Wegleitner, B. et al. (2012). Electromagnetic navigation bronchoscopy (ENB): increasing diagnostic yield. *Respir. Med.* 106: 710–715.

27 Pearlstein, D.P., Quinn, C.C., Burtis, C.C. et al. (2012). Electromagnetic navigation bronchoscopy performed by thoracic surgeons: one center's early success. *Ann. Thorac. Surg.* 93: 944–950.

28 Brownback, K.R., Quijano, F., Latham, H.E., and Simpson, S.Q. (2012). Electromagnetic navigational bronchoscopy in the diagnosis of lung lesions. *J. Bronchol. Interv. Pulmonol.* 19: 91–97.

29 Jensen, K.W., Hsia, D.W., Seijo, L.M. et al. (2012). Multicenter experience with electromagnetic navigation bronchoscopy for the diagnosis of pulmonary nodules. *J. Bronchol. Interv. Pulmonol.* 19: 195–199.

30 Karnak, D., Çiledag, A., Ceyhan, K. et al. (2013). Rapid on-site evaluation and low registration error enhance the success of electromagnetic navigation bronchoscopy. *Ann. Thorac. Med.* 8: 28.

31 Loo, F.L., Halligan, A.M., Port, J.L., and Hoda, R.S. (2014). The emerging technique of electromagnetic navigation bronchoscopy-guided fine-needle aspiration of peripheral lung lesions: promising results in 50 lesions. *Cancer Cytopathol.* 122: 191–199.

32 Bowling, M.R., Kohan, M.W., Walker, P. et al. (2015). The effect of general anesthesia versus intravenous. *J. Bronchol. Interv. Pulmonol.* 22: 5–13.

33 Steinfort, D.P., Bonney, A., See, K., and Irving, L.B. (2016). Sequential multimodality bronchoscopic investigation of peripheral pulmonary lesions. *Eur. Respir. J.* 47: 607–614.

34 Ozgul, G., Cetinkaya, E., Ozgul, M.A. et al. (2016). Efficacy and safety of electromagnetic navigation bronchoscopy with or without radial endobronchial ultrasound for peripheral lung lesions. *Endosc. Ultrasound* 5: 189–195.

35 Mukherjee, S. and Chacey, M. (2017). Diagnostic yield of electromagnetic navigation bronchoscopy using a curved-tip catheter to aid in the diagnosis of pulmonary lesions. *J. Bronchol. Interv. Pulmonol.* 24: 35–39.

36 Bhatt, K.M., Tandon, Y.K., Graham, R. et al. (2017). Electromagnetic navigational bronchoscopy versus CT-guided percutaneous sampling of peripheral indeterminate pulmonary nodules: a cohort study. *Radiology* 286: 170893.

37 Raval, A.A. and Amir, L. (2016). Lung cancer management community hospital experience using electromagnetic navigation bronchoscopy system integrating tidal volume computed tomography mapping. *Lung Cancer Manag.* 5: 9–19.

38 Flenaugh, E.L. and Mohammed, K.H. (2016). Initial experience using 4D electromagnetic navigation bronchoscopy system with tip tracked instruments for localization of peripheral lung nodules. *Internet J. Pulm. Med.* 18: 1–7.

39 Khan, A.Y., Berkowitz, D., Krimsky, W.S. et al. (2013). Safety of pacemakers and defibrillators in electromagnetic navigation bronchoscopy. *Chest J.* 143: 75–81.

40 Odronic, S.I., Gildea, T.R., and Chute, D.J. (2014). Electromagnetic navigation bronchoscopy-guided fine needle aspiration for the diagnosis of lung lesions. *Diagn. Cytopathol.* 42: 1045–1050.

41 Garwood, S.K., ClenDening, P., Hevelone, N.D. et al. (2016). Navigational bronchoscopy at a community hospital: clinical and economic outcomes. *Lung Cancer Manag.* 5: 131–140.

42 Yarmus, L.B., Arias, S., Feller-Kopman, D. et al. (2016).

Electromagnetic navigation transthoracic needle aspiration for the diagnosis of pulmonary nodules: a safety and feasibility pilot study. *J. Thorac. Dis.* 8: 186–194.
43 Copeland, S., Kambali, S., Berdine, G., and Alalawi, R. (2017). Electromagnetic navigational bronchoscopy in patients with solitary pulmonary nodules. *Southwest Respir. Crit. Care Chron.* 5: 12–16.
44 Saenghirunvattana, S., Bechara, R., Saenghirunvattana, C. et al. (2017). Electromagnetic navigation bronchoscopy. *Bangkok Med. J.* 13: 37–40.
45 Sun, J., Xie, F., Zheng, X. et al. (2017). Learning curve of electromagnetic navigation bronchoscopy for diagnosing peripheral pulmonary nodules in a single institution. *Transl. Cancer Res.* 6: 541–551.
46 Eberhardt, R., Anantham, D., Ernst, A. et al. (2007). Multimodality bronchoscopic diagnosis of peripheral lung lesions: a randomized controlled trial. *Am. J. Respir. Crit. Care Med.* 176: 36–41.
47 Eberhardt, R., Anantham, D., Herth, F. et al. (2007). Electromagnetic navigation diagnostic bronchoscopy in peripheral lung lesions. *Chest* 131: 1800–1805.
48 Wilson, D.S. and Bartlett, R.J. (2007). Improved diagnostic yield of bronchoscopy in a community practice: combination of electromagnetic navigation system and rapid on-site evaluation. *J. Bronchol.* 14: 227–232.
49 Bertoletti, L., Robert, A., Cottier, M. et al. (2009). Accuracy and feasibility of electromagnetic navigated bronchoscopy under nitrous oxide sedation for pulmonary peripheral opacities: an outpatient study. *Respiration* 78: 293–300.
50 Lamprecht, B., Porsch, P., Pirich, C., and Studnicka, M. (2009). Electromagnetic navigation bronchoscopy in combination with PET-CT and rapid on-site cytopathologic examination for diagnosis of peripheral lung lesions. *Lung* 187: 55–59.
51 Eberhardt, R., Morgan, R.K., Ernst, A. et al. (2009). Comparison of suction catheter versus forceps biopsy for sampling of solitary pulmonary nodules guided by electromagnetic navigational bronchoscopy. *Respiration* 79: 54–60.
52 Wang Memoli, J.S., Nietert, P.J., and Silvestri, G.A. (2012). Meta-analysis of guided bronchoscopy for the evaluation of the pulmonary nodule. *Chest* 142: 385–393.
53 Zhang, W., Chen, S., Dong, X., and Lei, P. (2015). Meta-analysis of the diagnostic yield and safety of electromagnetic navigation bronchoscopy for lung nodules. *J. Thorac. Dis.* 7: 799–809.
54 Gex, G., Pralong, J.A., Combescure, C. et al. (2014). Diagnostic yield and safety of electromagnetic navigation bronchoscopy for lung nodules: a systematic review and meta-analysis. *Respiration* 87: 165–176.
55 Ost, D.E., Ernst, A., Lei, X. et al. (2016). Diagnostic yield and complications of bronchoscopy for peripheral lung lesions: results of the AQuIRE registry. *Am. J. Respir. Crit. Care Med.* 193: 68–77.
56 Ali, M.S., Sethi, J., Taneja, A. et al. (2018). Bronchus sign and the diagnostic yield of guided bronchoscopy for peripheral pulmonary lesions: a systematic review and meta-analysis. *Ann. Am. Thorac. Soc.* 15 (8): 978–987.
57 McLemore, T.L. and Bedekar, A.R. (2007). Accurate diagnosis of peripheral lung lesions (Pll) in a private community hospital employing electromagnetic guidance bronchoscopy (Emb) coupled with radial endobronchial ultrasound (Rebus). *Chest* 132: 452A.
58 Shure, D. and Fedullo, P. (1983). Concise clinical study transbronchial needle aspiration of peripheral masses. *Am. J. Res.* 128: 1090–1092.
59 Wang, K.P., Haponik, E.F., Britt, E.J. et al. (1984). Transbronchial needle aspiration of peripheral pulmonary nodules. *Chest* 86: 819–823.
60 Wang, K.P., Marsh, B.R., Summer, W.R. et al. (1981). Transbronchial needle aspiration for diagnosis of lung cancer. *Chest* 80: 48–50.
61 Schenk, D.A., Bryan, C.L., Bower, J.H., and Myers, D.L. (1987). Transbronchial needle aspiration in the diagnosis of bronchogenic carcinoma. *Chest* 92: 83–85.
62 Gasparini, S., Ferretti, M., Secchi, E.B. et al. (1995). Integration of transbronchial and percutaneous approach in the diagnosis of peripheral pulmonary nodules or masses: experience with 1,027 consecutive cases. *Chest* 108: 131–137.
63 Katis, K., Inglesos, E., Zachariadis, E. et al. (1995). The role of transbronchial needle aspiration in the diagnosis of peripheral lung masses or nodules. *Eur. Respir. J.* 8: 963–966.
64 Reichenberger, F., Weber, J., Tamm, M. et al. (1999). The value of transbronchial needle aspiration in the diagnosis of peripheral pulmonary lesions. *Chest* 116: 704–708.
65 Franke, K.-J., Nilius, G., and Ruhle, K.-H. (2009). Transbronchial catheter aspiration compared to forceps biopsy in the diagnosis of peripheral lung cancer. *Eur. J. Med. Res.* 14: 13–17.
66 Li, D.R., Wan, T., Su, Y. et al. (2014). Liquid-based cytological test of samples obtained by catheter aspiration is applicable for the bronchoscopic confirmation of pulmonary malignant tumors. *Int. J. Clin. Exp. Pathol.* 7: 2508–2517.
67 Peschke, A., Wiedemann, B., Höffken, G., and Koschel, D. (2012). Forceps biopsy and suction catheter for sampling in pulmonary nodules and infiltrates. *Eur. Respir. J.* 39: 1432–1436.
68 Khandhar, S.J., Bowling, M.R., Flandes, J. et al. (2017). Electromagnetic navigation bronchoscopy to access lung lesions in 1,000 subjects: first results of the prospective, multicenter NAVIGATE study. *BMC Pulm. Med.* 17: 59.
69 Towe, C.W., Nead, M.A., Rickman, O.B. et al. (2018). Safety of electromagnctic navigation bronchoscopy in patients with COPD: results from the NAVIGATE study. *J. Bronchol. Interv. Pulmonol.* 00: 1–8.
70 Gilbert, C., Akulian, J., Ortiz, R. et al. (2014). Novel bronchoscopic strategies for the diagnosis of peripheral lung lesions: present techniques and future directions. *Respirology* 19: 636–644.
71 Santos, R.S., Gupta, A., Ebright, M.I. et al. (2010). Electromagnetic navigation to aid radiofrequency ablation and biopsy of lung tumors. *Ann. Thorac. Surg.* 89: 265–268.
72 Grand, D.J., Atalay, M.A., Cronan, J.J. et al. (2011). CT-

guided percutaneous lung biopsy: comparison of conventional CT fluoroscopy to CT fluoroscopy with electromagnetic navigation system in 60 consecutive patients. *Eur. J. Radiol.* 79: e133–e136.

73 Narsule, C.K., Sales Dos Santos, R., Gupta, A. et al. (2012). The efficacy of electromagnetic navigation to assist with computed tomography-guided percutaneous thermal ablation of lung tumors. *Innov. Technol. Tech. Cardiothorac. Vasc. Surg.* 7: 187–190.

74 Semaan, R.W., Lee, H.J., Feller-Kopman, D. et al. (2016). Same-day computed tomographic chest imaging for pulmonary nodule targeting with electromagnetic navigation bronchoscopy may decrease unnecessary procedures. *Ann. Am. Thorac. Soc.* 13: 2223–2228.

75 Furukawa, B.S., Pastis, N.J., Tanner, N.T. et al. (2018). Comparing pulmonary nodule location during electromagnetic bronchoscopy with predicted location on the basis of two virtual airway maps at different phases of respiration. *Chest* 153: e9–e12.

76 Andrade, R.S. (2010). Electromagnetic navigation bronchoscopy-guided thoracoscopic wedge resection of small pulmonary nodules. *Semin Thorac CardiovascSurg* 22: 262–265.

77 Hagmeyer, L., Priegnitz, C., Kocher, M. et al. (2016). Fiducial marker placement via conventional or electromagnetic navigation bronchoscopy (ENB): an interdisciplinary approach to the curative management of lung cancer. *Clin. Respir. J.* 10: 291–297.

78 Harley, D.P., Krimsky, W.S., Sarkar, S. et al. (2010). Fiducial marker placement using endobronchial ultrasound and navigational bronchoscopy for stereotactic radiosurgery: an alternative strategy. *Ann. Thorac. Surg.* 89: 368–374.

79 Schroeder, C., Hejal, R., and Linden, P.A. (2010). Coil spring fiducial markers placed safely using navigation bronchoscopy in inoperable patients allows accurate delivery of CyberKnife stereotactic radiosurgery. *J.*

80 *Thorac. Cardiovasc. Surg.* 140: 1137–1142. Steinfort, D.P., Siva, S., Kron, T. et al. (2014). Multimodality guidance for accurate bronchoscopic insertion of fiducial markers. *J. Thorac. Oncol.* 10: 324–330.

81 Minnich, D.J., Bryant, A.S., Wei, B. et al. (2015). Retention rate of electromagnetic navigation bronchoscopic placed fiducial markers for lung radiosurgery. *Ann. Thorac. Surg.* 100: 1163–1166.

82 Anantham, D., Feller-Kopman, D., Shanmugham, L.N. et al. (2007). Electromagnetic navigation bronchoscopy-guided fiducial placement for robotic stereotactic radiosurgery of lung tumors: a feasibility study. *Chest* 132: 930–935.

83 Trumm, C.G., Häußler, S.M., Muacevic, A. et al. (2014). CT fluoroscopy-guided percutaneous fiducial marker placement for cyberknife stereotactic radiosurgery: technical results and complications in 222 consecutive procedures. *J. Vasc. Interv. Radiol.* 25: 760–768.

84 Yousefi, S., Collins, B.T., Reichner, C.A. et al. (2007). Complications of thoracic computed tomography-guided fiducial placement for the purpose of stereotactic body radiation therapy. *Clin. Lung Cancer*.

85 Pennathur, A., Luketich, J.D., Heron, D.E. et al. (2009). Stereotactic radiosurgery for the treatment of lung neoplasm: experience in 100 consecutive patients. *Ann. Thorac. Surg.* 88: 1594–1600.

86 Pennathur, A., Luketich, J.D., Heron, D.E. et al. (2009). Stereotactic radiosurgery for the treatment of stage I non-small cell lung cancer in high-risk patients. *J. Thorac. Cardiovasc. Surg.* 137: 597–604.

87 Becker, H.D., McLemore, T., and Harms, W. (2008). Electromagnetic navigation and endobronchial ultrasound for brachytherapy of inoperable peripheral lung cancer – long-term results at two centers. *Chest.* 134 (4): 35S.

88 Harms, W., Krempien, R., Grehn, C. et al. (2006). Electromagnetically navigated brachytherapy as a new treatment option for peripheral pulmonary tumors. *Strahlenther. Onkol.* 182: 108–119.

89 Awais, O., Reidy, M.R., Mehta, K. et al. (2016). Electromagnetic navigation bronchoscopy-guided dye marking for thoracoscopic resection of pulmonary nodules. *Ann. Thorac. Surg.* 102: 223–229.

90 Ortega, P.R., Gutiérrez, J.G., Juárez, Á.O.R. et al. (2014). Diagnostic yield and complications associated with electromagnetic navigation bronchoscopy in peripheral lung lesions. *Eur. Respir. J.* 44 (Suppl 58): S686.

91 Zatloukal, J., Kolek, V., and Jakubec, P. (2014). Electromagnetic navigation-guided diagnostic bronchoscopy for small peripheral lung lesions: A prospective study. *Eur. Respir. J.* 44 (Suppl 58): 680.

92 Al-Jaghbeer, M., Marcus, M., Durkin, M. et al. (2016). Diagnostic yield of electromagnetic navigational bronchoscopy. *Therapeut. Adv. Respir. Dis.* 10 (4): 295–299.

93 Panchabhai, T.S., Roy, S.B., Madan, N. et al. (2018). Electromagnetic navigational bronchoscopy for diagnosing peripheral lung lesions in lung transplant recipients: a single-center experience. *J. Thorac. Dis.* 10 (8): S108–S114.

第 11 章

虚拟支气管镜导航

Swati Baveja[1], Wolfgang Hohenforst-Schmidt[2], J. Francis Turner, Jr.[1,3], and Ko-Pen Wang[4]

[1] Division of Pulmonary and Critical Care Medicine,
University of Tennessee Graduate School of Medicine, Knoxville, TN, USA

[2] Sana Clinic Group Franken, Department of Cardiology/Pulmonology/Intensive Care/Nephrology,
"Hof" Clinics, University of Erlangen, Hof, Germany

[3] National Supercomputing Institute, University of Nevada, Las Vegas, NV, USA

[4] Division of Pulmonary and Critical Care Medicine, Johns Hopkins Bayview Medical Center,
Johns Hopkins University School of Medicine, Baltimore, MD, USA

（译者：顾 晔 译者单位：同济大学附属上海市肺科医院）

11.1 概述

迄今为止，肺癌仍是世界上致死率最高的疾病之一。低剂量计算机体层成像（low-dose computed tomography，LDCT）是早期肺癌筛查的常用方法。随着 CT、正电子发射体层成像（positron emission tomography，PET）、磁共振成像（magnetic resonance imaging，MRI）的广泛使用，越来越多的肺外周病变被发现。即使有风险分级，大量的病灶仍需要持续随访、影像学检查或活检。

通过可弯曲支气管镜对肺外周结节进行活检评估的结果在不同报道中具有显著差异，诊断率为 36%~86%[1,2]。虚拟支气管镜导航（virtual bronchoscopic navigation，VBN）是一种有望提高可弯曲支气管镜诊断可靠性的新方法。

11.2 定义

VBN 是利用虚拟支气管影像建立支气管通向肺外周病变的路径，并通过导航引导支气管镜到达肺外周结节的一种方法。气管和支气管的 3D 影像来自完整的螺旋 CT 数据的重建，形成虚拟路径，引导实时支气管镜检查。

11.3 发展

2003 年，Asano 等在一篇病例报道中第一次描述了 VBN 技术的应用[3]。目前，在美国市场上可获得的 VBN 是 Bronchus 公司的 LungPoint® 系统和 Archimedes™ 系统（支气管旁路导航）[4]。在世界范围内，Bf-NAVI 系统（Olympus，东京，日本）是最常用的，大部分的研究数据是从 Olympus 系统中获取的。

11.4 技术

VBN 生成的图像依赖于所选定区域的 CT 值来区分气道和支气管腔。X 线图像是由许多屏幕上微小的二维发光区域所组成，这些区域被称为"像素"。这些像素有一个指定的数值，根据 X 线的密度，共同形成一幅图像。这些密度以"霍斯菲尔德单位（Hounsfield units,HU)"表示。使用线性变化的原始衰减系数,在标准压力和温度(standard pressure and temperature,STP)下测量蒸馏水辐射密度得出的结果定义为 0 HU。在STP下的空气辐射密度定义为–1 000 HU,血液为10~30 HU,实体器官为 30~150 HU,骨骼为 300 HU[5]。从 CT 影像中提取出三维立体像素,构建形成 3D 解剖结构影像,这个过程被称为"分割"。因此,为了确定在水平位、矢状位、冠状位支气管分支的存在与否,具有合适的 3D 设定值是非常重要的,而这主要取决于使用的 CT 设备。建议支气管镜医师自己制作 VBN 图像,并将它们与 CT 每个横截面图像进行比较,不准确的 3D 数值设置将会导致支气管镜路径错误。

另一问题是支气管镜插入时的旋转。当支气管镜旋转时,由于虚拟图像中深度和旋转信息的缺乏会扰乱基于图像和视频的追踪,误导真实图像的识别[6-8]。

VBN 的操作流程包括:①创建一个虚拟支气管镜(virtual bronchoscopy,VB)图像;②同步 VB 图像和真实支气管镜图像;③通过活检、刷检和灌洗取样肺外周病变。

VB 是一种非侵袭性的操作,它通过收集术前的 CT 数据完成,没有辐射暴露的风险。该系统的主要缺陷在于导航时缺乏真实的内镜可视化图像,无法实时确认支气管镜是否到达病灶内。所以,其他设备诸如 CT、透视和径向支气管内超声(radial endobronchial ultrasound,R-EBUS)经常和 VBN 结合在一起使用[9]。

近年来,锥形束 CT(cone beam CT,CBCT)已经成为重要的导航技术。Hohenforst-Schmidt 等进行了一项关于 CBCT 的可行性研究[10]。该研究中,大部分患者在镇静麻醉下使用双频高频喷射通气控制呼吸,以确保没有肺的运动,保持其稳定的过度充气状态。此时,以空气作为对比介质,形成类 CT 图像。在 3D 图像获取时肺部运动停止,同时比对 CBCT 与螺旋 CT 拍摄的图像质量。心跳可能是导致某些邻近心脏的区域产生图像模糊的原因(如右下叶的 B7)。3D 图像获得后,在 CBCT 处理系统中标记肺部病灶位置,使用活检工具沿路径进入。这种 3D 标记可以叠加在实时的 X 线透视影像上,当支气管镜医师向前推进器械时,可以直视活检工具朝向 3D 目标的移动,直至到达目标轮廓和覆盖目标(图 11.1)。所有的影像数据均可以在一次内镜操作中获得,并且在需要时可以随时重复操作。

另一项由 Hohenforst-Schmidt 等完成的 CBCT 研究结果显示,CBCT(DynaCT Artis Zee,西门子,福希海姆,德国)导航下经支气管活检钳活检肺外周结节,对小于 2 cm 的肺外周孤立性结节的诊断率高于传统 PNNs 腔内活检方式至少 2 倍。这项研究围绕 33 个体检发现的孤立性肺结节(solitary pulmonary nodules,SPN)开展,导航到达成功率为 91%,总诊断率(仅活检钳活检)为 70%,其中,恶性病变($n=28$)的诊断率为 82%。将结节大小以 2 cm 为界分为两个亚组,小于 2 cm 组总诊断率为 75%[15(±3)mm],大于

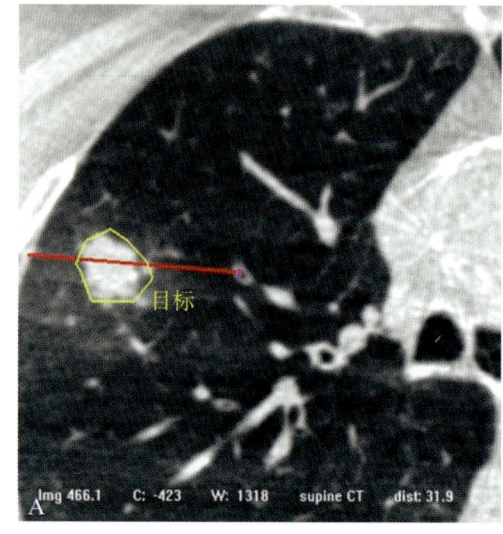 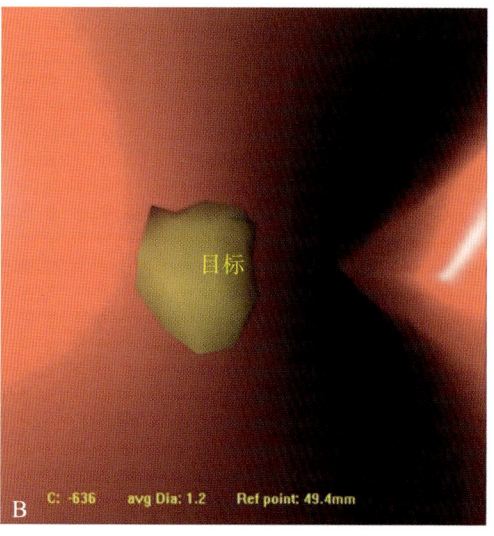

图 11.1　外周目标的获取与可视化路径的形成

A. VBN 系统在 CT 影像上获取外周目标;B. 在支气管镜下形成可视化路径[10]。详见视频 11.1。资料来源:Dr Wolfgang Hohenforst-Schmidt 提供。

2 cm 组为 67%[（30±11）mm]。在两个亚组中，恶性肿瘤的诊断敏感性均为 82%[11]。这项技术的风险因素之一是辐射暴露，但是暴露剂量（到达右上叶第 8 级支气管的 3D 数据收集和导航）在 0.98~1.15 mSv 之间（实际上优于其他肺部导航系统）[10]。

另一种成熟的方法是电磁导航（electromagnetic navigation，EMN）。它是利用磁场位置传感器的信息来推送引导鞘、活检工具以诊断肺外周病灶的方法。在后续章节中会详细讨论（表 11.1）。

表 11.1　VBN 与 EMN 的区别[12]

VBN	EMN
较便宜	因使用一次性传感器，价格更贵
X 线透视通常是必要的，除非在使用 EBUS-GS 情况下	可以不需要 X 线透视

VBN，虚拟支气管镜；EMN，电磁导航；EBUS-GS，经引导鞘管支气管内超声技术。表格来源：Eberhardt 等[12]。经美国呼吸与重症监护杂志许可转载。

视频 11.1　VBN 到达肺结节路径——来自锥形束 CT 数据集

11.5　讨论

关于使用 VBN 诊断肺外周病变（peripheral pulmonary lesion，PPL）的有效性的一些研究已经发表（表 11.2），其中包括 2 项前瞻性随机对照研究，但它们的研究结论是相互矛盾的。

Ishida 等进行的一项前瞻性多中心研究，探索了 VBN 辅助 EBUS 诊断肺外周小病变的价值。在这项研究中，将 199 例肺外周病变患者（直径 ≤ 30 mm）随机分配至 VBN 辅助（VBNA）组和非 VBN 辅助（NVBNA）组。在 VBNA 组中，支气管镜通过 VBN 系统引导进入目标支气管。VBNA 组的诊断率高于 NVBNA 组（80.4% 比 67.0%，$P=0.032$）。总操作时间和从检查开始到活检开始的操作时间，VBNA 组低于 NVBNA 组[中位数（范围），24.0（8.7~47.0）比 26.2（11.6~58.6）min，$P=0.016$；8.1（2.8~39.2）比 9.8（2.3~42.3）min，$P=0.045$]。发生的唯一不良事件是在 VNBNA 组中出现气胸 1 例[20]。

在 Asano 等发起的另一个研究中，将 350 例肺外周病变（直径 ≤ 30 mm）的患者分为 VBNA 组和 NVBNA 组。VBNA 组使用 2.8 mm 直径的超细支气管镜和 VBN 引导到达目标支气管；NVBNA 组则仅使用水平位 CT 作为参考，获取结节标本时使用 X 线透视来确认。研究者对 334 例患者的数据进行分析。

表 11.2　在不同研究中 VBN 的诊断率

作者	年份	病例数	结果
Tachihara 等[13]	2018	31	支气管镜联合 VBN 与 EBUS-GS 诊断肺外周病变[83.3%（X 线透视组）比 69.2%（未使用 X 线透视组）]
Kato 等[14]	2018	100	VBN 组诊断率高于非 VBN 组（84% 比 58%，$P=0.013$）
Maekura 等[15]	2017	45	联合 VBN、EBUS 和 ROSE 对肺外周病变的诊断率为 77.7%
Diez-Ferrer 等[16]	2017	63	VBN 组与非 VBN 组的诊断率为 75% 比 43.9%（$P=0.029$）
Asano 等[17]	2017	129	VBN 辅助组的诊断率为 76.9%（50/65），X 线透视辅助组的诊断率为 85.9%（55/64）
Winantea 等[18]	2016	19	VBN 支气管镜检查的诊断率为 66.7%（5 例良性，3 例恶性）
Asano 等[19]	2013	350	VBN 辅助组的诊断率高于非 VBN 辅助组：病灶位于右上叶（81.3% 比 53.2%，$P=0.004$）；病灶在后前位 X 线透视中可见（63.2% 比 40.5%，$P=0.043$）；病灶位于肺中外 1/3 区域（64.7% 比 52.1%，$P=0.047$）
Ishida 等[20]	2011	199	VBN 与非 VBN 的诊断率（80.4% 比 67.0%，$P=0.032$）
Shinagawa 等[21]	2007	69	从检查开始到第一次活检的时间和总检查时间，使用导航的方法明显短于使用模拟对照组（$P<0.05$）

VBN，虚拟支气管镜；EBUS-GS，经引导鞘管支气管内超声技术；ROSE，床旁快速评估。

VBNA 组的诊断率（67.1%）和 NVBNA 组（59.9%；$P=0.173$）没有显著差异。亚组分析显示，对于右上叶的病灶（81.3% 比 53.2%；$P=0.004$），后前位 X 线透视中可见的病灶（63.2% 比 40.5%；$P=0.043$），以及位于肺中外 1/3 区域的病灶（64.7% 比 52.1%；$P=0.047$），VBNA 组的诊断率均显著高于 NVBNA 组[19]。

其余的研究主要是小样本、单中心队列研究。

Shinagawa 等在 2001 年 6 月至 2002 年 10 月间在日本开展了一项探索性研究，共纳入了 25 例患者，共 26 个肺外周病变，使用螺旋 CT 数据重建 VB 影像，采用超细支气管镜在 CT 引导下经支气管活检（transbronchial biopsy，TBB），探讨直径≤20 mm 的肺外周病变的 VB 图像与超细支气管镜实时图像的一致性。结果显示 CT 引导下 TBB 操作是安全的，所有患者均未出现任何并发症。VB 影像下的支气管与超细支气管镜下的实时支气管图像高度一致。检查开始到第一次 CT 扫描、第一次活检、整个检查时间分别是 5.46 min、12.96 min 和 29.27 min。17 个病灶（65.4%）通过病理检测明确诊断（包括 13 例原发性肺癌；1 例非典型腺瘤样增生；1 例转移癌；1 例结节病和 1 例非结核分支杆菌感染）。其余的病灶未明确诊断，主要是由于标本量不足（6 块标本）或者超细支气管镜无法达到病灶（3 块标本）[21]。

Asano 等进行了一项应用 VB 辅助气管镜对 17 例患者，共 38 个病灶进行路径规划的早期研究。VB 影像可重建到平均 6 级支气管（3~9 级）。38 个病灶中有 36 个病灶（94.7%）可以通过超细支气管镜经计划路径到达。中位系统规划时间是 2.6 min，中位检查时间是 24.9 min。38 个病灶中有 33 个（86.8%）可以采用活检钳进入，其中 31 个病灶（81.6%）可明确诊断[22]。

Shinagawa 等在 2002 年 11 月至 2005 年 11 月间通过超细支气管镜经 CT 引导 TBB 诊断 69 例患者的 71 个肺外周结节（平均直径 13.7 mm）[23]。导航下 CT 引导的 TBB 是一种较安全的方法，所有的患者均未出现严重并发症。从检查开始到第一次扫描、第一次活检以及总操作时间分别是 5.3 min、8.5 min 和 24.5 min。15 个病灶（70%）可明确诊断。与模拟对照方法相比，导航下的诊断阳性率更高，但是差异并不显著。然而，检查开始到第一次活检的时间和总检查时间，导航组明显短于对照组（$P<0.05$）[23]。

Tachihara 等也通过超细支气管镜，连续评估了 94 例患者，共 96 个肺外周病变（最长径≤30 mm，中位最长径 16.2 mm）。该研究在 38 个病例中使用普通支气管镜，56 个病例中使用超细支气管镜。虚拟图像与真实支气管图像吻合度很高。平均总检查时间是 24.1（±7.4）min。总诊断率为 62.5%（60/96），常规支气管镜的诊断率为 71.1%（27/38），超细支气管镜的诊断率为 56.9%（33/58）。病灶<10 mm、10~20 mm、>20 mm 的诊断率分别为 35%、61.4% 和 94.7%。通过 CT 扫描发现 8 例磨玻璃结节（ground glass opacity，GGO），其中 7 例获得病理诊断。所有的病例均未发生并发症[13]。

另一项研究关注 VBN 联合 EBUS 在肺外周病变中的诊断价值。该研究纳入 31 例患者共 32 个肺外周病变，使用 EBUS-GS 联合 TBB 的诊断方法。在此研究中，EBUS 成功探查到 30 个病灶（93.8%），27 个病灶（84.4%）获得病理诊断。在直径≤30 mm 的病灶中，EBUS 的探查成功率达到 91.7%（22/24），诊断率为 79.2%（19/24）。中位总检查时间为 22.3 min（9.8~41.5）[24]。

2016 年，Winantea 等报道了 19 例采用 VBN 诊断的肺外周病变患者（直径≤35 mm，中位直径 20 mm）。其中 10 个病灶位于右上叶，1 个在右中叶，2 个在右下叶，5 个在左上叶，1 个在左下叶。VBN 支气管镜的诊断率为 66.7%（5 例良性，3 例恶性）。5 例（41.6%）病灶均可被 R-EBUS 发现。所有病灶通过支气管镜获得的组织学病理都能明确诊断，诊断率达到 100%[18]。

2017 年发表的两项研究回顾性地评估了 VBN 的效能。Maekura 等在 2014 年 6 月至 2015 年 7 月间评估了 50 例患者，结果无法证明联合 EBUS、VBN 与 ROSE 诊断肺外周病变的有效性[15]。Diez-Ferrer 等评估了 63 例肺外周病变患者，结果显示 VBN 与非 VBN 的诊断率分别为 75% 与 43.9%（$P=0.029$）。操作时间与并发症方面没有差异。他们还指出 VBN 对于位于肺外周且不能被透视发现的病灶诊断率更高。这项研究也表明使用 VBN 可以减少进一步诊断性操作的需求[16]。

Asano 等进行了一项随机研究来评估 VBN 能否替代 X 线透视。这项非劣效性研究纳入了 129 例患者，其中 VBN 组的诊断率为 76.9%（50/65），X 线透视组的诊断率为 85.9%（55/64）。两组的诊断率差异为 -9.0%（95% CI：-22.3%~4.3%）。EBUS 发现病灶的概率在 VBNA 组为 95.4%（62/65），而在 X 线透视组为 96.9%（62/64）。根据研究数据，VBN 辅助的非劣效性无法确立，因此作者的结论为 VBN 无法替代 X 线透视[17]。

在最近的一项研究中，Kato 等在 100 例患者中发现 VBN 对肺外周病变的诊断率相比 CT 引导的经支气管活检更高（84% 比 58%，$P=0.013$）[14]。

综上，VBN 的诊断率从 67% 到 86% 不等。

11.5.1 其他应用

VBN 被常用于注射钡剂标记肺外周结节，随后在胸外科手术中起到辅助定位的作用。2004 年开展了一项包含 23 例患者，共 31 个病灶的小型研究[14]。在此项研究中，使用超细支气管镜成功开展肺结节标记，未发生任何并发症。中位标记时间是 23.5 min，钡剂标记物与病灶的最短距离为 4 mm（27 个病灶均在 10 mm 之内）。在胸腔镜手术中，所有的钡剂标记位置均被术中放射透视所识别，所有的病灶均被切除[25]。病理检测证实 2 例为腺癌，12 例为非典型腺瘤样增生，2 例为肺部炎症。

11.5.2 新技术

全球首个关于 Archimedes™ VBN 系统的前瞻性研究已经完成。在此研究中，研究人员通过透壁的方法在 10 例患者中分别建立一条到达病灶的隧道通路，获得了足够的标本，其检测结果与外科切除后组织学检测一致。这项研究的结果提示该技术具有可行性[4]。

另一项关于 Archimedes™ VBN 在术中联合应用透视作为引导的前瞻性研究也已经完成[26]。

还有一项 VBN 研究尝试创建支气管腔与支气管壁之间的 3D 透视影像。这可以帮助我们预测气道阻塞、狭窄、支气管阻塞的直径与长度。这些 3D 透视影像可以从螺旋 CT 和 CBCT 中导出。

VBN 也常被用于胸腔内淋巴结的定位，在培训内科医师学习传统经支气管穿刺活检中具有一定的作用[27]。

11.6 结论

VBN 在肺外周病变诊断中能否提升诊断率仍存在争议。但可以确定的是，虚拟导航对于右上叶病变、透视下可见的病变、肺外周 1/3 的病变以及在 R-EBUS 显示支气管在病变中央的情况下可以提高诊断率[28]。大部分研究显示，虚拟导航有可能缩短操作时间。鉴于虚拟导航的价格低廉，且没有辐射暴露，我们推荐它作为一种额外的工具来诊断肺外周病变。但是它能否在其他的疾病中使用，仍需进一步评估[29,30]。

参考文献

1. Baaklini, W.A., Reinoso, M.A., Gorin, A.B. et al. (2000). Diagnostic yield of fiberoptic bronchoscopy in evaluating solitary pulmonary nodules. *Chest* 117: 1049–1054.
2. Schreiber, G. and McCrory, D.C. (2003). Performance characteristics of different modalities for diagnosis of suspected lung cancer: summary of published evidence. *Chest* 123: 115s–128s.
3. Asano, F., Matsuno, Y., Matsushita, T. et al. (2002). Transbronchial diagnosis of a pulmonary peripheral small lesion using an ultrathin bronchoscope with virtual bronchoscopic navigation. *J. Bronchol. Interv. Pulmonol.* 9: 108–111.
4. Herth, F.J., Eberhardt, R., Sterman, D. et al. (2015). Bronchoscopic transparenchymal nodule access (BTPNA): first in human trial of a novel procedure for sampling solitary pulmonary nodules. *Thorax* 70: 326–332.
5. Reynisson, P.J., Leira, H.O., Hernes, T.N. et al. (2014). Navigated bronchoscopy: a technical review. *J. Bronchol. Interv. Pulmonol.* 21: 242–264.
6. Asano, F. (2010). Virtual bronchoscopic navigation. *Clin. Chest Med.* 31: 75–85.
7. Luo, X., Kitasaka, T., and Mori, K. (2011). Bronchoscopy navigation beyond electromagnetic tracking systems: a novel bronchoscope tracking prototype. *Med. Image Comput. Comput. Assist. Interv.* 14: 194–202.
8. Luo, X. and Mori, K. (2013). Beyond current guided bronchoscopy: a robust and real-time bronchoscopic ultrasound navigation system. *Med. Image Comput. Comput. Assist. Interv.* 16: 388–395.
9. Touman, A., Vitsas, V., Koulouris, N. et al. (2017). Gaining access to the periphery of the lung: bronchoscopic and transthoracic approaches. *Ann. Thorac. Med.* 12: 162–170.
10. Hohenforst-Schmidt, W., Banckwitz, R., Zarogoulidis, P. et al. (2014). Radiation exposure of patients by cone beam CT during endobronchial navigation – a phantom study. *J. Cancer* 5: 192–202.
11. Hohenforst-Schmidt, W., Zarogoulidis, P., Vogl, T. et al. (2014). Cone beam computed tomography (CBCT) in interventional chest medicine – high feasibility for endobronchial realtime navigation. *J. Cancer* 5: 231–241.
12. Eberhardt, R., Anantham, D., Ernst, A. et al. (2007). Multimodality bronchoscopic diagnosis of peripheral lung lesions: a randomized controlled trial. *Am. J. Respir. Crit. Care Med.* 176: 36–41.
13. Tachihara, M., Tamura, D., Kiriu, T. et al. (2018). Bronchoscopy using virtual navigation and endobronchial ultrasonography with a guide sheath (EBUS-GS) with or without fluoroscopy for peripheral pulmonary lesions. *Kobe J. Med. Sci.* 63: E99–e104.
14. Kato, A., Yasuo, M., Tokoro, Y. et al. (2018). Virtual bronchoscopic navigation as an aid to CT-guided transbronchial biopsy improves the diagnostic yield for small peripheral pulmonary lesions. *Respirology* 23: 1049–1054.
15. Maekura, T., Sugimoto, C., Tamiya, A. et al. (2017).

Combination of virtual bronchoscopic navigation, endobronchial ultrasound, and rapid on-site evaluation for diagnosing small peripheral pulmonary lesions: a prospective phase II study. *J. Thorac. Dis.* 9: 1930–1936.

16 Diez-Ferrer, M., Morales, A., Cubero, N. et al. (2017). MA05.01 virtual bronchoscopic navigation-guided ultrathin bronchoscopy for diagnosing peripheral pulmonary lesions. *J. Thorac. Oncol.* 12: S364.

17 Asano, F., Ishida,T., Shinagawa, N. et al. (2017). Virtual bronchoscopic navigation without X-ray fluoroscopy to diagnose peripheral pulmonary lesions: a randomized trial. *BMC Pulm. Med.* 17: 184.

18 Winantea, J., Eisenmann, S., and Darwiche, K. (2016). Virtual bronchoscopic navigation: advantages and limitations for the diagnosis of peripheral pulmonary lesions. *Eur. Respir. J.* 48: PA4678.

19 Asano, F., Shinagawa, N., Ishida,T. et al. (2013). Virtual bronchoscopic navigation combined with ultrathin bronchoscopy. A randomized clinical trial. *Am. J. Respir. Crit. Care Med.* 188: 327–333.

20 Ishida,T., Asano, F., Yamazaki, K. et al. (2011). Virtual bronchoscopic navigation combined with endobronchial ultrasound to diagnose small peripheral pulmonary lesions: a randomised trial. *Thorax* 66: 1072–1077.

21 Shinagawa, N., Yamazaki, K., Onodera,Y. et al. (2004). CT-guided transbronchial biopsy using an ultrathin bronchoscope with virtual bronchoscopic navigation. *Chest* 125: 1138–1143.

22 Asano, F., Matsuno, Y., Shinagawa, N. et al. (2006). A virtual bronchoscopic navigation system for pulmonary peripheral lesions. *Chest* 130: 559–566.

23 Shinagawa, N., Yamazaki, K., Onodera,Y. et al. (2007). Virtual bronchoscopic navigation system shortens the examination time – feasibility study of virtual bronchoscopic navigation system. *Lung Cancer* 56: 201–206.

24 Asano, F., Matsuno, Y., Tsuzuku, A. et al. (2008). Diagnosis of peripheral pulmonary lesions using a bronchoscope insertion guidance system combined with endobronchial ultrasonography with a guide sheath. *Lung Cancer* 60: 366–373.

25 Asano, F., Shindoh, J., Shigemitsu, K. et al. (2004). Ultrathin bronchoscopic barium marking with virtual bronchoscopic navigation for fluoroscopy-assisted thoracoscopic surgery. *Chest* 126: 1687–1693.

26 Broncus Medical Announces New Study That Shows High Diagnostic Sensitivity for Archimedes Virtual Bronchoscopy Navigation System. (2018). www.businesswire.com/news/home/20180523005308/en/Broncus-Medical-Announces-New-Study-Shows-High

27 Wu, X., Shi, L., Xia,Y. et al. (2018). Intrabronchial display of hilar-mediastinal lymph nodes by virtual bronchoscopic navigation system. *Thorac. Cancer* 9: 415–419.

28 Belanger, A.R. and Akulian, J.A. (2017). An update on the role of advanced diagnostic bronchoscopy in the evaluation and staging of lung cancer. *Ther. Adv. Respir. Dis.* 11: 211–221.

29 Shepherd, R.W. (2016). Bronchoscopic pursuit of the peripheral pulmonary lesion: navigational bronchoscopy, radial endobronchial ultrasound, and ultrathin bronchoscopy. *Curr. Opin. Pulm. Med.* 22: 257–264.

30 Asano, F. (2018). Does virtual bronchoscopic navigation improve the diagnostic yield of transbronchial biopsy? *Respirology* 23: 970–971.

第 12 章

间接喉镜
咽喉解剖和可弯曲支气管镜的应用

Eric R. Carlson[1] and Thomas Schlieve[2]
[1] Oral/Head and Neck Oncologic Surgery Fellowship Program,
Department of Oral and Maxillofacial Surgery, University of Tennessee Medical Center,
University of Tennessee Cancer Institute, Knoxville, TN, USA
[2] Division of Oral and Maxillofacial Surgery, University of Texas Southwestern Medical School,
Parkland Memorial Hospital, Dallas, TX, USA
（译者：朱敏辉 译者单位：海军军医大学第一附属医院）

间接喉镜检查在头颈部手术中有许多应用，包括对已诊断为口腔/头颈癌的患者进行准确的临床分期，评估声音嘶哑患者的声带外展和内收功能，以及作为困难气道患者清醒插管中的一个重要应用环节。困难气道是指面罩通气困难、气管插管困难或同时出现这两种情况的气道[1]。在麻醉临床实践中，影响患者发病率和死亡率的一个重要且严峻的因素就是气管插管过程中的意外。Shiga 等[2]通过荟萃分析发现，在无气道病变的患者中，插管困难的发生率为 5.8%。降低困难气道插管过程中的发病率和死亡率，最重要的就是获取患者的气道病史，评估困难气道患者行直接喉镜检查的条件，并在检查前病理明确气道疾病的良恶性。为了更好保障患者的安全，最佳的处理办法就是进行间接喉镜检查前获取患者尽可能多的相关的临床资料。

12.1 气道病史

对准备行全身麻醉的患者来说，详细掌握气道病史是术前检查的一个重要环节。尽管如此，目前尚无文献充分证明通过询问患者病史或查阅患者的既往医疗资料可以预测困难气道的发生。目前，有病例报告表明，有阻塞性睡眠呼吸暂停和打鼾病史的患者出现插管困难的可能性更大[1]。此外，患有某些先天性或后天性疾病，如退行性骨关节炎、舌甲状腺或扁桃体肥大、特雷彻·柯林斯综合征、皮-罗综合征、唐氏综合征等，也与插管困难有关。因此，在进行麻醉时，有针对性地获取相关病史有利于识别困难气道和难以进行直接喉镜检查的气道。

了解气道病史的目的是明确哪些患者可能需要通过间接喉镜检查才可以进行全身麻醉。为此，对于可能难以进行直接喉镜检查的患者来说，Murphy[3]首先提出的纤维光镜可视下气管插管是目前进行选择性气道管理的公认标准[4]。表 12.1 列出了需要了解的气道病史要素。

表 12.1 预测需要进行间接喉镜检查的与困难气道相关的临床病史及气道病史要素

已知插管困难史
术前既往医疗记录提供的证据

(续表)

怀疑插管困难
病史证据表明患者有插管困难的倾向
颈椎不稳定
类风湿性关节炎，近期颈椎损伤
解剖异常及头颈部综合征
肢端肥大症（巨舌症、喉狭窄）
唐氏综合征（声门下狭窄、大舌门、寰枢关节不稳）
戈尔登哈尔综合征（半面部巨大儿）
特雷彻•柯林斯综合征（下颌后缩）
皮-罗综合征（下颌后缩）
克利佩尔-费尔综合征（颈椎融合及寰枕畸形）
贝-维综合征（巨舌症）
口腔/头颈部肿瘤
良性和恶性肿瘤伴舌部隆起
头颈部筋膜间隙感染
头颈部放射性组织损伤，特别是与牙关有关的损伤
颅面创伤

12.2 体格检查：重点评估气道

1956年，Cass等[6]发表了5名患者困难喉镜检查的结果，并对这些妨碍直接观察声门的解剖特征进行分析，这些特征包括：颈短、肌肉发达且牙列完整、下颌钝角、上颌门牙突出、颞下颌关节炎导致的下颌活动范围小、上腭高拱、牙槽-牙间距增大以及在直接喉镜检查时需要额外扩大下颌骨的开口等。

1983年，Mallampati等对美国麻醉师协会（ASA）体能状态评级为1级或2级的210例需要气管插管的患者进行了研究。女性163例，男性47例，其中199例患者的牙齿齐全，3例上颌没有牙齿，8例患者无牙齿，5名患者被诊断患有类风湿关节炎（rheumatoid arthritis，RA），1例患者患有骨关节炎。所有患者均无因颞下颌关节受累而导致三叉神经痛的情况。该研究中共22名工作人员参与气道评估和执行插管，其中包括6名麻醉护士、10名住院医师和6名麻醉医师。在术前气道评估时，医师指导患者处于坐位，最大程度地张开嘴巴并尽量伸出舌头。具体来说，麻醉医师应在术前访视中观察2次患者腭舌弓、腭咽弓、软腭和悬雍垂的情况。通过术前对患者气道的解剖评估，可以将患者分为3类：第1类：腭舌弓、腭咽弓、软腭及悬雍垂完全暴露；第2类：腭舌弓、腭咽弓、软腭均可见，但悬雍垂被舌根部分阻挡；第3类：仅软腭可见。

在该研究中，气管插管困难的定义是在直接喉镜检查过程中声门暴露不良。

暴露程度可分为1~4级：1级：声门完全可见，包括声门前后联合；2级：声门部分可见，前联合无法暴露；3级：声门未完全显露，只能看到杓状软骨。4级：无法显露声门及杓状软骨。

在该研究中，1级和2级表示声门暴露充分，3级和4级表示声门暴露不良。在155例Mallampati分级为1级的患者中，所有患者都能充分暴露声门，其中81%的患者暴露程度分级为1级。40名Mallampati分级为2级的患者中，65%的患者在直接喉镜下声门暴露充分，35%的患者在直接喉镜下声门暴露不充分。在15例3级气道患者中，均未实现声门完全暴露，60%的患者直接喉镜检查不充分，其中5例患者直接喉镜检查为4级。所有8例无牙患者和3例无上颌牙患者都能充分暴露声门。目前使用的改良版Mallampati分类将其分为4级而非3级（图12.1），由Samsoon和Young提出[7]，他们对1 980名患者中发生插管困难的7名产科患者（0.4%）进行了回顾性研究。

另一个用于评估直接喉镜检查难度的临床指标是甲颌间距，即甲状软骨的上缘到下颌骨完全伸展时前缘的距离。Frerk[8]在对244例成年患者的研究中证实，"甲颌间距小于7 cm"对预测直接喉镜检查困难的敏感性为90%，特异性为81.5%。他将这一测量结果与改良的Mallampati测试相结合，用于预测直接喉镜检查的难度。改良的Mallampati分级是基于最大程度张口时将舌头伸出，同时能看到的咽部结构来设计的。其咽部视野分级为：1级：软腭、悬雍垂和悬雍垂游离部可见；2级：悬雍垂游离部被舌根阻挡，只能看到悬雍垂根部；3级：仅可见软腭；4级：咽后壁不可见。在麻醉诱导和使用神经肌肉阻断剂后，尝试进行直接喉镜检查，并将检查结果分级如下：1级：声带完全显露。2级：只显露杓状软骨和后联合。3级：只显露会厌。4级：未显露声门结构。244例患者中，有11例插管困难，其中有9例咽部视野分级为3级或4级。此外，这11例患者中有9例甲颌间距为7 cm或更小。仅根据咽部视野分级3级或4级来预测困难气道的敏感性为81.2%，特异性为81.5%，有52名患者被预测为困难气道，43例为假阳性。基于甲颌间距≤7 cm预测气道困难的敏感性为90.9%，特异性为81.5%，有53例患者被预测为困难气道，43例为假阳性。在14例疑似困难气道和5例假阳性的患者中使用以上两种评估方法，敏感性为81.2%，特异性为97.8%。

作者的数据表明甲颌间距测定比改进的Mallampati

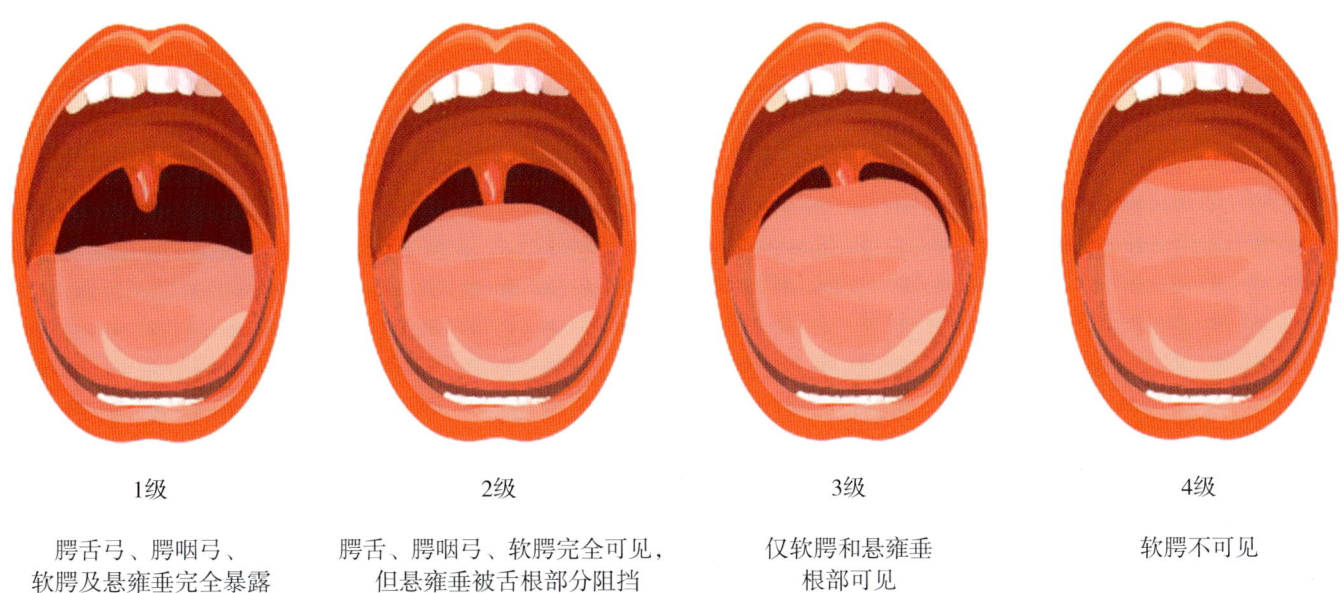

1级	2级	3级	4级
腭舌弓、腭咽弓、软腭及悬雍垂完全暴露	腭舌、腭咽弓、软腭完全可见，但悬雍垂被舌根部分阻挡	仅软腭和悬雍垂根部可见	软腭不可见

图 12.1 改良的气道 Mallampati 分类法

分级更敏感，比两种评估方法的结合更敏感。尽管如此，作者还是强调了这两项评估方法在术前评估直接喉镜检查可能存在困难的价值。

Wilson 等[9]评估了 633 例接受常规手术患者的数据，并确定了 5 个预测插管困难的危险因素：超重，尤其大于 90 kg 者；头部活动受限，尤其是小于 90°者；下颌骨活动障碍，切牙间隙小于 5 cm，下颌骨无法向前下移者；下颌骨严重后退者；门牙严重前突者。参照这一预测性评估方法，前瞻性队列观察 778 例患者，其中 1.5% 的患者存在插管困难。根据所选择的阈值不同，该评估规则可检测出 75% 的困难插管，而假阳性率为 12%。

在预测困难插管和是否需要纤维镜辅助检查时还需要考虑面罩通气是否困难这一因素。Langeron 等[10]对 1 502 例接受骨科、妇科、神经外科、泌尿外科和普通外科手术的患者进行为期 6 个月的前瞻性研究。据报道，75 例（5%）患者出现了面罩通气困难，其中 1 例无法进行通气。在 75 例患者中只有 13% 在预测时被认为会出现面罩通气困难。预计存在面罩通气困难的 56 例患者，但实际上并没有发生。

经多变量分析，面罩通气困难的危险因素包括：年龄＞55 岁、体重指数＞26 kg/m^2、无牙齿、有打鼾史等。作者还证实对于曾有过面罩通气困难的患者，困难插管和无法插管的发生率分别高出 4 倍和 12 倍。总的来说，与没有面罩通气困难的患者（8%）相比，存在面罩通气困难的患者（30%）插管困难的发生率明显更高。因此，面罩通气困难是插管困难的另一个危险因素，应及时采用纤维支气管辅助插管。

12.3 并发症

各种疾病可导致气道解剖结构扭曲，从而出现气管插管困难，具体可分为肿瘤性、非肿瘤性、感染性和非感染性情况[11]。

12.3.1 糖尿病

糖尿病与喉镜检查困难的关系已经得到证实。据了解，约 1/3 的 1 型糖尿病患者在喉镜检查时存在困难[11,12]。这种情况的出现被认为与身材矮小、关节僵硬、皮肤紧绷以及关节固定有关。关节固定被认为与长期高血糖导致组织蛋白的糖基化、胶原蛋白交联异常有关。其他导致插管困难的因素包括肥胖和颈围增大。Iseli 等[13]对 2 145 例直接喉镜检查中认为存在困难气道的 152 例患者进行前瞻性研究。清醒状态下纤维支气管镜辅助插管是困难气道插管最常用的方法，仅有 1.3% 的患者需要在清醒状态下行气管切开。首次插管失败的预测因素包括癌症、声门上病变以及既往进行过放射治疗。笔者认为，由头颈部病变导致的困难气道的处理需要包括外科团队在内的联合会诊。

Mudassir 等[12]对 357 例需要进行气管插管的择期手术的糖尿病患者进行研究，并评估"祈祷"征和

Mallampati 试验的结果。祈祷征的评估方法是让患者将手掌合拢，如果手掌之间存在间隙，则预示插管困难，如果手掌接触无困难，则预测插管无困难。总体而言，在研究的 357 例患者中有 125 例（35%）出现了插管困难，其敏感性为 30%，特异性为 94%。该体征在糖尿病患者中的准确率为 71%。这些统计数据与 Mallampati 测试相比，后者的敏感性为 79%，特异性为 99%，准确率为 92%。

Hashim 和 Thomas[14] 利用先前回顾的气道指数和掌纹征，对 60 名接受全身麻醉并气管插管的糖尿病患者进行了前瞻性评估。该测试是将惯用手的手指和手掌牢固地压在蓝色墨水垫上，然后将患者的手紧紧按在硬表面的白纸上。通过对印迹进行分级，将分级转化为困难插管的预测结果。60 例插管中有 13 例（21.7%）被确定为困难插管，掌纹征被认为是最重要的困难气道预测标志，其敏感性为 76.9%，特异性为 89.3%。

12.3.2 类风湿关节炎（RA）

RA 是普通人群中最常见的自身免疫性关节炎，据估计占成年人口的 0.5%~1.0%[15]。该疾病常见的分类为全身性、慢性和进行性 3 种，其影响关节滑膜并导致骨和软骨破坏，呈现不同程度畸形和对称的多发性关节炎，可累及颈部、肩部、手腕、手指、肘部、髋部、膝部、踝关节和足部。RA 通常会影响颈椎，导致 3 种特征性的不稳定结构：寰枢关节半脱位（atlantoaxial subluxation，AAS）、轴垂直半脱位（vertical subluxation，VS）和亚轴半脱位（subaxial subluxation，SAS）。对于有 RA 病史且计划行全身麻醉的患者，术前应通过 X 线检查颈椎半脱位的程度（图 12.2）。具体来说，这些半脱位可能导致不可逆的脊髓损伤、呼吸功能障碍和猝死。

对于计划行直接喉镜检查的该类患者，应考虑使用纤维支气管镜进行检查。特别是在插管期间要限制颈椎屈伸，即使理论上可行，实际上也很难进行常规的直接喉镜检查[16]。因此，对于有颈椎症状的患者，术前应行侧位颈椎屈伸平片，以评估是否存在颈椎半脱位[11]。研究认为，40%~85% 的 RA 患者如果伴有颈部疼痛可能与颈椎半脱位相关[17]。无症状的 RA 患者是否需要颈椎 X 线检查目前存在争议[11]，也没有证据表明行此类影像学检查具有明确价值[17]。尽管如此，对无症状 RA 患者，在接受直接喉镜检查和插管后，仍有出现术后神经损伤的病例报告。因此，术前需要对所有 RA 患者进行颈椎 X 线检查评估。除了 RA 患者的颈椎受累性外，在喉镜插管时，所有 RA 患者术前也须评估由于颞下颌关节受累导致开口受限的情况。当然，无论有无症状，只要术前有颈椎影像学证据显示颈椎下移，以及出现与颞下颌关节受累相关的张口受限的情况，都表明全身麻醉时需要间接喉镜检查和纤维支气管镜插管管理气道。

Terashima 等[15] 评估了 634 例 RA 患者，确定了 3 种类型的颈椎不稳定。他们对这些患者在完全屈曲、中位和完全伸展时的侧位颈椎 X 线检查进行了评估。颈椎不稳在寰枢前间隙（atlantodental interval，ADI）>3 mm、垂直半脱位（Ranawat 值<13 mm）和不可恢复的椎体平移 2 mm 或更多且无骨质增生的患者中表现为 AAS。ADI 为 10 mm 或更多的患者被定义为颈椎不稳并被认为是即将可能出现神经功能缺损的重危患者，Ranawat 值为 10 mm 或更低的患者被定义为 VS 者，不可恢复的椎体平移为 4 mm 或更多或在多个水平上为 2 mm 或更多的患者被定义为 SAS 患者[15]。在 503 例基线无严重颈椎不稳的 RA 患者中，143 例随访时间超过 10 年。其中，AAS、VS 或 SAS 任何程度颈椎不稳定的患者数量，在观察基线时为 59 例（41.3%），随访 5 年以上时增加到 97 例（67.8%），从而表明该疾病具有进展性。所有严重颈椎疾病患者，出现颈椎不稳定数量从基线时的 0 例（0%）增加到 5 年以上时的 35 例（24.5%）。就发生严重颈椎不稳定的预测风险因素而言，这类患者 C 反应蛋白（C-reactive protein，CRP）值往往较高，既往接受过关节手术，进行过皮质类固醇治疗。

Hakala 和 Randell[18] 回顾性地评估了 78 例总计接受过 89 次手术的 RA 患者。具体而言，他们根据插管困难程度对两组患者进行分析。对 1989—1992 年采用传统插管技术手术的 46 例患者中的 41 例（第 1 组）与 1993—1994 年采用清醒插管手术的 43 例患者中的 37 例（第 2 组）进行比较。第 1 组有 6 例患者（13%）遇到严重插管困难，其中 2 例需行气管切开。2 组中有 3 例（8%）患者出现严重插管困难。作者在该研究结论中指出，在 RA 患者气道管理中引入纤维支气管镜辅助插管技术有利于保障患者安全。

12.3.3 唐氏综合征

唐氏综合征是一种遗传性疾病，最常见的是 21-三体综合征。该综合征是人类最常见的染色体疾病，每 750~800 例婴儿中就有 1 例发生[19,20]。这些患者存在颅面和气道异常，其中 20%~30% 的患者出现寰

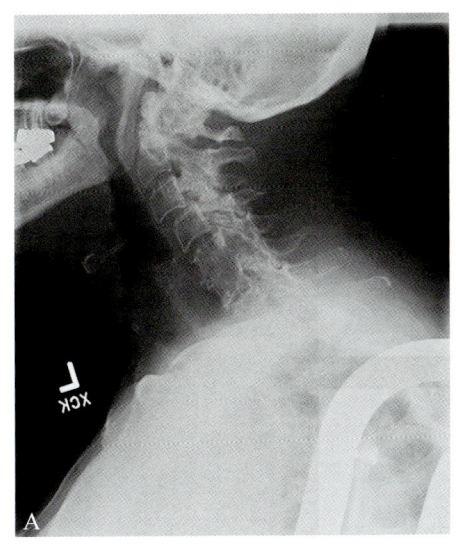 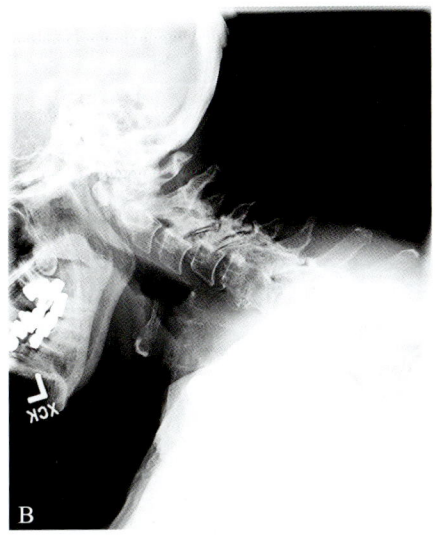 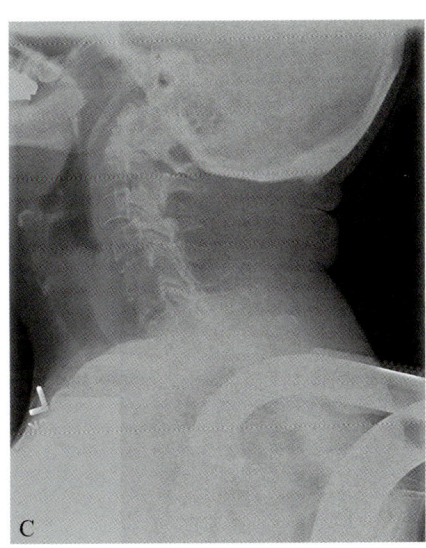

图 12.2　类风湿关节炎患者的颈椎 X 线侧位图

A. 中立位；B. 屈曲位；C. 伸展位。寰枢间隙在屈曲位时变宽至 4 mm，表明不稳定，在中立位和伸展位时不可见。C3 相对 C4 向前滑脱 4 mm，在屈曲位和伸展位时没有变化。C5~C6 节段存在骨融合。C1 和 C2 前方的椎前软组织及齿状突变宽，这与类风湿关节炎继发的淋巴结炎相对应。

枢椎不稳定，这是最常见的异常之一[21]。其他气道问题包括喉气管狭窄和声门下狭窄、舌扁桃体肥大、肿大腺样体的炎症和感染，以及近舌底软腭塌陷阻塞气道[19]。这些颅面和气道畸形提示需要使用纤维支气管镜联合间接喉气管插管。

Borland 等[19] 回顾性分析 1988 年 4 月至 1995 年 5 月在匹兹堡儿童医院接受非心脏手术麻醉的所有唐氏综合征患儿。其间共进行了 74 021 次麻醉，其中对 488 例唐氏综合征患儿进行了 930 次麻醉。这 488 例患儿中有 75 例（15.4%）有声门下狭窄史，33 例有扁桃体和腺样体肥大，10 例有颈椎缺陷，分别为 AAS 8 例和寰枢关节脱位 2 例。在该研究中，只有 0.54% 的唐氏综合征患儿发生了插管困难，而在其他人群中这一比例为 0.32%。BevilaCqua 等[22] 对 1992—1994 年接受心脏手术的 627 例唐氏综合征患儿进行了回顾性研究，这些患儿插管困难的发生率为 4.62%，并随年龄的降低而增加。

对唐氏综合征患者的寰枢椎不稳的情况已经进行了广泛的研究[21,23]，结果表明寰枢椎不稳定性有多种诱发因素，包括横韧带松弛和寰枢椎发育不全、畸形或完全缺失等。对颈椎不稳定的患者进行气管内插管的操作可能会对颈椎造成不良后果。唐氏综合征患者在气管插管中颈椎的伸展或屈曲都可能存在风险。因此，有必要在术前对颈椎的自然位、屈曲位和伸展位进行侧位成像，以避免出现不良的神经系统后遗症。

12.4　病理情况

上呼吸道的各种肿瘤性和非肿瘤性疾病都可能影响传统的气管插管，因此需要采用纤维支气管镜和间接喉镜插管。体格检查通常能够直接发现这些病理情况，从而决定采用间接喉镜和纤维支气管镜辅助插管来建立全身麻醉（视频 12.1）。有时，影像学检查也可意外地提示病理，表明全身麻醉和手术准备时通过间接喉镜检查行气管插管的必要性（图 12.3）。

在临床上常见的良性病变中，头颈部的硬皮样囊肿和表皮样囊肿通常对直接喉镜检查造成机械性障碍（图 12.4）。头颈部的恶性病变，尤其是直接累及喉部的恶性病变，通常需要纤维支气管镜辅助插管（图 12.5）。此外，感染性疾病导致气道阻塞时，偶尔也需要进行间接喉镜检查和纤支镜辅助插管，以建立全身麻醉，完成手术切开和引流（图 12.6）。最后，放射性组织损伤通常导致牙关紧闭，也是进行全麻手术时间接喉镜检查和纤维气管镜辅助插管的指征。

视频 12.1　间接喉镜和纤维支气管镜辅助插管

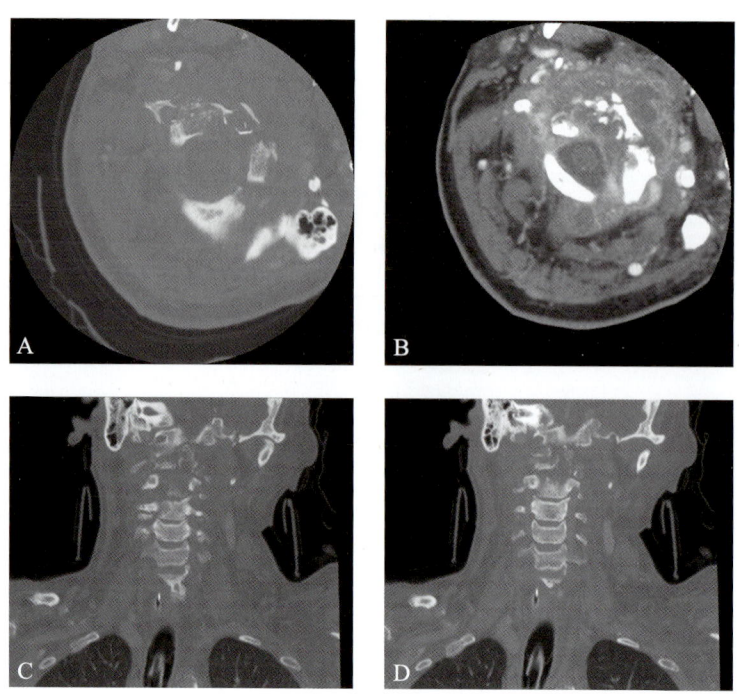

图 12.3 病例（一）

A~D. 患者，73 岁，女性，脊柱 CT，CT 血管造影显示右侧颈内动脉夹层。脊柱 CT 显示颅底、C1、C2 齿状突破坏性改变伴 C1~C2 脱位。在齿状突周围的左侧椎前间隙可见周围积液，并向左侧硬膜外间隙延伸。患者的影像学检查是重要检查的一部分，需要在间接喉镜插管前进行。

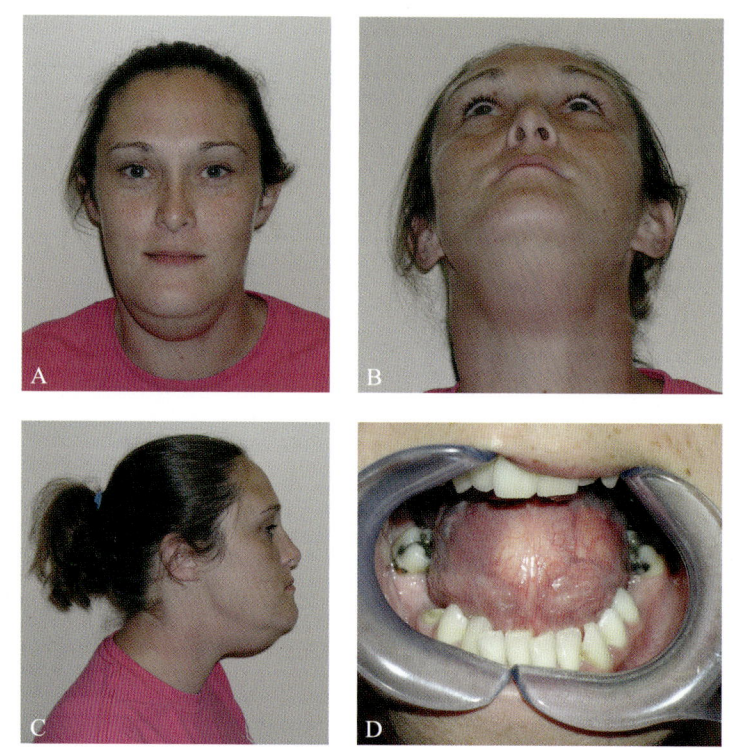

图 12.4 病例（二）

A~C. 患者，27 岁，女性，有 8 年的颌下肿胀和口前底肿胀史（D）。CT 检查（E~H）显示上颈部和口底低密度病变，最宽直径为 6.5 cm。因肿块及其舌部抬高引起部分气道阻塞，其术中须行间接喉镜和纤维支气管镜下气管插管进行气道管理（I）。

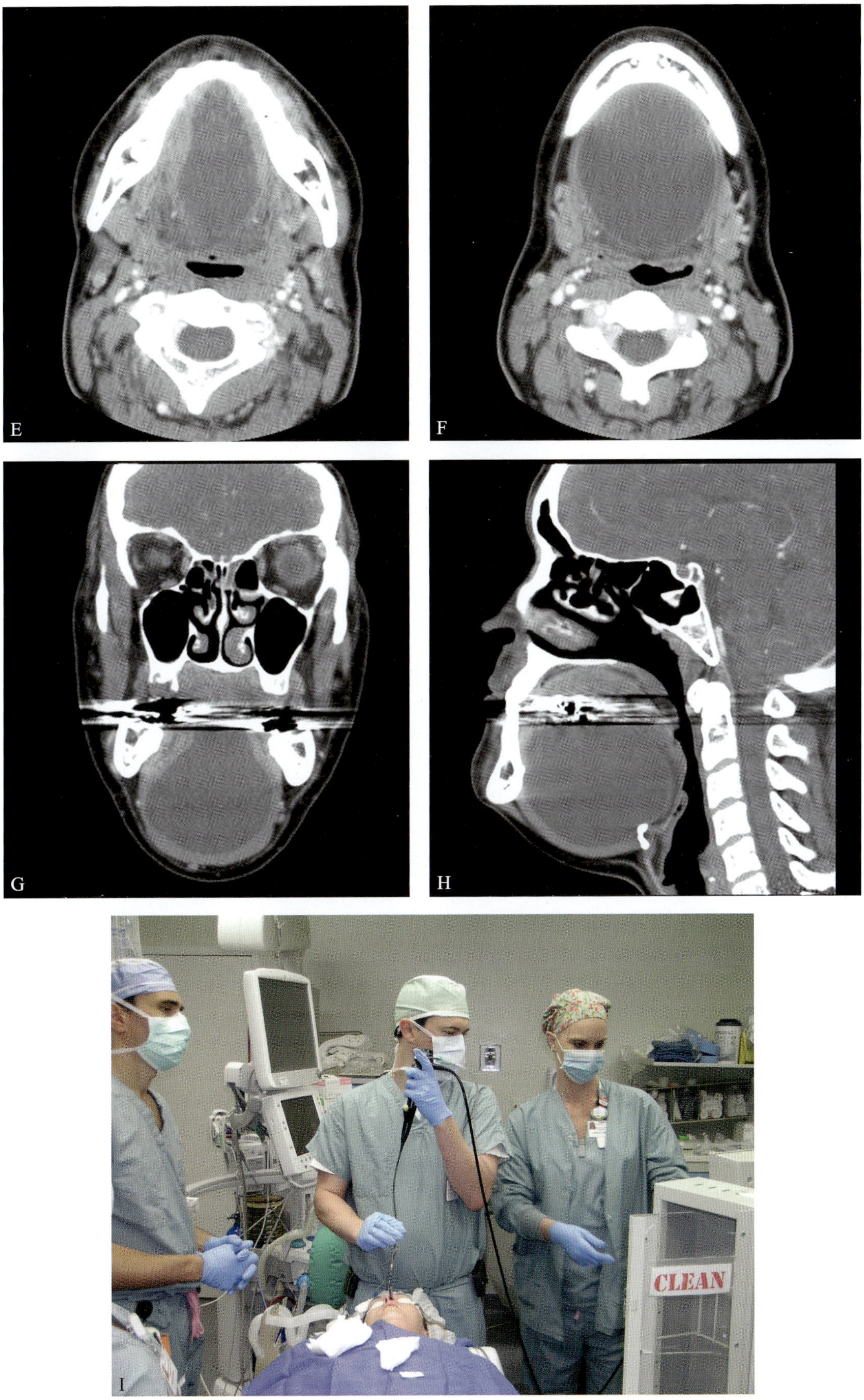

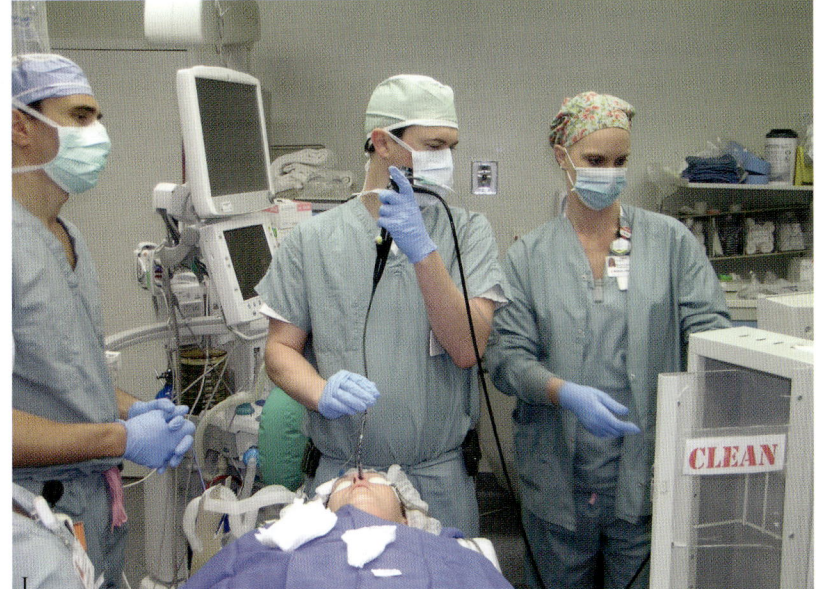

图 12.4 病例（二）（续图）

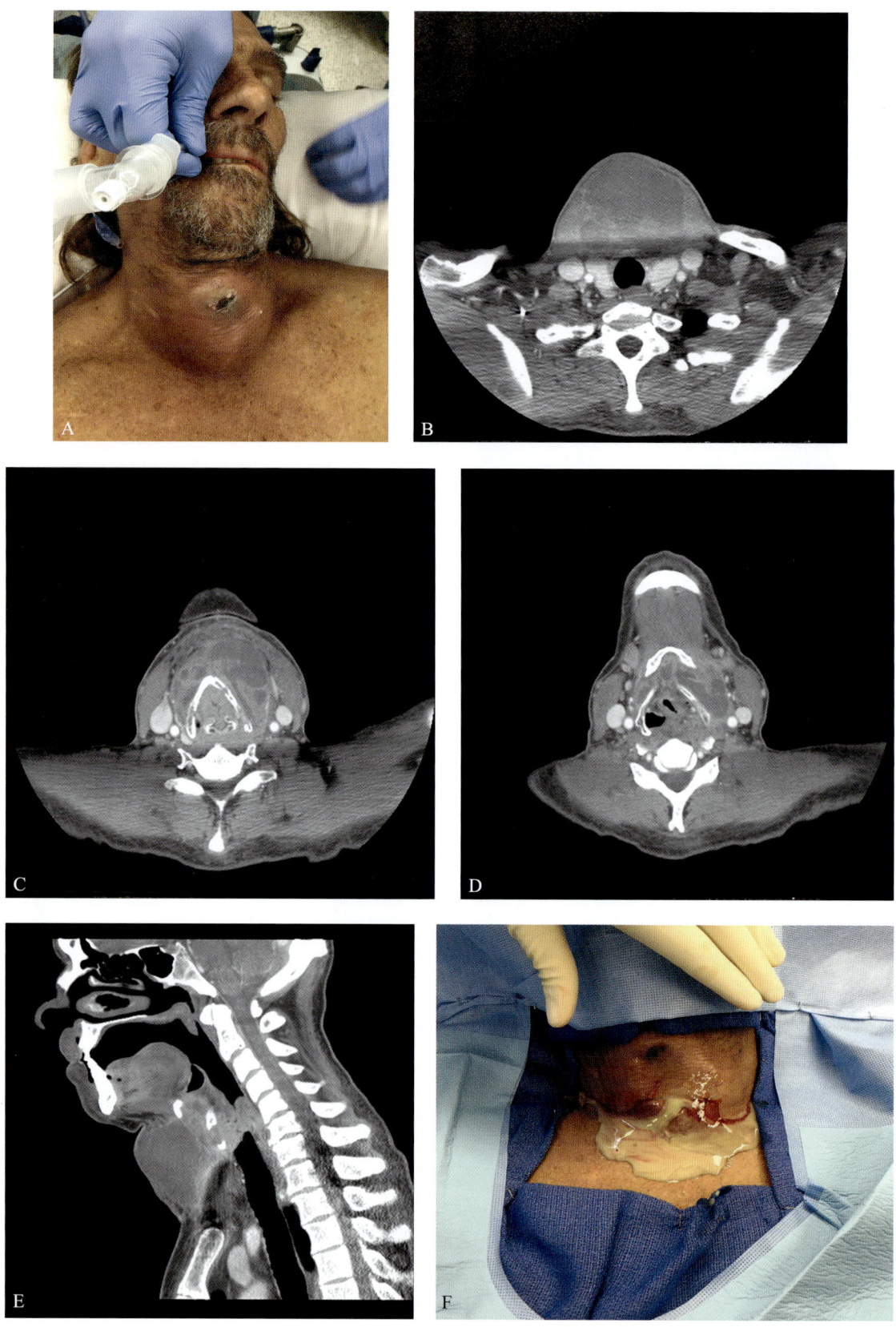

图 12.5　病例（三）

A. 患者，51岁，男性，上颈部感染、肿胀，气道受损；B～E. CT 扫描发现喉部一个阻塞气道的肿块，以及一个直径 7.3 cm 的脓肿，从左侧扁桃体延伸到梨状窝，累及喉部和气管前软组织。F. 通过间接喉镜和纤维气管镜下气管插管，并在全身麻醉下对其上颈部脓肿进行引流。

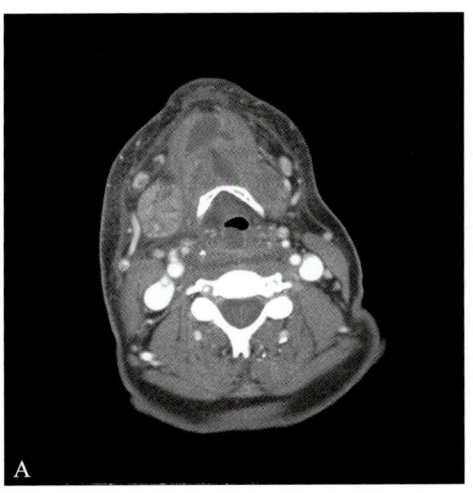
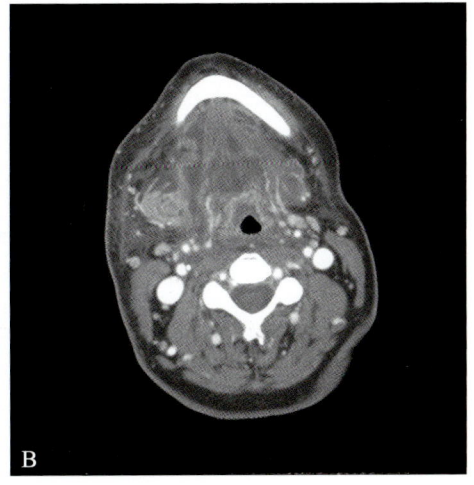

图 12.6 病例（四）：颈部轴位 CT 扫描

A、B. 患者，60 岁，女性，颈部脓肿导致气道狭窄和偏曲。出现颈部脓肿的患者，最好行增强 CT 扫描来评估气道，确定是否需要间接喉镜检查并在清醒气管插管下进行手术切开和引流。

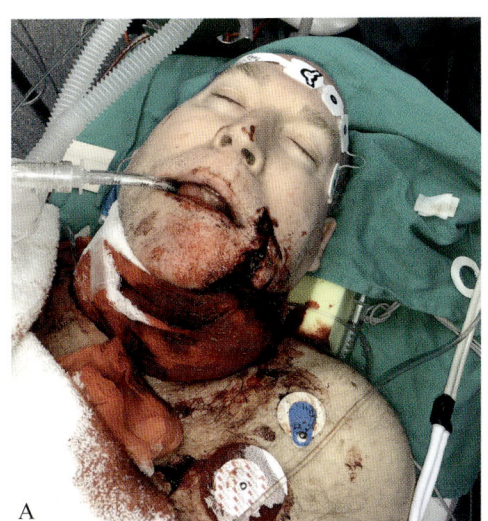
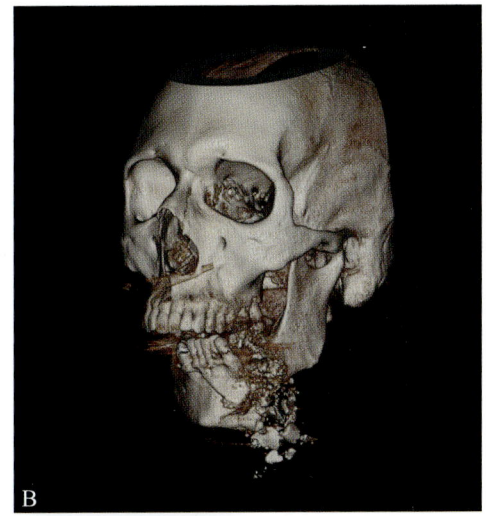
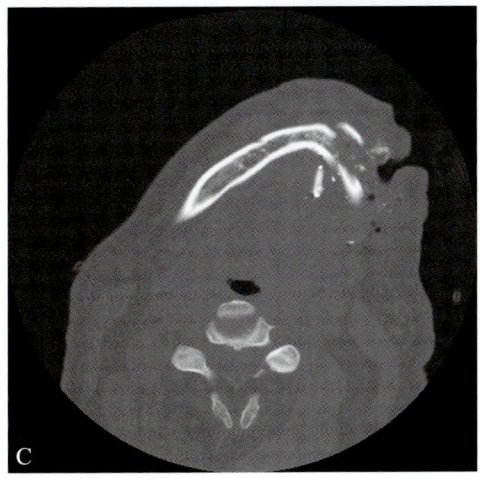

图 12.7 病例（五）

A~C. 患者，59 岁，男性，严重软硬组织损伤，左脸、上颈部、下颌骨和口腔黏膜遭受枪伤。在手术修复这些损伤时，建立气道时应考虑间接喉镜检查。

12.5 颅颌面外伤

严重的面部骨折（图 12.7），尤其是颅底骨折，经常伴有上呼吸道的损伤[24]。由于气管插管有穿透颅底的风险，对这些损伤患者进行鼻气管内盲插管可能会导致颅内感染和中枢神经系统损伤。Bahr 和 Stoll[25] 对 160 例前基底骨折合并脑脊液漏（cerebrospinal fluid leakage，CSFL）的患者进行了回顾性研究，其中对照组 80 例，患者存在 CSFL，但不存在需要修复的颌面骨折，并且只通过经口插管。试验组 80 例，患者存在颌面部骨折，采用经鼻腔气管插管。每组均有 2 例患者发生脑膜炎。两组比较表明插管方式对并发症发生率无影响，尤其没有病例发生直接脑膜损伤，经鼻气管插管相关脑膜炎的发生率为 2.5%，与经口气管插管相同。

颌面部骨折的另一个问题是可能会造成颈椎创伤，因此需要间接喉镜和纤支镜辅助插管来建立气道。Haug 等[26] 回顾了 563 例面部骨折患者，发现 11 例伴有颈椎骨折（2%）。Jamal 等[27] 检索了 6.5 年中因颈椎骨折入院的 701 例患者的病历，发现 44 例伴有面部骨折（6.3%）。笔者认为，需要假定所有面部骨折患者的颈椎都不稳定，并据此来建立气道。

12.6 咽部解剖

在讨论间接喉镜检查时，必须简要介绍咽部的解剖结构，因为要观察和检查喉部，必须通过此解剖区域。咽部最宽和最窄的部分分别位于舌骨和食管的水平面，咽从颅底延伸至环状软骨/第 6 颈椎，又细分为鼻咽部、口咽部和喉咽部。鼻咽内有咽鼓管的开口，在那里可见一个隆起组织，即咽鼓管圆枕。口咽部从软腭的下缘开始，延伸到会厌和舌骨的上缘。它由软腭、悬雍垂、舌根、前腭和舌骨组成。腭舌肌和腭咽肌分别组成扁桃体前弓和后弓，以及扁桃体窝。喉咽（又称下咽）位于会厌的下部至喉部后方的环状软骨水平处延伸至食管。

12.7 喉部解剖

喉保护气道免受误吸，参与发声，并通过维持气道通畅参与呼吸。女性和儿童的喉通常比成年男性的位置更高。在青春期之前，男性和女性的喉大小没有差别。在青春期，男性喉的前后径加倍，形成喉部突起，被称为喉结[28]。

喉的前部位于颈部的浅表，后部与喉咽相邻。喉的入口由会厌上缘，杓会厌襞和伸展于两个杓状软骨之间的黏膜襞（即杓间襞）形成。其向下延伸至环状软骨和气管[28]。整个喉部由鳞状上皮被覆，包括纤毛上皮、假复层上皮、柱状上皮或复层鳞状上皮。声带和会厌舌面受到磨损的风险较高，因此由弹性较好的复层鳞状上皮被覆[29]。

喉的解剖结构复杂，可分为成对和单个软骨、黏膜皱襞、固有肌和外在肌及其支配各自的神经[30]。黏膜皱襞是对被黏膜覆盖的韧带的一种解剖学描述[31]。尽管舌骨在连接上不属于喉的一部分，但由于其肌肉和韧带附着物较多，因此也被纳入喉的解剖学讨论范围内。

12.7.1 舌骨

舌骨悬吊喉部，并为喉部功能提供肌肉附件。其还为口底、舌、会厌和咽部的肌肉提供附着部位。舌骨是唯一参与喉功能和相关解剖的骨骼结构。

12.7.2 喉软骨

喉软骨是连接各种肌肉、韧带和黏膜皱褶的框架。喉软骨共有 9 块，其中 3 块成对（杓状软骨、角状软骨、楔形软骨）和 3 块不成对（甲状软骨、环状软骨和会厌软骨）。杓状软骨、甲状软骨和环状软骨由透明软骨组成，其他软骨为弹性软骨[32]。随着年龄的增长，透明软骨趋于骨化，因此在常规 X 线和 CT 中更容易被观察到。

甲状软骨是喉内最大的软骨结构，由 2 个独立的四边形椎板组成，它们向后分离，前中线在胚胎时融合，形成一个单一的盾状软骨，每一半称为甲状软骨板[33]。它形成喉的前壁和侧壁，以及在颈前部易触诊到的喉结。甲状软骨的内表面附着前庭韧带和声带韧带，上（大）角和整个软骨上缘通过甲状舌骨韧带（膜）与舌骨相连，下（小）角通过环甲关节与环状软骨相连。外表面为喉外肌（如胸骨甲状肌、甲状舌骨肌和咽下缩肌）提供附着，而甲状软骨下表面则通过前方的环甲膜（如环甲韧带）和前外侧环甲肌与环状软骨连接[28]。环甲关节运动可导致声带长度发生变化。

环状软骨位于第 6 颈椎的水平，是喉和气管的解剖分界[32]。由于它是唯一完整的软骨环，而且比甲状软骨更厚、更结实，因此在插管时对环状软骨施加压力时，它可以对喉后部保持支撑来维持气道通畅。环状软骨的前部高度仅为 3~4 mm，但更坚固的后部高度为 20~30 mm[28]。正是这种高度的急剧变化及相对无血管的环甲状软骨膜为环甲膜切开术进入气道创造了空间。环状软骨通过环气管韧带连接第一气管环，附着于环杓后肌，并与上外侧的环杓软骨相连。

会厌或会厌软骨呈叶状，被覆鳞状上皮。与甲状软骨和环状软骨不同，它不会骨化，并终生保持一定的弹性。会厌形成喉入口的屏障，以防止食物、液体或唾液吸入气道。它位于舌根和舌骨体的后面，以及喉入口的前面。在 1% 的成年人中，当嘴巴张开舌前倾时，可以看到会厌的尖端和后部[28]。会厌通过甲状会厌韧带连接到甲状软骨的中线内表面。从会厌前部延伸至舌后的是舌会厌中襞，并通过咽会厌外侧襞在咽部外侧成对附着。会厌谷，作为一个重要的成对结构，是由 3 个襞皱构成的。插管时，喉镜的尖端停顿在此，这也是异物嵌塞的常见部位。杓会厌褶从会厌外侧缘延伸至杓状软骨，其中包含杓会厌肌。成对的杓状软骨形状像一个三面金字塔，有底座、顶点和三个侧面。它们位于喉的后部，最重要的是，它们是假声带（前庭韧带）和声带肌的附着点。杓状软骨的基部与环状软骨衔接，形成环杓关节。该关节的运动会使声带内收和外展[29]。杓状软骨的后表面附有杓间肌，而杓状软骨的顶端与角状软骨相接。与其他关节一样，环杓状软骨关节也可能被 RA 累积，导致声音嘶哑、呼吸困难或危及生命的上气道阻塞[18]。角状软骨和楔形软骨加强并支撑着杓状软骨襞。角状软骨很小，呈三角形，位于杓状软骨的顶端。喉镜检查时可直接在杓状软骨上看到它们。楔状软骨呈圆柱形，位于杓状软骨前上方的杓会厌褶内[31]。喉镜检查时可看到黏膜内的白色隆起（图 12.8）。

12.7.3 黏膜皱襞

喉部的黏膜皱襞包括杓状皱襞、前庭皱襞和声带皱襞。杓会厌襞从杓状软骨延伸至会厌外侧，包含杓会厌肌肉和楔状软骨，并形成四角膜的上缘。该膜向下延伸，在此处变厚形成前庭韧带和前庭褶，也称为室带。室带可以防止误吸，保护声带，又称为假声带，有助于发音[30]。事实上，手术切除会厌的患者

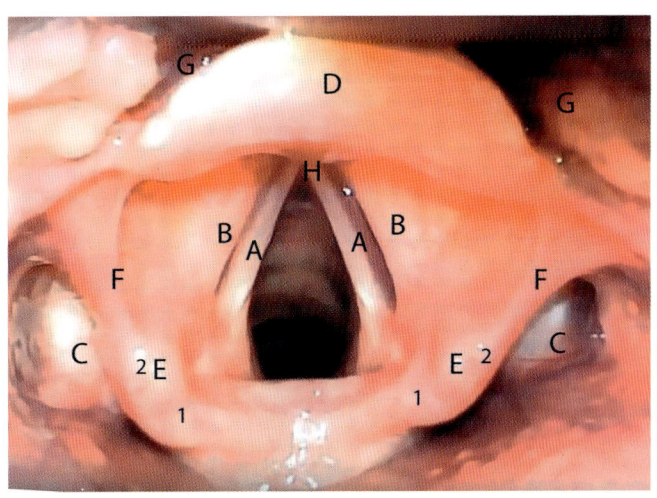

图 12.8　间接喉镜下喉部解剖标志

A. 声带（真声带）；B. 室带（假声带）；C. 梨状隐窝；D. 会厌；E. 杓状软骨（1. 角状软骨；2. 楔形软骨）；F. 杓会厌皱襞；G. 会厌谷；H. 前联合。

仅靠假声带就能防止误吸[28]。声带（真声带）包含声带肌，后部连接杓状软骨，前部连接甲状软骨。声带还包含弹性圆锥，与甲状软骨、杓状软骨和环状软骨相连。外缘与肌肉相连，而内缘是游离的，在喉镜检查时可以看到一条白色条形带，正上方是前庭褶[30]（图 12.8）。

12.7.4 喉部肌肉

喉部肌肉分为喉外肌群（连接喉部与邻近结构）和喉内肌群（喉软骨内）。喉外肌根据位置和功能分为舌骨上肌和舌骨下肌。舌骨上肌包括茎突舌骨肌、二腹肌、颏舌骨肌、下颌舌骨肌、茎突咽肌、舌骨舌肌和下咽缩肌。这群肌群的作用是抬高、支撑和固定喉部。舌骨下肌包括胸骨舌骨肌、胸骨甲状肌、甲状舌骨肌和肩胛舌骨肌。除了甲状舌骨肌能抬高甲状腺和压低舌骨外，它们都能稳定和压低喉部[29]。

喉内肌分为内收肌、外展肌和张肌/松弛肌。作为一个肌群，它们负责控制声带相关运动。它们通过改变甲杓状肌的肌肉长度、发声过程、固定会厌的方向来改变声带的形状、长度、张力和空间位置[30]。内收肌（如环状舌骨外侧肌、杓间肌等）使声带内收，以利于发音和吸气保护。外展肌（如环杓后肌）使声带外展，以利于空气流通和呼吸。张肌拉长并绷紧声带，松弛肌（如环甲肌、甲杓肌等）则缩短声带。

所有喉部固有肌作用都是成对的，可产生改变音调、音色和音质所需的精密运动，同时不影响呼

吸[29]。如上所述，环杓后肌是唯一的外展肌，因此也是唯一能够扩大声门以实现正常呼吸的肌肉。如果该肌肉受损或失去神经支配，则无法打开声门，就会影响正常呼吸，而双侧损伤可引起严重的呼吸困难。环甲外肌在发音时能使杓状软骨内收和内旋，以增加内侧压力。环甲肌可延长和绷紧声带，它位于喉的外侧，通过拉紧和拉长声带来控制发音，从而产生较高的音调。它是唯一由喉上神经外侧支支配的喉部肌肉。杓横肌可使杓状软骨内收，从而使声带内收。最后一块内收肌是杓斜状肌，它通过作用于杓状软骨来帮助杓横肌和环杓状外肌内收，从而使喉入口变窄。甲状舌骨肌群，可以放松、缩短和内收声带使讲话音调降低，其内部部分振动发声[32]。

12.7.5 喉部神经

迷走神经（第10颅神经）是一对支配喉部感觉和运动的神经。喉上神经从迷走神经分支出来，然后进一步分为外支和内支。喉的感觉神经由喉上神经的内支支配，而喉上神经的外支支配环甲肌。喉上神经的损伤会由于无法收紧声带而导致发音减弱，呼吸不畅。迷走神经的喉返神经分支产生内收支和外展支。喉返神经支配除环甲肌外的所有喉内肌。单侧喉返神经损伤，就会出现声音嘶哑。如果发生双侧喉返神经损伤，声音可能正常也可能嘶哑，但会出现呼吸窘迫和喘鸣，可能需要气管造口术以防止呼吸困难[30]。

在进行喉镜或支气管镜检查时，喉上神经阻滞是一种有效镇静辅助手段。由于喉上神经的内支支配喉部的感觉，局部麻醉阻滞该神经将消除呕吐反射并降低镇静需求。要进行喉上神经阻滞，必须熟悉喉上神经的解剖结构。喉上神经沿着咽部的外侧向下延伸，在颈内动脉后面，分为内外两支。内支下降到甲状舌骨膜，并在此穿过甲状舌骨膜，沿着环咽肌进入梨状隐窝。

在内支进入甲状舌骨膜处，有可触及的解剖标志来指导注射。双侧触诊舌骨大角，在手指压力下舌骨向准备注射的一侧移位。在刺穿甲状舌骨膜之前，喉上神经的内支走行在舌骨大角下方 2~4 mm 处[34]。插入一根 25 G 针头，接触舌骨大角，并向下和中线方向移动 2 mm，此处穿透甲状舌骨膜可对内支进行阻滞[34]。在注射前要抽吸注射器，以防止注射入动脉内或气管内，从而导致阻滞失败：2~3 mL 2% 利多卡因（含或不含肾上腺素）就足以实现阻滞[34]。然后在另一侧重复此过程以实现双侧阻滞。

参考文献

1 Apfelbaum, J.L., Hagberg, C.A., Caplan, R.A. et al. (2013). Practice guidelines for management of the difficult airway. An updated report by the American Society of Anesthesiologists Task Force on Management of the Difficult Airway. *Anesthesiology* 118: 251–270.

2 Shiga, T., Wajima, Z., Inoue, T., and Sakamoto, A. (2005). Predicting difficult intubation in apparently normal patients. *Anesthesiology* 103: 429–437.

3 Murphy, P. (1967). A fibre-optic endoscope used for nasal intubation. *Anaesthesia* 22: 489–491.

4 Collins, S.R. and Blank, R.S. (2014). Fiberoptic intubation: an overview and update. *Respir. Care* 59: 865–878.

5 Cass, N.M., James, N.R., and Lines, V. (1956). Difficult direct laryngoscopy complicating intubation for anaesthesia. *Br. Med. J.* 1: 488–489.

6 Mallampati, S.R., Gatt, S.P., Gugino, L.D. et al. (1985). A clinical sign to predict difficult tracheal intubation: a prospective study. *Can. Anaesth. Soc. J.* 32: 429–434.

7 Samsoon, G.L.T. and Young, J.R.B. (1987). Difficult tracheal intubation: a retrospective study. *Anaesthesia* 42: 487–490.

8 Frerk, C.M. (1991). Predicting difficult intubation. *Anaesthesia* 46: 1005–1008.

9 Wilson, M.E., Spiegelhalter, D., Robertson, J.A., and Lesser, P. (1988). Predicting difficult intubation. *Br. J. Anaesth.* 61: 211–216.

10 Langeron, O., Masso, E., Huraux, C. et al. (2000). Prediction of difficult mask ventilation. *Anesthesiology* 92: 1229–1236.

11 Doyle, D.J. and Arellano, R. (1995). Medical conditions with airway implications. *Anaesthesiol. Clin. NorthAm.* 13: 615–633.

12 Mudassir, M., Baig, A., and Khan, F.H. (2014). To compare the accuracy of Prayer's sign and Mallampati test in predicting difficult intubation in diabetic patients. *J. Pak. Med. Assoc.* 64: 879–883.

13 Iseli, T.A., Iseli, C.E., Golden, J.B. et al. (2012). Outcomes of intubation in difficult airways due to head and neck pathology. *Ear Nose Throat J.* 91: E1–E5.

14 Hashim, K.V. and Thomas, M. (2014). Sensitivity of palm print sign in prediction of difficult laryngoscopy in diabetes: a comparison with other airway indices. *Indian J. Anaesth.* 58: 298–302.

15 Terashima, Y., Yurube, T., Hirata, H. et al. (2017). Predictive risk factors of cervical spine instabilities in rheumatoid arthritis. *Spine* 42: 556–564.

16 Vieira, E.M., Goodman, S., and Tanaka, P.P. (2011). Anesthesia and rheumatoid arthritis. *Rev. Bras. Anestesiol.* 61: 367–375.

17 Aires, R.B., de Carvalho, J.F., and da Mota, L.M.H. (2014). Pre-operative anesthetic assessment of patients with rheumatoid arthritis. *Rev. Bras. Reumatol.* 54: 213–219.

18 Hakala, P. and Randell, T. (1998). Intubation difficulties in patients with rheumatoid arthritis. A retrospective study. *Acta Anaesthesiol. Scand.* 42: 195–198.

19 Borland, L.M., Colligan, J., and Brandom, B.W. (2004).

Frequency of anesthesia-related complications in children with Down syndrome under general anesthesia for noncardiac procedures. *Pediatr. Anaesthes.* 14: 733–738.

20 Harley, E.H. and Collins, M.D. (1994). Neurologic sequelae secondary to atlantoaxial instability in Down syndrome. Implications in otolaryngologic surgery. *Arch. Otolaryngol. Head Neck Surg.* 120: 159–165.

21 Nakamura, N., Inaba, Y., Aota, Y. et al. (2016). New radiological parameters for the assessment of atlantoaxial instability in children with Down syndrome. *Bone Joint J.* 98-B: 1704–1710.

22 Bevilacqua, S., Nicolini, A., DelSarto, P. et al. (1996). Difficult intubation in paediatric cardiac surgery. Significance of age. Association with Down's syndrome. *Minerva Anestesiol.* 62: 259–264.

23 Nargozian, C. (2004). The airway in patients with craniofacial abnormalities. *Pediatr. Anaesthes.* 14: 53–59.

24 Arrowsmith, J.E., Robertshaw, H.J., and Boyd, J.D. (1998). Nasotracheal intubation in the presence of frontobasal skull fracture. *Can. J. Anaesth.* 45: 71–75.

25 Bahr, W. and Stoll, P. (1992). Nasal intubation in the presence of frontobasal fractures: a retrospective study. *J. Oral Maxillofac. Surg.* 50: 445–447.

26 Haug, R.H., Wible, R.T., Likavec, M.J., and Conforti, P.J. (1991). Cervical spine fractures and maxillofacial trauma. *J. Oral Maxillofac. Surg.* 49: 725–729.

27 Jamal, B.T., Diecidue, R., Qutub, A., and Cohen, M. (2009). The pattern of combined maxillofacial and cervical spine fractures. *J. Oral Maxillofac. Surg.* 67: 559–562.

28 Coleman, L., Gold, J., and Zakowski, M. (2018). Functional anatomy of the airway. In: *Hagber and Benumof's Airway Management*, 4e (eds. C. Hagberg, A. Artime and M. Aziz), 2–18. St Louis: Elsevier.

29 Noordzij, J.P. and Ossoff, R.H. (2016). Anatomy and physiology of the larynx. *Otolaryngol. Clin. NorthAm.* 39: 1–10.

30 Pretterklieber, M.L. (2003). Functional anatomy of the human intrinsic laryngeal muscles. *Eur. Surg.* 35: 250–258.

31 Fried, M.P., Meller, S.M., and Rinaldo, A. (2009). Adult laryngeal anatomy. In: *The Larynx*, 3e (eds. M.P. Fried and A. Ferlito), 85–100. Plural Publishing.

32 DuFlo, S. and Thibeault, S. (2006). Anatomy of the larynx and physiology of phonation. In: *Textbook of Laryngology* (eds. A.L. Merati and S.A. Bielamowicz), 31–50. San Diego: Plural Publishing Inc.

33 Simpson, B. and Rose, C. (2008). Anatomy and physiology of the larynx. In: *Operative Techniques in Laryngology* (eds. C.A. Rosen, H. Leden and R.H. Ossoff), 3–8. New York: Springer.

34 Furlan, J.C. (2002). Anatomical study applied to anesthetic block technique of the superior laryngeal nerve. *Acta Anaesthesiol. Scand.* 46: 199–202.

第 13 章

气道病变的支气管镜检查
灌洗、刷检和支气管腔内活检

Heinrich D. Becker
Department of Interdisiplinary Endoscopy,
Thoraxclinic at Heidelberg University, Heidelberg, Germany
（译者：官振标　译者单位：海军军医大学第一附属医院）

13.1 引言

在"气道病变的支气管镜检查"章节中，对具有诊断意义的内镜下病变特征（症状）做了详细描述，这些特征本身极具特异性且无须其他操作检查。但进一步病理分析和确认通常是必要的，尤其高达 80% 的疑诊肺癌病例适合支气管镜检查[1]。为了明确病理诊断，已经形成了几种获取标本的侵袭性方法，如支气管肺泡灌洗、刷检和支气管腔内组织活检，以及这些方法的联合应用。由于"获取组织本身就是问题所在"，活检一直是最重要的环节，尤其个体化治疗的基础是对组织标本的进一步分子生物学分析。越来越先进的检验方法被应用于细胞学标本的检测，支气管镜灌洗和刷检得到广泛的应用，因为其可以替代高风险患者的活检，或者作为提高诊断准确度的附加手段。本章节根据个人经验和相关文献描述了当前的状况。

13.2 支气管病变发病率及内镜表现

尽管近年来肺癌的发生已趋向肺外周类型转变，但在更大规模的研究发现，有超过 30% 的肺癌位于支气管腔内可见范围内，其中 47% 呈腔内生长，53% 呈黏膜下生长[1]。关于活检技术，我们通常结合病变的气管壁不同浸润程度来区分腔内外生长、黏膜内和黏膜下肿瘤扩散、支气管壁内深层扩散和通常伴随气管压迫的外压型生长。通过普通白光支气管镜检查（white light bronchoscopy，WLB），可以评估病变的外部特征、气管黏膜的扭曲和颜色变化以及支气管壁受压情况。当然，为了进一步鉴别诊断和选择最佳取样方法，可以使用其他技术。

13.3 辅助成像技术

近年来，除了传统的电子支气管镜 WLB 检查外还发展了其他新技术。为了更详细地分析图像，放大内窥镜可以提供上皮和血管结构的可见图像。通过自荧光支气管镜（autofluorescence bronchoscopy，AFB）可以检测到早期和肉眼几乎不可见的肿瘤，以便定位获取标本的最佳部位。窄带成像（narrow-band imaging，NBI）可以更好地可视化作为肺癌早期征象的病变血管。由于 20 MHz 高分辨率经支气管镜腔内超声（endobronchial ultrasound，EBUS）探头现已上市，可以对支气管壁的复杂多层结构进行详细分析。

这些技术的应用有助于选择最佳活检位置和活检方法。

13.4 标本取样和制备技术

为了在不同的取样方法中获得最佳结果，除了选择最佳的活检位置和取样技术，与组织及细胞病理学家的密切沟通必不可少。很多文献研究为此提供了各种不同建议。此外，在某些取样困难部位，快速现场评估（rapid on-site evaluation，ROSE）可能是有益的。例如，经支气管针吸活检（transbronchial needle aspiration，TBNA）时，ROSE 可以避免反复操作。

13.4.1 活检技术

基于我们在经支气管镜肺活检上的良好经验，我们使用了可以通过至少 2.8 mm 活检通道进行支气管内活检的胃镜钳以获得最佳的活检标本[2]。为了减少取样失误，多次活检被证实是高效的；多项研究结果表明，进行 3~5 次活检可能是最优的[1,3-5]。文献报道仅一次活检的阳性率为 92%[5]。由于冷冻活检可以获得更大、保存更完整的标本，其应用越来越广泛。冷冻活检时应至少取样 2 次[3]。对于支气管壁内的病变、管外病变或者表面坏死严重，导致支气管腔内活检阴性的情况，应首选 TBNA。根据我们的经验，如果 EBUS 证实管壁内浸润或管外浸润，采用被称为纽扣洞口活检的技术通常会成功，该技术一直用于腔内肿瘤活检。该技术首先用活检钳去除覆盖病变的完整黏膜，然后打开活检钳从更深层活检。

13.4.2 标本制备

通常将标本直接固定在 10% 福尔马林中[1,3,6]。但我们更倾向于先用 0.9% 的生理盐水回收标本，以避免再次进入气道活检前福尔马林污染活检钳。研究证实，活组织印片的制备与细胞学刷检一样有效[7]。根据我们的经验，如果由专业细胞学家检查，使用上清液的离心细胞可以显著增加诊断成功率。一位研究者发现，在 5% 的组织学未能诊断的肿瘤病例中使用该方法，阳性诊断率从 66% 增加到 71%[8]。

13.4.3 细胞刷检

使用毛刷的细胞刷检比活检能够在更大的区域内获取细胞。可能是出于经济原因，可重复使用的鞘保护毛刷可能比一次性毛刷更受青睐，但毛刷和鞘管须彻底清洗以避免交叉污染。细胞刷检至少应采集两次标本[1,5]。涂片制备方法通常是对载玻片施加压力，然后将涂片固定在 95% 的乙醇中[1,5]。一些研究者会采用风干的方式制作涂片[6]。获得涂片后，用生理盐水洗涤毛刷，用于制备额外的细胞悬液或细胞蜡块。

13.4.4 支气管肺泡灌洗

通过灌洗获得细胞学标本，通常需缓慢滴入 0.9% 氯化钠溶液（10~40 mL），收集灌洗液进行离心和进一步处理。将收集的灌洗液离心并制备成 4 张优选涂片或细胞块。

13.5 操作结果及方法组合

在文献中，不同方法的敏感度存在显著差异，而特异度通常都很高。这可能与设备的可及性、机构的规模和经验相关。美国胸科医师学会的指南[9,10]制定基于对 MEDLINE、Healthstar 和 Cochrane 数据库以及印刷书目的广泛搜索，由于文献中的数据大多病例数较少，因此这些方法建议推荐级别大多为 IC（强推荐，低质量证据），少数为 IB（强推荐，中等质量证据）。这意味着获益明显大于风险和负担。在接下来的讨论中，我们将阐述单一方法以及不同方法的有序组合的结果。这些数据基于文献综述和个人经验，旨在总结合理的方法。

13.6 可见肿瘤的支气管腔内活检结果

显然，诊断结果因病变的类型和可及性而不同。其敏感性范围很广，从不到 70% 到超过 90%。大多数论文是基于回顾性数据，仅少数是前瞻性研究，其中随机研究更为少见。大多数文献报道敏感度范围在 70%~80% 之间[5,6,11-14]。从临床特征看，腔内肿瘤的活检阳性率为 70%~95%[1,15]，黏膜下和管壁内病变的活检阳性率为 55%~86%[1,16]。这些研究没有使用额外的内镜成像模式来选择最佳活检策略。关于活检位置，有一份研究显示，左舌叶和右中叶病灶的诊断阳性率低[17]。

13.7 刷检结果

刷检的结果差异较大，阳性率低至28%[14]，高至81%[5,7]，但总体上显著低于活检，大多数为50%~70%[1,2,6,11-13,17-19]。显然，黏膜下和管壁内病变的刷检阳性率比外生型腔内病变低，特别是当腔内型病变表现为黏膜不完整、病灶不规则或部分坏死时。

13.8 灌洗结果

支气管肺泡灌洗结果的差异更大，低至12%[7]，高至77%（与活检相当）。大多数阳性率在30%~50%之间[1,7,11-13,19-22]。

13.9 组合方法结果

可以预期的是，活检、刷检和灌洗技术之间组合运用优于单独活检。许多研究分析了增加刷检、灌洗或两种联合的效果，并研究了不同技术间应用顺序对结果的影响。联用其他方法的综合诊断率提高了4%~23%[1]。刷检对活检的贡献显著大于灌洗，诊断率从3%[11]增加到16%[1,11]。活检和刷检的组合诊断率达到85%~95%，腔内病变略高于黏膜下/管壁内病变[1,9,11-14,20,23]。然而，除活检和刷检外，肺泡灌洗对敏感度的贡献要小得多，0%~2%不等[1,11,14,20]。还有作者研究了活检/刷检之前或之后灌洗时间的影响。仅有1篇文献报道了外生型肿瘤和黏膜浸润的诊断率差异为32%~49.2%[17]，大多数研究者未找到它们之间的显著差异[6,7,13,24]。综上所述，活检联合刷检明显优于单纯刷检，而加用灌洗很少能提高支气管镜检查对支气管内病变的敏感度。在某些情况下，加用经支气管针吸活检略有益处，但并不比灌洗更有益处。

13.10 并发症

除可弯曲支气管镜检查的一般危险因素外，支气管腔内活检并未显著增加并发症，这也是ACCP指南将其作为IB和IC推荐的原因[9,10]。最常见的并发症是轻度出血，这可能会影响刷检的可视性[17]。此外，刷检后出血会模糊视野，此时活检必须更审慎地进行。出血发生率可高达30%，但大多可自行止血[16]。较严重出血的发生率为2%，予注入5~10 mL冰水、肾上腺素或行氩等离子凝固术（argon plasma coagulation，APC）后可止血。术后轻度咯血的发生率为3%[3,5]。就位置而言，中央支气管内病变较外周病变出血风险更高（52%比26%），但左右肺、各肺叶之间比较出血风险相似。鳞状细胞肺癌和小细胞肺癌比腺癌更容易发生出血，显然晚期肺癌比早期病变更容易出血。值得一提的是，使用活检钳活检和冷冻活检风险没有显著差异[3]。通常认为类癌更容易出血，有医生在活检前于瘤体内注射肾上腺素以减少出血，但根据我们的经验，这并没有降低出血风险。

13.11 成本效益

除了不同方法的有效性外，也需要考虑成本效益。活检和刷检的结果对诊断很重要，它们无疑具有成本高效益，但肺泡灌洗则是有争议的。这些观点在文献报道中存在争议。一篇印度的研究报告了在2名患者中为获得阳性结果进行了107次常规灌洗，通过灌洗获得阳性结果的2名患者的灌洗费用与2次重复支气管镜检查的费用（每次2 000卢比）进行了计算。根据作者的计算，常规灌洗的费用为3.2万卢比，被认为灌洗可能有获益，但不具有成本效益[20]。其他几篇文献得出了同样的结论[1,20]，相关研究发现，只有6%的患者可通过灌洗获得阳性结果，成本效益低[1,24]。

13.12 结论和建议

可弯曲支气管镜检查对支气管腔内病变的诊断具有较高的成功率。最有效的病理确诊方法是支气管镜腔内活检。因此，应该尽力使活检成功。包括AFB和NBI在内的方法有助于检测肉眼几乎不可见的早期病变和判断更晚期病变的边界，为外科手术做准备。在评估病变支气管壁浸润深度、黏膜下和壁内扩散以及管外肿瘤方面，EBUS已被证明是有益的。通过可视化血管有助于避免出血，特别是在大血管附近的坏死病灶。为了获得足够的标本，应多次活检。根据我们的经验，更大的活检钳是有益的。此外，对黏膜下/管壁内病变行 TBNA 也是有益的。为了充分利用标本，应从上清液中制备细胞学涂片和细胞蜡块。活检后刷检可显著提高诊断阳性率，获取组织学标本后应进一步用其他方法获取不同的标本。在病理医师指导下，用生理盐水冲洗刷检毛刷后的液体制备直接涂片和细胞离心涂片。在活检/刷检前后应分开准备洗涤液，尤其存在明显血液污染时。由于灌洗的工作量和成本相当大，而收益却往往微小，建议只在活检和刷检结果阴性的情况下进行肺泡灌洗。对于血供丰富的较脆病变，可以先进行灌洗和刷检，没有明显出血后再进行活检。在这种情况下，先行 ROSE 特别有益。如今甚至可以通过细胞学标本进行分子生物学特征鉴定，ROSE 阳性结果可以避免进一步活检。

参考文献

1. Jones, A.M., Hanson, I.M., Armstrong, G.R., and O'Driscoll, B.R. (2001). Diagnosis of lung cancer at flexible bronchoscopy. *Respir. Med.* 95: 374–378.
2. Becker, H.D. (1998). Transbronchial (transbronchoscopic) lung biopsy in the immunocompromised host. In: *Pulmonary Endoscopy and Biopsy Techniques*, vol. 9 (ed. J. Strausz), 193–208. Lausanne: European Respiratory Journals Monograph.
3. Wang, S., Ye, Q., Tu, J., and Son, Y. (2018). The location, histologic type, and stage of lung cancer are associated with bleeding during endobronchial biopsy. *Cancer Manag. Res.* 10: 1251–1257.
4. Popovich, J. Jr., Kvale, P.A., Eichenhorn, M.S. et al. (1982). Diagnostic accuracy of multiple biopsies from flexible fiberoptic bronchoscopy: a comparison of central versus peripheral carcinoma. *Am. Rev. Respir. Dis.* 125 (5): 521–523.
5. Fuladi, A.B., Munje, R.P., and Tayade, B.O. (2004). Value of washings, brushings, and biopsy at fibreoptic bronchoscopy in the diagnosis of lung cancer. *J. Indian Acad. Clin. Med.* 5 (2): 137–142.
6. Bandyopadhyay, A., Pal, M., Das, I. et al. (2016). A study of usefulness of washes and brush cytology with respect to histopathology in diagnosis of lung malignancy by using fiberoptic bronchoscopy. *Lung India* 5 (4): 293–298.
7. Bodh, A., Kaushal, V., Kashyap, S., and Gulati, A. (2013). Cytohistological correlation in diagnosis of lung tumors by using fiberoptic bronchoscopy: study of 200 cases. *Indian J. Pathol. Microbiol.* 56 (2): 84–88.
8. Rosell, A., Monsó, E., Lores, L. et al. (1998). Cytology of bronchial biopsy rinse fluid to improve the diagnostic yield for lung cancer. *Eur. Respir. J.* 12 (6): 1415–1418.
9. Rivera, M.P. and Mehta, A.C. (2007). Initial diagnosis of lung cancer: American College of Chest Physicians evidence-based clinical practice guidelines (2nd edition). *Chest* 132 (3 Suppl): 131S–148S.
10. Rivera, M.P., Mehta, A.C., and Wahidi, M.M. (2013). Establishing the diagnosis of lung cancer: diagnosis and management of lung cancer, 3rd ed: American College of Chest Physicians evidence-based clinical practice guidelines. *Chest* 143 (5 Suppl): e142S–e165S.
11. Karahalli, E., Yilmaz, A., Türker, H., and Özvaran, K. (2001). Usefulness of various diagnostic techniques during fiberoptic bronchoscopy for endoscopically visible lung cancer: should cytologic examinations be performed routinely? *Respiration* 68: 611–614.
12. Schreiber, G. and McCrory, D.C. (2003). Performance characteristics of different modalities for diagnosis of suspected lung cancer: summary of published evidence. *Chest* 123 (1 Suppl): 115S–128S.
13. Mathan, R.J. and Sowmiya, M. (2017). Does a routine post brush bronchial wash increase the yield in diagnosis of lung cancer? *Int. J. Res. Med. Sci.* 5 (7): 2878–2882.
14. Soler, T.V., Isamitt, D.D., and Carrasco, O.A. (2004). Yield of biopsy, brushing and bronchial washing through fiberbronchoscopy in the diagnosis of lung cancer with visible lesions. *Rev. Med. Chil.* 132 (10): 1198–1203.
15. Travis, W.D. and Rekhtman, N. (2011). Pathological diagnosis and classification of lung cancer in small biopsies and cytology: strategic management of tissue for molecular testing. *Semin. Respir. Crit. Care Med.* 32 (1): 22–31.
16. Liam, C.K., Pang, Y.K., and Poosparajah, S. (2007). Diagnostic yield of flexible bronchoscopic procedures in lung cancer patients according to tumour location. *Singapore Med. J.* 48 (7): 625.
17. Hou, G., Miao, Y., Hu, X-J. et al. (2016). The optimal sequence for bronchial brushing and forceps biopsy in lung cancer diagnosis: a random control study. *J. Thorac. Dis.* 8 (3): 520–526.
18. Bedrossian, C.W. and Rybka, D.L. (1976). Bronchial brushing during fiberoptic bronchoscopy for the cytodiagnosis of lung cancer: comparison with sputum and bronchial washings. *Acta Cytol.* 20 (5): 446–453.
19. Mak, V.H.F., Johnston, I.D.A., Hetzel, M.R., and Grubb, C. (1990). Value of washings and brushings at fibreopticbronchoscopy in the diagnosis of lung cancer. *Thorax* 45: 373–376.
20. Rawat, J., Sindhwani, G., Saini, S. et al. (2007). Usefulness and cost effectiveness of bronchial washing in diagnosing endobronchial malignancies. *Lung India* 24 (4): 139–141.
21. Liwsrisakun, C., Pothirat, C., Bumroongkit, C., and Deesomchok, A. (2004). Role of bronchial washing in the diagnosis of endoscopically visible lung cancer. *J. Med. Assoc. Thail.* 87 (6): 600–604.
22. Mufti, S.T. and Mokhta, G.A. (2015). Diagnostic value of bronchial wash, bronchial brushing, fine needle aspiration cytology versus combined bronchial wash and bronchial brushing in the diagnosis of primary lung carcinomas at a tertiary care hospital. *Biomed. Res.* 26 (4): 777–784.
23. Matsuda, M., Horai, T., Nakamura, S. et al. (1986). Bronchial brushing and bronchial biopsy: comparison of diagnostic accuracy and cell typing reliability in lung cancer. *Thorax* 41 (6): 475–478.
24. van der Drift, M.A., van der Wilt, G.-J., Thunnissen, F.B.J.M., and Janssen, J.P. (2005). Prospective study of the timing and cost-effectiveness of bronchial washing during bronchoscopy for pulmonary malignant tumors. *Chest* 128 (1): 394–400.

第 14 章

支气管肺泡灌洗术

Wei Zhang[1], Yi Huang[1], and Richard Helmers[2]
[1] Shanghai Changhai Hospital, Shanghai, China
[2] Mayo Clinic Health System, Eau Claire, WI, USA

（译者：张 伟 王 俊 黄 怡 译者单位：海军军医大学第一附属医院）

14.1 引言

支气管肺泡灌洗术（bronchoalveolar lavage，BAL）是指通过可弯曲支气管镜向远端气道内注入生理盐水，获取肺泡上皮细胞表面的细胞和非细胞成分进行分析的方法。BAL最早出现于20世纪70年代，与此同时，可弯曲支气管镜也几乎同时发展。BAL与支气管冲洗有本质区别，支气管冲洗是指从大气道吸出分泌物或少量灌注生理盐水。BAL是一种简单、安全、重要的方法，广泛应用于感染、肿瘤和许多其他疾病临床诊治过程等多个临床和科学领域[2,3]。本章将介绍BAL的关键技术要点，以及BAL在一些常见肺部疾病中的应用。

14.2 支气管肺泡灌洗术

从历史上看，不同研究机构之间的技术差异导致了BAL结果的相应差异。欧洲呼吸学会（ERS）于1989年和1999年发表了共识报告[4,5]。2012年，美国胸科学会发布了临床实践指南[6]。两份文档都包含完整的技术指导。

BAL最好在气道常规检查之后和活检/刷检之前进行，以避免回收的液体被过量的血液污染，这将影响灌洗液（BAL fluid，BALF）的细胞和非细胞分析的准确性。一些研究试图通过支气管刷检后进行灌洗来提高BALF中恶性细胞的检出率，但其他研究表明这并不能提高检出率。使用干净的吸引通道，支气管镜向远端推进，直到楔入亚节段支气管。应小心避免触壁和咳嗽，以防止回收的液体被分泌物和血块污染[7]。为了减少口咽污染，研究建议通过气管插管进行支气管镜检查[8]。然而，一些研究表明，这并不能增加BALF中恶性细胞的阳性率。

在弥漫性疾病中，常规在右中叶支气管或左舌段进行灌洗。这些区域的回收液量通常比其他肺叶大，这主要是由于支气管树的解剖结构和仰卧位重力的影响[2,3,9]。当影像学检查显示局部病变时，应在X线片显示的异常区域进行灌洗，因为这些区域的BALF可能是最异常的[4,5,10]。影像学和临床数据通常决定了支气管灌洗节段的数量和位置，以及标本是单独分析还是整体分析。

将支气管镜楔入后，用注射器将无菌生理盐水注入支气管镜负压吸引口。在BAL中使用温盐水仍有争议。盐水预热至37°C可减轻咳嗽和支气管痉挛，特别是气道高反应性患者，并可增加液体回收和有形细胞数量[3,5,7]。不同的机构使用的生理盐水量在20~60 mL不等，但目前的数据尚未支持特定的液体量。然后负压吸引并回收灌洗液。生理盐水总灌注量为100~300 mL[6]。

操作应轻柔，可经支气管镜注入1~2 mL 2%利多卡因于灌洗段局部麻醉。支气管镜的吸引通道应保持在管腔中央。如果在灌洗过程中，支气管镜尖端能够稳定地"楔塞入"，则患者不会咳嗽，因为灌洗液不应"漏"到支气管镜插入段近端以外[4]。在灌洗液自由流动减少之前，应该进行温和的吸引。ERS建议吸入负压应保持在100 mmHg（13.3 kPa）以下；50 mmHg（6.67 kPa）被证明容易导致呼吸道塌陷。吸入压力过大可导致气道塌陷和回收液体减少。

在肺总容量（total lung capacity，TLC）正常的健康人群中，一般灌洗段容积约为165 mL，该区域的残余容量约为45 mL[11]。有残余气体的肺泡会产生较高的细胞总数，但不能产生细胞计数差异[12]。成人每灌洗100 mL生理盐水，回收的40~60 mL液体中含有（5~10）×10^6细胞数和1~10 mg蛋白质。据估计，100 mL支气管肺泡灌洗液标本中含有约10^6个肺泡[3,11]。需要注意的是BAL细胞计数在气道内有脓性分泌物，支气管镜未稳定在"楔塞"位置或回收液体积占注入液体积的40%以下时是无效的[4]。

不同机构的生理盐水灌洗量不同。高容量（240~300 mL）已被使用，特别是当需要大量炎症细胞进行分析时。然而，大容量灌洗可能增加局部肺不张、发热和一过性低氧的风险[3,4,7]。相比之下，少量的BALF只能检测到较小的支气管或相对较少的肺泡。

一般认为，如果灌洗液量超过回收量100 mL以上，则必须终止灌洗[14,15]。对于远端气道的最佳采样，提取的总体积（汇总等分）应大于或等于总注入体积的30%。否则，回收的液体可能会导致细胞计数结果出现误差，特别是当总回收体积小于总注入体积的10%时。

对回收液的连续等分分析表明，初始灌洗液（如果液体体积较小，即20 mL）与后续灌洗液的不同之处在于，初始灌洗液中的细胞和蛋白质可能是从支气管而不是肺泡中回收的[7,16,19]。因此，在许多机构中最初的20 mL灌洗液通常被丢弃。然而，研究表明，含有最初的20 mL和随后的"主要是肺泡"的等分液的标本，包括最多只占总回收细胞10%的第一个等分液，在没有明显炎症的情况下，不太可能显著影响细胞分析。若存在明显的气道炎症，分析可能受到支气管气道分泌物的影响。

一般情况下，回收液体体积可达注入液体积的40%~60%，总细胞存活率可达80%以上[2,9,20]。回收量的减少通常是由以下因素造成的：年龄、吸烟、肺组织弹性回缩力丧失、阻塞性肺部疾病以及第一秒钟用力呼气量（forced expiratory volume in first second，FEV_1）与用力肺活量（forced vital capacity，FVC）之比（FEV_1/FVC）降低[2,3,7,21]。

由于BALF、肺泡液和血液之间的动态相互作用，准确评估肺泡成分非常困难且不确定。BAL过程本身可能对内源性稀释标志物（如尿素和白蛋白）有影响。肺泡上皮通透性改变的疾病，如急性呼吸窘迫综合征（acute respiratory distress syndrome，ARDS）也会影响这些标志物。巨噬细胞倾向于吸收外源性标志物，如亚甲基蓝。因此，在各种疾病中的应用将受到影响。这仍然是一个存在争议的领域[2,5,6,22]。

14.3 安全性和并发症

灌洗是相对安全的，可在常规可弯曲支气管镜检查期间进行。BAL没有绝对禁忌证，但某些危险因素和相对禁忌证仍然构成潜在威胁。例如，患者无法配合，FEV_1<800 mL，中、重度哮喘，高碳酸血症，缺氧（吸氧后氧饱和度不能达到90%），严重心律失常，6周内曾发生心肌梗死，未纠正的活动性出血和血流动力学不稳定等[2]。

BAL最常见的并发症是术后发热，发生率为10%~50%。这是一种由机体释放生物细胞活性介质（如细胞因子）引起[23-25]的一过性热原效应。BAL后发热很少与菌血症[26]相关，并可以用退热药[27]成功治疗。BAL后发热的发生率可能与灌洗过程中涉及的肺叶数量和每个特定部位的灌注总量成正比。

BAL的另一个常见并发症是一过性动脉血氧分压（partial pressure of oxygen，PaO_2）降低。Cole等发现，在BAL后PaO_2将会平均下降22.7 mmHg（3.02 kPa），持续至少2 h。PaO_2的降低已被证明与液体灌注量[29]成正比。在某些情况下，肺活量、FEV_1和呼气流量峰值（peak expiratory flow，PEF）也会短暂下降。无论肺功能水平如何，患者应在BAL[11]期间及术后立即给予补充氧。

BAL在哮喘和慢性阻塞性肺疾病（chronic obstructive pulmonary disease，COPD）患者中的安全性备受争议。大容量灌洗（500 mL）与FEV_1、FVC和PEF显著降低之间的相关性已经得到证实。在健康人群中，小容量（175 mL）灌洗未显示对肺功能测试结果[30]有显著影响。最近的文献综述证实了BAL在代偿性COPD和哮喘患者中的安全性，其并发症发生率与对照组相似[31,32]。虽然有报道质疑哮喘患者在不使用支气管扩张剂的情况下进行 BAL 的安全性，但大多数机构建议哮喘和 COPD 患者在 BAL 前雾化吸入支气管扩张剂。多项关于 BAL 在免疫抑制患者和血小板减少患者中的应用的研究显示其具有可接受的安全水平[34-38]。

BAL 术后高达 90% 的患者在灌洗区域影像学显示新的实变或渗出增多，这些渗出影的消退是逐渐的，在灌洗后 2 240 min 仍有 73% 的渗出影未消退。这些渗出影预计将在 24 h 内完全消退。渗出影的出现与生理盐水潴留量有关，仅限于灌洗区域，与临床并发症[39]无关。

只有极少例的气胸病例被报道为 BAL 的并发症，大多数病例发生在经支气管肺活检时进行 BAL。咳嗽可能是胸内压升高的主要原因，这在患有肺气肿、肺大泡的患者中尤其值得关注。

14.4 标本分析过程

回收的最小总体积应大于或等于注入等分体积的 5%（最佳采样回收率为 30%）。细胞分析需要 5 mL 的混合 BAL 样品。最佳体积为 10~20 mL[6]。典型的回收液容器应该由聚乙烯醇或聚碳酸酯等材料制成，细胞不能黏附在这些材料上。非硅化玻璃不适合使用[5,7]，因为巨噬细胞很容易附壁。时间和温度的控制是进一步保存和分析的关键决定因素。标本应在取得后 1 h 内进行评估。据报道，细胞在 25 ℃下可保存 4 h[39,40]，在 4 ℃下可保存 24 h[40]。蛋白质对温度敏感，通常在 −80 ℃下保存。

通过无菌纱布或尼龙网过滤灌洗液以去除多余黏液的传统做法会影响细胞计数和无菌性，并导致石棉接触患者的潜在有用信息（如含铁小体）和黏附性高的细胞（如活化的中性粒细胞[7]）丢失。因此，避免这样的过滤过程[41]在技术上是可取的。

与过滤相比，细胞离心是一种更常用，也更有利的分离细胞的方法。细胞离心可保持淋巴细胞浓度，减少细胞损伤和费用[42,43]。瑞特-吉姆萨染色法最常用于炎症细胞，而巴氏染色法通常用于分析感染细胞或癌症细胞。光学显微镜用于对染色的载玻片进行细胞计数。建议计数 300~500 个细胞核相关细胞，以确保标本[44]具有代表性。由于信息解释的差异很大，分析应由指定的实验室人员进行。

淋巴细胞亚群如 CD4 和 CD8 最常使用流式细胞术[45]进行测定。另一种方法是对细胞离心[46]制备的载玻片进行免疫组织化学染色。免疫荧光染色也用于评估感染和恶性肿瘤。

14.4.1 细胞分析

细胞分析在诊断、预后预测以及治疗评估中的价值已经被广泛认可。它在区分间质性疾病过程以及评估感染方面起到了关键作用。在健康的不吸烟人群中，每毫升肺泡灌洗液中的总细胞数为 10 万~15 万个细胞[15]。正常不吸烟成年人的肺泡灌洗液中，差异细胞计数表明细胞组成为巨噬细胞 80%~95%，淋巴细胞 5%~15%，CD4/CD8 比值为 1.5~1.8，中性粒细胞不到 3%，嗜酸性粒细胞、嗜碱性粒细胞和肥大细胞都不到 1%[2,20,47,48]。差异细胞计数中，淋巴细胞超过 15%、中性粒细胞超过 3%、嗜酸性粒细胞超过 1%、肥大细胞超过 0.5% 分别代表淋巴细胞型、中性粒细胞型、嗜酸性粒细胞型和组织细胞病变。每种情况都具有诊断意义。

肺泡灌洗液细胞分析的结果应以每毫升的细胞数及其占总细胞数的百分比（并应提供总细胞数的估算）2 种方式来表示[2,21]。将差异计数与总细胞计数相结合，允许对每种特定细胞类型在每个设定的体积中进行定量分析。正常的细胞计数不一定意味着没有炎症，而异常的细胞计数通常表明病理过程的存在和/或进展。研究人员已经证明，即使差异正常，肺部的细胞数量显著增加可能与炎症过程有关[20]。具体来说，一个细胞系的异常百分比可能会对其他系列的相对百分比产生影响。然而，肺泡灌洗液细胞分析的进一步应用可能受到灌洗体积标准化不足的限制。

吸烟、灌洗液回收的数量、灌洗处理以及年龄都会影响肺泡灌洗液的细胞分类。在吸烟者中，每单位体积的肺泡灌洗液中的总细胞数增加了 4~10 倍；巨噬细胞和中性粒细胞成比例增加，CD4/CD8 比值也会发生改变[21,49]。既往吸烟者和不吸烟者的细胞分类相似。年龄与淋巴细胞和中性粒细胞的百分比之间存在正相关关系[50]。

在大多数健康个体的肺泡灌洗液中，淋巴细胞的比例低于 10%，超过 15% 被视为异常。然而，在健康的不吸烟受试者中，也存在一过性升高，超过 20%[36]。在健康个体的肺泡结构中找到的淋巴细胞亚型与血液中的相似。CD3[+] T 细胞占肺泡淋巴细胞的大多数，而 B 细胞只占 4%~7%[21]。T 辅助细胞（CD4[+]）和 T 抑制细胞（CD8[+]）分别占总淋巴细胞的

39%~48% 和 23%~28%。因此，T 辅助细胞与 T 抑制细胞（CD4/CD8）的正常比值在 1.6~1.8 之间。

美国国立卫生研究院（NIH）的合作研究表明，淋巴细胞表型的变异与一系列因素密切相关，如年龄、性别和吸烟[21]。在数据分析和解释中应考虑这些因素：① 年龄在 50 岁以上的年龄组中，T 辅助细胞的平均百分比比 37 岁以下的年龄组高出 10% 以上；② 总 T 细胞、T 抑制细胞和 B 细胞的百分比在男性中明显高于女性，而 CD4/CD8 比值在男性中明显较低；③ 活跃吸烟者的 T 辅助细胞显著较低（32.2%）于既往吸烟者（46%）和不吸烟者（44.4%）。活跃吸烟者的 T 抑制细胞高于前吸烟者（20.7%）和不吸烟者（20.7%）。因此，吸烟者的 CD4/CD8 比例明显低于既往吸烟者和不吸烟者。

通常，中性粒细胞占总细胞数的比例低于 1%。血液污染、主动吸烟以及支气管的炎症性疾病是增加中性粒细胞水平的主要因素之一[2,4]。中性粒细胞水平的升高也出现在间质性疾病的晚期病例中（包括纤维化）。存在鳞状上皮细胞表明可能来自上呼吸道的污染。

14.4.2 无细胞分析：正常值

支气管肺泡灌洗液包含广泛的蛋白质、酶、细胞因子、趋化因子、脂质和电解质。由于对它们功能的深入理解以及难以定量和分析，无细胞物质的研究已经为细胞组分的研究所替代。缺乏明确的稀释标志物使得定量非细胞性肺泡组分变得非常困难。由于肺泡和血管空间之间的动态相互作用对细胞外组分（如细胞因子）产生影响，因此，BALF 可能不仅反映了肺泡空间的生理和病理情况，还反映了血流的情况，这使得准确评估肺泡物质的浓度变得非常困难。建议同时测量 BALF 和血清以便进行解释[51]。

14.5 临床应用

在大多数情况下，BAL 不能被视为具有高特异性和可靠性的独立诊断工具。然而，结合其他临床和实验室信息，它非常有价值。对于那些无法进行开胸肺活检的患者，BAL 在诊断过程中起到关键作用。此外，BAL 的结果可以成为决定是否应对那些呼吸症状明显但肺功能接近正常且胸部 X 线正常的患者进行开胸肺活检的重要因素[52]。还应注意，正常的 BALF 细胞计数并不排除肺组织中存在微观异常[6]。

14.5.1 肺结节病

BALF 提供了有关肺结节病病理学的宝贵信息。严重的肺泡炎症和 BAL 淋巴细胞升高严重质疑了肺结节病与免疫抑制之间的所谓关联[53,54]。关于将 BAL 作为肺结节病的诊断和预后工具的应用存在很多争议。然而，尽管已经确定 BAL 细胞分析可以帮助区分肺结节病与其他肉芽肿性和间质性疾病[55,56]，但目前的共识是，如果单独使用，它仍然不具备作为肺结节病的明确诊断工具的可信度。

目前的观点是，肺泡灌洗在预测疾病进展、持续时间和治疗反应方面发挥作用有限。肺泡灌洗细胞组分差异在变化很大的肺结节病中展示了当前肺泡炎症的水平。高度怀疑肺结节病的患者，即使没有肺部影像学证据，也可以出现 BAL 淋巴细胞数量增加[57]。典型的细胞计数是总细胞数正常或稍微升高，淋巴细胞升高，CD4/CD8 比值升高，嗜酸性粒细胞和中性粒细胞的百分比正常。值得注意的是，不出现"泡沫状巨噬细胞"和浆细胞[58,59]。

在肺结节病中，BALF 淋巴细胞增多的程度差异很大；在 10%~15% 的患者中，细胞计数可能正常，也可能显著增加到总细胞数的 80%[60,61]。重度吸烟者通常淋巴细胞计数降低。肺结节病患者的 CD4/CD8 比值也有相当大的变化。大约 60% 的患者中发现 CD4/CD8 比值升高。各种文献数据显示，当比值大于 3.5 时，敏感性为 52%~59%，特异性为 94%~96%[46,59,62]。

因此，淋巴细胞数量升高（具有良好的敏感性）与 CD4/CD8 比值升高（具有良好的特异性）结合起来作为联合诊断工具，值得进一步探讨。Costabel 等建议，在具有典型肺结节病临床表现的患者中，仅 CD4/CD8 比值升高可能足以作为明确的诊断工具，无须进一步进行活检[63]。预计淋巴细胞增多会预测疾病进程、持续时间和治疗反应。然而，尽管早期研究表明可能存在某些关联，后来的研究报道并没有明显的相关性[46,60,64]。

尽管肺结节病患者中 CD4/CD8 比值升高是常见的，但仅有这种升高并不能将肺结节病与其他间质性肺疾病（interstitial lung disease，ILD）区分开来。一些研究表明 CD103 可能是肺结节病的诊断工具。根据 Kolopp-Sarda 的研究，CD4/CD8 比值（≥2.5）和 CD103/CD4 比值（<0.31）的组合可能作为肺结节病诊断的高度敏感工具，敏感性高达 96%。由于在大多数肺部疾病中 CD8[+] 淋巴细胞同时表达 CD103，可能会产生

误导，因此与 CD103/CD4 比值相比，使用 CD103CD4/CD4 比值可能更可取[65]。其他研究建议重新定义 BALF CD103CD4/CD4 淋巴细胞比值<0.45 为肺结节病的满意诊断标志，尽管 CD4/CD8 比值<3.5[66]。

在肺结节病更为晚期的患者中，BALF 中的中性粒细胞计数可能高于正常水平[67]。Ziegenhagen 报告了中性粒细胞水平高于 3% 与疾病进展较快以及对类固醇治疗更为抵抗的关联[68]。另一项研究表明，与自发应答组相比，出现肺功能下降、影像学证据和功能障碍的患者 BALF 中的中性粒细胞水平升高[67]。在肺结节病患者的 BALF 中，表现出巨噬细胞活性水平增加[68]。巨噬细胞释放细胞因子，调节肉芽肿的形成，因此在肺结节病中发挥重要作用。然而，将 BALF 中的细胞因子作为诊断和预后工具的价值尚未得到证实。

14.5.2　特发性间质性肺炎

特发性间质性肺炎（idiopathic interstitial pneumonia，IIP）的诊断一直是一个棘手的临床问题。2002 年美国胸科学会/欧洲呼吸学会共识分类的发布确定了 7 种 IIP 类型[69]。2013 年，美国胸科学会/欧洲呼吸学会发表了一份官方声明，更新了 IIP 的国际多学科分类[70]。这个新的分类确定了 6 种主要 IIP［特发性肺纤维化、非特异性间质性肺炎（nonspecific interstitial pneumonia，NSIP）、呼吸性支气管炎-间质性肺病、脱屑性间质性肺炎、隐源性有组织性肺炎和急性间质性肺炎］、2 种罕见 IIP（特发性淋巴细胞性间质性肺炎和特发性胸膜间质纤维弹性组织病），以及不可分类的 IIP。在新声明中，传统的组织学诊断"金标准"被多学科讨论（MDD）使用的"动态综合方法"所取代。这使得 BAL 获取的数据在诊断中更有价值[70-72]。

特发性肺纤维化（idiopathic pulmonary fibrosis，IPF）患者的支气管肺泡灌洗细胞差异显示淋巴细胞水平降低（5%）和中性粒细胞水平升高（7%）[73,74]。IPF 患者的组织和 BALF 淋巴细胞亚群之间的相互关系也得到了证实[75]。BAL 的实用性不在于 IPF 的特征性 BALF 结果，而在于鉴别诊断排除最常见的其他病因：过敏性肺炎（hypersensitivity pneumonities，HP）、特发性 NSIP 以及与潜在结缔组织疾病相关的 ILD［结缔组织疾病-间质性肺疾病（connective tissue disease-interstitial lung disease，CTD-ILD）][76]。BALF 分析还有助于优化选择需要进行外科诊断性活检手术的患者。已经报道了伴随胶原血管性疾病的肺纤维化［普通型间质性肺炎（usual interstitial pneumonia，UIP）组织学模式］患者 BALF 细胞计数升高，这有助于区分非特发性病因的 IPF[73,74,77]。

BAL 的真正诊断价值在于 BALF 中是否存在以淋巴细胞增多为主的现象。这在 HP、NSIP、CTD-ILD 中常见[73,78,79]。IPF 和健康对照组中的 BALF 淋巴细胞含量相似[80]，而在 IPF 中（按传统诊断）的增加与中到重度的肺泡间质炎症相关[81]，增加了出现其他类型 UIP（如过敏性肺炎）的可能性。相比之下，过敏性肺炎、NSIP 和 CTD-ILD 中通常存在明显的 BALF 淋巴细胞增多。

在细胞型（非纤维化）NSIP 患者中，BALF 淋巴细胞通常升高至 40%，中性粒细胞略有增加，CD4/CD8 比值下降至低于 0.3[82]。BALF 具有正常水平的淋巴细胞亚群患者可能对类固醇治疗有反应。相比之下，非细胞型（纤维化）NSIP 表现出非特异性的淋巴细胞升高至 33% 和中性粒细胞升高至 14%[82]。这一组患者通常对类固醇治疗不产生反应。特异性的 NSIP 两个亚型的 BALF 细胞计数与由感染、结缔组织疾病、药物反应或其他非特异性病因引起的组织学表现为 NSIP 的患者相似。隐源性机化性肺炎（cryptogenic organizing pneumonia，COP）BALF 细胞计数通常可见淋巴细胞显著增多（>40%）和 CD4/CD8 比值降低[82]。与细胞型 NSIP 一样，对类固醇治疗有反应的患者，BALF 淋巴细胞水平可以恢复正常。COP 中的 BALF 细胞计数与组织病理提示机化性肺炎但没有特定病因的患者相似。对于那些影像学发现强烈提示 COP 但经纤支镜活检为阴性或无法进行活检的病例，分析 BALF 也具有诊断价值[83]。

急性间质性肺炎（acute interstitial pneumonia，AIP）中的 BALF 细胞组分与 IPF 恶化患者相似。典型的 AIP 细胞计数显示中性粒细胞升高，淋巴细胞稍有增加。与 IPF 恶化一样，还可能发现反应性肺细胞和透明膜碎片[69]。

对 IIP 的明确诊断需要排除其他间质性疾病的病因。分析 BALF 中特定物质和 BALF 培养在鉴别间质性肺炎的非特异性病因具有应用价值（例如，石棉体）。BALF 细胞分析可以区分具有明确病因的特发性和非特发性病因的患者，这些患者具有已确立的 UIP 组织学，但没有明确的病因。此外，BALF 细胞组分的分析有助于区分特发性组织学，特别是区分 IPF 和其他 IIP。BAL 不会排除需要活检的需求，但当活检不可行或组织学诊断不明确时，它可能会有所帮助。

在 HP 中，BAL 作为一种预后工具的价值存在极大争议。Veeraraghavan等对早期高效性的预测提出了严重怀疑[84]。然而，Ryu等在一项回顾性研究中，在122名患有UIP或NSIP的患者中进行支气管肺泡灌洗和高分辨率计算机断层扫描（HRCT）之后再进行活检，2年后的随访结果表明，BAL淋巴细胞增多反映了非UIP组织学模式和更好的预后[74]。

14.5.3 过敏性肺炎（HP）

HP也被称为外源性过敏性肺泡炎，是一种临床综合征，其表现多种多样（急性、亚急性和慢性/纤维化，这些形式常常有重叠）。由于缺乏明确的诊断标准，HP的诊断并不简单，它依赖于多个因素，包括暴露史、引发抗原的沉淀抗体、临床特征、BAL、放射学和病理特征[85,86]。HP表现出显著的类似其他IIP的倾向[87]。已经确立了BAL在HP中的诊断的价值，但BALF细胞分析并不是唯一的工具。它的特征是总细胞计数增加，淋巴细胞升高。从已发表的研究中可以看出，淋巴细胞增加超过50%支持诊断HP[88,89]。在这一人群中，CD4/CD8比值显示出变化，但通常低于1[90]。然而，这个比值可能根据暴露和疾病阶段而显著变化。此外，正常或升高的比值并不排除HP[91,92]，因此不再推荐进行比值测量。

关于细胞学细胞计数，需要注意的是，在急性暴露于相关抗原的情况下，可能会伴随中性粒细胞数量的增加，中性粒细胞在48 h后达到峰值，但在几天后恢复到以淋巴细胞为主的模式[92-94]。去除抗原后，这些水平可能会持续升高数月甚至数年。一些淋巴细胞呈异常的外观提示为原始细胞，具有明显凹凸多裂的细胞核和细胞质面积增大[95]。吸烟会导致淋巴细胞计数普遍下降。HP在不吸烟者中更常见，暗示了烟草的免疫抑制作用[96]。还有数据显示，已经发展成纤维化的HP患者的中性粒细胞水平升高[97]。

在HP中，BAL获得的总细胞中，巨噬细胞占比较低（通常低于40%），但实际数量与对照组相当[98]。巨噬细胞可能表现出泡沫状细胞质。暴露于HP患者的BALF标本中也可能含有数量增加的肥大细胞（多达10倍以上）[95,99]。在大多数患者中，当个体目前或最近暴露或在暴露后不久，肥大细胞的数量会增加，然后迅速下降[95]。在继续暴露和出现症状的情况下，肥大细胞和中性粒细胞可能保持升高[95]。

关于确立BALF细胞计数作为HP患者预后工具的实用性已经引发了很多争议。研究证实，在这些患者中，BALF中的淋巴细胞不能预测预后结果[100]。

14.5.4 尘肺病

尘肺病患者的BALF细胞分析通常反映肺泡炎，总细胞计数增加2~3倍，淋巴细胞增多，CD4/CD8比值升高。嗜中性粒细胞水平不稳定，但常常升高。单独进行细胞分析是不足作为诊断证明。然而，BAL在记录特定暴露方面仍然有用，如石棉纤维、硅粒子和铍敏感淋巴细胞。

石棉小体是一组由水合镁硅酸盐组成的天然纤维的商业术语。石棉纤维根据形状被分类为蛇纹状或角闪石状。石棉小体暴露会增加患肺纤维化、肺癌以及胸膜疾病如间皮瘤、纤维化、积液和斑块形成的风险[101]。石棉小体是吸入的镀铁石棉纤维颗粒，被含铁粘蛋白包裹并嵌入在肺组织中。石棉小体的形成是一种细胞内过程，发生在一个或多个肺泡巨噬细胞吞噬石棉纤维后。然后，纤维被包裹在细胞内液泡中，并覆盖有酸性黏多糖[102]。铁最初以含铁蛋白的形式积聚在包裹物中。在肺中只有很小一部分石棉纤维会形成含铁体[102,103]。石棉小体很少由蛇纹状纤维产生，主要由角闪石状纤维形成。因此，石棉小体的存在主要反映了长角闪石状纤维的数量，这些纤维最常与石棉肺和间皮瘤相关[104,105]。在没有职业石棉暴露但暴露于城市污染的人群中，大部分石棉纤维是蛇纹状的[106]。这些小纤维不会形成石棉小体，这可以解释为什么在支气管肺泡灌洗中找到石棉小体通常与职业暴露相关，并提示吸入了工业纤维。石棉小体仅代表了肺中和支气管肺泡灌洗中总石棉数量的一小部分[102,104]。

通过活检检测肺实质中的石棉小体仍然是检测石棉暴露的"金标准"[106]。研究证实，BALF中测得的石棉小体浓度为1 AB/mL可预测肺实质中石棉小体浓度为1 050~3 010 AB/g[104]。因此，BALF中浓度大于1 AB/mL表明存在显著的石棉暴露[107]，并与影像学病灶增多、呼吸症状加重以及肺功能降低相关[108]。在BALF中发现石棉小体是石棉暴露的最佳客观指标，但本身并不是疾病的诊断依据[103,105,106]。通过电子显微镜可以检测到BALF中的石棉、铁和磷颗粒[109]。在正确操作获取的BALF中未发现石棉小体也不能排除与石棉小体相关的胸膜疾病或石棉小体在肺实质广泛分布[106]。BALF中的石棉小体浓度可能与暴露的时长和强度呈正相关，与距离最后一次暴露的时间呈负相关。诱导痰液中的石棉小体进行筛查的敏感性较BAL低，仅限于严重石棉暴露的情况中使用[110,111]。

铍在现代工业中得到了广泛的应用。吸入铍金属粉尘、氧化铍或铍盐可以导致急性或慢性肺疾病。急性形式似乎对肺有毒性且呈剂量相关性，已经通过环境暴露控制基本被消除。慢性形式在1~20年内发展，占受暴露人群的1%~3%，是一种类似结节病的肺间质肉芽肿性疾病[20,112]。慢性铍肺病的诊断通常基于铍暴露史、典型的临床和组织学异常以及升高的肺铍水平[20,112]。长时间暴露于较高水平铍的工人临床症状更严重。BAL在评估疑似慢性铍肺病的患者中显示出价值。慢性铍肺病患者的BALF细胞计数类似于结节病患者[113]。巨噬细胞和T细胞的总数增加，淋巴细胞的百分比增加，其中大多数是T辅助细胞[20,112]。铍增加了慢性铍病患者肺中CD14（dim）CD16+亚群[114]。

在慢性铍肺病中，BAL的最大用途是评估铍的局部免疫反应。从慢性铍肺病患者的BALF中分离的淋巴细胞，在体外用可溶性铍盐刺激后出现增殖，其敏感性和特异性接近100%[98,99,115]。这种铍淋巴细胞增殖试验通常在血液或BALF标本上实施，是行业监测的常用工具。标本中单核细胞通常在不同浓度和时间间隔下与铍盐进行体外培养。细胞增殖的测量标准取决于实验室，尚未定义通用标准。先前具有铍暴露史和淋巴细胞增殖证据，但缺乏明确的肉芽肿组织学证据的患者可能被视为敏感个体。敏感患者的慢性铍肺病发展率每年高达6%~8%[116]。

14.5.5 嗜酸性肺疾病

来自健康非吸烟者的BAL标本显示，嗜酸性粒细胞占总细胞计数的不到1%。在吸烟者或曾吸烟者中，嗜酸性粒细胞浓度可能略有增加[2,20]。嗜酸性粒细胞计数>5%在临床上被认为具有重要意义[117]。各种病理过程，包括感染、药物反应、变态反应和特发性机制，可能导致血液和BALF中嗜酸性粒细胞浓度升高。嗜酸性粒细胞中度增多（5%~20%）是感染、变态反应和药物反应的典型表现[117-121]。

嗜酸性肺炎（eosinophilic pneumonia，EP）可能由感染性和非感染性因素引起，包括多种寄生虫感染、过敏、暴露于某些元素以及特发性原因。EP的经典定义是肺组织病理学上嗜酸性粒细胞占优势。然而，有明确的临床和放射学证据的情况下，BALF中嗜酸性粒细胞浓度升高可能也可以明确诊断，而无须进行肺活检。建议在具有放射学异常的区域进行技术合格的BAL，如果所取得的BALF标本中细胞计数正常，EP则可以被排除[122]。在EP中，嗜酸性粒细胞可能占BALF总细胞计数的90%[122]。还观察到超过80%的慢性嗜酸性肺炎病例，其嗜酸性粒细胞浓度超过BALF总细胞计数的40%。尽管嗜酸性粒细胞浓度的通用诊断标准尚未确立，Lazor等已建议将嗜酸性粒细胞浓度≥25%作为诊断标准[123]。

特发性急性嗜酸性肺炎的BALF嗜酸性粒细胞浓度平均在37%~54%，淋巴细胞和嗜中性粒细胞计数轻度升高[124,125]。Pope-Harmon等提出将最低嗜酸性粒细胞浓度的诊断标准设为25%。在特发性慢性嗜酸性肺炎中，嗜酸性粒细胞占BALF总细胞计数的平均值为58%，淋巴细胞和嗜中性粒细胞数量略微升高[125]。Marchand等提出将嗜酸性粒细胞浓度≥40%设为诊断标准[126,127]。

慢性嗜酸性肺炎（chronic EP，CEP）的BALF中包含细胞因子白细胞介素（interleukin，IL）-4、IL-5、IL-6、IL-10、IL-13和IL-18，这基本上与局部Th2炎症一致，尽管Th1细胞因子IL-2和IL-12也同时存在[128-130]。BALF中含有多种趋化因子，表明T细胞的募集在CEP的病理生理中起重要作用[130,131]。急性嗜酸性肺炎（acute EP，AEP）的潜在机制比CEP更难以捉摸，尽管在AEP患者的BALF中存在大致相似谱系的特定炎症介质。已经发现，在AEP患者的BALF中，包括IL-1ra、IL-2、IL-5、IL-10、IL-12、IL-13和IL-18在内的一系列Th2和Th1细胞因子升高，这可能反映嗜酸性粒细胞已知的分泌潜力[132]。与CEP一样，AEP中检测到趋化因子CCL17的水平较高，这可能与在AEP发病机制中招募的T细胞有关[130]。然而，Carmi等认为AEP和CEP可能共享共同的发病途径。因此，将EP分类为AEP或CEP的实用性有限，EP呈现的严重程度应是治疗的唯一决定因素[133]。

14.5.6 系统性硬化症

系统性硬化症患者的总BALF细胞计数通常是正常的，而淋巴细胞、嗜中性粒细胞和嗜酸性粒细胞的计数显示出不同程度的增加。通常，具有NSIP放射学和组织学典型表现的患者，嗜酸性粒细胞的升高水平通常高于组织学表现为UIP的患者。淋巴细胞浓度在细胞性NSIP中通常高于纤维性NSIP（前文已述）[134]。由于这种非特异性肺泡炎，BALF中细胞计数作为这类患者的诊断作用有限。

BAL肺泡炎是否可以作为一种预测预后和监测治疗反应的工具存在激烈争议。Silver等提出肺泡炎与肺功能测试（pulmonary function testing，PFT）结果恶化以及治疗反应不佳之间存在潜在相关性[135]。后续研究显示，嗜中性粒细胞占优势的肺泡炎与高分辨率计算机断层扫描（high-resolution computed tomography，HRCT）中纤维化疾病的严重程度以及 PFT 测量结果恶化之间存在相关性[136,137]。他们的发现强烈提示嗜中性粒细胞占优势的肺泡炎是疾病更晚期的指标，而不是疾病早期和不良预后的指标。还有证据表明，在 HRCT 上出现 ILD 进展证据的患者中，肺泡炎的存在可以用来预测预后[138]。

然而，Goh 等研究表明，当考虑到患者群体的基线疾病严重程度时，嗜中性粒细胞占优势的肺泡炎总体长期死亡率与淋巴细胞占优势的肺泡炎的总体长期死亡率之间没有相关性[136]。他们认为，首次发病时疾病严重程度可以更有价值地预测临床进程，而不是 BALF 的细胞计数。

14.5.6.1 肺朗格汉斯细胞组织细胞增多症

肺朗格汉斯细胞组织细胞增多症（pulmonary Langerhans cell histiocytosis，PLCH）是一种慢性肉芽肿性疾病。典型易感人群是年轻吸烟者。以前，它也被称为结缔组织细胞病和肺部嗜酸性肉芽肿。PLCH 的病理表现是抗原呈递细胞，即朗格汉斯细胞在间质中积聚[20]。在电子显微镜下，朗格汉斯细胞的特征是凹陷的细胞核和分散在细胞质中被称为 Birbeck 颗粒（直径 40~45 nm）的小型齿状细长体[2,20,139]。另一个特征是它们细胞表面上存在 CD1 抗原，以及在免疫染色中细胞质中存在 S100 蛋白[140]。在 PLCH 中，朗格汉斯细胞的增殖导致上叶网状结节浸润的形成，后期进展为囊性改变和蜂窝状改变。

BAL 作为 PLCH 可能的诊断工具具有潜在价值。BALF 细胞分析通常显示总细胞计数升高，包括吸烟患者在内的肺泡巨噬细胞包涵体的百分比升高，嗜中性粒细胞和嗜酸性粒细胞浓度轻度增加，淋巴细胞总数不确定[4]，突出的特征是 CD1+朗格汉斯细胞的存在，浓度为 5%。Soler 等证明，BALF 中朗格汉斯细胞浓度低于 5% 常见于其他间质性肺疾病、肺癌和健康吸烟者[141]。然而，Costabel 等建议浓度高于 4% 可以进行诊断，具有较高的特异性但敏感性较低[122]。目前，用于做出明确诊断的朗格汉斯细胞浓度仍存在争议。Helmers 等认为通过电子显微镜识别 Birbeck 颗粒在临床上并不实用[4]。

14.5.6.2 弥漫性肺泡出血

弥漫性肺泡出血（diffuse alveolar hemorrhage，DAH）是一种危及生命的紧急情况。传统上的定义包括咯血、贫血和弥漫性肺泡渗出三联征[142]。通常需要早期的支气管镜检查和 BAL 来明确诊断并排除感染[142]。然而，尽管肺泡内出血明显，多达 33% 的患者可能不出现咯血症状[143]。

DAH 可能由各种不同的病因引起，而血管炎是最常见的原因。仅基于临床和放射学很难做出明确的诊断，除非排除了感染和其他间质性疾病。BALF 呈明显的血性外观并不具有绝对诊断价值，因为它可能与支气管镜检查引起的损伤、感染或其他疾病相关[4]。在放射学异常的区域进行 BAL 对于 DAH 的诊断非常重要。在标准的 BAL 操作中，会注入和回收连续的小部分液体。回收的小部分液体中，出现出血逐渐增多（红细胞计数增加）与 DAH 的诊断一致[142,144]。需要注意的是，需要排除感染和癌症的可能性[6]。

通过对细胞进行铁染色分析检测携带含铁血黄素的巨噬细胞是 DAH 的一种非常有价值的诊断工具。De Lassence 等建议使用含铁血黄素巨噬细胞比例＞20% 作为诊断标准[145]。值得注意的是，巨噬细胞摄取含铁血黄素呈时间依赖性，在出血发生后的 48 h 内几乎无法检测到[146,147]。

与以前的 Golde 评分系统相比，使用含铁血黄素巨噬细胞计数作为诊断工具更简单[145]。需要排除多种其他肺部疾病，包括 IPF、心脏病、结节病、癌症、血管炎、肺泡蛋白沉积症（pulmonary alveolar proteinosis，PAP）和 PLCH[4,20,148]，因为在这些疾病过程中也发现了含铁血黄素巨噬细胞。在免疫受损、血小板减少和抗凝患者中，BAL 已经显示出作为 DAH 安全和准确的诊断工具的效用[148-151]。

14.5.7　肺泡蛋白沉积症（PAP）

PAP 是一种罕见的疾病，其特征是肺泡内异常聚积的肺表面活性剂，即肺泡内广泛充满一种可以用过碘酸-希夫（PAS）试剂染色的脂蛋白物质。这种脂蛋白物质的主要成分是肺表面活性剂磷脂和蛋白碎片。粒细胞-巨噬细胞集落刺激因子（GM-CSF）抗体的存在影响了巨噬细胞的清除能力，并导致这种物质在肺泡空间中的积聚[152-154]。有三种明确的疾病类别，其具有相似的组织学谱，即获得性 PAP、先天性 PAP 和继发性 PAP[155]。本文将重点介绍继发性 PAP。

BAL 已经证明在帮助了解这种疾病方面具有价值[152-154]。通过 BAL 获得的"乳白色"灌洗液的经典表现，可以确诊约 75% 的临床上怀疑 PAP 病例（图 14.1）[156,157]。这种液体含有大量颗粒状非细胞嗜酸性蛋白质物质，形态上异常的"泡沫状"巨噬细胞内充满了抗透明质酸酶的PAS阳性细胞内包涵物（图14.2）[60,157,158]，这些巨噬细胞巴氏染色后也显示出特征性特点[159,160]。在BALF的电子显微镜检查中出现的具有同心层状结构的磷脂体，称为片状体，可以确诊[161,162]。结合临床和影像学表现，典型的PAP BAL表现通常可以消除进一步活检的需求[158,163-165]。

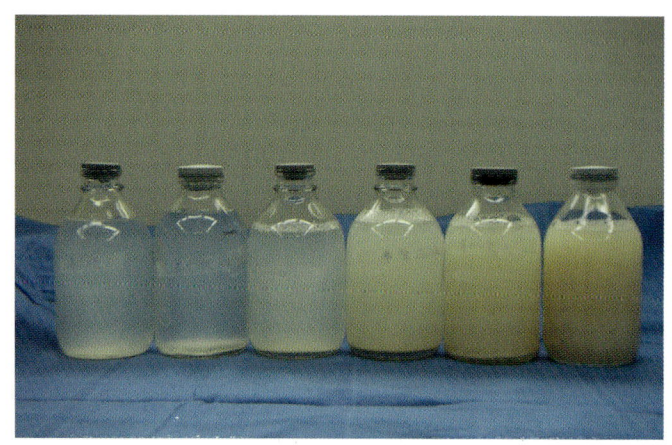

图14.3　肺泡蛋白沉积症患者的全肺灌洗液

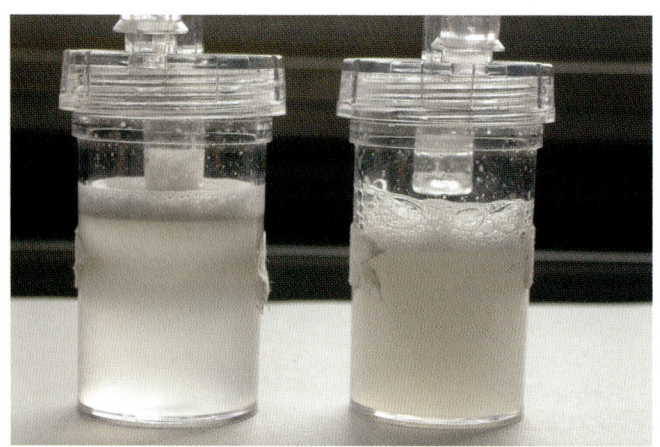

图14.1　牛奶样及云雾样支气管肺泡灌洗液

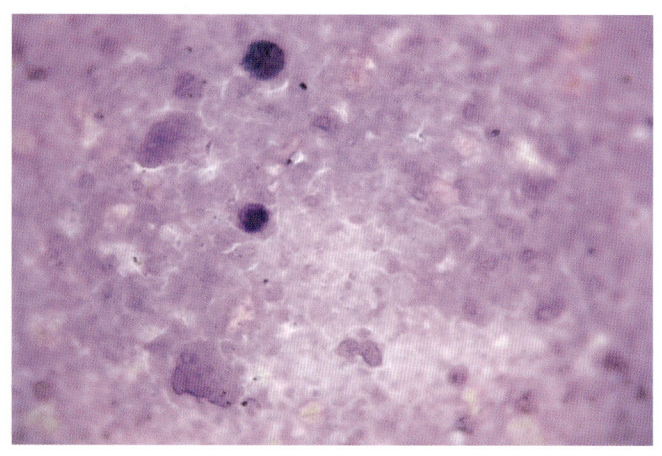

图14.2　支气管肺泡灌洗液PAS染色阳性

图片来源：周道银，上海长海医院，中国上海。

目前全麻下全肺灌洗（whole lung lavage，WLL）仍然是PAP的最有效治疗方法（图14.3）。最近的研究还证明了通过给予GM-CSF皮下注射和雾化吸入在某些PAP患者群体中的有效性。

14.5.8　药物诱导的肺疾病

药物诱导的肺毒性表现为多种临床、组织学和放射学病变。在肺泡水平，可能会发现变态反应和细胞毒性病变。BALF的细胞分析显示肺泡炎，以嗜酸性粒细胞、中性粒细胞或更常见的淋巴细胞为主。在大多数情况下，CD4/CD8比值低于正常水平，但接触甲氨蝶呤、硝基呋喃、氨苄青霉素的患者可能CD4细胞水平升高[166-169]。具有特定潜在组织学模式的药物反应，如NSIP和COP，显示了与相应组织学典型的BALF细胞计数（前文已述）[167,170,171]。

已经发现DAH与暴露于某些药物有关，这类患者BALF结果也是典型的[167]。尽管药物诱导的疾病不显示特征性的BALF细胞计数，但BAL可能有助于排除其他疾病过程，如感染。

BAL可作为评估可疑的胺碘酮肺毒性时的辅助检测方法[172]。肺泡巨噬细胞内的磷脂积聚导致胞浆片状体的形成，导致巨噬细胞"泡沫状"外观（图14.4）[172]。这是继发于胺碘酮药物效应的相对特征，约有50%的患者中可以找到"泡沫状"包涵物。因此，它们的存在不是毒性的专属诊断，但没有"泡沫状"包涵物则可以排除胺碘酮相关性肺炎[172,173]。

BAL还在评估药物诱发的嗜酸性肺炎中发挥作用。一项回顾性研究发现，在196例药物诱发的EP病例中，主要原因是达普霉素。这种综合征可分为AEP和CEP。AEP一般持续不到1个月，通常不到1周[174]。CEP起病逐渐，从起病到诊断的平均时间为5个月[133]。在这两种综合征中，嗜酸性粒细胞计数可能高于BALF中所有白细胞的25%[133]。

14.5.9　在恶性疾病中的应用

可弯曲支气管镜检查在肺部恶性肿瘤诊断中具有重要作用。通过支气管内活检，可见病变的诊断率高达90%[175]。通过支气管镜不可见的外周型病变经支气管活检、刷片和针吸的诊断率明显较低[175,176]。BAL在诊断这些外围病变方面显示出了一定的实用性。

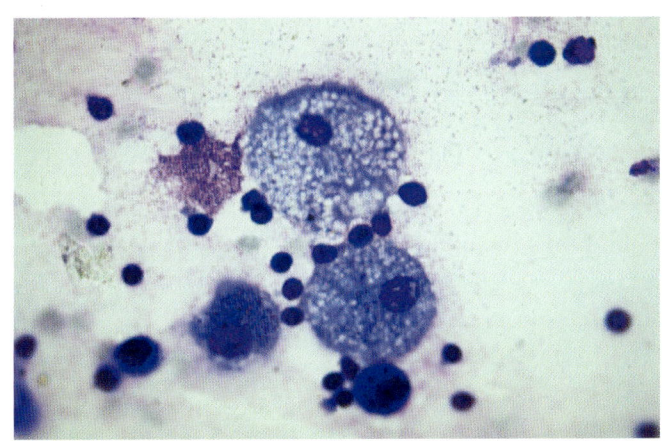

图 14.4　支气管肺泡灌洗液中的泡沫细胞
图片来源：周道银，上海长海医院，中国上海。

在肺部恶性肿瘤的诊断中，可弯曲支气管镜作为一种诊断工具的价值已得到证实。支气管镜下可见的病变诊断率高达 90%[145]。对于肺外周病变，支气管内超声引导鞘（endobronchial ultrasound with guide sheath，EBUS-GS）联合虚拟支气管镜显示出一定的实用性[177]。BAL 在诊断这些外周病变中作为一种辅助工具具有实际意义[177]。

BALF 的细胞分析通常显示出非特异性的肺泡炎[178]。淋巴细胞为主的肺泡炎可能与淋巴增生性疾病的肺部受累有关[179]。涉及肺部恶性肿瘤的免疫细胞化学和组织化学标志物是研究的热点。BALF 中有多种标志物可用，其实用性与特定的肿瘤类型相关[180]。

BAL 在诊断特定的原发性肺上皮肿瘤方面具有重要价值。在通过淋巴或鳞状上皮扩散的弥漫性疾病过程中，包括细支气管肺泡癌（bronchoalveolar cell carcinoma，BAC）和腺癌等肿瘤，诊断率最高。甚至仅凭 BAL 涂片就可以获得诊断性肿瘤细胞（图 14.5~14.7）[181]。根据 Ahmed 等的研究，与经支气管活检相比，BAL 细胞学在肺癌诊断中的敏感性为 93.44%，特异性为 100%[182]。然而，在一项 50 例的回顾性研究中，作为非小细胞肺癌的诊断工具，BAL 在支气管冲洗、支气管刷片涂片、胸腔积液、痰液、肺、转移淋巴结的引导细针吸取细胞学检查（fine needle aspiration cytology，FNAC）方面并未显示出优势[183]。黄海东等提出，基于 R-EBUS 的多种引导技术是诊断肺外周病变的安全有效的工具。采用活检结合支气管刷检和冲洗，诊断率得到改善[177]。还有研究表明，来自 BALF 的循环核酸（circulating free DNA，cfDNA）可用于表皮生长因子受体（epidermal growth factor receptor，EGFR）突变的分子检测和 p.T790M 突变的鉴定，且易于应用。这有助于对肺恶性肿瘤患者进行 EGFR 检测[184]。

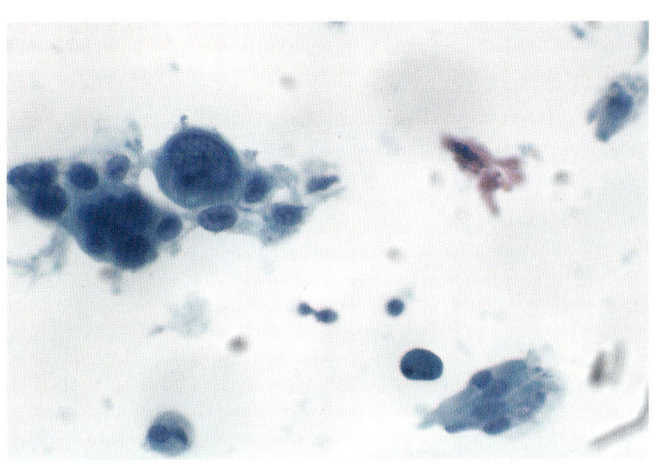

图 14.5　液基细胞学涂片显示鳞状细胞癌
图片来源：高莉，上海长海医院，中国上海。

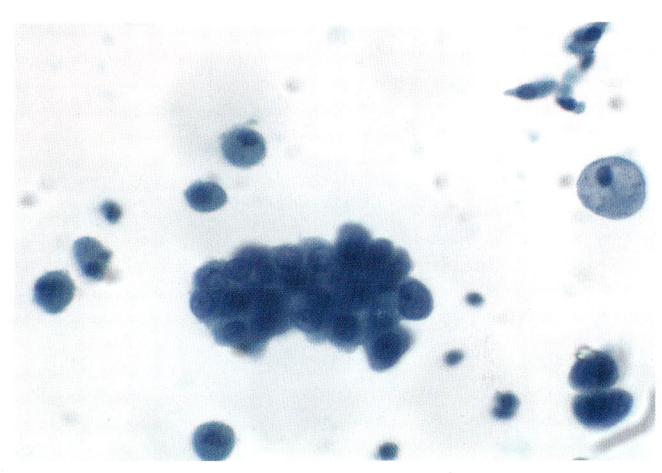

图 14.6　液基细胞学涂片显示腺癌
图片来源：高莉，上海长海医院，中国上海。

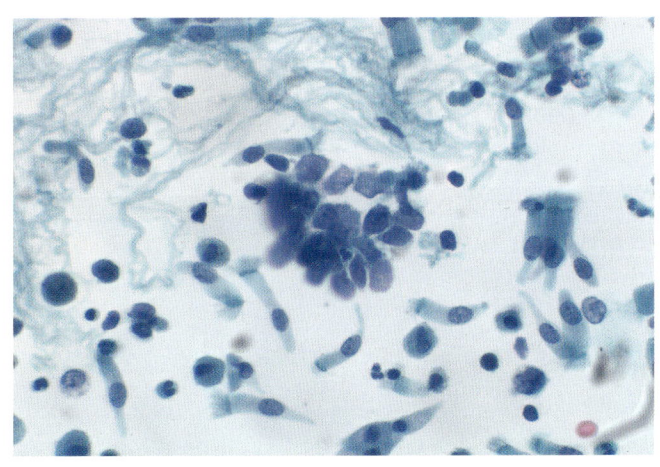

图 14.7　液基细胞学涂片显示小细胞癌
图片来源：高莉，上海长海医院，中国上海。

BAL 在诊断原发性肺非霍奇金淋巴瘤，如黏膜相关淋巴组织（mucosa-associated lymphoid tissue，MALT）和继发肺的非霍奇金淋巴瘤方面具有实用价值已得到证明[180,181,185]。据报道，BAL 对非霍奇金淋巴瘤的诊断率高达 67%[181]。较少见的是在 BAL 细胞学标本中发现 Reed-Sternberg 细胞可以明确霍奇金病的诊断[186,187]。

BAL 细胞学检测偶尔也可以检测到转移性疾病。已有报道的诊断病例包括转移性乳腺癌和黑色素瘤[181,188,189]。

总之，BAL 可作为活检的有效辅助工具，或者在活检不可行时作为肿瘤诊断的独立工具。然而，在解释检查结果之前，应认识到 BAL 在肿瘤诊断方面的局限性。在多种临床情况下，气道上皮细胞可能发生严重的异型性改变，很难与恶性改变区分。例如，肺炎、病毒感染、ARDS、IPF 恶化、胺碘酮肺损伤以及化疗后改变[190-192]。

肺癌诊治的进展，使得可以利用 BALF 中的 cfDNA 来测试 EGFR 突变，这也进一步促进了与肺部肿瘤相关的遗传突变的检测[184]。

14.5.10 在感染性疾病中的应用

在弥漫性间质或实质性肺部浸润、免疫抑制患者的肺部浸润、呼吸机相关性肺炎（ventilator-associated pneumonia，VAP）或治疗失败的肺炎中，BAL 技术仍然是病原微生物鉴定的基石[193-196]。关于疑似肺炎患者的 BAL 适应证，在文献中存在广泛的争议。尤其对 VAP 进行了大量的研究，研究表明，在这类患者中，早期识别和启动适当治疗与死亡率相关[197,198]。

多项研究比较了机械通气患者的支气管镜 BAL 标本和通过非侵入性采样（气管内吸痰）获得的 BAL 标本（图 14.8），结果发现两组患者在 28 天死亡率、总死亡率、ICU 住院时间、机械通气时间或抗生素更换方面没有显著差异[199-201]。因此，建议使用半定量培养的非侵入性采样（弱推荐，低质量证据）来诊断 VAP[202]。定量培养的侵入性采样可能会降低初期抗生素覆盖率不足的风险[203,204]，如果将生长低于规定的阈值（如 BAL 为 104 CFU/mL）作为停用抗生素的标准，则可能会减少抗生素暴露[205]。这一结果很重要，因为存在获得抗生素耐药性、药物副作用和不必要或过度使用抗生素的风险。BAL 较其他方法的优势仍然是一个持续争论的问题。

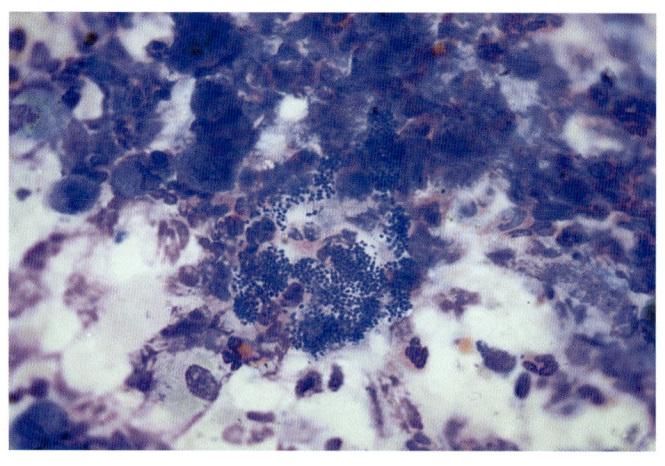

图 14.8　细菌性肺炎的支气管肺泡灌洗液

图片来源：周道银，上海长海医院，中国上海。

对于免疫受损患者的肺部浸润的鉴别诊断仍然具有挑战性。BAL 在这类患者中的实用性和安全性已经得到证实，BAL 是首选的诊断方法[206-210]。BALF 可通过培养、聚合酶链反应（polymerase chain reaction，PCR）和生物标志物（图 14.9）来检测各种病毒、细菌或真菌的种属。BALF 细胞学结果常常受到全血细胞减少、气道损伤以及频繁出血的限制。此外，BAL 标本的培养结果通常受到抗微生物药物治疗的影响。但在怀疑有侵袭性肺曲霉菌病（invasive pulmonary aspergillosis，IPA）的患者中建议进行 BAL。美国传染病学会建议使用标准化的 BAL 操作方法，BAL 标本应送检常规培养、细胞学检查以及非培养的检测方法［例如，半乳甘露聚糖（galactomannan，GM）］（强烈推荐；中等质量证据）[211]。当在特定患者亚群（血液系统恶性肿瘤、造血干细胞移植）中使用时，建议将 BAL 的 GM 检测作为成人和儿童诊断 IA 的准确标志物[211]，并建议在接受抗真菌药物治疗或预防的患者中进行常规筛查（强烈推荐；高质量证据）[211]。Guegan 等报告称，直接在 BAL 标本中进行曲霉分子检测可大大提高 IA 的诊断率，尤其在非血液病患者中（图 14.10）[212]。PCR 检测曲霉菌的敏感性在 61%~74% 之间，低于 GM（87%），但高于培养（47%）。将 PCR 与 EORTC/MSG 标准相结合，敏感性提高到 100%。有趣的是，非血液病患者的检测率在 60%~75% 之间，高于血液病患者和曾接触抗真菌药物的患者[15]。曲霉特异性侧流装置（lateral flow device，LFD）和 GM 在 BALF 中的诊断性能似乎相当[213]。

（图 14.11）。在某些病例中，可以观察到多种微生物和/或结核分枝杆菌的合并感染[219]。将 BALF 离心后，透射电子显微镜（×3 450）可以观察到肺泡巨噬细胞和具有扇形边缘的膜囊泡（图 14.12）。

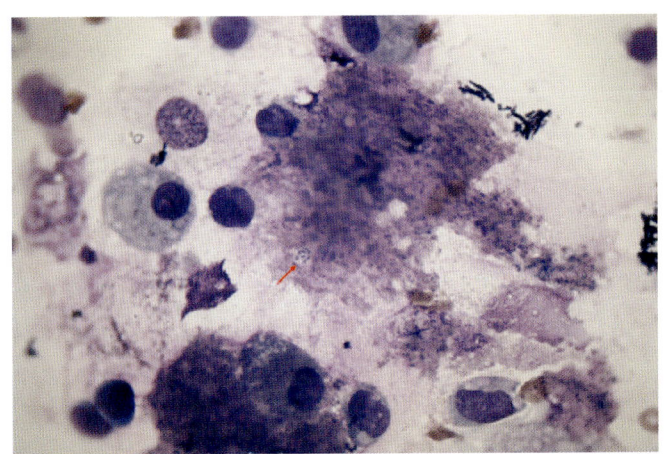

图 14.9　支气管肺泡灌洗液中显示肺囊虫（红色箭头示）
图片来源：周道银，上海长海医院，中国上海。

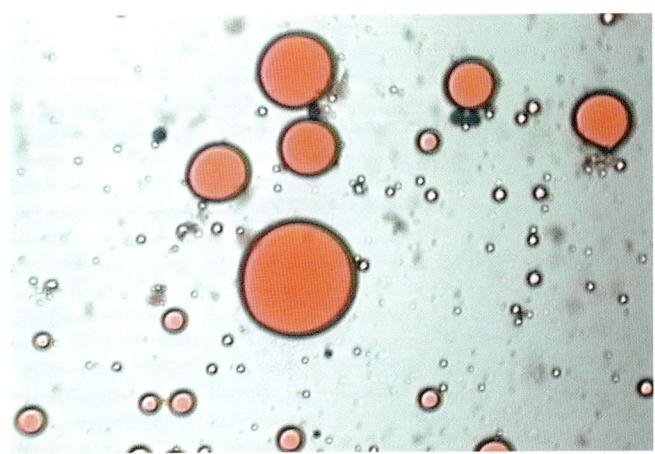

图 14.11　支气管肺泡灌洗液标本光镜下显示
油红-O 染色主要显示孤立的巨噬细胞吞噬胞外脂滴。

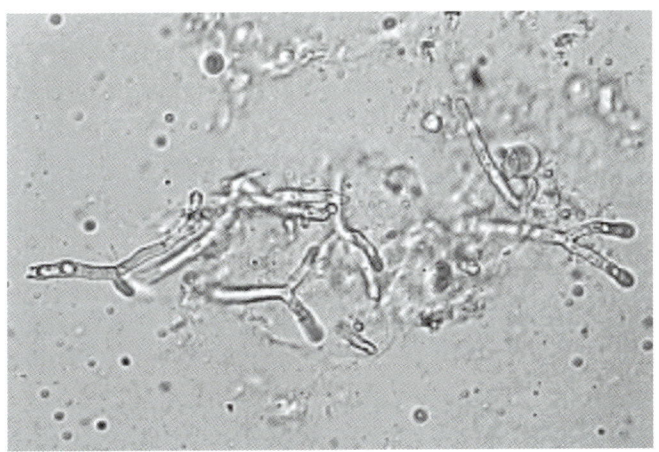

图 14.10　支气管肺泡灌洗液中曲霉菌菌丝
图片来源：周道银，上海长海医院，中国上海。

14.5.10.1　外源性脂质性肺炎

外源性脂质性肺炎（exogenous lipoid pneumonia，ELP），由 Laughlen 于 1925 年首次描述[214]，是一种罕见的良性疾病，没有特定的临床或影像学表现[215]。在胸部 CT 上，它可能呈现多种形式：合并症、磨玻璃密度影、"铺路石"征、间质增厚[3-5]或肿块[216-218]。在临床上，ELP 可以发生在所有年龄段，但老年人和儿童风险最大[215,219]。ELP 最常与矿物油吸入有关，而植物油、动物油和其他吸入物，如鼻膏/滴剂和与职业相关的物质也可能导致 ELP[220-228]。

对 ELP 的诊断可以通过两种方式进行：细胞病理学或手术病理学。细胞病理学标本可以通过 BAL 或细针穿刺获得。手术病理学标本也可以通过经支气管肺活检或手术活检获得[215]。ELP 的 BALF 呈混浊/乳状，在油红-O 染色时可见大量脂质巨噬细胞和细胞外脂质

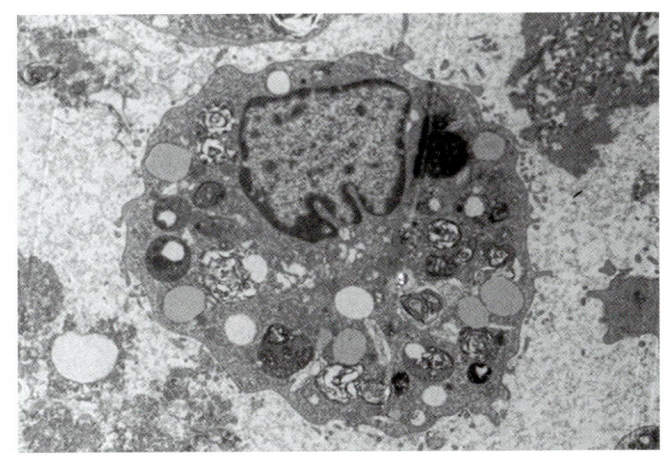

图 14.12　支气管肺泡灌洗液中肺泡巨噬细胞电镜下显示
可见有多个膜结合的扇形边缘膜囊泡。

主要治疗方法包括支持疗法和避免进一步暴露。糖皮质激素只在肺损伤严重且持续的情况下才作为治疗选择；其他治疗选择包括免疫球蛋白和反复进行全肺灌洗。手术仅在高度怀疑癌症的患者中进行[229]。

14.6　结论

40 年来，BAL 已经成为介入肺脏病学中最简单又最实用的技术之一。随着诊断技术的进步，BAL 将

继续在感染、肿瘤和其他肺部疾病领域发挥其独特的作用。

参考文献

1. Goldstein, R.A., Rohatgi, P.K., Bergofsky, E.H. et al. (1990). Clinical role of bronchoalveolar lavage in adults with pulmonary disease. *Am. Rev. Respir. Dis.* 142: 481–486.
2. Hunninghake, G.W., Gadek, J.E., Kawanami, O. et al. (1979). In ammatory and immune processes in the human lung in health and disease: evaluation by bronchoalveolar lavage. *Am. J. Pathol.* 97: 149–206.
3. Reynolds, H.Y. and Newball, H.H. (1974). Analysis of proteins and respiratory cells obtained from human lungs by bronchial lavage. *J. Lab. Clin. Med.* 84: 559–573.
4. European Society of Pneumology Task Group (1989). Technical recommendations and guidelines for bronchoalveolar lavage (BAL). *Eur. Respir. J.* 2: 561–585.
5. Haslam, P.L. and Baughman, R.P. (1999). Report of ERS task force: guidelines for measurement of acellular components and standardization of BAL. *Eur. Respir. J.* 14: 245–248.
6. Keith, C.M., Ganesh, R., Robert, P.B. et al. (2012). An official American Thoracic Society clinical practice guideline: the clinical utility of bronchoalveolar lavage cellular analysis in interstitial lung disease. *Am. J. Respir. Crit. Care Med.* 185: 1004–1014.
7. Haslam, P.L. (1984). Bronchoalveolar lavage. *Semin. Respir. Crit. Care Med.* 6: 55–70.
8. Pang, J.A., Cheng, A.F., Chan, H.S., and French, G.L. (1989). Special precautions reduce oropharyngeal contamination in bronchoalveolar lavage for bacteriologic studies. *Lung* 167: 261–267.
9. Pingleton, S.K., Harrison, G.F., Stechschulte, D.J. et al. (1983). Effect of location, pH, and temperature of instillate in bronchoalveolar lavage in normal volunteers. *Am. Rev. Respir. Dis.* 128: 1035–1037.
10. Helmers, R.A. and Hunninghake, G.W. (1989). Bronchoalveolar lavage in the nonimmunocompromised patient. *Chest* 96: 1184–1190.
11. Davis, G.S., Giancola, M.S., Costanza, M.C., and Low, R.B. (1982). Analyses of sequential bronchoalveolar lavage samples from healthy human volunteers. *Am. Rev. Respir. Dis.* 126: 611–616.
12. Carre, P., Laviolette, M., Belanger, J., and Cormier, Y. (1985). Technical variations of bronchoalveolar lavage (BAL): influence of atelectasis and the lung region lavaged. *Lung* 163: 117–125.
13. Kelly, C.A., Kotre, C.J., Ward, C. et al. (1987). Anatomical distribution of bronchoalveolar lavage fluid as assessed by digital subtraction radiography. *Thorax* 42: 624–628.
14. Baughman, R.P. (2007). Technical aspects of bronchoalveolar lavage: recommendations for a standard procedure. *Semin. Respir. Crit. Care Med.* 28: 475–485.
15. King, T.E. (1992). The handling and analysis of bronchoalveolar lavage specimens. In: *Bronchoalveolar Lavage* (ed. R.P. Baughman), 3–29. St Louis: Mosby Year Book.
16. Crystal, R.G., Reynolds, H.Y., and Kalica, A.R. (1986). Bronchoalveolar lavage. The report of an international conference. *Chest* 90: 122–131.
17. Dohn, M.N. and Baughman, R.P. (1985). Effect of changing instilled volume for bronchoalveolar lavage in patients with interstitial lung disease. *Am. Rev. Respir. Dis.* 132: 390–392.
18. Lam, S., Leriche, J.C., Kijek, K., and Phillips, D. (1985). Effect of bronchial lavage volume on cellular and protein recovery. *Chest* 88: 856–859.
19. Rennard, S.I., Ghafouri, M., Thompson, A.B. et al. (1990). Fractional processing of sequential bronchoalveolar lavage to separate bronchial and alveolar samples. *Am. Rev. Respir. Dis.* 141: 208–217.
20. Daniele, R.P., Elias, J.A., Epstein, P.E., and Rossman, M.D. (1985). Bronchoalveolar lavage: role in the pathogenesis, diagnosis, and management of interstitial lung disease. *Ann. Intern. Med.* 102: 93–108.
21. BAL Cooperative Group Steering Committee (1990). Bronchoalveolar lavage constituents in healthy individuals, idiopathic pulmonary fibrosis, and selected comparison groups. *Am. Rev. Respir. Dis.* 141: S169–S202.
22. Baughman, R.P. and Lower, E.E. (1999). New treatment for sarcoidosis: where's the proof? *Eur. Respir. J.* 14: 1000–1001.
23. Tilles, D.S., Goldenheim, P.D., Ginns, L.C., and Hales, C.A. (1986). Pulmonary function in normal subjects and patients with sarcoidosis after bronchoalveolar lavage. *Chest* 89: 244–248.
24. Von Essen, S.G., Robbins, R.A., Spurzem, J.R. et al. (1991). Bronchoscopy with bronchoalveolar lavage causes neutrophil recruitment to the lower respiratory tract. *Am. Rev. Respir. Dis.* 144: 848–854.
25. Krause, A., Hohberg, B., Heine, F. et al. (1997). Cytokines derived from alveolar macrophages induce fever after bronchoscopy and bronchoalveolar lavage. *Am. J. Respir. Crit. Care Med.* 155: 1793–1797.
26. Hemmers, T., Nusslein, T., Teig, N. et al. (2006). Prospective study of fever after bronchoalveolar lavage in children. *Klin. Padiatr.* 218: 74–78.
27. Laviolette, M., Carreau, M., and Coulombe, R. (1988). Bronchoalveolar lavage cell differential on microscope glass cover. A simple and accurate technique. *Am. Rev. Respir. Dis.* 138: 451–457.
28. Cole, P., Turton, C., Lanyon, H., and Collins, J. (1980). Bronchoalveolar lavage for the preparation of free lung cells: technique and complications. *Br. J. Dis. Chest* 74: 273–278.
29. Ognibene, F.P., Shelhamer, J., Gill, V. et al. (1984). The diagnosis of *Pneumocystis carinii* pneumonia in patients with the acquired immunodeficiency syndrome using subsegmental bronchoalveolar lavage. *Am. Rev. Respir. Dis.* 129: 929–932.
30. Lin, C.C., Wu, J.L., and Huang, W.C. (1988). Pulmonary function in normal subjects after bronchoalveolar lavage. *Chest* 93: 1049–1053.
31. Hattotuwa, K., Gamble, E.A., O'Shaughnessy, T. et al. (2002). Safety of bronchoscopy, biopsy, and BAL in research patients with COPD. *Chest* 122: 1909–1912.
32. Ouellette, D.R. (2006). The safety of bronchoscopy in a pulmonary fellowship program. *Chest* 130: 1185–1190.

33 Elston, W.J., Whittaker, A.J., Khan, L.N. et al. (2004). Safety of research bronchoscopy, biopsy and bronchoalveolar lavage in asthma. *Eur. Respir. J.* 24: 375–377.

34 Cordonnier, C., Bernaudin, J.F., Fleury, J. et al. (1985). Diagnostic yield of bronchoalveolar lavage in pneumonitis occurring after allogeneic bone marrow transplantation. *Am. Rev. Respir. Dis.* 132: 1118–1123.

35 Gurney, J.W., Harrison, W.C., Sears, K. et al. (1987). Bronchoalveolar lavage: radiographic manifestations. *Radiology* 163: 71–74.

36 Laviolette, M. (1985). Lymphocyte fluctuation in bronchoalveolar lavage fluid in normal volunteers. *Thorax* 40: 651–656.

37 Marcy, T.W., Merrill, W.W., Rankin, J.A., and Reynolds, H.Y. (1987). Limitations of using urea to quantify epithelial lining fluid recovered by bronchoalveolar lavage. *Am. Rev. Respir. Dis.* 135: 1276–1280.

38 Stover, D.E., White, D.A., Romano, P.A., and Gellene, R.A. (1984). Diagnosis of pulmonary disease in acquired immune deficiency syndrome (AIDS). Role of bronchoscopy and bronchoalveolar lavage. *Am. Rev. Respir. Dis.* 130: 659–662.

39 Thompson, A.B., Robbins, R.A., Ghafouri, M.A. et al. (1989). Bronchoalveolar lavage fluid processing. Effect of membrane filtration preparation on neutrophil recovery. *Acta Cytol.* 33: 544–549.

40 Rankin, J.A., Naegel, G.P., and Reynolds, H.Y. (1986). Use of a central laboratory for analysis of bronchoalveolar lavage fluid. *Am. Rev. Respir. Dis.* 133: 186–190.

41 Kelly, C., Ward, C., Bird, G. et al. (1989). The effect of filtration on absolute and differential cell counts in fluid obtained at bronchoalveolar lavage. *Respir. Med.* 83: 107–110.

42 Winquist, A.G., Orrico, M.A., and Peterson, L.R. (1997). Evaluation of the cyto-centrifuge gram stain as a screening test for bacteriuria in specimens from specific patient populations. *Am. J. Clin. Pathol.* 108: 515–524.

43 Armbruster, C., Pokieser, L., and Hassl, A. (1995). Diagnosis of *Pneumocystis carinii* pneumonia by bronchoalveolar lavage in AIDS patients. Comparison of Diff-Quik, fungifluorstain, direct immunofluorescence test and polymerase chain reaction. *Acta Cytol.* 39: 1089–1093.

44 De Brauwer, E.I., Jacobs, J.A., Nieman, F. et al. (2002). Bronchoalveolar lavage fluid differential cell count. How many cells should be counted? *Anal. Quant. Cytol. Histol.* 24: 337–341.

45 Smith, P.A., Kohli, L.M., Wood, K.L. et al. (2006). Cytometric analysis of BAL T cells labeled with a standardized antibody cocktail correlates with immunohistochemical staining. *Cytometry B Clin. Cytom.* 70: 170–178.

46 Welker, L., Jorres, R.A., Costabel, U., and Magnussen, H. (2004). Predictive value of BAL cell differentials in the diagnosis of interstitial lung diseases. *Eur. Respir. J.* 24: 1000–1006.

47 Emad, A. and Emad, Y. (2007). CD4/CD8 ratio and cytokine levels of the BAL fluid in patients with bronchiectasis caused by sulfur mustard gas inhalation. *J. Inflamm. (Lond.)* 4: 2.

48 Costabel, U. (1998). *Atlas of Bronchoalveolar Lavage*. London: Chapman & Hall Medical.

49 Costabel, U. and Guzman, J. (1992). Effect of smoking on bronchoalveolar lavage constituents. *Eur. Respir. J.* 5: 776–779.

50 Meyer, K.C. and Soergel, P. (1999). Variation of bronchoalveolar lymphocyte phenotypes with age in the physiologically normal human lung. *Thorax* 54: 697–700.

51 Rose, A.S. and Knox, K.S. (2007). Bronchoalveolar lavage as a research tool. *Semin. Respir. Crit. Care Med.* 28: 561–573.

52 Hunninghake, G.W., Kawanami, O., Ferrans, V.J. et al. (1981). Characterization of the inflammatory and immune effector cells in the lung parenchyma of patients with interstitial lung disease. *Am. Rev. Respir. Dis.* 123: 407–412.

53 Baughman, R.P. and Drent, M. (2001). Role of bronchoalveolar lavage in interstitial lung disease. *Clin. Chest Med.* 22: 331–341.

54 Hunninghake, G.W. and Crystal, R.G. (1981). Pulmonary sarcoidosis: a disorder mediated by excess helper T-lymphocyte activity at sites of disease activity. *N. Engl. J. Med.* 305: 429–434.

55 Costabel, U. and King, T.E. (2001). International consensus statement on idiopathic pulmonary fibrosis. *Eur. Respir. J.* 17: 163–167.

56 Drent, M., Grutters, J.C., Mulder, P.G. et al. (1997). Is the different T helper cell activity in sarcoidosis and extrinsic allergic alveolitis also reflected by the cellular bronchoalveolar lavage fluid profile? *Sarcoidosis Vasc. Diffuse Lung Dis.* 14: 31–38.

57 Takahashi, T., Azuma, A., Abe, S. et al. (2001). Significance of lymphocytosis in bronchoalveolar lavage in suspected ocular sarcoidosis. *Eur. Respir. J.* 18: 515–521.

58 Drent, M., Jacobs, J.A., Cobben, N.A. et al. (2001). Computer program supporting the diagnostic accuracy of cellular BALF analysis: a new release. *Respir. Med.* 95: 781–786.

59 Winterbauer, R.H., Lammert, J., Selland, M. et al. (1993). Bronchoalveolar lavage cell populations in the diagnosis of sarcoidosis. *Chest* 104: 352–361.

60 Costabel, U. and Guzman, J. (2001). Bronchoalveolar lavage in interstitial lung disease. *Curr. Opin. Pulm. Med.* 7: 255–261.

61 Drent, M., van Velzen-Blad, H., Diamant, M. et al. (1993). Relationship between presentation of sarcoidosis and T lymphocyte profile. A study in bronchoalveolar lavage fluid. *Chest* 104: 795–800.

62 Drent, M., Mansour, K., and Linssen, C. (2007). Bronchoalveolar lavage in sarcoidosis. *Semin. Respir. Crit. Care Med.* 28: 486–495.

63 Costabel, U. (1997). CD4/CD8 ratios in bronchoalveolar lavage fluid: of value for diagnosing sarcoidosis? *Eur. Respir. J.* 10: 2699–2700.

64 Grunewald, J. and Eklund, A. (2007). Sex-specific manifestations of Lofgren's syndrome. *Am. J. Respir. Crit. Care Med.* 175: 40–44.

65 Kolopp-Sarda, M.N., Kohler, C., de March, A.K. et al. (2000). Discriminative immunophenotype of bronchoalveolar lavage CD4 lymphocytes in sarcoidosis. *Lab. Invest.* 80: 1065–1069.

66 Patricia, C.M., Antonio, M., Carmo, P. et al. (2012). Diagnostic value of CD103 expression in bronchoalveolar lymphocytes in sarcoidosis. *Respir. Med.* 106: 104–120.

67 Drent, M., Jacobs, J.A., de Vries, J. et al. (1999). Does the cellular bronchoalveolar lavage fluid profile reflect the severity of sarcoidosis? *Eur. Respir. J.* 13: 1338–1344.

68 Ziegenhagen, M.W., Rothe, M.E., Zissel, G., and Muller-

Quernheim, J. (2002). Exaggerated TNFalpha release of alveolar macrophages in corticosteroid resistant sarcoidosis. *Sarcoidosis Vasc. Diffuse Lung Dis.* 19: 185–190.

69 American Thoracic Society/European Respiratory Society. International Multidisciplinary Consensus Classification of the Idiopathic Interstitial Pneumonias (2002). This joint statement of the American Thoracic Society (ATS), and the European Respiratory Society (ERS) was adopted by the ATS board of directors, June 2001 and by the ERS Executive Committee, June 2001. *Am. J. Respir. Crit. Care Med.* 165: 277–304.

70 William, D.T., Ulrich, C., David, M.H. et al. (2013). An official American Thoracic Society/European Respiratory Society statement: update of the international multidisciplinary classification of the idiopathic interstitial pneumonias. *Am. J. Respir. Crit. Care Med.* 188: 733–748.

71 Travis, W.D., Hunninghake, G., King, T.E. Jr. et al. (2008). Idiopathic nonspecific interstitial pneumonia: report of an American Thoracic Society project. *Am. J. Respir. Crit. Care Med.* 177: 1338–1347.

72 Raghu, G., Collard, H.R., Egan, J.J. et al. (2011). ATS/ERS/JRS/ALAT committee on idiopathic pulmonaryfibrosis. An official ATS/ERS/JRS/ALAT statement: idiopathic pulmonary fibrosis: evidence-based guidelines for diagnosis and management. *Am. J. Respir. Crit. Care Med.* 183: 788–824.

73 Nagao, T., Nagai, S., Kitaichi, M. et al. (2001). Usual interstitial pneumonia: idiopathic pulmonary fibrosis versus collagen vascular diseases. *Respiration* 68: 151–159.

74 Ryu, Y.J., Chung, M.P., Han, J. et al. (2007). Bronchoalveolar lavage in fibrotic idiopathic interstitial pneumonias. *Respir. Med.* 101: 655–660.

75 Papiris, S.A., Kollintza, A., Kitsanta, P. et al. (2005). Relationship of BAL and lung tissue CD4+ and CD8+ T lymphocytes, and their ratio in idiopathic pulmonary fibrosis. *Chest* 128: 2971–2977.

76 Athol, U.W. and Maria, A.K. (2017). Should BAL be routinely performed in the diagnostic evaluation of idiopathic pulmonary fibrosis? Yes. *Chest* 152: 917–919.

77 Flaherty, K.R., Travis, W.D., Colby, T.V. et al. (2001). Histopathologic variability in usual and nonspecific interstitial pneumonias. *Am. J. Respir. Crit. Care Med.* 164: 1722–1727.

78 Espoladore, L.M., Gregorio, B.B., Lima, M.S. et al. (2014). Cytological analysis of bronchoalveolar lavage in patients with interstitial lung diseases and the relation of cytological analysis to fibrosis in high-resolution computed tomography. *Anal. Quant. Cytopathol. Histpathol.* 36: 206–212.

79 Park, C.S., Jeon, J.W., Park, S.W. et al. (1996). Nonspecific interstitial pneumonia/fibrosis: clinical manifestations, histologic and radiologic features. *Korean J. Intern. Med.* 11: 122–132.

80 Boomars, K.A., Wagenaar, S.S., Mulder, P.G.H. et al. (1995). Relationship between cells obtained by bronchoalveolar lavage and survival in idiopathic pulmonary fibrosis. *Thorax* 50: 1087–1092.

81 Watters, L.C., Schwarz, M.I., Cherniack, R.M. et al. (1987). Idiopathic pulmonary fibrosis. Pretreatment bronchoalveolar lavage cellular constituents and their relationships with lung histopathology and clinical response to therapy. *Am. Rev. Respir. Dis.* 135: 696–704.

82 Nagai, S., Kitaichi, M., Itoh, H. et al. (1998). Idiopathic nonspecific interstitial pneumonia/fibrosis: comparison with idiopathic pulmonary fibrosis and BOOP. *Eur. Respir. J.* 12: 1010–1019.

83 Jara-Palomares, L., Gomez-Izquierdo, L., Gonzalez-Vergara, D. et al. (2010). Utility of high-resolution computed tomography and BAL in cryptogenic organizing pneumonia. *Respir. Med.* 104: 1706–1711.

84 Veeraraghavan, S., Latsi, P.I., Wells, A.U. et al. (2003). BAL findings in idiopathic nonspecific interstitial pneumonia and usual interstitial pneumonia. *Eur. Respir. J.* 22: 239–244.

85 Vasakova, M., Morell, F., Walsh, S. et al. (2017). Hypersensitivity pneumonitis: perspectives in diagnosis and management. *Am. J. Respir. Crit. CareMed.* 196 (6): 680–689.

86 Kouranos, V., Jacob, J., Nicholson, A. et al. (2017). Fibrotic hypersensitivity pneumonitis: key issues in diagnosis and management. *J. Clin. Med.* 6 (6): E62.

87 Ohshimo, S., Guzman, J., Costabel, U. et al. (2017). Differential diagnosis of granulomatous lung disease: clues and pitfalls: number 4 in the series "pathology for the clinician" edited by Peter Dorfmüller and Alberto Cavazza. *Eur. Respir. Rev.* 26 (145): 170012.

88 Gaxiola, M. and Buendia-Roldan, I. (2011). Morphologic diversity of chronic pigeon breeder's disease: clinical features and survival. *Respir. Med.* 105: 608–614.

89 Ohtani, Y. and Saiki, S. (2005). Chronic bird fancier's lung: histopathological and clinical correlation. An application of the 2002 ATS/ERS consensus classification of the idiopathic interstitial pneumonias. *Thorax* 60: 665–671.

90 Barrera, L. and Mendoza, F. (2008). Functional diversity of T-cell subpopulations in subacute and chronic hypersensitivity pneumonitis. *Am. J. Respir. Crit. Care Med.* 177: 44–55.

91 Caillaud, D.M. and Vergnon, J.M. (2012). Bronchoalveolar lavage in hypersensitivity pneumonitis: a series of 139 patients. *Inflamm. Allergy Drug Targets* 11: 15–19.

92 Selman, M. and Pardo, A. (2012). Hypersensitivity pneumonitis: insights in diagnosis and pathobiology. *Am. J. Respir. Crit. Care Med.* 186: 314–324.

93 Fournier, E., Tonnel, A.B., Gosset, P. et al. (1985). Early neutrophil alveolitis after antigen inhalation in hypersensitivity pneumonitis. *Chest* 88: 563–536.

94 Pereira, C.A., Gimenez, A., Kuranishi, L. et al. (2016). Chronic hypersensitivity pneumonitis. *J. Asthma Allergy* 9: 171–181.

95 Haslam, P.L., Dewar, A., Butchers, P. et al. (1987). Mast cells, atypical lymphocytes, and neutrophils in bronchoalveolar lavage in extrinsic allergic alveolitis. Comparison with other interstitial lung diseases. *Am. Rev. Respir. Dis.* 135: 35–47.

96 Mohr, L.C. (2004). Hypersensitivity pneumonitis. *Curr. Opin. Pulm. Med.* 10: 401–411.

97 Pardo, A., Barrios, R., Gaxiola, M. et al. (2000). Increase of lung neutrophilsin hypersensitivity pneumonitis is associated with lung fibrosis. *Am. J. Respir. Crit. Care Med.* 161: 1698–1704.

98 Haslam, P.L. (1987). Bronchoalveolar lavage in extrinsic allergic alveolitis. *Eur. J. Respir. Dis. Suppl.* 154: 120–135.

99 Bjermer, L., Engstrom-Laurent, A., Hallgren, R. et al. (1990). Bronchoalveolar lavage in persons acutely exposed to dust in the farm environment. *Am. J. Ind. Med.* 17: 106.

100 Cormier, Y., Belanger, J., and Laviolette, M. (1987). Prognostic significance of bronchoalveolar lymphocytosis in farmer's lung. *Am. Rev. Respir. Dis.* 135: 692–695.

101 Mossman, B.T., Bignon, J., Corn, M. et al. (1990). Asbestos: scientific developments and implications for public policy. *Science* 247: 294–301.

102 Rebuck, A.S. and Braude, A.C. (1983). Bronchoalveolar lavage in asbestosis. *Arch. Intern. Med.* 143: 950–952.

103 Dumortier, P., de Vuyst, P., and Yernault, J.C. (1988). Mineralogical analysis of bronchoalveolar lavage fluids. *Z. Erkr. Atmungsorgane* 171: 50–58.

104 De Vuyst, P., Dumortier, P., Moulin, E. et al. (1988). Asbestos bodies in bronchoalveolar lavage reflect lung asbestos body concentration. *Eur. Respir. J.* 1: 362–367.

105 De Vuyst, P., Jedwab, J., Dumortier, P. et al. (1982). Asbestos bodies in bronchoalveolar lavage. *Am. Rev. Respir. Dis.* 126: 972–976.

106 De Vuyst, P., Dumortier, P., Moulin, E. et al. (1987). Diagnostic value of asbestos bodies in bronchoalveolar lavage fluid. *Am. Rev. Respir. Dis.* 136: 1219–1224.

107 Churg, A. (1982). Fiber counting and analysis in the diagnosis of asbestos-related disease. *Hum. Pathol.* 13: 381–392.

108 Vathesatogkit, P., Harkin, T.J., Addrizzo-Harris, D.J. et al. (2004). Clinical correlation of asbestos bodies in BAL fluid. *Chest* 126: 966–971.

109 Kido, T., Morimoto, Y., Yatera, K. et al. (2017). The utility of electron microscopy in detecting asbestos fibers and particles in BALF in diffuse lung diseases. *BMC Pulm. Med.* 17 (1): 71.

110 Fireman, E. and Lerman, Y. (2006). Induced sputum in interstitial lung diseases. *Curr. Opin. Pulm. Med.* 12: 318–322.

111 Teschler, H., Thompson, A.B., Dollenkamp, R. et al. (1996). Relevance of asbestos bodies in sputum. *Eur. Respir. J.* 9: 680–686.

112 Epstein, P.E., Dauber, J.H., Rossman, M.D. et al. (1982). Bronchoalveolar lavage in a patient with chronic berylliosis: evidence for hypersensitivity pneumonitis. *Ann. Intern. Med.* 97: 213–216.

113 Mayer, A.S., Hamzeh, N., and Maier, L.A. (2014). Sarcoidosis and chronic beryllium disease: similarities and differences. *Semin. Respir. Crit. CareMed.* 35 (3): 316–329.

114 Li, L., Hamzeh, N., Gillespie, M. et al. (2015). Beryllium increases the CD14(dim)CD16+ subset in the lung of chronic beryllium disease. *PLoS One* 10 (2): e0117276.

115 Rossman, M.D., Kern, J.A., Elias, J.A. et al. (1988). Proliferative response of bronchoalveolar lymphocytes to beryllium. A test for chronic beryllium disease. *Ann. Intern. Med.* 108: 687–693.

116 Newman, L.S., Mroz, M.M., Balkissoon, R. et al. (2005). Beryllium sensitization progresses to chronic beryllium disease: a longitudinal study of disease risk. *Am. J. Respir. Crit. Care Med.* 171: 54–60.

117 Allen, J.N., Davis, W.B., and Pacht, E.R. (1990). Diagnostic significance of increased bronchoalveolar lavage fluid eosinophils. *Am. Rev. Respir. Dis.* 142: 642–647.

118 Bjermer, L., Lundgren, R., and Hallgren, R. (1989). Hyaluronan and type III procollagen peptide concentrations in bronchoalveolar lavage fluid in idiopathic pulmonary fibrosis. *Thorax* 44: 126–131.

119 Blaschke, E., Eklund, A., and Hernbrand, R. (1990). Extracellular matrix components in bronchoalveolar lavage fluid in sarcoidosis and their relationship to signs of alveolitis. *Am. Rev. Respir. Dis.* 141: 1020–1025.

120 O'Connor, C., Ward, K., van Breda, A. et al. (1989). Type 3 procollagen peptide in bronchoalveolar lavage fluid. Poor indicator of course and prognosis in sarcoidosis. *Chest* 96: 339–344.

121 Ward, K., O'Connor, C.M., Odlum, C. et al. (1990). Pulmonary disease progress in sarcoid patients with and without bronchoalveolar lavage collagenase. *Am. Rev. Respir. Dis.* 142: 636–641.

122 Costabel, U., Guzman, J., Bonella, F., and Oshimo, S. (2007). Bronchoalveolar lavage in other interstitial lung diseases. *Semin. Respir. Crit. Care Med.* 28: 514–524.

123 Lazor, R. and Cordier, J. (2007). Idiopathic eosinophilic pneumonias. In: *Diffuse Parenchymal Lung Disease*, vol. 36 (eds. U. Costabel and R.M. du Bois), 238–249. Basel: Karger.

124 Philit, F., Etienne-Mastroianni, B., Parrot, A. et al. (2002). Idiopathic acute eosinophilic pneumonia: a study of 22 patients. *Am. J. Respir. Crit. Care Med.* 166: 1235–1239.

125 Pope-Harman, A.L., Davis, W.B., Allen, E.D. et al. (1996). Acute eosinophilic pneumonia. A summary of 15 cases and review of the literature. *Medicine (Baltimore)* 75: 334–342.

126 Marchand, E., Etienne-Mastroianni, B., Chanez, P. et al. (2003). Idiopathic chronic eosinophilic pneumonia and asthma: how do they influence each other? *Eur. Respir. J.* 22: 8–13.

127 Marchand, E., Reynaud-Gaubert, M., Lauque, D. et al. (1998). Idiopathic chronic eosinophilic pneumonia. A clinical and follow-up study of 62 cases. The Groupe d'Etudes et de Recherche sur les Maladies "Orphelines" Pulmonaires (GERM"O"P). *Medicine (Baltimore)* 77: 299–312.

128 Katoh, S., Matsumoto, N., Matsumoto, K. et al. (2004). Elevated interleukin-18 levels in bronchoalveolar lavage fluid of patients with eosinophilic pneumonia. *Allergy* 59: 850–856.

129 Kita, H., Sur, S., Edell, E.S. et al. (1996). Cytokine production at the site of disease in chronic eosinophilic pneumonitis. *Am. J. Respir. Crit. Care Med.* 153: 1437–1441.

130 Miyazaki, E., Nureki, S., Fukami, T. et al. (2002). Elevated levels of thymus- and activation-regulated chemokine in bronchoalveolar lavage fluid from patients with eosinophilic pneumonia. *Am. J. Respir. Crit. CareMed.* 165: 1125–1131.

131 Katoh, S., Fukushima, K., Matsumoto, M. et al. (2003). Accumulation of CCR4-expressing CD4 T cells and high concentration of its ligands (TARC and MDC) in bronchoalveolar lavage fluid of patients with eosinophilic pneumonia. *Allergy* 58: 518–523.

132 Praveen, A. and Peter, F.W. (2012). Eosinophilic

133 Caimi, B., Iftach, S., and Leonid, B. (2018). Drug- induced eosinophilic pneumonia: a review of 196 case reports. *Medicine* 97: 1–6.

134 Bouros, D., Wells, A.U., Nicholson, A.G. et al. (2002). Histopathologic subsets of fibrosing alveolitis in patients with systemic sclerosis and their relationship to outcome. *Am. J. Respir. Crit. Care Med.* 165: 1581–1586.

135 Silver, R.M., Miller, K.S., Kinsella, M.B. et al. (1990). Evaluation and management of scleroderma lung disease using bronchoalveolar lavage. *Am. J. Med.* 88: 470–476.

136 Goh, N.S., Veeraraghavan, S., Desai, S.R. et al. (2007). Bronchoalveolar lavage cellular profiles in patients with systemic sclerosis-associated interstitial lung disease are not predictive of disease progression. *Arthritis Rheum.* 56: 2005–2012.

137 Wells, A.U., Hansell, D.M., Haslam, P.L. et al. (1998). Bronchoalveolar lavage cellularity: lone cryptogenic fibrosing alveolitis compared with the fibrosing alveolitis of systemic sclerosis. *Am. J. Respir. Crit. CareMed.* 157: 1474–1482.

138 Steen, V.D., Conte, C., Owens, G.R. et al. (1994). Severe restrictive lung disease in systemic sclerosis. *Arthritis Rheum.* 37: 1283–1289.

139 Basset, F., Soler, P., Jaurand, M.C., and Bignon, J. (1977). Ultrastructural examination of broncho-alveolar lavage for diagnosis of pulmonary histiocytosis X: preliminary report on 4 cases. *Thorax* 32: 303–306.

140 Casolaro, M.A., Bernaudin, J.F., Saltini, C. et al. (1988). Accumulation of Langerhans' cells on the epithelial surface of the lower respiratory tract in normal subjects in association with cigarette smoking. *Am. Rev. Respir. Dis.* 137: 406–411.

141 Soler, P., Moreau, A., Basset, F., and Hance, A.J. (1989). Cigarette smoking-induced changes in the number and differentiated state of pulmonary dendritic cells/Langerhans cells. *Am. Rev. Respir. Dis.* 139: 1112–1117.

142 Collard, H.R. and Schwarz, M.I. (2004). Diffuse alveolar hemorrhage. *Clin. Chest Med.* 25: 583–592.

143 Zamora, M.R., Warner, M.L., Tuder, R., and Schwarz, M.I. (1997). Diffuse alveolar hemorrhage and systemic lupus erythematosus. Clinical presentation, histology, survival, and outcome. *Medicine (Baltimore)* 76: 192–202.

144 Fontenot, A.P. and Schwarz, M.I. (2003). Diffuse alveolar hemorrhage. In: *Interstitial Lung Disease*, 4e (eds. T.E. King and S. Schwartz), 632–656. Hamilton, Canada: B.C. Decker.

145 De Lassence, A., Fleury-Feith, J., Escudier, E. et al. (1995). Alveolar hemorrhage. Diagnostic criteria and results in 194 immunocompromised hosts. *Am. J. Respir. Crit. Care Med.* 151: 157–163.

146 Springmeyer, S.C., Hoges, J., and Hammar, S.P. (1984). Significance of hemosiderin-laden macrophages in bronchoalveolar lavage fluid. *Am. Rev. Respir. Dis.* 131: A76.

147 Stover, D.E., Zaman, M.B., Hajdu, S.I. et al. (1984). Bronchoalveolar lavage in the diagnosis of diffuse pulmonary infiltrates in the immunosuppressed host. *Ann. Intern. Med.* 101: 1–7.

148 Drew, W.L., Finley, T.N., and Golde, D.W. (1977). Diagnostic lavage and occult pulmonary hemorrhage in thrombocytopenic immunocompromised patients. *Am. Rev. Respir. Dis.* 116: 215–221.

149 Finley, T.N., Aronow, A., Cosentino, A.M., and Golde, D.W. (1975). Occult pulmonary hemorrhage in anticoagulated patients. *Am. Rev. Respir. Dis.* 112: 23–29.

150 Huaringa, A.J., Leyva, F.J., Signes-Costa, J. et al. (2000). Bronchoalveolar lavage in the diagnosis of pulmonary complications of bone marrow transplant patients. *Bone Marrow Transplant.* 25: 975–979.

151 Sherman, J.M., Winnie, G., Thomassen, M.J. et al. (1984). Time course of hemosiderin production and clearance by human pulmonary macrophages. *Chest* 86: 409–411.

152 Bonfield, T.L., Russell, D., Burgess, S. et al. (2002). Autoantibodies against granulocyte macrophage colony-stimulating factor are diagnostic for pulmonary alveolar proteinosis. *Am. J. Respir. Cell Mol. Biol.* 27: 481–486.

153 Kitamura, T., Tanaka, N., Watanabe, J. et al. (1999). Idiopathic pulmonary alveolar proteinosis as an autoimmune disease with neutralizing antibody against granulocyte/macrophage colony-stimulating factor. *J. Exp. Med.* 190: 875–880.

154 Uchida, K., Nakata, K., Trapnell, B.C. et al. (2004). High-affinity autoantibodies specifically eliminate granulocyte-macrophage colony stimulating factor activity in the lungs of patients with idiopathic pulmonary alveolar proteinosis. *Blood* 103: 1089–1098.

155 John, F.S. and Jeffrey, J.P. (2002). Pulmonary alveolar proteinosis: progress in the first 44 years. *Am. J. Respir. Crit. Care Med.* 166: 215–235.

156 Shah, P.L., Hansell, D., Lawson, P.R. et al. (2000). Pulmonary alveolar proteinosis: clinical aspects and current concepts on pathogenesis. *Thorax* 55: 67–77.

157 Wang, B.M., Stern, E.J., Schmidt, R.A., and Pierson, D.J. (1997). Diagnosing pulmonary alveolar proteinosis: a review and update. *Chest* 111: 460–466.

158 Maygarden, S.J., Iacocca, M.V., Funkhouser, W.K. et al. (2001). Pulmonary alveolar proteinosis: a spectrum of cytologic, histochemical, and ultrastructural findings in bronchoalveolar lavage fluid. *Diagn. Cytopathol.* 24: 389–395.

159 Shen, H.Q., Duan, C.X., Li, Z.Y. et al. (1997). Effects of proteinosis surfactant proteins on the viability of rat alveolar macrophages. *Am. J. Respir. Crit. Care Med.* 156: 1679–1687.

160 Chou, C.W., Lin, F.C., Tung, S.M. et al. (2001). Diagnosis of pulmonary alveolar proteinosis: usefulness of papanicolaou-stained smears of bronchoalveolar lavage fluid. *Arch. Intern. Med.* 161: 562–566.

161 Costello, J.F., Moriarty, D.C., Branthwaite, M.A. et al. (1975). Diagnosis and management of alveolar proteinosis: the role of electron microscopy. *Thorax* 30: 121–132.

162 Gilmore, L.B., Talley, F.A., and Hook, G.E.R. (1988). Classification and morphometric quantification of insoluble materials from the lungs of patients with alveolar proteinosis. *Am. J. Pathol.* 133: 252–264.

163 Costabel, U. and Guzman, J. (2005). Pulmonary alveolar

proteinosis: a new autoimmune disease. *Sarcoidosis Vasc. Diffuse Lung Dis.* 22 (Suppl 1): S67–S73.

164 Danel, C., Israel-Biet, D., Costabel, U., and Klech, H. (1992). Therapeutic applications of bronchoalveolar lavage. *Eur. Respir. J.* 5: 1173–1175.

165 Mikami, T., Yamamoto, Y., Yokoyama, M., and Okayasu, I. (1997). Pulmonary alveolar proteinosis: diagnosis using routinely processed smears of bronchoalveolar lavage fluid. *J. Clin. Pathol.* 50: 981–984.

166 Brutinel, W.M. and Martin, W.J. 2nd. (1986). Chronic nitrofurantoin reaction associated with T-lymphocyte alveolitis. *Chest* 89: 150–152.

167 Costabel, U., Uzaslan, E., and Guzman, J. (2004). Bronchoalveolar lavage in drug-induced lung disease. *Clin. Chest Med.* 25: 25–35.

168 Fuhrman, C., Parrot, A., Wislez, M. et al. (2001). Spectrum of CD4 to CD8 T-cell ratios in lymphocytic alveolitis associated with methotrexate-induced pneumonitis. *Am. J. Respir. Crit. Care Med.* 164: 1186–1191.

169 Schnabel, A., Richter, C., Bauerfeind, S., and Gross, W.L. (1997). Bronchoalveolar lavage cell profile in methotrexate induced pneumonitis. *Thorax* 52: 377–379.

170 Costabel, U., Teschler, H., and Guzman, J. (1992). Bronchiolitis obliterans organizing pneumonia (BOOP): the cytological and immuno-cytological profile of bronchoalveolar lavage. *Eur. Respir. J.* 5: 791–797.

171 Akoun, G.M., Cadranel, J.L., Blanchette, G. et al. (1991). Bronchoalveolar lavage cell data in amiodarone-associated pneumonitis. Evaluation in 22 patients. *Chest* 99: 1177–1182.

172 Martin, W.J. 2nd and Rosenow, E.C. 3rd. (1988). Amiodarone pulmonary toxicity. Recognition and pathogenesis (partI). *Chest* 93: 1067–1075.

173 Coudert, B., Bailly, F., Lombard, J.N. et al. (1992). Amiodarone pneumonitis. Bronchoalveolar lavage findings in 15 patients and review of the literature. *Chest* 102: 1005–1012.

174 Katz, U. and Shoenfeld, Y. (2008). Pulmonary eosinophilia. *Clin. Rev. Allergy Immunol.* 34: 367–371.

175 Popovich, J. Jr., Kvale, P.A., Eichenhorn, M.S. et al. (1982). Diagnostic accuracy of multiple biopsies from flexible fiberoptic bronchoscopy. A comparison of central versus peripheral carcinoma. *Am. Rev. Respir. Dis.* 125: 521–523.

176 Shure, D. and Fedullo, P.F. (1983). Transbronchial needle aspiration of peripheral masses. *Am. Rev. Respir. Dis.* 128: 1090–1092.

177 Huang, H., Ning, Y., Zhang, W. et al. (2017). Multiple guided technologies based on radial probe endobronchial ultrasound for the diagnosis of solitary peripheral pulmonary lesions: a single-center study. *J. Cancer* 8: 3514–3521.

178 Bellocq, A., Antoine, M., Flahault, A. et al. (1998). Neutrophil alveolitis in bronchioloalveolar carcinoma: induction by tumor-derived interleukin-8 and relation to clinical outcome. *Am. J. Pathol.* 152: 83–92.

179 Poletti, V., Poletti, G., Murer, B. et al. (2007). Bronchoalveolar lavage in malignancy. *Semin. Respir. Crit. Care Med.* 28: 534–545.

180 Poletti, V., Romagna, M., Allen, K.A. et al. (1995). Bronchoalveolar lavage in the diagnosis of disseminated lung tumors. *Acta Cytol.* 39: 472–477.

181 Semenzato, G. and Poletti, V. (1992). Bronchoalveolar lavage in lung cancer. *Respiration* 59 (Suppl 1): 44–46.

182 Ahmed, A. and Ahmed, S. (2004). Comparison of bronchoalveolar lavage cytology and transbronchial biopsy in the diagnosis of carcinoma of lung. *J. Ayub Med. Coll. Abbottabad* 16 (4): 29–33.

183 Saumya, S., Kiran, P.M., Nuzhat, H. et al. (2015). The utility of cytology in the diagnosis of adenocarcinoma lung: a tertiary care center study. *J. Cytol.* 32 (3): 159–164.

184 Sojung, P., Jae, Y.H., Kye, Y.L. et al. (2017). Assessment of EGFR mutation status using cell-free DNA from bronchoalveolar lavage fluid. *Clin. Chem. Lab. Med.* 55 (10): 1489–1495.

185 Wislez, M., Massiani, M.A., Milleron, B. et al. (2003). Clinical characteristics of pneumonic-type adenocarcinoma of the lung. *Chest* 123: 1868–1877.

186 Morales, F.M. and Matthews, J.I. (1987). Diagnosis of parenchymal Hodgkin's disease using bronchoalveolar lavage. *Chest* 91: 785–787.

187 Wisecarver, J., Ness, M.J., Rennard, S.I. et al. (1989). Bronchoalveolar lavage in the assessment of pulmonary Hodgkin's disease. *Acta Cytol.* 33: 527–532.

188 Levy, H., Horak, D.A., and Lewis, M.I. (1988). The value of bronchial washings and bronchoalveolar lavage in the diagnosis of lymphangitic carcinomatosis. *Chest* 94: 1028–1030.

189 Radio, S.J., Rennard, S.I., Kessinger, A. et al. (1989). Breast carcinoma in bronchoalveolar lavage. A cytologic and immunocytochemical study. *Arch. Pathol. Lab. Med.* 113: 333–336.

190 Beskow, C.O., Drachenberg, C.B., Bourquin, P.M. et al. (2000). Diffuse alveolar damage. Morphologic features in bronchoalveolar lavage fluid. *Acta Cytol.* 44: 640–646.

191 Rennard, S.I. (1990). Bronchoalveolar lavage in the diagnosis of cancer. *Lung* 168 (Suppl): 1035–1040.

192 Stanley, M.W., Henry-Stanley, M.J., Gajl-Peczalska, K.J., and Bitterman, P.B. (1992). Hyperplasia of type II pneumocytes in acute lung injury. Cytologic findings of sequential bronchoalveolar lavage. *Am. J. Clin. Pathol.* 97: 669–677.

193 Sampsonas, F., Kontoyiannis, D.P., Dickey, B.F. et al. (2011). Performance of a standardized bronchoalveolar lavage protocol in a comprehensive cancer center: a prospective 2-year study. *Cancer* 117: 3424–3433.

194 Maschmeyer, G., Beinert, T., Buchheidt, D. et al. (2009). Diagnosis and antimicrobial therapy of lung infiltrates in febrile neutropenic patients: guidelines of the infectious diseases working party of the German Society of Haematology and Oncology. *Eur. J. Cancer* 45: 2462–2472.

195 Pereira Gomes, J.C., Pedreira, W.L. Jr., Araujo, E.M. et al. (2000). Impact of BAL in the management of pneumonia with treatment failure: positivity of BAL culture under

196 Velez, L., Correa, L.T., Maya, M.A. et al. (2007). Diagnostic accuracy of bronchoalveolar lavage samples in immunosuppressed patients with suspected pneumonia: analysis of a protocol. *Respir. Med.* 101: 2160–2167.

197 Iregui, M., Ward, S., Sherman, G. et al. (2002). Clinical importance of delays in the initiation of appropriate antibiotic treatment for ventilator-associated pneumonia. *Chest* 122: 262–268.

198 Luna, C.M., Aruj, P., Niederman, M.S. et al. (2006). Appropriateness and delay to initiate therapy in ventilator-associated pneumonia. *Eur. Respir. J.* 27: 158–164.

199 Canadian Critical Care Trials Group (2006). A randomized trial of diagnostic techniques for ventilator-associated pneumonia. *N. Engl. J. Med.* 355: 2619–2630.

200 Fagon, J.Y., Chastre, J., Wolff, M. et al. (2000). Invasive and noninvasive strategies for management of suspected ventilator-associated pneumonia. A randomized trial. *Ann. Intern. Med.* 132: 621–630.

201 Sole, V.J., Fernandez, J.A., Benitez, A.B. et al. (2000). Impact of quantitative invasive diagnostic techniques in the management and outcome of mechanically ventilated patients with suspected pneumonia. *Crit. Care Med.* 28: 2737–2741.

202 Kalil, A.C., Metersky, M.L., Klompas, M. et al. (2016). Management of adults with hospital-acquired and ventilator-associated pneumonia: 2016 clinical practice guidelines by the Infectious Diseases Society of America and the American Thoracic Society. *Clin. Infect. Dis.* 63 (5): e61–e111.

203 Dalhoff, K., Braun, J., Hollandt, H. et al. (1993). Diagnostic value of bronchoalveolar lavage in patients with opportunistic and non-opportunistic bacterial pneumonia. *Infection* 21: 291–296.

204 Chung, D.R., Song, J.H., Kim, S.H. et al. (2011). High prevalence of multidrug-resistant nonfermentersin hospital-acquired pneumonia in Asia. *Am. J. Respir. Crit. Care Med.* 184: 1409–1417.

205 Raman, K., Nailor, M.D., Nicolau, D.P. et al. (2013). Early antibiotic discontinuation in patients with clinically suspected ventilator-associated pneumonia and negative quantitative bronchoscopy cultures. *Crit. Care Med.* 41: 1656–1663.

206 Pisani, R.J. and Wright, A.J. (1992). Clinical utility of bronchoalveolar lavage in immunocompromised hosts. *Mayo Clin. Proc.* 67: 221–227.

207 Johnson, P.C., Hogg, K.M., and Sarosi, G.A. (1990). The rapid diagnosis of pulmonary infections in solid organ transplant recipients. *Semin. Respir. Infect.* 5: 2–9.

208 Kahn, F.W. and Jones, J.M. (1988). Analysis of bronchoalveolar lavage specimens from immunocompromised patients with a protocol applicable in the microbiology laboratory. *J. Clin. Microbiol.* 26: 1150–1155.

209 Martin, W.J. 2nd, Smith, T.F., Sanderson, D.R. et al. (1987). Role of bronchoalveolar lavage in the assessment of opportunistic pulmonary infections: utility and complications. *Mayo Clin. Proc.* 62: 549–557.

210 Xaubet, A., Torres, A., Marco, F. et al. (1989). Pulmonary infiltrates in immunocompromised patients. Diagnostic value of telescoping plugged catheter and bronchoalveolar lavage. *Chest* 95: 130–135.

211 Patterson, T.F., Thompson, G.R., Denning, D.W. et al. (2016). Practice guidelines for the diagnosis and management of aspergillosis: 2016 update by the Infectious Diseases Society of America. *Clin. Infect. Dis.* 63 (4): e1–e60.

212 Guegan, H., Robert-Gangneux, F., Camus, C. et al. (2018). Improving the diagnosis of invasive aspergillosis by the detection of Aspergillus in broncho-alveolar lavage fluid: comparison of non-culture-based assays. *J. Infect.* 76 (2): 196–205.

213 Castillo, C.G., Kauffman, C.A., Zhai, J. et al. (2018). Testing the performance of a prototype lateral flow device using bronchoalveolar lavage fluid for the diagnosis of invasive pulmonary aspergillosis in high-risk patients. *Mycoses* 61 (1): 4–10.

214 Laughlen, G.F. (1925). Studies on pneumonia following nasopharyngeal injection of oil. *Am. J. Pathol.* 1: 407–414.

215 Sung, S., Tazelaar, H.D., Crapanzano, P. et al. (2018). Adult exogenous lipoid pneumonia: a rare and under recognized entity in cytology – a case series. *Cytojournal* 15: 17.

216 Baron, S.E., Haramati, L.B., and Rivera, V.T. (2003). Radiological and clinical findings in acute and chronic exogenous lipoid pneumonia. *J. Thorac. Imaging* 18: 217–224.

217 Laurent, F., Philippe, J.C., Vergier, B. et al. (1999). Exogenous lipoid pneumonia: HRCT, MR, and pathologic findings. *Eur. Radiol.* 9: 1190–1196.

218 Betancourt, S.L., Martinez-Jimenez, S., Rossi, S.E. et al. (2010). Lipoid pneumonia: spectrum of clinical and radiologic manifestations. *Am. J. Roentgenol.* 194: 103–109.

219 Marangu, D., Pillay, K., Banderker, E. et al. (2018). Exogenous lipoid pneumonia: an important cause of interstitial lung disease in infants. *Respirol. Case Rep.* 6 (7): e00356.

220 Brown, A.C., Slocum, P.C., Putthoff, S.L. et al. (1994). Exogenous lipoid pneumonia due to nasal application of petroleum jelly. *Chest* 105: 968–969.

221 de Albuquerque Filho, A.P. (2006). Exogenous lipoid pneumonia: importance of clinical history to the diagnosis. *J. Bras. Pneumol.* 32: 596–598.

222 Ganso, M., Goebel, R., Melhorn, S. et al. (2016). Lipoid pneumonia associated with lipid-containing nasal sprays and nose drops. *Laryngorhinootologie* 95: 534–539.

223 Gattuso, P., Reddy, V.B., and Castelli, M.J. (1991). Exogenous lipoid pneumonitis due to vicks vaporub inhalation diagnosed by fine needle aspiration cytology. *Cytopathology* 2: 315–316.

224 Glynn, K.P. and Gale, N.A. (1990). Exogenous lipoid pneumonia due to inhalation of spray lubricant (WD-40 lung). *Chest* 97: 1265–1266.

225 Lizarzábal Suárez, P.C., Núñez Savall, E., and Carrión, V.F. (2015). Lipoid pneumonia due to accidental aspiration of paraffin in a "fire-eater". *Arch. Bronconeumol.* 51: 530–531.

226 Majori, M., Scarascia, A., Anghinolfi, M. et al. (2014). Lipoid pneumonia as a complication of Lorenzo's oil therapy in a patient with adrenoleukodystrophy. *J. Bronchology Interv. Pulmonol.* 21: 271–273.

227 Osman, G.A., Ricci, A., Terzo, F. et al. (2016). Exogenous lipoid pneumonia induced by nasal decongestant. *Clin. Respir. J.* 12: 524–531.

228 Yampara Guarachi, G.I., Barbosa Moreira, V., Santos Ferreira, A. et al. (2014). Lipoid pneumonia in a gas station attendant. *Case Rep. Pulmonol.* 2014: 358761.

229 Hadda, V. and Khilnani, G.C. (2010). Lipoid pneumonia: an overview. *Expert Rev. Respir. Med.* 4: 799–807.

第 15 章

支气管镜肺活检术

Sean McKay[1], Robert F. Browning Jr.[1], J. Francis Turner, Jr.[2,3], and Ko-Pen Wang[4]

[1] Interventional Pulmonology, Walter Reed National Military Medical Center;
Uniformed Services University of Health Sciences, Bethesda, MD, USA
[2] Division of Pulmonary and Critical Care Medicine,
University of Tennessee Graduate School of Medicine, Knoxville, TN, USA
[3] National Supercomputing Institute, University of Nevada, Las Vegas, NV, USA
[4] Division of Pulmonary and Critical Care Medicine, Johns Hopkins Bayview Medical Center,
Johns Hopkins University School of Medicine, Baltimore, MD, USA

（译者：刘庆华　译者单位：同济大学附属东方医院）

15.1　引言

多年来，用于局灶性和弥漫性肺部疾病的诊断性肺活检一直是通过开胸手术完成。对于间质性肺疾病的早期调查，这些大标本的肺实质组织病理学结果特别有用[1,2]。使用经皮切割针和穿刺针活检快速获取肺组织的方法也曾用于获取肺实质标本，但由于该方法死亡率和并发症发生率高，在很大程度上已被摒弃[3-9]。1965 年，梅奥诊所的 Andersen 等报道了 13 例支气管镜肺活检（bronchoscopic lung biopsy, BLB）或经支气管镜肺活检术（transbronchial lung biopsy, TBLB）的技术和研究结果，他们的团队采用硬质支气管镜技术完成活检[10]。随后的研究支持了这些初步结果，并证明了最初的 450 例患者，其中 84% 可以通过硬质支气管镜检查成功获得肺组织[10-13]。

20 世纪 60 年代末，引入了可弯曲支气管镜，加大了支气管镜技术的普及，并正式使用可弯曲支气管镜进行经支气管活检术（transbronchial biopsy, TBBX），死亡率和并发症发生率较低[14-16]。1974 年 Levin 等首次描述了纤维支气管镜下 TBLB 的应用，Andersen 等证实 82% 的病例活检结果阳性[14,15]。因此，通过可弯曲支气管镜进行 TBBX，已在很大程度上取代了外科手术肺活检。几项观察性文献也参考引用了使用可弯曲支气管镜和活检器械进行经支气管肺活检技术。本章我们将这些活检技术称为 TBBX 或经支气管镜针吸活检术（transbronchial needle aspiration, TBNA）。

随着支气管镜的发展，通过可弯曲支气管镜进行肺活检的器械范围也在不断发展，诸如钳子大小和设计的不同差异，TBNA 在肺外周取样的临床应用也相应增加，温度依赖的肺外周活检技术也逐步开展应用，如近年来开展的肺外周冷冻活检技术。

自本书上一版 2012 年出版以来，文献检索显示，已经超过 8 500 篇参考文献关注 BLB 一词。因此，本章中我们综述了 BLB 最常见的适应证和技术要点，以及 TBNA 和冷冻肺活检在获取外周标本的作用和最新进展。

15.2　适应证

15.2.1　弥漫性肺疾病

影像学上表现为弥漫性肺疾病可能是 TBLB 的指征，与其他任何诊断性操作一样，在进行侵入性手术之前，应考虑操作临床相关性和其他侵入性较小的诊断性检查。例如，表15.1列举的高分辨率计算机断层扫描（high-resolution computed tomography，HRCT）在疾病诊断方面的重要价值[16-18]。由于影像学不能对许多弥漫性疾病做出明确的诊断，传统上，用TBBX可以帮助评估弥漫性肺疾病小叶中心性病灶[6-8]。此外，虽然TBBX在某些情况下可以帮助确诊某些间质性肺疾病（如结节病、嗜酸性粒细胞性肺炎、过敏性肺炎、淋巴管癌等），但它对诊断普通型间质性肺炎（特发性肺纤维化）价值不大[19-24]。

表15.1 经支气管镜肺活检可有更高诊断率的肺部疾病

结节病
肺朗格汉斯细胞组织细胞增多症（histiocytosis X）
淋巴管癌
肺泡蛋白沉积症
分枝杆菌和真菌引起的弥漫性肺部感染
弥漫性肺泡细胞癌
肺淋巴管平滑肌瘤病
矽肺病

TBBX也可能有助于鉴别感染和诊断肺外周病变（peripheral pulmonary lesion，PPL），也可以使用其他侵入性较小的技术，如支气管肺泡灌洗（bronchoalveolar lavage，BAL）和刷检。在表15.1列出的所有检查中，TBBX具有更高的诊断率[22-28]。所有诊断技术相结合，BAL、刷检和TBBX，可能是互补的，可提高总体诊断率[19,29,30]。此外，随着免疫抑制药物在血液和实体恶性肿瘤、移植医学中的广泛使用，以及生物制剂在风湿病治疗中的使用增加，导致患者免疫抑制的发生率增加，从而导致非典型感染增加。在免疫抑制患者中非典型病原微生物感染（如真菌感染）的识别和诊断困难，也是治疗的挑战。BAL和TBBX联合检查有助于确定诊断并确定是否存在侵袭性疾病，这将直接影响治疗计划[31]。

估计TBBX的死亡率<0.05%，最常见的并发症是气胸（<2%）和出血>50 mL（<4%）[19,22,24-26]。大多数患者的出血风险较低，但服用氯吡格雷的患者出血风险可高达89%[31]。如果服用氯吡格雷的患者必须进行TBBX，目前的建议是在与患者医生讨论后，在手术前至少停药5天[32,33]。

15.2.2 局灶性肺病

随着CT的广泛使用、国家肺部筛查试验建议以及最近的NELSON研究，局灶性病变或PPL的识别和定位需求明显增加[34,35]。随着透视下经支气管镜直接活检以及新的导航技术的发展，如径向超声、虚拟支气管镜导航（virtual bronchoscopic navigation，VBN）、电磁导航（electromagnetic navigation，EMN）支气管镜、CT和锥形束CT的引导，利用可弯曲支气管镜进行肺外周病变采样可能性显著增加。对局灶性或肺外周性病变活检，不仅可以通过传统支气管活检钳活检，还可以通过本章后面介绍的TBNA和其他技术完成。

15.3 禁忌证

通过可弯曲支气管镜进行TBBX绝对禁忌证包括患者无法配合手术、心血管状态不稳定、呼吸支持状态下仍存在严重低氧血症、哮喘发作状态以及缺乏训练有素的医生和缺少可以正常运行的手术设备[36]。相对禁忌证包括无法控制的咳嗽、无法控制的凝血功能障碍、晚期肾衰竭、广泛肺大疱或计划活检部位附近有血管畸形。

肺动脉高压以前被认为是TBBX的禁忌证，2005年对227名肺科医师的调查显示，28.7%的受访者认为这是绝对禁忌证，58.6%的受访者认为这是相对禁忌证[37]。尽管如此，Morris等的研究首次证明肺动脉高压羊模型出血风险没有增加，随后在间质性肺疾病和潜在肺动脉高压患者的队列研究中也证明了这一点[38,39]。2019年，Ishiwata等完成并发表的一项10年回顾性最新研究发现，与无肺动脉高压患者相比，肺动脉高压患者的BLB风险并未增加[40]。这支持了Diaz-Fuentes等之前的研究，他们在2016年对100多名接受BLB治疗的肺动脉高压患者进行了同样的安全性研究[41]。在常规临床实践中，对于潜在肺动脉高压患者，准备和实施BLB时仍要谨慎。

15.4 术前评估

在详细说明支气管镜检查和TBBX的操作细节、目的和风险后，应获得患者签署的知情同意书。此外，应获得完整的病史和体格检查资料，特别强调了解可能在术中或术后造成并发症风险的患者特征（表15.2）。了解患者是否存在家族性或获得性凝血障碍也很重要。

表 15.2 支气管镜检查前清单

1) 是否具有支气管镜检查的适应证？
2) 既往是否做过支气管镜检查？
3) 如果以上问题的答案为"是"，那么是否有并发症？
4) 是否患者及其近亲（如果患者无法沟通或同意）完全了解支气管镜操作的风险、目的、益处和并发症？
5) 患者既往病史（对药物和局部麻醉过敏情况）和目前的临床状况是否存在特殊问题或并发症倾向？
6) 是否完成了术前所需检查并获得了结果？
7) 前期处理是否正确，药物剂量是否合理？
8) 患者术前（如哮喘急性发作时需要的皮质类固醇激素，治疗糖尿病需要的胰岛素，或预防细菌性心内膜炎的措施）或术中（氧气或额外的镇静）是否需要特殊考虑？
9) 支气管镜检查术后护理的计划是否合适？
10) 是否有适当的器械和人员来辅助操作和处理潜在的并发症？

其他健康人计划接受支气管镜检查时，不论是否进行TBBX，不需要常规行全血细胞计数、血生化、尿液分析和凝血检查[42,43]。此外，没有任何单项凝血系统检查结果可以预测手术期间的出血风险[44,45]，即使凝血试验常规组合也不能预测TBBX术后出血的风险[46-49]。

由于抗血小板聚集药物（如氯吡格雷和新型口服抗凝剂）的使用增加，这些患者进行BLB时，应认识其潜在凝血障碍和仔细进行凝血功能检查。这些药物会增加操作出血的发生率。因此，应仔细了解病史，术前及时停用这些药物或进行桥接治疗，正如最近美国胸科医师学会关于抗凝治疗的指南所概述的那样[50]。

血小板减少和血小板功能障碍被认为是支气管镜活检的相对禁忌证。血小板减少症，即血小板计数小于50 000，出血风险增加，应进行术前评估，并可能输注血小板以获得血小板绝对水平大于50 000[51]。尽管血小板计数正常，但对使用上述抗血小板药物和尿毒症患者，血小板功能障碍可能是一个更值得关注的问题。血小板功能障碍（尽管血小板计数正常）与出血风险增加有关，可能表现为出血时间延长。Zavala报道了尿毒症患者TBBX术后显著出血的发生率为45%，并指出"尿毒症患者因存在较大出血风险应尽可能避免任何活检"[46,47]。如果在尿毒症患者血小板

功能障碍的情况下绝对必要进行TBBX时，则术前可以进行透析或给予1-去氨基-8-D-精氨酸血管加压素（DDAVP）药物。血小板功能障碍会导致临床潜在的活检后大出血的发生率显著增加，基于这一观察结果，血清肌酐水平≥3 mg/dL或血清尿素氮水平为30 mg/dL被认为是TBBX的相对禁忌证[48,49,51-53]。许多接受TBBX的弥漫性肺病患者有明显的肺功能障碍，通常为低氧血症，但如果有适当的人员和支持设备，则不应禁忌进行BLB。常规肺功能检查和动脉血气分析在经支气管镜肺活检前不是必需的，但如果计划进行BLB，肺功能检查和动脉血气分析检查应在支气管镜操作前进行，因为BLB后可能出现黏膜水肿和支气管痉挛，这可能会影响肺功能检查结果[54]。术前应常规评估影像学检查，以确定在何处活检以获得最高的诊断率和最少的并发症。可以通过X线断层扫描或HRCT识别病灶特殊影像特征及其病灶位置，优化支气管镜操作，提高诊断率，识别活检时应避开的区域，如连续性肺大疱、异常的血管和胸膜病变。

15.5 操作技术

可弯曲支气管镜下经TBBX可以采用多种麻醉辅助手段，从仅局部镇静到全身麻醉，取决于患者、术者和拟进行的支气管镜活检方式。第5章对可弯曲支气管镜的麻醉方式问题进行了充分的讨论，可作为参考。肺周围病灶TBBX的目的是获取肺结节、肺肿块或弥漫性肺疾病的肺实质标本。对弥漫性肺病变进行肺实质活检时，活检钳向前推进过程中需通过肺中央区域较大的支气管动脉时，采用透视引导是非常重要的，以减少出血风险。如果对肺结节或肿块进行活检，在闭合活检钳之前，用透视或其他成像方式确认活检钳是否在病变内也同样重要。在透视下TBBX时，通过旋转C形臂45°~90°来确认活检钳位于病灶内部，活检过程中如果病灶和活检钳在同一方向上一起移动，说明活检钳通常"位于病灶内"，如果无同向移动，则提示活检钳不在病灶内。仔细规划操作路径和选择目标病灶，也可以降低气胸和出血的风险。

历史文献上TBLB有两种类型：无引导辅助和有引导辅助。在没有引导辅助情况下进行活检，通常是针对肺弥漫性疾病，被称为"经支气管镜盲检"。这种方式不常被使用，因为这种方式要依赖中度镇静患者的感觉反馈，会增加相当大的额外风险。但在某

些特殊情况下可能需要这种技术。该技术描述如下：① 在气管内向前推进活检钳，直到遇到阻力；② 一旦感觉到阻力，撤回活检钳 1~2 cm，并嘱咐患者深吸气；③ 患者吸气时，嘱咐助手打开活检钳；④ 然后嘱咐患者呼气，并关闭活检钳；⑤ 然后询问患者是否感到疼痛；如果答案是否定的，则迅速将活检钳取出完成活检，并获得肺组织标本。如果答案是肯定的，则打开活检钳并重复该步骤，但活检钳不能被向前推进至肺外周；⑥ 把活检钳取出的组织放入福尔马林溶液进行组织学检查或放入无菌生理盐水中进行培养。如果将标本放入福尔马林中，则需用无菌水冲洗活检钳的尖端，以防止在随后的活检中将福尔马林溶液带入肺部。

使用透视引导下 TBBX 是目前的标准方法，透视引导下 TBBX 的正确步骤如下：

1）患者无须保持清醒，也不需要听从命令或回答问题。

2）在持续透视引导下将活检钳向前推进，直至活检钳抵达位于距离胸膜边缘 1~2 cm 的远端气道内。

3）一旦到达正确位置，将活检钳回撤 1 cm，并嘱咐助手打开活检钳。

4）然后将活检钳向前推进 1 cm，随后闭合。技师关闭活检钳时应注意，强行打开或关闭活检钳会由于导管张力变化，从而导致活检钳的位置移动，这可能会改变活检的准确性。

5）在两个平面上旋转 C 形臂 45°~90°，以确保活检钳位于目标病灶。即使 C 形臂轴向旋转，但在透视图像中活检钳和目标病变应保持在一起。

6）只需轻轻用力，活检钳就可以轻轻收回。如果阻力很小，则迅速将其拉回，并获得肺组织标本。如果阻力很大，则应释放活检钳上的张力，打开活检钳，释放肺组织，并将活检钳轻轻闭合后拉回。一旦活检钳在闭合时可以自由移动，则需重复活检。这种情况通常发生在活检钳过度靠近支气管近端，在支气管分嵴处闭合或在较大的支气管血管区域闭合时。更外周的肺活检通常不会显示出明显的阻力，除非在活检钳内有胸膜或瘢痕组织。

7）从支气管镜中将带标本的活检钳拔出，把标本放入福尔马林中进行组织学检查，或放入无菌生理盐水中进行培养。如果将标本置于福尔马林中，则用无菌生理盐水冲洗活检钳的尖端，以防止在随后的活检中将福尔马林溶液带入肺部。

上述技术也可以用于能够通过支气管镜工作通道的任何其他柔性活检工具。在透视引导下，使用活检钳、毛刷和穿刺针对 CT 上显示的肺外周结节进行活检（图 15.1）。其他引导工具如 VBN、EMN、CT-TBBX 或径向超声探头，可以在使用或不使用透视引导的情况下应用。这些不同活检技术的诊断率将在后面的章节中讨论。

TBBX 的并发症主要有两种：出血和气胸。在取出活检钳的过程中，如果遇到明显出血，则可将支气管镜楔塞在出血的支气管位置并保持一段时间[48]。这种"楔塞"技术有双重优点：它将支气管镜的尖端保持在最佳位置，这样就可以获取更多次的活检，而不必取出支气管镜清洁镜头；最重要的是，如果活检后发生出血，楔形位置将出血限制在活检后的肺段或亚段。"楔塞"技术的主要局限性在于：一旦血块覆盖气管镜镜头，支气管镜医师将无法看清气道。活检初次出血后，需要通过透视或其他实时外部成像观察出血的程度和进展。在透视检查中，活检处的出血增加时会增加靶病灶的密度和大小。

如果出血持续或不能减少，术者可以采取以下几种镜下操作方法来减少和控制出血。首先，在较长时间内保持气管镜置于"楔塞"位置以在局部形成血栓，这是有效的止血措施，"楔塞"可将血液完全封堵在出血的肺段或亚段。如有需要，可保持支气管镜尖端在"楔塞"的位置进行持续或长时间的间歇性吸引判断出血控制情况，也可通过支气管镜将 10~15 mL 的冰生理盐水轻轻注入出血部位，有助于止血。在缓慢灌注冰生理盐水过程中，内镜医师透过生理盐水能够看到出血支气管叶段远端情况，并应保持支气管树远端"盐水灌注状态"数秒。如果镜下见到从支气管远端流出的新鲜血液混合有刚刚注入的生理盐水，通常表明活检部位存在持续性出血。此时，则应采用支气管镜吸引清理出血，并重复上述冰盐水灌注。此方法可重复数次，直至出血停止。在许多患者中，该技术可减少并最终终止 TBBX 引起的出血[48]。

其他控制 TBBX 并发出血的技术包括：灌注肾上腺素帮助血管收缩、灌注凝血酶帮助形成血块、球囊填塞、应用纤维蛋白胶、硬质支气管镜下吸引出血和出血支气管内填塞、插入双腔气管内插管隔离支气管树以及最后的手术切除出血肺段[48]。报道的较新方法，如通过支气管镜采用可吸收明胶与凝血酶悬液的混合物，成功治疗了活检后的出血[53]。

当出血严重时，应将患者翻身处于患侧卧位，防止血液溢至未出血的一侧肺。需要注意的是，气道死

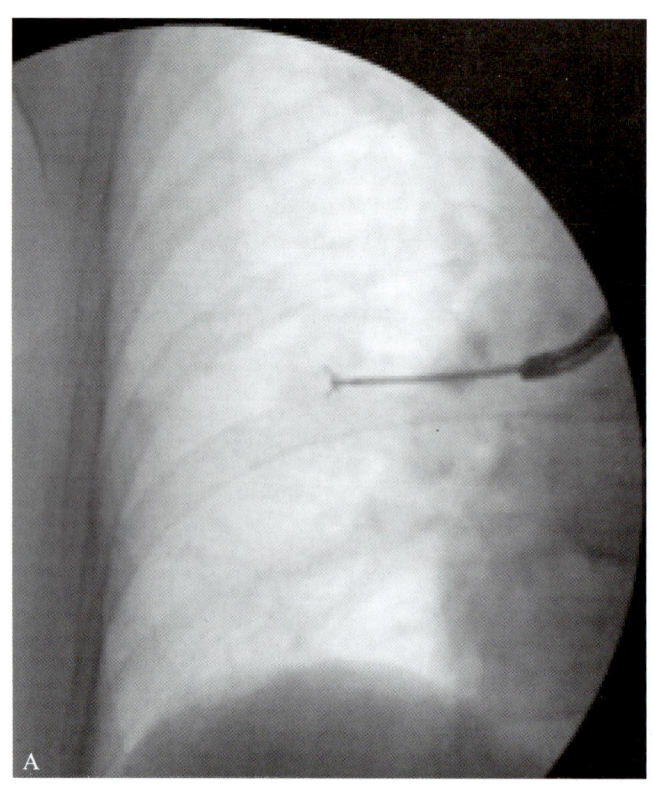
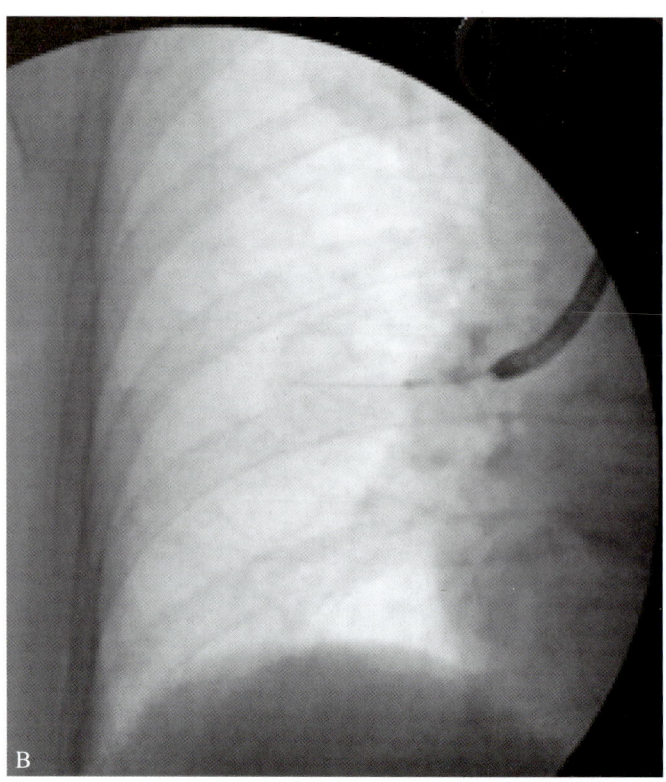
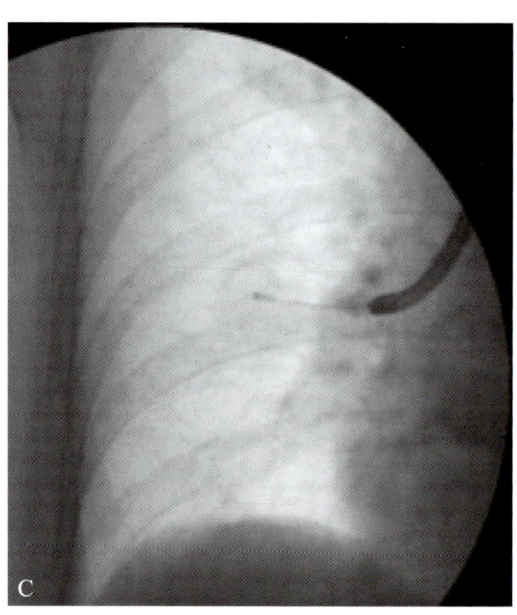
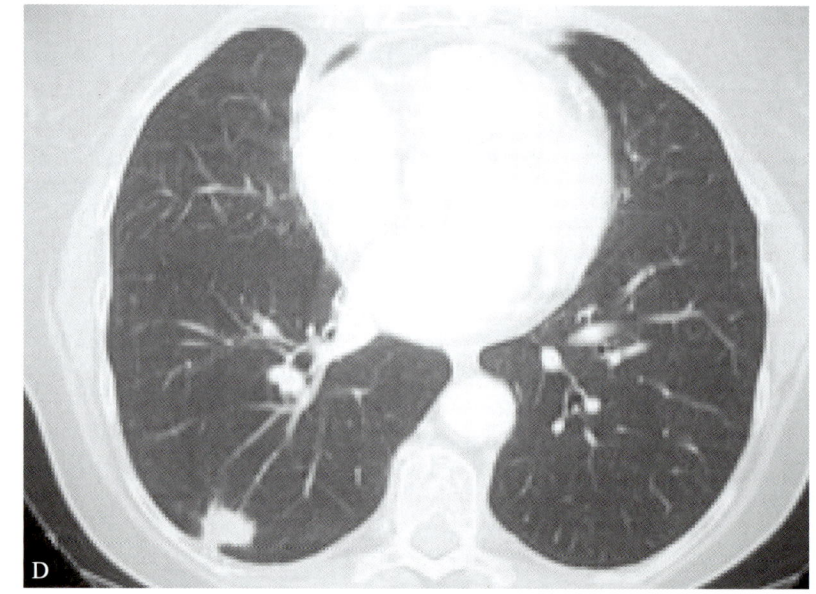

图 15.1　透视引导下经支气管镜活检右下叶病变

透视引导下，术者从选定的区域获得肺标本。A. 活检钳活检；B. 刷检；C. 针吸活检；D. 右下叶病灶 CT 图像。

腔容积较小（150~350 mL），因此，少量血液即可因血凝块形成导致窒息。本文所描述的这些技术很少使用，但随着最近一些活检技术的出现，支气管镜检查团队需要积极掌握这些技术。

　　完成 TBBX 检查并确认无出血后，从气道中撤出支气管镜。如果已经采用透视或胸部超声筛查排除了气胸，则 TBBX 术后不需要常规胸部 X 线检查[55-57]。如 TBBX 期间患者过度咳嗽或反复主诉疼痛，或出现其他肺部症状（如呼吸困难、胸闷、胸痛等），应进行胸部 X 线检查。TBBX 后临床怀疑出现气胸或有气胸临床表现、严重出血，不明原因的呼吸困难或其他明显的心肺症状是住院治疗的指征。

如果在接下来的 24 h 内出现新的症状,应告知患者和医生联系或去急诊科就诊。

随着诊断性支气管镜检查的应用增加,出现了新型设计的活检钳。标准的活检钳有杯形钳和鳄鱼形钳两种类型。通常鳄鱼钳能提供更大体积的标本,但诊断率并不一定会提高[58-60]。

在支气管镜室内,常常会观察肺活检标本放入福尔马林容器时是否可以"漂浮"评判标本质量。"漂浮"迹象被认为是存在较多含气肺泡的标志,并且可能更能代表标本量足够。然而,这一迹象并不可靠,因为不含气的病变也会"漂浮"。一项对 44 例接受 BLB 的患者的前瞻性研究发现,"漂浮"迹象的存在并不能预测获得的组织是否足够[61]。

对局灶性病变、肺外周结节或均匀受累的弥漫性肺疾病患者,标本活检次数取决于目标病灶的获取情况,Descombes 等评估了 516 例免疫功能正常的慢性弥漫性肺浸润患者的肺活检,观察到 TBBX 标本量与总体诊断率之间存在直接相关性(1~3 次钳夹获取的组织碎片诊断率为 38%,6~10 次钳夹诊断率为 69%,$P<0.01$)。基于这些发现,他们建议 TBBX 至少采集 5~6 次活检钳钳夹[61]。

细支气管周围性疾病(如结节病、淋巴管癌或感染等)更容易通过 TBBX 诊断,且标本数量与总体诊断率相关。Ⅰ期结节病可能需要多达 10 次 TBBX 才能明确诊断,而Ⅱ期或Ⅲ期结节病在至少进行 4~5 次 TBBX 活检时,其诊断敏感性才能达到 95%[58-60,62]。

BLB 标本的处理是该操作的重要组成部分。应小心处理标本,避免形成挤压伪影。将活检钳中的标本简单冲洗到福尔马林里,标本采用轻轻拂拭的方式较用镊子拣取更可取,因为后者可能导致挤压假象。

进行 BLB 的弥漫性肺疾病患者,通常因潜在的免疫抑制状态而接受评估,并与感染、血液系统恶性肿瘤和干细胞移植后状态、实体恶性肿瘤和应用化疗药物或肺移植后引起的免疫抑制有关。Gilbert 等回顾了使用可弯曲支气管镜评估伴有肺浸润的造血干细胞移植人群的 14 年经验,结果显示 BAL 的总体诊断率为 52.5%,TBBX 阳性率为 18/22(81.8%)。经 TBBX 诊断的患者最常见的病因是非特异性间质性肺炎、移植物抗宿主病、特发性肺炎、弥漫性肺泡损伤、机化性肺炎和葡萄球菌性肺炎。接受 TBBX 的患者中无气胸发生。作者得出结论:根据现有数据纤维支气管镜检查是弥漫性肺病首选的初始诊断方法,具有较高的诊断率,使用 BAL 和保护性标本刷分别可以给 53.5% 和 44% 的患者带来治疗变化,如果初始支气管镜检查结果无法明确诊断,再次进行支气管镜检查,则应考虑 TBBX[63,64]。

15.5.1 经支气管穿刺针吸活检

以前,"经支气管"一词专用于在支气管镜下对纵隔淋巴结针吸活检。正如在其他章节中所讨论的,支气管镜超声(endobronchial ultrasound,EBUS)的出现提高了 TBNA 诊断的准确性,降低了并发症的发生率,这对于纵隔淋巴结肿大的患者来说是件好事,但对于肺外周结节、肿块、空腔和其他异常的患者来说又该是什么情况呢?新的成像技术(如 HRCT、锥形束 CT、透视、径向超声等)和电磁导航支气管镜的出现,大大提高了支气管镜医师发现更小、更外周病变的能力,但其活检的准确性如何?

支气管镜医师对肺外周实质病变传统上采用支气管肺泡灌洗、刷检和经支气管活检钳活检获取组织标本,但成功率有限。单项技术的成功率分别为 24%、27% 和 38%,如果联合使用,诊断率通常为 46%[65]。TBNA 是指在透视或电磁引导下,使用 19~22 G 长度 0.5~3 cm 的穿刺针,经支气管镜的活检工作通道进入肺外周病变。一旦确认针尖位于病变内,则用注射器进行抽吸,并在病变内来回移动针尖,收集细胞,然后撤出穿刺针,将标本涂抹在载玻片上以备评估[66]。单独 TBNA 对肺外周病变的诊断率为 53%,优于毛刷和灌洗联合活检钳活检的诊断率[67]。如果 TBNA 与刷检、活检和灌洗相结合,诊断率可提高到 70% 以上[68]。

TBNA 联合纵隔淋巴结 EBUS 可以提高肺癌诊断的敏感性和准确性[69]。提高诊断率的其他因素包括病变大小(直径>20 mm)、细胞学快速现场评估(rapid on site evaluation,ROSE)、CT 影像存在支气管征以及径向 EBUS 图像呈现中央型同心圆视图[70-74]。超声显示同心视图的肺外周病灶 TBNA 与 CT 引导下 TBNA 诊断率相似,但气胸的风险降低[74]。支气管镜活检的额外好处是对纵隔淋巴结病变能够进行 EBUS 检查,不仅可以提高诊断敏感度和准确性,也可为肺癌分期提供依据。

气胸是与肺活检最相关的并发症,但支气管镜活检并发气胸的发生率低于经皮肺穿刺活检[75]。这些因素将在本书其他章节中单独讨论。

早期肺癌筛查发现,23% 的 60 岁以上胸部 CT 筛查患者会出现肺结节,其中只有 2.7% 被确定为恶性[76]。这些结节通常很小(直径<10 mm),并且位于活检工具难以抵达的位置,这对病灶活检可能具有

挑战性。以前，可供选择的评估方法限于连续 CT 扫描观察随访或手术切除，其中 60% 的结节证实为良性[77]。为提高对肺小结节评估的能力，开启了 TBNA 和经皮活检临床应用的研究。Wang 等报道了一项涉及 329 例患者的前瞻性研究，如果患者初始 TBNA 未能确诊，则进行经皮肺穿刺活检（transthoracic needle aspiration，TTNA）[78]，在其研究中，TBNA 确诊了部分不伴纵隔淋巴结肿大的肺外周肺结节患者（45.6%；73/160），对 TBNA 后未能确诊的患者（105 例），TTNA 确诊率为 69.5%。这两种方法都是在中度镇静下使用标准支气管镜技术完成的，在 TTNA 时使用 C 形臂透视或 CT 引导，两种方法联合的诊断率为 90.3%。作者建议，顺次使用这些技术是诊断 PPL 的合理策略。最近，也有类似的研究，该研究首先使用支气管镜检查，然后使用 EMN 引导的 TTNA[79] 及随访观察等待，与单纯使用 C 形臂或 CT 的标准检查技术进行了比较。

上述针对肺结节顺次使用不同穿刺技术明确病理的结果，能够让患者相信，有时对肺结节密切随访观察可能也是一种安全和谨慎的方法，而不是继续进行更具侵入性的手术，手术可能会导致肺储备有限的患者严重并发症发生率显著增加。

为支持这一临床实践策略，Welker 等发表了一项前瞻性观察性研究，对 118 例孤立性肺病变患者进行了为期 4 年的分期活检和观察。在这一组连续观察的患者中，重复穿刺活检结合临床观察和连续 CT 扫描，确定孤立性肺结节是否为恶性肿瘤准确率为 100%。实施这样的方案可将良性结节的不必要手术切除降低 50% 以上[80]。建议这种方法只能在拥有经验丰富的多学科团队的医疗中心使用，团队成员在先进的支气管镜技能、经皮肺活检技能和外科手术方面都训练有素。这些技术将在本书相关章节进行讨论。另外，该研究还建议能有专职人员来处理检查结果并安排合理的患者随访。

15.6 新技术

研发的新技术和辅助技术包括 EMN 和锥形束 CT，旨在增强支气管镜活检成功率和安全性，提高诊断准确性。新数据报道最多的技术是冷冻肺活检。自 2009 年以来，在弥漫性肺实质疾病的评估中，冷冻活检已被用作获取组织学标本的非手术方法。使用可弯曲冷冻探头获取标本，探头温度可达到 $-89.5℃$ [81]。探头通过导管中心的管道在高压下施加制冷剂（通常为二氧化碳）来获得低温。由于导管尖端的大气和喷嘴之间存在压力差，气体膨胀，导致温度下降（焦耳-汤姆逊效应）。向前推进冷冻探头进入肺实质后冷冻，然后撤出携带被冻切取出的黏附有肺组织的冷冻探头。

冷冻肺活检诊断率为 51%~89%，并发症发生率为 3%~33%[82-89]。最常见的并发症是出血（轻至中度）和气胸。诊断率和并发症发生率的差异可能和操作医师的经验和技术差异有关。

为了提高对冷冻活检的认识和安全性，在第三届弥漫性肺间质疾病经支气管冷冻活检国际会议上提出了一份专家声明并于最近发表于《呼吸病学》杂志（*Respiration*）[83]。该专家声明的要点主要包括以下几点：

1）经支气管冷冻肺活检应在气管插管、深度镇静或全身麻醉下进行。

2）如果使用柔性气管内插管，应预置支气管内阻滞器/Fogarty 球囊以预防性控制出血（如果使用硬质支气管镜，该措施属于可选择性措施）。

3）在透视引导下，距离脏层胸膜 1 cm 处活检 3~5 次。

4）经支气管冷冻活检应由接受过冷冻活检专门培训和具有处理气道内出血、气胸和呼吸衰竭能力的呼吸内镜医师进行。

5）该操作应在手术室或配备急救设备的支气管镜室中进行。应具备将患者送入 ICU 和处理并发症的能力。

此外，在冷冻活检成为标准化方案之前，还需要做更多的工作。如果冷冻活检操作由接受过培训的个人操作并遵循专家组列出的建议，冷冻肺活检可以成为替代外科手术肺活检并在门诊实施的用于评估弥漫性肺间质疾病的可选方法。

15.7 特殊患者群体

最后，再谈一下两类特殊移植患者群体的活检：实体器官移植患者，特别是肺移植患者，以及造血干细胞移植（hematopoietic stem cell transplantation，HSCT）患者。

约有 50% 接受造血干细胞移植的患者会出现肺部相关并发症，死亡率可高达 60%[90-96]。对 HSCT 患者，虽然BAL在感染性肺炎的早期识别中发挥了作用，但TBBX可提高诊断率并调整治疗方案，但受限于回顾性研究和小样本的研究结果[97-105]。O'Dwyer等最近进行了一项大型回顾性分析，对130例HSCT后出现肺部并发症患者，给予TBBX[106]，他们发现最常见的组织学改变是非特异性间质性肺炎（18%），检出病原体的概率不到5%。此外，接受TBBX患者出现与手术相关的并发症风险增加。作者得出结论：支气管镜检查期间TBBX与调整抗生素治疗或提高感染病原体的诊断率无关，与BAL相比未能增加额外价值，并指出会增加手术相关并发症风险。因此，TBBX在合并肺部并发症的HSCT患者中的应用价值，需要进一步的前瞻性研究。

肺移植患者较其他任何患者进行肺活检操作更为常见[107]。主要适应证是识别同种异体移植排斥反应、机会性感染和气道并发症，如伤口裂开、瘘或吻合口狭窄。对肺移植患者实施监测性支气管镜操作（surveillance bronchoscopy，SB）或基于临床适应证的支气管镜操作（clinically indicated bronchoscopy，CB），是评估组织排异反应的标准方法[108-110]。

尽管经常会应用CB，但文献中关于SB的价值并没有达成共识[109]。CB一般用于出现咳嗽、呼吸困难等新发症状或新出现的影像学改变或FEV_1减少10%及以上的患者[111]。相比之下，SB则用于定期评估可能发生的术后吻合口缺血、坏死、破裂、狭窄形成，TBBX联合BAL以评估急性细胞排斥反应（acute cellular rejection，ACR）和同种异体移植慢性肺功能障碍（chronic lung allograft dysfunction，CLAD）。

虽然各中心对SB的应用和具体方案有所不同，但最近发表的文献都支持实施SB。2014年，Inoue等回顾性分析了生前进行SB的肺移植受者尸解结果[112]，在该项研究中，92例次（49%）SB支气管镜操作有阳性发现，并发症发生率低，如中度出血（11%）、气胸（1%）和低氧血症（0.5%）。总体来说，他们认为SB确实有助于识别排斥反应、气道感染或定植，特别是在移植后的12个月内。2018年，Tosi等对110例TBBX患者进行了为期4年的回顾性分析[110]，结果发现，TBBX可以识别8%需要药物干预的急性排斥反应，并发症发生率只有4%，他们认为这是可以接受的，监测方案中没有去掉CB的必要性。因此，TBBX在HSCT、实体器官移植和肺移植患者中的作用仍需继续评估。我们还注意到了最近一项在移植患者中关于冷冻肺活检的研究，如前文所述，该技术需要进一步的标准化和前瞻性研究[113]。

参考文献

1. Gaensler, E.A. and Carrington, C.B. (1980). Open biopsy for chronic diffuse interstitial lung disease: clinical, roentgenographic, and physiological correlations in 502 patients. *Ann. Thorac. Surg.* 30: 411-426.
2. Blewett, C.J., Bennett, F., Miller, J.D. et al. (2001). Open lung biopsy as an outpatient procedure. *Ann. Thorac. Surg.* 71: 1113-1115.
3. Andersen, H.A., Miller, W.E., and Bernatz, P.E. (1973). Lung biopsy: transbronchoscopic, percutaneous, open. *Surg. Clin. NorthAm.* 53: 785-793.
4. Vitums, V.C. (1972). Percutaneous needle biopsy of the lung with a new disposable needle. *Chest* 62: 717-719.
5. Zavala, D.C. and Bedell, G.N. (1972). Percutaneous lung biopsy with a cutting needle. An analysis of 40 cases and comparison with other biopsy techniques. *Am. Rev. Respir. Dis.* 106: 186-193.
6. Mehnert, J.H. and Brown, M.J. (1978). Percutaneous needle core biopsy of peripheral pulmonary masses. *Am. J. Surg.* 136: 151-156.
7. Feist, J.H. (1976). Letter: cutting needle biopsies. *Chest* 69: 244-245.
8. Castellino, R.A. (1976). Percutaneous pulmonary needle diagnosis of *Pneumocystis carinii* pneumonitis. *Natl. Cancer Inst. Monogr.* 43: 137-140.
9. Elliot, T.L., Lynch, D.A., Newell, J.D. Jr. et al. (2005). High-resolution computed tomography features of nonspecific interstitial pneumonia and usual interstitial pneumonia. *J. Comput. Assist. Tomogr.* 29: 339-345.
10. Andersen, H.A., Fontana, R.S., and Harrison, E.G. Jr. (1965). Transbronchoscopic lung biopsy in diffuse pulmonary disease. *Dis. Chest* 48: 187-192.
11. Andersen, H.A. and Fontana, R.S. (1972). Transbronchoscopic lung biopsy for diffuse pulmonary diseases: technique and results in 450 cases. *Chest* 62: 125-128.
12. Palojoki, A. and Sutinen, S. (1972). Transbronchoscopic lung biopsy as aid in pulmonary diagnostics. *Scand. J. Respir. Dis.* 53: 120-124.
13. Andersen, H.A. (1977). Transbronchial lung biopsy in diffuse pulmonary disease. *Ann. Thorac. Surg.* 24: 1.
14. Andersen, H.A. (1978). Transbronchoscopiclug biopsy for diffuse pulmonary diseases. Results in 939 patients. *Chest* 73: 734-736.
15. Asai, M., Samayoa, A.X., and Hodge, C. (2017). Elective intubation and positive pressure ventilation for transbronchial lung biopsy. *J. Surg. Res.* 219: 296-301.
16. Levin, D.C., Wicks, A.B., and Ellis, J.H. Jr. (1974). Transbronchial lung biopsy via the fiberoptic bronchoscope. *Am. Rev. Respir. Dis.* 110: 4-12.
17. Nishimura, K., Izumi, T., Kitaichi, M. et al. (1993). The diagnostic accuracy of high-resolution computed tomography in diffuse infiltrative lung diseases. *Chest* 104: 1149-1155.
18. Sundaram, B., Gross, B.H., Martinez, F.J. et al. (2008).

Accuracy of high- resolution CT in the diagnosis of diffuse lung disease: effect of predominance and distribution of findings. *Am. J. Roentgenol.* 191: 1032–1039.

19 Bradley, B., Brabanley, H.M., Egan, J.J. et al. (2008). Interstitial lung disease guideline: the British Thoracic Society in collaboration with the Thoracic Society of Australia and New Zealand anthem the Irish Thoracic Society. *Thorax* 63 (suppl 5): v1.

20 Ensminger, S.A. and Prakash, U.B. (2006). Is bronchoscope lung biopsy helpful in the management of patents with diffuse lung disease? *Eur. Respir. J.* 28 (6): 1081.

21 Leslie, K.O., Gruden, J.F., Parish, J.M., and Scholand, M.D. (2007). Transbronchial biopsy interpretation in the patient with diffuse parenchymal lung disease. *Arch. Pathol. Lab. Med.* 131 (3): 407–423.

22 Sehgal, I.S., Bal, A., Dhooria, S. et al. (2016). A prospective randomized controlled trial comparing the efficacy and safety of cup vs alligator forceps for performing Transbronchial lung biopsy in patients with sarcoidosis. *Chest* 149 (6): 1584–1586.

23 Raj, R., Raparia, K., Lynch, D.A., and Brown, K.K. (2017). Surgical lung biopsy for Intersitial lung diseases. *Chest* (5): 1131.

24 Glaspole, I.N., Wells, A.U., and du Bois, R. (2001). Lung biopsy in diffuse parenchymal lung disease. *Monaldi Arch. Chest Dis.* 56 (3): 225–232.

25 Sindhwani, G., Shirazi, N., Sodhi, R. et al. (2015). Transbronchial lung biopsy in patients with diffuse parenchyma lung disease without "idiopathic pulmonary fibrosis patter" on HRCT scan-experience from a tertiary care center in North India. *Lung India* 32 (5): 453–456.

26 Pue, C.A. and Pacht, E.R. (1995). Complications of fiberoptic bronchoscopy at a university hospital. *Chest* 107 (2): 430.

27 Rennard, S.I. and Spurzem, J.R. (1992). Bronchoalveolar lavage in the diagnosis of lung cancer. *Chest* 102: 331–332.

28 Jain, P., Sandur, S., Meli, Y. et al. (2004). Role of flexible bronchoscopy in immunocompromised patients with lung infiltrates. *Chest* 125: 712–722.

29 Prakash, U.B., Barham, S.S., Carpenter, H.A. et al. (1987). Pulmonary alveolar phospholipoproteinosis: experience with 34 cases and a review. *Mayo Clin. Proc.* 62: 499–518.

30 Linder, J., Radio, S.J., Robbins, R.A. et al. (1987). Bronchoalveolar lavage in the cytologic diagnosis of carcinoma of the lung. *Acta Cytol.* 31: 796–801.

31 Ernst, A., Eberhard, R., Wahidi, M. et al. (2006). Effect of routine clopidogrel use on bleeding complications after trans bronchial biopsy in humans. *Chest* 129 (3): 734.

32 Pernasconi, M., Casutt, A., Koutsokera, A. et al. (2016). Radial ultrasound-assisted transbronchial biopsy: a new diagnostic approach for non resolving pulmonary infiltrates in neutropenic hemato-oncological patients. *Lung* 194 (6): 917–921.

33 Fleisher, L.A., Beckman, J.A., Brown, K.A. et al. (2007). ACC/AHA 2007 Guidelines on perioperative cardiovascular evaluation and care for noncardiac surgery: executive summary: a report of the American College of Cardiology/American Heart Association Task Force on Practice Guidelines (Writing Committee to Revise the 2002 Guidelines on Perioperative Cardiovascular Evaluation for Noncardiac Surgery)Developed in Collaboration With the American Society of Echocar diography, American Society of Nuclear Cardiology, Heart Rhythm Society, Society of Cardiovascular Anesthesiologists, Society for Cardiovascular Angiography and Interventions, Society for Vascular Medicine and Biology, and Society for Vascular Surgery. *J. Am. Coll. Cardiol.* 50: 1707–1732.

34 National Lung Screening Trial Research Team (2011). Reduced lung-cancer mortality with low-dose computed tomography screening. *N. Engl. J. Med.* 365: 395–409.

35 Horeweg, N., van Rosmalen, J., Heuvelmans, M.A. et al. (2014). Lung cancer probability in patients with CT-detected pulmonary nodules: a prespecified analysis of data from the NELSON trial of low-dose CT screening. *Lancet Oncol.* 15: 1332–1341.

36 McDougall, J.C. (1994). Bronchscopic Lung Biopsy. New York: Raven Press.

37 Wahidi, M.M., Rocha, A.T., Holligsworth, J.W. et al. (2005). Contraindications and safety of transbronchial lung biopsy via flexible bronchoscopy. *Respiration* 72 (3): 285–295.

38 Morris, M.J., Peacock, P.M., Lloyd, W.C. III, and Blanton, H.M. (1996). The effect of pulmonary hypertension upon bleeding in sheep undergoing bronchoscopic biopsy. *J. Bronchol.* 3: 11–16.

39 Morris, M.J., Peacock, P.M., Mego, D.M. et al. (1998). The risk of hemorrhage from bronchoscopic lung biopsy due to pulmonary hypertension in interstitial lung disease. *J. Bronchol.* 5: 115–121.

40 Ishiwata, I., Abe, M., Kasai, H. et al. (2019). Safety of diagnostic flexible bronchoscopy in patients with echocardiographic evidence of pulmonary hypertension. *Respir. Invest.* 57 (1): 73–78.

41 Diaz-Fuentes, G., Bajantri, B., and Adrish, M. (2016). Safety of bronchoscopy in patients with echocardiographic evidence of pulmonary hypertension. *Respiration* 92 (3): 182–187.

42 Fleisher, L.A., Beckman, J.A., Brown, K.A. et al. (2008). ACC/AHA 2007 guidelines on perioperative cardiovascular evaluation and care for noncardiac surgery: executive summary: a report of the American College of Cardiology/American Heart Association Task Force on Practice Guidelines (Writing Committee to Revise the 2002 Guidelines on Perioperative Cardiovascular Evaluation for Noncardiac Surgery). *Anesth. Analg.* 106: 685–712.

43 Prakash, U.B. and Stubbs, S.E. (1991). The bronchoscopy survey. Some reflections. *Chest* 100: 1660–1667.

44 Prakash, U. (1994). Optimal Bronchoscopy. New York: Raven Press.

45 Rodgers, R.P. and Levin, J. (1990). A critical reappraisal of the bleeding time. *Semin. Thromb. Hemost.* 16: 1–20.

46 Lind, S.E. (1991). The bleeding time does not predict surgical bleeding. *Blood* 77: 2547–2552.

47 Bjortuft, O., Brosstad, F., and Boe, J. (1998). Bronchoscopy with transbronchial biopsies: measurement of bleeding volume and evaluation of the predictive value of coagulation tests. *Eur. Respir. J.* 12: 1025–1027.

48 Zavala, D.C. (1976). Pulmonary hemorrhage in fiberoptic transbronchial biopsy. *Chest* 70: 584–588.

49 Zavala, D.C. (1978). Transbronchial biopsy in diffuse lung

disease. *Chest* 73: 727–733.

50 Karen, C., Akl, E.A., Ornelas, J. et al. (2016). Antithrombotic therapy for VTE disease: chest guideline and expert panel report. *Chest* 149 (2): 315–352.

51 Papin, T.A., Lynch, J.P. 3rd, and Weg, J.G. (1985). Transbronchial biopsy in the thrombocytopenic patient. *Chest* 88: 549–552.

52 Prakash, U.B.S. and Freitag, L. (1994). Hemoptysis and Bronchoscopy-Induced Hemorrhage. New York: Raven Press.

53 Peralta, A.R., Chawla, M., and Lee, R.P. (2018). Novel bronchoscopic management of airway bleeding with absorbable gelatin and thrombin slurry. *J. Bronchol. Interv. Pulmonol.* 25 (3): 204–211.

54 Matsushima, Y., Jones, R.L., King, E.G. et al. (1984). Alterations in pulmonary mechanics and gas exchange during routine fiberoptic bronchoscopy. *Chest* 86: 184–188.

55 Ahmad, M., Livingston, D.R., Golish, J.A. et al. (1986). The safety of out-patient transbronchial biopsy. *Chest* 90: 403–405.

56 Frazier, W.D., Pope, T.L. Jr., and Findley, L.J. (1990). Pneumothorax following transbronchial biopsy. Low diagnostic yield with routine chest roentgenograms. *Chest* 97: 539–540.

57 Bensted, K., McKenzie, J., Havryk, A. et al. (2018). Lung ultrasound after transbronchial biopsy for pneumothorax screening in post-lung transplant patients. *J. Bronchol. Interv. Pulmonol.* 25 (1): 42–47.

58 Wang, K.P., Wise, R.A., Terry, P.B. et al. (1980). Comparison of standard and large forceps for transbronchial lung biopsy and the diagnosis of lung infiltrates. *Endoscopy* 12: 151–154.

59 Alice, S., Seaquist, M., and Schillaci, R.F. (1985). Comparison no forceps used for transbronchial lung biopsy. Bigger may not be better. *Chest* 87: 574–576.

60 Almadani, A., Ping, M.N.Y., Deenadayalu, A. et al. (2019). The effect of using different types of forceps and the efficacy of transbronchial lung biopsy. *Lung* 197: 61–66.

61 Anders, G.T., Linville, K.C., Johnson, J.E. et al. (1991). Evaluation of the float sign for determining adequacy of specimens obtained with transbronchial biopsy. *Am. Rev. Respir. Dis.* 144: 1406–1407.

62 Curley, F.J., Johal, J.S., Burke, M.E. et al. (1998). Transbronchial lung biopsy: can specimen quality be predicted at the time of biopsy? *Chest* 113: 1037–1041.

63 Gilbert, C.R., Lerner, A., Baram, M. et al. (2013). Utility of flexible bronchoscopy in the evaluation of pulmonary infiltrates in the hematopoietic stem cell transplant population – a single center fourteen year experience. *Arch. Bronchopneumol.* 49 (5): 189–195.

64 Sirithanakul, S., Salloum, A., Klien, J.L. et al. (2005). Pulmonary complications following hematopoietic stem cell transplantation: diagnostic approach. *Am. J. Hematol.* 80: 137–146.

65 Katis, K., Inglesos, E., Zachariadis, E. et al. (1995). The role of transbronchial needle aspiration in the diagnosis of peripheral lung masses or nodules. *Eur. Respir. J.* 8: 963–966.

66 Tsuboi, E., Ikeda, S., Tajiks, M. et al. (1967). Transbronchial biopsy smear for diagnosis of peripheral pulmonary carcinomas. *Cancer* 20: 687.

67 Shure, D. and Fedullo, P.F. (1983). Transbronchial needle aspiration of peripheral masses. *Am. Rev. Respir. Dis.* 128 (6): 1090.

68 Mondoni, M., Sotgiu, G., Bonifazi, M. et al. (2016). Transbronchial needle aspiration in peripheral pulmonary lesions: a systemic review and meta-analysis. *Eur. Respir. J.* 48 (1): 196–204.

69 Gasparini, S., Ferretti, M., Secchi, E.B. et al. (1995). Integration of transbronchial and percutaneous approach in the diagnosis of peripheral nodules or masses. Experience with 1,027 consecutive cases. *Chest* 108: 131.

70 Paone, G., Nicastri, E., Lucantoni, G. et al. (2005). Endobronchial ultrasound-driven biopsy in the diagnosis of peripheral lung lesions. *Chest* 128: 3551.

71 Ost, D.E., Ernst, A., Lei, X. et al. (2016). Diagnostic yield and complications of bronchoscopy for peripheral lung lesions: results of the AQuIRE registry. *Am. J. Respir. Crit. Care Med.* 193 (1): 68–77.

72 Milam, M.G., Evins, A.E., and Sahn, S.A. (1989). Immediate chest roentgenography following fiberoptic bronchoscopy. *Chest* 96: 477–479.

73 Seijo, L.M., de Torres, J.P., Lozano, M.D. et al. (2010). Diagnostic yield of electromagnetic navigation bronchoscopy is highly dependent upon the presence fo a bronchus sign on CT imaging: results from a protective study. *Chest* 138: 1316–1321.

74 Brownback, K.R., Quijano, F., Latham, H.E., and Simpson, S.Q. (2012). Electromagnetic navigation bronchoscopy in the diagnosis of lung lesions. *J. Bronchol. Interv. Pulmonol.* 19 (2): 91–97.

75 Chen, A., China, P., Loiselle, A. et al. (2014). Radial probe endobronchial ultrasound for peripheral lesions. A 5-year institutional experience. *Ann. Am. Thorac. Soc.* 11 (4): 578–582.

76 Henschke, C.I., McCauley, D.I., Yankelevitz, D.F. et al. (1999). Early Lung Cancer Action Project: overall design and findings from baseline screening. *Lancet* 354: 99–105.

77 Midthun, D.E. (2000). Solitary pulmonary nodule: time to think small. *Curr. Opin. Pulm. Med.* 6 (4): 364–370.

78 Wang, K.P., Gonullu, U., and Baker, R. (1994). Transbronchial needle aspiration versus transthoracic needle aspiration in the diagnosis of pulmonary lesions. *J. Bronchol.* 1: 199–204.

79 Yarmus, L.B., Arias, S., Feller-Kopman, D. et al. (2016). Electromagentic navigation transthoracic needle aspiration for the diagnosis of pulmonary nodules: a safety and feasibility study. *J. Thorac. Dis.* 8 (1): 186–194.

80 Welker, J.A., Alattar, M., and Gautam, S. (2005). Repeat needle biopsies combined with clinical observation are safe and accurate in the management of a solitary pulmonary nodule. *Cancer* 103: 599–607.

81 River, M.P., Mehta, A.C., and Wahidi, M.M. (2013). Establishing the diagnosis of lung cancer: diagnosis and management of lung cancer, 3rd ed: American College of Chest Physicians evidence-based clinical practice guidelines. *Chest* 143: e142S.

82 Franke, K.J., Szyrach, M., Nilius, G. et al. (2009). Experimental study on biopsy sampling using new flexible cryoprobes: influence of activation time, probe size, tissue consistency, and contact pressure of the probe on the size of the biopsy specimen. *Lung* 187 (4): 253–259.

83 Hetzel, J., Maldonado, F., Ravaglia, C. et al. (2018). Transbronchial cryobiopsies for the diagnosis of diffuse

parenchymal lung diseases: expert statement from the cryobiopsy working group on safety and utility and a call for standardization of the procedure. *Respiration* 95 (3): 188–200.

84 Lentz, R.J., Taylor, T.M., Kropski, J.A. et al. (2018). Utility of flexible bronchoscopic cryobiopsy for diagnosis of diffuse parenchymal lung diseases. *J. Bronchol. Interv. Pulmonol.* 25 (2): 88–96.

85 Bango-Álvarez, A., Ariza-Prota, M., Torres-Rivas, H. et al. (2017). Transbronchial cryobiopsy in interstitial lung disease: experience in 106 cases – how to do it. *ERJ Open Res.* 3 (1): ii.

86 Ussavarungsi, K., Kern, R.M., Roden, A.C. et al. (2017). Transbronchial cryobiopsy in diffuse parenchymal lung disease: retrospective analysis of 74 cases. *Chest* 151 (2): 400.

87 Gershman, E., Fruchter, O., Benjamin, F. et al. (2015). Safety of cryo-transbronchial biopsy in diffuse lung diseases: analysis of three hundred cases. *Respiration* 90 (1): 40–46.

88 Tomassetti, S., Wells, A.U., Costabel, U. et al. (2016). Bronchoscopiclung cryobiopsy increases diagnostic confidence in the multidisciplinary diagnosis of idiopathic pulmonary fibrosis. *Am. J. Respir. Crit. Care Med.* 193 (7): 745–752.

89 Schumann, C., Hetzel, J., Babiak, A.J. et al. (2010). Cryoprobe biopsy increases the diagnostic yield in endobronchial tumor lesions. *J. Thorac. Cardiovasc. Surg.* 140 (2): 417–421.

90 Krowka, M.J., Rosenow, E.C. 3rd, and Hoagland, H.C. (1985). Pulmonary complications of bone marrow transplantation. *Chest* 87 (2): 237–246.

91 Soubani, A.O., Miller, K.B., and Hassoun, P.M. (1996). Pulmonary complications of bone marrow transplantation. *Chest* 109 (4): 1066–1077.

92 Harris, B., Lowy, F.D., Stover, D.E., and Arcasoy, S.M. (2013). Diagnostic bronchoscopy in solid-organ and hematopoietic stem cell transplantation. *Ann. Am. Thorac. Soc.* 10 (1): 39–49.

93 Dunagan, D.P., Baker, A.M., Hurd, D.D., and Haponik, E.F. (1997). Bronchoscopic evaluation of pulmonary infiltrates following bone marrow transplantation. *Chest* 111 (1): 135–141.

94 Lucena, C.M., Torres, A., Rovira, M. et al. (2014). Pulmonary complications in hematopoietic SCT: a prospective study. *Bone Marrow Transplant.* 49 (10): 1293–1299.

95 Allareddy, V., Roy, A., Rampa, S. et al. (2014). Outcomes of stem cell transplant patients with acute respiratory failure requiring mechanical ventilation in the United States. *Bone Marrow Transplant.* 49 (10): 1278–1286.

96 Yadav, H., Nolan, M.E., Bohman, J.K. et al. (2016). Epidemiology of acute respiratory distress syndrome following hematopoietic stem cell transplantation. *Crit. Care Med.* 44 (6): 1082–1090.

97 Shannon,V.R., Andersson, B.S., Lei,X. et al. (2010). Utility of early versus late fiberoptic bronchoscopy in the evaluation of new pulmonary infiltrates following hematopoietic stem cell transplantation. *Bone Marrow Transplant.* 45 (4): 647–655.

98 Chellapandian, D., Lehrnbecher, T., Phillips, B. et al. (2015). Bronchoalveolar lavage and lung biopsy in patients with cancer and hematopoietic stem-cell transplantation recipients: a systematic review and meta-analysis. *J. Clin. Oncol.* 33 (5): 501–509.

99 Patel, N.R., Lee, P.S., Kim, J.H. et al. (2005). The influence of diagnostic bronchoscopy on clinical outcomes comparing adult autologous and allogeneic bone marrow transplant patients. *Chest* 127 (4): 1388–1396.

100 White, P., Bonacum, J.T., and Miller, C.B. (1997). Utility of fiberoptic bronchoscopy in bone marrow transplant patients. *Bone Marrow Transplant.* 20 (8): 681–687.

101 Soubani, A.O., Qureshi, M.A., and Baynes, R.D. (2001). Stem cell transplantation. Flexible bronchoscopy in the diagnosis of pulmonary infiltrates following autologous peripheral stem cell transplantation for advanced breast cancer. *Bone Marrow Transplant.* 28 (10): 981–985.

102 Gilbert, C.R., Lerner, A., Baram, M., and Awsare, B.K. (2013). Utility of flexible bronchoscopy in the evaluation of pulmonary infiltrates in the hematopoietic stem cell transplant population – a single center fourteen year experience. *Arch. Bronconeumol.* 49 (5): 189–195.

103 Qualter, E., Satwani, P., Ricci, A. et al. (2014). A comparison of bronchoalveolar lavage versus lung biopsy in pediatric recipients after stem cell transplantation. *Biol. Blood Marrow Transplant.* 20 (8): 1229–1237.

104 Springmeyer, S.C., Silvestri, R.C., Sale, G.E. et al. (1982). The role of transbronchial biopsy for the diagnosis of diffuse pneumonias in immunocompromised marrow transplant recipients. *Am. Rev. Respir. Dis.* 126 (5): 763–765.

105 Campbell, J.H., Blessing, N., Burnett, A.K., and Stevenson, R.D. (1993). Investigation and management of pulmonary infiltrates following bone marrow transplantation: an eight year review. *Thorax* 48 (12): 1248–1251.

106 O'Dwyer, D.N., Duvall, A.S., Xia, M. et al. (2018). Transbronchial biopsy in the management of pulmonary complications of hematopoietic stem cell transplantation. *Bone Marrow Transplant.* 53 (2): 193–198.

107 Patel, R.R. and Utz, J.P. (2012). Bronchoscopiclung biopsy. In: Flexible Bronchoscopy, 3e (eds. K.P. Wang, A. Mehta and J.F. Turner), 117–131. Ames: Blackwell Science.

108 Higenbottam, T., Stewart, S., Penketh, A., and Wallwork, J. (1988). Transbronchial lung biopsy for the diagnosis of rejection in heart-lung transplant patients. *Transplantation* 46: 532–539.

109 Glanville, A.R. (2010). Bronchoscopic monitoring after lung transplantation. *Semin. Respir. Crit. Care Med.* 31: 208–221.

110 Tosi, D., Carrinola, R., Morlacchi, L.C. et al. (2019). Surveillance transbronchial biopsy program to evaluate acute rejection after lung transplantation: a single institution experience. *Transplant. Proc.* 51: 198–201.

111 Benzimra, M. (2018). Surveillance bronchoscopy: is it still relevant? *Semin. Respir. Crit. Care Med.* 39: 219–226.

112 Inoue, M., Minami, N., Wada, N. et al. (2014). Results of surveillance bronchoscopy after cadaveric lung transplantation: a Japanese single-institution study. *Transplant. Proc.* 46: 944–947.

113 Montero, M.A., de Gracia, J., Culebras, A.M. et al. (2018). The role of transbronchial cryobiopsy in lung transplantation. *Histopathology* 73: 593–600.

第 16 章

经支气管针吸活检术获取细胞学和组织学标本

Yang Xia[1], J. Francis Turner, Jr.[2,3], Atul C. Mehta[4], and Ko-Pen Wang[5]

[1] Division of Pulmonary and Critical Care Medicine,
Second Affiliated Hospital of Zhejiang University School of Medicine, Hangzhou, China

[2] Division of Pulmonary & Critical Care Medicine,
University of Tennessee Graduate School of Medicine, Knoxville, TN, USA

[3] National Supercomputing Institute, University of Nevada, NV, USA

[4] Lerner College of Medicine, Buoncore Family Endowed Chair in Lung Transplantation,
Department of Pulmonary Medicine, Respiratory Institute, Cleveland Clinic, Cleveland, OH, USA

[5] Division of Pulmonary and Critical Care Medicine, Johns Hopkins Bayview Medical Center,
Johns Hopkins University School of Medicine, Baltimore, MD, USA

（译者：夏　旸　周凌霄　陈来娟　译者单位：浙江大学医学院附属第二医院）

16.1 引言

经支气管针吸活检术（transbronchial needle aspiration，TBNA）的应用在文献中已有详细记载[1-5]。自 2012 年《可弯曲支气管镜技术》第 3 版出版以来，已有超过 1 400 篇论文对该技术的有效性进行了评论。然而，尽管 TBNA 很有用，但美国胸科医师学会早期对北美肺科专家的调查显示，只有 11.8% 的受访肺科专家在恶性疾病中常规使用 TBNA，49.4% 的专家很少使用该技术[6]。1999 年，美国气管镜学会的一项后续研究再次证实了 TBNA 的少用性，54%（n=270）的专家在 12 个月内使用 TBNA 的次数少于 10 次，18%（n=136）的专家在前 1 年中从未使用过 TBNA[7]。《欧洲呼吸杂志》（European Respiratory Journal）于 2002 年发表了一项关于英国可弯曲支气管镜使用情况的研究。该研究采用问卷的方式调研 328 名成人呼吸内科主任医师[8]。在这次调研中，发现可弯曲支气管镜的总体使用情况参差不齐，尤其是 TBNA，在过去 12 个月中仅有 27% 的从业人员使用过该技术，并且文章也注意到了他们的诊断率比较低。

2018 年发表的印度支气管镜调查报告显示，在接受调查的 669 名支气管镜医师中，74% 的医师正在进行常规经支气管针吸活检术（conventional TBNA，C-TBNA），这反映了 TBNA 技术国际上的重要性[9]。此外，超声支气管镜（endobronchial ultrasound，EBUS）、计算机断层扫描（computed tomography，CT）透视和电磁导航等工具也越来越普及，激发了人们对 TBNA 的新兴趣[8-12]。我们支持 EBUS 等辅助器械的协同使用，并继续提倡联合使用多种成像系统支持 TBNA，以提高取样的可靠性和活检量[13-15]。EBUS 和电磁导航支气管镜（electromagnetic navigation bronchoscopy，ENB）等辅助器械的使用详见本书其他章节。

我们认为 TBNA 是诊断胸部恶性和非恶性疾病的有力工具，尤其是在支气管恶性肿瘤的诊断和分期方面[3,16,17]。随着 EBUS 协同技术的应用，支气管镜医师对 TBNA 取样技术的兴趣激增，开始探索各种 TBNA

取样技术,并重新认识了 TBNA 技术在肺部疾病中的重要作用。

因此,本综述旨在概述常规 TBNA 技术的历史,并讨论器械、活检技术、相关解剖学、适应证、并发症,以及该技术在可弯曲支气管镜时代的局限性和前景[18]。

16.2 历史概述

1949 年,Eduardo Schieppati 在阿根廷支气管食管大会上发表了 TBNA 历史上的一个里程碑式的报告。Schieppati 于 1949 年发表了他的数据,随后于 1958 年在英文文献《外科、妇科和产科杂志》(*Journal of Surgery, Gynecology, and Obstetrics*)上发表了他的研究成果[19,20]。他的技术是将一根 1 mm 的钢针通过硬质支气管镜对隆突进行 TBNA,以协助诊断食管癌或支气管恶性肿瘤。后续的文献中仍有少量关于使用硬质支气管镜进行 TBNA 的报道[21-25]。这一技术得到的关注极其有限,直到 Ko-Pen Wang 使用硬质支气管镜和 23G 食管静脉曲张针在气管旁肿块中进行了 TBNA[1]。

1970 年,Shigeto Ikeda 在美国支气管食管协会上发表了另一个具有历史意义的演讲。Ikeda 的演讲和随后发表的有关他使用柔性光纤的开创性工作的文章,不仅对检查支气管树的技术产生了影响,还使 TBNA 的应用更加实用[26,27]。随着可弯曲支气管镜的出现,巴尔的摩约翰霍普金斯医院的 Ko-Pen Wang 设计并使用了一种新型可通过这种可弯曲支气管镜的穿刺针来实行 TBNA[2]。

此后,其他机构的支气管镜医师证实了 TBNA 的有效性。

16.3 器械

16.3.1 常规 TBNA 针(C-TBNA)

1978 年,Ko-Pen Wang 等在美国首次报道了使用改良食管静脉曲张针进行 C-TBNA 的经验[1]。随后,该研究小组开发了一种用于可弯曲支气管镜的原型针,并对其设计进行了不断的修改,以便在不同情况下使用。最初的王氏 TBNA 针包括 3 种类型:Ⅰ 型(MW-122)是单腔活检针,Ⅱ 型(MW-222)是双腔可伸缩设计活检针(图 16.1),Ⅲ 型(MW-322)由一种双腔微型套管组成。3 种类型的活检针均为长 1.3 cm,针尖为斜面或平端的 22G 针。

Ⅰ 型穿刺针适用于中央病变,与 MW-222 相比,其针腔更大,抽吸力更强。Ⅱ 型穿刺针对气管镜和气道的保护更好,功能更全面,因此推荐用于中央和外周病变。Ⅲ 型穿刺针通过双腔微型套管设计避免了针头堵塞。由于 MW-222 在抽吸前需要移除导丝,造成不便,因此后续推出了改良型号 MW-522 用于开展外周病变 TBNA 和收集细胞学标本。

除 MW TBNA 针外,还开发了一系列新的 SW TBNA 针,以方便制备涂片。SW-121 专为中央病变设计;SW-221 既可用于中央型病变,也可用于外周型病变(图 16.1);SW-321 主要用于外周型病变。SW 系列的活检针为带有内芯的长度为 1.56 cm 的 21G 针。与 MW 针相比,SW 针的诊断率更高。为了获取病理组织,

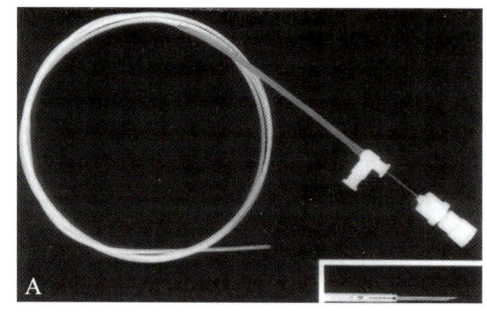 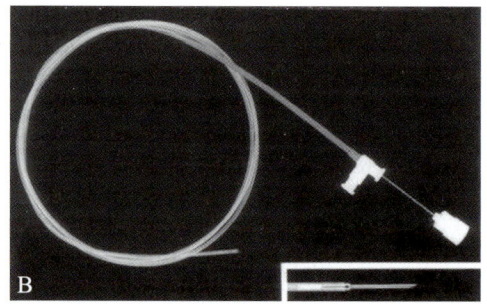

图 16.1 SW-221 和 MW-222 经支气管穿刺针

A. MW-222 经支气管穿刺针,近端部分即"导丝鞘",抽吸时不需要回缩,但在处理外周病变时也可部分回缩以增加针的柔韧性,这一操作应该在进入气管镜之前完成,此时,抽吸时无需重新推进导丝帽;B. SW-221 针,近端只有两个部件,当针头处于缩回位置时,远端是柔软的可弯曲的,当针头推进并锁定以进行穿刺时,远端较硬,所有其他细胞学穿刺针,无论用于中央病灶(MW-122 和 SW-121)还是外周病灶(MW-522 和 SW-521),在外观上都与该针相似,在所有带弹簧的针中,如在缩回状态时针尖仍暴露在外,只需使用前将其抵住无菌硬物推进去即可。

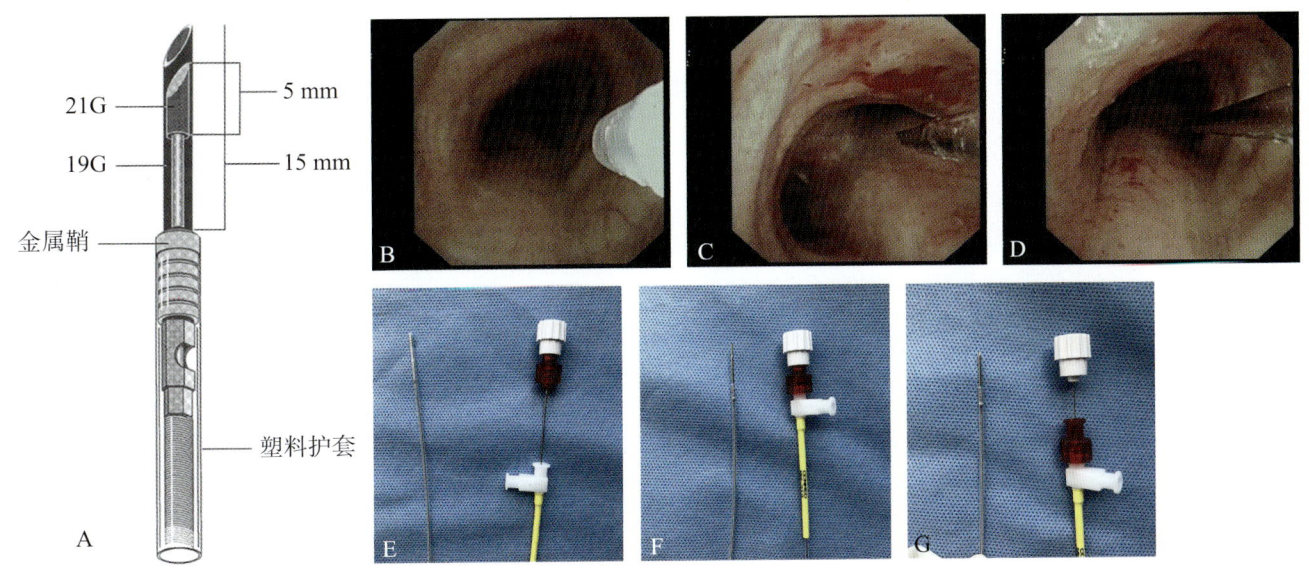

图 16.2 TBNA 针与 MW-319 穿刺针
A. 用于采集组织学标本的 TBNA 针远端示意图；B~D. 不同状态下的 MW-319 穿刺针在支气管内视图；E~G. 操作示意图。

最早推出 MW-418，内针为 21G，外针为 18G；后来改进为 MW-319，内针为 21G，外针为 19G，由于外针较小，使用更方便（图 16.2）。MW-319 至今仍是中央和外周病变的首选 TBNA 针，而对于尖段等特殊部位，建议可使用单腔设计并具有更柔性导管的 MWF-319 针。

最近，Ko-Pen Wang 在原有 Wang 氏针的基础上设计了一系列新的 TBNA 针。新系列针被称为 DT 新 Wang 氏针（中国德天），使用更简便、更安全。就 DT 新 Wang 氏针 I 型（单腔可伸缩）而言，其抽吸是通过金属丝和外鞘之间的空隙进行的，并通过针头近端的侧切孔传输到针尖。DT 新 Wang 氏针 III 型与原 Wang 氏针 II 型类似，都是双腔回缩设计，只是导丝连接在注射器的活塞上（图 16.3）。DT 新式 Wang 氏针 IV 型与

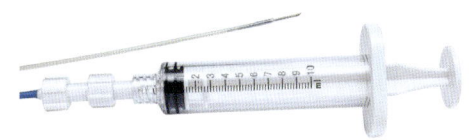

图 16.3 经支气管或经食管针抽吸系统（DT 新 Wang 氏针）
斜面针与半透明鞘相连。内有钢针穿过鞘，在抽吸过程中提供硬性支撑，直接连接到 TBNA 针近端的注射器上。

原 Wang 氏针 III 型相似，只是导丝连接到一个近端带有"Y"形双向适配器的鞘上[18]。

总的来说，MW-122、SW-121 和 MW-319 的设计目的是穿刺纵隔病变，MW-122 和 SW-121 用于采集细胞学标本，MW-319 用于采集组织学标本。MW-522

表 16.1 Wang 氏 TBNA 针

规格	细胞学标本			组织学标本		
	C	C+P	P	C	C+P	P
22G	MW-122 MW-223	MW-222 DT-EN-W122 DT-EN-W322	MW-522	−	−	−
21G	SW-121	SW-221 DT-EN-W322	SW-521	−	−	−
20G	W-120	W-220 DT-EN-W320	W-520	−	DT-EN-W420	−
19G	−	DT-EN-W319		MW-319		MWF-319

TBNA，经支气管针吸活检术；W，Wang；MW，改良 Wang 或 Mill-Rose Wang；SW，Spring Wang；C，中央，纵隔和肺门淋巴结；C+P，中央和外周都适用；3，在 MW-322 和 MW-319 使用外鞘管；P，肺外周结节或肿块；-1，一针（如 SW-221-1）；-4，四针（如 MW-319-4）。

和 SW-521 的设计是用于外周病变 TBNA 并采集细胞学标本。SW-221 可用于中央和外周病变（表 16.1）。

16.3.2 EBUS-TBNA

2002 年，奥林巴斯公司开发出第一代气道超声设备。该凸式超声探头 CP-EBUS 可形成纵隔和肺门淋巴结的实时图像，从而推动 TBNA 广泛应用于临床。2009 年，奥林巴斯公司推出了带有超声图像处理器（EU-M1）的第二代 EBUS 支气管镜（BF-UC260FW）。2013 年，新型超声图像处理器（EU-M2）投入临床实践。与 EU-M1 相比，EU-M2 配备了更强大的功能。例如，组织谐波回声（tissue harmonic echo，THE）、对比谐波超声 CH-EUS 和弹性成像（图 16.4），它提供了一种额外的成像模式来绘制组织弹性图，这有助于显示病灶并突出活检的新区域，从而提高操作质量。

富士公司也开发了一种 EBUS 支气管（EB530 US）。它的前方斜视角度（10°）和外径都相对较小，确保在进行 EBUS-TBNA 的同时获得更好的内窥镜视野。使用富士 EBUS 支气管镜可减少使用常规支气管镜进行第 2 次支气管检查的需要，并简化了 TBNA。波士顿科学公司近年来推出了一种新的 25G 针头，其作用不亚于传统的 22G 针头[28]。库克医疗公司开发了带侧孔的 EchoTip®，旨在从 TBNA 中获取更多组织（图 16.5）。

16.3.3 穿刺技术

使用 TBNA 技术进行细胞或组织学采样在技术上是相似的，只是根据所用穿刺针类型和取样位置略有调整。在将导管和穿刺针交给支气管镜医生之前，支气管镜技术人员应测试设备，以确保导丝插入"锁定位置"后，针头会从保护性外导管和远端金属鞘中伸出。测试完成后，技术人员应再次将针头缩回保护性外导管，确保针尖斜面被半透明外导管末端的金属鞘包围。然后可将穿刺导管远端交给支气管镜操作者。操作者应再次检查保护性套管和鞘远端是否有针斜面尖端突出，检查导管远端的金属鞘是否覆盖斜面尖端。这种双重检查有助于避免在随后的插入过程中损坏支气管镜工作通道，避免推出穿刺针的针尖至远端鞘时，斜面尖端穿透外部导管。

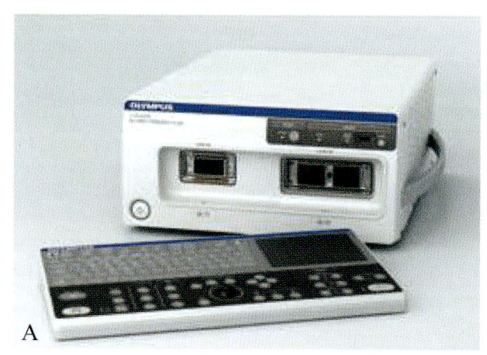
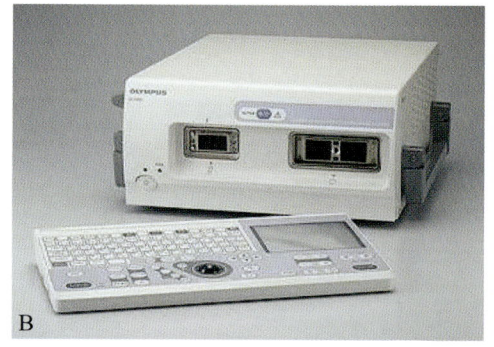
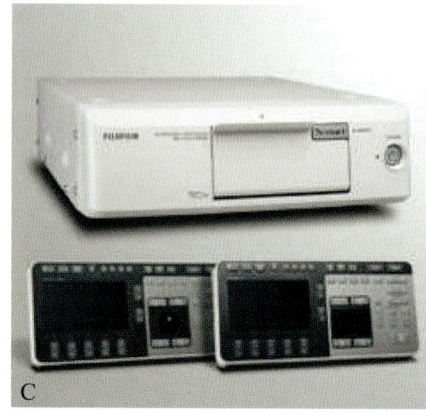
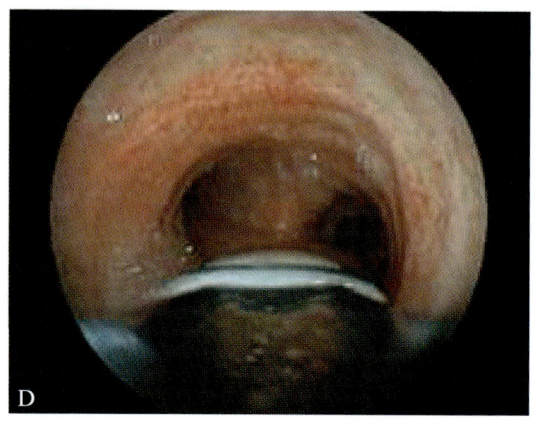

图 16.4 EBUS-TBNA

A. 日本奥林巴斯公司超声图像处理器 EU-M1；B. 日本奥林巴斯公司超声图像处理器 EU-M2；C. 日本富士公司超声图像处理器；D. 日本富士公司 EBUS 支气管镜的支气管腔内视图。

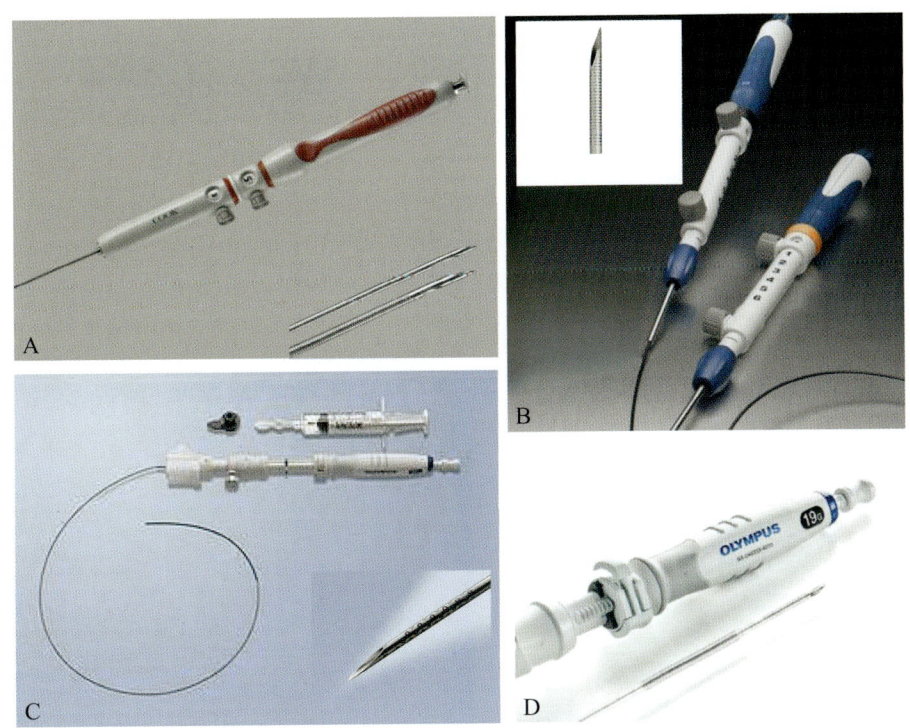

图 16.5 市售 EBUS-TBNA 针

A. 库克医疗公司的 EchoTip®，针尖上有一个侧孔（嵌入）；B. 波士顿科学公司的 25G TBNA 针；C. 奥林巴斯的 21G 和 22G EBUS-TBNA 针；D. 最近出现的 19G 组织学穿刺针。

将导管装置置入支气管镜的工作通道，直到看到导管远端的金属鞘伸出于支气管镜的远端并处于视野内。此操作应在支气管镜远端平直且大约位于气管管腔中央位置进行，因为这将有助于防止在支气管镜尖端处于弯曲或伸展位置时不慎刺穿导管和工作通道（图 16.6）。此外，将针头置于气管管腔中央将有助于防止针尖远端碰到黏膜，从而避免在确定穿刺部位之前，标本被支气管黏膜污染。

在看到金属鞘后，推出针头并锁定到位。然后轻轻后撤，直到支气管镜视野中只能看到针头的最远端。对于中央型病变，可使用 MW 和 SW-121、221 和 222 型针，因为这些针的导丝更加坚硬，提高了穿刺气管旁、隆突或肺门等中央型病变的能力。确定穿刺部位后，将露出针尖的支气管镜推进到目标部位，并将支气管镜的顶端向穿刺部位弯曲。气管镜操作助手将气管镜固定在患者的鼻子或嘴上，然后操作者快速推进导管，使穿刺针从软骨环间隙中穿过。克利夫兰诊所的 Mehta 简要介绍了 4 种插入技术（图 16.7）[29]。

16.3.4 突刺法

当助手将气管镜固定在鼻部或口腔时，将针尖快速且有力地刺入（视频 16.1，视频 16.2）。

视频 16.1　C-TBNA 突刺法进针（1）

视频 16.2　C-TBNA 突刺法进针（2）

16.3.5 推进法

针头推进并锁定位置后，用固定器或示指将 TBNA 导管和镜子一起固定，以稳定的力量将支气管镜和导管作为一个整体推动，直至针头完全插入。

16.3.6 金属鞘贴壁法

在针头回缩的情况下，将导管远端（金属鞘）与目标物接触并牢牢固定，然后将针头推出导管以穿透气管支气管壁（视频 16.3）。

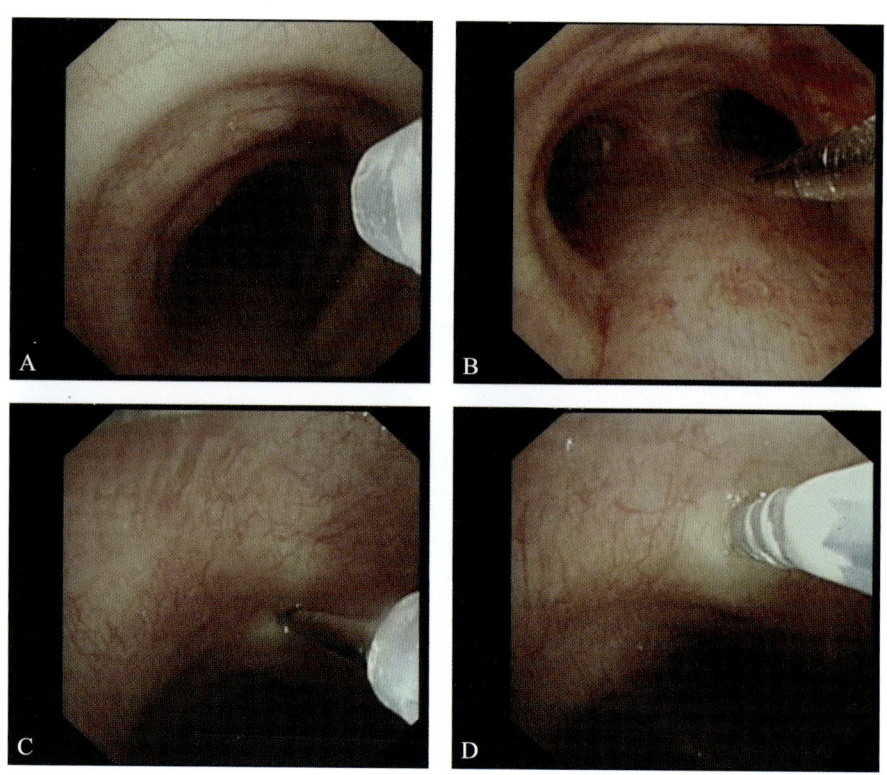

图 16.6 Wang 氏 TBNA 针（MW-319）

A. 导管定位；B. 出针；C. 确定活检位置；D. 插入活检针。

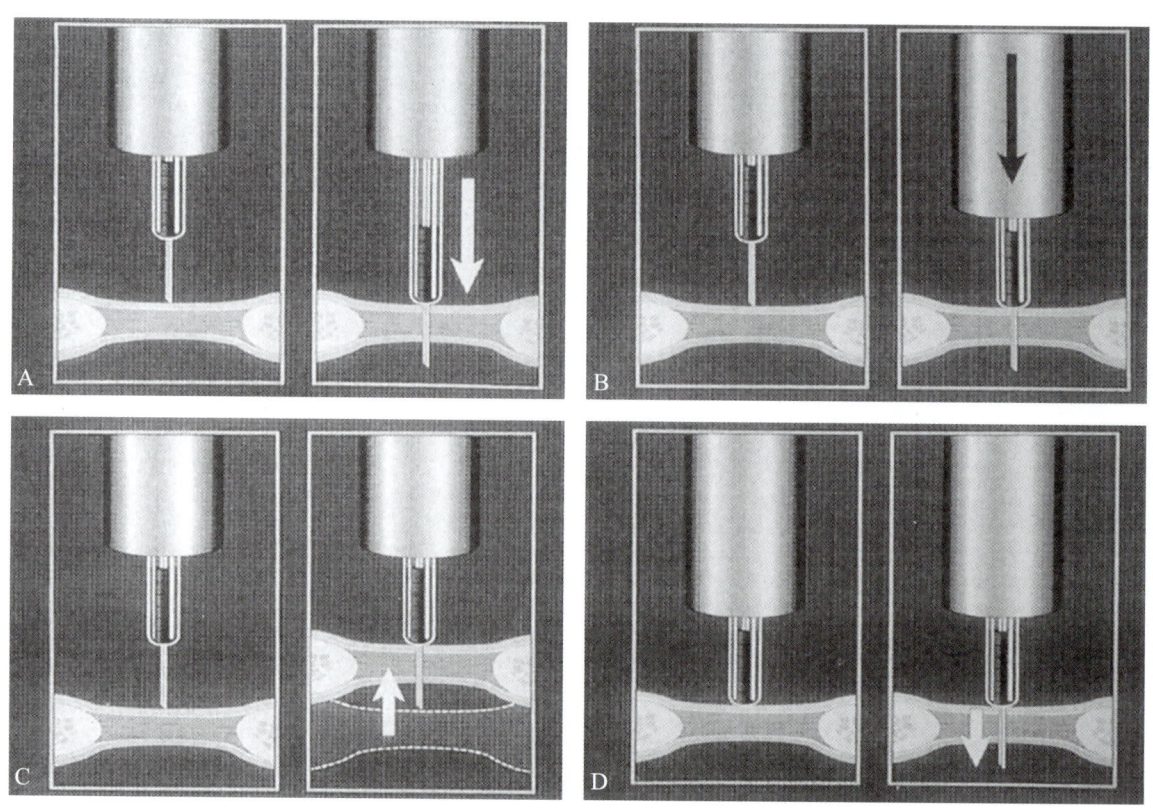

图 16.7 TBNA 用于穿透气管支气管壁的不同技术

A. 突刺法；B. 推进法；C. 咳嗽法；D. 金属鞘贴壁法。来源：经 Dasgupta 和 Mehta[29] 授权转载。

视频 16.3　C-TBNA 金属鞘贴壁法进针

16.3.7 咳嗽法

这种方法应作为刺入法或推入法的辅助方法。支气管镜医师应要求患者有意咳嗽，因为咳嗽有助于穿刺和清理支气管镜视野。

试图穿透软骨环会遇到更多阻力，应调整穿刺点以避免这种情况。穿刺时经常会遇到纤维组织，使得穿刺变得困难。有时还可以采用另外一种技术，即针尖固定在穿刺点的黏膜组织后，将导管推进到几乎整个针头都位于气管镜末端之外。使用这种技术时，当支气管镜被推开时，针尖已经嵌入黏膜，针头将以更加垂直的方向穿透支气管壁。这种垂直角度可以增加针头在目标部位的穿刺深度，并避开下方毗邻的软骨环。这也适用于主动脉-肺动脉窗肿大淋巴结的活检，因为这需要垂直插入针头，以便穿透主动脉和肺动脉之间（图 16.8）。

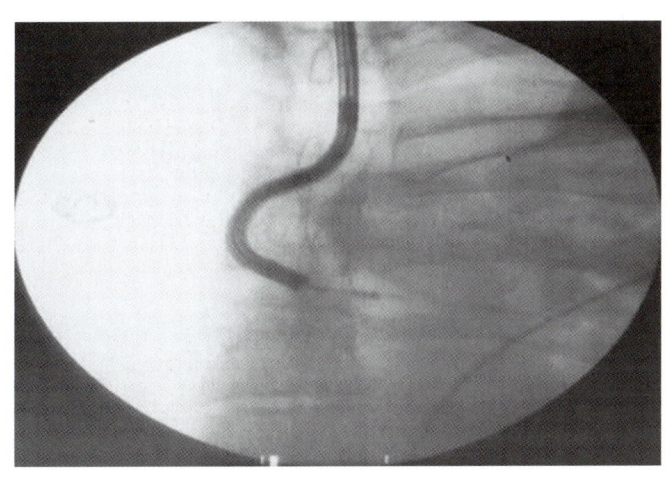

图 16.8　将 Wang 氏针经支气管推进主动脉-肺动脉窗

当穿刺针刺穿支气管壁并完全插入后，操作者会指导支气管镜助手在近端抽吸口进行抽吸。产生的负压可使细胞滞留在针头内腔。有些操作者在保持抽吸的情况下，会部分拔出针头，然后用这种穿刺技术重新扎入针头，来回抽动数次，而不让针头完全抽出，从而导致被支气管上皮污染。停止穿刺后，将注射器从导管近端鲁尔接口分离。再将针头从穿刺部位退出，支气管镜再次保持平直，将导管和针从支气管镜的工作通道中抽出。

然后，气管镜助手或操作者拿起伸出的针头，将针尖置于载玻片的上方并与之垂直。然后用注射器通过导管近端鲁尔接口导入正压，将针腔中收集的标本"吹"到载玻片上。然后用另一张载玻片对标本进行按压和涂片，并立即将载玻片放入 95% 乙醇中。然后将这些涂片送至细胞学实验室进行染色，无须再做其他准备。

一项比较涂片技术与微孔过滤技术的研究表明，涂片技术在获得诊断结果方面更胜一筹[30]。在获取外周病变的标本时，技术略有改进。可以先通过工作通道导入导管，直到在支气管镜的视野中看到导管鞘。当导管鞘出现在视野中，此时针头仍在鞘内，支气管镜和导管同时进入段和亚段支气管，接近外周靶病灶。然后在胸透引导下，将导管推进至靶病灶。注意将针头推出导管时，针头将凸出导管顶端 15 mm。然后将胸部透视旋转到不同的斜视角度，以更好地确保导管以及针头在两个视角下确实接触靶病灶[4]。在呼吸和标本采集的过程中，可以看到针头在与病灶同向"舞动"。如果没有这种同向移动，穿刺针远端就有可能伸向了病灶的前方或后方，但在后前位胸透下却似乎处于正确位置。确认位置正确后，将针头推进并抽吸，以便取回标本。关闭抽吸后，把穿刺针收回导管，使针头刚好收回支气管镜的远端。然后放松支气管镜操纵杆，以便在不损伤支气管镜工作通道的情况下轻松抽出。然后按照标准涂片方式准备切片。

从中央和外周位置获取组织学标本的技术亦如上述（图 16.9）。中央病灶组织学活检使用的是 MW-319 穿刺针。如上所述，该针内部有一个 21G 针芯，可轻松穿透支气管黏膜，同时避免 19G 管腔受到支气管上皮的污染。

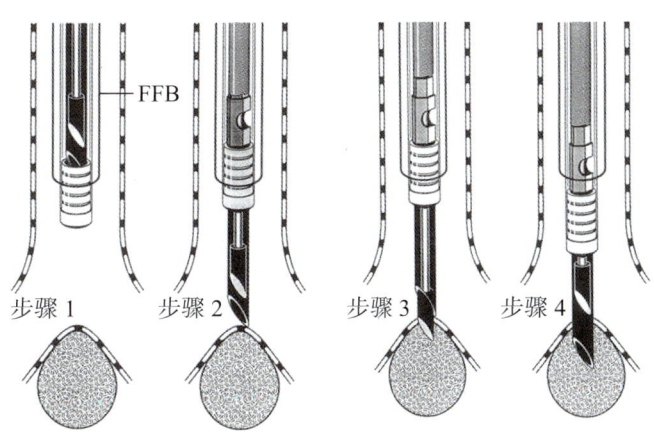

图 16.9　获取组织学标本的 TBNA 技术

步骤 1：看到套管；步骤 2：推出并锁定针头，推进 21G 或 19G 针头；步骤 3：将针尖插入黏膜；步骤 4：推动套管穿透支气管壁。来源：Dasgupta 和 Mehta[29] 授权转载。

通过支气管镜推进导管后，可在支气管视野中看到导管的远端鞘。然后推出针头针芯组合并锁定，随后撤导管直到只看到针头尖端。然后接近目标区域，穿刺针尖嵌入支气管黏膜。由助手将支气管镜固定在鼻子或嘴上，然后操作员将 19G 针头刺入黏膜，穿透针头的长度。当整个针头长度都刺入后，支气管镜助手解开针芯固定旋钮，从近端抽出 21G 针芯。在此过程中，不要移动导管，这样在抽出针芯的同时，19G 针会留在目标病灶中。这样，针芯抽出后，19G 针内的管道就形成了切割并留存标本的空腔。在支气管镜的直视下，反复将穿刺针的长度拔出到其长度的 1/2~2/3，然后重新送入病灶，这个动作需要一些练习后，操作员才能"取到" 19G 的组织学标本。注意穿刺过程中不拔出组织学针头，这样可避免标本受到支气管上皮的污染。

与上述细胞学抽吸一样，在组织学标本采集过程中也要进行抽吸。保持抽吸状态反复推进数次后，将针头从活检部位完全抽出，此时已获得一定大小的组织条（图 16.10）。移除注射器并将针头从支气管壁上拔出后，确认针头收回导管，然后将导管从支气管镜中取出。然后用 3~5 mL 生理盐水经导管近端的鲁尔接口施加正压，从穿刺针内冲出穿刺组织，然后将活检组织放入福尔马林中，分离其中的生理盐水并送检细胞学检查。如果所得组织为多个小碎片，可在倾去生理盐水后，在组织标本中滴入几滴患者的血液，使碎片凝结在一起，形成一个组织块。然后，将这种"果冻"样组织块放入福尔马林中进行组织学处理[5]。

MWF-319 比 MW-319 更柔软，适用于更为外周病灶的组织学活检。这种穿刺针所用的穿刺技术与中央病灶组织学技术相同，不同之处在于病变的识别和接近是在透视引导下进行的，这一点在获取外周病灶细胞学标本时已经讨论过。

16.4 相关解剖学

成功开展 TBNA 不仅需要充分了解器械、技术和细胞学切片的制备，还要求支气管镜医师详细了解气管支气管树与相关纵隔和血管结构之间的关系。淋巴结图被广泛用于描述肺癌淋巴结受累的临床和病理情况。第一个淋巴结图由 Naruke 于 1967 年绘制，在日本、北美和欧洲被广泛采用[31]。随后，美国胸科学会（ATS）于 1983 年制定了新的淋巴结图[32]，1997 年推出了对 ATS 淋巴结图的 Mountain-Dresler 修改版（MD-ATS）[33]。1996 年，美国癌症联合委员会（AJCC）和国际抗癌联盟（UICC）采用了 MD-ATS 图，并在北美得到广泛认可。

随着 CT 扫描和 TBNA 的发展，需要一个国际统一的系统来评估肺癌。因此，1994 年，Wang 推出了以支气管镜为导向的分期系统——Wang 氏 TBNA 分期系统[3]。为了帮助支气管镜医师确定支气管内位置，选择了支气管树 4 个标志性水平：隆突、右上叶支气管、中间支气管和左上叶支气管（图 16.11、表 16.2）。这 4 个标志性水平不仅在胸部 CT 扫描中很容易识别，而且在支气管镜检查中也很容易识别。这 4 个标志对应 11 个淋巴结站点，可通过 TBNA 轻易取样。这 11 个部位分别是隆突前淋巴结（1 站）、隆突后淋巴结（2 站）、右气管旁淋巴结（3 站）、左气管旁淋巴结（4 站）、右主支气管淋巴结（5 站）、左主支气管淋巴结（6 站）、右上肺门淋巴结（7 站）、隆突下淋巴结（8 站）、右下肺门淋巴结（9 站）、隆突远端淋巴结（10 站）和左肺门淋巴结（11 站）。这 11 个淋巴结站与转移性肿瘤最常见和最常累及的淋巴结站点相对应[3]。该系统结合了 CT 扫描和支气管镜检查的优势，允许支气管镜医师利用气道内标志确定穿刺部位。

需指出的是，这 11 个站点并不包括 AJCC/UICC 结节分期系统[34]所定义的一些常见转移部位。

1998 年，国际肺癌研究协会（IASLC）成立了肺癌分期项目，制定了一套国际肺癌分期系统，即现在的 IASLC 淋巴结绘图系统。IASLC 淋巴结图于 2009 年提出，它协调了 Naruke 和 MD-ATS 淋巴结图之间的差异，并重新定义了淋巴结站。第 8 版肺癌 TNM 分期法进一步修订了与预后相关的 N 分期描述[35]。根

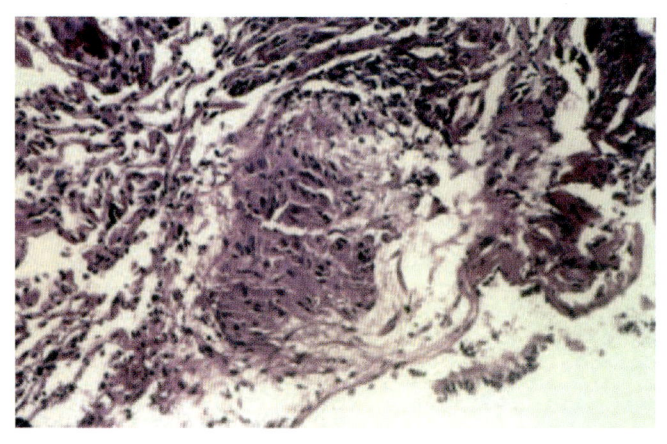

图 16.10 通过 19G 经支气管针吸取的组织学标本
来源：经 Dasgupta 和 Mehta[29] 授权转载。

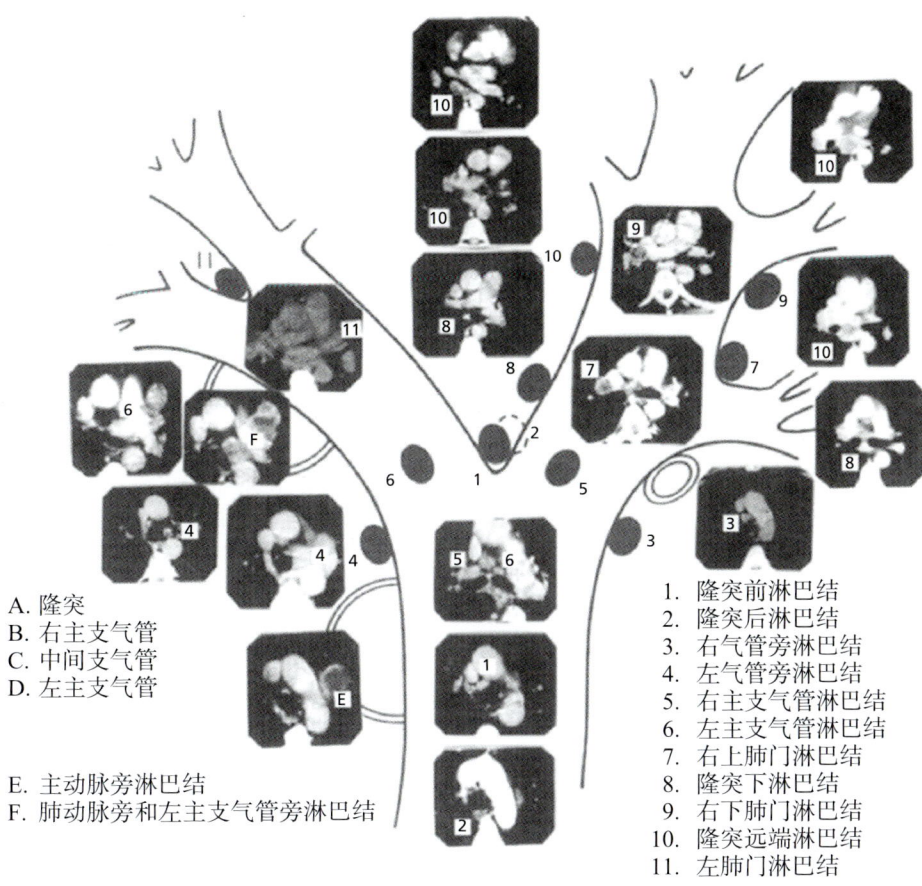

图 16.11　经 TBNA 纵隔和肺门淋巴结的命名

表 16.2　Wang 氏 TBNA 分期系统：纵隔和肺门淋巴结 TBNA 的部位（通过支气管镜确定）

序号	淋巴结	部位
1	隆突前	从气管下端开始的第 1 和第 2 软骨间隙，位于 12 点钟至 1 点钟位置
2	隆突后	隆突后部位于 5~6 点钟位置
3	右气管旁	下气管的第 2 至第 4 软骨间隙，约 12 点钟位置
4	左气管旁	下气管的第 1 或第 2 软骨间隙，约 9 点钟位置
5	右主支气管	从右主支气管近端开始的第 1 或第 2 软骨间隙，约 12 点钟位置
6	左主支气管	距左主支气管近端开始的第 1 或第 2 软骨间隙，约 12 点钟位置
7	右上肺门	右上肺叶分支的前部
8	隆突下	右主支气管内壁，约 9 点钟位置，右上叶开口近端水平
9	右下肺门	中间支气管侧壁或前壁，约在 3 点钟和 12 点钟位置，靠近右中叶开口或与之相平
10	隆突远端	中间支气管内壁，约 9 点钟位置，接近右中叶开口水平
11	左肺门	左下叶支气管侧壁，约 9 点钟位置，位于左下叶上段开口水平处

资料来源：经 Wang[3] 授权转载。

据 IASLC 淋巴结图，胸部淋巴结被划分为 14 个站：颈下、锁骨上和胸骨切迹淋巴结（1 站）、上气管旁淋巴结（2 站）、血管前和气管后淋巴结（3 站）、下气管旁淋巴结（4 站）、主动脉下淋巴结（5 站）、主动脉旁淋巴结（6 站）、隆突下淋巴结（7 站）、食管旁淋巴结（8 站）、肺韧带淋巴结（9 站）、肺门淋巴结（10 站）、叶间淋巴结（11 站）、肺叶淋巴结（12 站）、肺段淋巴结（13 站）和亚段淋巴结（14 站）[36]。IASLC 图被纳

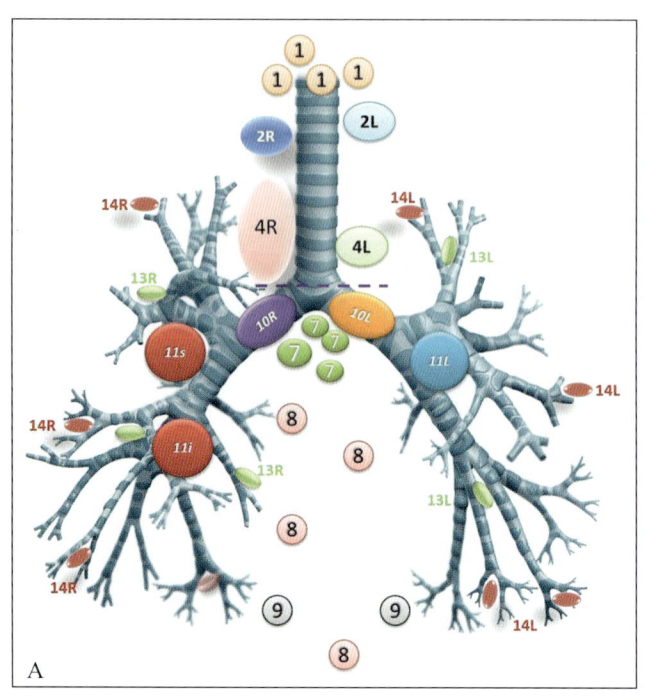
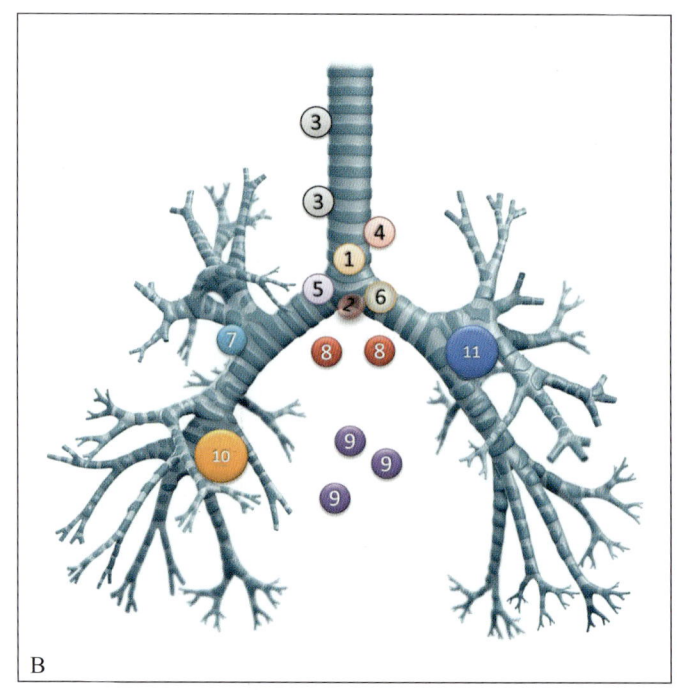

图 16.12　IASLC 淋巴结图（A）与 Wang 氏淋巴结图（B）的比较

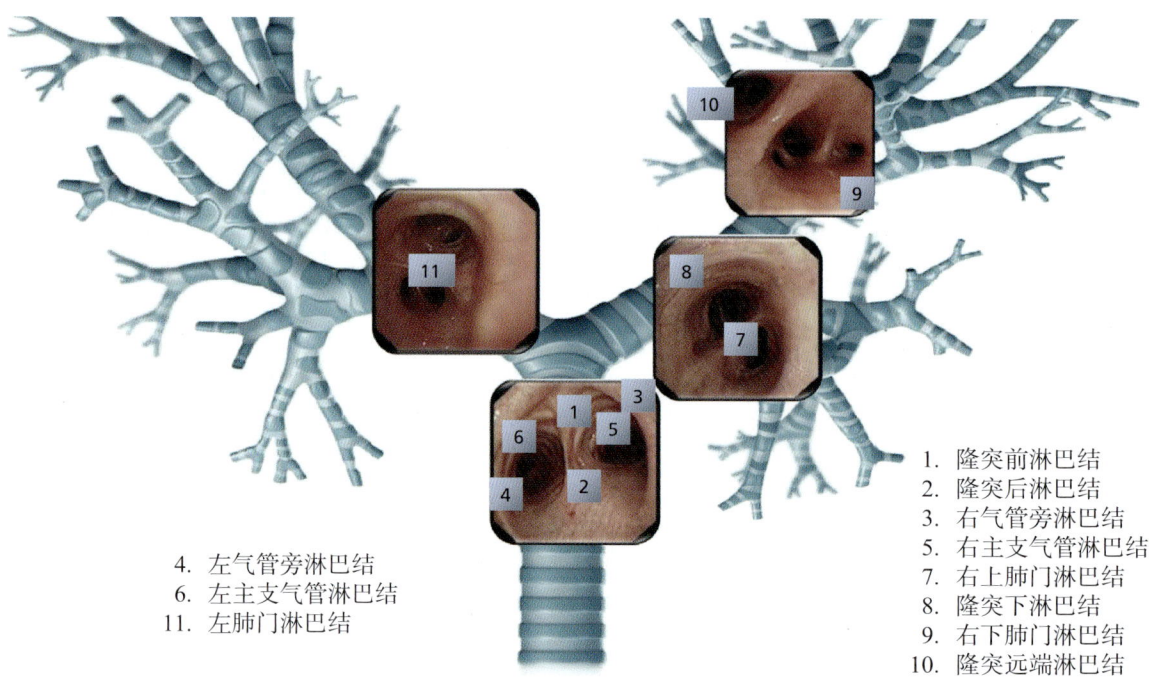

1. 隆突前淋巴结
2. 隆突后淋巴结
3. 右气管旁淋巴结
4. 左气管旁淋巴结
5. 右主支气管淋巴结
6. 左主支气管淋巴结
7. 右上肺门淋巴结
8. 隆突下淋巴结
9. 右下肺门淋巴结
10. 隆突远端淋巴结
11. 左肺门淋巴结

图 16.13　根据 Wang 氏淋巴结图（由支气管镜下确定）确定经支气管针吸术的纵隔和肺门淋巴结位置　数字表示 11 个淋巴结站。

入肺癌分期系统，而 Wang 氏图在 TBNA 实践中发挥着重要作用（图 16.12）。

通过 CT 扫描和气管镜下图像，描述了 11 个淋巴结站点与其支气管镜下水平的关系（图 16.13、表 16.3）。在隆突水平有 6 个淋巴结站点：① 隆突前；② 隆突后；③ 右气管旁；④ 左气管旁；⑤ 右主支气管；⑥ 左主支气管。

隆突前淋巴结是指位于隆突前方的淋巴结。这一

表 16.3　Wang 氏 TBNA 分期系统：用于 TBNA 的纵隔和肺门淋巴结定位（由 CT 扫描确定）

序号	淋巴结	部位
1	隆突前	左右主支气管近端的前方和之间的位置
2	隆突后	左右主支气管近端之间的后面，或在右主支气管的正后方
3	右气管旁	上腔静脉后方及气管下段前外侧前方，靠近奇静脉弓
4	左气管旁	气管外侧，靠近气管支气管成角处，主动脉弓下方，左主肺动脉上方
5	右主支气管	右主支气管前方
6	左主支气管	左主支气管前方
7	右上肺门	右上肺叶支气管和中间支气管前方和之间
8	隆突下	右主和左主支气管之间，在右上叶支气管水平处或附近
9	右下肺门	中间支气管的外侧或前方，在右中叶支气管水平处或附近
10	隆突远端	中间支气管和左主支气管之间，在右中叶支气管水平或附近
11	左肺门	左上叶和左下叶支气管之间

资料来源：经 Wang[3] 授权转载。

层面常位于奇静脉弓层面。当出现这种情况时，该淋巴结可能被称为"奇静脉淋巴结"，通常位于中线稍外侧，偏向奇静脉。要穿刺隆突前淋巴结，可将穿刺针置于气管下部 12 点钟至 1 点钟位置的第 1 或第 2 软骨间隙中。第 2 站是隆突后淋巴结，位于气管后方的隆突水平处。CT 扫描将显示该淋巴结通常位于右主支气管的后方，TBNA 的穿刺点位于右主支气管内侧后壁 5~6 点钟位置。虽然该区域没有大血管，但应注意在没有肿大淋巴结的情况下，可能会穿刺到奇静脉食管隐窝，从而产生气胸。

第 3 站是右气管旁淋巴结。它位于气管的前方和外侧，在奇静脉弓上缘，上腔静脉后方。要对该站进行采样，应在隆突上方第 2 气管软骨间隙处前外侧或大约 1 点钟位置进行穿刺。第 4 站是左气管旁淋巴结，位于气管左下缘外侧。它位于主动脉弓下方，紧靠肺动脉上方，因此也被称为肺动脉窗淋巴结。肺动脉窗淋巴结的取样方法是将穿刺针置于紧邻气管支气管转角的位置，尽可能与气管保持水平，大约在 9 点钟的位置。

第 5 站和 6 站分别是右主支气管淋巴结和左主支气管淋巴结。主支气管淋巴结位于隆突前的下方和外侧。右主支气管淋巴结取样时将针头放在右主支气管近端的第 1 或第 2 软骨间隙中约 12 点钟位置，而左主支气管淋巴结取样时则放在左主支气管近端的第 1 或第 2 软骨间隙中 12 点钟位置。

在 CT 扫描或气管镜下观察到的第 2 个水平是右主支气管靠近右上叶开口的位置。这样就可以看到第 7 站

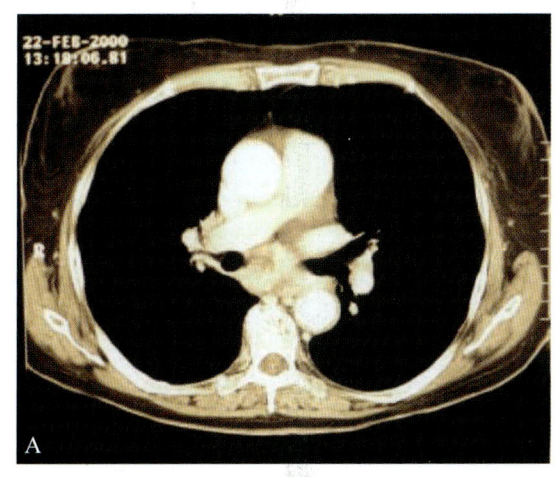 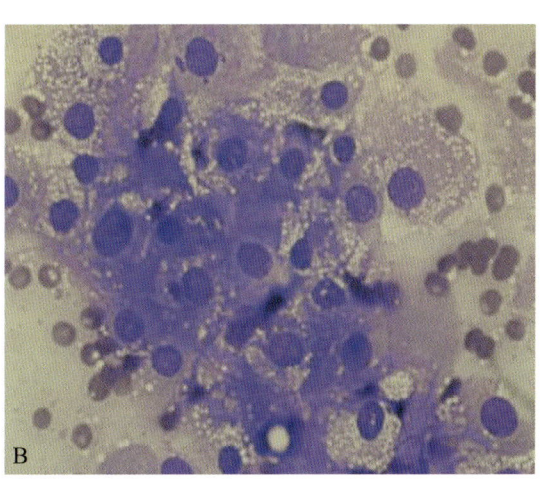

图 16.14　隆突下淋巴结 CT 图像及病理涂片

A. CT 扫描显示隆突下淋巴结肿大（第 8 站）；B. 第 8 站的病理涂片显示转移性肾细胞癌。

淋巴结（右上肺门淋巴结）和第8站淋巴结（隆突下淋巴结）(图16.14)。在CT扫描中，右上肺门淋巴结（第7站）位于右上叶支气管和中间支气管的前方和中间，而隆突下淋巴结（第8站）则位于右主支气管和左主支气管之间，右上叶支气管开口的水平或附近。在支气管镜检查过程中，当看到右上叶支气管时，就可以锁定这两个部位。在第7站取样时，将针头放在右上叶支气管的前部，在第8站取样时，将针头放在右主支气管内侧壁上，大约在右上叶支气管开口近端9点钟位置。

确定的第3个水平是在右中叶开口附近的中间支气管层次。在这一层面，确定了第9站（右下肺门淋巴结）和第10站（隆突远端淋巴结）。在CT扫描中，右下肺门淋巴结（第9站）位于右中叶支气管水平或附近的中间支气管外侧或前方，而隆突远端淋巴结（第10站）位于右中叶支气管水平或附近的中间支气管和左主支气管之间。支气管镜检查过程中，在中间支气管的视野内，可确定并锁定第9和第10站。要对第9站取样，应在中间支气管前壁或侧壁约3点钟位置和12点钟位置靠近或位于右中叶开口水平处进行穿刺，而第10站的取样则是在中间支气管内侧壁约9点钟位置，即靠近右中叶开口水平处进针。第4个标志水平也是最后一个气管内标志，位于左主支气管左上叶和左下叶之间嵴处。

通过CT扫描，在左上叶和左下叶之间发现了左肺门淋巴结，并标记为第11站。要对11站进行取样，应在左下叶支气管上段开口水平，沿左下叶支气管侧壁约9点钟位置进行穿刺。

在AJCC系统中，不包括在上述11个站中的淋巴结包括主动脉下淋巴结（第5站）、主动脉旁淋巴结（第6站）、食管旁淋巴结（第8站）和肺韧带淋巴结（第9站）。在这些情况下，不建议对主动脉周围、肺动脉周围淋巴结或AP窗淋巴结进行TBNA采样，因为这些淋巴结位于气管外侧。经皮肺穿刺活检（transthoracic needle aspiration，TTNA）更容易对其他这些经常受累的淋巴结进行取样[4]。

虽然对11站进行常规取样不会出现严重并发症（第2站除外），特别是已存在支气管内异常（如黏膜不规则或隆突/第2隆突增宽）的情况下，但将拟行TBNA的穿刺点与胸部CT联系起来还是很有帮助的。有时在核查时会发现，所描述的解剖结构有关的位置会存在细微差别。然后，胸部CT也将描述各站淋巴结受累的情况。还需要注意的是，被定义为右侧纵隔淋巴结的第1、第3和第5站通常都会受转移性病变

的影响，很难将它们相互区分开来。另外，在肺动脉窗取样时，如果穿刺针放置过高，可能会穿刺到主动脉，如果放置过低，可能会穿刺到肺动脉，因此穿刺第4站时选择准确的位点非常重要。穿刺右上和右下肺门淋巴结有时可能会导致出血，因为右上肺门淋巴结靠近上肺静脉，右下肺门淋巴结靠近右主肺动脉。

如上所述，每个站点的范围可以改变的。第1站和2站的重要标志是位于隆突的前方或后方，但也可从隆突延伸至左右主支气管的近端，偶尔也可延伸至右上叶支气管的水平。右气管旁淋巴结（第3站）可向上部延伸至头臂干。左侧气管旁淋巴结站（肺动脉，第4站）可位于气管支气管转角处，也可位于左主支气管。当CT扫描可见右上叶支气管时，右上叶支气管前方的任何淋巴结都被定义为右上肺门淋巴结。此外，CT扫描中还经常可以看到第9和第10站淋巴结延伸至右中叶支气管下方。左侧肺门淋巴结（第11站）可高达左上肺门附近，也可低至左下叶上段[3,37]。

Wang氏所定义的11站系统并不是对现有IASLC系统的重大修改[3]。相反，它将被用作一个框架，据此气管镜观察结果可能与现有传统定义的淋巴结站相关，也可能与CT结果相关。由于AJCC系统中的第1、第2、第3站淋巴结很少会累及第4站淋巴结。因此，在本系统中的第1、第2、第3、第4站淋巴结合并为Wang氏的第3站淋巴结。AJCC第5站和第6站只能通过TTNA或纵隔切开术取样，因此在Wang氏系统中被取消。第7站扩大到包括纵隔前和纵隔后以及隆突下和隆突远端淋巴结，因为这些淋巴结被认为是中纵隔N_2站。第8站和第10站可能代表一些食管旁或肺韧带淋巴结。只有第7、第9和第11站被视为N_1肺门淋巴结，相当于AJCC和ATS系统中的第11站叶间淋巴结。第5和第6站，即左右主支气管淋巴结，在我们的系统中被视为N_2纵隔淋巴结，而在ATS系统和最新的AJCC系统中被视为N_2（表16.4）。

表16.4 Wang氏图与IASLC图的比较

Wang氏图	IASLC	LN分期
第1、3、5站	4R	N_2
第4、6站	4L	N_2
第2、8、10站	7	N_2
第7、9站	11R	N_1
第11站	11L	N_1

IASLC，国际肺癌研究协会；LN，淋巴结。

16.5 适应证

16.5.1 支气管来源恶性肿瘤的分期

我们认为该技术最大的潜力可应用于支气管来源恶性肿瘤的分期。众所周知，肿瘤扩散到纵隔淋巴结对预后有很大影响。肺癌最常见的转移方式是首先转移到紧邻的周围淋巴结和支气管淋巴结，最终转移到肺门、纵隔淋巴结，最后转移到对侧淋巴结。这种扩散的评估价值不仅对患者个人，而且对肺癌的研究都很重要，因此多年来已经形成了一套详细的分期系统[38-42]。1983 年，Wang 使用 21G TBNA 针和纤维支气管镜（奥林巴斯 BF-B3R 大通道支气管镜）诊断肺癌的纵隔转移[43]。1984 年，Deborah Shure 采用同样的方法对 134 名疑似肺癌患者进行了 TBNA 检查，证实了该技术的安全性和有效性。此外，Shure 还确定了两类最有可能阳性的人群：支气管内肿瘤患者和支气管镜检查中出现隆突病变的患者[44]。此后，TBNA 被广泛应用，并逐渐取代了诊断纵隔淋巴结肿大的其他侵入性手术。

TBNA 的成功率取决于以下几个因素：取样淋巴结的大小、淋巴结的位置、淋巴结的受累情况、进行的穿刺次数以及细胞学快速现场评估（rapid on site evaluation，ROSE）的使用[45]。需要指出的是，在 TBNA 过程中，可能会发生跳跃性淋巴结转移，因此即使 N_1 阴性，也建议检查 N_2 和 N_3 淋巴结。淋巴结活检应依次按照 N_3、N_2、N_1 站的顺序进行，每个淋巴结站点都应考虑是否可能进行针吸，以提高 TBNA 的准确性[46,47]。在预后分析方面，根据最新的 IASLC 分期系统，N_1 分为单站点 N_1（N_{1a}）和多站点 N_1（N_{1b}）；N_2 分为无 N_1 受累的单站 N_2（"跳过"转移，N_{2a1}）、有 N_1 受累的单站点 N_2（N_{2a2}）和多站点 N_2（N_{2b}）[35]。

第 7 版 TNM 系统现已过渡到第 8 版[34,48]。这一修订版分期系统已被 AJCC 和国际抗癌联盟采用。他们建议每位支气管癌患者都应接受临床诊断分期，以帮助治疗并评估预后。如以上部分所述，11 站淋巴结分期系统与第 8 版 IASLC 分期系统并不冲突，而是进行了修改，使支气管镜医师能够轻松地将气管镜下表现与 CT 成像关联起来，以提高 TBNA 的诊断率，从而在不进行纵隔切开术或胸廓切开术等更具侵入性手术的情况下进行分期。

尽管有人认为 CT 或磁共振成像（magnetic resonance imaging，MRI）可能是对疾病程度进行无创分期的方法，但 Grover 于 1994 年对文献进行了系统回顾，发现使用 CT 对 N_2 进行分期的敏感性为 70%~90%，特异性为 60%~90%，准确性仅为 66%~90%[49]。在核医学和 CT 成像技术进步的基础上，正电子发射计算机体层成像（positron emission tomography，PET）与 CT 的整合显示，T、N 和 M 分期的无创分期效果有所改善。对 N 分期汇总数据的回顾显示，其准确率为 87%，而单 PET 为 82%，单 CT 为 73%[50]。正如美国胸科医师学会（ACCP）于 2013 年发布的《肺癌诊治指南》中指出的，CT 和 PET 成像为肺癌的无创分期提供了重要信息[51]。CT 扫描可提供解剖细节，而 PET 扫描的灵敏度和特异性均优于 CT。然而，正如指南中指出的，异常成像必须经由组织学证实，以确保准确分期。

由于"组织是问题所在"，通过可弯曲支气管镜进行 TBNA 在纵隔病灶取样方面兼具了敏感性和特异性[52,53]。文献[44,54-58]对 TBNA 的灵敏度和特异性进行了详细记录。在 Wang 等的一项开创性前瞻性研究中，纵隔病变的诊断率为 89.3%，纵隔或肺门区无异常的肺部病变的诊断率为 45.6%[57]。总体诊断率为 68.1%。尽管有报告称 TBNA 的诊断率较低，但印第安纳大学和鲍曼-格雷医学院通过为期 3 年的干预措施以提高 TBNA 操作的一致性，使得 TBNA 的诊断率从 21.4% 显著提高到 47.6%[59]。随后的研究也证实，TBNA 经验的增加会提升诊断率[60,61]。

因此，通过辅助成像技术和内窥镜评估所收集的信息，首先对假定原发灶的最对侧淋巴结站点进行取样。这样可以在尝试采样的过程中尽量减少工作通道和穿刺针可能受到的污染。最对侧淋巴结的阳性诊断将有效地对患者进行分期。虽然从手术的敏感性来看，在某一特定部位活检阴性并不能完全排除该淋巴结部位受累的可能性，但假阳性的报道也很少[62]。我们相信，正确应用 TBNA 是肺癌分期的可靠、有效的微创工具。

16.5.2 黏膜下和腔内病变

经支气管针吸术有助于诊断腔内肿块、坏死或黏膜下病变[43,63]。适用于富含血管或容易出血的肿瘤（如类癌）。在这种情况下，针刺比刷检或活检技术出血更少。TBNA 也可用于黏膜坏死或黏膜下病变的取样，而无需反复活检表层坏死区或正常黏膜（图 16.15）。

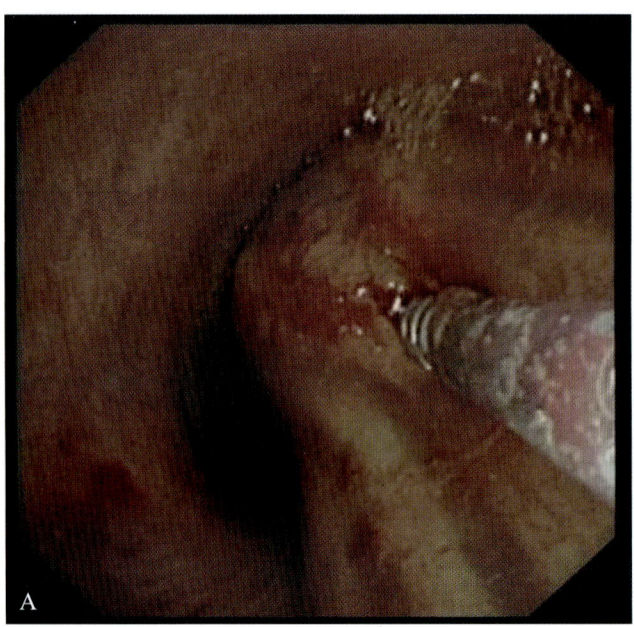
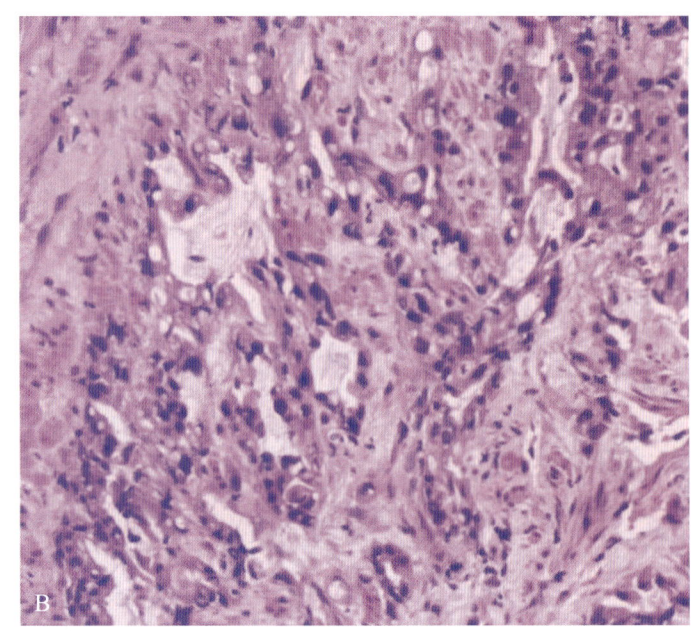

图 16.15　支气管内息肉样病变
A. 支气管内息肉样病变阻塞右主支气管；B. 通过 TBNA 得出的支气管内病变组织学显示为腺癌。

Shure 和 Fedullo 研究了 31 例支气管腔内病变患者，他们综合使用了冲洗、刷取、钳取和 TBNA 技术。他们发现，71% 的患者仅通过 TBNA 就能确诊腺癌[54]。随后，Dasgupta 等在 Mehta 支气管镜室医疗组的指导下进行的一项研究显示，TBNA 能够为 95.6% 的支气管内病变患者提供诊断结果，超过了所有其他手术的综合结果[64]。2005 年，美国医学会再次回顾了常规诊断程序（conventional diagnostic procedures，CDT），包括活检钳活检、冲洗、刷检术，对外生性肿块病变、黏膜下疾病和支气管周围疾病患者联合使用 TBNA 的情况进行了比较[65]。该研究对 2001—2003 年间的 115 例肺癌病例进行了回顾，结果表明，在 CDT 的基础上使用 TBNA，诊断率总体上有显著提高（$P<0.001$）。此外，TBNA 对支气管周围疾病的敏感性从 52% 提高到 87%（$P<0.001$），具有显著的统计学意义，对外生性肿块病变和黏膜下疾病的敏感性也有明显提高，分别从 85% 提高到 100%，从 84% 提高到 97%。

随后对 1 194 例患者进行了更大规模的回顾性研究，将支气管内病变分为 3 组，即支气管腔内肿块、黏膜下病变和支气管周围疾病。在传统诊断方法（如活检钳活检、支气管刷检、支气管灌洗等）的基础上增加 TBNA，黏膜下病变组的诊断率有显著性统计学意义（$P=0.008$），所有组别的诊断敏感性均提高了 60%～82%（$P=0.001$）[66]。一项针对 150 例腔内生长病变的前瞻性研究再次证实了包括 TBNA 在内的综合诊断率的重要性。TBNA、常规联合诊断方法、常规诊断方法加 TBNA 的诊断率差别具有统计学意义（$P<0.001$），TBNA、CDT 和 TBNA 加 CDT 的诊断率分别为 60.66%、79.33% 和 84.66%[67]。

16.5.3　淋巴瘤

经支气管针吸术可用于伴有纵隔淋巴结肿大患者的淋巴瘤诊断。Kennedy 等对 25 例接受 EBUS-TBNA 检查的累及纵隔淋巴结的淋巴瘤患者进行了回顾性分析，结果显示 EBUS-TBNA 诊断纵隔淋巴瘤的敏感性为 90.9%，特异性为 100%，阳性预测值为 100%，阴性预测值为 92.9%[68]。

16.5.4　肉芽肿性疾病

肉芽肿性疾病如结节病，可通过 TBNA 进行有效诊断。Garwood 等使用细胞学 TBNA 针（22G），连续对 50 例结节病患者进行了评估[69]。在这项研究中，共穿刺了 82 个淋巴结，中位直径为 16 mm，85% 的淋巴结显示为非干酪样肉芽肿，最终诊断为结节病。

据 Mehta 和 Meeker 在克利夫兰诊所的经验，因肉芽肿性疾病有时需要较大的活检标本，以便观察到适当的结构进行诊断，因此他们建议用 TBNA 获取组织学标本[45]。组织学活检的 TBNA 使用的是 18G 或较新的 19G 穿刺针（MW-319）。在他们的经验中，25例患者的组织学标本被判定为合格，16 例达到诊断性标本。其中有 9 例定性为良性疾病；9 例活检中有 4 例确诊，其中 2 例"完全确诊"为结节病。剩下的阳性标本被诊断为组织胞浆菌病。在 4 份"非诊断性"标本中，1 例患者被诊断为结节病，3 例患者被发现合并其他良性疾病（如间皮瘤、矽肺和脓胸）。没有假阳性，检验的总体阳性预测值（包括良性和恶性疾病）为 100%，特异性为 100%，灵敏度为 61%。

Morales 等连续对 51 例疑似患有结节病的患者采用 TBNA 检查。在Ⅰ期和Ⅱ期患者中，TBNA 的诊断率分别为 53%、48%。Leonard 等将经支气管活检、支气管肺泡灌洗（bronchoalveolar lavage，BAL）和 TBNA 技术相结合，使结节病的诊断敏感性达到 100%[70,71]。Agarwal 等对 1980—2012 年发表的数据进行的荟萃分析表明，C-TBNA 的总有效率为 62%，当与经支气管活检相结合时，诊断率为 83%[72]。Trisolini 等在 2008 年再次发表文章称，标准 TBNA 几乎可以成功地对所有患者进行淋巴结取样，79% 的患者可观察到非坏死性肉芽肿[73]。

随着 EBUS 的引入，已经有一些研究比较了 EBUS-TBNA 与 C-TBNA。在 2013 年进行的 GRANULOMA 试验中，主要结果是在最终确诊为结节病的患者中发现非干酪样肉芽肿的诊断率。在这项对 304 例连续患者进行的研究中，超声内镜组对Ⅰ/Ⅱ期结节病病患的诊断率明显更高（80% 比 53%）[74]。2014 年，Gupta 等再次研究了这些技术之间的比较，其主要结果是检测出肉芽肿[75]。在随后对 Gupta 等的研究进行的回顾中，作者评论说，C-TBNA 与支气管腔内活检和经支气管活检的诊断率与 EBUS-TBNA 联合经支气管活检的收益率相似，并敦促操作者应尽量增加所有可用的技术以达到最佳诊断率[76]。Gasparini 小组最近的一项研究调查了 253 例随机接受 C-TBNA 与 EBUS-TBNA 检查的患者[77]。

尽管 EBUS-TBNA 可能是最佳的单一诊断工具，但考虑到成本效益及标准程序的序列组合具有极高的成功率，在临床实践中可考虑采用分阶段策略。另外，随着 19G 组织活检针的引入，TBNA 已被证明可用于良性肉芽肿病症的诊断，一位作者评论说，它可能会成为肉芽肿病、淋巴瘤和其他表现为纵隔肿块的首选诊断方式[1,78,79]。

16.5.5 囊性病变

高达 20% 的成人纵隔肿块是由囊性病变引起的，主要起源于心包、支气管和肠道[80,81]。支气管源性囊肿和食管囊肿以及可能存在的纵隔脓肿可以很容易地取样诊断；使用具有良好抽吸能力的 TBNA 针（如 MW-122）还可以进行治疗性抽吸[1,79,82-84]。

纵隔囊肿是由先天性前肠和早期气管支气管树的异常出芽引起的，在外科系列手术中占所有原发性纵隔肿瘤的 9%[85-87]。每种类型的前肠囊肿都有典型的组织学特征和胸腔内的解剖位置特征，并可能在胸片或常规食管造影检查中偶然发现[88]。但不同类型的先天性囊肿有时很难区分，因为它们的解剖位置和组织学特征有重叠[81]。此外，当前肠囊肿发生炎症和出血时，特异性内膜可能会被非特异性肉芽组织取代，非特异性囊肿占所有前肠囊肿的 17%~20%[85,89]。

支气管源性囊肿是最常见的胸内前肠囊肿，占外科手术病例的 54%~63%[85,88,89]。在胚胎发育早期，肺是从原始前肠产生的腹侧憩室开始发育的。憩室随后经过一系列的发育，形成气管支气管树和肺泡。异常的出芽会产生囊性结构，这些结构可能与支气管树相通，也可能不相通，而且很少发生在支气管腔内[81,89]。这些支气管源性囊肿通常由纤毛柱状上皮和假层状鳞状上皮排布，也可能含有支气管腺体或支气管软骨[81,88,89]。支气管源性囊肿的位置可以是肺实质或纵隔，最常发生在气管旁、隆突、肺门和食管旁等部位。

食管重复囊肿并不常见，占所有食管肿块的 0.5%~2.5%，占所有消化道重复畸形的 10%~15%[90,91]。大多数食管重复囊肿是在儿童时期发现的，但也有高达 25%~30% 的食管重复囊肿直到成年才被发现[90]。

原始前肠在胚胎发育的第 4 周左右开始伸长，随着内膜细胞的增殖，形成一个近似实心的管道。不过，到第 6 周时，管内开始出现小孔或空泡，并聚集在一起形成肠腔。当孤立的空泡无法与管腔的其他部分融合在一起时，就会出现重复囊肿[86,88,90,91]。

组织学上，食管重复囊肿包含双层平滑肌，没有软骨[81]。它们还可能含有胃黏膜，导致消化性溃疡或出血[81,88]。锝-99m 过硫酸钠扫描显示某些重复囊肿吸收示踪剂，表明存在异位胃黏膜[92]。食管重复囊肿可出现在食管附近，其中 60% 位于食管下段 1/3 处。其余的位于食管上 1/3 或中 1/3 附近，两者数量相当[90]。虽然食管旁位置是重复囊肿的常见位置，但它们也可能位于食管内。

神经管原肠囊肿是脊索分裂综合征的一部分。当卵黄囊和原始前肠的一部分从缝裂隙中游离出并附着在背侧外胚层或原始皮肤组织上时，就会出现这种现象[88]。

神经源性囊肿具有与胃肠道类似的平滑肌壁，但其上皮内膜可变。伴发的脊柱缺陷（如半椎体、蝶形椎体和脊柱侧弯）很常见，通常囊肿位于椎体畸形的下方[88,93]。神经管原肠囊肿与胸椎脑膜之间可能有联系，也可能没有联系，但与实际蛛网膜下腔的联系并不常见。

纵隔囊肿可能会通过压迫邻近结构而产生症状，如压迫食管导致吞咽困难，或压迫气管、支气管导致呼吸困难或持续咳嗽。出血或感染也可能导致囊肿增大，加重症状[90]。

大多数良性纵隔囊肿的特征性 CT 表现为界限清楚的囊性肿块，CT 值在水密度（0~20 HU）范围内（图 16.16）。囊性肿块的壁较薄或难以分辨，静脉注射造影剂后无强化。其他一些疾病过程也可能产生 CT 值较低的纵隔肿块。例如，睾丸肿瘤转移、卵巢癌或胃癌的囊性转移、脓肿、可消散的血肿、治疗或未治疗的淋巴瘤、包虫囊肿、淋巴管瘤、黏液肿和一些神经源性肿瘤[94,95]。这些肿块的 CT 衰减很少低至水样密度，纵隔肿块也很少符合诊断良性纵隔囊肿的其他 CT 标准[79,96,97]。虽然大多数良性纵隔囊肿的 CT 显示衰减值在 0~20 HU 范围内，但偶尔也会发现 CT 密度高于水的纵隔囊肿。这通常是由于囊肿内存在钙乳、蛋白液、黏液或红细胞[98-100]。然而，即使在这些病例中，虽然病变具有特征性形状和位置、均匀的外观以及完全没有造影剂增强，人们通常也会做出疑似良性纵隔囊肿的诊断[101]。

纵隔囊肿的 MRI 表现包括中纵隔和后纵隔出现界限清楚的圆形肿块[102,103]。MRI 还可显示某些纵隔囊肿存在出血。

通过影像学检查推测诊断为良性纵隔囊肿时，可对无症状者或老年患者进行保守随访，并进行连续 CT 检查，以确保囊肿大小和性质不随时间改变。但当患者出现症状、体征，提示恶性肿瘤可能，或是囊肿的大小或形状随时间发生变化，就需要进一步检查。气管旁和隆突部位的异常曾经需要通过纵隔镜检查或开胸手术进行诊断和治疗，但如今经支气管或经食道针吸术已可以进行诊断和治疗[1,79,82,83,96,104]。McDougal 和 Fromme 很好地描述了 TBNA 的应用。他们报告了 1 例在全身麻醉期间因隆突下囊肿导致严重气道阻塞的患者。他们选择通过可弯曲支气管镜对囊肿进行减压，从而在全身麻醉期间实现了更有效的通气[84]。1 例纵隔囊肿继发中央气道狭窄的患者也使用了这种技术，使用的是 22G 的 TBNA 针，随访 1 年未见复发[105]。2015 年有关支气管源性囊肿使用 TBNA 的综述整合了 26 项研究共计 32 名患者，均使用了常规 TBNA 或 EBUS-TBNA[106]。其中 14 名患者的随访时间达 14 个月，均无复发。并发症发生率为 16.1%，其中 4 例感染，1 例 TBNA 术后心动过缓，均未危及生命。

这项操作在手术室或内镜室进行，使用阿片类药物和苯二氮䓬（如芬太尼和咪达唑仑）镇静，同时使用 2% 的利多卡因对鼻腔、鼻咽和口咽进行连续的局部麻醉[107]。

根据 CT 检查结果，将可弯曲支气管镜导入适当位置。活检鞘系统包括一个 120 cm 长的半透明聚乙烯鞘，鞘内附有 18G、21G 或 22G 针，长度为 12 mm（ConMed，Utica，NY），让针尖伸出刚好超出气管镜末端。稍稍回撤内芯导丝，将针尖穿刺入目标部位，然后进一步回撤内芯导丝，用 30 mL 或 50 mL 注射器抽吸囊肿，注射器的近端鲁尔接口连接有 3 mL 生理盐水或汉克（Hank's）平衡溶液。对抽吸出的物质进行细胞病理学检查和培养[107]。术后对纵隔病灶进行 CT 复查，以确定抽吸手术是否成功，并排除出血、脓肿或气胸等并发症。

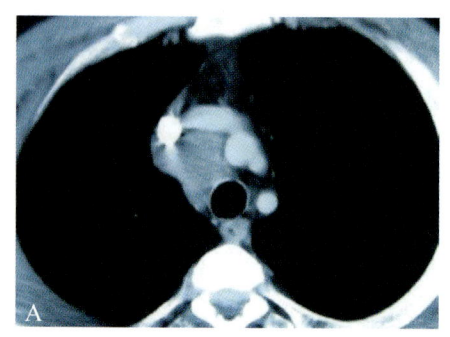
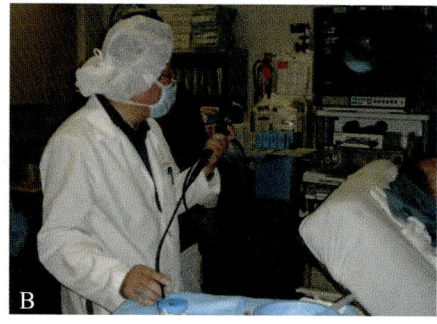
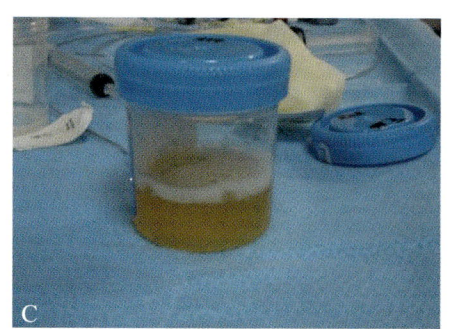

图 16.16　良性纵隔囊肿的 TBNA 诊断治疗
A. 发现右侧气管旁肿块，CT 表现为良性纵隔囊肿，衰减均匀，CT 值为 10~20 HU；B. Ko-Pen Wang 教授准备使用支气管镜对右侧气管旁肿块行 TBNA 检查，明确诊断并治疗；C. 气管旁囊肿引流，通过 TBNA 抽吸获得浆液。来源：Robert Browning 博士提供。

16.5.6 感染性疾病

TBNA 在诊断感染性疾病方面也很有价值（图 16.17）[108-110]。1998 年，Harkin 等对 41 例患有纵隔或肺门淋巴结肿大的 HIV 感染者进行了 44 次手术。其中 52% 的患者存在分枝杆菌病，87% 的患者通过 TBNA 得到诊断。2006 年的一项后续研究回顾了 15 年来的经验，结果显示 TBNA 对分枝杆菌病的诊断率为 82%，对真菌病的诊断率为 75%，并为其中的 35% 的病例提供了唯一的诊断依据[111,112]。TBNA 还有助于诊断其他感染，包括卡氏肺孢子菌、组织胞浆菌和隐球菌[5,113]。

16.5.7 在肺部外周病变中的应用

自《可弯曲支气管镜技术》第 3 版出版以来，TBNA 在肺外周病变（peripheral pulmonary lesion，PPL）诊断中的应用更加广泛，并辅以影像引导技术，如径向超声、电磁导航支气管镜和虚拟导航（图 16.18）。外周病变尤其是无纵隔受累证据的单发肺结节，最常采用 TTNA 或通过电视胸腔镜外科手术（video-assisted thoracoscopic surgery，VATS）或传统开胸手术进行切除活检来诊断。

1984 年，Wang 对 20 例不明原因肺结节和肿块患者进行了 TBNA 检查，以确定 TBNA 在诊断肺外周病变中的作用。首先用刷子和活检钳接近病灶，然后进行 TBNA。TBNA 的诊断率明显高于活检钳活检、支气管刷检或两者结合的综合诊断率[114,115]。有趣的是，Wang 发现针刷的诊断率明显高于常规刷检和镊子活检，甚至高于 TBNA[115]。与普通的刷检相比，针刷的顶端被削尖，从而具有穿透能力和更大的捕获细胞的表面。

随后在 1994 年，Wang 等发表了一项前瞻性研究，对 329 例接受 TBNA 的患者进行细胞学或组织学检查，发现 68% 的患者通过 TBNA 确诊为恶性或良性疾病[57]。在局限于外周且未累及纵隔的病变中，TBNA

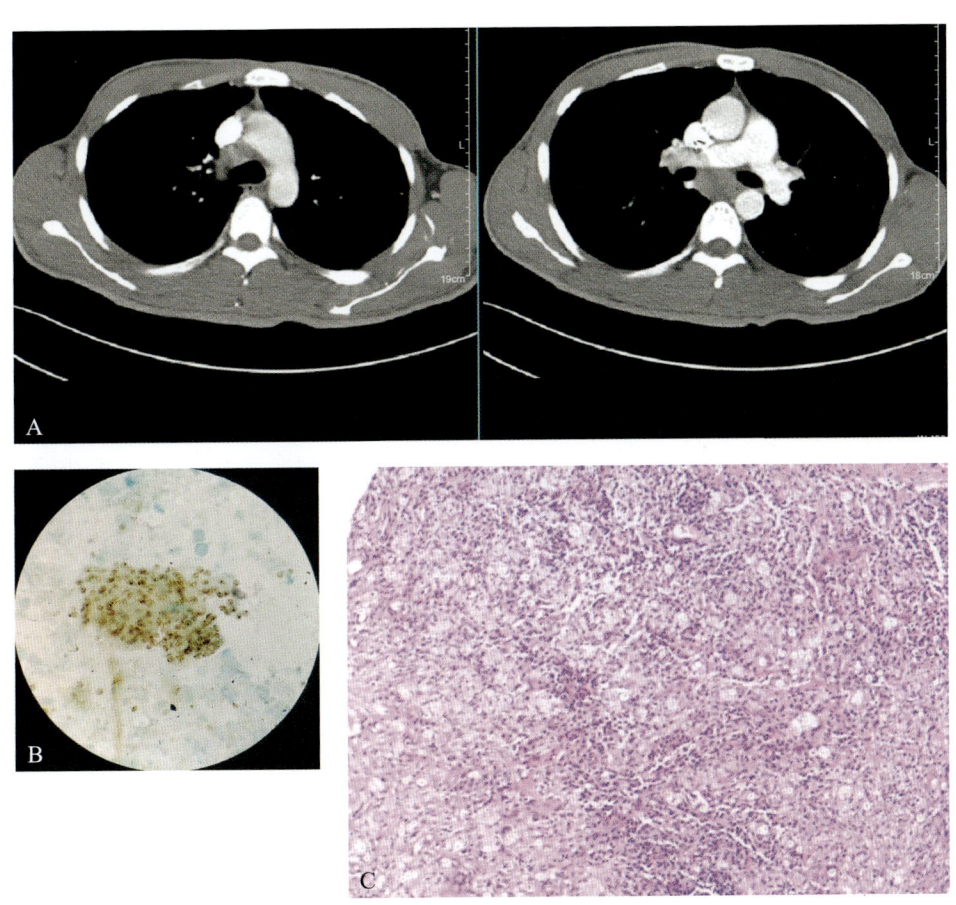

图 16.17　感染性纵隔病变的 TBNA 诊断

A. CT 扫描显示第 4R 站和第 7 站纵隔淋巴结肿大，随后对第 4R 站淋巴结进行 TBNA；B. 第 4R 站的 TBNA 涂片；C. 组织学检查显示球孢子菌病。

的诊断率为45.6%。虽然与TBNA相比，TTNA对纵隔或肺门未受累的肺部病变的诊断率更高（66.7%），但气胸并发症的发生率却更高。因此，作者认为，对于纵隔或肺门未受累的肺部病变患者，应首先考虑TBNA。该研究还指出，通过TBNA诊断出的良性病变占8.8%。在这20个良性诊断中，结节病16例（80%），支气管源性囊肿2例（10%），曲菌球1例（5%），结核病1例（5%）。在评估外周病变是否适用TBNA时，该技术的灵敏度通常与肿瘤与支气管的关系、病灶的大小以及在肺野中的位置有关。

Tsuboi根据肺癌与支气管的关系将其分为4种类型（图16.19）[116]。在Ⅰ型中，支气管管腔与肿瘤块相通，肿瘤组织暴露在管腔中。在Ⅱ型中，肿瘤组织暴露于狭窄的支气管腔内。在Ⅲ型中，支气管被肿瘤压迫，管腔变窄，肿瘤组织不直接暴露于支气管管腔。在Ⅳ型中，受累支气管的近端因肿瘤浸润而狭窄，刮匙无法伸入远端支气管[116]。在Ⅰ型和Ⅱ型中，毛刷、活检钳、刮匙和针都可以直接接近肿瘤块，因此这些技术可以提供诊断。在Ⅲ型和Ⅳ型中，TBNA在无法进行直接手术时显示出诊断优势。在Ⅲ型中，穿刺针可穿透肿瘤块，而在Ⅳ型中，穿刺针可穿透近端阻塞的支气管并到达远端肿瘤[114]。TBNA在上述每种分类

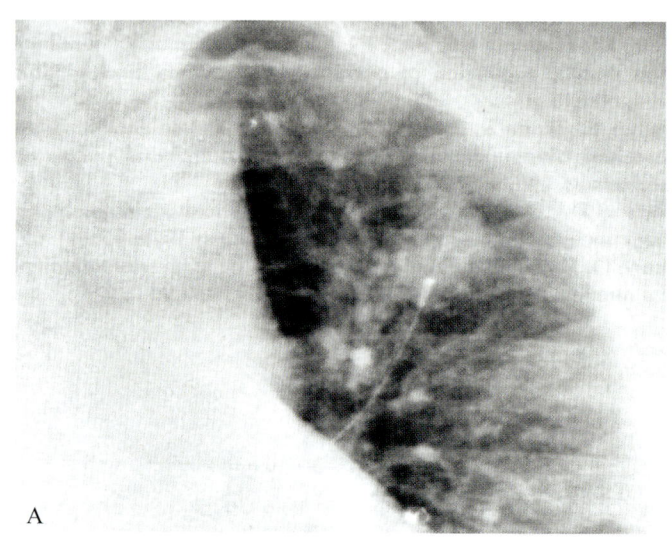
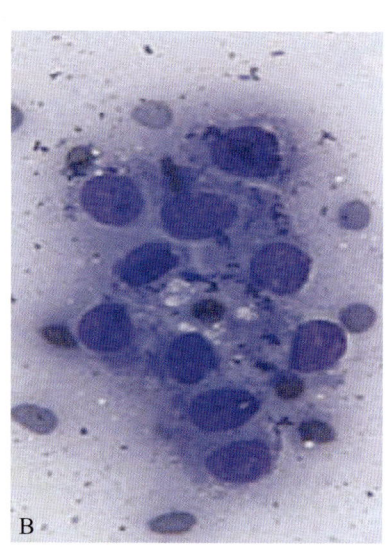

图16.18 肺周围病灶的TBNA诊断

A. 胸部X线片显示左上叶结节，行TBNA进行诊断；B. 细胞学涂片显示腺癌。

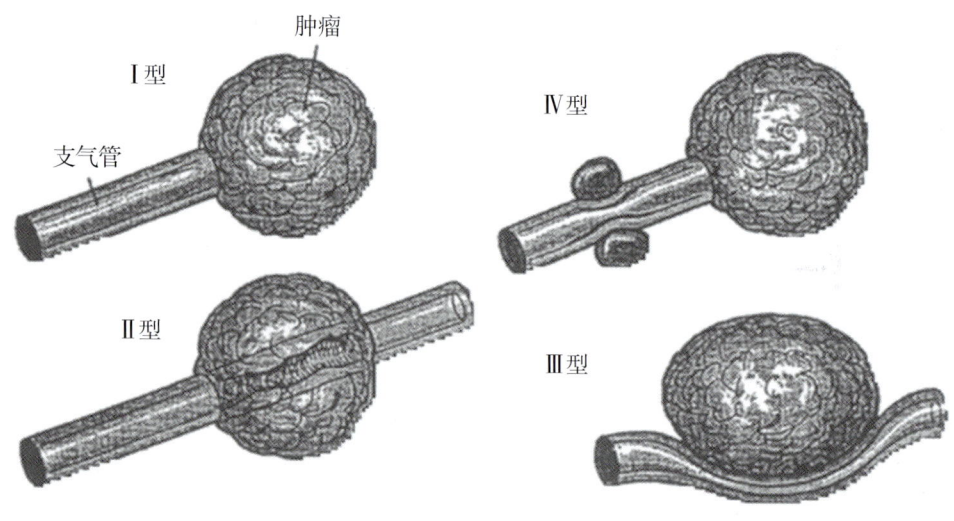

图16.19 肿瘤与支气管的关系

来源：Dasgupta和Mehta[29]授权转载。

中的作用都是有益的，是对传统细胞学检查和经支气管钳夹病理的补充，因为传统细胞学检查和经支气管钳无法穿透支气管壁。结节大小也与 TBNA 的诊断率相关。支气管镜对直径 <2 cm 的病灶的诊断率低于 >2 cm 的病灶[114]。

Baaklini 等对 TBNA 的有效性进行了研究，同时考虑了病变在肺实质中的位置（外 1/3 与内 2/3）以及病变的大小[117]。他们发现，总体而言，支气管镜检查对恶性和良性病变的诊断准确率分别为 64%（97/151）和 35%（9/26）。诊断率与病变的大小（P<0.001）和与肺门的距离有关。<2 cm 的病灶位于肺外周 1/3 处时，诊断率为 14%（2/14），而位于肺内侧 2/3 处时，诊断率为 31%（5/16）。

1999 年，瑞士巴塞尔大学医院的 Reichenberger 等利用 TBNA 诊断了 172 例患者的肺外周病变[118]。有 87 例患者（51%）的最终诊断是通过支气管镜检查而确诊，而在 172 例患者中，有 152 例（89%）使用了 TBNA。35% 的病例 TBNA 结果呈阳性，而相比之下，经支气管活检为 17%，支气管灌洗为 22%，支气管刷检为 30%。TBNA 在直径 <3 cm 的恶性病变中的诊断率为 27.5%，在直径 >3 cm 的病变的诊断率为 65%。TBNA 的使用将支气管镜检查的诊断率从 35% 提高到 51%，且不会增加并发症风险。

16.5.8 导航技术引导的 TBNA

近年来，新兴成像模式的发展使人们对 TBNA 重新产生了兴趣。EBUS、ENB、虚拟支气管镜（virtual bronchoscopy, VB）和支气管镜下经肺实质结节抵达术（bronchoscopic transparenchymal nodule access, BTPNA）进一步完善了 TBNA 的诊断技术。

2009—2013 年，研究人员利用 AQuIRE（ACCP 质量改进登记、评估和教育）登记系统对接受经支气管活检的患者进行了一项多中心研究[119]。该研究纳入了 15 个中心的 581 例患者。ENB 和径向支气管内超声（radial EBUS, r-EBUS）用于指导外周病灶 TBNA（表 16.5）。在这项研究中，传统支气管镜检查的诊断率优于引导支气管镜检查，为 63.7% 比 38.5%~57%[119]。与诊断率增加相关的因素包括外周 TBNA、病变较大、非上叶位置和吸烟，而 ENB 与诊断率降低相关[119]。这一结果似乎与直觉相反，因此研究人员提出了多种可能的原因。首先，支气管镜医师倾向于选择他们最熟悉的技术，这意味着当肿块或结节容易触及时，最有可能通过常规支气管镜进行诊

断。其次，出于同样的原因，最难诊断的患者被转移到导航引导下支气管镜组。更重要的是如果导航哪怕有细微的不准确，医生也可能会得不到合适的标本。这项研究揭示了传统支气管镜检查和导航引导下支气管镜检查在现实环境中的应用。虽然结果并不令人满意，但我们仍应不断创新先进技术，提高诊断性能。

表 16.5 单个手术及其组合的诊断率

	支气管镜诊断率		
	否（n=269）	是（n=312）	P 值
外周结节/肿块的 TBNA，n(%)			
无	236（48.6）	250（51.4）	
有	33（34.7）	62（65.3）	0.01
常规无引导下外周 TBNA，n(%)			
无	268（46.9）	303（53.1）	
有	1（10）	9（90）	0.02
引导下外周 TBNA：凸面 EBUS，n(%)			
无	263（47）	296（53）	
有	6（27.3）	16（72.7）	0.07
引导下外周 TBNA：透视，n(%)			
无	251（47.4）	278（52.6）	
有	18（34.6）	34（65.4）	0.08
引导下外周 TBNA：ENB，n(%)			
无	251（46.7）	286（53.3）	
有	18（40.9）	26（59.1）	0.45
引导下外周 TBNA：径向 EBUS，n(%)			
无	251（47）	283（53）	
有	18（38.3）	29（61.7）	0.25
现场细胞学检查，n(%)			
无	254（46）	298（54）	
有	15（51.7）	14（48.3）	0.55

TBNA，经支气管针吸活检；EBUS，经支气管腔内超声；ENB，电磁导航支气管镜；来源：经授权，转载自 Ost 等[119]。

16.5.9 EBUS-TBNA

使用径向探头的支气管内超声是一种能够检测纵隔小淋巴结的技术，据报道，在纵隔淋巴结诊断和肺癌分期方面，其敏感性为 88%~95%，特异性为 100%[120-122]。

与 C-TBNA 相比，EBUS-TBNA 有几个优点。首先，EBUS-TBNA 可实时定位淋巴结，在采集标本前即可确认针尖定位是否成功[120,123]。其次，针头更长，活检范围更大，可收集更多活检材料[123]。EBUS-TBNA 的主要缺点是对主动脉弓下淋巴结和食管旁淋巴结的取材受到限制[120]。穿刺针系统较笨重，抽吸前需要完全拔出导丝也是潜在风险[123]。与 C-TBNA 相比，EBUS-TBNA 需要更多镇静剂，而且 TBNA 必须在 EBUS 的基础上使用，使手术更加复杂。EBUS-TBNA 无法替代 C-TBNA。我们建议在以下情况下优先选择 EBUS-TBNA：① C-TBNA 无法确诊；② 疑似淋巴结直径<1 cm；③ 气管高位淋巴结受累。

与 PET 和 CT 相比，EBUS-TBNA 的灵敏度最高，为 92.3%，而 CT 的灵敏度最低。在肺癌的纵隔淋巴结分期中，EBUS-TBNA 的灵敏度最高，为 92.3%，特异性为 100%，诊断准确率为 98.0%[124]。当检测范围在 5~10 mm 的小淋巴结，其保持较高的敏感性和特异性，可用于对 Ⅰ 期肺癌患者进行准确分期[123,125]。

16.6 电磁导航支气管镜（ENB）

ENB 于 2006 年首次应用于人体[126]。它主要用于诊断肺部外周病变[126-128]。ENB 对周围病变的诊断率为 60%~75%，而对淋巴结的诊断率为 100%[12,129]。诊断率与周围病变或淋巴结的大小或位置无明显相关性[12]。一般来说，ENB 是一种检测外周和纵隔病变的安全方法。

16.7 虚拟支气管镜检查（VB）

VB 能准确显示主要的支气管内解剖结构[130]。多项研究证实，VB 引导下 TBNA 在诊断肺结节方面具有较高的灵敏度和特异性、阳性预测值、阴性预测值和诊断率[131-133]。与 C-TBNA 相比，VB 可显著提高对远离隆突的淋巴结（如气管旁病变）取样的敏感性和诊断准确性[131]。

16.8 支气管镜下经肺实质肺结节抵达术（BTPNA）

利用患者的 CT 图像，BTPNA 可以计算出最佳的气道壁穿刺点，以及避开血管从穿刺点到单发肺结节的肺组织穿刺路径[134]。这种技术不需要气道进入病灶，而是直接穿过肺实质建立穿刺路径。Herth 首次在人体中应用该技术，并得出结论：单发肺结节的 BTPNA 是可行的[134]。事实上，BTPNA 也是 TBNA 的延伸。

16.8.1 并发症和局限性

TBNA 总体上非常安全，没有重大并发症的报道。TBNA 的主要并发症是支气管镜工作通道穿孔。只要密切注意技术细节和穿刺针的位置，就能成功避免这种情况。尽管有报告称 TBNA 术后会出现轻微发热，温度约为 38 ℃（100.4 °F），但在 TBNA 后 5 min 和 30 min 抽取的血培养与临床上可检测到的菌血症无关，也无须进行抗菌预防[135]。一项前瞻性研究对 67 例患者进行了总共 351 次细针穿刺，随后进行了血液培养，结果显示无明显菌血症，仅有 3% 的患者发热[136]。有报道称，1 例多发性骨髓瘤患者在接受隆突下肿块 TBNA 后，因口腔多种微生物菌群感染而引发化脓性心包炎，但患者在感染后存活了下来[137]。2008 年以摘要形式发表的第 2 例纵隔炎和脓胸性心包炎病例，推测或继发于 EBUS-TBNA[138]。虽然有极少数气胸发生于隆突后淋巴结或外周病变 TBNA 后，也有 1 例 TBNA 后发生血气胸，但均未造成严重后遗症[139]。

该手术的主要局限有两类，与设备和操作者的经验有关。据报道，在最初使用不可伸缩针头时，支气管镜的工作通道会受到损坏。虽然也有使用 19G 针造成镜体损坏的报道，但只要小心使用器械，这一问题并不常见[140,141]。

TBNA 的诊断敏感性低也被认为限制了该技术的实用性。但操作者对靶病灶的详细了解以及对现有技术的充分应用也有助于提高活检效果。Rong 和 Cui 对 CT 引导的纵隔病灶 TBNA 也进行了评估，他们建议在患者接受支气管镜检查时使用多张静态 CT 图像来定位针尖位置[142]，称这将显著提高该技术的敏感性，诊断率从 20% 提高至 60%，TBNA 的特异性也有所提高。

当然，EBUS 技术的协同应用也对医疗行业产生了巨大的影响，这一点在本书的其他章节也有讨论。此外，正如 Haponik 所指出的，最初使用 C-TBNA，现在许多中心使用 EBUS-TBNA，培训支气管镜医师早期掌握这些技术，成功地提高了操作人员的水平[59,143-145]。因此，支气管镜医师有责任了解 TBNA 对良性和恶性疾病以及肺癌分期的诊断和预后意义，并与病理科医师密切合作来分析这些结果。笔者所在的支气管镜室的标准做法是，支气管镜技术人员要接受涂片技术的专门培训，支气管镜医师要与病理科医师就病例的实际情况进行协商，并随后审查复核自己的细胞学和组织学材料。这样做，是为了确保支气管镜医师和细胞病理学家了解标本的来源以及规范使用标本。

Diette 和 Davenport 认为，细胞病理学医师使用 ROSE 可以提高肺结节或肺门及纵隔肿物取样的诊断率[146,147]。Baram 等随后对 44 例带有 TBNA 的支气管镜操作进行了研究，结果显示使用和不使用 ROSE 的手术在诊断敏感性（79%~98%）、准确度（85%~99%）和手术时间方面相似；但是，由于减少了额外的活检次数，从而减少了放射和病理资源的消耗[148]。

也有学者对使用 TBNA 技术获得最大量病理的穿刺次数进行了调查。Shure 建议每个目标部位至少进行 3 次 TBNA 穿刺，这与 Wang 的原始报告一致[55,149]。在一项针对 79 例患者的前瞻性研究中，Chin 等进行了 451 次穿刺，平均每位患者穿刺 5.7 次，57% 的患者获得了恶性肿瘤的阳性诊断[150]。值得注意的是，在使用 ROSE 的患者中（55 例患者），71% 获得了阳性诊断，而未使用 ROSE 的患者中，25%（6 例患者）获得了阳性诊断。重要的是，77% 的恶性肿瘤诊断是在前 4 次尝试中获得的，93% 的诊断率是在前 4 次尝试中的单一结节位置获得的。这项研究表明，隆突下（64%）和右气管旁（38%）淋巴结的活检率有所提高。与非小细胞癌相比，诊断小细胞癌所需的标本更少。Herth 和 Becker 在比较 c-TBNA 和 EBUS-TBNA 时指出，EBUS-TBNA 所需的平均抽吸次数为 4 次，在统计学上提高了穿刺率[151]。

Lee 等前瞻性地招募了 106 例经轴向 CT 扫描淋巴结在 5~20 mm 之间且经判断可以进行活检的患者，并进行 EBUS-TBNA[152]。选取的部位为左右气管旁淋巴结和隆突下淋巴结（AJCC 2R、2L、4R、4L、7）。CT 扫描的平均短轴直径为 8.6 mm。1 次穿刺的取样阳性率为 90.1%，3 次穿刺的取样阳性率达到 100%。该研究的阳性预测值为 100%，预测纵隔转移的敏感性和特异性分别为 93.8% 和 100%，结论是非小细胞癌纵隔分期的 EBUS-TBNA 穿刺 3 次即可获得最佳结果。此外，Kanoh 等发现，使用 R-EBUS 和双工作通道的支气管镜（可同时在 r-EBUS 下实施 C-TBNA），诊断所需的平均穿刺次数仅为 1.24 次[153]。

在进行 TBNA 时，还必须清楚了解该技术本身的敏感性和特异性。如前所述，通过正确的技术和标本处理，假阳性结果可能性很低，但根据手术的总体敏感性，假阴性结果还是有可能出现的。因此，如果 TBNA 结果为阴性，但临床上仍怀疑是恶性肿瘤，则应将患者转为纵隔切开术或开胸手术等更具侵入性的诊断或治疗操作。

16.9 结论

TBNA 是准确诊断良恶性疾病的重要手段，它对肺癌的分期也起到举足轻重的作用。

参考文献

1　Wang, K.P., Terry, P., and Marsh, B. (1978). Bronchoscopic needle aspiration biopsy of paratracheal tumors. *Am. Rev. Respir. Dis.* 118 (1): 17–21.

2　Wang, K.P., Gupta, P.K., Haponik, E.F., and Erozan, Y.S. (1984). Flexible transbronchial needle aspiration: technical considerations. *Ann. Otol. Rhinol. Laryngol.* 93 (3): 233–236.

3　Wang, K.P. (1994). Staging of bronchogenic carcinoma by bronchoscopy. *Chest* 106 (2): 588–593.

4　Wang, K.-P. (1994). How I do it: transbronchial needle aspiration. *J. Bronchol.* 1 (1): 63–68.

5　Wang, K.-P. (1994). Transbronchial needle aspiration to obtain histology specimen. *J. Bronchology Interv. Pulmonol.* 1 (2): 116–122.

6　Prakash, U.B., Offord, K.P., and Stubbs, S.E. (1991). Bronchoscopy in North America: the ACCP survey. *Chest* 100 (6): 1668–1675.

7　Colt, H.G., Prakash, U.B., and Offord, K.P. (2000). Bronchoscopy in North America: survey by the American Association for Bronchology, 1999. *J. Bronchology Interv. Pulmonol.* 7 (1): 8–25.

8　Smyth, C.M. and Stead, R.J. (2002). Survey of flexible fibreoptic bronchoscopy in the United Kingdom. *Eur. Respir. J.* 19 (3): 458–463.

9　Madan, K., Mohan, A., Agarwal, R. et al. (2018). A survey of flexible bronchoscopy practices in India: the Indian bronchoscopy survey (2017). *Lung India* 35 (2): 98–107.

10　Herth, F.J., Becker, H.D., and Ernst, A. (2003). Ultrasound-guided transbronchial needle aspiration: an experience in 242 patients. *Chest* 123 (2): 604–607.

11　Ost, D., Shah, R., Anasco, E. et al. (2008). A randomized trial of CT fluoroscopic-guided bronchoscopy vs conventional bronchoscopy in patients with suspected lung cancer. *Chest* 134 (3): 507–513.

12　Gildea, T.R., Mazzone, P.J., Karnak, D. et al. (2006).

12. Electromagnetic navigation diagnostic bronchoscopy: a prospective study. *Am. J. Respir. Crit. Care Med.* 174 (9): 982–989.
13. Turner, J. (2002). Endobronchial ultrasound and peripheral pulmonary lesions: localization and histopathologic correlates using a miniature probe and the flexible bronchoscope. *Chest* 122 (6): 1874.
14. Arias, S., Liu, Q.H., Frimpong, B. et al. (2016). Role of the endobronchial landmarks guiding TBNA and EBUS-TBNA in lung cancer staging. *Can. Respir. J.* 2016: 1652178.
15. Cordovilla, R., Torracchi, A.M., and Garcia-Macias, M.C. (2014). Enhancement of conventional TBNA outcome after EBUS training. *J. Bronchology Interv. Pulmonol.* 21 (4): 322–326.
16. Fuso, L., Varone, F., Smargiassi, A. et al. (2015). Usefulness of conventional transbronchial needle aspiration for sampling of mediastinal lymph nodes in lung cancer. *J. Bronchology Interv. Pulmonol.* 22 (4): 294–299.
17. Alberts, W.M. (2007). Diagnosis and management of lung cancer executive summary: ACCP evidence-based clinical practice guidelines. *Chest* 132 (3): 1S–19S.
18. Yang, H., Zhang, Y., Wang, K.-P., and Ma, Y. (2015). Transbronchial needle aspiration: development history, current status and future perspective. *J. Thorac. Dis.* 7 (Suppl 4): S279.
19. Schieppati, E. (1949). Mediastinal puncture thru the tracheal carina. *Rev. Asoc. Med. Argent.* 63 (663-664): 497–499.
20. Schieppati, E. (1958). Mediastinal lymph node puncture through the tracheal carina. *Surg. Gynecol. Obstet.* 107 (2): 243.
21. Versteegh, R.M. and Swierenga, J. (1963). Bronchoscopic evaluation of the operability of pulmonary carcinoma. *Acta Otolaryngol.* 56: 603–611.
22. Fox, R.T., Lees, W.M., and Shields, T.W. (1965). Transcarinal bronchoscopic needle biopsy. *Ann. Thorac. Surg.* 1: 92–96.
23. Simecek, C. (1966). Cytological investigation of intrathoracic lymph nodes in carcinoma of the lung. *Thorax* 21 (4): 369–371.
24. Bridgman, A.H., Duffield, G.D., and Takaro, T. (1968). An appraisal of newer diagnostic methods for intrathoracic lesions. *Dis Chest.* 53 (3): 321–327.
25. Atay, Z. and Brandt, H.-J. (1977). Die Bedeutung der Zytodiagnostik der perbronchialen Feinnadelpunktion von mediastinalen oder hilären Tumoren. *Dtsch. Med. Wochenschr.* 102 (10): 345–348.
26. Ikeda, S. (1970). Flexible bronchofiberscope. *Ann. Otol. Rhinol. Laryngol.* 79 (5): 916–923.
27. Ikeda, S. (1988). The development and progress of endoscopes in the field of bronchoesophagology. *Nihon Kikan Shokudoka Gakkai Kaiho* 39 (2): 85–96.
28. Sakairi, Y., Nakajima, T., Yonemori, Y. et al. (2017). P2.12-006 evaluation of new 25G needle in EBUS-TBNA comparing conventional 22G needle in diagnosis for nodal metastasis of lung cancer. *J. Thorac. Oncol.* 12 (11): S2165.
29. Dasgupta, A. and Mehta, A.C. (1999). Transbronchial needle aspiration. An underused diagnostic technique. *Clin. Chest Med.* 20 (1): 39–51.
30. Wang, K.P., Selcuk, Z.T., and Erozan, Y. (1994). Transbronchial needle aspiration for cytology specimens. *Monaldi Arch. Chest Dis.* 49 (3): 265–267.
31. Naruke, T. (1967). The spread of lung cancer and its relevance to surgery. *Nippon Kyobu Geka Gakkai Zasshi* 68: 1607–1621.
32. American Thoracic Society. Medical Section of the American Lung Association (1983). Clinical staging of primary lung cancer. *Am. Rev. Respir. Dis.* 127 (5): 659–664.
33. Mountain, C.F. and Dresler, C.M. (1997). Regional lymph node classification for lung cancer staging. *Chest* 111 (6): 1718–1723.
34. Detterbeck, F.C., Boffa, D.J., Kim, A.W., and Tanoue, L.T. (2017). The eighth edition lung cancer stage classification. *Chest* 151 (1): 193–203.
35. Asamura, H., Chansky, K., Crowley, J. et al. (2015). The International Association for the Study of Lung Cancer lung cancer staging project: proposals for the revision of the N descriptors in the forthcoming 8th edition of the TNM classification for lung cancer. *J. Thorac. Oncol.* 10 (12): 1675–1684.
36. Rusch, V.W., Asamura, H., Watanabe, H. et al. (2009). The IASLC lung cancer staging project: a proposal for a new international lymph node map in the forthcoming seventh edition of the TNM classification for lung cancer. *J. Thorac. Oncol.* 4 (5): 568–577.
37. Wang, K.P. (1995). Transbronchial needle aspiration and percutaneous needle aspiration for staging and diagnosis of lung cancer. *Clin. Chest Med.* 16 (3): 535–552.
38. Naruke, T., Goya, T., Tsuchiya, R., and Suemasu, K. (1988). Prognosis and survival in resected lung carcinoma based on the new international staging system. *J. Thorac. Cardiovasc. Surg.* 96 (3): 440–447.
39. Mountain, C.F. (1986). A new international staging system for lung cancer. *Chest* 89 (4 Suppl): 225S–233S.
40. Mountain, C.F. (1997). Revisions in the international system for staging lung cancer. *Chest* 111 (6): 1710–1717. Epub 1997/06/01.
41. Mountain, C.F. (1988). Prognostic implications of the international staging system for lung cancer. *Semin. Oncol.* 15 (3): 236–245.
42. Mountain, C.F. (1989). Value of the new TNM staging system for lung cancer. *Chest* 96 (1 Suppl): 47S–49S. Epub 1989/07/01.
43. Wang, K.P. and Terry, P.B. (1983). Transbronchial needle aspiration in the diagnosis and staging of bronchogenic carcinoma. *Am. Rev. Respir. Dis.* 127 (3): 344–347.
44. Shure, D. and Fedullo, P.F. (1984). The role of transcarinal needle aspiration in the staging of bronchogenic carcinoma. *Chest* 86 (5): 693–696.
45. Mehta, A.C. (2013). *Interventional Bronchoscopy: A Clinical Guide.* New York: Springer.
46. Jin, X.R., Ye, M., Cai, Z.Z. et al. (2015). Standardized transbronchial needle aspiration procedure for intrathoracic lymph node staging of non-small cell lung cancer. *J. Thorac. Dis.* 7 (Suppl 4): S266–S271.
47. Xia, Y., Zhang, B., Zhang, H. et al. (2015). Evaluation of lymph node metastasis in lung cancer: who is the chief justice? *J. Thorac. Dis.* 7 (Suppl 4): S231–S237.
48. Goldstraw, P. (2009). The 7th edition of TNM in lung cancer: what now? *J. Thorac. Oncol.* 4 (6): 671–673.

49 Grover, F.L. (1994). The role of CT and MRI in staging of the mediastinum. *Chest* 106 (6 Suppl): 391S–396S.

50 De Wever, W., Stroobants, S., Coolen, J., and Verschakelen, J.A. (2009). Integrated PET/CT in the staging of nonsmall cell lung cancer: technical aspects and clinical integration. *Eur. Respir. J.* 33 (1): 201–212.

51 Silvestri, G.A., Gonzalez, A.V., Jantz, M.A. et al. (2013). Methods for staging non-small cell lung cancer: diagnosis and management of lung cancer, 3rd ed: American College of Chest Physicians evidence-based clinical practice guidelines. *Chest* 143 (5 Suppl): e211S–e250S.

52 Turner, J. Jr. and Wang, K.-P. (1996). Staging of mediastinal involvement in lung cancer by bronchoscopic needle aspiration: pro bronchoscopic needle aspiration. *J. Bronchology Interv. Pulmonol.* 3 (1): 74–76.

53 Turner, J.F., del Rosario, A.D., Simoff, M. et al. (2008). Staging of bronchogenic carcinoma: an interventional pulmonary perspective. In: *Thoracic Endoscopy: Advances in Interventional Pulmonology* (eds. M.J. Simoff, D. Sterman and A. Ernst), 279–297. Oxford: Blackwell.

54 Shure, D. and Fedullo, P.F. (1985). Transbronchial needle aspiration in the diagnosis of submucosal and peribronchial bronchogenic carcinoma. *Chest* 88 (1): 49–51.

55 Shure, D. (1989). Transbronchial biopsy and needle aspiration. *Chest* 95 (5): 1130–1138.

56 Schenk, D.A., Bryan, C.L., Bower, J.H., and Myers, D.L. (1987). Transbronchial needle aspiration in the diagnosis of bronchogenic carcinoma. *Chest* 92 (1): 83–85.

57 Wang, K.-P., Gonullu, U., and Baker, R. (1994). Transbronchial needle aspiration versus transthoracic needle aspiration in the diagnosis of pulmonary lesions. *J. Bronchology Interv. Pulmonol.* 1 (3): 199–204.

58 Utz, J.P., Patel, A.M., and Edell, E.S. (1993). The role of transcarinal needle aspiration in the staging of bronchogenic carcinoma. *Chest* 104 (4): 1012–1016. Epub 1993/10/01.

59 Haponik, E.F., Cappellari, J.O., Chin, R. et al. (1995). Education and experience improve transbronchial needle aspiration performance. *Am. J. Respir. Crit. Care Med.* 151 (6): 1998–2002.

60 Rodriguez de Castro, F., Diaz Lopez, F., Serda, G.J. et al. (1997). Relevance of training in transbronchial fine-needle aspiration technique. *Chest* 111 (1): 103–105.

61 Hsu, L.H., Liu, C.C., and Ko, J.S. (2004). Education and experience improve the performance of transbronchial needle aspiration: a learning curve at a cancer center. *Chest* 125 (2): 532–540.

62 Schenk, D.A., Bower, J.H., Bryan, C.L. et al. (1986). Transbronchial needle aspiration staging of bronchogenic carcinoma. *Am. Rev. Respir. Dis.* 134 (1): 146–148.

63 Buirski, G., Calverley, P.M., Douglas, N.J. et al. (1981). Bronchial needle aspiration in the diagnosis of bronchial carcinoma. *Thorax* 36 (7): 508–511.

64 Dasgupta, A., Jain, P., Minai, O.A. et al. (1999). Utility of transbronchial needle aspiration in the diagnosis of endobronchial lesions. *Chest* 115 (5): 1237–1241.

65 Caglayan, B., Akturk, U.A., Fidan, A. et al. (2005). Transbronchial needle aspiration in the diagnosis of endobronchial malignant lesions: a 3-year experience. *Chest* 128 (2): 704–708.

66 Uskul, B.T., Turker, H., Melikoglu, A. et al. (2007). Value of transbronchial needle aspiration in the diagnosis of endobronchial malignant lesions. *Tuberk. Toraks* 55 (3): 259–265.

67 Shital, P., Rujuta, A., and Sanjay, M. (2014). Transbronchial needle aspiration cytology (TBNA) in endobronchial lesions: a valuable technique during bronchoscopy in diagnosing lung cancer and it will decrease repeat bronchoscopy. *J. Cancer Res. Clin. Oncol.* 140 (5): 809–815.

68 Kennedy, M.P., Jimenez, C.A., Bruzzi, J.F. et al. (2008). Endobronchial ultrasound-guided transbronchial needle aspiration in the diagnosis of lymphoma. *Thorax* 63 (4): 360–365.

69 Garwood, S., Judson, M.A., Silvestri, G. et al. (2007). Endobronchial ultrasound for the diagnosis of pulmonary sarcoidosis. *Chest* 132 (4): 1298–1304.

70 Morales, C.F., Patefield, A.J., Strollo, P.J. Jr., and Schenk, D.A. (1994). Flexible transbronchial needle aspiration in the diagnosis of sarcoidosis. *Chest* 106 (3): 709–711.

71 Leonard, C., Tormey, V.J., O'Keane, C., and Burke, C.M. (1997). Bronchoscopic diagnosis of sarcoidosis. *Eur. Respir. J.* 10 (12): 2722–2724.

72 Agarwal, R., Aggarwal, A.N., and Gupta, D. (2013). Efficacy and safety of conventional transbronchial needle aspiration in sarcoidosis: a systematic review and meta-analysis. *Respir. Care* 58 (4): 683–693.

73 Trisolini, R., Tinelli, C., Cancellieri, A. et al. (2008). Transbronchial needle aspiration in sarcoidosis: yield and predictors of a positive aspirate. *J. Thorac. Cardiovasc. Surg.* 135 (4): 837–842.

74 von Bartheld, M.B., Dekkers, O.M., Szlubowski, A. et al. (2013). Endosonography vs conventional bronchoscopy for the diagnosis of sarcoidosis: the GRANULOMA randomized clinical trial. *JAMA* 309 (23): 2457–2464.

75 Gupta, D., Dadhwal, D.S., Agarwal, R. et al. (2014). Endobronchial ultrasound-guided transbronchial needle aspiration vs conventional transbronchial needle aspiration in the diagnosis of sarcoidosis. *Chest* 146 (3): 547–556.

76 Mondoni, M., Radovanovic, D., Valenti, V. et al. (2015). Bronchoscopy in sarcoidosis: union is strength. *Minerva Med.* 106 (2 Suppl 2): 1–7.

77 Bonifazi, M., Tramacere, I., Zuccatosta, L. et al. (2017). Conventional versus ultrasound-guided transbronchial needle aspiration for the diagnosis of hilar/mediastinal lymph adenopathies: a randomized controlled trial. *Respiration* 94 (2): 216–223.

78 Trisolini, R., LazzariAgli, L., Cancellieri, A. et al. (2003). The value of flexible transbronchial needle aspiration in the diagnosis of stage I sarcoidosis. *Chest* 124 (6): 2126–2130.

79 Kuhlman, J.E., Fishman, E.K., Wang, K.P., and Siegelman, S.S. (1985). Esophageal duplication cyst: CT and transesophageal needle aspiration. *Am. J. Roentgenol.* 145 (3): 531–532.

80 Silverman, N.A. and Sabiston, D.C. Jr. (1980). Mediastinal masses. *Surg. Clin. North Am.* 60 (4): 757–777.

81 Salyer, D.C., Salyer, W.R., and Eggleston, J.C. (1977). Benign developmental cysts of the mediastinum. *Arch. Pathol. Lab. Med.* 101 (3): 136–139.

82 Wang, K.P., Nelson, S., Scatarige, J., and Siegelman, S. (1983). Transbronchial needle aspiration of a mediastinal mass: therapeutic implications. *Thorax* 38 (7): 556–557.

83 Schwartz, D.B., Beals,T.F., Wimbish, K.J., and Hammersley, J.R. (1985). Transbronchial fine needle aspiration of bronchogenic cysts. *Chest* 88 (4): 573–575.

84 McDougall, J.C. and Fromme, G.A. (1990). Transcarinal aspiration of a mediastinal cyst to facilitate anesthetic management. *Chest* 97 (6): 1490–1492.

85 Wychulis, A.R., Payne, W.S., Clagett, O.T., and Woolner, L.B. (1971). Surgical treatment of mediastinal tumors: a 40 year experience. *J. Thorac. Cardiovasc. Surg.* 62 (3): 379–392.

86 Morrison, I.M. (1958). Tumours and cysts of the mediastinum. *Thorax* 13 (4): 294–307.

87 Heithoff, K.B., Sane, S.M., Williams, H.J. et al. (1976). Bronchopulmonary foregut malformations. A unifying etiological concept. *Am. J. Roentgenol.* 126 (1): 46–55.

88 Kirwan, W.O., Walbaum, P.R., and McCormack, R.J. (1973). Cystic intrathoracic derivatives of the foregut and their complications. *Thorax* 28 (4): 424–428.

89 Sirivella, S., Ford, W.B., Zikria, E.A. et al. (1985). Foregut cysts of the mediastinum. Results in 20 consecutive surgically treated cases. *J. Thorac. Cardiovasc. Surg.* 90 (5): 776–782.

90 Whitaker, J.A., Deffenbaugh, L.D., and Cooke, A.R. (1980). Esophageal duplication cyst. Case report. *Am. J. Gastroenterol.* 73 (4): 329–332.

91 Hocking, M. and Young, D.G. (1981). Duplications of the alimentary tract. *Br. J. Surg.* 68 (2): 92–96.

92 Ferguson, C.C., Young, L.N., Sutherland, J.B., and Macpherson, R.I. (1973). Intrathoracic gastrogenic cyst – preoperative diagnosis by technetium pertechnetate scan. *J. Pediatr. Surg.* 8 (5): 827–828.

93 Reed, J.C. and Sobonya, R.E. (1974). Morphologic analysis of foregut cysts in the thorax. *Am. J. Roentgenol. Radium Ther. Nucl. Med.* 120 (4): 851–860.

94 Yousem, D.M., Scatarige, J.C., Fishman, E.K., and Siegelman, S.S. (1986). Low-attenuation thoracic metastases in testicular malignancy. *Am. J. Roentgenol.* 146 (2): 291–293.

95 Glazer, H.S., Siegel, M.J., and Sagel, S.S. (1989). Low-attenuation mediastinal masses on CT. *Am. J. Roentgenol.* 152 (6): 1173–1177.

96 Kuhlman, J.E., Fishman, E.K., Wang, K.P. et al. (1988). Mediastinal cysts: diagnosis by CT and needle aspiration. *Am. J. Roentgenol.* 150 (1): 75–78.

97 Weiss, L.M., Fagelman, D., and Warhit, J.M. (1983). CT demonstration of an esophageal duplication cyst. *J. Comput. Assist. Tomogr.* 7 (4): 716–718.

98 Nakata, H., Sato, Y., Nakayama, T. et al. (1986). Bronchogenic cyst with high CT number: analysis of contents. *J. Comput. Assist. Tomogr.* 10 (2): 360.

99 Nakata, H., Nakayama, C., Kimoto, T. et al. (1982). Computed tomography of mediastinal bronchogenic cysts. *J. Comput. Assist. Tomogr.* 6 (4): 733–738.

100 Mendelson, D.S., Rose, J.S., Efremidis, S.C. et al. (1983). Bronchogenic cysts with high CT numbers. *Am. J. Roentgenol.* 140 (3): 463–465.

101 Salonen, O. (1987). CT characteristics of expansions in the middle and posterior mediastinum. *Comput. Radiol.* 11 (2): 95–100.

102 Lupetin, A.R. and Dash, N. (1987). MRI appearance of esophageal duplication cyst. *Gastrointest. Radiol.* 12 (1): 7–9.

103 Rhee, R.S., Kravetz, M., Langer, B. et al. (1988). Cervical esophageal duplication cyst: MR imaging. *J. Comput. Assist. Tomogr.* 12 (4): 693–695.

104 Schwartz, A.R., Fishman, E.K., and Wang, K.P. (1986). Diagnosis and treatment of a bronchogenic cyst using transbronchial needle aspiration. *Thorax* 41 (4): 326–327.

105 Nakajima, T., Yasufuku, K., Shibuya, K., and Fujisawa, T. (2007). Endobronchial ultrasound-guided transbronchial needle aspiration for the treatment of central airway stenosis caused by a mediastinal cyst. *Eur. J. Cardiothorac. Surg.* 32 (3): 538–540.

106 Maturu, V.N., Dhooria, S., and Agarwal, R. (2015). Efficacy and safety of transbronchial needle aspiration in diagnosis and treatment of mediastinal bronchogenic cysts. *J. Bronchology Interv. Pulmonol.* 22 (3): 195–203.

107 Scatarige, J.C.W.K. and Siegelman, S.S. (1984). Transbronchial needle aspiration biopsy of the mediastinum. In: *Contemporary Issues in Computed Tomography* (ed. S.S. Siegelman), 59–79. New York: Churchill Livingstone.

108 Simecek, C. (1992). Diagnosis of mycobacterial mediastinal lymphadenopathy by transbronchial needle aspiration. *Chest* 102 (6): 1919.

109 Serda, G.J., de Castro, F.R., Sanchez-Alarcos, J.F. et al. (1990). Transcarinal needle aspiration in the diagnosis of mediastinal adenitis in a patient infected with the human immunodeficiency virus. *Thorax* 45 (5): 414.

110 Baron, K.M. and Aranda, C.P. (1991). Diagnosis of mediastinal mycobacterial lymphadenopathy by transbronchial needle aspiration. *Chest* 100 (6): 1723–1724.

111 Herscovici, P., Harkin, T.J., Naidich, D.P. et al. (2006). Transbronchial needle aspiration in HIV-infected patients with intrathoracic adenopathy: a 15-year experience at a major teaching hospital. *Chest* 130 (4): 275S.

112 Harkin, T.J., Ciotoli, C., Addrizzo-Harris, D.J. et al. (1998). Transbronchial needle aspiration (TBNA) in patients infected with HIV. *Am. J. Respir. Crit. Care Med.* 157 (6): 1913–1918.

113 Malabonga, V.M., Basti, J., and Kamholz, S.L. (1991). Utility of bronchoscopic sampling techniques for cryptococcal disease in AIDS. *Chest* 99 (2): 370–372.

114 Wang, K.P., Haponik, E.F., Britt, E.J. et al. (1984). Transbronchial needle aspiration of peripheral pulmonary nodules. *Chest* 86 (6): 819–823.

115 Wang, K.P. and Britt, E.J. (1991). Needle brush in the diagnosis of lung mass or nodule through flexible bronchoscopy. *Chest* 100 (4): 1148–1150.

116 Tsuboi, E., Ikeda, S., Tajima, M. et al. (1967). Transbronchial biopsy smear for diagnosis of peripheral pulmonary carcinomas. *Cancer* 20 (5): 687–698.

117 Baaklini, W.A., Reinoso, M.A., Gorin, A.B. et al. (2000). Diagnostic yield of fiberoptic bronchoscopy in evaluating solitary pulmonary nodules. *Chest* 117 (4): 1049–1054.

118 Reichenberger, F., Weber, J., Tamm, M. et al. (1999). The value of transbronchial needle aspiration in the diagnosis of peripheral pulmonary lesions. *Chest* 116 (3): 704–708.

119 Ost, D.E., Ernst, A., Lei, X. et al. (2016). Diagnostic yield and complications of bronchoscopy for peripheral lung lesions. Results of the AQuIRE registry. *Am. J. Respir. Crit. Care Med.* 193 (1): 68–77.

120 Yasufuku, K., Chiyo, M., Koh, E. et al. (2005). Endobronchial ultrasound guided transbronchial needle aspiration for staging of lung cancer. *Lung Cancer* 50 (3): 347–354.

121 Gu, P., Zhao, Y.Z., Jiang, L.Y. et al. (2009). Endobronchial ultrasound-guided transbronchial needle aspiration for staging of lung cancer: a systematic review and meta-analysis. *Eur. J. Cancer* 45 (8): 1389–1396.

122 Adams, K., Shah, P.L., Edmonds, L., and Lim, E. (2009). Test performance of endobronchial ultrasound and transbronchial needle aspiration biopsy for mediastinal staging in patients with lung cancer: systematic review and meta-analysis. *Thorax* 64 (9): 757–762.

123 Wang, K.P. and Browning, R. (2010). Transbronchial needle aspiration with or without endobronchial ultrasound. *Thorac Cancer* 1 (2): 87–93.

124 Yasufuku, K., Nakajima, T., Motoori, K. et al. (2006). Comparison of endobronchial ultrasound, positron emission tomography, and CT for lymph node staging of lung cancer. *Chest* 130 (3): 710–718.

125 Herth, F.J., Eberhardt, R., Krasnik, M., and Ernst, A. (2008). Endobronchial ultrasound-guided transbronchial needle aspiration of lymph nodes in the radiologically and positron emission tomography-normal mediastinum in patients with lung cancer. *Chest* 133 (4): 887–891.

126 Schwarz, Y., Greif, J., Becker, H.D. et al. (2006). Real-time electromagnetic navigation bronchoscopy to peripheral lung lesions using overlaid CT images: the first human study. *Chest* 129 (4): 988–994.

127 Becker, H.D., Herth, F., Ernst, A., and Schwarz, Y. (2005). Bronchoscopic biopsy of peripheral lung lesions under electromagnetic guidance: a pilot study. *J. Bronchology Interv. Pulmonol.* 12 (1): 9–13.

128 Schwarz, Y., Mehta, A.C., Ernst, A. et al. (2003). Electromagnetic navigation during flexible bronchoscopy. *Respiration* 70 (5): 516–522.

129 Makris, D., Scherpereel, A., Leroy, S. et al. (2007). Electromagnetic navigation diagnostic bronchoscopy for small peripheral lung lesions. *Eur. Respir. J.* 29 (6): 1187–1192.

130 Vining, D.J., Liu, K., Choplin, R.H., and Haponik, E.F. (1996). Virtual bronchoscopy. Relationships of virtual reality endobronchial simulations to actual bronchoscopic findings. *Chest* 109 (2): 549–553.

131 Fiorelli, A., Raucci, A., Cascone, R. et al. (2017). Three-dimensional virtual bronchoscopy using a tablet computer to guide real-time transbronchial needle aspiration. *Interact. Cardiovasc. Thorac. Surg.* 24 (4): 567–575.

132 Hopper, K.D., Lucas, T.A., Gleeson, K. et al. (2001). Transbronchial biopsy with virtual CT bronchoscopy and nodal highlighting. *Radiology* 221 (2): 531–536.

133 McAdams, H.P., Goodman, P.C., and Kussin, P. (1998). Virtual bronchoscopy for directing transbronchial needle aspiration of hilar and mediastinal lymph nodes: a pilot study. *Am. J. Roentgenol.* 170 (5): 1361–1364.

134 Herth, F.J., Eberhardt, R., Sterman, D. et al. (2015). Bronchoscopic transparenchymal nodule access (BTPNA): first in human trial of a nove6-332procedure for sampling solitary pulmonary nodules. *Thorax* 70: 326–332.

135 Witte, M.M.C., Opal, M.S.M., Gilbert, M.J.G. et al. (1986). Incidence of fever and bacteremia following transbronchial needle aspiration. *Chest* 89 (1): 85–87.

136 Compère, C., Duysinx, B., Dediste, A. et al. (2007). Prospective risk assessment of bacteremia and other infectious complications associated with real-time ultrasound-guided transbronchial needle aspiration (EBUS-TBNA). *Chest* 132 (4): 439A.

137 Epstein, S.K., Winslow, C.J., Brecher, S.M., and Faling, L.J. (1992). Polymicrobial bacterial pericarditis after transbronchial needle aspiration. *Am. Rev. Respir. Dis.* 146: 523–525.

138 Ostman, H. (ed.) (2008). Mediastinitis and purulent pericarditis following endobronchial ultrasound transbronchial needle aspiration of lymph node. *Chest* 134: 26C.

139 Kucera, R.F., Wolfe, G.K., and Perry, M.E. (1986). Hemomediastinum after transbronchial needle aspiration. *Chest* 90 (3): 466.

140 Sherling, B.E. (1990). Complication with a transbronchial histology needle. *Chest* 98 (3): 783.

141 Mehta, A.C., Curtis, P.S., Scalzitti, M.L., and Meeker, D.P. (1990). The high price of bronchoscopy. Maintenance and repair of the flexible fiberoptic bronchoscope. *Chest* 98 (2): 448–454.

142 Rong, F. and Cui, B. (1998). CT scan directed transbronchial needle aspiration biopsy for mediastinal nodes. *Chest* 114 (1): 36–39.

143 Zhang, W.C., Chen, W., Zhou, J.P. et al. (2017). A comparison of different training methods in the successful learning of endobronchial ultrasound-guided transbronchial needle aspiration. *Respiration* 93 (5): 319–326.

144 Naur, T.M.H., Konge, L., Nayahangan, L.J., and Clementsen, P.F. (2017). Training and certification in endobronchial ultrasound-guided transbronchial needle aspiration. *J. Thorac. Dis.* 9 (7): 2118–2123.

145 Farr, A., Clementsen, P., Herth, F. et al. (2016). Endobronchial ultrasound: launch of an ERS structured training programme. *Breathe* 12 (3): 217.

146 Diette, G.B., White, P. Jr., Terry, P. et al. (2000). Utility of on-site cytopathology assessment for bronchoscopic evaluation of lung masses and adenopathy. *Chest* 117 (4): 1186–1190.

147 Davenport, R.D. (1990). Rapid on-site evaluation of transbronchial aspirates. *Chest* 98 (1): 59–61.

148 Baram, D., Garcia, R.B., and Richman, P.S. (2005). Impact of rapid on-site cytologic evaluation during transbronchial needle aspiration. *Chest* 128 (2): 869–875.

149 Wang, K.P., Brower, R., Haponik, E.F., and Siegelman, S. (1983). Flexible transbronchial needle aspiration for staging of bronchogenic carcinoma. *Chest* 84 (5): 571–576.

150 Chin, R. Jr., McCain, T.W., Lucia, M.A. et al. (2002). Transbronchial needle aspiration in diagnosing and staging lung cancer: how many aspirates are needed? *Am. J. Respir. Crit. Care Med.* 166 (3): 377–381.

151 Herth, F., Becker, H.D., and Ernst, A. (2004). Conventional vs endobronchial ultrasound-guided transbronchial needle aspiration: a randomized trial. *Chest* 125 (1): 322–325.

152 Lee, H.S., Lee, G.K., Lee, H-S. et al. (2008). Real-time endobronchial ultrasound-guided transbronchial needle aspiration in mediastinal staging of non-small cell lung cancer: how many aspirations per target lymph node station? *Chest* 134 (2): 368–374.

153 Kanoh, K., Miyazawa, T., Kurimoto, N. et al. (2005). Endobronchial ultrasonography guidance for transbronchial needle aspiration using a double-channel bronchoscope. *Chest* 128 (1): 388–393.

第 17 章

支气管肺癌的分期

J. Francis Turner, Jr.[1,2] and Ko-Pen Wang[3]

[1] Division of Pulmonary and Critical Care Medicine,
University of Tennessee Graduate School of Medicine, Knoxville, TN, USA
[2] National Supercomputing Institute, University of Nevada, Las Vegas, NV, USA
[3] Division of Pulmonary and Critical Care Medicine, Johns Hopkins Bayview Medical Center,
Johns Hopkins University School of Medicine, Baltimore, MD, USA

（译者：石 荟 译者单位：海军军医大学第一附属医院）

1994年，《胸部疾病》杂志（Chest）[1]发表了一篇具有里程碑式的论著《支气管镜下支气管肺癌的分期》。这是一份向美国胸科医师学会提交的特别报告，是理解和应用经支气管镜针吸活检术（transbronchial needle，TBNA）在肺癌分期方面的一项里程碑式成果，也是多年来这项强大技术的研究和实践经验的高峰。

与许多其他创新想法和发明一样，支气管肺癌分期技术飞跃发展的历史和创新发现始于更早的时期。在吸烟流行之前，原发性肺癌并不常见，早在1761年，它就被认为是一种独特的疾病，威廉·奥斯勒在1892年出版的第一版《医学原理与实践》（Principles and Practice of Medicine）中将其描述为罕见病[2,3]。1950年，理查德·多尔和奥斯汀·布拉德福德·希尔在《英国医学杂志》（British Medical Journal）上发表文章，首次指出吸烟与肺癌之间的关系[4,5]。

1964年1月11日，在美国举行了一次具有里程碑意义的听证会，当时的卫生总监路德·特里报告称，吸烟者的死亡率比不吸烟者高出70%[6]。1986年，外科医生埃弗雷特·库普就被动吸烟对健康的影响发表声明，指出持续暴露于二手烟中相当于每天吸两支香烟，这是一个非常适中的吸烟率，但增加了罹患肺癌和其他疾病的风险[7]。

自1950年以来，吸烟与肺癌之间的关系以及氡等物质导致肺癌的其他环境因素得到充分证实[8]。随之而来的是，美国肺癌死亡人数呈现出惊人的上升趋势，每天有433名美国人死于肺癌。中国的统计数据也反映了全球肺癌死亡率的趋势。在过去30年中，中国的肺癌死亡率增加了465%[9,10]。

在现代外科技术出现之前，肺癌曾被视为一种无法治愈的疾病。希波克拉底曾断言："最好不要尝试治疗隐藏的癌症，因为治疗的人死得更快，而没有治疗的人反而活得更长"[11]。1951年，Cahan医生建议将肺切除术加上肺门和纵隔淋巴结清扫术作为肺癌患者的标准手术[12]。随后，1960年，他在《胸腔和心血管外科杂志》（Journal of Thoracic and Cardiovascular Surgery）上报告了他的肺叶切除术和区域淋巴结清扫术。该技术已成为局限性肺癌的标准外科治疗方法[13,14]。

1978年，在东京国立癌症中心医院工作了30多年的胸腔镜手术先驱Tsuguo Naruke描述了一幅解剖图，其中概述了淋巴结站的编号系统，该系统后来被广泛用于指导肺癌手术中的淋巴结清扫[15]。Naruke的工作深刻地改变了我们对肺癌的认知和治疗策略的理解与实践。

1983年，一个偶然的事件催生了可弯曲支气管镜下 TBNA 原型穿刺针的设计完成，并首次发表了其应用案例[16]。虽然早在 1949 年，阿根廷的 Eduardo Schieppatti 就已研发出硬质支气管镜下使用的 TBNA 穿刺针，但真正改变支气管癌诊断和分期标准的是 1964 年池田茂人推出的可弯曲支气管镜样机和可弯曲经支气管穿刺针[17-25]。

从 20 世纪 70 年代初到 80 年代的 20 年间，美国癌症联合委员会、Naruke 和 Mountain 等人继续根据肺门和纵隔淋巴结的解剖位置，描述了肺癌的临床分期系统[26-29]。正是在这一时期，人们广泛认识到对支气管肺癌及纵隔疾病进行充分分期的必要性，并首次报道了可弯曲支气管镜与 TBNA 技术的协同作用[30-34]。

上述简短的历史回顾，有助于我们理解 1994 年发表的那份具有里程碑意义的文献。该文献详细介绍了支气管镜对支气管源性肿瘤的分期[1]。这份特别报告旨在融合现有分期系统的理念和不同观点，为通过可弯曲支气管镜进行经支气管针吸术的应用提供实用方法。该报告描述了一个详细的淋巴结分期系统，通过该系统，可以从放射成像［尤其是胸部计算机断层扫描（computed tomography，CT）］、支气管镜成像以及对相关解剖结构和气管支气管标志的了解中收集信息，从而获得更精确、更准确的分期技术，为选择治疗方法和进行更多临床检查提供指导。这个分期系统包括根据支气管镜视图和之前的 CT 成像建立的 4 个支气管镜下解剖断面：① 气管下端靠近隆突；② 右主支气管靠近右上叶开口；③ 中间支气管靠近中叶开口；④ 左主支气管靠近下叶和上叶支气管。这 4 个断面包括 11 个淋巴结站点，可通过可弯曲支气管镜到达，比国际肺癌研究协会（IASLC）后来描述的 7 个淋巴区和 14 个淋巴结站点更早[35]。虽然可弯曲支气管镜下常规 TBNA（conventional TBNA，C-TBNA）在训练有素的医生手中应用后，可具备高度的诊断敏感性和特异性，但由于不同研究结果存在差异，因此并未在呼吸科医生中得到广泛应用。然而，随着操作设备的不断更新，气管镜技术进步与 TBNA 核心技术的协同使用在随后的 30 年中迅速发展。20 世纪 80 年代末，德国的 Becker 和日本的 Miyazawa 等创新者与奥林巴斯公司合作，开发了微型径向超声扫描探头，并将其应用于内镜下各种杂交操作技术。2004 年，Yasufuku 发表了利用凸式超声支气管镜进行淋巴结分期的论文[36-48]。

随着经支气管镜腔内超声（endobronchial ultrasound，EBUS）的引入和使用，TBNA 技术现在被认为是肺部恶性肿瘤和纵隔疾病患者最可靠的诊断、分期和再分期工具。然而，使用这项技术的医师必须明白，"TBNA 就是 TBNA"，如果没有针吸术获得的细胞学和组织学材料，相伴使用的超声波没有任何益处。与任何新技术一样，额外医疗设备的使用也需要根据上述原则进行验证。我们认为，支气管镜腔内超声推进了 TBNA 技术的应用和使用，这种协同使用和 TBNA 诊断效能的显著提高归因于以下几个原因。

首先，EBUS 的使用类似于拥有一辆装有 GPS 的新车。当你开车去一个熟悉的目的地时，你可能不会使用这个功能，但如果你必须导航到城市中一个更精确的目的地或某个你从未去过的地方，那么 GPS 可能是无价的。这类似于了解纵隔解剖和淋巴结分布有固定的关系，就像街上的邮局不会移动一样，所以在这种情况下 GPS 是多余的。然而，当你尝试定位一个 0.5 cm 12R 组淋巴结时则需要支气管超声的辅助。因此，如果你的目标是 2 cm 的隆突下淋巴结，那么常规或超声辅助技术在训练有素的医生面前可能同样有效。但如果目标很小，或者你很少进行针吸操作，那么 EBUS 可以在解剖学和心理学上都保证你是在一个最佳的位置进行针吸。纵隔和肺门肿大的淋巴结间固定毗邻关系，使得开展传统 TBNA 不存在重大的并发症，而食管穿刺针吸术则不然，因为内镜下难以区分正常食管和纵隔淋巴结肿大的表现，此时超声是必需的。

其次，EBUS 内镜有助于简化 TBNA 的穿刺技术。与常规的可弯曲支气管镜相比，EBUS 镜的远端部分更大、更硬，且出镜时针头呈 30° 角。这有助于稳定穿刺针，引导和提供穿刺角度，以更好地定位针在软骨环之间穿刺。此外，与常规支气管镜的工作通道出口在 3 点钟或 9 点钟位置不同，EBUS 镜工作通道出口在中线，允许针直接刺入靶病灶的中心位置。

第三，在超声的帮助下，已经开发了许多课程来培训 TBNA 技术。在 TBNA 应用历史上，超声增加了在某点进行 TBNA 时的可视性及其临床应用场景。随着胸外科技术［如电视辅助胸腔镜手术（video-assisted thoracoscopic surgery，VATS）和亚肺叶切除术］的发展，以及肿瘤免疫治疗等新疗法，正确分期和描述细胞类型已被公认为至关重要。

因此，EBUS 技术可以更容易地辅助应用 TBNA 进行明确诊断和分期，提高了对经支气管针吸技术的认识和表现。

随着支气管镜检查和图像引导的针吸活检技术步

入新千年时代，我们也进入了一个从基因和分子生物学特征认识肺癌的新时代。随着对肺癌的常规治疗和靶向治疗期望的增加，支气管镜检查和TBNA技术在常规或图像引导下诊断和分期的效能，使其成为疑诊肺癌和胸部CT异常[51]患者的首选检查手段。

肺癌分期和分子诊断在支持肺癌患者个体化治疗中的地位越来越重要。支气管镜操作医生需理解镜下检查淋巴结的解剖位置、超声及其他成像特征（如弹性成像），正确对待技术的适宜性和局限性，以及能获得的标本量。

认识到C-TBNA和超声图像引导的经支气管针吸技术都存在学习曲线，我们相信，通过以下流程步骤结合使用两种技术，将为患者提供更好的服务。

1）仔细检查术前影像，全面了解纵隔解剖结构和制订取到靶病灶的计划；

2）同时使用Wang氏支气管胸内淋巴结图谱和C-TBNA或EBUS引导的TBNA技术；

3）深入了解Wang氏支气管胸内淋巴结图谱和国际肺癌研究协会（IASLC）淋巴结图谱在纵隔和肺门淋巴结分类上的差异；

4）请病理科或呼吸科医生通过快速现场评估（rapid on site evaluation，ROSE）对细胞学标本进行实时判定；

5）恰当的标本加工和处理。

以上第1~3步骤需要了解本章开头所简要描述的淋巴结解剖学描述的历史，以及了解实时支气管镜下纵隔解剖、淋巴结分期和超声显示[24,48,52,53]。历史上，随着不同淋巴结分站图谱系统的发展，美国胸科学会（ATS）制定的Mountain-Dresler MDATS修改版与日本制定的Naruke淋巴结图谱之间存在差异，导致日本、美国和欧洲使用不同淋巴结图谱进行数据分析[52,54-60]。具体而言，在日本进行手术分期的患者使用的是日本肺癌协会Naruke淋巴结图谱，而在日本以外的患者一般采用MDATS分期系统[61,62]。这两个不同淋巴结图谱之间的主要区别在于N_1和N_2淋巴结区交界处，主要的不一致出现在主支气管下缘。Naruke图谱认为隆突下间隙主支气管下缘淋巴结为10组，因此为N_1分期。相比之下，MDATS图谱将这些淋巴结定义为7组，因此为N_2分期。

随后，IASLC与国际抗癌联盟（UICC）和美国癌症联合委员会（AJCC）合作，整合了每个淋巴结站点解剖边界之间的差异，其成果最新发表于AJCC第8版癌症分期手册[35]。Wang氏胸内淋巴结图谱描述了11个TBNA穿刺术的淋巴结站点，IASLC淋巴结图谱第8版详细描述了7区和14个淋巴结站点。应用Wang氏胸内淋巴结图谱和详细的IASLC分期系统，结合所有可用的影像、视觉和超声成像TBNA，有助于理解淋巴结分期与支气管肺癌预后和治疗的相关性。因此，我们认为了解Wang氏淋巴结图谱和IASLC定义的淋巴结图谱之间的区别是非常重要的。

11个淋巴结站点对应容易识别的支气管内标志[57]（图17.1）。当这些支气管内站点组合在一起时，形成了相应穿刺位点路径，类似于IASLC图谱的特定分期系统。这种目视识别的路径和位点可以通过C-TBNA获取，或进一步使用EBUS进行扫描。特别是右上区纵隔淋巴结（4R站）被Wang氏淋巴结图谱第1、3、5站合并和左上区纵隔淋巴结（4L站）被第4和6站合并（图17.1、图17.2）。Wang氏淋巴结图谱中纵隔淋巴结，第2、8、10站在IASLC图谱中被指定为隆突下及隆突下更低的区域，代表隆突下及食管旁淋巴结（第7、8站）（图17.3）。

深入理解支气管内和纵隔解剖的重要性，反映了当前对精准分期的持续重视，包括确认纵隔胸膜包膜内外是否有淋巴结受累，有无其他淋巴结转移，淋巴结位置与原发病灶的关系等[62,63]。无论使用常规、超声或导航图像引导的TBNA，首先必须将支气管镜远端置于感兴趣的支气管内区域。我们详细利用Wang氏胸内淋巴结图谱，可以让支气管镜操作医生准确地定位在如IASLC图谱中所详细描述的"区域所在"。一旦"进入该区域"，如果继续进行C-TBNA，则所描述的特定穿刺部位就可以被识别。如果使用EBUS，那么相关的血管标志和淋巴结就可能更快及更有效地被识别。

无论是通过支气管内成像还是超声成像识别定位标志，重要的是要注意到血管和淋巴结的位置与气道的关系可能会变化。如图17.4所示，纵隔或肺门淋巴结肿大的一些病例，会因患者的淋巴结而上调分期或下调分期，这也是之前讨论的一个原因[64]。

随着胸部影像学和肺癌分期技术的发展，我们对不同诊断方法的局限性和优势的理解也在不断发展。CT扫描已成为肺结节检查前的标准检查手段，汇总数据显示纵隔分期的敏感性为0.60，特异性为0.81。正电子发射体层成像（positron emission tomography，PET）的加入提高了图像引导分期的准确性、敏感性和特异性分别为0.85和0.88[5,65,66]。随着影像学敏感性的提高，Fisher等前瞻性随机将患者分为常规分期

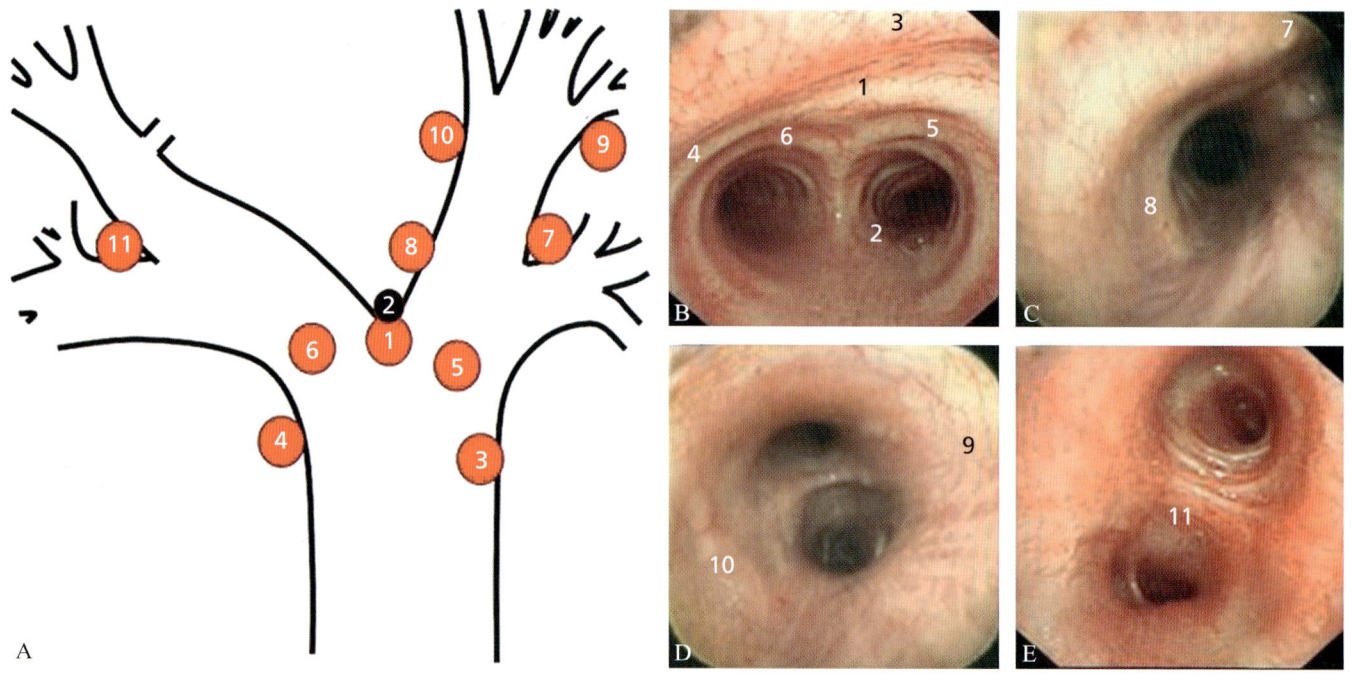

图 17.1　Wang 氏淋巴结图谱及经支气管吸针穿刺部位

A. Wang 氏淋巴结图；B. 隆突水平；C. 右主支气管水平；D. 右中间支气管水平；E. 左主支气管水平。1. 前隆突淋巴结；2. 后隆突淋巴结；3. 右气管旁淋巴结；4. 左气管旁淋巴结；5. 右主支气管淋巴结；6. 左主支气管淋巴结；7. 右上肺门淋巴结；8. 隆突下淋巴结；9. 右下肺门淋巴结；10. 隆突远端淋巴结；11. 左肺门淋巴结。资料来源：Li 等[57]，经《胸外科疾病》杂志（Journal of Thoracic Disease）许可转载。

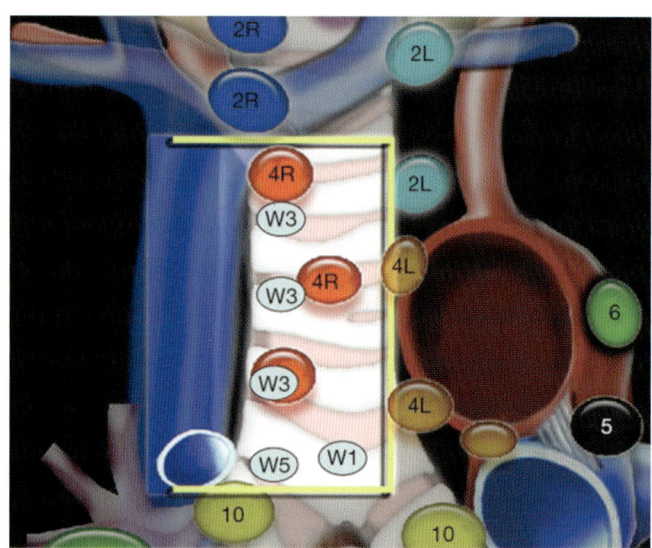

图 17.2　Wang 氏胸内淋巴结图谱与 IASLC 图谱右侧淋巴结的相关性

IASLC 图谱中的 4R 站包括 Wang 氏胸内淋巴结图谱中的 1、3、5 站，属于纵隔淋巴结。资料来源：Li 等[57]，经《胸外科疾病》杂志（Journal of Thoracic Disease）许可转载。

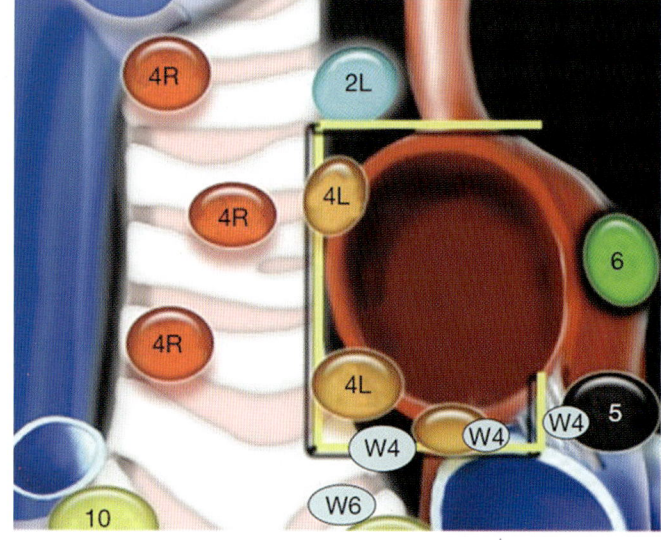

图 17.3　IASLC 图谱上隆突下淋巴结与 Wang 氏胸内淋巴结图谱上关于中纵隔淋巴结的相关性

IASLC 图中隆突下淋巴结（7 站）与 Wang 氏图中的 2、8、10 站淋巴结重合。资料来源：Li 等[57]，经《胸外科疾病》杂志（Journal of Thoracic Disease）许可转载。

加 PET-CT 或单纯常规分期。2009 年发表在《新英格兰医学杂志》（New England Journal of Medicine）上的一篇关于 98 名患者的报告发现，PET-CT 应用的增加，减少了总开胸次数和无效开胸次数，但不影响总死亡率[67]。

随着 PET-CT 的联合成像技术越来越容易获得，

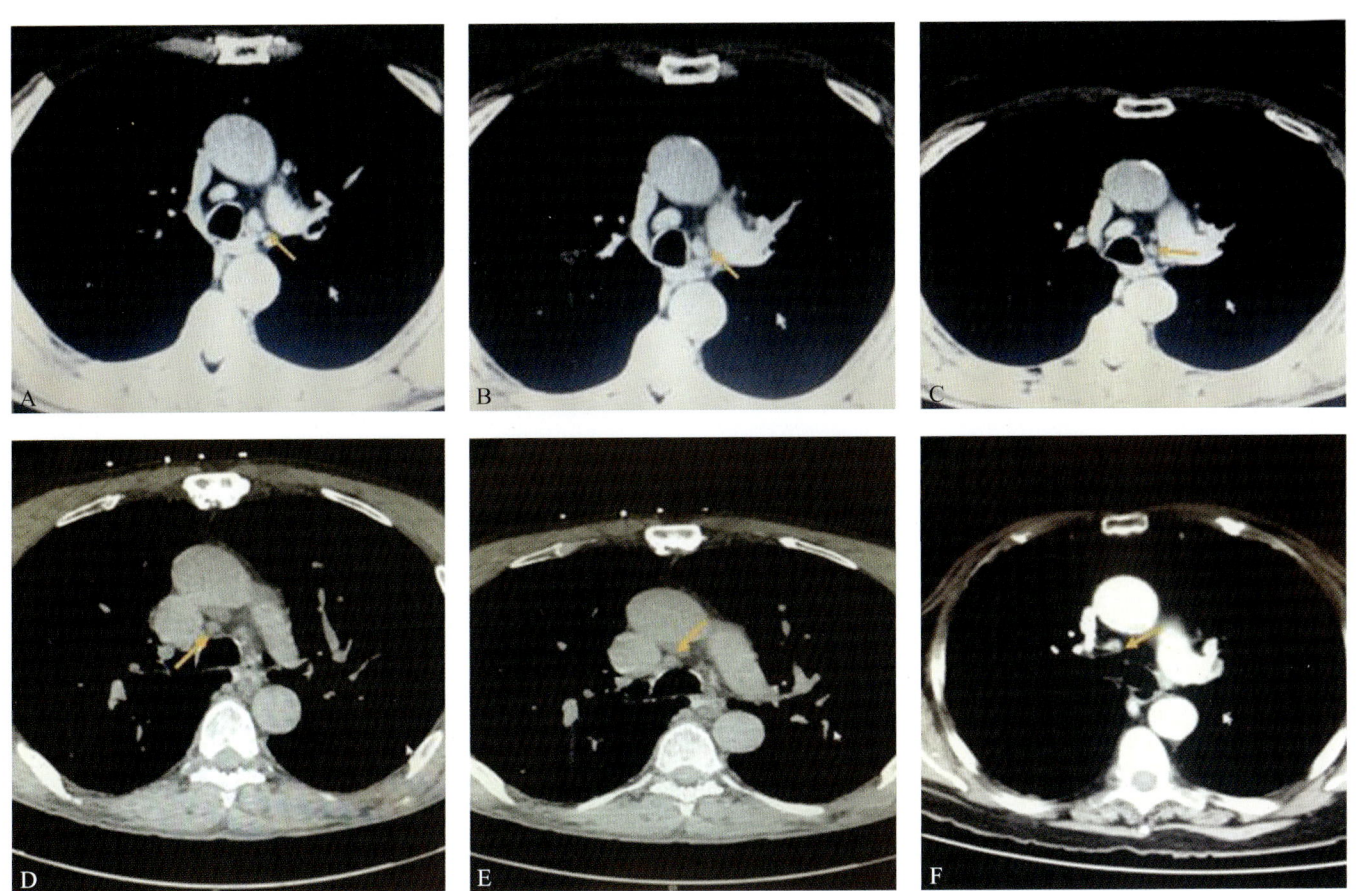

图 17.4　血管和淋巴结相对于气道的位置可能不同（A~C）

当以左侧肺动脉为分期标志时，左侧淋巴结（黄色箭头）为 10 L（A）。然而，在 Wang 氏的图谱上，这些是在 4R 和 6 组。D 和 E 中的淋巴结（黄色箭头）如果以奇静脉弓作为分期标志，应归类为 10R；然而，这些在 IASLC 图谱上被划分为 4R 组，或者在 Wang 氏的图谱上被划分为 1 和 5 组。如果用血管作为分期标志，F 中的淋巴结（黄色箭头）可能会被误认为 4R 组；但它在支气管右上叶管腔的水平，实际上 10R 组也是如此。如果只观察血管，A~E 所示患者的淋巴结将被下调分期，F 所示患者的淋巴结将被上调分期。资料来源：Li 等[57]，经《胸外科疾病》杂志（Journal of Thoracic Disease）许可转载。

成像与经支气管针吸微创技术的协同作用使得改进的淋巴结分期的应用变得越来越普遍。在修订的欧洲胸外科学会 ESTS 术前纵隔淋巴结分期指南中，deLyn 等正确地指出，有几种技术可以用于原发性纵隔淋巴结分期，这取决于当地医疗资源可及性和专业水平[68,69]。这些技术具体包括：① 成像技术；② 内窥镜技术；③ 手术技术。

ESTS 标准工作组指出，未预见到 pN$_2$ 在 10% 以内是可以接受的，因为经过彻底纵隔分期后，这种未预见的 pN$_2$ 多为单站可切除淋巴结肿大，并提出了术前纵隔淋巴结分期的算法指南（图 17.5）[69]。

那么，为什么自 1994 年以来，对淋巴结分期的重视程度越来越高？

这个问题的答案在于我们对淋巴结累及定义的不断探索，因为它与疾病的分期、淋巴结累及的特征改变、对肺癌不同生物学和遗传学的理解都有关系，进而改变了手术技术和免疫治疗相关的治疗策略。

首先，关于淋巴结受累的解剖学定义，淋巴结转移的位置是决定预后和治疗的关键。随着 IASLC 分期系统对淋巴结区域和淋巴站点的修改，值得我们注意的是解剖学中线的重要定义从纵隔中线偏移向左气管旁边缘，即所谓的纵隔肿瘤中线[66,69]。这条肿瘤中线主要影响上区淋巴结，即 2R、2L、4R 和 4L。根据这一修改后的解剖学定义，如果伴有中线右侧淋巴结受累的右侧原发病灶将被归类为 N$_2$ 期疾病，而起源于左肺且肿瘤中线右侧淋巴结受累的肿瘤将被归类为 N$_3$ 期疾病[69]。因此，这可能被视为ⅢA 期和ⅢB 期肿瘤之间的区别，并可能改变放化疗和/或手术治疗策略的选择。

此外，淋巴结站的数目和淋巴结受累的特征

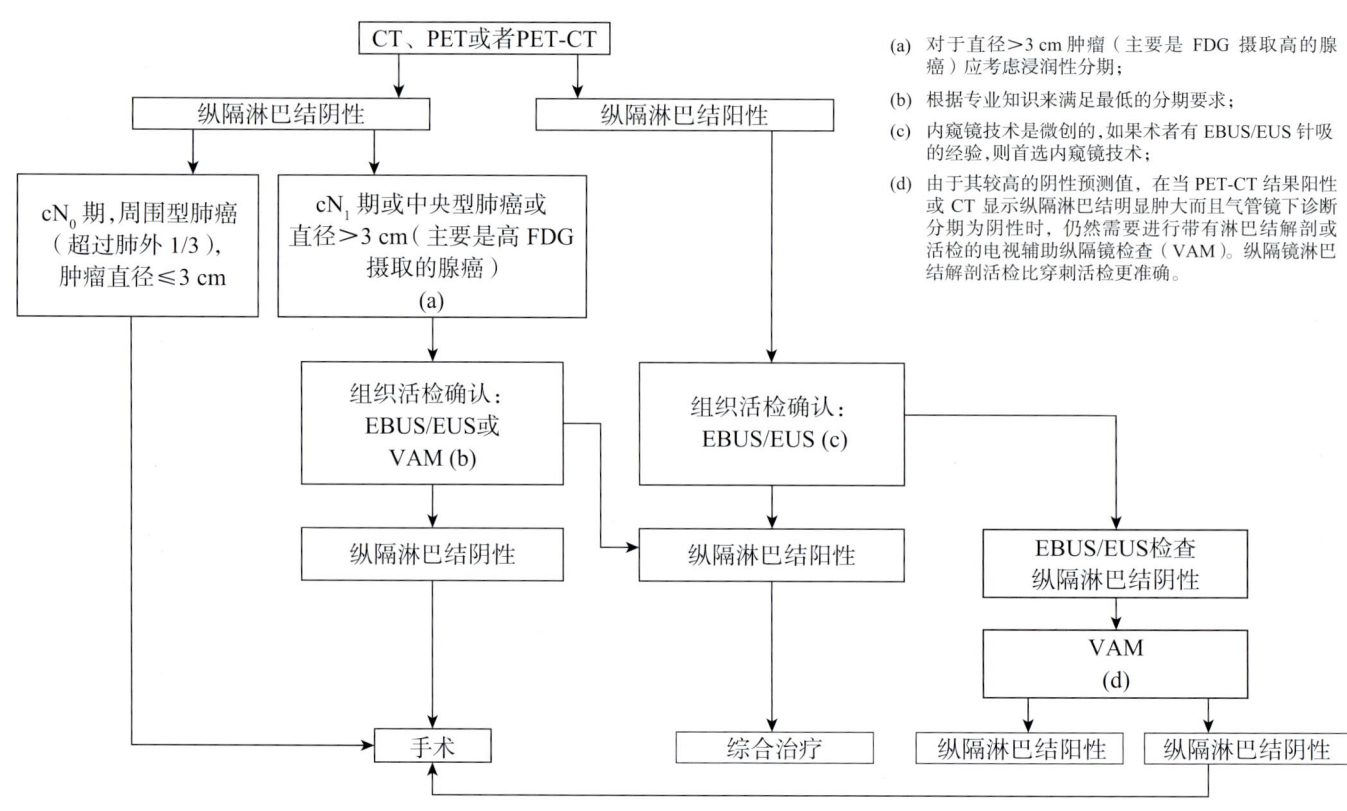

图 17.5 修订后的原发性纵隔分期的 ESTS 指南

来源：获得牛津大学出版社 de Leyn 等作者许可[69]。

可能有预后意义。Wei 等在 2011 年和 Saji 在 2013 年[63,70]回顾性分析了淋巴结站受累的数量。Wei 回顾了 1 659 例患者，将转移淋巴结的数量分为 4 类，从无淋巴结转移（nN_0）到累及 7 个或 7 个以上淋巴结（nN_3）。虽然他们的研究存在局限性，但他们确实得出结论：仅基于 pN 分期的定位对非小细胞肺癌的预后具有较差的预测能力。他们继续注意到 pN_1 和 pN_2 患者在预后方面有异质性，并同意总体疾病负担而不是淋巴结受累的解剖位置提供了最重要的预后信息。他们的结论是，尽管研究具有局限性，但 N 分期是一个更好的预测预后的因素，并与总体疾病负担相关。此外，还对特定的淋巴结站进行了描述，纵隔淋巴结 N_2 受累是一个预后多样化的人群[71-75]。事实上，Sakao 等在 2010 年回顾了 106 例多水平 N_2 期疾病患者，并得出结论：患者预后较差，且多水平 N_2 期病变也是隐匿性肺内转移的先兆[76]。值得注意的是，在他们的研究中，排除了较大纵隔淋巴肿大的患者（短轴直径＞2.0 cm），因为这些患者已经接受了放化疗治疗。

除了淋巴结转移的解剖位置和水平外，肺腺癌中跳过 N_2 转移的诊断识别也被重点提及[77]。当发现患者有纵隔淋巴结转移，但与原发肿瘤无同侧支气管周围或肺门淋巴结累及时，就会出现这种情况。20%~30% 的 N_2 患者会发生跳跃转移，且预后较好[78-80]。在 Li 对 177 例肺腺癌患者的研究中，45 例患者发现跳跃转移。跳跃转移也与腺泡亚型、分化良好和右侧肺癌相关。跳跃组的无复发生存率和总生存率明显更好，跳跃组和对照组 5 年无复发生存率分别为 37.4% 和 5.7%（$P=0.005$），总生存率分别为 60.7% 和 32.1%（$P=0.024$）。Li 得出结论，跳跃性转移与无跳跃性转移在临床病理特征及预后方面存在明显差异，这对肺腺癌患者可能具有临床意义。

Asamura 等在 IASLC 肺癌第 8 版分期提案中进一步提及了这一点。对 pN 进行细分，pN_{1a} 为单站转移，pN_{1b} 为多站 N_1 淋巴结转移，pN_{2a} 和 pN_{2b} 类似。跳跃转移进一步细分为 pN_{2a1}（N_2 单跳过，无 pN_1 累及）、pN_{2a2}（pN_1 和 pN_2 累及，无跳过）和 pN_{2b}（多淋巴结转移）。值得注意的是，pN_{2a1} 和 pN_{2a2}、pN_{2a2} 和 pN_{2b} 的生存率有统计学差异，但 pN_{1b} 和 pN_{2a1} 的预后无差异。这表明在相应 N_1 区未累及淋巴结的 pN_{2a1} 累及（跳过

转移）患者的预后与在 N_2 站未累及淋巴结的 pN_{1b} 患者的预后接近[61]。

最后，随着对肺癌不同生物学和遗传学的理解的深入以及免疫治疗等治疗策略的进步，经支气管镜下穿刺活检进行充分采样技术从未像现在这样显得如此重要。

1994年，人们明确认识到支气管肺癌的组织学诊断和分期对肺癌患者的预后至关重要。在那个年代，区分小细胞肺癌和非小细胞肺癌的特征病理学表现并据此指导后续患者手术或放化疗是治疗的标准流程。在过去的20年里，快速发展的科研给我们打开了生物学上了解肿瘤基因组学的窗口，并提供了个性化的治疗机会。尽管立体定向消融放疗在局限期肺癌中的作用正在增加[81,82]，但在患者肿瘤分期允许时，手术仍然是"金标准"。随着 VATS 等更加微创手术的加入，以及放疗靶标定位和能量输送技术的进步，这两种治疗方式也在经历飞速的进步。尽管如此，直到最近，晚期非小细胞肺癌的标准治疗仍一直集中在以铂为基础的两药联合化疗。然而，随着不断地研究深入，我们现在知道肿瘤可以通过可溶性因子改变其微环境，逃避免疫监测和破坏[83,84]。基于此，再加上对肿瘤特异性抗原的更深入理解，抗体和免疫检查点抑制剂的应用在晚期肺癌的治疗中发挥了越来越重要的作用[85]。依据肿瘤分期和患者个体化驱动基因的差异，靶向治疗和免疫检查点抑制剂这些突破性疗法已占据了非小细胞肺癌药物治疗的舞台中央。因此，组织取样技术和充足的标本量变得越来越重要。

经支气管镜下针吸早已被证实可以获取足够的细胞学和组织学标本，这在非感染性肉芽肿疾病和淋巴增殖性疾病（如肉瘤和淋巴瘤）中得到了进一步证明，其中获取组织学病理是关键[24,86-88]。

因此，获得足够的组织病理学标本的重要性，不仅体现在呼吸病学家需要足够的组织标本来进行免疫组化分析，而且还体现在组织获取、标本观察和处理的一系列连续过程中，并且谨慎、细致管理可用的细胞和组织标本，以识别它们可能包含的关键信息[89,90]。目标采样的中心原则是，操作者应首先从最近端、对侧的病灶处获取标本，以允许同时诊断和分期。标本的后续处理已在本书的其他地方进行了讨论，但应特别注意肿瘤细胞的数量和质量，选择待评估标本的标志物，以及对所获标本结果的仔细解读[91-93]。随着可用标志物的大量发展，相应的诊断算法也应运而生，从而使对可获得标本的使用更加仔细和有效[94-96]。

总之，当我们回顾从1994年到现在利用 TBNA 诊断和分期支气管肺癌时，我们比20多年前发展初始阶段怀有更多期待和热情。TBNA 的关键作用在于肺癌的诊断和分期，目前认为 TBNA 在患者选择最佳初始治疗计划、再分期和治疗性应用中更为重要。我们希望本章不仅带领大家回望过去，更期望能和大家一起展望未来[97-100]。

参考文献

1　Wang, K.P. (1994). Staging of bronchogenic carcinoma by bronchoscopy. *Chest* 106:588–593.

2　Yang, P. (2011). Lung cancer and never smokers. *Semin. Respir. Crit. Care Med.* 32 (1): 10–21.

3　Hosler, W. (1978). *New Growths in the Lungs. The Principles and Practice of Medicine. The Classics of Medicine Library*, 556–557. Omaha: Gryphon Editions Ltd.

4　Doll, R. and Hill, A.B.G. (1950). Smoking and carcinoma of the lung. *BMJ* 2:739–748.

5　Spiro, S.G. and Silvestri, G.A. (2005). One hundred years of lung cancer. *Am. J. Respir. Crit. Care Med.* 172:523–529.

6　US Public Health Service (1964). *Surgeon General's Advisory Committee on Smoking and Health*, Publication No. 1103. Washington DC: US Government Printing Office.

7　C. Everett Koop Papers. Tobacco, Second-Hand Smoke, and the Campaign for a Smoke-Free America. www.profiles.nlm.nih.gov

8　Krewski, D., Lubin, J.H., Zielinski, J.M. et al. (2005). Radon and risk of lung cancer: a combined analysis 7 North American case controlled studies. *Epidemiology* 16:137–145.

9　National Cancer Institute (2016). *Surveillance, Epidemiology, and End Results (SEER), US Cancer Mortality, 1975–2013*. Bethesda: National Cancer Institute.

10　Wen, C. and Dehnel, T. (2011). China wrestles with lung cancer. *Lancet Oncol.* 12 (1): 15.

11　Hippocrates (1982). *The Aphorisms of Hippocrates*. Omaha: Gryphon Editions Ltd.

12　Cahan, W.G., Watson, W.L., and Pool, J.L. (1951). Radical pneumonectomy. *J. Thorac. Surg.* 22: 449–473.

13　Cahan, W.G. (1960). Radical lobectomy. *J. Thorac. Cardiovasc. Surg.* 39: 555–572.

14　Watanabe, S. (2014). Lymph node dissection for lung cancer: past, present, and future. *Gen. Thorac. Cardiovasc. Surg.* 62: 407–414.

15　Naruke, T., Suemasu, K., and Ishikawa, S. (1978). Lymph node mapping and curability at various level of metastasis in resected lung cancer. *J. Thorac. Cardiovasc. Surg.* 76: 832–839.

16　Wang, K.P. and Terry, P. (1983). Transbronchial needle aspiration in the diagnosis and staging of bronchogenic carcinoma. *Am. Rev. Respir. Dis.* 127: 344–347.

17　Schiepatti, E. (1949). La puncion mediastinal atraves del espolon traquea reveiw. *Rev. Asoc. Med. Argent.* 663: 497–499.

18　Versteegh, R.M. and Swierenga, J. (1963). Bronchoscopic evaluation of the operability of pulmonary carcinoma. *Acta*

Otolaryngol. 56: 603–611.

19 Fox, R.T., Lees, W.M., and Shields, T.W. (1965). Transcarinal bronchoscopic needle biopsy. *Ann. Thorac. Surg.* 1: 92–966.

20 Simecek, C. (1966). Cytological investigation of intrathoracic lymph nodes in carcinoma of the lung. *Thorax* 21: 369–371.

21 Bridgeman, A.H., Duffield, G.D., and Takaro, T. (1968). An appraisal of newer diagnostic methods for intrathoracic lesions. *Dis. Chest* 53: 321–327.

22 Atay, Z. and Brandt, H.J. (1977). Die Bedeutung Der Zytodiagnostik Der Perbronchialen Feinnadelpunktion von mediastinalen oder ilaren Tumoren. *Dtsch. Med. Wochenschr.* 102: 345–348.

23 Lemer, J., Malberger, E., and Konig-Nativ, R. (1982). Transbronchial fine needle aspiration. *Thorax* 37: 270–274.

24 Wang, K.P., Mehta, A., and Turner, J.F. (2012). Transbronchial needle aspiration for cytology and histology specimens. In: *Flexible Bronchoscopy*, 3e (eds. K.P. Wang, A. Mehta and J.F. Turner), 147–169. Hoboken: Blackwell Science.

25 Ikeda, S., Yawai, N., and Ishikawa, S. (1968). Flexible bronchofiberscope. *Keio J. Med.* 17: 1–133.

26 American Joint Committee on Cancer (1973). *Clinical Staging System for Carcinoma of the Lung: American Joint Committee for Cancer Staging and end Results Reporting*. Philadelphia: JB Lippincott.

27 American Joint Committee on Cancer (1977). *Manual for Staging of Cancer*, 2e, 99–105. Philadelphia: JB Lippincott.

28 Mountain, C.F. (1986). A new international staging system for lung cancer. *Chest* 89 (suppl): 225S–233S.

29 American Joint Committee on Cancer (1988). *Staging of Cancer*, 3e, 115–121. Philadelphia: JB Lippincott.

30 Zerhouni, E.A. and Stitik, F.P. (1985). Controversies in computed tomography of the thorax: the pulmonary nodule-lung cancer staging. *Radiol. Clin. NorthAm.* 23: 407–426.

31 Templeton, P.A., Caskey, C.I., and Zerhouni, E.A. (1990). Current uses of CT and MR imaging in the staging of lung cancer. *Radiol. Clin. N. Am.* 28: 631–646.

32 Wang, K.P., Brower, R., Haponik, E.F., and Siegelman, S. (1983). Flexible transbronchial needle aspiration for staging of bronchogenic carcinoma. *Chest* 84: 671–676.

33 Shure, D. and Fedullo, P.F. (1984). The role of transcarinal needle aspiration in the staging of bronchogenic carcinoma. *Chest* 86: 693–696.

34 Schenk, D.A., Bower, J.H., Bryan, C.L. et al. (1986). Transbronchial needle aspiration staging of bronchogenic carcinoma. *Am. Rev. Respir. Dis.* 134: 146–148.

35 Rami-Porta, R., Asamura, H., Travis, W., and Rusch, V.W. (2017). Lung cancer-major changes in American Joint Committee on Cancer eighth edition cancer staging manual. *CA Cancer J. Clin.* 67: 138–155.

36 Becker, H.D. (2006). EBUS – a new dimension in bronchoscopy. *Respiration* 73: 583–586.

37 Koga, T., Ogata, K., Hayashida, R., and Hattori, R. (1994). Usefulness of transluminal ultrasonography in the evaluation of bronchial stenosis secondary to tuberculosis. *Int. J. Jpn. Sociol.* 16: 477–482.

38 Frank, N., Holzapfel, P., and Wenk, A. (1994). Neue Endoschall Minisonde in der täglichen Praxis. *Endosk Heute* 3: 238–244.

39 Becker, H.D. (2006). Endobronchial ultrasound with miniprobe radial scanning. In: *Endoscopic Ultrasound – An Introductory Manual and Atlas* (ed. C.F. Dietrich), 334–351. New York: Thieme.

40 Hürther, T. and Hanrath, P. (1990). Endobronchial sonography in the diagnosis of pulmonary and mediastinal tumors. *Dtsch. Med. Wochenschr.* 115: 1899–1905.

41 Hürther, T. and Hanrath, P. (1992). Endobronchial sonography: feasibility and preliminary results. *Thorax* 47: 565–567.

42 Kurimoto, N., Murayama, M., Yoshioka, S. et al. (1999). Assessment of usefulness of endobronchial ultrasonography in determination of depth of tracheobronchial tumor invasion. *Chest* 115: 1500–1506.

43 Miyazu, Y., Miyazawa, T., Kurimoto, N. et al. (2002). Endobronchial ultrasonography in the assessment of centrally located early-stage lung cancer before photodynamic therapy. *Am. J. Respir. Crit. Care Med.* 165: 832–837.

44 Shaw, T.J., Wakely, S.L., Peebles, C.R. et al. (2004). Endobronchial ultrasound to assess airway wall thickening: validation in vitro and in vivo. *Eur. Respir. J.* 23: 813–817.

45 Becker, H.D. (1995). Bronchoscopy for airway lesions. In: *Flexible Bronchoscopy* (eds. K.P. Wang and A.C. Mehta), 136–159. Ames: Blackwell Scientific Publications.

46 Omori, S., Takiguchi, Y., Hiroshima, K. et al. (2002). Peripheral pulmonary diseases: evaluation with endobronchial US; initial experience. *Radiology* 24: 603–608.

47 Herth, F., Becker, H.D., Manegold, C., and Drings, P. (2001). Endobronchial ultrasound (EBUS): assessment of a new diagnostic tool in bronchoscopy for staging of lung cancer. *Onkologie* 24: 151–154.

48 Yasufuku, K., Chiyo, M., Sekine, Y. et al. (2004). Real-time endobronchial ultrasound- guided Transbronchial needle aspiration of mediastinal and hilar lymph nodes. *Chest* 126: 122–128.

49 Wang, K.P. and Turner, J.F. (2007). TBNA versus TENA in the diagnosis and staging of bronchogenic carcinoma: "a comparative study". *J. Broadcast.* 14: 246–250.

50 Carbone, D.P., Gandara, D.R., Antonia, S.J. et al. (2015). Non-small cell lung cancer: role of the immune system and potential for immunotherapy. *J. Thorac. Oncol.* 10 (7): 974–984.

51 Navani, N., Nankivell, M., Lawrence, D.R. et al. (2015). Lung cancer diagnosis and staging with endobronchial ultrasound-guided needle aspiration compared with conventional approaches: an open-labe, pragmatic, randomized controlled trial. *Lancet Respir. Med.* 3 (4): 282–289.

52 Kavuru, M.S., Mehta, A.C., and Turner, J.F. (2012). Applied anatomy of the airways. In: *Flexible Bronchoscopy*, 3e (eds. K.P. Wang, A. Mehta and J.F. Turner), 46–52. Hoboken: Blackwell Science.

53 Yasufuku, K. (2009). EBUS-TBNA bronchoscopy. In: *Endobronchial Ultrasound. An Atlas and Practical Guide* (eds. A. Ernst and F.J.F. Herth), 119–144. New York: Springer

Science+Business Media, LLC.

54. Ryan, B., Yendamuri, K., and Yendamuri, S. (2017). Anatomical considerations in bronchoscopy. *J. Thorac. Dis.* 9 (suppl 10): S1123–S1127.
55. Lin, C.K., Lai, C.L., Chang, L.Y. et al. (2018). Learning curve and advantages of endobronchial ultrasound-guided transbronchial needle aspiration as a first-line diagnostic and staging procedure. *Thorac. Cancer* 9: 75–82.
56. Haponik, E.F., Cappellari, J.O., Chin, R. et al. (1995). Education and experience improved transbronchial needle aspiration performance. *Am. J. Respir. Crit. Care Med.* 141: 1998–2002.
57. Li, Y.Q., Wang, K.P., and Ben, S.Q. (2015). Insight into the differences in classification of mediastinal and hilar lymph nodes between Wang's lymph node map in the International Association for the Study of Lung Cancer lymph node map. *J. Thorac. Dis.* 7 (S4): S246–S255.
58. Wang, K.P. (1989). *Biopsy Techniques in Pulmonary Disorders*. New York: Raven Press.
59. Bonifazi, M., Sediari, M., Ferretti, M. et al. (2014). The role of the pulmonologist and rapid on-site cytologic evaluation of transbronchial needle aspiration. A prospective study. *Chest* 145 (1): 60–65.
60. Rusch, V.W., Crowley, J., Giroux, D.J. et al. (2007). The IASLC lung cancer staging project: proposals for the revision of the N descriptors in the forthcoming seventh edition of the TNM classification for lung cancer. *J. Thorac. Oncol.* 2: 603–612.
61. Asamura, H., Chansky, K., Crowley, J. et al. (2015). The International Association for the Study of Lung Cancer lung cancer staging project. Proposals for the revision of the N descriptors in the forthcoming 8th edition of the TNM classification for lung cancer. *J. Thorac. Oncol.* 10 (12): 1675–1684.
62. Rusch, V.W., Asamura, H., Watanabe, H. et al. (2009). A proposal for a new international lymph node map in the forthcoming seventh edition of the TNM classification for lung cancer. *J. Thorac. Oncol.* 4 (5): 568–577.
63. Wei, S., Asamura, H., Kawachi, R. et al. (2011). Which is the better prognostic factor for resected non-small cell lung cancer – the number of metastatic lymph nodes or the currently used nodal stage classification? *J. Thorac. Oncol.* 6 (2): 310–318.
64. Irion, K.L., Fewins, H., and Binukrishana, S. (2009). Comments on the proposed new international lymph node International Association for the Study of Lung Cancer map. *J. Thorac. Oncol.* 4 (11): 1445–1446.
65. Toloza, E., Harpole, L., and McCrory, D.C. (2003). Non-invasive clinical staging of non-small cell lung cancer: radiographic and clinical evaluation of intra- and extrathoracic disease. *Chest* 123 (1 suppl): 137s–146s.
66. Silvestri, G.A., Tanoue, L.T., Margolis, M.L. et al. (2003). The noninvasive staging of non-small cell lung cancer: the guidelines. *Chest* 123: 147s–156s.
67. Fischer, B., Lassen, U., and Mortensen, J. (2009). Preoperative staging of lung cancer with combined PET-CT. *N. Engl. J. Med.* 361: 32–39.
68. De Leyn, P., Dooms, C., Kuzdzal, J. et al. (2014). Preoperative mediastinal lymph node staging for non-small cell lung cancer: 2014 update of the 2007 ESTS guidelines. *Trans. Lung Cancer Res.* 3 (4): 225–233.
69. De Leyn, P., Dooms, C., Kuzdzal, J. et al. (2014). Revised ESTS guidelines for preoperative mediastinal lymph node staging for non-small-cell-lung cancer. *Eur. J. Cardiothorac. Surg.* 45: 787–798.
70. Saji, H., Tsuboi, M., Shimada, Y. et al. (2013). A proposal for combination of total number in anatomical location of involved lymph nodes for nodal classification in non-small cell lung cancer. *Chest* 143: 1618–1625.
71. Daly, B.D., Mueller, J.D., Faling, L.J. et al. (1993). N2 lung cancer: outcome in patients with false negative computed tomography scans of the chest. *J. Thorac. Cardiovasc. Surg.* 105: 904–911.
72. Cybulsky, I.J., Lanza, L.A., Ryan, M.B. et al. (1992). Prognostic significance of computed tomography in resected N2 lung cancer. *Ann. Thorac. Surg.* 54: 533–537.
73. Vansteenkiste, J.F., de Leyn, P.R., Deneffe, G.J. et al. (1997). Survival and prognostic factors in resected N2 non-small cell lung cancer: a study of 140 cases: Leuven Lung Cancer Group. *Ann. Thorac. Surg.* 63: 1441–1450.
74. Sakao, K., Miyamoto, H., Oh, S. et al. (2007). Clinicopathological factors associated with unexpected N3 in patients with mediastinal lymph node involvement. *J. Thorac. Oncol.* 2: 1107–1111.
75. Andre, F., Grunewald, D., Pignon, J.P. et al. (2000). Survival of patients with resected N2 non-small cell lung cancer: evidence for a subclassification and implications. *J. Clin. Oncol.* 18: 2981–2989.
76. Sakao, Y., Okumura, S., Mun, M. et al. (2010). Prognostic heterogeneity and multilevel N2 non-small cell lung cancer patients: importance of lymphadenopathy and occult intrapulmonary metastasis. *Ann. Thorac. Surg.* 89: 1060–1063.
77. Li, H., Hu, H., Wang, R. et al. (2015). Lung adenocarcinoma: are skipped N2 metastasis different from non-skip? *J. Thorac. Cardiovasc. Surg.* 150: 790–795.
78. Ricquet, M., Assouad, J., Bagan, P. et al. (2005). Skip mediastinal lymph node metastasis and lung cancer: a particular N2 subgroup with a better prognosis. *Ann. Thorac. Surg.* 79: 225–233.
79. Yoshino, I., Yokoyama, H., Yano, T. et al. (1996). Skip metastasis to the mediastinal lymph nodes and non-small cell lung cancer. *Ann. Thorac. Surg.* 62: 1021–1025.
80. Misthos, P., Sepsas, E., Athanassiadi, K. et al. (2004). Skip metastasis: analysis of their clinical significance and prognosis in the IIIa stage of non-small cell lung cancer. *Eur. J. Cardiothorac. Surg.* 25: 502–508.
81. Verstegen, N.E., Oosterhuis, J.W.A., Palma, D.A. et al. (2013). Stage I-II non-small cell lung cancer treated using either stereotactic ablative radiotherapy (SABR) or lobectomy via video-assisted thoracoscopic surgery (VATS): outcomes of a propensity score-matched analysis. *Ann. Oncol.* 24: 1543–1548.
82. Chang, J.Y., Senan, S., Paul, M.A. et al. (2015). Stereotactic ablative radiotherapy versus lobectomy for operable stage I non-small-cell lung cancer: a pooled analysis of two randomized

trials. *Lancet Oncol.* 16 (6): 630–637.

83 Masters, F.A., Temin, S., Azzoli, C.G. et al. (2015). Systemic therapy for stage IV non-small-cell lung cancer: American Society of Clinical Oncology clinical practice guideline update. *J. Clin. Oncol.* 33: 3488–3515.

84 Kirkwood, J.M., Butterfield, L.H., Tarhini, A.A. et al. (2012). Immunotherapy of cancer in 2012. *CA Cancer J. Clin.* 62 (5): 309–335.

85 Lu, J. and Ramirez, R.A. (2017). The role of checkpoint inhibition in non-small cell lung cancer. *Oschner J* 17: 379–387.

86 Wang, K.P. (1985). Flexible transbronchial needle aspiration biopsy for histologic specimens. *Chest* 88 (6): 860–863.

87 Wang, K.P., Johns, C.J., and Fuenning, C. (1989). Felxible transbronchial needle aspiration for the diagnosis of sarcoidosis. *Ann. Otol. RhinolLayrngol.* 98 (4, 1): 298–300.

88 Mehta, A.C. and Wang, K.P. (2013). Teaching conventional transbronchial needle aspiration: a continuum. *Ann. Am. Thorac. Soc.* 10 (6): 685–689.

89 Righi, L., Freacesca, F., Montarolo, F. et al. (2017). Endobronchial ultrasound-guided transbronchial needle aspiration (EBUS-TBNA)– from morphology to molecular testing. *J. Thorac. Dis.* 9 (Suppl 5): S395–S404.

90 Heijden, E.H., Casal, R.F., Trisolini, R. et al. (2014). Guideline for the acquisition and preparation of conventional and endobronchial ultrasound-guided transbronchial needle aspiration specimens for the diagnosis and molecular testing of patients with known or suspected lung cancer. *Respiration* 88: 500–517.

91 Casakio, C., Guarize, J., Donghi, S. et al. (2015). Molecular testing for targeted therapy and advanced non-small cell lung cancer: suitability of endobronchial ultrasound transbronchial needle aspiration. *Am. J. Clin. Pathol.* 144: 629–634.

92 Trisolini, R., Cancelliere, A., Tinelli, C. et al. (2015). A randomized trial of endobronchial ultrasound-guided transbronchial needle aspiration with and without rapid on-site evaluation for lung cancer genotyping. *Chest* 148: 1430–1437.

93 Jeyabalan, A., Bhatt, N., Plummeridge, M.J. et al. (2016). Adequacy of endobronchial ultrasound-guided transbronchial needle aspiration samples processed as histopathological samples for genetic mutation analysis and lung adenocarcinoma. *Mol. Clin. Oncol.* 4: 119–125.

94 Travis,W.D., Brambilla, E., Burke, E. et al. (2015). *WHO Classification of Tumors of the Lung, Pleura, Thymus, and Heart*, 4e. Lyon: IARC Press.

95 Whithaus, K., Fukuoka, J., and Prihoda,T.J. (2012). Evaluation of napsin A, cytokeratin 5/6, p63, and thyroid transcription factor 1 in adenocarcinoma versus squamous cell carcinoma of the lung. *Arch. Pathol. Lab. Med.* 136: 155–162.

96 Righi, L., Vavala, T., Rapa, I. et al. (2014). Impact of non-small cell lung cancer not otherwise specified immunophenotyping on treatment outcome. *J. Thorac. Oncol.* 9: 1540–1546.

97 Kunst, P.W.A., Lee, P., Paul, M.A. et al. (2007). Restaging of mediastinal nodes with transbronchial needle aspiration after induction chemoradiation for locally advanced non-small cell lung cancer. *J. Thorac. Oncol.* 10 (2): 912–915.

98 Çetinkaya, E., Usluer, O., Yilmaz, A. et al. (2017). Is endobronchial ultrasound-guided transbronchial needle aspiration an effective diagnostic procedure in restaging of non-small cell lung cancer patients? *Endosc. Ultrasound* 6 (3): 162–167.

99 Hohenforst-Schmidt,W., Zarogoulidis, P., Darwiche, K. et al. (2013). Intratumoral chemotherapy for lung cancer: re-challenge current targeted therapies. *Drug Des. Devel. Ther.* 7: 571–583.

100 Khan, F., Anker, C.J., Garrison, G. et al. (2015). Endobronchial ultrasound-guided transbronchial needle injection for local control of recurrent non-small cell lung cancer. *Ann. Am. Thorac. Soc.* 12 (1): 101–104.

第 18 章

介入肺脏病学的未来

Ala Eddin Sagar[1] and David E. Ost[2]
[1] Banner MD Anderson Cancer Center, Phoenix, AZ, USA
[2] Division of Internal Medicine, Department of Pulmonary Medicine,
MD Anderson Cancer Center, University of Texas, Houston, TX, USA

（译者：白 冲 译者单位：海军军医大学第一附属医院）

18.1 引言

1968年，池田茂人发明了可弯曲性支气管镜，随后支气管镜技术取得了重大飞跃[1]。目前，基于支气管镜检查平台，大量新技术不断涌现，以提高诊断率[如径向探头-支气管腔内超声（radial-probe endobronchial ultrasound，RP-EBUS）、凸式支气管腔内超声（endobronchial ultrasound，EBUS）、电磁导航（electromagnetic navigation，EMN）]和提供新的治疗方式（如气道支架置入、消融技术、肺气肿的支气管镜治疗）。本章将提供一个概念性框架，深入分析如何利用基础科学的进步来促进介入肺脏病学（interventional pulmonology，IP）领域的诊疗[2]；讨论将基础科研成果转化为改善患者和人类健康的临床实践所涉及的研究过程和步骤；通过纵隔淋巴结分期和周围肺结节的诊断为例，来说明该框架如何应用于识别知识空白，从而推进未来的工作。

18.2 转化性研究理念框架

Dougherty等曾发表过一份对转化过程进行分类的框架性文献（图18.1）[2]。医学能力的发展需要启动基础科研工作。在许多医学领域，这些基础研究往往侧重于分子生物学技术，但在介入肺脏病领域，则需要更广泛的研究视野。影响介入肺脏病领域的基础科学发展是多方面的，成像技术、机器人技术和材料科学的进步都可能有助于进一步推进介入肺脏病领域的发展。

转化的第一个阶段（T1）旨在利用这些基础科学的发展来解决临床问题。这一阶段的研究目的在于确立临床疗效，即需要解决一个基本问题：这种干预措施是否能够真的达到目的？最开始的初步研究可能会侧重于可行性，随后的研究将衡量新的干预措施与标准诊疗效果之间的差异。在这个阶段，恰当的对照是至关重要的，需要通过严格的临床研究方法来证明其临床疗效。

诊断和治疗的临床有效性是不同的。对诊断而言，目标是确定干预措施明确某特定疾病的敏感性和特异性；而治疗的有效性是通过明确有意义的临床结果（如呼吸困难的改变、生活质量和长期死亡率的改变）以及比较不同干预措施之间的风险差异来确定的。

一旦确立有临床疗效，转化下一阶段（T2）的重点是积累证据，证明该项干预措施在临床实践中确切有效。这里包括要证明该项干预措施对特定患者群体是有效的。这一阶段的研究类型包括临床有效性研究、有效性比较研究和制定循证实践指南的研究。这一阶段的研究强调对特定人群的临床结果。不同个体间的比较也是一个重要的考虑因素，因为不同的临床情况可能采用完全不同的诊断方法（如经支气管镜活检与经皮CT引导下活检）。重要的是要强调临床疗效（在T1阶段评估）和临床有效性（在T2阶段评估）之间的差异。临床疗效决定了在理想情况下，干预措施是否能达到预期的结果。鉴于研究的理想条件，这种初步研究的结果不能外推到一般人群。临床有效性是评估在实际临床环境中的获益程度。比较有效性旨在确定在给定的临床环境中哪种干预措施效果最好。这些研究应被视为一个连续的过程，而不是相互排斥的不同研究。

一旦确立了临床有效性，接下来的转化阶段是想办法开发能可靠适用于所有临床情况的干预措施（T3）。为了让研究能切实帮助到患者，必须将从T1和T2研究中获得的知识应用于更大的患者群体。但是，在各种不同的环境中以经济、有效的方式可靠地提供新的干预措施，以改善个别患者以及整体人群的健康并不容易。这就需要在不同的具体层面对结果进行测试，对质量进行测试，对成本进行测试。科学实施是一个关键的考量因素，因为有效干预措施的规模和传播受到许多因素的影响，包括医护人员培训、数量-质量关系、成本效益、激励机制、转诊模式和医护协调，而研发企业通常并不能全部解决这些因素。

18.3　开展转化研究的挑战

严格的流行病学和生物统计学对有效的转化研究至关重要。关于适当的研究设计、混淆、建模和分析的全面讨论超出了本章的范围，但是有许多合适的专业书籍会涵盖这一领域。当然，强调避免以下一些与介入肺脏病研究特别相关的临床研究陷阱是有益的：

1）样本量；
2）选择偏倚；
3）研究中诊断率的应用；
4）外部有效性有限；
5）发表偏倚。

18.3.1　样本量

小样本量的研究往往效力不足，与类似的大样本量研究相比，其结果有较大的变异性[3]。因此，即便是统计上有显著差异，其结果也可能存在很宽的置信区间（confidence interval，CI），这反过来可能会妨碍我们准确判断其真实的有效性和效果的强度。例如，在IP领域，曾尝试在肺癌筛查中实施自荧光（autofluorescence，AF）支气管镜检查。较早的小型研究结果显示，敏感性和特异性变化很大，CI很宽[4-6]。随后进行了一项设计良好的前瞻性观察性试验，纳入了更多的受试者[7]。该研究考察了在高危人群中单独进行AF支气管镜检查以及AF联合低剂量CT进行肺癌筛查时的有效性。共有2 537名患者被纳入该研究，其中一半的患者（1 300例）接受了AF支气管镜检查和低剂量CT检查。在这1 300例患者中，有333例（占25.6%）在自荧光支气管镜下进行了776次支气管腔内活检。在这些活组织检查中，AF支气管镜检出

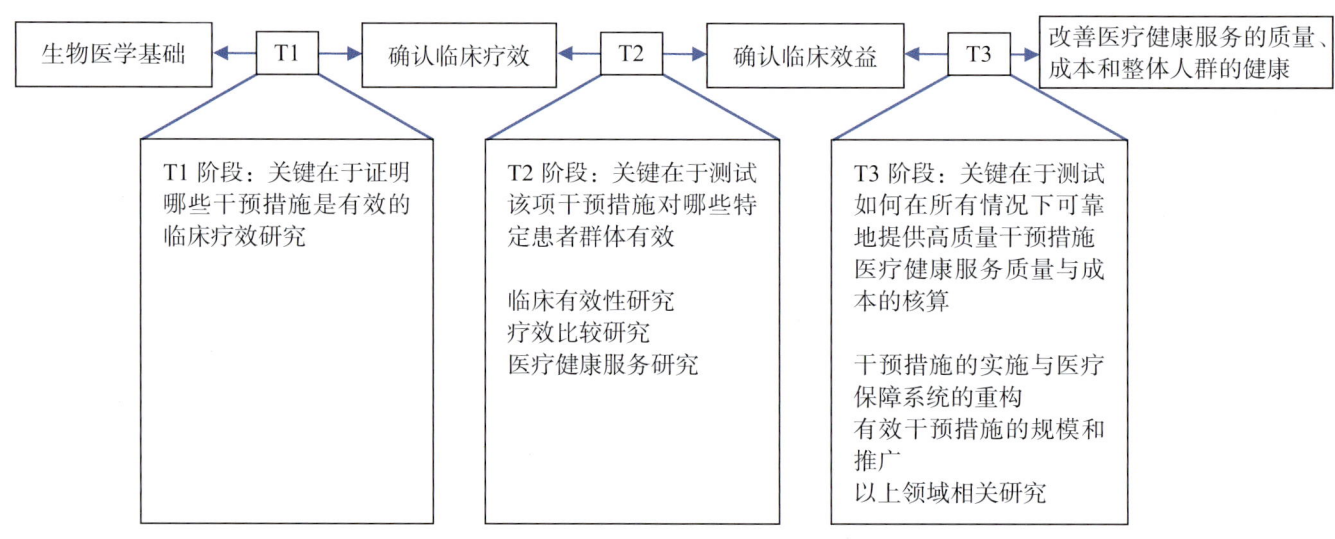

图18.1　转化研究概念框架

资料来源：Dougherty 等[2]，经《美国医学会杂志》(the Journal of the American Medical Association，JAMA) 许可转载。

1例原位癌和4例肺癌。而低剂量CT仅漏诊1例类癌和1例原位癌。当AF与低剂量CT联合使用时，AF支气管镜检查的增量值为2/1 300或0.15%（95% CI：0.0%~0.6%）。结果显示，使用AF的额外收益非常小，这对于肺癌筛查来说不具有成本效益[7]。

就IP领域而言，样本量是一个突出的问题。因为对于任何单个医院来说，针对特定疾病的操作量可能都很小，这使得纳入研究患者的入组速度缓慢且繁琐。克服这一问题的解决方案是建立多中心协作组。

18.3.2 选择偏倚

当一个结论是基于一个并不能充分代表要分析的总体的样本时，就会出现选择偏倚。这种情况下所研究的干预措施与结果之间的关系，对于所研究的样本和拟分析的人群可能是不同的。选择偏倚也可能导致研究之间的比较是无效的。例如，一项对恶性中央气道阻塞患者接受气道支架并发症的回顾性分析表明，与Ultraflex™支架相比，应用硅酮支架患者的死亡率较低[8]。然而，硅酮支架降低死亡率的结论并不一定正确。所观察到的支架类型与死亡率之间的关联可能受到选择偏倚的影响，因为硅酮支架在技术上比金属支架更难放置，但更容易取出。由于医生知道硅酮支架更容易取出，硅酮支架也许更可能用于那些被认为有可能长时间生存的患者，或者那些被认为对放疗和化疗反应更好的患者。因此，两组患者（硅酮支架组和Ultraflex支架组）可能一开始就没有那么相似。因此，观察到的死亡率差异可能并非仅由使用不同的支架类型所导致。在讨论支气管镜检查应用于肺外周病变时，我们会进一步强调这一概念。

18.3.3 使用诊断率而非敏感性/特异性

在研究诊断干预措施时，一个重要的问题是报告研究结果的指标是诊断率，而不是诊断的敏感性和特异性。虽然诊断率和诊断效率听起来可能是同义词，但它们实际上是不同的结果。敏感性描述的是一种检测方法在患有疾病的患者中检测出疾病的能力。敏感性方程为真阳性/（真阳性＋假阴性）。由于分母是每个患有该疾病的人，因此特定测试的真正敏感性不受疾病流行程度的直接影响。另一方面，诊断率反映了在人群中，通过检测可以诊断的患者所占的百分比。诊断可能是对的，也可能是错的，此外，诊断的疾病可能不是我们感兴趣的疾病。例如，当对外周病变进行支气管镜检查时，一些患者可能患有肺癌，而另一些可能患有分枝杆菌疾病，另一些可能患有真菌感染。肺癌的诊断敏感性的分母为肺癌的患者，分子为肺癌检测呈阳性的患者。诊断率的分母为队列中的所有患者，而分子包括所有（如肺癌或结核病或真菌感染）检测呈阳性的患者。请注意，如果支气管镜检查对结核病和肺部感染的敏感性不同于恶性肿瘤，则该检查的诊断结果将会根据人群中相应疾病的潜在分布而变化。如果许多患者根本没有疾病，那么诊断率就会降低。如果支气管镜检查对感染的敏感性高于恶性肿瘤，那么在感染高流行率的研究中，诊断率将高于其他感染低流行率的研究。

因此，诊断率受到人群中疾病类型、每种疾病的患病率以及测试方法性能特征的影响。正是由于诊断率的差异可能是群体差异、测试方法性能的差异，或两者兼而有之，所以，在比较研究之间的诊断率时存在困难。相比之下，诊断敏感性是测试和识别特定疾病能力的函数，因此研究之间的比较是有效的。

18.3.4 外部有效性

研究的结果并不总是足以得出关于其有效性的结论。外部有效性反映了研究结果在其他情况下可以推广的程度。当看到一项研究的结果时，医生应该问这样一个问题：这个结果是否适用于我的情况和我的诊疗对象？例如，一项由一名技能娴熟的医生完成的随机对照试验，评估镇静类型是否影响超声支气管镜引导下经支气管针吸活检术（EBUS-guided Transbronchial Needle Aspiration，EBUS-TBNA）的诊断率，如果同一试验由多名技能熟练程度不同的医生进行，就可能无法复制出该试验的结果[9]。因此，这样的研究结论不宜推广到其他医生。外部有效性是T1研究的局限性之一，在T2研究中则得到了一定程度的解决。

18.3.5 发表偏倚

发表偏倚是指与方法无关的因素影响了对某一研究报告的接受发表和传播。发表偏倚的一种特别常见的偏倚形式，发生在研究结果影响了结果的发表与否。例如，研究A和B用同样严格的方法解决了同样的问题，但研究A报告了很大的效应量（如治疗方案之间的生存差异很大），而研究B报告了差异不显著的统计学结果，被认为是一项"阴性"研究。结果，研究A比研究B更有可能被发表，这就导致了发表偏倚，因为文献中的证据总量将表现为不对等（不能代表结果为"阴性"的研究）。

这一点很重要，因为即使是对高质量研究进行了良好的荟萃分析，也会受到这种形式的偏倚的影响，因为荟萃分析主要是总结已发表的文献。这种由于倾向于发表更大效应量的文献所引起的发表偏倚，将导致荟萃分析的结果的不准确，这反过来又影响了循证指南（T2）的质量（循证指南通常在很大程度上受到荟萃分析结论的影响）。

上述例子强调了临床研究中一些陷阱，可能影响结果和研究价值。采用一个清晰的研究框架（将在下一节中强调），可以引导研究人员在不同的转化阶段正确前行，确保每个阶段的研究都严谨的。

18.4 转化研究理念在介入肺脏病学中的应用

为了说明这个转化研究理念如何应用于IP，我们将评估两个常见的IP问题：非小细胞肺癌（nonsmall cell lung cancer，NSCLC）的纵隔淋巴结分期和支气管镜诊断肺外周结节。

18.4.1 纵隔淋巴结分期

纤维成像技术、细胞学和影像学的进步为支气管镜技术的蓬勃发展提供了必要的条件（图18.2）。这些技术进步有助于解决纵隔采样的挑战。过去，对纵隔淋巴结尝试通过硬质支气管镜进行TBNA取样[10]。1966年，池田茂人发明的纤维支气管镜，提供了一种用于纵隔取样的工具[1]。Ko Pen Wang开发了一种用于可弯曲支气管镜的原型针，可以对隆突下淋巴结进行采样[11]。然而，当时这种技术的主要限制是无法看到病变，而导致无法进行采样。RP-EBUS开发后，实现了纵隔淋巴结的实时可视化[12]。

同样，在具体操作时，因为必须移除RP-EBUS设备，以便穿刺针可以执行TBNA。这为凸式EBUS的发展铺平了道路。因为凸式EBUS可以让医生实时看到病变同时进行针吸活检操作，这改变了纵隔淋巴结分期的方式，目前凸式EBUS是纵隔分期的首选方式（优于纵隔镜检查）[13]。

超声探头的小型化和成像技术的进步促进了凸式EBUS的发展。T1期开始于评估凸式EBUS在纵隔淋巴结取样中的可行性和有效性的研究[14-16]。最开始的研究常常错误地将纵隔镜检查作为"金标准"，但后续其他研究使用了更严格的手术作为"金标准"[17,18]。随后其他T1研究比较了凸式EBUS-TBNA与不带超声的常规TBNA，后者是当时支气管镜引导下纵隔淋巴结取样的首选诊断标准[19]。

在确立了EBUS的优势后，在各种临床背景下进行了多项T2转化研究，进一步明确其作用。除了已经

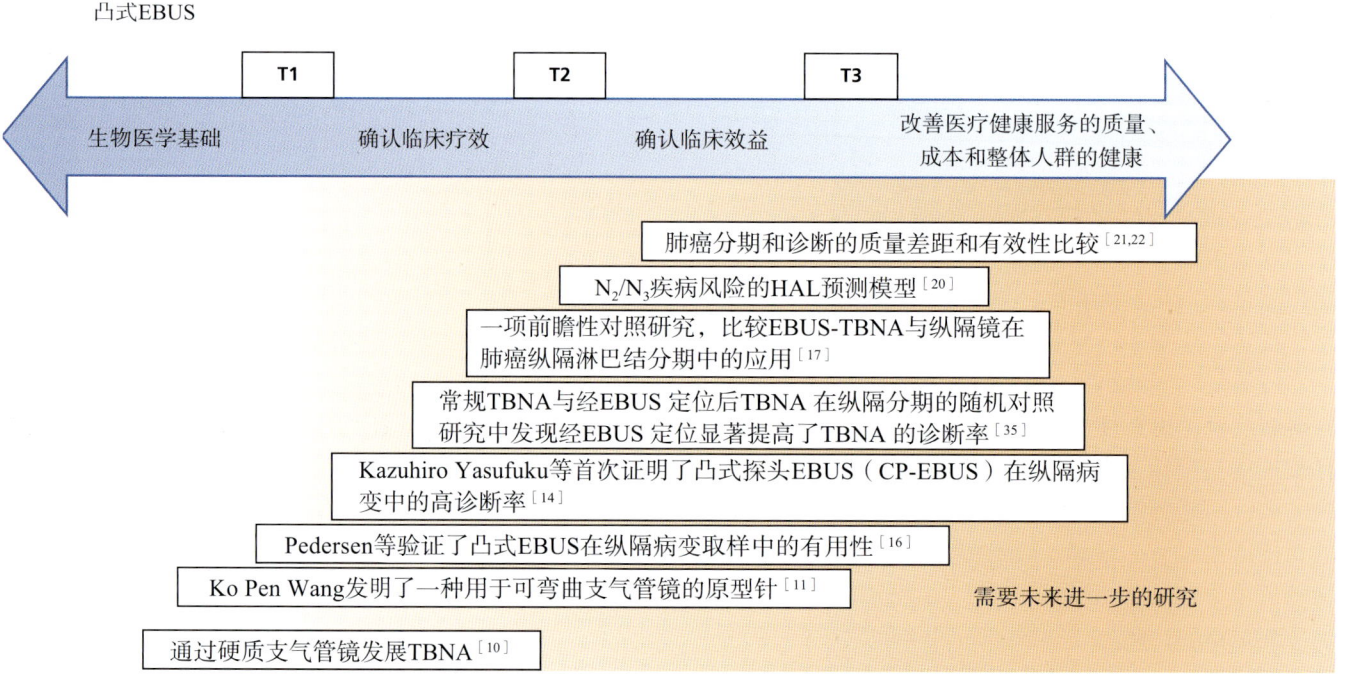

图18.2 转化科学：凸阵扫描EBUS纵隔取样的发展

验证的EBUS-TBNA自身特点外，它的临床应用场景也很重要。也就是说，EBUS-TBNA的价值取决于N_2或N_3疾病的先验概率。如果N_2或N_3疾病的先验概率非常低，如CT和/或正电子发射体层成像（positron emission tomography，PET）未发现淋巴结病变的外周T1结节，则EBUS-TBNA可能不那么有用[12]。

因此，有必要利用预测工具对N_2/N_3疾病发生的概率提供更精确的估计。这种预测工具使我们能够根据患N_2/N_3疾病的可能性对患者进行分层，并评估EBUS-TBNA是否会提供可能改变治疗过程的额外信息。如果预测点参与的概率极低，则EBUS-TBNA不太可能改变临床诊疗过程，也不具有良好的成本效益。例如，HAL模型是一个预测模型，该模型显示组织学、年龄、肿瘤中心位置和PET/CT N 分期可以准确预测EBUS-TBNA识别为N_2或N_3疾病的概率[17]。因为肺癌患病率的差异和可能存在PET扫描的假阳性（如结节病、组织胞浆菌病），所以该模型可能并不完美，需要在中心之间进行校准，但它仍然有价值，并有可能促进是否使用EBUS-TBNA进行NSCLC分期的临床决策。

需要强调的另一个重要问题是在T2阶段当前的知识体系应用。一些研究表明，并不需要总是遵循与指南一致的肺癌分期和诊断方法[18-20]。这些差异包括：对于疑似肺癌合并纵隔淋巴结转移但无远处转移的患者未能首先进行纵隔取样，未能对NSCLC患者进行纵隔取样，以及过度使用开胸手术。与指南不一致的方法会导致进行更多的检查，增加了不必要的治疗费用并导致更多并发症。虽然这些研究发现了现有知识在实施方面的差异，但它们没有为这些问题提供任何解决方案。因此，这些知识体系不被视为T3阶段研究。凸式EBUS需要更多的T3阶段研究来评估如何适当地传播和实施该技术，以改善整体人群的诊断水平。这应该是未来研究的重点。

18.4.2 外周支气管镜检查

外周支气管镜检查仍然是未来研究的一个感兴趣的领域，因为我们目前从外周病变中获取标本的能力还有改进的空间。支气管镜诊断周围病变有4个主要挑战：导航、可操作性、定位确认和足量的组织标本。为了到达周围病变，必须确定支气管镜或活检工具、导航的气道路径。在确定了清晰的路径之后，下一个挑战是通过该路径到达预定的目标病灶。一种验证正确定位的方法，通常是通过结节可视化来实现，然后允许医生最大限度地提高成功活检的机会。最后，活检工具必须能够准确地获得足量的标本。正如RP-EBUS对纵隔淋巴结分期所证明的那样，即使我们能够导航和操纵到达该部位，并验证我们的位置，但如果最后一步组织获取无效，就会出现问题。理解这4个基本目标，使我们能够分析当前可用方法的优势和局限性。

传统的方法，仅仅依靠透视来导航到病变并验证其位置是不理想的。虽然可能已经根据先前的CT扫描规划了一个潜在的路径，但由于气道大小或靶病灶所处的角度，支气管镜可能无法通过预定的路径进行操作。此外，虽然支气管镜可能具有足够的可操作性，但活检工具，如TBNA针，可能无法达到病变。因为分辨率有限，透视在位置验证方面也不太理想。

与凸式EBUS的情况一样，基础科学研究，包括超声探头的小型化以及成像和导航技术的进步，促进了几种工具的发展，以解决上述局限性（图18.3）。在这些工具中，EMN支气管镜检查和RP-EBUS是应用最广泛的。EMN和RP-EBUS已经作为提供更精确的外周病变靶向的潜在手段被引入到外周支气管镜检查中。EMN通过利用CT信息，提供通往目标的虚拟路径来解决导航问题。EMN还通过在电磁场中绘制的病变位置，在一定程度上解决了位置验证问题。与EMN相比，RP-EBUS提供了实时信息，解决了位置验证问题。

初步研究（T1期）探讨了EMN和RP-EBUS在肺周围病变诊断中的可行性和临床疗效[15,21-23]。随后的研究受到几个方法学问题的困扰，这些问题可能导致在现实的实践中，其结果低于预期[21]。一些先前强调的临床研究缺陷可以解释这种差异。

18.4.2.1 研究中诊断率的应用

大多数检查EMN和RP-EBUS效用的研究报告了这两种方法的诊断率，而不是它们的诊断敏感性和特异性。报道的EMN诊断率为33%~96.8%，RP-EBUS为46%~86.2%[22,24-26]。如前所述，很难比较研究之间的诊断率，因为诊断率的差异可能是由于群体差异，或检测性能的差异，或两者兼而有之。诊断率的使用可能是研究结果差异很大及发表的结果与临床实践中的实际表现之间不一致的部分原因。

18.4.2.2 缺少对照组

缺少对照组是研究外周支气管镜检查工具的主要限制之一。如果没有适当的比较，一种新的诊断工具的边际效益程度是难以评估的。如果没有适当的对照，则无法确定是否值得为该边际效益付出相应成本。大多

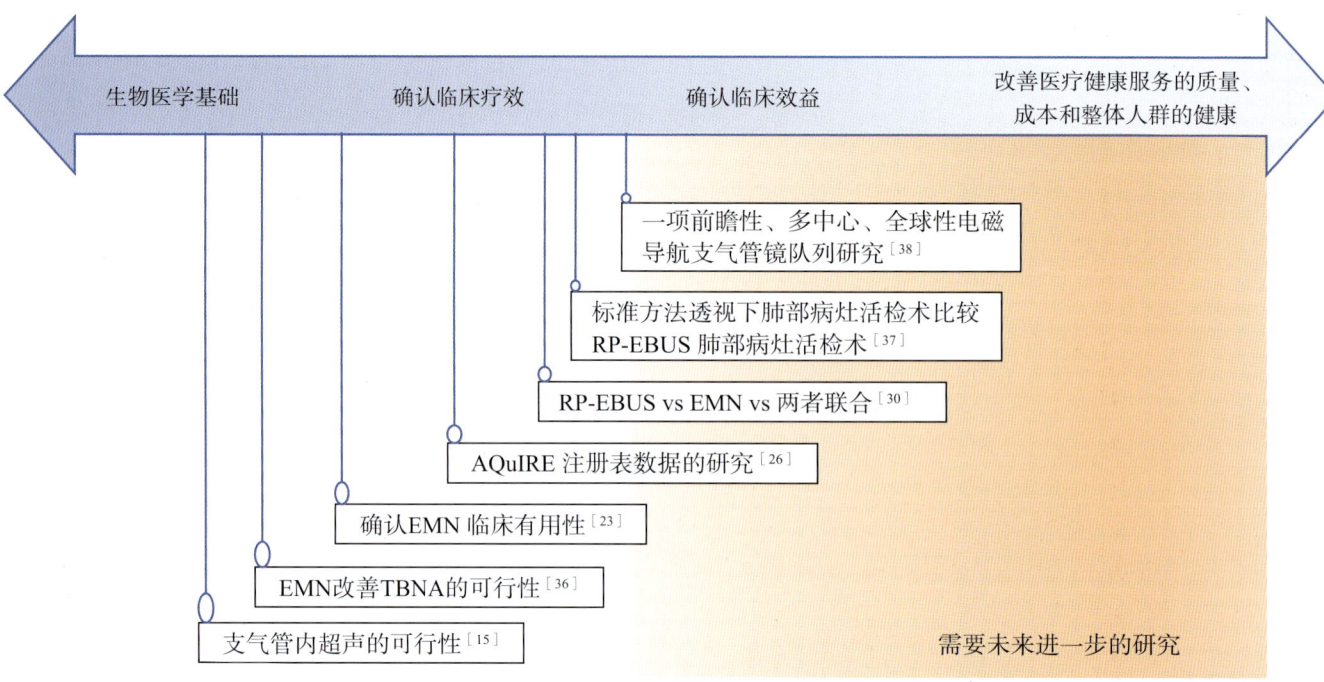

图 18.3 转化科学：EMN 和 RP-EBUS 应用于周围型肺部病变中的发展

数 EMN 研究将 EMN 的诊断率与文献报道的诊断率进行了比较，但没有直接与对照组比较。使用历史对照会受到前面提到的所有缺陷的影响，主要是选择偏倚和发表偏倚，并可能给人一种优越的误导性印象。只有少数 EMN 和 RP-EBUS 研究解决了这个问题[27-29]。

18.4.2.3 选择偏倚

检验 EMN 和 RP-EBUS 效用的研究，大多是在高度特定或选择的人群中进行的，选择标准和病变特征都很狭窄。因此，这些干预措施与结果之间的关系对于所研究的样本和拟分析的人群可能是不同的。例如，大多数报告 RP-EBUS 诊断率的数据来自实性肺结节。将这些结果外推到亚实性或磨玻璃结节可能不会简单地获得相同的结果。事实上，有报道称 RP-EBUS 对亚实性病变和磨玻璃结节的诊断率低于实性病变[30,31]。这并不一定意味着这项技术是无用的，它仅仅意味着在决定最佳方法之前，我们需要回过头来重新测量该方法在这一人群中的性能特征。

18.5 结论

新技术通常伴随着高昂的价格标签。一项技术是否会占据主导地位，不仅取决于它的可行性和实用性，

还取决于它与传统方法相比是否具有成本效益。为了评估这一点，唯一的方法就是进行严格的研究，涵盖转化研究的不同阶段。提供一个框架来对研究的不同阶段进行适当的分类，有助于确定知识差距，并有助于指导未来的研究。它还可以有助于理解为什么技术从实验室应用到临床后没有达到预期效果的可能原因。

参考文献

1 Ikeda, S., Yanai, N., and Ishikawa, S. (1968). Flexible bronchofiberscope. *Keio J. Med.* 17 (1): 1–16.

2 Dougherty, D. and Conway, P.H. (2008). The "3T's" road map to transform US health care: the "how" of high-quality care. *JAMA* 299 (19): 2319–2321.

3 Ioannidis, J.P. (2005). Contradicted and initially stronger effects in highly cited clinical research. *JAMA* 294 (2): 218–228.

4 McWilliams, A.M., Mayo, J.R., Ahn, M.I. et al. (2006). Lung cancer screening using multi-slice thin-section computed tomography and autofluorescence bronchoscopy. *J. Thorac. Oncol.* 1 (1): 61–68.

5 Edell, E., Lam, S., Pass, H. et al. (2009). Detection and localization of intraepithelial neoplasia and invasive carcinoma using fluorescence-reflectance bronchoscopy: an international, multicenter clinical trial. *J. Thorac. Oncol.* 4 (1): 49–54.

6 Lam, S., Kennedy, T., Unger, M. et al. (1998). Localization of bronchial intraepithelial neoplastic lesions by fluorescence bronchoscopy. *Chest* 113 (3): 696–702.

7 Tremblay, A., Taghizadeh, N., McWilliams, A.M. et al. (2016). Low prevalence of high-grade lesions detected with autofluorescence bronchoscopy in the setting of lung cancer

screening in the pan-Canadian lung cancer screening study. *Chest* 150 (5): 1015–1022.

8 Ost, D.E., Shah, A.M., Lei, X. et al. (2012). Respiratory infections increase the risk of granulation tissue formation following airway stenting in patients with malignant airway obstruction. *Chest* 141 (6): 1473–1481.

9 Casal, R.F., Lazarus, D.R., Kuhl, K. et al. (2015). Randomized trial of endobronchial ultrasound-guided transbronchial needle aspiration under general anesthesia versus moderate sedation. *Am. J. Respir. Crit. Care Med.* 191 (7): 796–803.

10 Schieppati, E. (1949). Mediastinal puncture thru the tracheal carina. *Rev. Asoc. Med. Argent.* 63 (663–664): 497–499.

11 Wang, K.P., Terry, P., and Marsh, B. (1978). Bronchoscopic needle aspiration biopsy of paratracheal tumors. *Am. Rev. Respir. Dis.* 118 (1): 17–21.

12 Becker, H.D. (1996). Endobronchial ultrasound–a new perspective in bronchology. *Ultraschall. Med.* 17 (3): 106–112.

13 Lewis, S.Z., Diekemper, R., and Addrizzo-Harris, D.J. (2013). Methodology for development of guidelines for lung cancer: diagnosis and management of lung cancer, 3rd ed: American College of Chest Physicians evidence- based clinical practice guidelines. *Chest* 143 (5 Suppl): 41S–50S.

14 Yasufuku, K., Chiyo, M., Sekine, Y. et al. (2004). Real-time endobronchial ultrasound-guided transbronchial needle aspiration of mediastinal and hilar lymph nodes. *Chest* 126 (1): 122–128.

15 Hurter, T. and Hanrath, P. (1992). Endobronchial sonography: feasibility and preliminary results. *Thorax* 47 (7): 565–567.

16 Pedersen, B.H., Vilmann, P., Folke, K. et al. (1996). Endoscopic ultrasonography and real-time guided fine-needle aspiration biopsy of solid lesions of the mediastinum suspected of malignancy. *Chest* 110 (2): 539–544.

17 Yasufuku, K., Pierre, A., Darling, G. et al. (2011). A prospective controlled trial of endobronchial ultrasound-guided transbronchial needle aspiration compared with mediastinoscopy formediastinal lymph node staging of lung cancer. *J. Thorac. Cardiovasc. Surg.* 142 (6): 1393–1400.

18 Ernst, A., Anantham, D., Eberhardt, R. et al. (2008). Diagnosis of mediastinal adenopathy – real-time endobronchial ultrasound guided needle aspiration versus mediastinoscopy. *J. Thorac. Oncol.* 3 (6): 577–582.

19 Trisolini, R., LazzariAgli, L., and Patelli, M. (2004). Conventional vs endobronchial ultrasound-guided transbronchial needle aspiration of the mediastinum. *Chest* 126 (3): 1005–1006.

20 O'Connell, O.J., Almeida, F.A., Simoff, M.J. et al. (2017). A prediction model to help with the assessment of adenopathy in lung cancer: HAL. *Am. J. Respir. Crit. Care Med.* 195 (12): 1651–1660.

21 Ost, D.E., Niu, J., Elting, L.S. et al. (2014). Quality gaps and comparative effectiveness in lung cancer staging and diagnosis. *Chest* 145 (2): 331–345.

22 Almeida, F.A., Casal, R.F., Jimenez, C.A. et al. (2013). Quality gaps and comparative effectiveness in lung cancer staging: the impact of test sequencing on outcomes. *Chest* 144 (6): 1776–1782.

23 Asano, F., Matsuno, Y., Shinagawa, N. et al. (2006). A virtual bronchoscopic navigation system for pulmonary peripheral lesions. *Chest* 130 (2): 559–566.

24 Gildea, T.R., Mazzone, P.J., Karnak, D. et al. (2006). Electromagnetic navigation diagnostic bronchoscopy: a prospective study. *Am. J. Respir. Crit. Care Med.* 174 (9): 982–989.

25 Makris, D., Scherpereel, A., Leroy, S. et al. (2007). Electromagnetic navigation diagnostic bronchoscopy for small peripheral lung lesions. *Eur. Respir. J.* 29 (6): 1187–1192.

26 Ost, D.E., Ernst, A., Lei, X. et al. (2016). Diagnostic yield and complications of bronchoscopy for peripheral lung lesions. Results of the AQuIRE registry. *Am. J. Respir. Crit. Care Med.* 193 (1): 68–77.

27 Yarmus, L.B., Arias, S., Feller-Kopman, D. et al. (2016). Electromagnetic navigation transthoracic needle aspiration for the diagnosis of pulmonary nodules: a safety and feasibility pilot study. *J. Thorac. Dis.* 8 (1): 186–194.

28 Mukherjee, S. and Chacey, M. (2017). Diagnostic yield of electromagnetic navigation bronchoscopy using a curved-tip catheter to aid in the diagnosis of pulmonary lesions. *J. Bronchol. Interv. Pulmonol.* 24 (1): 35–39.

29 Wang Memoli, J.S., Nietert, P.J., and Silvestri, G.A. (2012). Meta-analysis of guided bronchoscopy for the evaluation of the pulmonary nodule. *Chest* 142 (2): 385–393.

30 Eberhardt, R., Anantham, D., Ernst, A. et al. (2007). Multimodality bronchoscopic diagnosis of peripheral lung lesions: a randomized controlled trial. *Am. J. Respir. Crit. Care Med.* 176 (1): 36–41.

31 Roth, K., Eagan, T.M., Andreassen, A.H. et al. (2011). A randomised trial of endobronchial ultrasound guided sampling in peripheral lung lesions. *Lung Cancer* 74 (2): 219–225.

32 Fielding, D.I., Robinson, P.J., and Kurimoto, N. (2008). Biopsy site selection for endobronchial ultrasound guide-sheath transbronchial biopsy of peripheral lung lesions. *Intern. Med. J.* 38 (2): 77–84.

33 Ikezawa, Y., Sukoh, N., Shinagawa, N. et al. (2014). Endobronchial ultrasonography with a guide sheath for pure or mixed ground-glass opacity lesions. *Respir. Int. Rev. Thorac. Dis.* 88 (2): 137–143.

34 Izumo, T., Sasada, S., Chavez, C., and Tsuchida, T. (2013). The diagnostic utility of endobronchial ultrasonography with a guide sheath and tomosynthesis images for ground glass opacity pulmonary lesions. *J. Thorac. Dis.* 5 (6): 745–750.

35 Herth, F.J., Ernst, A., Eberhardt, R. et al. (2006). Endobronchial ultrasound-guided transbronchial needle aspiration of lymph nodes in the radiologically normal mediastinum. *Eur. Respir. J.* 28 (5): 910–914.

36 Solomon, S.B., White, P. Jr., Acker, D.E. et al. (1998). Real-time bronchoscope tip localization enables three- dimensional CT image guidance for transbronchial needle aspiration in swine. *Chest* 114 (5): 1405–1410.

37 Tanner, N.T., Yarmus, L., Chen, A. et al. (2018). Standard bronchoscopy with fluoroscopy vs thin bronchoscopy and radial endobronchial ultrasound for biopsy of pulmonary lesions: a multicenter, prospective, randomized trial. *Chest* 154: 1035–1043.

38 Folch, E.E., Bowling, M.R., Gildea, T.R. et al. (2016). Design of a prospective, multicenter, global, cohort study of electromagnetic navigation bronchoscopy. *BMC Pulm. Med.* 16 (1): 60.

第 19 章

可弯曲支气管镜下的激光、电凝、氩等离子体凝固术及冷冻治疗

Danai Khemasuwan[1] and Semra Bilaceroglu[2]

[1] Tufts University School of Medicine and St Elizabeth's Medical Center, Boston, MA, USA

[2] Izmir Dr Suat Seren Training and Research Hospital for Thoracic Medicine and Surgery, Health Sciences University, Izmir, Turkey

（译者：徐 浩 译者单位：浙江大学医学院附属第二医院）

19.1 引言

处理中央气道阻塞是介入呼吸病医师需要掌握的一项重要技能。根据病变位置和范围的不同，中央气道阻塞可表现为出血、阻塞性肺炎、呼吸窘迫及肺不张。支气管镜下治疗可以作为良恶性气道疾病根治前的缓解性或过渡性治疗手段。对支气管腔内病变，介入呼吸病医师可以采取一系列消融策略，如氩等离子体凝固术（argon plasma coagulation，APC）、高频电（electrocautery，EC）、激光切除和冷冻疗法（图19.1）等。上述手术策略，联合硬质支气管镜镜身机械铲切、钳夹、球囊扩张、支架置入等方法，往往可以成功治疗且并发症较少[1]。本章重点介绍这些治疗方法在中央性气道病变管理策略中的适应证、禁忌证、设备、技术和结局。

19.2 激光

自1960年以来，激光在治疗方面的作用已逐渐得到学界认可。激光技术利用了辐射能和光放大的特性。

必须有足够数量的激发态电子释放光子来产生激光，这种现象被称为"粒子数反转"，这需要通过一个外部的能量源激发某个指定的介质。几乎任何固体、液体或气体都可以作为介质。将介质置于一个两端有镜子的腔体中，将进一步促进激发（即"粒子数反转"现象）的发生。

激光的有效性与3个重要特性有关：波长、空间相干性和时间相干性，这与自然产生的光有所不同[2]。自然光包含不同波长的光，而激光则只发出一种颜色或

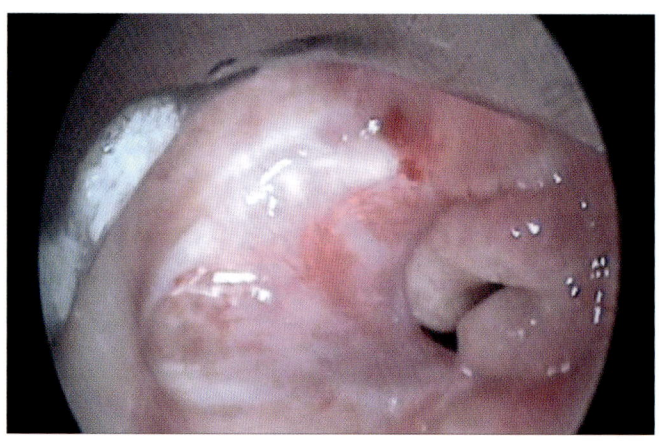

图 19.1 支气管腔内病变

插管后膜状狭窄导致50%以上的管腔阻塞和呼吸功能不全。资料来源：由塞尔维亚贝尔格莱德大学 Spasoje Popevic 提供。

窄波段波长的光。由于激光与光源的距离很小，其强度几乎可保持不变，从而确保了空间相干性的实现。由于激光产生的能量在均匀时间内以稳定的频率排列和移动，这形成了时间相干性。无论介质是固体、气体还是液体，上述3种特性均可适用。

传递到病变的能量取决于激光器的功率设置（以W为单位）、激光尖端与目标之间的距离以及激光作用的持续时间[3]。指向表面的光也可能被反射、散射、透射或吸收[2]。因此，光穿透的深度不仅取决于光的性质，还取决于组织的固有性质、所产生的光的特性和所使用的介质。介入呼吸病学中最常用的激光类型包括：钕∶钇-铝-石榴石（Nd:YAG）、钕∶钇-铝-钙钛矿（Nd:YAP）和钬∶钇-铝-石榴石（Ho:YAG）3种。不同类型的激光及其对组织影响的比较见表19.1。

发症[4]。在上述研究中，最常见的激光功率设置为20 W/30 Hz。

Ho:YAG激光的工作波长为2 100 nm，其在水中的吸收效率大约是Nd:YAG激光器的100倍。因此，Ho:YAG激光以类似于二氧化碳激光的方式切割组织，并限制附近组织的热坏死效应。有趣的是，Ho:YAG保持了与Nd:YAG激光器相似的凝血特性。这种类型的激光在恶性和良性支气管内疾病[5]中都显示出了安全性和有效性。Ho:YAG激光纤维可以被放置在距离目标几毫米的地方，以快速气化组织。

19.2.1 适应证和禁忌证

激光治疗的适应证取决于梗阻性病变的解剖特征和临床情况（表19.2）。

表19.1 常见医用激光的特性

激光	单位（nm）	输送装置	穿透深度	凝血作用	切割效果
氩	516	石英纤维	1.0~2.0 mm	++	+
KTP	532	石英纤维	1.0 mm	++	+
二极管	808	石英纤维	1.0 mm	++	+++
Nd:YAG	1 060	石英纤维	0.5~1.5 cm	+++	+
Nd:YAP	1 340	石英纤维	0.5~1.0 cm	++++	+
Ho:YAG	2 100	石英纤维	0.5~1.0 cm	+++	++
二氧化碳	10 600	耦合器和波导	0.23 mm	+	+++

KTP，磷酸钛钾激光；Nd:YAG，钕∶钇-铝-石榴石激光；Nd:YAP，钕∶钇-铝-钙钛矿激光；Ho:YAG，钬∶钇-铝-石榴石激光。

目前，在介入呼吸病中最常用的激光是Nd:YAG，其介质是钕（一种掺入钇的粉红色稀土）、铝，以及石榴石。Nd:YAG激光的波长为1 064 nm。有趣的是，这种波长的激光在组织中的水和血红蛋白成分中的吸收率很低，使其能够在组织中深入渗透（最高可达15 mm）。因此，这一特性使其可在气道内进行有效凝血。然而，由于穿透深度很难预测，激光束应该始终向视野下可见的管腔方向发射。由于Nd:YAG激光波长在人眼可见范围之外，因此在其基础上增加了一个可见波长的激光，为操作者提供可视化激光束参考。

近年来，一种更高效且更便携式的热激光技术被引入医学领域。Nd:YAP激光的波长是1 340 nm，它在水中的吸收系数是Nd:YAG的20倍。理论上，由于Nd:YAP的波长较Nd:YAG稍长，因此可能具有更强凝血和血管毁损能力。在一项回顾性研究中，使用Nd:YAP激光可有效恢复气道通畅且未出现严重并

表19.2 激光、高频电、冷冻治疗的适应证

良性或恶性气道病变，并伴有：
呼吸困难
不受控制的咳嗽
吸气延长
喘鸣
气道阻塞所致脱机困难
阻塞性肺炎
有症状且未处理的肺不张
主支气管几乎完全性阻塞（>50%）
复发性咯血
闭合常规治疗无效的支气管胸膜瘘

考虑到病灶的毗邻结构以及患者的相关临床状况，气管-支气管树的激光治疗在一些情况下存在禁忌（表19.3）。如病灶组织破坏的深度达到食管腔、纵隔和血

管等结构的边界，此时即存在解剖相关禁忌。对于因严重的心肺疾病而无法耐受清醒状态下操作或不耐受全身麻醉，或有不可纠正的凝血功能障碍的患者，则考虑存在临床相关禁忌。此外，梗阻远端肺不张持续超过4周的患者可能不会从内镜下激光治疗中获益，因为受累的肺不太可能复张。

表 19.3　激光、高频电、冷冻治疗的禁忌证

解剖学禁忌证
支气管内无病变的外压性闭塞
病变侵犯邻近大血管结构
病变侵犯邻近食管
病变侵犯邻近纵隔，可能有瘘管形成
临床禁忌证
可行手术切除者
短期预后不良，无症状缓解的可能性
不能耐受镇静或全麻
凝血障碍
闭塞总时间超过4周

19.2.2　并发症

激光治疗在经验丰富的医师手中是非常安全的，严重的并发症包括解剖边界评估不当、气道控制失败、视野不佳（表19.4）。为防止气道内失着火，吸入氧浓度（fraction of inspired oxygen，FiO_2）被维持在较低水平，同时采用负压吸引来清除分泌物、血液和烟雾，这些可能导致患者出现周围毛细血管血氧饱和度（SpO_2）和呼气末二氧化碳（end-tidal carbon dioxide，$ETCO_2$）的显著波动。因此，持续的心电监测及指脉氧监测对保障患者的安全极为重要。

表 19.4　激光气道治疗的并发症

患者	设备和医疗保健人员
出血	视网膜损伤
支气管内着火	接触探头尖端断裂
气胸	
纵隔气肿	
空气栓塞	
激光烟尘	
感染	
呼吸心血管系统并发症	

气管内燃烧是激光治疗中最可怕的并发症之一，这通常发生在气管内导管、可弯曲支气管镜、抽吸导管等易燃物质被激光束照射时。通过确保FiO_2始终低于40%，可以避免在激光发射模式下出现气道内起火。激光治疗时，麻醉气体或氧气可产生"火炬效应"，对患者和手术室人员构成即时危险，即可能发生气管内爆炸。气管插管起火可引起黏膜脱落、气道内肉芽组织阻塞及下气道吸入性损伤，这些可能引起长期并发症。同样地，在使用激光之前，也应该移除硅酮支架。

如激光治疗导致大血管穿孔，则可发生大出血，这是较为常见的并发症，原因在于无法准确判断激光的穿透深度。高功率（>40 W）或长脉冲持续时间（>1秒）是发生大血管穿孔的危险因素。Nd:YAG激光也可引起气管壁的损伤，从而导致气管狭窄的形成。径向EBUS已被用来探测靶部位的气管解剖结构，以减少激光损伤，但仍需要进一步研究[6]。

空气栓塞也偶见报道，这可能与使用高流量的空气冷却系统有关。因此，建议尽量减少冷却系统中的空气流量，并使用非接触式探头，以避免发生空气栓塞[7]。

19.2.3　技术要点

医师更喜欢在全麻、硬质支气管镜下来进行激光治疗操作，尽管该操作也可以在局部麻醉下使用可弯曲支气管镜完成[8]。给氧和通气可以采用自发性辅助通气、喷气通气或喉部面罩辅助通气等。

激光治疗的第一步是对肿瘤进行光凝固治疗。然后，通过使用硬质支气管镜斜面边缘、活检钳和吸引器来取出凝固的组织。也可以选择进行完全激光气化，但有支气管内着火的高风险。激光束应始终平行于支气管壁，且绝不应与气道壁形成垂直角度发射。激光脉冲的持续时间往往控制在1 s以内。使用可弯曲支气管镜时，由于镜腔及钳子较小，切除脱落的组织可能较为缓慢和困难。此外，可弯曲支气管镜本身可能是可燃的。

19.2.4　注意事项

为避免意外激光散射伤害，应使用盐渍垫和铝箔来保护患者眼睛，同时所有工作人员均应佩戴护目镜。应采取以下预防措施以尽量降低着火风险：保持FiO_2在40%以下；移除气管内导管等易燃材料；在使用激光前移除硅酮支架；当组织从支气管镜中取出时，保持激光处于待机模式；使用可弯曲支气管镜时，保持激光在距离支气管镜尖端足够远的距离；激光能量设置不应超过40 W。

19.2.5 转归

大多数与激光治疗相关转归的研究为非随机非对照研究，对于死亡率的比较多来自经验分享和历史对照。同时，病例研究中的大多数恶性疾病都采用了多种方式治疗，包括放疗和化疗等。一项研究通过历史对照比较了外照射放疗联合 Nd:YAG 激光治疗与单独接受紧急放疗患者的结局，发现联合放疗患者在死亡率方面显著获益（150 天比 267 天，$P=0.04$）[9]。在一项比较 Nd:YAG 激光单独或联合其他治疗方式的回顾性研究中，在非小细胞肺癌患者人群中，联合治疗组第 2 次干预的中位时间显著延长了 1.7 个月，而在所有形式的癌症人群中显著延长了 3.2 个月[10]。对于特定类型的恶性肿瘤（如类癌），使用 Nd:YAG 激光也取得了较好的效果[11]。

激光治疗也被用于处理长期插管造成的气道狭窄[12]，分枝杆菌感染引起炎性肉芽组织增生所造成的气道狭窄，肺移植后吻合口肉芽组织增生[13]、缝合处肉芽肿[14]，结缔组织疾病如韦格纳肉芽肿、白塞综合征、复发性多软骨炎等引起的系统性炎性疾病等[15,16]。另外，支气管内激光还可用于继发于支气管结石的症状性梗阻[17]。

在 Ramser 和 Beamis 对支气管镜下激光治疗的回顾性研究中[18]，100 例患者中有 85% 症状缓解并达到了术前目标；87% 病灶位于主支气管内；总体并发症发生率为 6.5%，无死亡病例。虽然以生存期为终点的研究大多采用历史对照，但症状的缓解和使一些患者脱离机械通气的能力为激光治疗的疗效提供了证据。Mehta 的研究纳入了采用 Nd:YAG 激光治疗及随后的外照射放射联合治疗或外照射放射治疗联合近距离放射治疗的患者[19]。虽然患者数量较少（300 例患者中有 17 例），但他们的生存率明显高于仅接受放疗的历史对照组。

19.2.6 结论

对于经验丰富的操作者而言，激光是治疗中央气道阻塞的有效工具，它可作为其他支气管内治疗方式的辅助手段之一。Nd:YAG 是目前最常用的激光。多项研究证明，在气道良恶性阻塞性病变的治疗中，采用激光治疗可以显著获益。

19.3 高频电凝（EC）治疗

EC 利用电流来产生热量，并切割、凝固及气化组织。Strauss 等在 1913 年使用 EC 治疗胃肠道肿瘤，并在 1935 年报告了他们治疗 40 多例患者的经验[20]。EC 装置的功率（以 W 为单位）对应于组织中产生的热量，计算公式：功率 =（电流）^{2} × 电阻。

EC 治疗时，使组织凝固需采用高电流和低电压，而使组织气化则要采用高电压和低电流。切割具有凝固能力的组织时则可以混合这两种设置。在温度约为 60℃时，组织开始失活，超过 150℃会发生碳化，超过 300℃则将开始气化。组织破坏的程度取决于所施加的功率、组织的电特性、设备-组织接触时间和接触表面积。EC 会在切口边缘形成凝固区，从而减少了组织的机械损伤。

EC 治疗有两种形式：单极和双极电极。介入支气管镜操作中最常使用的是单极 EC，此时电流从发生器通过主动电极进入目标组织，并通过患者到达接地垫，然后返回发生器。在双极 EC 中，电流只通过钳形电极两条臂之间的组织。

19.3.1 适应证

EC 的适应证和禁忌证与 Nd:YAG 激光相似[21,22]（表 19.2、表 19.3）。与激光治疗类似，EC 可快速削减肿瘤的体积，并以较低的成本用于缓解即将发生的呼吸衰竭。

19.3.2 设备和技术

常用的 EC 钝性探头和 EC 圈套均可通过可弯曲支气管镜的 2.0 mm 工作通道，此外也可以使用电刀和电活检钳。电发生器应具备调节高频电流的能力，以便操作者可以调整设置来进行凝固、切割、混凝或气化。单极 EC 必须通过电极垫接地，以允许电子离开患者身体。

操作者可以使用闭合的活检钳或钝性 EC 探头来探测病变，以评估其大小、活动性、脆性及出血可能，并定位气道上的任何附着物。钝性探头可能更适用于长条形或扁平的病变，而圈套器更适用于息肉样病变。圈套器用于切割和去除组织，采用混合电流用于切割和凝固，但不使组织气化。当圈套环打开时，圈套应被放置在尽可能靠近组织的基底部。当圈套环被收紧时，控制圈套器的手柄会有一种拉紧的感觉。此时激活电路，圈套环将慢慢地收紧。采用这种方式，组织的切割和凝固是通过电流产生的热量而不是圈套器钢丝的机械作用完成的。当操作结束时，控制圈套器手柄上的拉紧感就消失了，这时将环回收至导管中，被切断的组织可以用圈套或活检钳取出。内切方式是一种具有交替切割和凝固的分步切割方式。凝固的持续时间和强度可以在该设置下进行调整。

EC 推荐的功率设置为 20~40 W，并具有混合波形，可以同时用来切割和凝固。这种混合设置允许在切割组织时同时止血。

19.3.3 转归

在一项纳入 56 例患者的研究中，Homasson 指出，经过 EC 治疗后，75% 的患者控制了咯血，67% 的患者呼吸困难缓解，55% 的患者咳嗽或喘鸣得到缓解[23]。Petrou 等报道，29 例患者中有 28 例在使用圈套器切除病变后症状有所改善[24]。Sutedja 等的研究结果显示，17 例接受治疗的患者中有 15 例立即恢复了气道通畅；8 例患者呼吸困难得到缓解，4 例患者的咯血得到控制[25]。大多数研究主要涉及恶性肿瘤[26-28]。手术的成功率（定义为切除超过 50% 的肿瘤）据报道为 70%~95%。EC 已被证明比 Nd:YAG 激光器更具成本效益优势[29]。一项回顾性病例系列研究提示，EC 在良性和恶性气道阻塞的治疗中是安全且有效的[30]。EC 也可用于对支气管内病变进行"热活检"，采用凝固可以减少出血风险[31]。虽然热量可能造成一定程度的组织学损伤，带来一定的人为影响[32]，但所获标本的质量仍足以进行病理学判断和解释[31,33]。

19.3.4 并发症

EC 的并发症相对罕见。有少数病例报告了支气管内燃烧事件，这些与吸入氧浓度过高及硅酮支架相关[34]。患者的烧伤和电击常被认为是可能的并发症之一，但缺少发表数据的支持。另一项顾虑是在带有起搏器或自动植入式除颤器的患者中使用 EC，因为可能使这些设备出现故障并导致心律失常。如果有必要，可采用以下措施来降低干扰：

1）采用双极技术而不是单极技术。
2）使用低功率设置。
3）在手术前停用起搏器。
4）将平板放置得尽可能靠近操作区域，距离起搏器最少为 15 cm。
5）避免长时间激活。

短时间的激活时间类似心律失常，从而无意中导致除颤器的电击。当用于动物模型时，EC 已被证明会导致气道狭窄和软骨损伤。这种软骨损伤可导致支气管软化症[23]。然而，EC 引起的气道狭窄、软骨损伤和穿孔是罕见的，通常与应用功率、接触时间和面积以及采用环绕电凝相关。凝固模式的使用可以减少这些并发症[32,35]。

19.3.5 结论

与激光治疗一样，EC 是一种有效治疗支气管内病变的方式。它是激光治疗之外的一种更便宜的替代疗法。EC 的并发症的数量较少，严重程度较轻。

19.4 氩等离子体凝固术

APC 是一种类似于激光或 EC 的电外科技术，可用于清除阻塞性病变和/或实现止血。APC 是一种单极电外科手术，电能通过电离的氩气（等离子体）转移到组织中。氩等离子体流向电阻最小的区域，如生物组织或任何可燃物体。这种现象为内窥镜的应用提供了实际的好处，因为氩等离子体既可以实现通电氩气所在区域接触面上的热治疗，也可以实现气体喷射方向上的热切割治疗。

氩等离子体凝固术早在 20 多年前就发展起来，以改善手术止血。在 20 世纪 90 年代早期，可弯曲探头的引入方便了 APC 在内窥镜手术中的使用。APC 最初用于胃肠道内窥镜息肉切除术中止血[36]，目前已被用于清除恶性气道肿瘤、控制咯血、从支架或吻合口去除肉芽组织，以及在支气管镜手术中治疗各种其他良性疾病（图 19.2）[37-40]。它是一种 EC 的非接触性形式，其适应证和禁忌证与激光和 EC 类似。

19.4.1 过程

与 EC 类似，应在患者的背部或大腿上部放置一个接地垫。设置应为 30~50 W 的功率，氩气流量应为 0.8~1 升/分。主要有 3 种模式：强力 APC、脉冲 APC 和精细 APC。强力 APC 提供高频电压，这与输出设置（瓦特）直接相关。对于脉冲 APC，有两种设置："效应 1"，提供较高的能量输出，脉冲间隔更长（大约 1 个脉冲/秒）；"效应 2"，提供更多的脉冲（16 个脉冲/秒），较低的能量输出。精细 APC 则具有自动调节控制功能，其电离等离子体的强度与效应设置和与目标组织的距离直接相关。

探头尖端应超过支气管镜尖端 1~1.5 cm，以确保支气管镜不受损坏。探针尖端应在目标病灶 1 cm 以内。如果探头离目标病灶更远，则电流将无法介导至靶目标。氩气从探头中排出，然后高压电流通过探头传

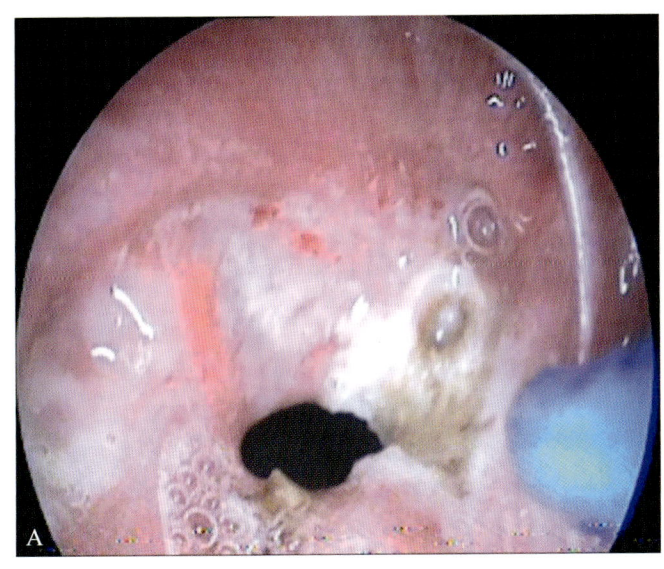 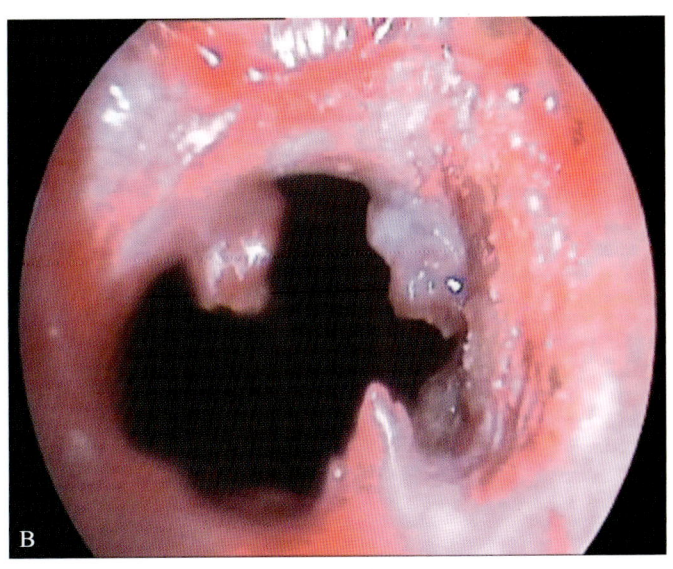

图 19.2　氩等离子体凝固术（APC）在插管后气管网状狭窄患者中的应用

A. 使用 APC 在狭窄段前壁和侧壁上进行切割；B. 硬质支气管镜和球囊扩张后管腔明显增大。资料来源：由塞尔维亚贝尔格莱德大学 Spasoje Popevic 提供。

递，电离氩气，并将单极电流传导到目标病灶[41]。目前，有 3 种探头尖端设计（垂直发射、侧向发射和圆周发射）。

在 APC 清除支气管内病变的过程中，由于组织的破坏而形成焦痂和碎片（图 19.2），此时用活检钳或冷冻治疗探针取出，然后将 APC 应用于下面的新鲜组织，将比应用于碎片和焦痂更有效。重复这个过程，直到肿瘤被切除。如果遇到快速出血，APC 也可以用于凝固和止血，而不会产生烟雾，从而改善视野。

APC 在目标组织表面以下几毫米处引起的表面热损伤会导致碳化和气化。APC 应该通过像移动画笔一样移动探头动态应用在目标区域，同时要密切监测靶组织的效应。热损伤的程度取决于影响凝固深度的 3 个最重要的因素：应用时间、功率/效应和探头到目标组织的距离。

19.4.2　转归

一项纳入 364 例接受 APC（482 次操作）患者的前瞻性队列研究显示，APC 的成功率为 67%，"成功"定义为止血和/或完全或部分气道再通[40]。APC 最常见的应用为气道阻塞（51%）和止血（33%），其中近 90% 的根本病因是恶性肿瘤。值得注意的是，90% 的操作都使用了硬质支气管镜。在一项对 60 例接受 APC（70 次操作）的患者进行的回顾性研究中[38]，59 例患者的治疗立即成功。所有患者均有咯血或气道阻塞，治疗成功的定义为咯血缓解和/或气道阻塞减少。平均随访 97 天，咯血没有复发，并且平均随访 53 天，呼吸困难持续得到改善。95% 的患者存在恶性疾病，所有手术均采用可弯曲支气管镜。一项针对 47 例患者的类似研究报告成功率为 92%[37]，且平均随访 6.7 个月，治疗效果保持不变。然而，平均每个患者需要 3 次以上的治疗才能达到这个结果。APC 也被成功用于良性疾病的治疗，如支架或气道吻合的肉芽组织增生[40,42]。

19.4.3　并发症

APC 的并发症并不常见（<1%），主要包括气道灼伤和气道穿孔，可导致纵隔气肿、皮下气肿和气胸[40]。气体栓塞可发生于气道腔内压力高于静脉压时，此时气体可从 APC 探头进入静脉系统。在一项回顾病例系列研究中，气体栓塞导致 3 例发生心力衰竭和 1 例死亡[43]。这种并发症的预防措施包括最大限度地减少达到组织效果所需的氩气流，应用 APC 时避免探头与组织之间的直接接触，避免探头持续垂直于组织，避免将探头直接对准大的、开放的血管。

由于单极电路配置和使用电压较高，氩等离子体凝固术可与植入式心脏设备间产生电磁干扰。由于电压可达 2.58 ± 0.34 mV，APC 被认为是电磁干扰植入式心脏设备的"高危"技术[44]。因此，如果可能的话应在治疗前关闭植入式心脏设备。否则，应考虑采用替代的治疗方式。

与激光和EC类似，在应用APC的过程中应限制吸入氧浓度、应用功率（<80 W）和应用时间（<5 s），这对于降低气道穿孔或着火的风险来说非常重要。保持探头尖端远离任何可燃材料几厘米，对于防止气道点燃也是必要的。同样地，为了防止支气管镜的着火，探头的尖端应与支气管镜的尖端保持几厘米的距离。

19.4.4　结论

在所有的方法中，只有支气管镜热治疗（APC、EC和激光）有即时的效果，因此可以迅速清除组织。APC在稳定性方面优于EC和激光治疗。然而，APC消融和止血的效果非常表浅（仅1~2 mm深度）。APC的并发症是罕见的，发生在不到1%的操作中。

19.5　冷冻疗法

一篇公元前3 500年的文献描述了使用冷冻作为一种治疗肿胀和战伤的方法[45]。希波克拉底提到了如何使用冷冻治疗骨科损伤[45]。Arnott描述了使用-8℃至-12℃含有碎冰的盐溶液来冷冻晚期肿瘤，从而缩小肿瘤大小，改善疼痛[46,47]。焦耳-汤姆逊效应是指气体从高压向低压环境变化时，气体突然膨胀形成低温，这是低温探头发挥作用的基础，在呼吸病领域中尤为常用。

Neel证明了冷冻的破坏性作用[48]。冷冻后，黏膜、黏膜下腺体和浆膜会被完全破坏，而结缔组织和软骨的框架仍然可以保持完整，在冷冻后的14天内，气管-支气管树和上皮开始再生和愈合[48-55]。关于冷冻治疗的第一项研究纳入了来自梅奥诊所的28例支气管内肿瘤患者，该研究发现冷冻疗法是缓解肿瘤的一个很好的替代方法[56-59]。

冷冻疗法通过冷冻的细胞毒性作用来破坏生物物质。冷冻引起的损伤发生在多个水平上，包括分子、细胞和结构水平以及整体组织水平。冷冻的效果受到多种因素的影响，细胞的存活取决于冷却速率[60-62]、解冻速率[63]、达到的最低温度[64]和反复冻融循环的次数[65,66]。某些组织对于低温更加敏感（如皮肤、黏膜、肉芽组织等），而另一些组织则不敏感（如脂肪、软骨、纤维或结缔组织等）。低温敏感性取决于细胞的含水量。肿瘤细胞可能比正常细胞更敏感[66]。

在美国，目前有两种冷冻剂输送的方法。

1）采用一氧化二氮（N_2O）减压冷却的尖端接触式冷冻探头。尖端的温度可以降低到-89.5℃（Erbe Elektromedezin，德国）。冷冻探针有1.9 mm和2.4 mm两种尺寸。

2）冷冻喷雾，其中导管尖端输送气体液氮（N_2）产生一种出口温度为-196℃（CSA Medical，Baltimore，MD）的冷冻喷雾。该系统为非接触式，有一个7 F导管，至少需要2.8 mm的工作通道[67-69]。和冷冻探针相比，使用冷冻喷雾来进行支气管镜下冷冻治疗的经验和文献较少。然而，支气管镜下冷冻喷雾治疗恶性气道阻塞[69]和良性气道疾病[68,70]似乎是安全有效的。

19.5.1　设备

冷冻机有3个部分：控制台、冷冻探头以及连接控制台和气瓶到探针的传输线。冷冻探针可以是硬质、半硬质或可弯曲的；硬质和半硬质冷冻探针只能通过硬质支气管镜使用，但可弯曲冷冻探头可以通过可弯曲支气管镜或硬质支气管镜使用。光学设备并不会因低温而变形，然而，整个支气管镜在冷冻期间温度将下降，如果冷冻探头有缺陷，这种降温则可能随着反复冻融而愈发增大[67]。

冷冻的监测仍然是一个问题[71]，目前仍没有理想的解决方案。这依赖于操作者的经验，而操作者则依赖于冷冻组织的颜色或一致性和冷冻区域长度的变化。在临床研究中[72]，使用硬质、半硬质或可弯曲的冷冻探头，每个冻融周期被设定为30秒左右。对于硬质探头，解冻速度非常快，但对于可弯曲探头，解冻速度由体温决定，从而增加了冻融循环的时间。

19.5.2　适应证

冷冻治疗适用于腔内良性或恶性气管支气管阻塞或狭窄。选择标准类似于激光、APC或EC（表19.2、表19.3），但不适用于紧急治疗。此外，冷冻疗法可用于取出异物（特别是有机异物）、血凝块或黏液栓[67,68]。

19.5.3　技术

可使用可弯曲冷冻探头来开展内镜下治疗[59]，其可通过支气管镜的工作通道。从支气管镜下可以看到冷冻探头的尖端，然后直接施加到肿瘤所在区域。

一旦在气道腔内，即距离支气管镜尖端约4 mm处，就可以用脚踏板激活冷冻探头。探头尖端30 s内出现一个冰球；1~3个冻融循环，每次持续1 min，应用于同一区域或其相邻区域（图19.3）。探头的尖端可以垂直、正切或进入肿瘤肿块。在-30℃至-40℃，冷冻组织的破坏很容易看到。通过将脚从踏板上移除，冷冻探头就会解除冷冻。在每个冷冻周期中，在从病变中移除尖端之前，都要等待冰球完全解冻。对于浸润性病变，冷冻疗法可采用侧向正切接触法。

最适合冷冻治疗的病变类型是良性或恶性的息肉样病变。将冷冻探针的金属尖端放置在肿块上或推入其中会产生最大体积的圆周型冻结。在每个位点都进行3次冻融循环，然后将探头移动5~6 mm，并在相邻区域再进行3个循环。

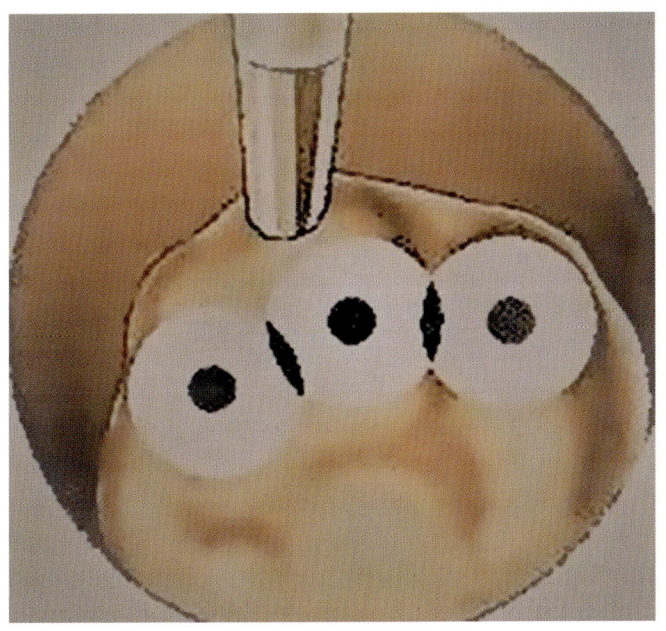

图19.3 冷冻疗法应用
1~3次冻融循环，每次持续1 min，在同一或邻近区域重叠使用。

19.5.4 转归

Walsh等报道了冷冻疗法对呼吸困难、咯血、咳嗽和喘鸣等症状的治疗效果[73]。在该研究中，33例患者，共实施了81次冷冻治疗，记录治疗前后的症状、肺功能、胸片和支气管镜检查结果。大多数患者的整体症状、喘鸣和咯血有所改善，呼吸困难总体较前改善。同样，Maiwand等报告了600例采用冷冻治疗的患者[74]。在冷冻治疗后，78%的患者表示他们的症状有了主观上的改善，其咳嗽（64%）、呼吸困难（66%）、咯血（65%）和嘶鸣（70%）等症状较前减轻。Homasson等研究提示，经冷冻治疗后，80%的患者咯血停止，50%的患者呼吸困难较前减轻[75]。Mathur等则在小样本人群中使用纤维支气管镜进行冷冻治疗，获得了类似的结果[59,76]。Walsh研究显示，58%的患者肺功能得到客观改善，且肺功能的改善与症状改善是相关联的[73]。

Hetzel等对60例腔内型肿瘤患者进行了低温冻切再通[77]，在这些病例中冷冻疗法迅速起效，并避免了二次操作影响再通的可能（图19.4）。冷冻探头尖端接触肿瘤组织，冷冻后回拉探头从而将整个肿块从气道中切除。在本研究中，83%的患者的治疗完全或部分成功，其中6例患者发生出血，进行了APC治疗。随后，Hetzel等在225例有症状的气道狭窄患者中推广了他们的经验[78]。91.1%的患者成功进行冷冻冻切再通，其中16.4%的患者使用了APC治疗出血，而8%的患者出血较严重，需要使用支气管封堵术。可弯曲冷冻探头可以成功治疗有症状的支气管内肿瘤引起的阻塞，并立即起效，但其安全性有待进一步研究。没有经验的操作者，可能会有潜在的危险。冻切也有助于获得更大的活检样本[70]。

由于常规经支气管肺活检（transbronchial lung biopsy, TBLB）标本数量有限，且获取时遭受人为挤压，影响质量，冷冻探头冻切活检术已被用于获取TBLB组织来辅助弥漫性肺疾病的诊断。在一项研究中，选取41例弥漫性肺病患者进行TBLB治疗。在可弯曲支气管镜检查中，首先使用活检钳进行常规的经支气管活检。然后，在透视引导下，将可弯曲冷冻探头引入选定的支气管。一旦进入拟定位置，探头随即降温，然后将冷冻的肺组织附着在尖端完成冻切检。相较于冷冻探头（15.11 mm^2，2.15~54.15 mm^2），活检钳取下的标本明显更小（5.82 mm^2，0.58~20.88 mm^2）。2例患者出现气胸，经留置胸腔引流管后得到缓解[79]。然而，需要进一步研究来比较冷冻-TBLB和电视辅助胸腔镜手术，以及更好地评估其并发症。

人们对早期肺癌冷冻治疗重新产生了兴趣。法国GECC（冷冻外科研究组）报道了针对36例患者44个病变（原位或微浸润性肿瘤）的治疗经验[80]，其中42%的患者曾因侵袭性耳鼻喉癌症或支气管癌接受治疗。1年后，88.8%的患者其肿瘤达到了临床和组织学完全控制，平均随访时间为32个月。该人群的平均生存时间为30个月。此外，支气管内冷冻治疗与症状改善、Karnofsky评分和肺功能测试均相关。两次冷冻治疗后的平均生存时间为15个月[81]。

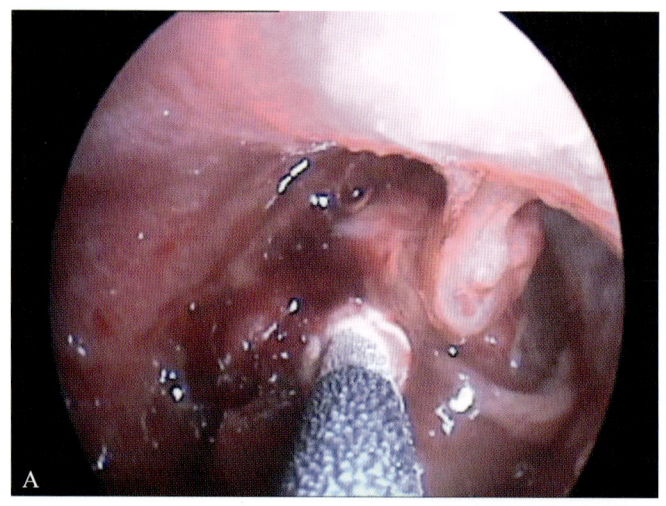
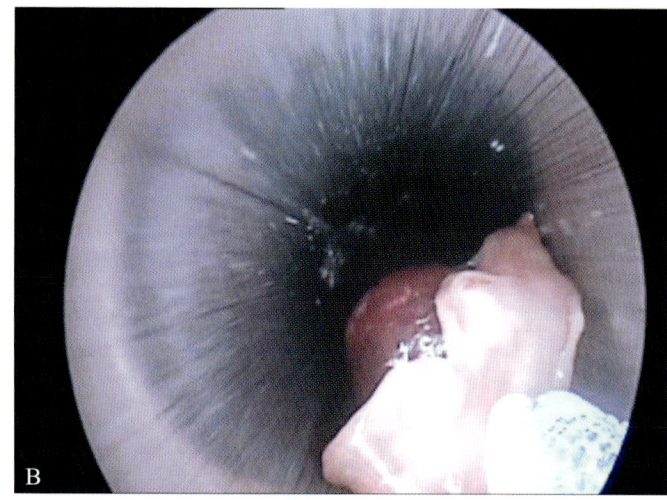
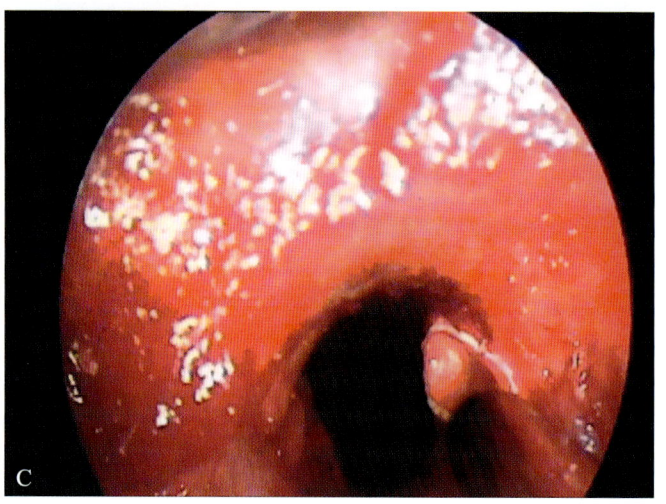

图 19.4　冷冻疗法

A. 用冷冻探头冷冻气管内恶性肿瘤；B. 冻切冷冻肿瘤碎片并取出；C. 治疗后气管实现再通。资料来源：由塞尔维亚贝尔格莱德大学 Spasoje Popevic 提供。

19.5.5　冷冻治疗−放疗的联合疗效研究

与激光或 EC 治疗类似，冷冻治疗可以缓解支气管阻塞，防止局部并发症，而这是大多数死亡的原因。某些研究表明，由于血流的影响，冷冻治疗和外照射放疗之间可能存在协同作用[74]。在两项类似的前瞻性研究中，Vergnon[82]和 Homasson[56]均利用冷冻治疗联合放疗对患者进行了治疗。大于 50% 的肿瘤破坏定义为治疗满意。Vergnon 的研究纳入了 29 例患者，他们因局部或功能原因出现症状性、不可切除的阻塞。每例患者进行了 1~2 次冷冻治疗，其中 16 例治疗满意；13 例治疗不满意，肿瘤病变持续生长。在放疗剂量方面，21 例患者接受 65 Gy，8 例一般情况较差的患者接受 45 Gy。在不满意的冷冻治疗组中，患者迅速死于局部并发症，中位生存期仅为 5 个月；在满意的冷冻治疗组中，患者中位生存期为 11 个月，生存期有显著改善。

19.5.6　良性气管支气管病变

良性病变已通过冷冻治疗取得了非常好的效果。特别是对于肉芽肿性组织，治疗后疗效达到 100%，且数月甚至数年均无复发。肉芽状组织对冷的反应非常敏感。冷冻疗法比热消融疗法的明显优势是没有支气管内着火的风险。

因此，冷冻疗法已越来越多地用于治疗声门下、气管和支气管狭窄。冷冻治疗联合球囊扩张可导致气道直径增加和瘢痕组织坏死。气管切除术是复杂气管狭窄（长度>1 cm 或<1 cm 但伴有软化）的治疗方

法。然而，单纯性狭窄（长度<1 cm，无软化，通常呈膜状）更适合使用支气管腔内治疗，如冷冻治疗、球囊扩张、支架置入术或热治疗[67,68]。此外，如果由于狭窄的解剖程度和/或患者的状态而不能进行手术，则复杂气管狭窄也可以采用支气管腔内治疗。

当类癌、圆柱瘤和喉气管乳头状瘤等肿瘤不可进行手术时，冷冻治疗可能取得成功。目前，冷冻喷雾的安全性/有效性数据有限[83,84]。

19.5.7 取出异物

冷冻治疗已被成功地用来取出异物。它最常用于去除如下异物或生物材料，如药丸、花生、牙齿、鸡骨头等。它对去除血凝块、黏液栓和糜烂组织等也非常有帮助。

19.5.8 冷冻治疗的未来

冷冻治疗除了在阻塞性或狭窄性支气管内病变的气道重建中表现出良好的疗效外，还能对气道免疫系统产生刺激和抑制作用。存在于消融区外边缘的凋亡细胞不释放细胞内容物，并可能诱导免疫耐受。此外，大量的凋亡细胞可能具有组织保护作用，同时坏死细胞可能作为免疫刺激剂。利用气道冷冻治疗的保护作用，可能将其用于早期和晚期癌症的治疗中[67,85]。

19.5.9 结论

冷冻治疗良恶性支气管内病变已被证明是一种有效和安全的治疗方法。该技术尤其对肺癌和气道阻塞的患者非常有用。超过一半患者的症状和呼吸功能都得到了改善。除了上述优点以外，冷冻疗法安全性高，易于操作，价格低廉，且并发症少。

19.6 实践要点和建议

1）在所有介入支气管镜操作中，应该始终牢记"可以做，不代表就需要做"原则。

2）当选择最佳的支气管镜消融治疗方法时，应该合理、实际地仔细考虑如下内容：
    a. 合适的能量设置和持续时间；
    b. 病灶的类型、位置和性质；
    c. 安全的吸入氧浓度；
    d. 消融治疗的可及性；
    e. 支气管镜操作者的培训及经验；
    f. 立即进行消融的必要性。

3）恶性和良性腔内病变可采用姑息性或治愈性治疗。

4）对于严重的中央气道症状性阻塞，通常建议立即进行支气管镜下热治疗——激光或EC。冷冻治疗的效果往往有所延迟，但冻切可以提供即刻的气道再通效果。

5）EC更经济，其功效可与激光相媲美。

6）应选择合适的EC探头来针对特定的支气管内病变进行个性化治疗。

7）APC是理想的迅速凝血的方法，但不能在短时间内消融一个较大的肿块。

8）EC和APC可通过电流使心脏起搏器和其他植入的心脏设备发生功能失调，而激光则没有这种影响[86]。

9）在热治疗（如激光、EC、APC）期间，应通过保持$FiO_2<40\%$来降低气管内着火的风险，放置喉罩而不是气管插管和/或使用硬质支气管镜。

10）在冷冻疗法中，不存在由于FiO_2水平引起气道着火的风险。

11）支气管镜下消融治疗可与其他消融方法（如冷冻疗法+APC、EC/激光+APC）、内镜治疗技术（球囊支气管成形术和/或支架植入术）或疾病治疗方案（如化疗、放疗或手术）联合使用，以改善预后和减少并发症。

12）要进行支气管镜下消融治疗，需要对操作者进行严格的培训、手术流程和能力的确认。操作者应不但能够提供最佳的、个体化的、高效安全的治疗，且应具备处理并发症的能力。

参考文献

1 Scarlata, S., Fuso, L., Lucantoni, G. et al. (2017). The technique of endoscopic airway tumor treatment. *J. Thorac. Dis.* 9: 2619–2639.

2 Herd, R.M., Dover, J.S., and Amdt, K.A. (1997). Lasers in dermatology. *Dermatol. Clin.* 15: 355–373.

3 Dumon, M.C. and Dumon, J.F. (1995). Laser bronchoscopy. In: Textbook of Bronchoscopy (eds. S.H. Feinsilver and A.M. Fein), 393–399. Baltimore: Williams & Wilkins.

4 Lee, H.J., Malhotra, R., Grossman, C. et al. (2011). Initial report of neodymium: yttrium-aluminum-perovskite (Nd: YAP) laser use during bronchoscopy. *J. Bronchol. Interv. Pulmonol.* 18 (3): 229–232.

5 Squiers, J.J., Teeter, W.A., Hoopman, J.E. et al. (2014). Holmium: YAG laser bronchoscopy ablation of benign and malignant airway obstructions: an 8-year experience. *Lasers*

Med. Sci. 29 (4): 1437–1443.

6 Murgu, S.D., Colt, H.G., Mukai, D. et al. (2010). Multimodal imaging guidance for laser ablation in tracheal stenosis. *Laryngoscope* 120 (9): 1840–1846.

7 Golish, J.A., Pena, C.M., Mehta, A.C. et al. (1992). Massive air embolism complicating Nd-YAG laser endobronchial photoresection. *Lasers Surg. Med.* 12 (3): 338–342.

8 Prakash, U.B.S., Offord, K.P., and Stubbs, S.E. (1991). Bronchoscopy in North America: the ACCP survey. *Chest* 100: 1668–1675.

9 Desai, S.J., Mehta, A.C., Medendorp, S.V. et al. (1988). Survival experience following Nd YAG laser photoresection for primary bronchogenic carcinoma. *Chest* 94 (5): 939–944.

10 Han, C.C., Prasetyo, D., and Wright, G.M. (2007). Endobronchial palliation using Nd: YAG laser is associated with improved survival when combined with multimodal adjuvant treatments. *J. Thorac. Oncol.* 2 (1): 59–64.

11 Fuks, L., Fruchter, O., Amital, A. et al. (2009). Long-term follow-up of flexible bronchoscopic treatment for bronchial carcinoids with curative intent. *Diagn. Ther. Endosc.* 2009: 782961.

12 Toty, L., Personne, C., Colchen, A. et al. (1981). Bronchoscopic management of tracheal lesions using the neodymium yttrium aluminum garnet laser. *Thorax* 36: 175–178.

13 Madden, B.P., Kumar, P., Sayer, R. et al. (1997). Successful resection of obstructing airway granulation tissue following lung transplan-tation using endobronchial (Nd: YAG) therapy. *Eur. J. Cardiothorac. Surg.* 12: 480–485.

14 Brutinel, W.M., Cortese, D.A., Edell, E.S. et al. (1988). Complications of Nd: YAG laser therapy. *Chest* 94: 903–904.

15 Sacco, O., Fregonese, B., Oddone, M. et al. (1997). Severe endobronchial obstruction in a girl with relapsing polychondritis: treatment with Nd YAG laser and endobronchial silicon stent. *Eur. Respir. J.* 10: 494–496.

16 Witt, C., John, M., Martin, H. et al. (1996). Bechet's syndrome with pulmonary involvement – combined therapy for endobronchial stenosis using neodymium- YAG laser, balloon dilation and immunosuppression. *Respiration* 63: 195–198.

17 Cahill, B.C., Harmon, K.R., Sumway, S.J. et al. (1992). Tracheobronchial obstruction due to silicosis. *Am. Rev. Respir. Dis.* 145: 719–721.

18 Ramser, E.R. and Beamis, J.F. (1995). Laser bronchoscopy. *Clin. Chest Med.* 16: 415–426.

19 Mehta, A.C., Lee, F.Y.W., and GE, D.B. (1995). Flexible bronchoscopy and the use of lasers. In: Flexible Bronchoscopy (eds. K.P. Wang and A.C. Mehta), 274. Cambridge: Blackwell Science.

20 Strauss, A.A., Strauss, S.F., and Crawford, R.A. (1935). Surgical diathermy of carcinoma of the rectum, its clinical end results. *JAMA* 104: 1480–1404.

21 Hooper, R.G. and Jackson, F.N. (1985). Endobronchial electrocautery. *Chest* 87: 712–714.

22 Hooper, R.G. and Jackson, F.N. (1988). Endobronchial electrocautery. *Chest* 94: 595–598.

23 Homasson, J.P. (1997). Endobronchial electrocautery. *Semin. Respir. Crit. Care Med.* 18: 535–543.

24 Petrou, M., Kaptan, D., and Goldstraw, P. (1993). Bronchoscopic diathermy resection and stent insertion: a cost effective treatment for tracheobronchial obstruction. *Thorax* 48: 1156–1159.

25 Sutedja, C., van Kralingen, K., Schramet, F.M.N.H. et al. (1994). Fiberoptic bronchoscopic electrosurgery under local anesthesia for rapid palliation in patients with central airway malignancies: a preliminary report. *Thorax* 49: 1243–1246.

26 Carpenter, R.J., Neel, T., and Sanderson, D.R. (1977). Comparison of endoscopic cryosurgery and electrocoagulation of bronchi. *Trans. Am. Acad. Ophthalmol. Otolaryngol.* 84: 313–323.

27 Sutedja, C., Schramel, P.M.N.H., Smit, H.J.F. et al. (1996). Bronchoscopic electrocautery as an alternative for Nd: YAG laser in patients with intraluminal tumor. *Eur. Res.* 9 (Suppl 23): 258–259.

28 Lavandier, M., Carre, T., Rivoire, B. et al. (1996). High frequency electrocautery in the management of tracheobronchial disorders. *Respir. Crit. Care Med.* 75: A477.

29 Boxem, T.V., Muller, M., Venmans, B. et al. (1999). Nd-YAG laser vs bronchoscopic electrocautery for palliation of symptomatic airway obstruction: a cost- effectiveness study. *Chest* 116 (4): 1108–1112.

30 Wahidi, M.M., Unroe, M.A., Adlakha, N. et al. (2011). The use of electrocautery as the primary ablation modality for malignant and benign airway obstruction. *J. Thorac. Oncol.* 6 (9): 1516–1520.

31 Tremblay, A., Michaud, G., and Urbanski, S.J. (2007). Hot biopsy forceps in the diagnosis of endobronchial lesions. *Eur. Respir. J.* 29 (1): 108–111.

32 van Boxem, T.J., Westerga, J., Venmans, B.J. et al. (2000). Tissue effects of bronchoscopic electrocautery: bronchoscopic appearance and histologic changes of bronchial wall after electrocautery. *Chest* 117 (3): 887–891.

33 Firoozbakhsh, S., Seifirad, S., Safavi, E. et al. (2011). Comparison of hot versus cold biopsy forceps in the diagnosis of endobronchial lesions. *Arch. Bronconeumol.* 47: 547–551.

34 Yankauer, S. (1922). Two cases of lung tumor treated bronchoscopically. *N. Y. Med. J.* 21: 741–742.

35 Mudambi, L., Miller, R., and Eapen, G.A. (2017). Malignant central airway obstruction. *J. Thorac. Dis.* 9 (Suppl 10): S1087–S1110.

36 Grund, K.E., Storek, D., and Farin, G. (1994). Endoscopic argon plasma coagulation (APC): first clinical experiences in flexible endoscopy. *Endosc. Surg. Allied Technol.* 2: 42–46.

37 Crosta, C., Spaggiari, L., de Stefano, A. et al. (2001). Endoscopic argon plasma coagulation for palliative treatment of malignant airway obstructions: early results in 47 cases. *Lung Cancer* 33: 75–80.

38 Morice, R.C., Ece, T., Ece, F., and Keus, L. (2001). Endobronchial argon plasma coagulation for treatment of hemoptysis and neoplastic airway obstruction. *Chest* 119: 781–787.

39 Reichle, G., Freitag, L., Kullmann, H.J. et al. (2000). Argon plasma coagulation in bronchology: a new method – alternative or complementary? *Pneumologie* 54: 508–516.

40 Platt, R.C. (1997). Argon plasma electrosurgical coagulation. *Biomed. Sci. Instrum.* 34: 332–337.

41 Vonk-Noordegraaf, A., Postmus, P.E., and Sutedja, T.G.

42 Colt, H.G. (1998). Bronchoscopic resection of Wallstent-associated granulation tissue using argon plasma coagulation. *J. Bronchol.* 5: 209.

43 Reddy, C., Majid, A., Michaud, G. et al. (2008). Gas embolism following bronchoscopic argon plasma coagulation: a case series. *Chest* 134: 1066–1069.

44 Paniccia, A., Rozner, M., Jones, E.L. et al. (2014). Electromagnetic interference caused by common surgical energy-based devices on an implanted cardiac defibrillator. *Am. J. Surg.* 208 (6): 932–936.

45 Breasted, J.H. (1930). The Edwin Smith Surgical Papyrus, vol. 3, 217. Chicago: University of Chicago Oriental Institute.

46 Arnott, J. (1851). On the Treatment of Cancer by Regulated Application of an Anaesthetic Temperature. London: J. Churchill.

47 Arnott, J. (1855). On the Treatment of Cancer by Congelation and an Improved Mode of Pressure. London: J. Churchill.

48 Neel, H.B., Farrell, K.H., DeSanto, L.W. et al. (1973). Cryosurgery of respiratory structures 1. Cryonecrosis of trachea and bronchus. *Laryngoscope* 83: 1062–1071.

49 Grana, L., Kidd, J., and Swenson, O. (1969). Cryogenic techniques within tracheobronchial tree. *J. Cryosurg.* 2: 62.

50 Thomford, N.R., Wilson, W.H., Blackburn, E.D., and Pace, W.G. (1970). Morphological changes in canine trachea after freezing. *Cryobiology* 7: 19–26.

51 Skivolocki, W.P., Pace, W.G., and Thomford, N.R. (1971). Effect of cryotherapy on tracheal tumors in rats. *Arch. Surg.* 103: 341–343.

52 Gorenstein, A., Neel, H.B., and Sanderson, D.R. (1976). Transbronchoscopic cryosurgery of respiratory strictures. Experimental and clinical studies. *Ann. Otol. Rhinol. Laryngol.* 85: 670–678.

53 Carpenter, R.J., Neel, H.B., and Sanderson, D.R. (1977). Cryosurgery of bronchopulmonary structures. An approach to lesions inaccessible to the rigid bronchoscope. *Chest* 72: 279–284.

54 Gage, A.A. (1968). Cryotherapy for cancer. In: Cryosurgery (eds. R. Rand, R. Rinfret, A. Rinfret and H. von Leden), 376–387. Springfield: Charles C. Thomas.

55 Sanderson, D.R., Neel, H.B., Payne, W.S., and Woolner, L.B. (1975). Cryotherapy of bronchogenic carcinoma. Report of a case. *Mayo Clin. Proc.* 50: 435–437.

56 Homasson, J.P., Renault, P., Angebault, M. et al. (1986). Bronchoscopic cryotherapy for airway strictures caused by tumors. *Chest* 90: 159–164.

57 Maiwand, M.O. (1986). Cryotherapy for advanced carcinoma of the trachea and bronchi. *Br. Med. J.* 293: 181–182.

58 Astesiano, A., Aversa, S., Ciotta, D. et al. (1986). Distruzione crioterapica dei tumori invasivi tracheobronchiali. Casistica personale. *Min. Med.* 77: 2159.

59 Mathur, P.N., Wolf, K.M., Busk, M.F. et al. (1996). Fiberoptic bronchoscopic cryotherapy in the management of tracheobronchial obstruction. *Chest* 110: 718–723.

60 Fahy, G.M., Saur, J., and Williams, R.J. (1990). Physical problems with the vitrification of large biological systems. *Cryobiology* 27: 492–510.

61 Gage, A.A., Guest, K., Montes, M. et al. (1985). Effect of varying freezing and thawing rates in experimental cryosurgery. *Cryobiology* 22: 175–182.

62 Smith, J.J. and Fraser, J. (1974). An estimation of tissue damage and thermal history in cryolesion. *Cryobiology* 11: 139–147.

63 Miller, R.H. and Mazur, P. (1976). Survival of frozen-thawed human red cells as a function of cooling and warming velocities. *Cryobiology* 13: 404–414.

64 Gage, A.A. (1982). Critical temperature for skin necrosis in experimental cryosurgery. *Cryobiology* 19: 273–282.

65 Rand, R.W., Rand, R.P., Eggerding, F.A. et al. (1985). Cryolumpestomy for breast cancer: an experimental study. *Cryobiology* 22: 307–318.

66 Rubinsky, B. and Ikeda, M. (1985). A cryomicroscope using directional solidification for the controlled freezing of biological tissue. *Cryobiology* 22: 55.

67 Ratwani, A., Fernando, H., Khandhar, S.J., and Mahajan, A.K. (2017). Review of advanced airway cryosurgical techniques. *Curr. Respir. Med. Rev.* 13: 1–6.

68 DiBardino, D.M., Lanfranco, A.R., and Haas, A.R. (2016). Bronchoscopic cryotherapy: clinical applications of the cryoprobe, cryospray, and cryoadhesion. *Ann. Am. Thorac. Soc.* 13: 1405–1415.

69 Browning, R., Turner, J.F. Jr., and Parrish, S. (2017). Spray cryotherapy (SCT): institutional evolution of techniques and clinical practice from early experience in the treatment of malignant airway disease. *J. Thorac. Dis.* 9 (8): 2619–2639.

70 Franke, K.J., Szyrach, M., Nilius, G. et al. (2009). Experimental study on biopsy sampling using new flexible cryoprobes: influence of activation time, probe size, tissue consistency, and contact pressure of the probe on the size of the biopsy specimen. *Lung* 187: 253–259.

71 Homasson, J.P., Thiery, J.P., Angebault, M. et al. (1994). The operation and efficacy of cryosurgical, nitrous oxide-driven cryoprobe. Cryoprobe physical characteristics: their effects on cell cryo destruction. *Cryobiology* 31: 290–304.

72 Le Pivert, P.J., Binder, P., and Ougier, T. (1977). Measurement of intratissue bioelectrical low frequency impedance: a new method to predict per-operatively the destructive effect of cryosurgery. *Cryobiology* 14: 245–250.

73 Walsh, D.A., Maiwand, M.O., Nath, A.R. et al. (1990). Bronchoscopic cryotherapy for advanced bronchial carcinoma. *Thorax* 45: 509–513.

74 Maiwand, M.O. and Homasson, J.P. (1995). Cryotherapy for tracheobronchial disorders. *Clin. Chest Med.* 16: 427–443.

75 Homasson, J.P. (1989). Cryotherapy in pulmonology today and tomorrow. *Eur. Respir. J.* 2: 799–801.

76 Sheski, F.D. and Mathur, P.N. (1998). Endobronchial cryotherapy for benign tracheobronchial lesions. *Chest* 114: 261s–262s.

77 Hetzel, M., Hetzel, J., Schumann, C. et al. (2004). Cryorecanalization: a new approach for the immediate management of acute airway obstruction. *J. Thorac. Cardiovasc. Surg.* 127: 1427–1431.

78 Schumann, C., Hetzel, M., Babiak, A.J. et al. (2010). Endobronchial tumor debulking with a flexible cryoprobe for immediate treatment of malignant stenosis. *J. Thorac. Cardiovasc. Surg.* 139: 997–1000.

79 Babiak, A., Hetzel, J., Krishna, G. et al. (2009). Transbronchial cryobiopsy: a new tool for lung biopsies. *Respiration* 78: 203–208.

80 Deygas, N., Froudarakis, M.E., Ozenne, G. et al. (1998). Cryotherapy in early superficial bronchogenic carcinoma. *Eur. Respir. J.* 12 (Suppl 28): 266S.

81 Asimakopoulos, G., Beeson, J., Evans, J. et al. (2005). Cryosurgery for malignant endobronchial tumors: analysis of outcome. *Chest* 127 (6): 2007–2014.

82 Vergnon, J.M., Schmitt, T., Alamartine, E. et al. (1992). Initial combined cryotherapy and irradiation for unresectable non-small cell lung cancer. *Chest* 102: 1436–1440.

83 Fernando, H.C., Dekeratry, D., Downie, G. et al. (2011). Feasibility of spray cryotherapy and balloon dilation for non-malignant strictures of the airway. *Eur. J. Cardiothorac. Surg.* 40 (5): 1177–1180.

84 Finley, D.J., Dycoco, J., Sarkar, S. et al. (2012). Airway spray cryotherapy: initial outcomes from a multiinstitutional registry. *Ann. Thorac. Surg.* 94 (1): 199–203.

85 Sabel, M.S. (2009). Cryo-immunology: a review of the literature and proposed mechanisms for stimulatory versus suppressive immune responses. *Cryobiology* 58 (1): 1–11.

86 Kumar, A., Dhillon, S.S., Patel, S. et al. (2017). Management of cardiac implantable electronic devices during interventional pulmonology procedures. *J. Thorac. Dis.* 9 (Suppl 10): S1059–S1068.

第 20 章

可弯曲支气管镜技术在支气管腔内近距离放射治疗、标记物定位、射频消融和微波消融中的应用

Michael A. Jantz

Division of Pulmonary, Critical Care, and Sleep Medicine,
University of Florida, Gainesville, FL, USA

（译者：许 菲 张 楠 译者单位：应急总医院）

据估计，2018 年美国有 234 030 人被诊断为肺癌，154 050 人死于支气管肺癌[1]。由于大多数患者在诊断时已处于疾病的Ⅲ期或Ⅳ期，许多患者需接受放射治疗（简称放疗）作为治疗的一部分。无论是否进行体外放疗，近距离放疗都可用于治疗支气管肺癌，也可用于治疗肺外恶性肿瘤的支气管内转移患者。一些患有早期肺癌或其他原发性疾病寡转移瘤的患者，可能由于肺功能不全或其他合并症，无法进行手术切除。影像引导放疗在这些患者的治疗中发挥着重要作用。其中一些影像引导放疗系统需要使用示踪肿瘤的标记物。支气管镜下放置标记物的技术正在持续发展。射频消融术（radiofrequency ablation，RFA）也被用于治疗无法接受手术切除的早期肺癌及肺转移癌患者。尽管支气管镜下 RFA 的经验非常有限，但结合导航支气管镜进行 RFA 治疗还是有很大的应用前景。本章将对上述主题进行介绍和综述。

20.1 近距离放疗

大多数肺癌患者确诊时已处于局部晚期或出现肺转移肿瘤，不适合进行根治性手术切除。许多患者的肿瘤位于中央气道，导致呼吸困难、咳嗽、咯血、肺不张和/或阻塞性肺炎。体外放疗（外放疗）逆转肺不张，对 21%~74% 患者是有效的[2,3]。高达 50% 的患者在外放疗后可能会出现肿瘤复发[4]。这些患者中大多数将没有指征接受额外的外放疗。支气管内近距离放疗可用于缓解支气管内阻塞症状，控制局部病变，并为原位癌患者提供根治性治疗方案。鉴于近距离放疗的局部效果，其可为已接受最大剂量体外放疗的患者提供治疗机会。近距离放疗可与外放疗或其他支气管镜技术联合应用，如激光治疗、高频电治疗、冷冻治疗和支架置入，以缓解恶性气道阻塞的症状。

近距离放疗，源自希腊语"short"，指的是在肿瘤内或肿瘤附近放置高放射源。本章将重点讨论支气管内近距离放疗，而不是在手术切除或经皮将放射源放置在肿瘤肿块内（组织间近距离放疗）。

1922 年，Yankauer 描述了 2 例通过硬质支气管镜置入氡胶囊治疗肺癌[5]。在 20 世纪 60 年代，钴-60 经常被用作放射源。除了氡-222 和钴-60，用于支气管内近距离放疗的其他放射性核素还包括铯-137、金-198、碘-125 和钯-103。医务人员暴露于辐射的风险以及需要硬质支气管镜置入放射源阻碍了支气管内近距离放疗的广泛采用。20 世纪 80 年代，两个重要

的事件使人们对支气管内近距离放疗重新产生了兴趣。首先是可弯曲支气管镜的发展，其可以实现在每个支气管段插入小直径后装导管。其次是高活性铱-192 的可用性，以及将铱-192 放射性粒子放入导管的远程后装机的发展。

与传统的外放疗相比，近距离放疗提供了一个潜在的优势，即在保留正常组织的同时，为肿瘤提供更高剂量的照射。放射性同位素的特征是平方反比定律，这意味着辐射剂量率的降低与辐射源中心距离平方成反比函数。辐射吸收剂量的标准单位是戈瑞（Gy）。支气管内近距离放疗可分为 3 个剂量率区域。低剂量率（low dose rate，LDR）定义为每小时<2 Gy，中剂量率（intermediate dose rate，IDR）为每小时 2~12 Gy，高剂量率（high dose rate，HDR）为每小时>12 Gy。LDR 近距离放疗通常需要 8~48 h 的治疗时间，而 HDR 可以在几分钟的治疗时间内实现。

一般来说，考虑近距离放疗的患者应具备以下特征：

1）具有恶性肿瘤的组织学诊断。
2）较大的支气管内肿瘤阻塞导致呼吸困难、咯血、咳嗽和/或阻塞性肺炎等症状。
3）近端气道受累，如气管、支气管或叶支气管。
4）能够将导管插入阻塞的支气管内病变，最好能穿过阻塞性支气管内病变。
5）由于癌症分期或肺功能障碍而无法进行手术切除。
6）有足够的预期寿命可以从姑息治疗中获益，通常情况下超过 3 个月。

不可切除的、复发的和合并气道转移的肺癌患者具有支气管内近距离放疗的指征。病灶应位于支气管镜下可见的近端气道。支气管镜检查人员应将导管插入阻塞性病灶，最好能穿过病灶。虽然近距离放疗可用于治疗外源性气道压迫，但内源性肿瘤性气道阻塞是更为常见的治疗指征。外源性气道压迫可通过支架置入获得更好的治疗。支气管完全狭窄时可能需要行再通术（如激光、高频电切除或球囊扩张），使导管能够穿过阻塞病灶。但需警惕激光切除联合支气管内近距离放疗可能造成瘘形成的高风险。因此，有些作者建议在激光再通术和近距离放疗之间间隔 1~2 周，而另一些作者则建议将这两种手术在一次支气管镜检查中完成[6-8]。

近距离放疗的主要指征是缓解因肿瘤阻塞气道引起的症状。近距离放疗也被用作非小细胞肺癌外放疗的辅助手段。它在外照射之前、其间和之后都被用作疗效巩固治疗。在主支气管阻塞致肺不张时，近距离放疗有助于减少大范围辐射区域对正常肺组织的辐射量。在一项研究中，支气管内近距离放疗平均减少了 32% 的正常组织辐射量[9]。此外，支气管内近距离放疗是支气管原位癌的根治性治疗方法。

支气管内近距离放疗的禁忌证包括气道食管瘘、气道纵隔瘘和支气管胸膜瘘。近距离放疗可能不适用于无症状患者，除非有根治的目的。主气道阻塞和接近呼吸衰竭的患者在开始近距离放疗前，应使用其他支气管镜技术进行治疗。这些技术可能包括机械性消瘤、激光治疗、氩等离子体凝固术、高频电凝术、冷冻治疗和/或支架置入。由于担心放疗后水肿导致完全性气道阻塞，在近距离放疗之前，应采用可供选择的其他方法治疗严重气道阻塞性病变。

LDR 近距离放疗可使用尼龙带包裹的低活性铱-192 放射性粒子。由放射肿瘤学家手动定位并输送导管到目标支气管。导管和放射性粒子留置在原位 24~72 h。虽然 LDR 近距离放疗不需要昂贵的设备，但主要缺点包括患者需要住院治疗和不耐受留置导管。

HDR 近距离放疗使用高活性铱-192 放射源。HDR 远程后装近距离放疗系统由放射源的外壳组件、放射源驱动器和治疗计划计算机系统组成。通过计算机控制的电缆沿着输送导管驱动放射源。放射源将在停留点停留指定的时间，以输出规定的剂量。由计算机来计算停留点的数量和停留点之间的间隔时间，以提供肿瘤体积的最佳放射量。患者应在有辐射防护的房间中接受治疗。HDR 近距离放疗的治疗时间非常短，通常持续 5~20 min。尽管初始设备成本较高，但 HDR 近距离放疗具有使患者感觉更舒适，门诊即可提供治疗，医务人员没有辐射暴露的优点。鉴于这些优势，在大多数机构 HDR 近距离放疗已经取代了 LDR 近距离放疗。

20.1.1 技术和治疗计划

近距离放疗处方包括每次的辐射剂量、次数和预定深度，即处方剂量的放射源辐射距离。辐射过程的生物效应不仅由总辐射剂量决定，还由每次剂量、剂量率和整个辐射过程的总时间决定[10]。对于给定的总辐射剂量，相比较小的分段剂量，对肿瘤使用较大的分段剂量会获得更高的有效辐射剂量。然而，随着分段剂量的增加，延迟反应组织的放射性生物学效应会比肿瘤细胞增加得更快。较大辐射剂量可能会提高治疗效果，但也会增加并发症风险，需两者权衡[10]。

HDR 近距离放疗的剂量和频次方案可能因机构

而异。治疗方案从单次 15 Gy，到治疗 4~5 次，每次 4 Gy 不等。总剂量超过 30 Gy 似乎并非充分控制肿瘤的必要剂量，而且可能与较高的致命性出血风险有关[11]。治疗间隔时间为 1~3 周，最常用的间隔时间是 1 周。美国近距离放疗学会推荐，当 HDR 近距离放疗作为姑息治疗的唯一方式时，在距放射源 1 cm 的位置，每周 3 次，每次 7.5 Gy；或每周 2 次，每次 10 Gy；或每周 4 次，每次 6 Gy[12]。当用作增强外放疗的姑息治疗时，建议 HDR 近距离放疗每 1~2 周在 1 cm 处 2 次，每次 7.5 Gy；或 3 次，每次 5 Gy；或 4 次，每次 4 Gy。当作为根治目的时，推荐采用在距放射源 1 cm 处进行 3 次，每次 5 Gy；或 2 次，每次 7.5 Gy 的 HDR 近距离放疗，以及 30 次，每次 60 Gy；或 15 次，每次 45 Gy 的外放疗。如果 HDR 近距离放疗仅用于先前未经照射的患者，建议在 1 cm 处进行 5 次，每次 5 Gy；或 3 次，每次 7.5 Gy 治疗。

关于 LDR 近距离放疗，美国近距离治疗学会推荐，当用作主要治疗方式时，1 cm 处的总剂量为 30 Gy；当用作辅助外放疗时，1 cm 处的总剂量为 20 Gy[12]。根据先前的照射情况或位置（如左上叶支气管）可以减少预定深度或照射次数。如果患者接受了放射增敏性化疗，则应考虑减少近距离放疗的剂量。支气管内近距离放疗的范围应在肿瘤靶点的每一端至少留有 1 cm 的边缘。

支气管内近距离放疗的第一步是评估近期影像学检查。支气管镜检查按照常规标准检查方法，以局部麻醉结合镇静方式开展，通常经鼻入路，以便在患者转运和治疗期间保持导管的稳定性。应注意对喉部和导管置入部位进行充分的局部麻醉，以减少咳嗽和导管移位的可能性。如果可能的话，肿瘤靶点的近端和远端都可以借助支气管镜观察。放置多个导管可以有助于隆突位置复杂肿瘤的治疗。

对肿瘤检查并确定所需导管数量后，将一根或多根导管（5~6 F）通过支气管镜工作通道置入，并在支气管镜直视下穿过支气管内肿瘤区域（图 20.1）。不透射线的内部导丝可以帮助放置导管并通过透视确认导管位置。当支气管镜医生或助手将导管/导丝推进时，需与支气管镜缓慢退出的长度相等，并且导管/导丝在鼻子处固定。然后重新插入支气管镜，并对导管位置进行可视化确认。在导丝就位的情况下，透视检查也可用于确认定位（图 20.1）。

在确定合适的位置后，将导管用胶带固定在鼻子

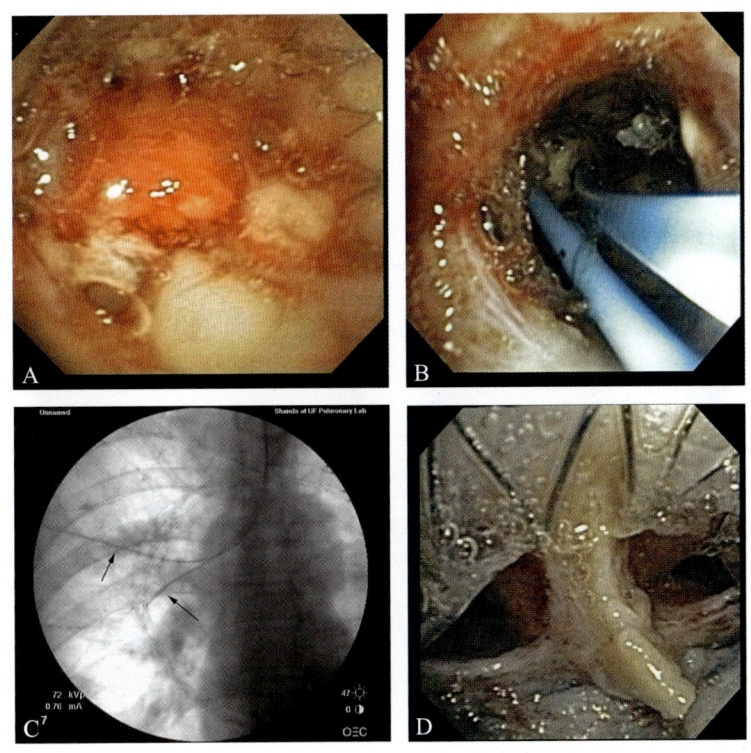

图 20.1　近距离放疗导管放置

A. 支气管支架末端肿瘤复发；B. 氩等离子体凝固术后插入近距离放疗导管；C. 使用导丝放置导管后的透视图像（箭头示）；D. 支气管镜随访时的气道表现。

上。如果需要增加导管，重复此过程，通常将增加的导管放入另一个支气管段。导管尖端可以放置在超过肿瘤远端 2 cm 的位置，或者将其楔入更小的外周支气管，放置在尽可能远的位置。当支气管镜无法观察到肿瘤的远端时，可能需要根据既往的胸片或计算机断层扫描（computed tomography，CT）来估计照射靶点远端的长度。与放射科的诊疗室相比，支气管镜室可能更利于放置更远端的导管，以减少患者转运过程中导管移位的可能。如果进行 LDR 近距离放疗，考虑到治疗时间较长，楔入导管可能也是有用的。对于远端肺外周位置放置，插入导管/导丝时应注意不要过度用力，以免导致气胸。如前所述，可能需要再通技术才能将导管置入完全闭塞的气道中（图 20.1）。尽管已经设计出各种外鞘、球囊和网篮，将导管固定在气道中心并避免"照射点"置于支气管黏膜上，但大多数医生通常不会使用这些工具。

在支气管镜下放置导管并将患者转运至肿瘤放射治疗区后，将由不透射线标记物构成的模拟放射粒子插入导管。拍摄 X 线片来确定放置位置正确并便于制定治疗计划，使用软件制订治疗计划（图 20.2）。然后移除模拟放射粒子后，将放射性粒子装载到导管中在预先设定的时间内进行照射。每次治疗结束后取出导管，患者出院回家。治疗过程中可能出现的急性不良反应包括咳嗽、支气管痉挛、支气管分泌物增加、肿瘤破坏引起的咯血以及导管/导丝刺破肺部引起的气胸。

20.1.2 恶性疾病的疗效

目前已经发表了一些关于使用 HDR 的随机试验。在对 HDR 近距离放射治疗的不同治疗方案进行评估的研究中，Huber 等将肺癌患者随机分为两组，第 1 组（$n=44$）接受 1 cm，每周 1 次，每次 3.8 Gy 共 4 次的 HDR 近距离放疗，第 2 组（$n=49$）接受 1 cm，每 3 周 1 次，每次 7.2 Gy 共 2 次的 HDR 近距离放疗[13]；第 1 组 88.9% 的患者和第 2 组 92.7% 的患者既往接受过治疗，其中分别有 47.2% 和 39.0% 的患者接受过外放疗。第 1 组中 12 名患者和第 2 组中 7 名患者因死亡或疾病恶化而未接受全身治疗。两组平均 KPS（Karnofsky performance scores）评分变化很小：分别为 60.7~63.8（第 1 组）和 60.0~65.7（第 2 组）。两组的中位生存时间基本相等，分别为 19 周和 18 周。两组 1 年生存率分别为 11.4%（第 1 组）和 20.4%（第 2 组）（P=ns，差异无统计学意义）。致死性咯血发生率分别为 22%（第 1 组）和 21%（第 2 组）；第 1 组中 18.2% 的患者和第 2 组中 22.4% 的患者需要进一步治疗。

Niomoeller 等将 142 名中央型肺癌患者随机分 2 组：一组每周 1 次，每次 3.8 Gy，共 4 次治疗，另一组每 3 周一次，每次 7.2 Gy，共 2 次治疗[14]。经支气管镜检查证实，局部病灶控制的平均持续时间分别为 11 周（4 次组）和 37 周（2 次组）（$P=0.015$）。中位生存期分别为 19 周和 18 周（P=ns，差异无统计学意义）。致死性咯血发生率分别为 18.3%（4 次组）和 12.2%（2 次组）。

Mallick 等在一项针对晚期非小细胞肺癌患者的随机对照研究中，比较了有或无外照射的 3 种不同剂量的 HDR 近距离放疗[15]。15 名患者接受了 1 cm 深度，每次 8 Gy，共 2 次近距离放疗和 30 Gy 外放疗；另 15 名患者接受了 1 cm 深度，1 次 10 Gy 的近距离放疗和 30 Gy 外放疗；还有 15 名患者接受了 1 cm 深度，1 次 15 Gy 的近距离放疗，没有外放疗。阻塞评分的降低率分别为 57.7%、55.8% 和 44.4%（$P=0.54$）。总症状缓解率分别为呼吸困难 91%、咳嗽 84%、咯血 94% 和阻塞性肺炎 83%。3 组患者上述症状的改善情况相似，但仅近距离放疗组的咯血缓解时间明显更短。3 组患者 EORTC QLQ-C30（欧洲癌症研究与治疗组织生活质量问卷）总体健康状况评分的改善情况相似，QLQ-LC13 评分也相似。QLQ-C30 总体健康状况评分从 35 分提高到 67 分，QLQ-LC13 呼吸困难评分从 30 分改善到 10 分。

一些随机研究将 HDR 近距离放疗（有或没有外放疗）与单独的外放疗进行了比较。Huber 等对不能手术的非小细胞肺癌（non-small cell lung cancer，NSCLC）患者进行了一项随机试验，将单独的外放疗与外放疗加 HDR 近距离放疗进行比较[16]。仅接受外部照射的患者（$n=42$）接受 50 Gy 治疗，每周 4~5 次，外加 10 Gy 强化治疗。接受外放疗和近距离放疗的患者（$n=56$），接受相同剂量的体外照射并在外照射前 1 周，接受 1 cm 深度 4.8 Gy 剂量的近距离放疗，在完成外照射后 3 周接受第 2 次照射。25 名患者（44.6%）未接受第 2 次近距离放疗。根据作者的说法，这种偏离治疗方案的主要原因是来自外地的门诊治疗患者结束了外照射治疗后，由于症状完全缓解，3 周后没有再就诊。两组的 KPS 评分无差异。外放疗组的总中位生存期为 28 周，外放疗加近距离放疗组为 27 周（$P=0.42$）。在按照方案治疗的患者中，外放疗组中

第20章 可弯曲支气管镜技术在支气管腔内近距离放射治疗、标记物定位、射频消融和微波消融中的应用

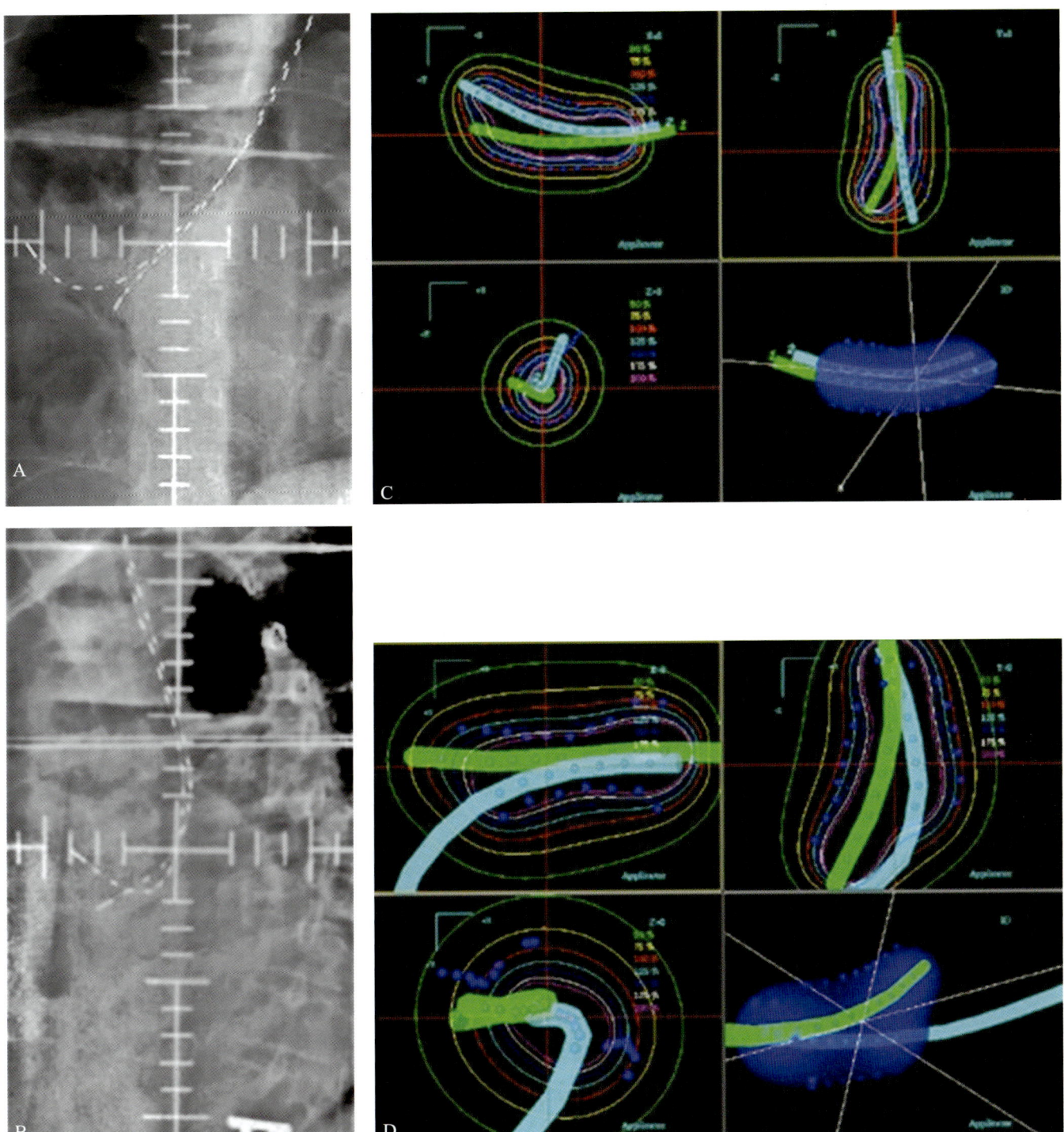

图 20.2 治疗计划

A、B. 在两个导管和模拟导线（靶区）放置好的情况下进行胸部 X 线检查；C、D. 利用等剂量分布和等剂量云进行治疗规划。资料来源：美国佛罗里达大学 Robert Zlotecki 博士提供。

位生存时间为 33 周，外放疗加近距离放疗组的中位生存时间为 43 周（$P=0.08$）。在鳞状细胞癌患者亚组（$n=68$）中，外放疗加近距离放疗组的中位生存时间为 40 周，外放疗组是 33 周，两组之间没有统计学差异趋势。外放疗组中 6 例患者和外放疗加近距离放疗组中 11 例患者发生了致命性咯血。

Langendijk 等[17]报道了第 2 项随机研究，将无法手术的 NSCLC 患者接受 HDR 近距离放疗联合外放疗

与单独外照射疗法相比较。在根治性外照射疗法中，体力状况（performance status，PS）评分≤2且没有锁骨上淋巴结受累（79%）的患者接受60 Gy的根治性外照射治疗，而PS评分为3或锁骨上淋巴结受累（21%）的患者接受30 Gy的姑息性外照射治疗。在接受近距离放疗组中，第1天和第8天的剂量为7.5 Gy。随机分组，共48例患者接受单独的外照射放疗，47例接受外放疗加近距离放疗。在放疗前有肺不张的患者组中，26例中有9例（35%）仅使用外照射治疗后改善，30例中有17例（57%）接受外照射联合近距离放疗后得到改善。外放疗组和外放疗加近距离放疗组的呼吸困难有效改善率分别为37%和46%（$P=0.29$），咳嗽有效改善率为38%和24%，咯血有效改善率为82%和86%。仅外放疗的中位生存期为8.5个月，外放疗联合近距离放疗的中位生存期为7个月（$P=0.21$）。接受外放疗加近距离放疗中的7名患者（15%），以及仅接受外放疗中的6名患者死于大咯血（13%）。

第3项随机研究由Sur等以摘要的形式发表[18,19]，研究比较了支气管内膜受累的局部晚期NSCLC患者的外照射放疗联合近距离放疗与单独外照射放疗的效果。65名患者在接受30~40 Gy的10~20次外照射后，被随机分为接受10次，20 Gy的进一步外照射治疗；或接受1 cm深度，每次6 Gy，每周2次的HDR近距离放疗。单独外放疗组的无症状生存期为129天，外放疗加近距离放疗组的无症状生存期为77天（$P=0.009$）。1年总生存率相似，分别为29.4%和29.7%。

Stout等的一项随机试验比较了HDR支气管内近距离放疗和外照射治疗对99名无法手术的NSCLC患者的姑息治疗效果[20]。49名患者接受了1 cm深度15 Gy剂量的单次近距离放疗，50名患者接受了30 Gy的10~12次外照射治疗。临床医生在8周时评估，近距离放疗组与外放疗组症状终点的阳性反应率分别为：呼吸困难59%和78%，咳嗽50%和67%，咯血78%和89%，胸痛61%和80%，疲劳57%和74%，厌食63%和78%。尽管临床医生评估的外放疗组各项改善情况指标较好，但结果并无统计学差异。近距离放疗组和外放疗组的患者在8周时自我评估对阳性反应率分别为：呼吸困难38%和49%，咳嗽45%和65%，咯血71%和90%，胸痛43%和77%（$P<0.05$），疲劳30%和65%（$P<0.05$）以及厌食43%和77%。在临床医生（91%比76%，$P=0.09$）和患者（83%比59%，$P=0.029$）的评估中，外放疗组中有更

高比例的患者获得了良好的症状整体缓解。近距离放疗组中51%的患者需要在中位时间125天（从15到511天）后接受外照射治疗，而外放疗组中28%的患者需要在中位时间304天（从98到1 037天）后接受近距离放疗。外放疗组的中位生存期为287天，而近距离放疗组中位生存时间为250天，1年生存率分别为38%和22%（$P=0.04$）。

许多非随机研究评估了HDR近距离放疗不同剂量方案及HDR近距离放疗有无外放疗方案的不同。Muto等的一项研究中，320名ⅢA或ⅢB期NSCLC患者接受了10 Gy 1次（$n=84$）、7 Gy 2次（$n=47$）或5 Gy 3次（$n=189$）的治疗[21]。患者还接受了60 Gy的外放疗。呼吸困难改善率分别为80%、85%和94%；咳嗽改善率分别为58%、72%和89%；咯血改善率分别为100%、99%和99%。平均生存期为9.7个月，各组之间没有差异。在6个月时，80%的10 Gy单次组、48%的7 Gy×2次组和17%的5 Gy×3次组发现放射性支气管炎，伴或不伴支气管狭窄。3组中分别有2.5%、6.5%和3.2%的患者发生了致命性咯血。1%~2%的患者出现支气管食管瘘。

Mallick等对95名ⅢA或ⅢB期NSCLC患者进行了HDR近距离放疗加外放疗或仅用HDR近距离放疗治疗[22]。65名患者接受了1 cm深度的每次8 Gy×2次的HDR近距离放疗和30 Gy×10次外放疗，15例患者接受1 cm深度的10 Gy单次HDR近距离放疗和30 Gy×10次外放疗，还有15例患者仅仅接受1 cm深度15 Gy单次HDR近距离放疗。3组阻塞评分的变化率分别为57%、54%和44%（$P=0.066$）。呼吸困难、咳嗽、咯血、阻塞性肺炎的总有效率分别是93%、81%、97%和91%。3组患者呼吸困难、咳嗽和阻塞性肺炎的症状反应是相似的，但仅接受近距离治疗组患者咯血症状改善较少（83.3%比100%，$P=0.041$）。EORTC QLQ-30从35分提高到67分，QLQ-LC13呼吸困难评分从30分改善到10分。症状进展的中位时间为6~11个月。

Skowronek等对648例局部晚期NSCLC患者采用了2种不同剂量方案的HDR近距离放疗，具体取决于临床分期和ECOG（东部合作肿瘤组）评分[23]。303例患者接受1 cm深度每周7.5 Gy×3次的治疗，345例大多数评分>2分的患者接受1 cm深度每周10 Gy单次治疗。在接受3次7.5 Gy治疗的患者中有改善生存时间的趋势，但在多变量分析中并无统计学意义。

Mantz 等对 HDR 近距离放疗联合外照射放疗或单纯外照射放疗的效果进行比较，在无法手术的 NSCLC 患者中进行配对分析[24]。39 例患者接受了分 2~4 次进行，总剂量为 10~30 Gy 的近距离放疗，和总剂量为 54.0~75.6 Gy 的外照射放疗。每位患者与 2 例分期和外照射剂量相似的患者匹配。5 年后，接受近距离放疗联合外照射治疗的患者实现了 58% 的局部控制率，而仅接受外照射治疗的患者局部控制率为 32%。3 年总生存率分别为 15% 和 9%。急性毒性和晚期毒性无统计学差异。

目前，已经公开发表了许多关于近距离放疗的案例报告（表 20.1）。患者呼吸困难的改善率在 24%~100% 之间。咳嗽改善率在 24%~88% 之间。与呼吸困难或咳嗽相比，咯血得到控制的患者比例更高，有效率在 69%~100% 之间。肺不张或阻塞性肺炎的改善情况差异较大，影像学反应在 20%~85% 之间。中位生存时间为 5~21 个月，这取决于治疗目的是姑息性还是根治性治疗。如表 20.1 所示，在一些研究中，不同患者组中观察到了不同的生存时间，这与既往治疗、未曾治疗、同时使用外放疗以及近距离放疗的剂量或次数有关。一些研究除了评估近距离放疗后症状的变化，还评估了 PS 的变化。

表 20.1 HDR 近距离放疗描述性病例系列研究

作者，年份（参考文献）	例数	治疗方案[a]	症状改善（例数）					PS 评分	中位生存期[b]
			总改善率	咳嗽	呼吸困难	咯血	肺不张/肺炎		
Manali 等[25]	34	7.1 Gy×1~3 ± EBRT	56%						7.8 个月
Hauswald 等[26]	41	5 Gy×1~5	58%						6.7 个月
Ozkok 等[27]	158	5~7.5 Gy q1w×2~3 ± EBRT		57%	85%	88%			6~11 个月
Hennequin 等[28]	106	5~7 Gy qw×6							21.4 个月
Escobar-Sacristán 等[29]	81	5 Gy q1w×4	85%	88%（30/34）	75%（18/24）	96%（23/24）			
Gejerman 等[30]	41	5~7.5 Gy q1~2w×1~5 ± EBRT	72%						5.2 个月
Anacak 等[31]	30	5 Gy q2w×3+EBRT		43%（12/28）	80%（12/15）	95（20/21）			11 个月
Petera 等[32]	67	5~7.5 Gy q1~2w×1~5 ± EBRT	52%（23/44）	59%（29/51）	76%（13/17）	50%（27/54）			5.0~8.2 个月
Harms 等[33]	55	5 Gy×2~5 ± EBRT	75%						5，20 个月
Kelly 等[34]	175	15 Gy q2w×1~3	66%						6 个月
Marsiglia et 等[35]	34	5 Gy q1w×6							2 年内 78%
Taulelle 等[36]	189	8~10 Gy q1w×3~4		54%	54%	74%			7 个月
Ofiara 等[37]	30	8 Gy q2w×3		46%（11/24）	33%（8/24）	79%（11/14）	43%（9/21）		
Ornadel 等[38]	117	15 Gy×1 ± LR		59%	73%	73%		75% 改善	
Nomoto 等[39]	39	6 Gy q1w×3+EBRT 或 10 Gy×1							8 个月
Pérol 等[40]	19	7 Gy q1w×3~5							28 个月
Delclos 等[41]	81	15 Gy×@6~7.5 mm q2w×1~3	84%（68/81）						5
Hernandez 等[42]	29	7.5~10 Gy q2w×1~3		24%（7/29）	24%（7/29）	69%（11/16）	28%（5/18）	24% 改善	
Macha 等[43]	365	5 Gy q2w×1~6							5~9 个月
Trédaniel 等[44]	51	连续 2 天 7 Gy q2w×3	70%（21/30）	85%	55%	85%			5 个月，未达到

（续表）

作者，年份（参考文献）	例数	治疗方案[a]	症状改善（例数）					PS评分	中位生存期[b]
			总改善率	咳嗽	呼吸困难	咯血	肺不张/肺炎		
Chang 等[45]	76	7 Gy q2w×3±EBRT		79%（37/47）	87%（47/54）	95%（20/21）	88%（15/17）		5个月
Goldman 等[46]	19	15 Gy×1	89%（17/19）	37%（7/19）	89%（17/19）	100%（6/6）	69%（9/13）		
Gollins 等[47]	406	10~20 Gy×1±EBRT		45%（172/380）	45%（172/380）	84%（128/152）	43%（89/207）		4.3~6.6个月
Speiser, Spratling[48]	342	7.5~10 Gy@0.5~1cm q1w×3±EBRT		85%	86%	99%			5.6~9.5个月
Pisch 等[49]	39	10 Gy q2w×1~2		80%（16/20）		93%（13/14）	20%（3/15）		
Nori 等[50]	32	5 Gy q1w×3±EBRT		86%（6/7）	100%（10/10）	100%（15/15）	44%	14个ECOG≥2患者中11个改善	7.5，17.5个月
Bedwinek 等[51]	38	6 Gy q1w×3	76%（29/38）				64%（9/14）		6.5个月
Gauwitz 等[52]	24	15 Gy@ 6 mm q2w×3	88%（21/24）				83%（15/18）		7.4个月
Mehta 等[53]	31	4 Gy@2 cm×4 over 2d	79%（19/26）	73%（18/24）	75%（10/10）	100%（12/14）	85%	ECOG 2.1 → 1.6	
Sutedja 等[54]	31	10 Gy q2w×1~3±LR			82%（18/22）				3，7个月
Aygun 等[55]	62	5 Gy q1w×3~5+EBRT							10，20个月
Burt 等[56]	50	15~20 Gy×1		50%（9/18）	64%（21/33）	86%（24/28）	33%（11/24）		

Gy，辐射吸收剂量标准单位；ECOG，东部肿瘤合作组；EBRT，体外放射治疗；LR，激光切除；q，每个；w，周。
[a] 1 cm 深度治疗，除非特殊提示。
[b] 中位生存期会因不同病例组治疗剂量的不同而不同，或因根治性治疗和姑息性治疗的不同而不同。

Nori 等用近距离放疗治疗了 32 例恶性气道阻塞患者[50]。17 例患者接受了近距离放疗和外放疗辅助照射（第1组），15 例患者在既往外放疗后接受了支气管内复发治疗（第2组）。大多数患者接受了 3~4 次 HDR 近距离放疗，剂量为 1 cm 深度每次 4~5 Gy。治疗 1 个月后评估，ECOG 评分从 2.2 分改善到 1.2 分。干预前，14 例患者为 3 级或 4 级，而干预后 5 名患者 ECOG 评分严重下降。第1组的中位生存期为 17.7 个月，第2组为 7.5 个月。

Hernandez 等对 29 例接受最大剂量外照射后出现症状性支气管内复发的肺癌患者行 HDR 近距离放疗[42]。患者每 2 周接受 3 次治疗，1 cm 深度每次剂量 7.5~10 Gy。26 例患者完成了该方案。PS 评分（研究开始时 PS 评分平均为 1.9 分）改善的患者占 24%，保持不变的患者占 42%，恶化的患者占 34%。

Mehta 等采用 HDR 近距离放疗治疗 31 例原发性肺癌和转移性恶性肿瘤患者，2 天内在 1 cm 深度提供 4 Gy×4 次剂量[53]。PS 评分从 2.1 分改善到 1.6 分。Cotter 及其同事评估了 65 例原发性肺癌致气道阻塞患者的 PS 评分[57]。患者接受了 55~66 Gy 剂量的外照射放疗，17 例患者接受 IDR 近距离放疗（135~300 cGy/h），48 例患者接受 HDR 近距离放疗（15~74 cGy/s），总剂量范围从 2.7~10 Gy 不等。总体而言，66% 的患者的 PS 评分有所改善。总剂量低于 70 Gy 的患者中有 39%（5/13）、总剂量在 70~84 Gy 之间的患者中有 72%（13/18）和总剂量≥85 Gy 的患者中有 74%（20/27）出现了 PS 改善。所有患者的平均生存期为 12.4 个月，根据放疗总剂量分层分析后没有统计学差异。

一些研究还评估了近距离放疗后肺功能的变化。Goldman 等评估了 19 例患者 HDR 近距离放疗后肺功能、通气和灌注的变化[46]。患者接受 1 cm 深度单次 15 Gy 照射。6 周后肺功能检查显示，第 1 秒用力呼气量（FEV_1）从 1.45 L 平均增加到 1.61 L（预测值的 55.5%~62.3%），用力肺活量（FVC）从 2.17 L 平均增加至 2.48 L（预测值的 63.9%~74.0%）（两者均 $P<0.05$）。总肺活量、残余容量或弥散能力没有显著变化。治疗后 6 周的放射性核素肺扫描显示，异常肺的通气改善率从 17.0% 提高到 27.7%，灌注率从 15.1% 提高到 21.9%（$P<0.005$）。平均 5 min 步行距离从 305 m 增加到 329 m（$P<0.01$）。主支气管阻塞患者比叶支气管阻塞患者有更大的改善。

Macha 等评估了 40 例主支气管阻塞患者接受 HDR 近距离放疗后的肺功能，HDR 近距离放疗剂量为 1 cm 深度每次 5 Gy 剂量，每 2 周治疗 1~6 次[43]。FEV_1 从 1.50 L 增加到 2.15 L，FVC 从 2.61 L 增加到 3.41 L。Mehta 等对 38 名患者 LDR 近距离放疗后的肺功能进行评估[58]。平均 FEV_1 从 1.47 L 提高到 1.88 L，FVC 从 2.21 L 提高到 3.09 L。

近距离治疗已被用于治疗不适合手术切除的患者。Skowronek 等对 13 例术后局部残端复发和 21 名术后组织病理学边缘阳性的患者进行治疗[59]。25 例患者接受了 7.5 Gy 的 4 次治疗，9 例接受了 6 Gy 的 2 次治疗和 50 Gy 的外照射治疗。1 个月后的完全缓解率为 73.5%，边缘阳性组的缓解率为 100%。1 年后，支气管残端组的总无病生存率为 30.8%，切缘阳性组为 71.4%。Kawamura 等对 13 例患有 16 种支气管肺癌的患者进行了 20~25 Gy 的 HDR 近距离放疗（$n=6$）或 20 Gy 的 HDR 近距离放疗联合 40~61 Gy 的外放疗[60]。2 年局部控制率为 86.2%，2 年总生存率为 92.3%。

Aumont-Le-Guilcher 等用 24~35 Gy 分 4~6 次治疗了 226 名支气管肺癌患者[61]。3 个月后，支气管镜检查完全缓解率为 93.6%。2 年无病生存率为 68%，5 年无病生存率为 50%，37% 的患者出现局部复发。中位生存期为 28.6 个月。并发症包括支气管狭窄（9.5%），支气管壁坏死（3.5%）、咯血（6.6%），6% 的患者死于并发症。Macha 等对 14 名患有局限性支气管内疾病的患者（包括 11 名术后支气管残端阳性的患者），在 1 cm 深度用 5 Gy 共 4 次治疗[43]。平均生存时间为 23 个月。Trédaniel 等治疗了 29 名局限于支气管壁和管腔的肺癌患者[44]。患者连续 2 天接受 1 cm 深度 7 Gy 分次治疗，每 15 天重复治疗一次，最多 6 次。在接受支气管镜检查评估的患者中，25 例中有 18 例患者出现了组织学完全缓解。随访 23 个月后患者中位总存活率并未达到预期效果。

Pérol 等对 19 例病灶≤1 cm 的局限性非小细胞支气管肺癌患者进行了 HDR 近距离放疗[40]。患者接受 1 cm 深度，每周 7 Gy，共 3~5 次的照射。16 例患者中有 12 例在 1 年后通过支气管镜检查得到肿瘤控制的组织学证据。1 年和 2 年的总生存率分别为 78% 和 58%，中位数为 28 个月。18 例患者中 10 例患者治疗后出现了支气管的部分纤维性狭窄，其中 12 例患者中有 8 例接受了 5 次治疗。2 例患者接受了 5 次治疗进展为支气管壁坏死。Hennequin 等对 106 例局限于支气管的肺癌患者进行治疗，这些患者手术或（$n=43$）外放疗（$n=27$）后出现复发，或因呼吸功能不全而无法接受其他治疗（$n=36$），每周接受 6 次 7 Gy（初始方案）或 5 Gy（后续方案）的治疗[28]。5 年的局部控制率、总生存率和病因特异性存活率分别为 51.6%、24% 和 48.5%。2 例患者死于咯血，3 例死于支气管坏死。

Marsiglia 等发现，34 例早期支气管非小细胞肺癌患者接受每周 6 次 5 Gy 治疗后，2 年局部控制率达 85%，生存率为 78%[33]。Aygun 等在 19 名 I 期 NSCLC 患者的亚组分析中发现，这些患者在接受 1 cm 深度，每次 5 Gy，每周 3~5 次的 HDR 近距离放疗联合 50~60 Gy 外放疗后，中位生存时间为 20 个月[55]。在接受外放疗和 LDR 近距离放疗的肺癌患者中，发现了与上述相似的结果[62,63]。

近距离治疗也被用作支气管内转移恶性肿瘤的姑息治疗。在一项研究中，35 例支气管内转移癌患者接受了 1~3 次 5~8 Gy 的治疗[64]。75% 咳嗽的患者、76.4% 咯血的患者和 25.7% 疼痛的患者症状得到改善，中位持续时间为 3 个月；60% 的患者呼吸困难得到改善，中位持续时间为 6 个月。在随后进行影像学检查的 22 例肺不张患者中，有 7 例（32%）出现复张。中位总生存期为 112 天。在另一项研究中，11 例支气管内转移癌患者在 1 cm 处接受了每周 3~4 次的 5~6 Gy 治疗[65]。8 例患者的梗阻症状和体征有所改善。支气管镜检查评估显示，3 例完全缓解，5 例部分缓解（梗阻减少≥60%）。还有一项研究中，37 例支气管内转移癌患者接受 1 cm 深度单次 10~15 Gy 治疗[66]。42% 的患者呼吸困难得到改善，50% 的患者咳嗽得到改善，67% 的患者咯血得到改善。生存期从 9 天到 1 145 天不等，中位生存时间 280 天。没有明显支气管外转移的患者生存期更长。尽管在研究中没有进行具体评估，但各种近距离放疗的病例系列中也包括支气管内转移患者。

其他支气管镜下治疗方式已经与近距离放疗相结合。Chella 等对 15 例中央型 NSCLC 患者随机分组，其中 15 例患者单独接受 Nd:YAG 激光治疗，14 例患者接受 Nd:YAG 激光切除后再进行 HDR 近距离放疗[67]。近距离放疗剂量为 0.5 cm 深度，每周 5 Gy，总剂量为 15 Gy，在激光治疗后 15~18 天开始。仅激光切除组的中位生存期为 7.4 个月，激光切除联合 HDR 近距离放疗组的中位生存期为 10.3 个月（P=ns，差异无统计学意义）。两组患者的 Speiser 阻塞指数改善程度相似。Nd:YAG 治疗组和 Nd:YAG 和 HDR 联合治疗组患者无症状期分别为 2.8 个月和 8.5 个月（$P<0.05$）。两组肺活量测定的改善情况相似：FEV_1 分别为 1.35~2.16 L 和 1.43~2.32 L；FVC 分别为 2.08~3.34 L 和 2.11~3.47 L。单独使用 Nd:YAG 激光治疗的 15 例需要进一步的支气管镜干预，而 Nd:YAG 联合近距离放疗组只有 3 例需要进行支气管镜干预。

Jang 等对接受激光切除（n=22）、HDR 近距离放疗（n=37）或联合治疗（n=21）的原发性肺癌（n=67）或转移性癌症（n=13）患者进行了回顾性研究[68]。绝大多数患者接受了平均剂量为 12.5 Gy 的单次近距离放疗。激光治疗组的总中位生存时间为 111 天，近距离放疗组为 115 天，联合治疗组为 264 天，在近距离放疗与联合治疗组之间具有统计学意义，但在激光治疗与联合治疗之间没有统计学意义。Shea 等对 33 例单独接受 Nd:YAG 激光治疗的鳞状细胞癌患者和 13 例接受 Nd:YAG 激光联合 LDR 近距离放疗的患者进行了回顾性研究[69]。中位生存时间分别为 16.4 周和 40.8 周（P=0.001）。

还有作者提出，激光治疗和近距离放疗的联合可能会延长无进展生存期，尽管是在非对照的病例研究中[7,38]。Kohek 等对 79 例原发性肺癌患者进行了 HDR 近距离放疗[8]。患者每次接受 5 Gy 治疗，总剂量为 5~25 Gy（平均 11.6 Gy）。在 26 名完全或几乎完全梗阻的患者中，进行 Nd:YAG 激光切除以放置导管。48 名患者在近距离放疗后接受了外照射放疗，总剂量为 50~70 Gy。79 例患者中有 58 例的 KPS 评分从 68.2 分提高到 77.2 分。67% 的患者呼吸困难得到缓解（41/61），86% 的患者咯血得到缓解（6/7），70% 的患者咳嗽得到缓解（50/71）。在 41 例肺不张患者中，有 29 例（70%）放射学证据显示肺复张。48 例接受外照射放疗的患者的中位生存期为 13 个月，而 31 例未接受外照射的患者的中位生存期为 6 个月（$P<0.01$）。

Ornadel 等评估了 117 例接受 HDR 近距离放疗后复发的恶性气道阻塞的患者[38]。除了 4 例接受了额外的治疗外，其余均仅接受 1 cm 深度单次 15 Gy 的治疗。51 例在近距离放疗前进行了 Nd:YAG 激光切除术。54% 的患者的 ECOG 评分至少改善了一个级别（P=0.0417）。50% 的患者呼吸困难症状改善（P=0.0063），平均 FEV_1 从 1.30 L 增加到 1.38 L（P=0.0504），平均 FVC 从 1.92 L 增加到 2.06 L（P=0.041）。中位生存期为 12 个月。Macha 等对 56 例气管或主支气管恶性阻塞的患者接受 1 cm 深度，每次 7.5 Gy，共 3 次的 HDR 近距离放疗治疗后的情况进行评估[70]。29 例主支气管闭塞患者在放置导管前接受 Nd:YAG 激光切除术。进行肺功能检查的 20 名患者中（没有具体说明其中有多少人接受了激光切除），证实 FEV_1 的平均值从 1.62 L 增加到 2.13 L，FVC 的平均值由 2.61 L 增加到 3.31 L（两者 $P<0.001$）。44 例（79%）患者的呼吸困难程度减轻。在 25 例肺不张患者中，有 22 例（88%）患者的放射学证据显示肺复张。

近距离放疗也与光动力疗法（photodynamic therapy，PDT）相结合。Freitag 等对 32 例无法手术或复发的支气管内 NSCLC 患者进行 PDT，并在完成 PDT 5~6 周进行 HDR 近距离放疗[71]。HDR 近距离放疗方案是在 PDT 后 6 周开始，在 1 cm 深度，每周 5 次，每次 4 Gy 剂量。24 例（75%）患者在初次 PDT 后获得完全缓解，除 1 名患者外，所有患者在近距离放疗后获得完全缓解（97%）。6 例患者 6~26 个月内肿瘤复发。在治疗后 2~3 个月通常会观察到支气管的中度瘢痕形成，但无需干预。未发现其他并发症。Weinberg 等对 9 例 NSCLC 患者进行了 PDT 联合 HDR 近距离放疗[72]。7 例接受 0.5 cm 深度，每周 3 次，5 Gy 的照射后进行 PDT 治疗，而 2 例患者先接受 PDT 治疗。两种治疗间隔时间为 9~63 天。7 例获得了局部控制。8 例出现支气管瘢痕和/或良性局部组织反应。

Allison 等也描述了 HDR 近距离治疗联合支架置入术的情况[73]。10 例经化疗和放疗的 Ⅲ 期 NSCLC 患者出现支气管内复发症状，在同一次支气管镜检查中接受了自膨胀金属支架置入和 HDR 近距离放疗。患者接受了 0.5 cm 深度，每周 3 次，每次 6 Gy 治疗。所有患者的 KPS 都有所改善。所有患者均获得局部控制，生存时间为 4~18 个月，无并发症发生。

经支气管镜的近距离放疗已被用于治疗周围型早期肺癌。Kobayashi 等在 CT 引导下对 2 例周围型肺癌患者进行 HDR 近距离放疗[74]。第 1 例患者为左上叶 2.3 cm×2.2 cm 的腺癌，在 CT 引导下，经支气管镜在临近脏层胸膜的病灶周边支气管内灌注钡来标记病变。9天后，患者再次接受了支气管镜检查，透视下，在钡标记物的位置放置一个 5 F 的放射源。接受 1 cm 深度 8 Gy 剂量的近距离放疗。每周重复 2 次。第 2 例患者为右上叶 2.6 cm×1.8 cm 腺癌，接受 1 cm 深度 15 Gy 单次治疗。该病例未进行钡剂标记，在 CT 引导下，经支气管镜置入近距离放疗导管。18 个月和 10 个月的随访中显示出良好的治疗效果。

Imamura 等[75]应用透视和 CT 引导，对 7 例 T_1~T_2 周围型肺癌患者进行经支气管近距离放疗。第 8 例患者曾尝试经支气管近距离放疗，但由于无法通过肿瘤而失败。近距离放疗方案包括 5 Gy×5 次、7 Gy×3 次和 12.5 Gy×2 次。本研究还包括 5 名经皮进行近距离放疗的患者。3 例患者出现完全缓解，4 例患者部分缓解，5 例患者病情稳定。3 例患者在治疗后 12~32 个月疾病复发，包括 1 例 T_2 肿瘤患者和 1 例在适形体外放疗后接受近距离放疗的患者。接受经支气管近距离放疗与经皮近距离放疗患者的结果没有单独报告。

Harms 等描述了联合导航支气管镜与近距离放疗治疗 1 例右上叶肺癌患者的报告[76]。导航支气管镜应用 SuperDimension™ 系统（美国明尼苏达州明尼阿波利斯市，美敦力公司）将延长工作通道导管定位到肿瘤，使用径向探头支气管内超声（radial-endobronchial ultrasound, R-EBUS）（奥林巴斯公司，东京，日本）确认延长工作通道导管的位置。然后穿过延长工作通道导管放置 6 F 近距离放疗导管，随后移除延长工作通道导管。近距离放疗剂量为每周 5 Gy，共 3 次，在治疗期间保留近距离放疗导管。患者对导管的耐受性良好，治疗前重复成像显示导管无移位。反复支气管镜下活检结果均为阴性。海德堡大学的同一研究人员和德克萨斯大学泰勒分校的合作者采用相似的方法，应用电磁导航支气管镜联合径向 EBUS 确认导管位置，以摘要形式报告了 32 名周围型肺癌患者的治疗情况[77]。患者接受了总剂量 15~30 Gy 的 HDR 近距离放疗。在海德堡大学接受治疗的患者将近距离放疗导管放置长达 8 天，而德克萨斯大学泰勒分校的患者在 2 周内分别接受了 2 次的近距离放疗导管置入。1 例患者导管无法放置，另 1 例患者出现了无需治疗的气胸。随访至少 2 年后，32 例患者中 27 例经组织学证实病情完全缓解。

20.1.3　良性疾病的疗效

HDR 近距离放疗也被用于治疗肺移植和良性疾病支架置入后支气管内阻塞性肉芽组织。Kennedy 等对 2 例患者左主支气管复发性肉芽组织进行了 1 cm 深度 3 Gy 近距离放疗，尽管他们之前曾接受过支架置入（Wallstent™，波士顿科学公司，马萨诸塞州纳蒂克）、Nd:YAG 激光切除术和球囊扩张术[78]。患者分别在肺移植后 3 个月和 4 个月接受支架置入，并在支架置入后 4 个月和 7 个月接受近距离放疗。为了在近距离放疗前治疗狭窄，1 例患者需要每 10~14 天进行 1 次支气管镜检查，而另 1 例患者则需要每 28~35 天进行 1 次支气管镜检查。1 例患者由于肉芽组织复发，需要在第 1 次治疗 3 周后进行第 2 次治疗（3 Gy）。随访 6 个月和 7 个月时，所有患者均未再出现肉芽组织。

Halkos 等在 1~30 个月的时间内，对 4 例气道狭窄患者进行了 1 cm 深度，每次 3 Gy 的 2~4 次治疗[79]。这些患者在移植后 4~12 个月因吻合口狭窄接受了支架置入；硅酮支架 2 例，金属支架（Wallstent）1 例，金属支架（Walltent）后硅酮支架 1 例，以及 Nd:YAG 激光治疗、高频电治疗和球囊扩张。近距离放疗在移植后 9 个月至 5 年内进行。3 例治疗成功，而 1 例患者尽管接受近距离放疗 4 次，但没有任何获益，死于肺炎和呼吸衰竭。Madu 等治疗了 5 例复发性阻塞性肉芽组织的患者：4 例患者因肺移植吻合口狭窄，1 例患者因气管切开插管而出现复发性气管肉芽组织[80]。首次狭窄的时间从 1 个月到 10 个月不等，既往介入治疗方法包括支架置入、球囊扩张、支气管内类固醇注射、Nd:YAG 激光、高频电治疗和局部应用丝裂霉素-C。肺移植患者接受每周 2~3 次、每次 7 Gy 的近距离放疗，气管造口术后患者接受每周 2 次、每次 5 Gy 的近距离放疗。在 12 个月的中位随访中，近距离放疗后介入手术的次数从 11 次（范围 6~17）减少到 3 次（范围 0~7）。4 例肺移植患者 FEV_1 在近距离放疗后均有所升高。1 例患者在随后的支气管镜支架置入手术中死亡，可能是继发于脑空气栓塞。

Kramer 等对 6 例因声门下/气管狭窄（$n=5$）和右主支气管狭窄（$n=2$）而置入 Wallstent 金属支架后出现肉芽组织的患者进行了 HDR 近距离放疗[81]。其中 5 例患者因复发性肉芽组织需要多次手术和治疗，2 例患者接受了预防性治疗。近距离放疗在 Nd:YAG 激光切除肉芽组织后进行，1 cm 深度单次 10 Gy 治疗。在 4~30 个月的随访中，2 例患者没有肉芽组织，4 例患者只有极小的肉芽组织，1 例患者在近距离放疗后 5~30 个月出现复发性中度肉芽组织。1 例患者出现放射性组织坏死。在接受预防性治疗的 2 例患者中，1 例没有肉芽组织，1 例有很少的肉芽组织。

同一研究人员在一项针对 115 例良性气管狭窄接受治疗的研究中报告，在 33 例金属支架置入（Wallstent 和 SMART™，镍钛诺支架，Cordis 公司，美国新泽西州布里奇沃特）的患者中，有 28 名患者接受 1 cm 深度、10 Gy 单次 HDR 近距离放疗来治疗复发性肉芽组织。所有患者在近距离放疗后需要较少的治疗性支气管镜检查，但没有提供进一步的细节证据。未见并发症。

Tendulkar 等治疗了 8 例因肺移植吻合口问题（n=6）、气管支气管软化症（n=1）和韦格纳肉芽肿病（n=1）而置入支架后出现难治性支气管内肉芽组织的患者[82]。患者接受 1 cm 深度每次 7.1 Gy×1~2 次的 HDR 近距离放疗。肺移植和近距离放射治疗的间隔时间为 7~50 个月。最后一次支气管镜检查和近距离放疗之间的间隔时间为 1~215 天不等。在近距离放疗后的前 6 个月内，6 例患者被判定为反应良好至极好，而 2 例患者的反应是一般至较差。治疗前后 6 个月的平均手术次数从 3.1 次下降至 1.8 次。FEV₁ 从预计值 36% 增加到预计值 46%。在 1 年后存活的 4 例患者中，只有 1 例保持了极好的效果。值得注意的是，该患者在接受近距离放疗前接受了肉芽组织的电切术。研究人员推测，如果去除肉芽组织 24~48 h，进行近距离放疗可能有效。就并发症而言，1 例患者在近距离放疗后 5 个月出现吻合口裂开，1 例患者在近距离治疗后 4 个月因支气管动脉瘘引起致命性咯血。

20.1.4 并发症

支气管内近距离放疗是一种总体上耐受性良好、急性并发症很少的治疗方式。大多数急性并发症与支气管镜下放置导管和近距离放疗导管放置期间的咳嗽有关。大咯血是最常见的危及生命的并发症。大咯血的发生率在 0%~32% 之间，大多数文献报告的发生率在 3%~10% 之间。肿瘤进展可能是许多患者的并发症之一，因此很难区分肿瘤进展与近距离放疗直接造成大咯血的关系。

已经报道了发生大咯血的不同危险因素，包括肿瘤位置来自上叶、支气管内肿瘤长度、既往放疗、既往激光治疗、大分段剂量以及治疗前是否存在咯血。Bedwinek 等分析 38 例先前接受过外照射放疗后的患者时发现，12 例患者（32%）在接受 3 次 6 Gy HDR 近距离放疗 2~56 周后出现致命性肺出血[51]。这种并发症主要出现在接受上叶和右主支气管治疗的患者中。其他研究员还注意到，接受肺上叶治疗会增加大咯血的风险。出现这种情况的部分原因可能是右肺动脉直接位于右主和右上叶支气管的前表面，而左肺动脉则直接位于左主和左上叶支气管前面。近距离放疗导管在上叶支气管向上的角度时，可能会沿着支气管壁和邻近的肺动脉产生一个"热点"。

Ornadel 等对 117 例患者进行 HDR 近距离放疗，其中 51 例患者曾接受 Nd:YAG 激光切除术[38]。有 11 例出现致命性咯血。患有严重支气管疾病导致肺不张或严重的呼吸窘迫患者接受 Nd:YAG 激光治疗时更有可能出现致命性咯血，因此可能存在肿瘤相关因素的差异。在对 406 例接受单剂量 15 Gy 或 20 Gy HDR 近距离放疗患者的分析中，Gollins 等证实 32 例（8%）患者在治疗后 7 天至 26 个月死于大咯血[11]。Cox 多元回归分析显示，增加近距离放疗剂量（20 Gy 比 15 Gy）、激光治疗后近距离放疗以及同一部位第二次近距离放疗会增加致命性大咯血的风险。在回归分析中，同时使用近距离放疗和外照射并没有达到统计学意义（$P=0.08$）。在对死于大咯血的 25 例患者的评估中发现，有 20 例（80%）患者有肿瘤残留或复发的证据。

Hennequin 等对接受了 4~7 Gy 共 2~6 次 HDR 近距离放疗后 149 例患者的并发症进行了回顾性研究[83]。近距离治疗 1~48 周后，11 例（7.4%）患者出现咯血，其中 10 例致命性咯血。除 1 例患者外，其他患者均考虑存在疾病进展。在因素分析中，姑息治疗（而非根治性治疗）和支气管内肿瘤长度与咯血显著相关，肿瘤位置、治疗量参数和相关的支气管镜治疗与咯血无关。在多因素分析中，只有治疗组具有统计学意义。在 Hara 等的一项研究中，36 例接受 HDR 近距离放疗的患者中有 7 例出现了致命性咯血[84]。发现局部治疗失败或恶性肿瘤存在和激光切除与大咯血有明显统计学意义，导管和大血管附近的气管支气管壁直接接触也有统计学相关性。近距离治疗次数和总剂量、治疗支气管段长度以及同时或既往外照射治疗没有相关性。

Carvalho 等的一系列研究中，84 例患者中有 8 例（9.5%）在 HDR 近距离放疗后 0.5~8 个月出现致命性咯血[85]。与致命性咯血唯一显著相关的因素是较大的照射量。Langendijk 等回顾了 938 例接受外放疗和/或 HDR 近距离放疗的患者[86]。在接受外照射患者中致命性大咯血发生率为 4.3%（18/421），在接受外照射放疗但曾经接受过近距离治疗的患者（55/419）中为 13.1%，接受外照射联合近距离放疗患者中为 25.8%（16/62），仅接受近距离放疗患者中为 15.4%（2/13），在外照射后复发而又接受近距离放疗的患者中为 43.4%（10/23）。在多变量分析中，照射量大小（15 Gy

比 10 Gy 或 7.5 Gy)(相对风险 5.3)、上叶位置(相对风险 2.7)、支气管内肿瘤延伸至主支气管(相对风险 2.7)和放疗前咯血(相对风险 2.1)与接受近距离治疗患者的致命性咯血相关。关于并发症(包括大咯血)的研究总结见表 20.2。

放射性支气管炎和狭窄已被报告为近距离放疗的并发症之一(表 20.2)。Speiser 和 Spratling 于 1993 年首次对此进行描述[88]。他们对接受 HDR 近距离放疗的患者进行评估,在接受 5 mm 深度,每次 10 Gy,共 3 次治疗的患者中,发生率为 9%,在接受 1 cm 深度,每次 10 Gy,共 3 次治疗的患者中发生率为 12%,在接受 1 cm 深度,每次 7.5 Gy,共 3 次治疗的患者发生率为 13%。与风险增加相关的因素包括根治性治疗目的、既往激光切除、同步外照射放疗和更长的生存期。表 20.3 列出了 Speiser 和 Spratling 提出的分级系统,美国近距离放疗协会随后对其进行了修改。在所有可观察到的病例中,49% 的病例出现 Ⅲ 级或 Ⅳ 级放射性支气管炎。

表 20.2 高剂量率(HDR)近距离放疗并发症

作者,年份(参考文献)	例数	治疗方案a	治疗前/同步外放疗	治疗前激光治疗	大咯血	放射性支气管炎(任何级)	放射性支气管炎(Ⅲ/Ⅳ级)	瘘	气管狭窄
Manali 等[25]	34		68%	26%	3%	21%			
Hauswald 等[26]	41	5 Gy×1~5	100%		15%	5%		5%	
Weinberg 等[72]	9	5 Gy@5 mm q1w×3+PDT	36%	11%	0%	78%		0%	22%
Ozkok 等[27]	158	5~7.5 Gy q1w×2~3	100%		11%	5%			
Carvalho 等[85]	84	5~7.5 Gy×1~5	55%	24%	10%				
Hennequin 等[28]	106	5~7 Gy q1w×6	47%		8%	4%			
Escobar-Sacristán 等[29]	81	5 Gy q1w×4	63%	2%	0%	1%	1%	1%	
Mantz 等[24]	39	4~9 Gy q1w×2~4	100%	0%	0%				2.6%
Langendijk 等[17]	47	7.5 Gy q1w×2	100%	0%	15%				4%
Hara 等[84]	36	4~45 Gy 总剂量	81%	22%	19%				
Anacak 等[31]	30	5 Gy q2w×3	100%	11%	70%	7%		13%	
Petera 等[32]	67	5~7.5 Gy q1~2w×1~5	84%	3%	7%	1.5%	1.5%	4%	
Muto 等[21]	84	10 Gy×1	100%	5%	2.5%	80%	37%	1%	
	47	7 Gy×2			6.5%	48%	13%	2%	
	50	5 Gy×3			5.5%	22%	17%	3%	
	139	5 Gy@5 mm×3			2.5%	16%	8%	0%	
Stout 等[20]	49	15 Gy×1	0%	0%	8%				
Marsiglia 等[35]	34	5 Gy q1w×6	0%		3%				
Kelly 等[34]	175	15 Gy q2w×1~3	NS	11%	5%			0.5%	0.5%
Taulelle 等[36]	189	8~10 Gy q1w×3~4	62%	14%	7%	22%	6%	1.6%	6%
Hennequin 等[83]	149	4~7 Gy×2~6	75%	6%	7%	9%			1%
Langendijk 等[86]	98	7.5 Gy×2 或 10~15 Gy×1	87%	NS	29%				
Ornadel 等[38]	117	15 Gy×1	79%	44%	9%				
Huber 等[16]	56	4.8 Gy×2	100%	16%	19%				
Pérol 等[40]	19	7 Gy q1w×3~5	0		11%	56%	11%		
Nomoto 等[39]	39	6 Gy q1w×3+EBRT 或 10 Gy×1	NS		8%				
Delclos 等[41]	81	15 Gy @ 6~7.5mm q2w×1~3	100%	NS	1%	2%		1%	2%
Gollins 等[11]	406	15 Gy×1	20%	2%	6%	44%	13%	0%	2%
		20 Gy×1			16%	60%	20%		

(续表)

作者，年份（参考文献）	例数	治疗方案[a]	治疗前/同步外放疗	治疗前激光治疗	大咯血	放射性支气管炎（任何级）	放射性支气管炎（Ⅲ/Ⅳ级）	瘘	气管狭窄
Hernandez 等[42]	29	7.5~10 Gy q2w×1~3	100%	10%	4%	0%			0%
Gustafson 等[87]	46	7 Gy q1w×3	30%	0%	7%				
Huber 等[13]	44	3.8 Gy q1w×4	47%	33%	22%				
	49	7.2 Gy q3w×2	39%	46%	21%				
Macha 等[43]	365	5 Gy q2w×1~6	Most	Most	21%			2%	
Trédaniel 等[44]	51	连续 2 天 7 Gy q2w×3	63%	8%	10%	14%			
Chang 等[45]	76	7 Gy q2w×3	80%	3%	4%				
Speiser and Spratling[88]	47	10 Gy@5 mm×3	41%	24%	4%	9%	9%		
	144	10 Gy×3			7%	12%	9%		
	151	7.5 Gy×3			9%	13%	2%		
Cotter 等[57]	65	6~35 Gy 总剂量 HDR 或 IDR	100%		1.5%	8%		5%	1.5%
Pisch 等[49]	39	10 Gy q2w×1~2	85%	23%	3%				6%
Bedwinek 等[51]	38	6 Gy q1w×3	100%	22%	32%		0%	0%	0%
Sutedja 等[54]	31	10 Gy q2w×1~3	100%	45%	30%			10%	
Gauwitz 等[52]	24	15 Gy @ 6mm q2w×3	100%	0%	4%	4%	4%		
Aygun 等[55]	62	5 Gy q1w×3~5	100%		15%			0%	1.7%
Khanavkar 等[89]	12	8 Gy@5 mm q1~2w×2~8	92%	42%	50%			17%	

EBRT，体外照射放疗；Gy，gray 放疗剂量单位；HDR，高剂量频率；IDR，中剂量频率；PDT，光动力疗法；q，每个；w，周。
[a] 1 cm 深度治疗，除非特殊提示。
来源：Yao 和 Koh[10]。

表 20.3 美国近距离放疗协会修订的放射性支气管炎和狭窄分级

分级	具体表现
Ⅰ级	黏膜轻度炎症反应伴肿胀，表现为薄而白色的环形伪膜，无显著的管腔阻塞，无需干预
Ⅱ级	白色纤维渗出伪膜，引起咳嗽和/或阻塞，需要治疗干预
Ⅲ级	严重炎症反应伴明显黏膜渗出，需要多次进行清理或其他干预措施来恢复管腔通畅
Ⅳ级	严重的纤维化伴环形狭窄导致管腔直径缩小
Ⅴ级	狭窄，气管和/或支气管软化，或与肿瘤侵犯无关的治疗相关大咯血

来源：Nag 等[12]。

在 Gollins 等对并发症的分析中，55% 的随访支气管镜检查中出现了一定程度的黏膜反应[11]。在 6 个月及以后的大多数支气管镜检查中都发现了一定程度的纤维化，并发现了与放射相关的变化。然而，406 例患者中只有 2 例需要支气管镜介入治疗。Hennequin 等在他们的 149 例患者中观察到 13 例（8.7%）放射性支气管炎[83]。其中 2 例死亡患者继发于纤维蛋白碎片完全阻塞气管和随后的感染。在单变量分析中，根治性治疗、肿瘤位于气管或主支气管、近距离放疗剂量和治疗的肿瘤体积与放射性支气管炎有关，而在多变量分析中只有肿瘤位置具有统计学意义。在一项对 189 例予 1 cm 深度，8~10 Gy，3~4 次治疗的患者的研究中，Taulelle 等发现 12 例患者（13%）支气管狭窄[36]。Muto 等在比较不同近距离放疗分段方案联合外照射放

表 20.4 放射性支气管炎可能的治疗方法

分级	治疗
Ⅰ级	观察
Ⅱ级	口服类固醇激素和/或吸入支气管扩张剂 麻醉性止咳药
Ⅲ级	多次支气管镜清理
Ⅳ级	清理 球囊或硬镜扩张 激光切除 氩等离子体凝固/电切 冷冻治疗 支架置入

来源：Speiser 和 Spratling 修订[88]。

疗时发现，Ⅲ级或Ⅳ级放射性支气管炎出现在24%接受1 cm深度单次10 Gy放疗的患者中，13%接受2次1 cm深度7 Gy治疗的患者中，17%接受3次1 cm深度5 Gy治疗的患者中，8%接受3次0.5 cm深度5 Gy治疗的患者中[21]。表20.4列出了放射性支气管炎和狭窄的潜在治疗方法。

其他潜在并发症包括气道瘘、气道坏死、气管/支气管软化、气胸、放射性肺炎和支气管痉挛[21,29,35,36,40-42,45,53,54,56,60]。

基于以上讨论，很明显，近距离放疗可以成为一种缓解支气管内肿瘤相关症状的有效方式。对于那些曾接受过外照射放疗但因疾病复发而出现支气管内浸润或支气管阻塞症状的患者，可以强烈推荐考虑近距离放疗。根据Huber等[16]和Langendijk等[17]的随机试验，在外照射的基础上增加近距离放疗，在症状控制、表现状态或生存方面似乎没有带来额外的益处。根据Stout等进行的支气管内近距离放疗与外照射放疗随机比较试验[20]，作为NSCLC相关症状的初始治疗，外照射放疗似乎优于近距离放疗。虽然Nd:YAG激光治疗是否联合近距离放疗在生存率方面相似，但联合治疗可改善无症状进展和对额外支气管镜治疗的需求。近距离放疗可考虑用于根治局部支气管内早期肺癌。

关于近距离放疗治疗支架置入后复发性肉芽组织的数据是令人感兴趣的，尽管需要进一步研究以确定这种治疗的作用。随着导航支气管镜技术的出现，治疗无法手术周围型肺癌患者将有更多的可能性，但同样需要更多的数据。由于随机对照试验中患者人数较少而且试验中使用的剂量和方案各不相同，近距离放疗的最佳剂量和分段剂量尚不清楚。临床医生也应该意识到近距离放疗带来的致命性咯血风险，以及短期放射性支气管炎或长期放射性纤维化和狭窄导致的进行性气道阻塞。

20.2 标记物置入

很多早期肺癌患者由于基础肺部疾病引起的呼吸系统损害（如慢性阻塞性肺疾病）、严重心脏病或其他疾病，或因个人偏好不愿手术，从而无法接受根治性手术切除。一篇综述报道，传统外照射放疗的5年生存率在6%~31%之间，平均生存率为21%[90]。图像引导放疗，包括立体定向放疗（stereotactic body radiotherapy，SBRT）和调强放疗（intensity-modulated radiation therapy，IMRT），可以向局限性癌症进行集中、高剂量的放疗。一项文献调查显示，SBRT对早期肺癌的1年局部控制率平均为92.7%（范围64%~100%），3年为86.7%（范围40%~98%）[91]。1年和3年的总生存率分别为87%（范围78%~100%）和60%（范围32%~95%）。平均中位生存期为38.4个月（范围27~57个月）。SBRT和IMRT靶区勾画的主要障碍是呼吸导致的靶区运动，也称肿瘤靶区运动。

包括呼吸控制、呼吸门控、机载成像系统和实时肿瘤追踪在内的各种技术已被用于更精准地指导肺癌放疗[92]。一些实时肿瘤追踪系统，如CyberKnife®同步技术（Accuray公司，加利福尼亚州森尼韦尔），利用在肿瘤内或肿瘤附近放置的致密金属金或铂标记物（称为靶标），以实现系统跟踪和射束调整[93-96]。通常需要3个靶标，每个靶标在不同平面上相距2 cm，但为防止靶标移动，一些临床医生可能会额外放置1~2个靶标。靶标最初在CT引导下经皮置入。由于放置靶标需要多次穿刺，而且许多接受此类手术的患者都有严重的肺气肿，据报道气胸发生率在6%~25%之间[94-96]。随着导航支气管镜技术的出现，及其有助于提高早期周围型肺癌的检出得到验证，人们对支气管镜下放置靶标产生了极大的兴趣。

支气管镜置入各种标记物及置入方法已经使用。Harada等使用1~2 mm大小的球形金标记物在透视引导下通过一根聚四氟乙烯导管，使用硬塑料丝将标记物插入导管完成置放[97]。20例患者中，16例为周围型肺癌，4例为中央型肺癌，1例中央型肺癌患者无法放置标记物。14例患者的标记物治疗中固定在同一位置，5例患者的标记物从插入位置脱落（包括3例中央型肺癌患者）。在另一随访研究中，使用相同的置入技术将154个球形金标记物插入57例周围型肺癌患者病灶中[98]。154个标记物中，在插入后0~5天的CT检查可检测到122个（79%），在整个治疗周期中（6~15天，中位数10天）可检测到115个，在最后一次随访（16~181天，中位数44天）中可检测到104个（占初始置入的68%）。个别患者咳出了标记物，部分患者通过腹部X线片可显示脱落的标记物。放置的标记物越靠外周，观察到的移位越少。一例患者出现了无须干预的气胸。值得注意的是，在这项研究中观察到了一条学习曲线。对于进行了<20次、20~50次和>50次置入操作的医生，固定率分别为58%、64%和75%（$P=0.05$）。

Reichner 等使用矩形金靶标（货号 351-1；Best Medical International 公司，美国伊利诺伊州）[99]。将标记物放置在的 Wang 氏 19/21G 支气管穿刺针（MW-319，CONMED 公司，美国纽约）的 19G 穿刺针中。然后将针尖浸入无菌手术润滑剂中，以提高标记物对针头的黏附性。将装有标记物的 19G 针缩回鞘内，鞘穿过可弯曲支气管镜。在所需位置，将 19G 针伸出刺入肿瘤。然后拧紧 21G 针头组件，释放标记物，在透视引导下放置。在 15 例肺癌或转移性恶性肿瘤的患者中共放置了 54 个标记物，每例患者平均 3.6 个。放置位置包括上叶、左下叶、气管旁 2 站和 4 站、隆突下淋巴结、左肺门、左主和右中间支气管。12 个标记物在置入前掉到气道中；其中 7 个用活检钳取出，其余的可能是咳出来的。无气胸发生。一个标记物通过肺动脉放置于隆突下淋巴结，没有不良后果发生。

随后的研究利用导航支气管镜和/或径向 EBUS 进行标记点定位。Anantham 等使用 SuperDimension 电磁导航支气管镜系统成功地在 9 例 T1/T2 周围型原发性或转移性肺恶性肿瘤患者中的 8 例置入标记物[100]。使用 0.8 mm×5 mm 大小的金放射性粒子（型号 SMG0242-025，Alpha-Omega Services 公司，美国加州）作为标记物。将标记物楔入微生物标本刷（货号 1650，波士顿科学公司）的蜡尖中（图 20.3）。成功导航到肿瘤后，将传感器探针从延长工作通道中取出，并更换为装载的微生物刷。当刷子导管到达延长工作通道的远端时，将刷子推出蜡尖以置入标记物。然后将延长工作通道导航到肿瘤附近的另一个区域，并重复上述过程。每个患者放置 4~6 个标记物，在 8 例患者中有 7 例患者的标记物可直接放置在肿瘤内。在 1 周后放疗计划进行中，观察到 39 个插入的标记物中有 35 个仍在原位。1 例患者在放置后出现慢性阻塞性肺疾病的急性加重，未见气胸发生。

Kupelian 等详细介绍了他们使用 SuperDimension 导航系统在 8 名患者身上经支气管镜置入标记物以及在 15 名患者身上进行经皮穿刺置入标记物的经验[101]。在支气管镜插入时，双腔 Wang 氏经支气管针中装载 0.8 mm×3 mm 固体金标记物或 1 cm 长 Visicoil™ 金植入物（IBA Dosimetry，Bartlett，美国田纳西州）(图 20.4)。所有患者在 16~188 天内标记物都

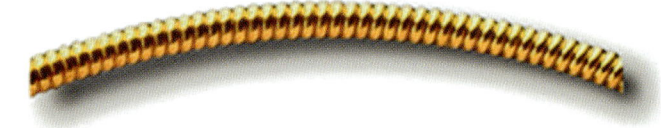

图 20.4　Visicoil 标记物

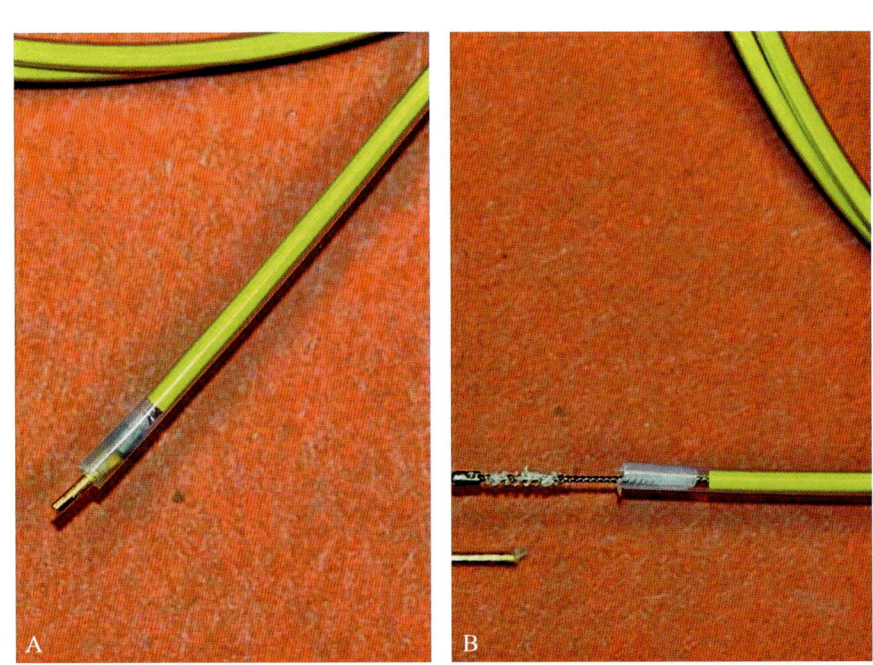

图 20.3　金放射性粒子标记物

A. 金放射粒子装载到微生物标本刷蜡尖上；B. 标本刷推出时放置标记物。资料来源：Anantham 等[100]。经美国胸科医师学会许可转载，版权所有 2007。

保持原位。1例患者在进行支气管镜活检和标记物的放置中，出现了气胸。在15例行经皮穿刺标记物置入术的患者中，有8例患者出现了气胸。作者指出，他们目前使用1~2 cm的Visicoil标记物，因为更大、更灵活的标记物会楔入气道或肿瘤内，而且大小和黏附性会阻碍其移位，所以应该更稳定。

Harley等报道了在43例患者中使用径向EBUS以及SuperDimension导航系统置入标记物的情况[102]。将20 MHz EBUS径向探头（UM-S20-20R，奥林巴斯公司）插入引导鞘，推进到目标支气管中。当定位到外周病灶后，取出探头，将引导鞘留在肿瘤内或靠近肿瘤的区域。如果周围病变难以到达，可进行电磁导航支气管镜检查。将0.8 mm×5 mm或0.8 mm×3 mm大小的金标记物（351-2、351-1，Best Medical International公司）装入针刷鞘（NB-120，CONMED公司）或Wang氏19/21G穿刺针（MW-319）的尖端。使用骨蜡将标记物密封到置入系统中，防止释放前标记物丢失。将针刷和支气管穿刺针插入引导鞘或延长的工作通道，到达远端后，在透视引导下使用细胞刷或Wang氏针的内针置入标记物。为了确保标记物嵌入远端气道或肺实质中，在透视引导下使用细胞刷（Cellebrity 1601，波士顿科学公司）。9个肿瘤位于中心，34个位于外周，大小在0.9~6.5 cm之间。共置入了161个标记物（每位患者平均3.7个）。在2周后的CT扫描中，39例患者（90.6%）的肿瘤内或肿瘤周围共检测到139个标记物。30例患者（69.7%）未观察到任何标记物的丢失或明显移动。移位的标志物距离目标肿瘤平均距离1.67 cm（0.5~4.56 cm）。1例患者发生了少量气胸，需要放置猪尾导管。

Steinfort等应用虚拟支气管镜和径向EBUS在15例患者的16个病变中置入标记物，径向EBUS无法定位的肿瘤使用电磁导航[103]。使用的标记物是10 mm×0.75 mm线性Visicoil标记物或13 mm×0.9 mm双带superLock™标记物（美敦力公司，美国明尼苏达州）（图20.5）。根据不同手术流程将标记物插入引导鞘或延长工作通道，然后使用取样器械将其推进到引导鞘末端。12例患者由EBUS定位置入。4个病灶中，通过电磁导航的引导实现了6 mm的中位标记物-病灶的距离。在放置Visicoil标记物的8例患者中，有2例患者发现早期标记物移位，而superLock标记物没有发现移位。

Lachkar等报道了使用径向EBUS对34例结节直径为20 mm的患者放置标记物的情况[104]。结节长轴

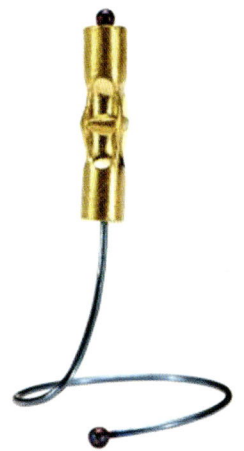

图20.5　SuperLock标记物

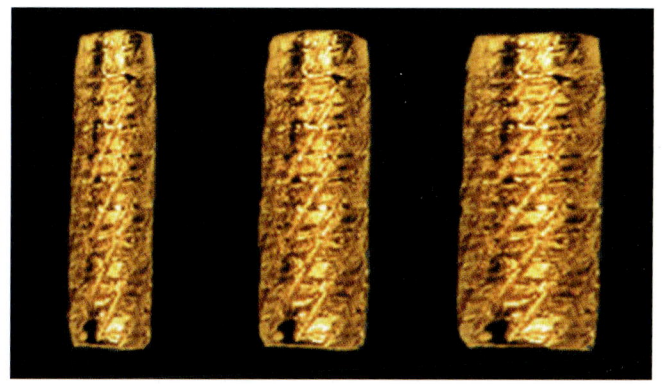

图20.6　Civco标记物

平均直径15 mm，范围9~20 mm；将5 mm×0.8 mm的标记物（Best Medical International公司）使用利多卡因凝胶粘在支气管刷的远端；然后将该刷插入引导鞘到达结节。32个结节通过径向EBUS定位。6例（18%）发生了标记物移位，其中2例发生在置入当天，4例发生在开始放疗前1周。

螺旋弹簧标记的使用已经由众多学者报道。在Schroeder等的一项研究中，最初的4例患者接受了1 mm×5 mm线性金标记物（CyberMark™ MT-NW-887~853，Civco Medical Solutions，Orange City，美国爱荷华州）（图20.6）。随后放置的56个标记物使用3 mm×3.3 mm金字塔形铂金螺旋弹簧圈（VortX®18，波士顿科学公司）完成（图20.7）[105]。将SuperDimension电磁导航系统的延长工作通道定位在目标处后，使用蜡尖微生物样本刷（型号130，CONMED）通过延长工作通道输送2个标记物。在装载标记物的运输刷定位前移除蜡塞，然后用黏性无菌

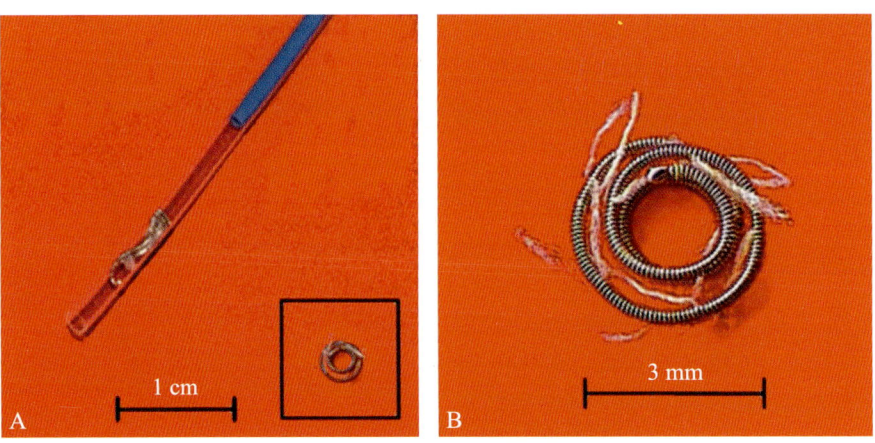

图 20.7　金字塔形铂金螺旋弹簧图

A. 装在微生物标本刷尖端的铂金螺旋弹簧圈；B. 放大的金字塔形的螺旋弹簧标记物，附有促进血栓形成的纤维。来源：经 Elsevier 许可，转载自 Schroeder 等[105]。

润滑剂临时密封。每次放置后，将延长工作通道导航到肿瘤邻近的不同区域。共有 52 名患者接受了 60 个标记物放置。在放置 1~2 周后进行计划放疗中，17 个线性标记物中只有 8 个（47%）仍在原位，接受线性标记物置入的 4 例患者中有 2 例需要额外的放置手术。在 217 个螺旋弹簧标记物中，215 个（99%）在放疗计划时仍然在原位（图 20.8）。肿瘤平均直径为 23.7 mm（范围为 8~53 mm）。3 例患者出现了气胸，其中 2 例患者在同一手术中进行了经支气管活检。作者认为，螺旋弹簧标记物具有更大的稳定性，这是因为其自身可被反冲力楔入周围的肺组织，而且附着在金属线圈上的致密聚酯纤维会促进血栓形成并固定在相邻组织中。

Nabavizadeh 等还使用电磁导航支气管镜对 31 例患者 34 个结节放置螺旋弹簧标记物[106]。在他们的研究中，使用标记物放置套件（SuperDimension，美敦力公司）放置 4 mm VortX 35 纤维铂线圈（波士顿科学公司）。在放置的 105 个标记物中，103 个（98.1%）在 CT 模拟定位机上被确认；86% 的标记物放置在距结节 1 cm 内，52% 直接放置在结节表面。在 SBRT 治

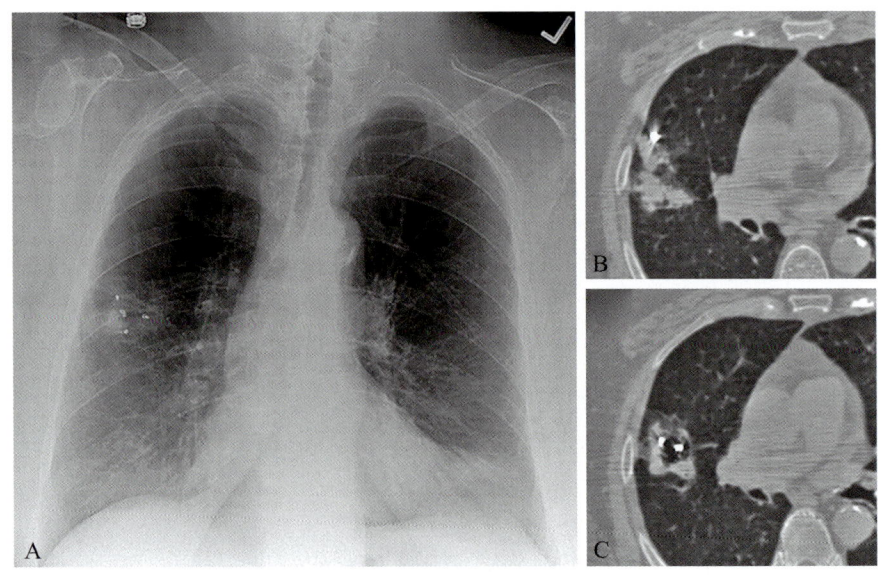

图 20.8　经电磁导航支气管镜置入标记物后的胸片（A）和胸部 CT 扫描（B、C）

可见右肺病变及其周围的不透射线标记物。来源：经 Elsevier 许可，转载自 Schroeder 等[105]。

疗期间，锥形束CT评估标记物移位<7 mm的患者占98%，<5 mm的患者占96%，<2 mm的患者为67%。

McGuire等报道了另一种标记物置入方法[107]。他们使用的是0.75 mm的Visicoil螺旋金标记，通常长度为20 mm，但10 mm和30 mm的长度也使用。一种方法是使用MW-319 19/22G的Wang氏支气管针，在导航支气管镜引导下，将延长的工作通道定位在病变处，将Wang氏支气管针推到延长的工作通道，并在透视引导下将针插入病变中。将内部21G针完全移除，留下19G针和引导鞘。Visicoil标记物被反向装到引导鞘中，使用一根0.66 mm导丝（ChoICE PT Extra Support；波士顿科学公司）将标记物推过鞘的长度，然后，将针头慢慢拉回，同时保持导丝上的压力以推出标记物。第2种方法中，将延长工作通道定位在适当位置后，将一根5 F JB1的导管（Benton Hanafee Wilson Glidecath®，波士顿科学公司）通过延长的工作通道推进到病变中。将Visicoil标记物装入导管的近端，然后将0.66 mm导丝穿过导管，在透视引导下，通过导丝从导管中挤出标记物。Glidecath导管可以向不同的方向转动，由于导管的角度特性，可以放置在肿瘤的不同平面上。作者指出后一种方法是他们的首选。报告中没有提供任何一种方法的成功或移位的数据。

Minnich等评估了他们机构电磁导航支气管镜引导下放置标记物的无移位率[108]。48例患者使用的标记物包括3 mm金放射粒子、superLock双带标记物和VortX 35闭塞线圈。VortX 35的保留率最高，为96.7%（59/61），而superLock的保留率为72.7%（24/33），金放射粒子的保留率则为69.7%（23/33）。VortX 35和其他标记物之间的保留率差异具有统计学意义。

最近，凸探头式EBUS（convex-probe EBUS，cp-EBUS）已被报道用于中央型病变放置标记物。Casutt等在转移性黑色素瘤继发左肺门肿块中放置了一个5 mm×0.5 mm的Visicoil标记物[109]。将标记物装载到针手柄处的通道中，用针芯将其穿过针尖推入肿瘤中。Chambers等将Cook Medical Hilal 微栓塞线圈（Cook公司）放入右下叶和左下叶，用于治疗放射学上隐匿的支气管内膜鳞状细胞癌[110]。将线圈反向装到EBUS针中，并用骨蜡固定。Belanger等报道了5例患者的病例系列，其中3例患者使用cp-EBUS在淋巴结中放置标记物，1例患者放置在左下叶结节，1例患者放置在左下叶肿块中[111]。当使用21G EBUS针时，放置0.5 mm×5 mm的Visicoil标记物；当使用22G EBUS针时，放置0.35 mm×5 mm的Viscoil标记物。将探针向后拉回5~10 cm，首先将标记物装到针的末端。用无菌手术润滑剂封住针头，以避免丢失标记物。在将针插入目标病变后，然后向前推进针芯，直到与针夹齐平，将标记物置入病变中。

Seides等对8例患者通过支气管镜置入标记物；其中5例放置在淋巴结，3例放置在支气管周围病变[112]。手术使用21G针。用剪刀将0.75 mm×5 mm的Visicoil标记物分割成较短的片段。将碎片反向载到针头中，尖端用骨蜡密封以防止移位。穿刺病变后，推进探针，放置标记物。

从以上发表文章中可以推测，关于肺癌和转移性肺部恶性肿瘤的图像引导置入放疗标记物，目前还没有"金标准"，也没有通过支气管镜放置标记物的标准方法。笔者使用的方法与Harley等[96]的报道类似，使用Wang氏经支气管针或Olympus引导鞘（奥林巴斯公司，日本东京）和活检钳，联合Broncus LungPoint®虚拟导航支气管镜系统（Broncus Technologies公司，美国加州）和径向EBUS（图20.9至图20.11）进行标记物放置。线圈标记物似乎比线性标记物有更少的移位，但价格更贵。使用导航支气管镜系统和/或外周EBUS来确保更外周的标记物置入，可以降低线性标记物的移位率。应将标记物楔入小的外周气道或肺实质，以减少移位。对于淋巴结和中央型肿块，可以使用cp-EBUS将标记物直接放置在淋巴结或肿块中，笔者使用这种方法取得了成功。如前所述，通常会放置3个标志物，但一些临床医生喜欢放置更多，以防其

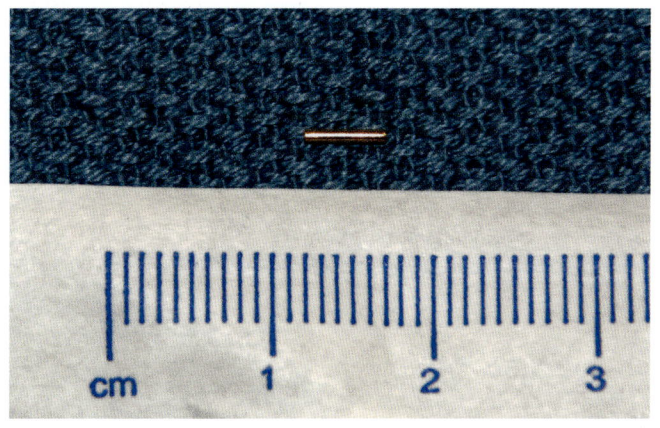

图20.9 Alpha-Omega 标记物
型号SMG0242-025，Alpha-Omega Services公司，美国加州。

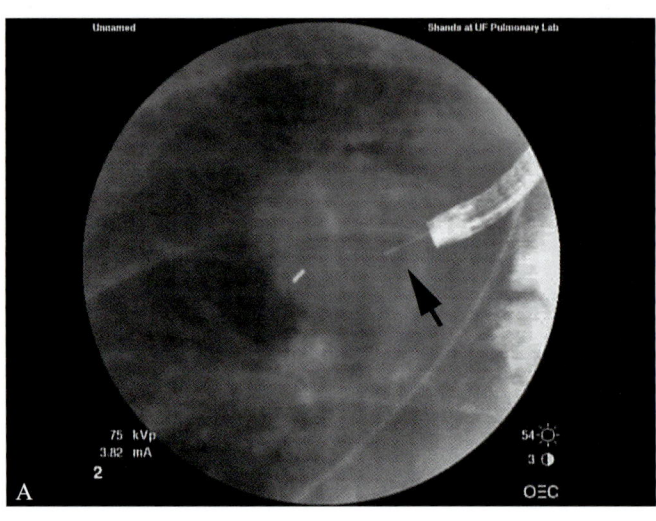
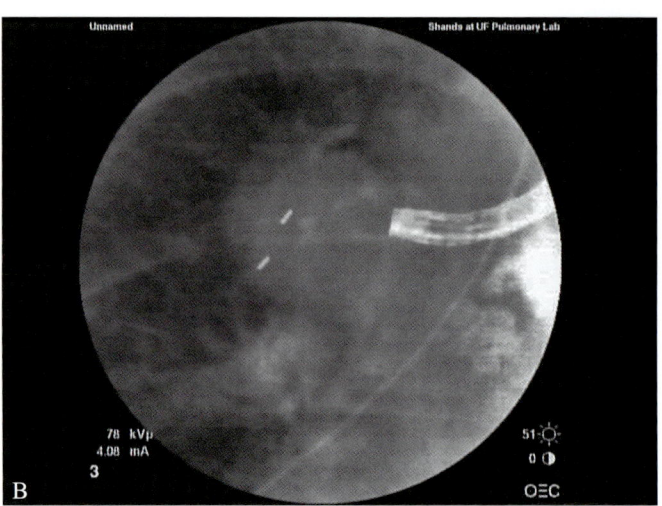

图 20.10　肺门肿块中的标记物

A. 肺门肿块和经支气管针置入肺门肿块的标记物（箭头示）；B. 在肺门肿块中放置第 2 个标记物。

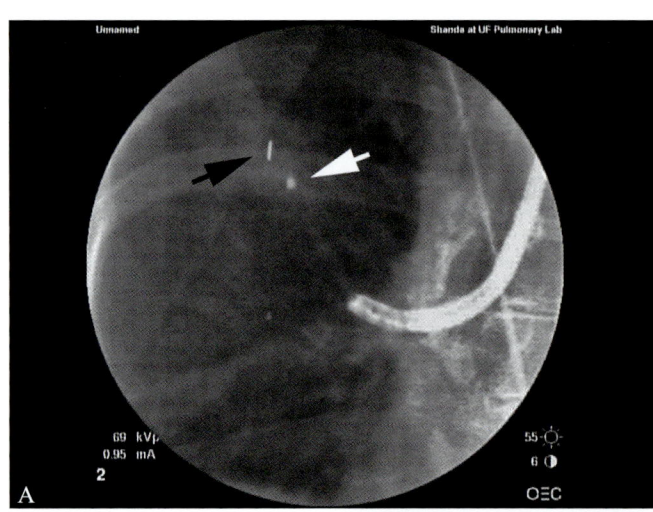
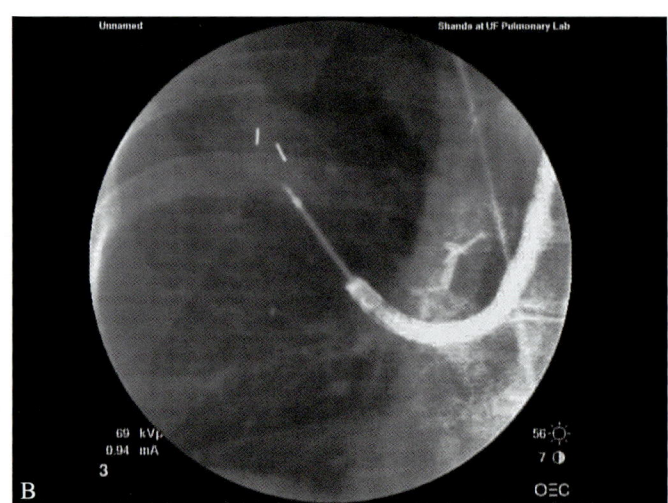
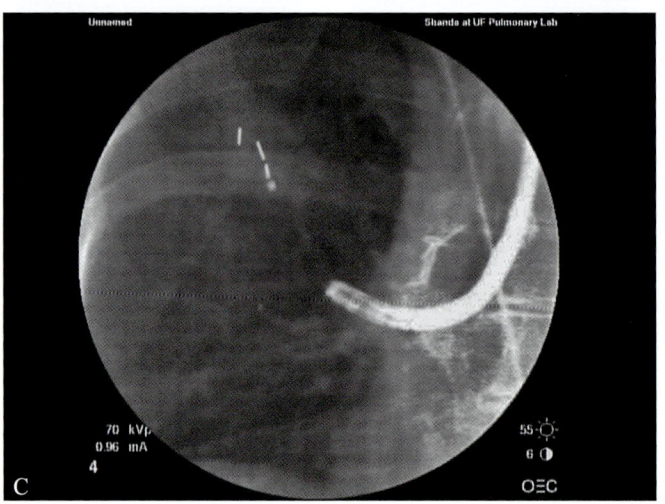

图 20.11　在外周结节周围放置标记物

A. 结节附近的引导鞘末端（白色箭头示）及放置的标记物（黑色箭头示）；B. 从引导鞘末端伸出的活检钳和标记物，以及 2 个已放置的标记物；C. 引导鞘末端附近的置入的第 3 个标记物。

中一个标志物发生移位。考虑到标记物在置入后大约5天开始纤维化反应[113]，并且大多数标记物丢失似乎发生在置入后的第1周内。因此，应在标记物放置1周后进行CT扫描。随着定位周围型肺癌技术的改进和气胸发生率的降低，支气管镜下放置标记物可能会取代许多机构的经皮穿刺置入术。

20.3 射频消融

射频消融（radiofrequency ablation，RFA）已成为手术或放疗的替代疗法，用于治疗无法手术的原发性肺癌或转移性肺部恶性肿瘤患者[114,115]。在RFA期间，射频发生器产生交变流电，从肿瘤内的活性电极向接地电极移动。快速变化的交变电流导致组织内的离子随着电流的变化方向而振荡。这些高速离子振荡对组织产生摩擦加热。加热至50°C以上的组织会发生蛋白质变性和凝固性坏死。加热至105°C以上的组织会发生烧焦和炭化，并产生小气孔。组织过热引起的碳化和汽化会增加组织阻抗，从而导致电流减少和凝固性坏死受制。因此，在RFA过程中，组织内的温度最好在60~105°C之间。肺内的肿瘤可能非常适合RFA，因为在所谓的"烤箱效应"中，肺内恶性肿瘤周围充满空气的肺组织可充当绝缘体，将输送的热能截留在肿瘤内，并保护邻近正常结构[116]。

RFA是在CT引导下，在全身麻醉或深度麻醉下经皮操作的。目前可用的RFA系统有单针电极、由3根平行针组成的集束探针，还有具有7~9根可扩展针头的探针，以增加治疗的表面积。目前的RFA系统可根据治疗组织的温度和/或阻抗监测在手术过程中提供关于治疗效果的反馈。在2014年发表的一项关于RFA治疗NSCLC的调查研究中，Ⅰ期NSCLC经RFA治疗后局部肿瘤进展率在各研究中相似（31%~42%）[117]。Ⅰ期NSCLC的1年、2年、3年和5年总生存率分别为78%~100%、53%~86%、36%~88%和25%~61%。1年、2年、3年的癌症特异性生存率分别为89%~100%、92%~93%和59%~88%。中位生存时间从29个月到67个月不等。在2018年发表的一项评估肺癌RFA治疗的荟萃分析中，汇总的局部肿瘤进展率为26%[118]。在一项文献调查中，最常见的并发症是气胸，发生率为28.3%（范围0%~90%），还有胸腔积液（14.8%，范围0%~87%）和胸痛（14.1%，范围0%~100%）[119]。其他报告的并发症还有咯血、肺炎、肺脓肿、支气管胸膜瘘、血胸和急性呼吸窘迫综合征[114,115,119]。

Tsushima等对绵羊进行了一项支气管镜引导下RFA的可行性研究[120]。研究中使用自行设计的具有4 mm活性电极的标准非冷循环电极和带有4 mm活性电极的内部冷循环电极。冷循环RFA电极的功率输出设定为30 W，持续60秒，使用室温水可产生40 mm×45 mm的烧伤病变，而使用冷水冷循环产生

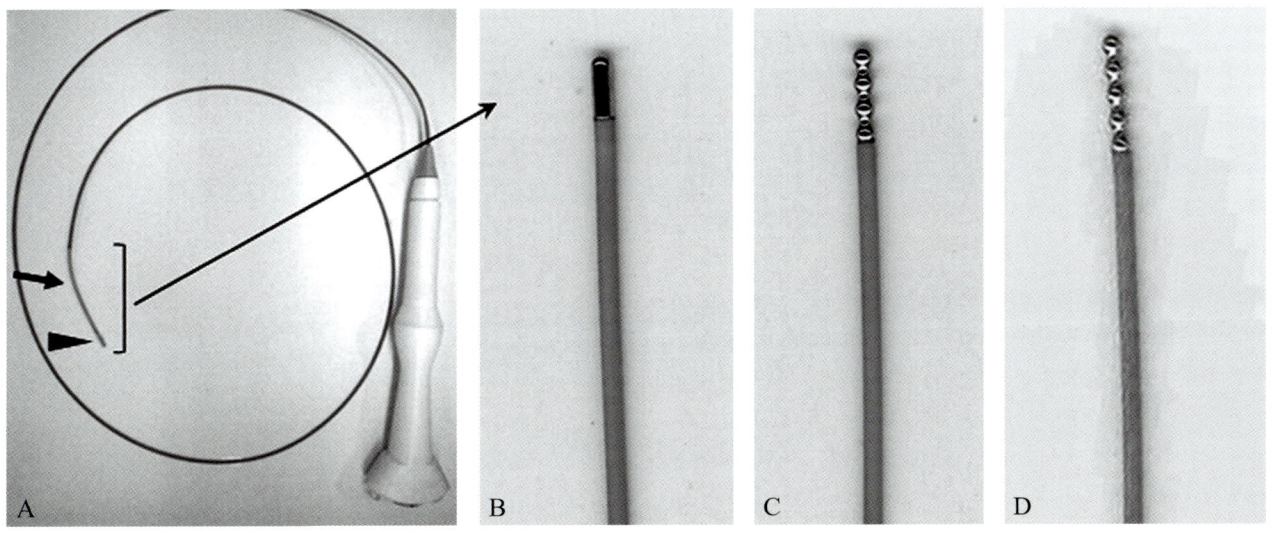

图20.12　内部冷循环射频消融（RFA）电极

A. 电极轴（长箭头示）和尖端（三角箭头示），顶部电极产生功率输出并测量尖端温度和阻抗，使用了3种类型的电极头：5 mm圆柱形活性电极（B）；8 mm具有4枚串珠状的活性电极（C）；10 mm具有5枚串珠状的活性电极（D）。资料来源：Tanabe等[121]。经美国胸科医师学会许可，版权所有2010。

20 mm×15 mm 的烧伤病变。随后，又对 10 例 T_1 期 NSCLC 患者进行 CT 引导下支气管镜 RFA 的初步试验，随后进行了标准的手术切除和分析[121]。使用了 3 种类型的电极：内部冷循环的 5 mm 活性电极、8 mm 带有 4 枚串珠状活性电极和 10 mm 带有 5 枚串珠状的活性电极，直径均为 1.67 mm（图 20.12）。RFA 前用低剂量胸部 CT 确认电极尖端在肿瘤内的位置。对每位患者使用 3 次 RFA。在功率输出为 20 W、输送时间为 50 秒的情况下，使用 10 mm 活性电极可获得令人满意的结果，消融面积从 13 mm×8 mm 到 16 mm×12 mm 不等。然而，在组织学检查时，外围区域还存在一些肿瘤细胞。

同一研究小组随后发表了 2 篇论文，一篇是 2 个病例的报告，另一篇是病例系列研究，介绍了他们在支气管镜 RFA 方面进一步的经验。在病例报告中，1 例病灶为 20 mm 肺腺癌的患者和 1 例未公开大小的肺腺癌患者使用电极长度 10 mm 带有 5 个串珠状的冷循环导管进行治疗[122]。在 CT 透视检查确认导管位置，RFA 输出功率为 30 W，消融间隔为 50 秒。在第 1 例患者中，治疗后 4 年内的放射学检查结果稳定，随后肿瘤体积增大。因推测疾病进展患者再次接受支气管镜 RFA 治疗，第 2 次治疗后的放射学检查结果稳定至 12 个月。第 2 例患者治疗后放射学检查结果在 40 个月内保持稳定。在病例研究中，纳入了 20 例无法手术或拒绝手术的患者，有 23 个 $T_1 \sim T_2$ 期 NSCLC 病灶[123]。研究中使用具有电极长度 10 mm 带有 5 枚串珠状的冷循环导管（直径 1.67 mm）。最初，输出功率和温度上限设置为 20 W 和 60℃，但随后分别更改为 30 W 和 70℃。经低剂量 CT 证实导管电极位置合适。中位随访时间为 46 个月，从 23 个月到 93 个月不等。11 个病灶的肿瘤大小显著缩小，有效率为 47.8%。在研究过程中，12 个病灶出现局部进展，因此局部肿瘤控制率为 47.8%。5 例患者再次进行了支气管镜 RFA 治疗。中位无进展期为 35 个月，5 年生存率为 61.5%。

另一研究团队报告了 3 例接受支气管镜 RFA 治疗患者的情况[124]。手术中使用电磁或虚拟支气管镜导航，并使用径向 EBUS 来确认导管或引导鞘的位置。病例 1：患者患有大小为 13.3 mm 的肺癌，使用线性电极（图 20.13）进行治疗，输出功率为 20 W，持续 5 min。病例 2：患者患有大小为 14.8 mm 的肺癌，使用可扩张的锥形导管治疗，以 20 W 消融 220 s，以 40 W 进行第 2 次近端消融 10 min。病例 3：患者患有大小为 21.8 mm 的肾细胞癌转移瘤，使用扩张的锥形

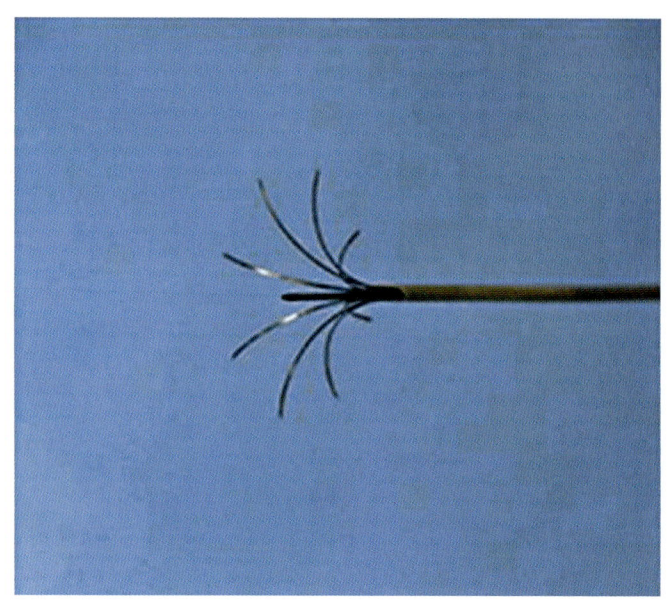

图 20.13　可伸缩的尖齿型射频消融（RFA）导管
资料来源：谢等[124]。

导管进行治疗，消融从 20 W 开始，在 400 s 内增加到 50 W。病例 2 和病例 3 在 1 年内治疗效果极好，无疾病迹象。病例 1 在治疗后 3 个月的 PET/CT 上显示肿瘤体积和摄取量减少，但治疗后 6 个月的 CT 显示肿瘤进展。

目前，经支气管镜行 RFA 治疗的潜力是令人鼓舞的。导航支气管镜技术的出现，联合径向 EBUS，使 RFA 靶向周围型肺癌成为一个有吸引力的想法。经支气管镜放置 RFA 电极，并发症发生率可能会低得多，尤其是气胸。还需要进行更多的研究来评估经支气管镜 RFA 的疗效。此外，有必要对不同的电极配置进行比较。

20.4　微波消融

微波辐射是指 300~3 000 MHz 之间的电磁频谱区域。临床使用的微波探头通常在 900~2 450 MHz 范围内工作[125]。水分子是有极性的，分子的氢侧带正电荷，氧侧带负电荷。微波探针周围快速变化的电场导致水分子快速旋转，试图与相反极性的电磁电荷对齐[125]。旋转的水分子与周围组织相互作用，传递其部分动能，从而产生热量，随后周围组织通过凝固性坏死而死亡。

与 RFA 相比，微波消融具有潜在的优势。由于微

波场能均匀地穿透组织，因此微波消融通常会产生更大、更球形和可预测的消融区[126]。RFA 受到肺组织高电阻率的阻碍。此外，消融引起的组织变化，如炭化和干燥，也会增加组织电阻率，从而进一步阻碍消融区的扩大。肺的高电阻率和消融引起的组织不均匀性使得消融区的扩大特别依赖于热传导，尤其在消融区的外围，这使得 RFA 产生的热量容易被周围的血管带走，这种现象被称为热沉降效应[126]。另一方面，微波消融具有加热沉积能力，这得益于水的存在，并且已被证明不太容易受到热沉降效应的影响，因为它能使大多数直径 <6 mm 的血管完全血栓化[126]。

已经发表了几项关于微波消融治疗肺部肿瘤的研究。下面介绍两篇代表性文章。Yang 等用微波消融术治疗了 47 例无法手术的 I 期 NSCLC 患者[127]。1 年、3 年和 5 年的局部控制率分别为 96%、64% 和 48%。术后 1 年、2 年、3 年和 5 年的总生存率分别为 89%、63%、43% 和 16%。癌症特异性中位生存期和中位总生存期分别为 47.4 和 33.8 个月。Zheng 等用微波消融治疗 184 例患者，其中 75% 为原发性肺癌，25% 为肺转移癌[128]。局部进展率为 19.1%。1 年、2 年、3 年和 5 年局部无进展率分别为 81.8%、76.1%、74.1% 和 74.1%。癌症特异性中位生存期和总生存期分别为 24.9 个月和 23.7 个月。

两项微波消融动物模型的研究以摘要形式发表。第 1 项研究中，经支气管镜使用可弯曲 17G 微波针，在 3 只猪身上设置不同的功率和时间进行 4 次消融[129]。消融区在短轴上的范围为 1.2~3.7 cm，大致对应于所使用的功率。在第 2 项研究中，经支气管镜使用 Emprint™ 消融导管套装（美敦力公司）对 8 只动物分别进行 3 次微波消融[130]。Emprint 系统利用 3 种空间技术来控制消融能量：热控制、场控制和波长控制。功率设置分别为 45 W、75 W 和 100 W。在 45 W 时，可产生高达 2.7 cm 的消融区，而在 75 W 和 100 W 时，分别产生高达 3.4 cm 和 3.5 cm 的消融区域。

已有 1 例经支气管镜对患者进行微波消融治疗的病例报告[131]。该患者由于鳞状细胞癌导致隆突下的肿块，压迫主支气管。微波消融术是通过一根专用的针形导管穿过左右主支气管的内壁进行的，消融后肿块缩小。摘要中没有提供针形导管的详细信息。

与 RFA 一样，微波消融作为经支气管镜肿瘤消融技术具有潜力[132]。与 RFA 相比，微波消融有一些理论上的优势，可能形成更大的消融区。一些公司正在开发经支气管镜微波消融探针，我们很可能在不久的将来看到人体研究的结果。

参考文献

1 https://seer.cancer.gov/statfacts/html/lungb.html
2 Reddy, S.P. and Marks, J.E. (1990). Total atelectasis of the lung secondary to malignant airway obstruction. Response to radiation therapy. *Am. J. Clin. Oncol.* 13: 394–400.
3 Chetty, K.G., Moran, E.M., Sassoon, C.S. et al. (1989). Effect of radiation therapy on bronchial obstruction due to bronchogenic carcinoma. *Chest* 95: 582–584.
4 Perez, C.A., Stanley, K., Grundy, G. et al. (1982). Impact of irradiation technique and tumor extent in tumor control and survival of patients with unresectable non-oat cell carcinoma of the lung: report by the Radiation Therapy Oncology Group. *Cancer* 50: 1091–1099.
5 Yankauer, S. (1922). Two cases of lung cancer treated bronchoscopically. *NY Med. J.* 21: 741–742.
6 Mehta, M., Shahabi, S., Jarjour, N. et al. (1990). Effect of endobronchial radiation therapy on malignant bronchial obstruction. *Chest* 97: 662–665.
7 Miller, J.I. Jr. and Phillips, T.W. (1990). Neodymium: YAG laser and brachytherapy in the management of inoperable bronchogenic carcinoma. *Ann. Thorac. Surg.* 50: 190–196.
8 Kohek, P.H., Pakisch, B., and Glanzer, H. (1994). Intraluminal irradiation in the treatment of malignant airway obstruction. *Eur. J. Surg. Oncol.* 20: 674–680.
9 Bastin, K.T., Mehta, M.P., and Kinsella, T.J. (1993). Thoracic volume radiation sparing following endobronchial brachytherapy: a quantitative analysis. *Int. J. Radiat. Oncol. Biol. Phys.* 25: 703–707.
10 Yao, M.S. and Koh, W.J. (2001). Endobronchial brachytherapy. *Chest Surg. Clin. North Am.* 11: 813–827.
11 Gollins, S.W., Ryder, W.D., Burt, P.A. et al. (1996). Massive haemoptysis death and other morbidity associated with high dose rate intraluminal radiotherapy for carcinoma of the bronchus. *Radiother. Oncol.* 39: 105–116.
12 Nag, S., Kelly, J.F., Horton, J.L. et al. (2001). Brachytherapy for carcinoma of the lung. *Oncology (Williston Park)* 15: 371–381.
13 Huber, R.M., Fischer, R., Hatmann, H. et al. (1995). Palliative endobronchial brachytherapy for central lung tumors. A prospective, randomized comparison of two fractionation schedules. *Chest* 107: 463–470.
14 Niemoeller, O.M., Pöllinger, B., Niyazi, M. et al. (2013). Mature results of a randomized trial comparing two fractionation schedules of high dose rate endoluminal brachytherapy for the treatment of endobronchial tumors. *Radiat. Oncol.* 8: 1–8.
15 Mallick, I., Sharma, S.C., Behera, D. et al. (2006). Optimization of dose and fractionation of endobronchial brachytherapy with or without external radiation in the palliative management of non-small cell lung cancer: a prospective randomized study. *J. Cancer Res. Ther.* 2: 119–125.
16 Huber, R.M., Fischer, R., Hautmann, H. et al. (1997). Does additional brachytherapy improve the effect of external

irradiation? A prospective, randomized study in central lung tumors. *Int. J. Radiat. Oncol. Biol. Phys.* 38: 533–540.

17 Langendijk, H., de Jong, J., Tjwa, M. et al. (2001). External irradiation versus external irradiation plus endobronchial brachytherapy in inoperable non-small cell lung cancer: a prospective randomized study. *Radiother. Oncol.* 58: 257–268.

18 Sur, R., Ahmed, S.N., Donde, B. et al. (2001). Brachytherapy boost vs teletherapy boost in palliation of symptomatic, locally advanced non-small cell lung cancer: preliminary analysis of a randomized, prospective trial. *J. Brachyther. Intl.* 17: 309–315.

19 Sur, R., Donde, B., Mohuiddin, M. et al. (2004). Randomized prospective study on the role of high dose rate intraluminal brachytherapy (HDRILBT) in palliation of symptoms in advanced non small cell lung cancer (NSCLC) treated with radiation alone. *Int. J. Radiat. Oncol. Biol. Phys.* 60 (suppl 1): S205.

20 Stout, R., Barber, P., Burt, P. et al. (2000). Clinical and quality of life outcomes in the first United Kingdom randomized trial of endobronchial brachytherapy (intraluminal radiotherapy) vs. external beam radiotherapy in the palliative treatment of inoperable non-small cell lung cancer. *Radiother. Oncol.* 56: 323–327.

21 Muto, P., Ravo, V., Panelli, G. et al. (2000). High-dose rate brachytherapy of bronchial cancer: treatment optimization using three schemes of therapy. *Oncologist* 5: 209–214.

22 Mallick, I., Sharma, S.C., and Behera, D. (2007). Endobronchial brachytherapy for symptom palliation in non-small cell lung cancer – analysis of symptom response, endoscopic improvement and quality of life. *Lung Cancer* 55: 313–318.

23 Skowronek, J., Kubaszewska, M., Kanikowski, M. et al. (2009). HDR endobronchial brachytherapy (HDRBT) in the management of advanced lung cancer – comparison of two different dose schedules. *Radiother. Oncol.* 93: 436–440.

24 Mantz, C.A., Dosoretz, D.E., Rubenstein, J.H. et al. (2004). Endobronchial brachytherapy and optimization of local disease control in medically inoperable non-small cell lung carcinoma: a matched-pair analysis. *Brachytherapy* 3: 183–190.

25 Manali, E.D., Stathopoulos, G.T., Gildea, T.R. et al. (2010). High dose-rate endobronchial radiotherapy for proximal airway obstruction due to lung cancer: 8-year experience of a referral center. *Cancer Biother. Radiopharm.* 25: 207–213.

26 Hauswald, H., Stoiber, E., Rochet, N. et al. (2010). Treatment of recurrent bronchial carcinoma: the role of high-dose-rate endoluminal brachytherapy. *Int. J. Radiat. Oncol. Biol. Phys.* 77: 373–377.

27 Ozkok, S., Karakoyun-Celik, O., Goksel, T. et al. (2008). High dose rate endobronchial brachytherapy in the management of lung cancer: response and toxicity evaluation in 158 patients. *Lung Cancer* 62: 326–333.

28 Hennequin, C., Bleichner, O., Trédaniel, J. et al. (2007). Long-term results of endobronchial brachytherapy: a curative treatment? *Int. J. Radiat. Oncol. Biol. Phys.* 67: 425–430.

29 Escobar-Sacristán, J.A., Granda-Orive, J.I., Gutiérrez Jiménez, T. et al. (2004). Endobronchial brachytherapy in the treatment of malignant lung tumours. *Eur. Respir. J.* 24: 348–352.

30 Gejerman, G., Mullokandov, E.A., Bagiella, E. et al. (2002). Endobronchial brachytherapy and external-beam radiotherapy in patients with endobronchial obstruction and extrabronchial extension. *Brachytherapy* 1: 204–210.

31 Anacak, Y., Mogulkoc, N., Ozkok, S. et al. (2001). High dose rate endobronchial brachytherapy in combination with external beam radiotherapy for stage III non-small cell lung cancer. *Lung Cancer* 34: 253–259.

32 Petera, J., Spásová, I., Neumanová, R. et al. (2001). High dose rate intraluminal brachytherapy in the treatment of malignant airway obstructions. *Neoplasma* 48: 148–153.

33 Harms, W., Schraube, P., Becker, H. et al. (2000). Effect and toxicity of endoluminal high-dose-rate (HDR) brachytherapy in centrally located tumors of the upper respiratory tract. *Strahlenther. Onkol.* 176: 60–66.

34 Kelly, J.F., Delclos, M.E., Morice, R.C. et al. (2000). High-dose-rate endobronchial brachytherapy effectively palliates symptoms due to airway tumors: the 10-year M. D. Anderson cancer center experience. *Int. J. Radiat. Oncol. Biol. Phys.* 48: 697–702.

35 Marsiglia, H., Baldeyrou, P., Lartigau, E. et al. (2000). High-dose-rate brachytherapy as sole modality for early-stage endobronchial carcinoma. *Int. J. Radiat. Oncol. Biol. Phys.* 47: 665–672.

36 Taulelle, M., Chauvet, B., Vincent, P. et al. (1998). High dose rate endobronchial brachytherapy: results and complications in 189 patients. *Eur. Respir. J.* 11: 162–168.

37 Ofiara, L., Roman, T., Schwartzman, K., and Levy, R.D. (1997). Local determinants of response to endobronchial high-dose rate brachytherapy in bronchogenic carcinoma. *Chest* 112: 946–953.

38 Ornadel, D., Duchesne, G., Wall, P. et al. (1997). Defining the roles of high dose rate endobronchial brachytherapy and laser resection for recurrent bronchial malignancy. *Lung Cancer* 16: 203–213.

39 Nomoto, Y., Shouji, K., Toyota, S. et al. (1997). High dose rate endobronchial brachytherapy using a new applicator. *Radiother. Oncol.* 45: 33–37.

40 Pérol, M., Caliandro, R., Pommier, P. et al. (1997). Curative irradiation of limited endobronchial carcinomas with high-dose rate brachytherapy. Results of a pilot study. *Chest* 111: 1417–1423.

41 Delclos, M.E., Komaki, R., Morice, R.C. et al. (1996). Endobronchial brachytherapy with high-dose-rate remote afterloading for recurrent endobronchial lesions. *Radiology* 201: 279–282.

42 Hernandez, P., Gursahaney, A., Roman, T. et al. (1996). High dose rate brachytherapy for the local control of endobronchial carcinoma following external irradiation. *Thorax* 51: 354–358.

43 Macha, H.N., Wahlers, B., Reichle, C., and von Zwehl, D. (1995). Endobronchial radiation therapy for obstructing malignancies: ten years' experience with iridium-192 high-dose radiation brachytherapy afterloading technique in 365 patients. *Lung* 173: 271–280.

44 Trédaniel, J., Hennequin, C., Zalcman, G. et al. (1994). Prolonged survival after high-dose rate endobronchial radiation

for malignant airway obstruction. *Chest* 105: 767–772.

45 Chang, L.F., Horvath, J., Peyton, W., and Ling, S.S. (1994). High dose rate afterloading intraluminal brachytherapy in malignant airway obstruction of lung cancer. *Int. J. Radiat. Oncol. Biol. Phys.* 28: 589–596.

46 Goldman, J.M., Bulman, A.S., Rathmell, A.J. et al. (1993). Physiologic effect of endobronchial radiotherapy in patients with major airway occlusion by carcinoma. *Thorax* 48: 110–114.

47 Gollins, S.W., Burt, P.A., Barber, P.V., and Stout, R. (1994). High dose rate intraluminal radiotherapy for carcinoma of the bronchus: outcome of treatment of 406 patients. *Radiother. Oncol.* 33: 31–40.

48 Speiser, B.L. and Spratling, L. (1993). Remote afterloading brachytherapy for the local control of endobronchial carcinoma. *Int. J. Radiat. Oncol. Biol. Phys.* 25: 579–587.

49 Pisch, J., Villamena, P.C., Harvey, J.C. et al. (1993). High dose-rate endobronchial irradiation in malignant airway obstruction. *Chest* 104: 721–725.

50 Nori, D., Allison, R., Kaplan, B. et al. (1993). High dose-rate intraluminal irradiation in bronchogenic carcinoma: technique and results. *Chest* 104: 1006–1011.

51 Bedwinek, J., Petty, A., Bruton, C. et al. (1992). The use of high dose rate endobronchial brachytherapy to palliate symptomatic endobronchial recurrence of previously irradiated bronchogenic carcinoma. *Int. J. Radiat. Oncol. Biol. Phys.* 22: 23–30.

52 Gauwitz, M., Ellerbroek, N., Komaki, R. et al. (1992). High dose endobronchial irradiation in recurrent bronchogenic carcinoma. *Int. J. Radiat. Oncol. Biol. Phys.* 23: 397–400.

53 Mehta, M., Petereit, D., Chosy, L. et al. (1992). Sequential comparison of low dose rate and hyperfractionated high dose rate endobronchial radiation for malignant airway occlusion. *Int. J. Radiat. Oncol. Biol. Phys.* 23: 133–139.

54 Sutedja, G., Baris, G., Schaake-Koning, C., and van Zandwijk, N. (1992). High dose rate brachytherapy in patients with local recurrences after radiotherapy of non-small cell lung cancer. *Int. J. Radiat. Oncol. Biol. Phys.* 24: 551–553.

55 Aygun, C., Weiner, S., Scariato, A. et al. (1992). Treatment of non-small cell lung cancer with external beam radiotherapy and high dose rate brachytherapy. *Int. J. Radiat. Oncol. Biol. Phys.* 23: 127–132.

56 Burt, P.A., O'Driscoll, B.R., Notley, H.M. et al. (1990). Intraluminal irradiation for the palliation of lung cancer with the high dose rate micro-Selectron. *Thorax* 45: 765–768.

57 Cotter, G.W., Lariscy, C., Ellingwood, K.E., and Herbert, D. (1993). Inoperable endobronchial obstructing lung cancer treated with combined endobronchial and external beam irradiation: a dosimetric analysis. *Int. J. Radiat. Oncol. Biol. Phys.* 27: 531–535.

58 Mehta, M.P., Shahabi, S., Jarjour, N.N., and Kinsella, T.J. (1989). Endobronchial irradiation for malignant airway obstruction. *Int. J. Radiat. Oncol. Biol. Phys.* 17: 847–851.

59 Skowronek, J., Piorunek, T., Kanikowski, M. et al. (2013). Definitive high-dose-rate endobronchial brachytherapy of bronchial stump for lung cancer after surgery. *Brachytherapy* 12: 560–566.

60 Kawamura, H., Ebara, T., Katoh, H. et al. (2012). Long-term results of curative intraluminal high dose rate brachytherapy for endobronchial carcinoma. *Radiat. Oncol.* 7: 112.

61 Aumont-le Guilcher, M., Prevost, B., Sunyach, M.P. et al. (2011). High-dose-rate brachytherapy for non-small-cell lung carcinoma: a retrospective study of 226 patients. *Int. J. Radiat. Oncol. Biol. Phys.* 79: 1112–1116.

62 Fuwa, N., Kodaira, T., Tachibana, H. et al. (2008). Long-term observation of 64 patients with roentgenographically occult lung cancer treated with external irradiation and intraluminal irradiation using low-dose-rate iridium. *Jpn. J. Clin. Oncol.* 38: 581–588.

63 Saito, M., Yokoyama, A., Kurita, Y. et al. (2000). Treatment of roentgenographically occult endobronchial carcinoma with external beam radiotherapy and intraluminal low-dose-rate brachytherapy: second report. *Int. J. Radiat. Oncol. Biol. Phys.* 47: 673–680.

64 Donovan, E., Timotin, E., Farrell, T. et al. (2017). Endobronchial brachytherapy for metastasis from extrapulmonary malignancies as an effective treatment for palliation of symptoms. *Brachytherapy* 16: 630–638.

65 Stranzl, H., Gabor, S., Mayer, R. et al. (2002). Fractionated intraluminal HDR 192Ir brachytherapy as palliative treatment in patients with endobronchial metastases from non-bronchogenic primaries. *Strahlenther. Onkol.* 178: 442–445.

66 Quantrill, S.J., Burt, P.A., Barber, P.V., and Stout, R. (2000). Treatment of endobronchial metastases with intraluminal radiotherapy. *Respir. Med.* 94: 369–372.

67 Chella, A., Ambrogi, M.C., Ribechini, A. et al. (2000). Combined Nd-YAG laser/HDR brachytherapy versus Nd-YAG laser only in malignant central airway involvement: a prospective randomized study. *Lung Cancer* 27: 169–175.

68 Jang, T.W., Blackman, G., and George, J.J. (2002). Survival benefits of lung cancer patients undergoing laser and brachytherapy. *J. Korean Med. Sci.* 17: 341–347.

69 Shea, J.M., Allen, R.P., Tharratt, R.S. et al. (1993). Survival of patients undergoing Nd: YAG laser therapy compared with Nd: YAG laser therapy and brachytherapy for malignant airway disease. *Chest* 103: 1028–1031.

70 Macha, H.N., Koch, K., Stadler, M. et al. (1987). New technique for treating occlusive and stenosing tumours of the trachea and main bronchi: endobronchial irradiation by high dose iridium-192 combined with laser cannalisation. *Thorax* 42: 511–515.

71 Freitag, L., Ernst, A., Thomas, M. et al. (2004). Sequential photodynamic therapy (PDT) and high dose brachytherapy for endobronchial tumour control inpatients with limited bronchogenic carcinoma. *Thorax* 59: 790–793.

72 Weinberg, B.D., Allison, R.R., Sibata, C. et al. (2010). Results of combined photodynamic therapy (PDT) and high dose rate brachytherapy (HDR) in treatment of obstructive endobronchial non-small cell lung cancer (NSCLC). *Photodiagn. Photodyn. Ther.* 7: 50–58.

73 Allison, R., Sibata, C., Sarma, K. et al. (2004). High-dose-rate brachytherapy in combination with stenting offers a rapid

and statistically significant improvement in quality of life for patients with endobronchial recurrence. *Cancer J.* 10: 368–373.

74 Kobayashi, T., Kaneko, M., Sumi, M. et al. (2000). CT-assisted transbronchial brachytherapy for small peripheral lung cancer. *Jpn. J. Clin. Oncol.* 30: 109–112.

75 Imamura, F., Ueno, K., Kusunoki, Y. et al. (2006). High-dose-rate brachytherapy for small-sized peripherally located lung cancer. *Strahlenther. Onkol.* 182: 703–707.

76 Harms, W., Krempien, R., Grehn, C. et al. (2006). Electromagnetically navigated brachytherapy as a new treatment option for peripheral pulmonary tumors. *Strahlenther. Onkol.* 182: 108–111.

77 Becker, H.D., McLemore, T., and Harms, W. (2009). Electromagnetic navigation and endobronchial ultrasound for brachytherapy of peripheral lung cancer-experience and long term results at two centers. *Am. J. Respir. Crit. Care Med.* 179: A6167.

78 Kennedy, A.S., Sonett, J.R., Orens, J.B., and King, K. (2000). High dose rate brachytherapy to prevent recurrent benign hyperplasia in lung transplant bronchi: theoretical and clinical considerations. *J. Heart Lung Transplant.* 19: 155–159.

79 Halkos, M.E., Godette, K.D., Lawrence, E.C., and Miller, J.I. Jr. (2003). High dose rate brachytherapy in the management of lung transplant airway stenosis. *Ann. Thorac. Surg.* 76: 381–384.

80 Madu, C.N., Machuzak, M.S., Sterman, D.H. et al. (2006). High-dose-rate (HDR) brachytherapy for the treatment of benign obstructive endobronchial granulation tissue. *Int. J. Radiat. Oncol. Biol. Phys.* 66: 1450–1456.

81 Kramer, M.R., Katz, A., Yarmolovsky, A. et al. (2001). Successful use of high dose rate brachytherapy for non-malignant bronchial obstruction. *Thorax* 56: 415–416.

82 Tendulkar, R.D., Fleming, P.A., Reddy, C.A. et al. (2008). High-dose-rate endobronchial brachytherapy for recurrent airway obstruction from hyperplastic granulation tissue. *Int. J. Radiat. Oncol. Biol. Phys.* 70: 701–706.

83 Hennequin, C., Tredaniel, J., Chevret, S. et al. (1998). Predictive factors for late toxicity after endobronchial brachytherapy: a multivariate analysis. *Int. J. Radiat. Oncol. Biol. Phys.* 42: 21–27.

84 Hara, R., Itami, J., Aruga, T. et al. (2001). Risk factors for massive hemoptysis after endobronchial brachytherapy in patients with tracheobronchial malignancies. *Cancer* 92: 2623–2627.

85 Carvalho Hde, A., Gonçalves, S.L., Pedreira, W. Jr. et al. (2007). Irradiated volume and the risk of fatal hemoptysis in patients submitted to high dose-rate endobronchial brachytherapy. *Lung Cancer* 55: 319–327.

86 Langendijk, J.A., Tjwa, M.K., de Jong, J.M. et al. (1998). Massive haemoptysis after radiotherapy in inoperable non-small cell lung carcinoma: is endobronchial brachytherapy really a risk factor? *Radiother. Oncol.* 49: 175–183.

87 Gustafson, G., Vicini, F., Freedman, L. et al. (1995). High dose rate endobronchial brachytherapy in the management of primary and recurrent bronchogenic malignancies. *Cancer* 75: 2345–2350.

88 Speiser, B.L. and Spratling, L. (1993). Radiation bronchitis and stenosis secondary to high dose rate endobronchial irradiation. *Int. J. Radiat. Oncol. Biol. Phys.* 25: 589–597.

89 Khanavkar, B., Stern, P., Alberti, W., and Nakhosteen, J.A. (1991). Complications associated with brachytherapy alone or with laser in lung cancer. *Chest* 99: 1062–1065.

90 Qiao, X., Tullgren, O., Lax, I. et al. (2003). The role of radiotherapy in treatment of stage I non-small cell lung cancer. *Lung Cancer* 41: 1–11.

91 Murray, P., Franks, K., and Hanna, G.G. (2017). A systematic review of outcomes following stereotactic ablative radiotherapy in the treatment of early-stage primary lung cancer. *Br. J. Radiol.* 90: 20160732.

92 Chang, J.Y., Dong, L., Liu, H. et al. (2008). Image-guided radiation therapy for non-small cell lung cancer. *J. Thorac. Oncol.* 3: 177–186.

93 Brown, W.T., Wu, X., Fayad, F. et al. (2009). Application of robotic stereotactic radiotherapy to peripheral stage I non-small cell lung cancer with curative intent. *Clin. Oncol.* 21: 623–631.

94 van der Voort van Zyp, N.C., Prévost, J.B., Hoogeman, M.S. et al. (2009). Stereotactic radiotherapy with real-time tumor tracking for non-small cell lung cancer: clinical outcome. *Radiother. Oncol.* 91: 296–300.

95 Collins, B.T., Vahdat, S., Erickson, K. et al. (2009). Radical cyberknife radiosurgery with tumor tracking: an effective treatment for inoperable small peripheral stage I non-small cell lung cancer. *J. Hematol. Oncol.* 2: 1.

96 Le, Q.T., Loo, B.W., Ho, A. et al. (2006). Results of a phase I dose-escalation study using single-fraction stereotactic radiotherapy for lung tumors. *J. Thorac. Oncol.* 1: 802–809.

97 Harada, T., Shirato, H., Ogura, S. et al. (2002). Real-time tumor-tracking radiation therapy for lung carcinoma by the aid of insertion of a gold marker using bronchofiberscopy. *Cancer* 95: 1720–1727.

98 Imura, M., Yamazaki, K., Shirato, H. et al. (2005). Insertion and fixation of fiducial markers for setup and tracking of lung tumors in radiotherapy. *Int. J. Radiat. Oncol. Biol. Phys.* 63: 1442–1447.

99 Reichner, C.A., Collins, B.T., Gagnon, G.J. et al. (2005). The placement of gold fiducials for CyberKnife stereotactic radiosurgery using a modified transbronchial needle aspiration technique. *J. Bronchol.* 12: 193–195.

100 Anantham, D., Feller-Kopman, D., Shanmugham, L.N. et al. (2007). Electromagnetic navigation bronchoscopy-guided fiducial placement for robotic stereotactic radiosurgery of lung tumors: a feasibility study. *Chest* 132: 930–935.

101 Kupelian, P.A., Forbes, A., Willoughby, T.R. et al. (2007). Implantation and stability of metallic fiducials within pulmonary lesions. *Int. J. Radiat. Oncol. Biol. Phys.* 69: 777–785.

102 Harley, D.P., Krimsky, W.S., Sarkar, S. et al. (2010). Fiducial marker placement using endobronchial ultrasound and navigational bronchoscopy for stereotactic radiosurgery: an alternative strategy. *Ann. Thorac. Surg.* 89: 368–373.

103 Steinfort, D.P., Siva, S., Kron, T. et al. (2015). Multimodality

guidance for accurate bronchoscopic insertion of fiducial markers. *J. Thorac. Oncol.* 10: 324–330.

104 Lachkar, S., Guisier, F., Roger, M. et al. (2018). Assessment of per-endoscopic placement of fiducial gold markers for small peripheral lung nodules <20 mm before stereotactic radiation therapy. *Chest* 153: 387–394.

105 Schroeder, C., Hejal, R., and Linden, P.A. (2010). Coil spring fiducial markers placed safely using navigation bronchoscopy in inoperable patients allows accurate delivery of CyberKnife stereotactic radiosurgery. *J. Thorac. Cardiovasc. Surg.* 2010 (140): 1137–1142.

106 Nabavizadeh, N., Zhang, J., Elliott, D.A. et al. (2014). Electromagnetic navigational bronchoscopy-guided fiducial markers for lung stereotactic body radiation therapy: analysis of safety, feasibility, and interfraction stability. *J. Bronchol. Interv. Pulmonol.* 2: 123–130.

107 McGuire, F.R., Kerley, M., Ochran, T. et al. (2007). Radiotherapy monitoring device implantation into peripheral lung cancers: a therapeutic utility of electromagnetic navigational bronchoscopy. *J. Bronchol.* 14: 189–192.

108 Minnich, D.J., Bryant, A.S., Wei, B. et al. (2015). Retention rate of electromagnetic navigation bronchoscopic placed fiducial markers for lung radiosurgery. *Ann. Thorac. Surg.* 100: 1163–1165; discussion 1165–1166.

109 Casutt, A., Koutsokera, A., Peguret, N., and Lovis, A. (2017). Linear-endobronchial ultrasound-guided insertion of a fiducial marker: a new tool for tracking central lesions. *J. Bronchol. Interv. Pulmonol.* 24: 166–169.

110 Chambers, D.M., Pfister, G.J., and Gauhar, U.A. (2017). Linear EBUS-guided fiducial marker placement to guide radiotherapy for endobronchial, radiographically occult synchronous primary squamous cell carcinoma of the lung. *Respir. Med. Case Rep.* 22: 60–63.

111 Belanger, A.R., Zagar, T., and Akulian, J.A. (2016). Convex endobronchial ultrasound-guided fiducial placement for malignant central lung lesions: a case series. *J. Bronchol. Interv. Pulmonol.* 23: 46–50.

112 Seides, B.J., Egan, J.P. 3rd, French, K.D. et al. (2018). Fiducial marker placement for stereotactic body radiation therapy via convex probe endobronchial ultrasound: a case series and review of literature. *J. Thorac. Dis.* 10: 1972–1983.

113 Imura, M., Yamazaki, K., Kubota, K.C. et al. (2008). Histopathologic consideration of fiducial gold markers inserted for real-time tumor-tracking radiotherapy against lung cancer. *Int. J. Radiat. Oncol. Biol. Phys.* 70: 382–384.

114 Casal, R.F., Tam, A.L., and Eapen, G.A. (2010). Radiofrequency ablation of lung tumors. *Clin. Chest Med.* 31: 151–163.

115 Abbas, G., Pennathur, A., Landreneau, R.J., and Luketich, J.D. (2009). Radiofrequency and microwave ablation of lung tumors. *J. Surg. Oncol.* 100: 645–650.

116 Roy, A.M., Bent, C., and Fotheringham, T. (2009). Radiofrequency ablation of lung lesions: practical applications and tips. *Curr. Probl. Diagn. Radiol.* 38: 44–52.

117 Hiraki, T., Gobara, H., Iguchi, T. et al. (2014). Radiofrequency ablation for early-stage nonsmall cell lung cancer. *Biomed. Res. Int.* 2014: 152087.

118 Li, G., Xue, M., Chen, W., and Yi, S. (2018). Efficacy and safety of radiofrequency ablation for lung cancers: a systematic review and meta-analysis. *Eur. J. Radiol.* 100: 92–98.

119 Chan, V.O., McDermott, S., Malone, D.E., and Dodd, J.D. (2011). Percutaneous radiofrequency ablation of lung tumors: evaluation of the literature using evidence-based techniques. *J. Thorac. Imaging* 26: 18–26.

120 Tsushima, K., Koizumi, T., Tanabe, T. et al. (2007). Bronchoscopy-guided radiofrequency ablation as a potential novel therapeutic tool. *Eur. Respir. J.* 29: 1193–1200.

121 Tanabe, T., Koizumi, T., Tsushima, K. et al. (2010). Comparative study of three different catheters for CT imaging-bronchoscopy-guided radiofrequency ablation as a potential and novel interventional therapy for lung cancer. *Chest* 137: 890–897.

122 Koizumi, T., Kobayashi, T., Tanabe, T. et al. (2013). Clinical experience of bronchoscopy-guided radiofrequency ablation for peripheral-type lung cancer. *Case Rep. Oncol. Med.* 2013: 515160.

123 Koizumi, T., Tsushima, K., Tanabe, T. et al. (2015). Bronchoscopy-guided cooled radiofrequency ablation as a novel intervention therapy for peripheral lung cancer. *Respiration* 90: 47–55.

124 Xie, F., Zheng, X., Xiao, B. et al. (2017). Navigation bronchoscopy-guided radiofrequency ablation for nonsurgical peripheral pulmonary tumors. *Respiration* 94: 293–298.

125 Wasser, E.J. and Dupuy, D.E. (2008). Microwave ablation in the treatment of primary lung tumors. *Semin. Respir. Crit. Care Med.* 29: 384–394.

126 Vogl, T.J., Nour-Eldin, N.A., Albrecht, M.H. et al. (2017). Thermal ablation of lung tumors: focus on microwave ablation. *RöFo* 189: 828–843.

127 Yang, X., Ye, X., Zheng, A. et al. (2014). Percutaneous microwave ablation of stage I medically inoperable non-small cell lung cancer: clinical evaluation of 47 cases. *J. Surg. Oncol.* 110: 758–763.

128 Zheng, A., Ye, X., Yang, X. et al. (2016). Local efficacy and survival after microwave ablation of lung tumors: a retrospective study in 183 patients. *J. Vasc. Interv. Radiol.* 27: 1806–1814.

129 Ferguson, J., Egressy, K., Schefelker, R. et al. (2013). Bronchoscopically-guided microwave ablation in the lung. *Chest* 144: 87A.

130 Howk, K., Dickhans, W., Rooks, K. et al. (2016). Characterization of a bronchoscopic thermal ablation catheter in porcine lung. *Am. J. Respir. Crit. Care Med.* 193: A6019.

131 Bezzi, M., Trigiani, M., Novali, M. et al. (2016). "Cooking the beast" microwaves: a new fast method for reopening the airways. *Eur. Respir. J.* 48: PA3838.

132 Brenner, B., Kramer, M.R., Katz, A. et al. (2003). High dose rate brachytherapy for nonmalignant airway obstruction: new treatment option. *Chest* 124: 1605–1610.

第 21 章

气道异物吸入与可弯曲支气管镜技术

Erik E. Folch[1], Alexander S. Rabin[1], and Atul C. Mehta[2]

[1] Division of Pulmonary and Critical Care Medicine,
Massachusetts General Hospital, Boston, MA, USA

[2] Lerner College of Medicine, Buoncore Family Endowed Chair in Lung Transplantation,
Department of Pulmonary Medicine, Respiratory Institute, Cleveland Clinic, Cleveland, OH, USA

（译者：吴晓东　译者单位：同济大学附属东方医院）

21.1　引言

可弯曲支气管镜是诊断气道异物吸入的最常用工具，也是移除成人气道内异物的首选器械[1,2]。

气道异物吸入发生的年龄呈两极分化，常见于低幼及高龄人群[3-5]。尽管症状不具特异性，但详细的病史询问、查体以及胸部影像学检查对诊断极有价值。很多病例均是经支气管镜的直视检查才最终确诊。在大多数成人病例中，首次支气管镜操作过程中便可移除异物。

每例异物吸入都各有不同。这些差异包括吸入异物的类型、吸入后的反应以及位置。异物的物理特性、患者临床表现以及支气管镜医师的专业水平通常会决定最终临床转归。移除异物是一个非常有成就感的过程，因为该操作的成功率高，而并发症率通常较低。然而，在进行该操作前，如果准备不足，也可能会导致灾难性的结果。

对于儿童患者，通常在硬质支气管镜下移除异物，有时也结合使用可弯曲支气管镜操作[6]。然而，近年来研究数据表明在儿科患者中使用可弯曲支气管镜也是有效且安全的[7-9]。本章将综述在成人和儿童人群中使用可弯曲支气管镜取气道异物的应用价值。

21.2　危险因素

气道异物所致窒息是造成意外伤害死亡的第四大原因，2015 年度累计死亡人数达 5 051 人[10]。异物吸入在幼儿（＜5 岁）和老年人中最为常见，但两组人群的危险因素有所不同。

在儿童中，异物吸入通常是因为儿童天性好奇，喜欢将物品放入口中。他们用门齿咬物品，这可能会猛力将物体推送到咽喉深处，引起吞咽反射。儿童还经常会在进食时大笑、说话、哭闹或玩耍而致异物吸入。

成人异物吸入的高危因素包括长居护理院、精神障碍、使用安眠药和帕金森病。成人吸入异物后窒息死亡的风险更高，超过一半的死亡病例发生在 74 岁以上的患者中[11]。这些窒息导致的致命事件通常发生在居所（41%）、餐馆（29%）、养老院或精神病院里（14%）[11]。成人异物吸入的其他风险因素见表 21.1。

表 21.1　成人异物吸入的危险因素

酒精中毒
使用镇定或催眠药物
口腔健康状况差

(续表)

高龄
智力障碍
帕金森病
主要影响吞咽或意识状态的神经系统疾病
外伤后意识丧失
癫痫
全身麻醉

21.3 临床表现

异物吸入的临床表现与异物的类型、阻塞部位，以及患者的整体年龄和临床状况密切相关。发生窒息后，约1/3的气道异物位于声门近端。这些物体通常较大，极易阻塞喉部。意识清醒的患者在声门近端异物吸入后会出现严重的咳嗽、窒息、声音嘶哑和作呕。

在儿童中，亲眼所见或报告出现窒息是最常见的表现。儿童可能出现极度危急的情况，放射学检查示放射性不透明异物或单侧肺过度充气。相比之下，成人往往表现为慢性咳嗽的症状，这是由于吸入异物慢性刺激所致[12]，可能没有明显的窒息史[13]。在异物突发吸入的过程中，患者会突然出现窒息和难以控制的咳嗽，伴或不伴有呕吐。较少见的症状可能包括发热、呼吸困难或喘息（表21.2）[14]。需要注意的是，39%的异物吸入患者无阳性体征[15]，6%~38%患者的胸部X线检查可能正常[6,15-20]。

表21.2 异物吸入的体征和症状

咳嗽史
慢性咳嗽
单侧呼吸音减弱
肺不张
单侧肺过度充气
反复性肺炎
单侧或双侧哮鸣音
咯血
纵隔气肿
气胸
皮下气肿
支气管扩张
肺脓肿
胸膜炎性胸痛

在就医之前，很多患者已咳出异物。即便临床症状提示异物吸入，但仍有约50%有窒息史的儿童的气道内找不到异物。这是异物被无意咳出、被吞咽还是误诊，目前尚不清楚。

由于气管支气管解剖结构的差异，成年人和儿童气道内异物滞留的部位有所不同。儿童的气道解剖结构更对称，与之相比，成人左主支气管起始部的角度更锐利，右主支气管更粗，因而异物更可能被吸入至右下叶。儿童两侧则无明显差异[21]。

21.4 异物类型

异物分为有机和无机两类。有机异物诱发的炎症反应常较无机异物重。例如，花生或草在吸入后几小时内会引起强烈的宿主反应。这对临床具有重要意义，因为随着时间的推移，有机异物周边会形成肉芽组织，这将使得异物的移除变得更困难。取异物会导致出血和其他并发症。

儿童最常吸入的异物是花生、种子、谷物和坚果等食物颗粒[15,22]。儿童中最常见的无机异物包括玩具、小塑料块或金属。这些物体吸入后通常宿主反应小，可以在吸入部位停留数周到数年。实际上，一些吸入的异物可能是在儿童因其他原因接受支气管镜检查时偶然被发现的[23]。

在成人中，肉类是最常吸入的异物，通常（30%）会卡在声门或声门下区域[11]。大块食物特别危险，因为它们可能阻塞上呼吸道最狭窄的部位——声门下，导致危及生命的窒息。所幸的是，它们通常可以通过体位引流（头低足高位）、患者的有力咳嗽或腹部用力等动作后被排出[24,25]。使用麦氏插管钳和其他直接喉镜检查工具可能会有效。

成人还常吸入其他食物颗粒，如坚果、瓜子[26-28]。吸入的无机异物包括牙齿修复物[29]、牙齿填充物、硬币、安全别针、耳塞、玻璃、气管切开管碎片或气切管发声阀[30,31]以及药片[32]等。文化、生活方式和饮食习惯不同，吸入异物的种类也有所不同。例如，沿海地区可见到吸入蜗牛[33]，而在某些族群中还可见到吸入念珠或头巾别针的患者[28,34-36]。

21.5 影像学评估

怀疑异物吸入时，常先行胸部 X 线检查。如前所述，大多数吸入的异物可透过 X 线，这限制了常规胸片诊断气道异物的能力。然而，吸气和呼气相片可能显示出一些细微的征象，如气体潴留、肺不张、纵隔移位或肺部浸润等。在已发表的研究中，胸部 X 线片异常诊断异物吸入的效能存在较大差异（敏感性 70%~82%，特异性 44%~74%，阳性预测值 72%~83%，阴性预测值 41%~73%）[6,17,37]。因此，在胸部 X 线片上出现放射性异物可能是诊断的依据，但细微的影像学异常必须结合患者的临床病史和体格检查进行解释。

异物吸入的其他放射学发现包括纵隔气肿（通常见于儿童）[38]，颈部侧位片显示声门下水肿（提示喉-气管异物）[39]，以及存在被称为支气管结石的钙化物[40]。支气管结石可由压迫并最终侵入邻近支气管腔内的钙化淋巴结形成。淋巴结钙化可继发于慢性感染或组织炎症性疾病（如组织胞浆菌病、结核病或结节病）。支气管结石也可能代表了直接吸入异物中的钙化物质（图 21.1）。

在慢性阻塞情况下，胸部计算机断层扫描（computed tomography，CT）可以显示异物吸入的远期并发症，包括支气管狭窄、支气管扩张、支气管腔内新生物或肉芽组织形成等。目前已探索了使用基于多层螺旋 CT 的虚拟支气管镜检查来诊断异物吸入的研究。虚拟支气管镜检查的优点包括确定异物的存在与否，以及术前定位异物。但虚拟支气管镜检查并非治疗性的，在大多数医院无法开展，且可能会因此延误干预措施。

21.6 气道异物诊断的延误

虽然现在有了越来越灵敏的成像技术，但需谨记异物吸入常会因症状或仅依赖影像而被漏诊或误诊。由于症状不典型、胸部 X 线片阴性和医师误诊，儿童异物吸入诊断常会被延迟（24 h 到 3 天不等）[45,46]。儿童异物吸入易与哮吼（喉气管支气管炎）、复发性咽喉炎、哮喘或原发性气道肿瘤[47-49]相混淆。成人异物吸入的诊断同样也常会被延误[50]，异物吸入可能会与其他疾病，如恶性肿瘤[51]、哮喘[52]、结核病和反复性肺炎等混淆。鉴于异物吸入诊断的不确定性，可弯曲支气管镜技术仍然是疑诊异物吸入的首选确诊手段。

21.7 并发症

异物吸入的并发症可急可缓。急性并发症包括窒息、气胸、纵隔气肿、肺不张、肺叶塌陷，甚至死亡。慢性并发症包括阻塞性肺炎、支气管扩张、肺脓肿、进行性呼吸衰竭、支气管狭窄、肉芽组织形成和咯血。

21.8 取异物的方法

疑诊异物吸入时，应密切观察患者，直到确诊（或排除），并且异物被移除。即便临床稳定的患者，也可能会因为异物移位，或气道内出血或气胸等继发性损害而突发临床状况变化[53,54]。

异物在气道内停留的时间越长，就越会增加组织反应和相关炎症的程度[18,22,55]。在吸入后的最初 24 h 内，支气管黏膜可能会出现炎症、红肿和肉芽组织增生的迹象[18]。除非为了协调必要的人员和设备，或者为了将患者及时转移到能够安全取出异物的其他机构时，否则不宜推迟移除异物。可通过以下 3 种方式来

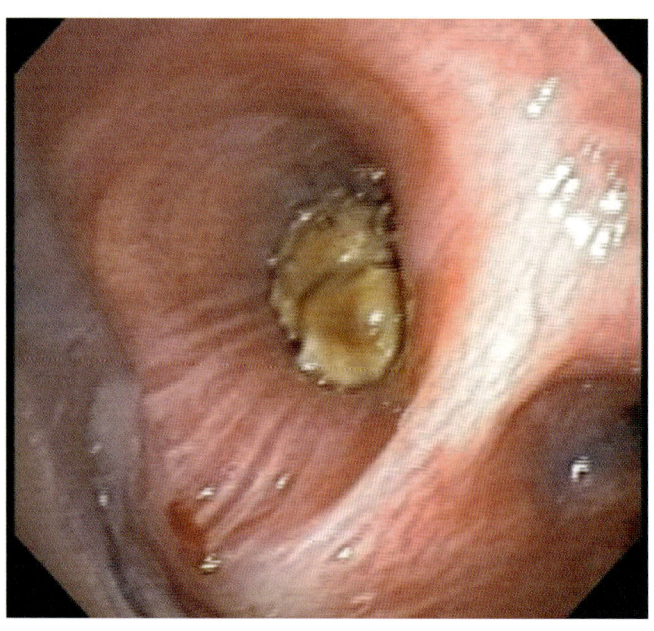

图 21.1　硬质支气管镜检查发现慢性组织胞浆菌病引起的支气管结石

移除异物,包括:体位引流、可弯曲支气管镜和硬质支气管镜。

21.8.1 体位引流和其他非内镜治疗方法

初诊异物吸入时,不建议吸入支气管扩张剂及进行体位引流,因为异物向近端移位可能导致气道阻塞和其他并发症[56]。延迟实施支气管镜检查会增加肺炎、肺不张和心肺骤停等并发症的风险,同时降低了气道异物成功取出的概率[55-57]。

针对因气道完全阻塞而无法言语或呼吸的危及生命的异物吸入,现推荐对婴儿患者进行背部拍击和胸部压迫,而对较大儿童和成人患者则进行腹部冲击(海姆立克急救法)。对于疑似近端气道阻塞导致危及生命的窒息,推荐进行喉镜评估。有资质的医务人员还应尝试通过高浓度面罩通气、气管插管与心肺复苏的方式来保护气道。当患者病情稳定后,再进行支气管镜检查并取出异物。

21.8.2 硬质支气管镜

硬质支气管镜诞生于针对异物吸入的诊疗过程中。1897年,古斯塔夫·基利安首次通过从一位患者气道内取出猪骨,展示出了硬质内窥镜的实用性[58]。1936年,谢瓦利尔·杰克逊报道气道异物移除的成功率达98%,异物吸入的死亡率也因此显著降低(从24%降至2%)[59]。更近期的病例系列报道显示,硬质支气管镜下气道异物移除的成功率为95%~99%[22,26-28,53,60,61]。

硬质支气管镜在移除气道异物上有诸多优势,它能通过标准的容量通气或高频喷射通气实现充分通气,具有良好的视野和吸引能力,同时配备多种取异物器械。这些器械包括光学钳、四爪钩、网篮、冷冻探头和球囊等。通常根据异物的类型和位置选取最合适的器械,有些病例可能需要配合使用多种器械。

在全麻下或内镜技术使用得当时,硬质支气管镜下取异物安全且有效,对许多儿科患者而言,这依然是取异物的首选方法[62]。其使用的局限性包括:全麻及其相关风险,对操作人员资质和技能的要求(在美国,只有少数普通肺病专家能开展硬质支气管镜操作)和医疗花费。

21.8.3 可弯曲支气管镜

对于成人患者,可弯曲支气管镜已成为初步评估和移除气道异物的首选手段。在专家手中,使用可弯曲支气管镜取异物安全且有效。它使患者和术者避免了上述硬质支气管镜检查中的种种不便。近来的数据显示,经验丰富的术者使用可弯曲支气管镜取气道异物的成功率超过90%[63]。此外,可弯曲支气管镜在取出牙齿、挡风玻璃碎片、耳塞、别针、钉子、鱼刺、花生和硬币等难以取出的异物方面也表现出色[35,36,64-69]。表21.3列出了在可弯曲支气管镜下成功取出的异物。

表21.3 经可弯曲支气管镜取气道异物的病例系列报道

第一作者	病例数	成功移除	成功率(%)
Hiller[70]	7	6	86
Cunanan[71]	300	267	89
Clark[72]	3	3	100
Nunez[73]	17	12	71
Lan[74]	33	32	97
Limper[60]	23	14	61
Chen[75]	43	32	74
Moura e sa[76]	2a	2a	100
Ali Ali[36]	16	9	56
Gencer[35]	23	21	91
Dong[50]	200	193	97
Fang[12]	94	85	90
Tenenbaum[9]	28	28	100

a 77名患者中,有2例患者,通过硬质支气管镜也无法取出异物。

虽然使用可弯曲支气管镜取异物的成功率很高,但该操作需经充分培训及准备。使用可弯曲支气管镜检查寻找气道异物时,必须全面、细致,因为吸入的异物可能被血液或肉芽组织覆盖,异物碎片可能分散到多支支气管内。

一旦明确了气道异物的类型、大小和位置,就可以尝试取出。建议术者在制订异物移除计划时,多准备几种器械。目前已开发了一系列取异物器械,包括可弯曲异物钳、鼠齿钳、圈套器、异物网篮、渔网篮、冷冻探头、球囊导管(Fogarty)和磁性抓取器等。

可弯曲与硬质支气管镜应用于异物取出时何者更优,当前仍存在着争论。随着可弯曲支气管镜技术的进步,笔者认为可弯曲支气管镜在成人气道异物的诊断和移除中至关重要。值得注意的是,并非每位肺科医师都能够熟练自如地操作可弯曲支气管镜以及应对异物取出失败的后果。如有疑问,应首先稳定患者的一般情况,并转诊至能够熟练开展可弯曲和硬质支气管镜相关操作的医疗机构。我们认为硬质支气管镜是一个候补工具，在进行异物取出过程中，应保证其随时可用。

21.8.3.1 可弯曲支气管镜下取异物的技术原则

要成功地解除气道梗阻，建议遵循以下基本的支气管镜技术原则。

21.8.3.1.1 原则一：支气管镜操作需有恰当指征

术前应认真审视支气管镜操作的目的和流程。为了错误的目的而实施支气管镜操作，往往会造成并发症和失误，并因而一错再错。

例如，尝试在局麻、可弯曲支气管镜下对儿童实施异物取出术就不甚恰当。儿童的气道较窄，异物位置变动后造成窒息的风险高。此外，儿童患者往往难达到充分镇静和配合，这增加了异物取出的难度。虽然可弯曲支气管镜是有用的诊断工具，但当明确有气道异物后，推荐使用硬质支气管镜取异物。

21.8.3.1.2 原则二：充分的准备是成功移除异物的关键

当试图走"捷径"时，一些问题和并发症往往会接踵而至。因此，在开展操作之前，应确保需要用到的所有支气管镜配件准备齐全，并逐一测试，同时备好各种可能用到的异物移除器械。操作者应随时准备好应对可能出现的困难和突发情况，在处理困难气道梗阻时需做到随机应变并灵活使用各种支气管镜介入技术[70,79]。

此外，仔细阅读影像学检查是非常重要的。有些情况下，需要与胸部放射科医师一起解读影像学检查结果。

21.8.3.1.3 原则三：支气管镜下异物移除术需有"第三双手"参与

一个常见的错误是尝试独自进行支气管镜操作。在支气管镜下取异物时，我们往往需要多一双手（如受过培训的助手）来插入并管理支气管镜过程中所需要的器械（如抓钳、异物网篮等），这样能确保操作者集中注意力操控支气管镜及相关工具到达目标部位。

21.8.3.1.4 原则四：顺利、安全的操作离不开培训良好的团队

有经验的术者都知道成功的支气管镜操作是团队合作的成果。一项研究表明，由经验丰富的医师和护士组成的团队协助取异物时，操作者耗时更少，感觉更轻松。支气管镜操作团队必须有明确的角色分工。可安排护士负责镇静并监测生命体征。接受过支气管镜辅助器械使用培训的助手可协助操作者进行内镜操作。此外，胸外科和麻醉师应能随时支援以应对并发症事件。

21.8.3.1.5 原则五：时间和奉献至关重要

多数失败的支气管镜操作往往是因为临床医师有其他工作安排，因而匆忙结束操作。耐心是必不可少的，医师应该奉献出必要的时间，直至取出异物。一次失败的支气管镜操作将增加患者再次内镜操作的风险。在患者没有急性呼吸窘迫的情况下，花费几个小时去准备一场组织良好、配合顺畅的支气管镜异物移除术也是值得的，这样能确保操作成功。如果在 24 h 内未取出异物，组织反应和继发气道炎症的风险将增加[18,22,55]。

21.8.3.1.6 原则六：认清自身局限性

取异物可能是最具挑战性的可弯曲支气管镜操作，这项任务可能需移交给团队中或其他医疗机构中经验更丰富、技能更熟练的成员来完成。经验欠缺的医师在取异物时更容易导致并发症[14]。无论是硬质支气管镜还是可弯曲支气管镜，异物移除的成功率主要取决于操作者的经验和技能，而不是器械本身。

21.8.3.1.7 原则七：每个病例都应被视为一个教学或培训机会

经验更丰富、技能更熟练的操作者需要将他们的技能传授给初级工作人员。应鼓励肺科住院医师和助理医师积极参与所有气道梗阻物的移除操作。这样做，医师不仅参与了对患者的照护，也确保了支气管镜技术的传承和完善。

21.8.3.2 麻醉和镇痛

可弯曲支气管镜取异物在中度镇静及局麻下就可开展，而硬质支气管镜则需要全身麻醉。在取异物时，镇静的一个显著优势是保留了咳嗽反射，这可以进一步促进异物的取出。通过支气管镜技术将异物移向气管，然后可以嘱患者咳出。

过去，对在缺乏气道保护的情况下实施中度镇静下的异物取出术颇具争议。其焦点在于异物在被移除的过程中可能会脱落至狭窄的声门下区域，从而增加窒息的风险。然而据我们所知，文献中并未报告过此类事件。

在困难病例中，当无法实现中度镇静时，采取全身麻醉下的硬质支气管镜检查是最佳选择。如异物位于气道远端，硬质支气管镜无法探及时，可在气管插管下使用可弯曲支气管镜来取异物。如果异物的大小超过气管插管的直径，可将异物固定住后，将其与气

管插管和支气管镜一起取出[80,81]。然后及时进行重新气管插管。另一个方案是使用喉罩来代替全麻下气管插管。即使在更深的镇静状态下，通过合理的气道管理，也可以实现可弯曲支气管镜操作[82,83]。

21.8.3.3 可弯曲支气管镜的辅助工具

用于可弯曲支气管镜异物取出的器械种类繁多。器械的选择在很大程度上取决于异物的位置、类型以及伴随的机体组织反应。

21.8.3.3.1 异物钳

异物钳是用于处理气道梗阻最常用和最广泛使用的器械。不同设计包括不同的钳口大小和形状、旋转机制、是否有齿以及其他附件，如中央开孔或细针等。选择的异物钳的钳口应足够大，需超过异物的整体直径。如需紧咬以防止硬质异物滑动，建议使用鳄鱼钳、鼠齿钳或鲨齿钳。对于更精细的操作，可以使用"W"形或尖端有包被的异物钳。一般而言，异物钳仅用于移除扁平或薄的无机异物（如硬币、别针、螺丝、夹子等）或坚硬的有机异物（如骨头）。而尝试使用异物钳来夹取易碎的有机异物可能会导致异物的断裂和散落。

21.8.3.3.2 球囊导管

充气式球囊导管可能是最有用但也未被充分利用的取异物器械。经支气管镜的工作通道置入 Fogarty 导管（尺寸 4~7 号），然后注入 1~3 mL 的生理盐水以使球囊膨胀。球囊可以逆行方式将异物从气道远端拉至近端（图 21.2）。其他一些专为支气管镜设计的充气式球囊导管也能找到。我们将在异物移除技术细节详述球囊导管的使用步骤。

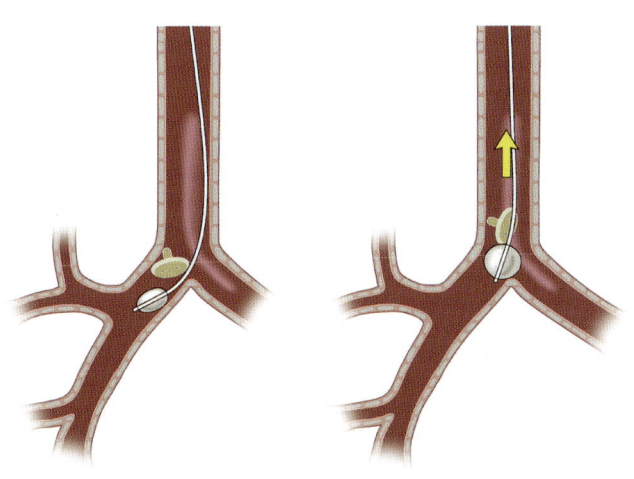

图 21.2 使用 Fogarty 球囊导管将异物移至近端气道

21.8.3.3.3 无尖端或改进型 Dormia 网篮

胃肠科和泌尿科医师从胆总管或输尿管中取结石的 Dormia 网篮的改进版本，也可用于支气管镜检查中移除气道异物。网篮的侧翼可收入聚酰胺/聚四氟乙烯外套内。网篮在气道中打开后，其镍钛合金丝"侧翼"可包绕并捕获住异物。这种网篮尤其适合移除较大的异物。它有 12 mm 和 16 mm 两种规格，对于移除形状不规则的异物非常有效。

21.8.3.3.4 渔网形网篮

渔网形网篮由电切圈套器改进而来，由一层细丝网与圈套器环相连而成，易于折叠和展开。网篮可回缩在鞘管内，以便轻松通过可弯曲支气管镜的工作通道。当圈套器环向前推进时，渔网会慢慢释放以包住异物。然后，慢慢回收圈套器环以将异物包裹在渔网内。完成后，网篮、被捕获的异物和支气管镜会作为一个整体取出。渔网形网篮在移除大块异物时也非常有用。

21.8.3.3.5 三爪/四爪圈套器

圈套器是一种非常灵活的器械，可用于抓取异物或肿瘤。圈套器通常收紧在鞘管内。操作时，圈套器的开口端被打开，从而包住异物。当操作者捏紧器械的手柄时，圈套器的远端会合拢，捕获异物。固定好后，可将异物、圈套器和可弯曲支气管镜小心地作为一个整体取出。由于圈套器相对脆弱，因此不建议在移除坚硬的、实心异物时使用此器械。一些特定的气道肿瘤可能会使用外科电圈套器来移除。

21.8.3.3.6 磁性抓取器

磁性抓取器由尖端带有磁性圆柱体的柔性探头组成。该器械专门设计成可通过支气管镜工作通道。使用此器械可以轻松地移除小型、可移动的金属异物，如断裂的镊子或细胞刷等。

21.8.3.3.7 冷冻治疗导管

支气管腔内冷冻疗法是应用超低温治疗气道内良恶性疾病的一种介入技术。冷冻探头的黏附性使其成为许多异物移除的理想工具。该系统含一个制冷剂罐（如一氧化二氮或氮气），通过将气体快速减压而在冷冻探头的尖端产生超低温（-40~-15 ℃）（图 21.3）。当冷冻探头直接接触到异物后，会将其黏附在探头上，然后操作者将可弯曲支气管镜连同冷冻探头和异物一起小心地取出。这种技术对于移除血块、黏液栓、有机物质和小型无机异物非常有效。根据我们的经验，这是移除有机物最有用的器械之一。操作时，支气管镜医师应当小心保持视野的清晰，以避免探头与周围黏膜接触而损伤正常组织。

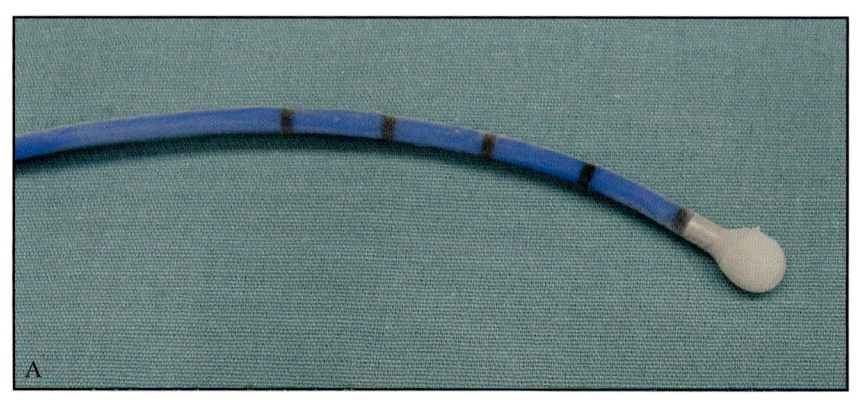
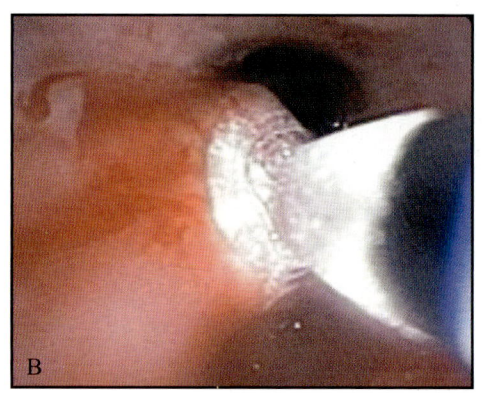

图 21.3 冷冻治疗

A. 冷冻探头；B. 冷冻探头在良性气道疾病中的应用。

21.8.4 可弯曲支气管镜

使用可弯曲支气管镜移除异物分为 3 个步骤：移动、固定和取出。取异物时，应经口途径置入可弯曲支气管镜，以避开狭窄的鼻腔通道。首先，应进行全面的气道检查。可先从未受影响侧肺叶开始检查。最后再对异物侧进行检查。进行全面、仔细地检查，确保只有一个异物且其碎片未分散到其他气道中。如能直接观察到异物，在尝试取出之前，应该仔细检查异物周围的毗邻关系。当在支气管镜视野下无法观察到异物的全貌时，需要在手术过程中查看放射学影像，以明确异物看不见部分所在位置。然后根据异物的大小、形状、位置和密度确定适当的移除器械。

在操作可弯曲支气管镜时，应避免将异物推至更远端的气道。通常，我们的策略是使用 Fogarty 球囊移动异物，并将其移动至气管近端，然后尝试固定以准备取出[64,92]。如图 21.2 所示，Fogarty 球囊导管被定位于异物的稍远端位置，然后充气，将异物（逆行拖动）从段支气管移动至气管。一旦异物移至气管中，将很容易取出。当将异物移动到上气道后，我们有时会要求患者坐起来，通过咳嗽将异物咳出。通常我们会对小而软的异物采用这种策略。

一个常见的误区是经支气管镜的工作通道来移除异物。移除异物的关键在于能够通过支气管镜相关器械来充分固定异物，无论是夹持还是套扎。一旦异物被夹持或套扎住，三者（支气管镜、夹持工具和异物）将可作为一个整体从支气管树中同时取出。在移除过程中，操作医师必须密切观察异物，始终保持其位于气道中央。

异物周围的组织反应也是影响异物取出的一个重要因素。如果异物隐藏在大量的肉芽组织中，移除将会很困难。这时，需要在取异物之前清理周围的肉芽组织。在这些情况下，可能需要全身麻醉配合，以进行支气管镜下的异物移除。此外，可以利用激光光切割将大的异物打碎成小块来取出[93,94]，或通过烧灼气化来清理包绕异物的肉芽组织。其他方式，如支气管镜下电凝治疗术，也可以用于清理周围的肉芽组织。一些学者建议在取异物操作前可以给予短程皮质激素治疗[19,78]。

咯血是取异物的一个罕见并发症，这在硬质支气管镜下很好处理。对于熟练的医生而言，咯血更为罕见。Rees 在对 2 500 例患者的回顾性研究中描述了 1 例异物取出导致的咯血事件[94]。故不必过度担心大咯血而用硬质支气管镜取代可弯曲支气管镜取异物[74,92]。

一旦出现咯血，我们的做法是通过支气管镜注入 1:10 000 稀释的肾上腺素腔内局部注入，以使局部血管收缩而达到止血目的。我们还发现局部使用冰生理盐水（4℃），也可通过低温血管收缩起到非常好的止血效果。

取锐器是一个不容犯错的挑战。取这类异物的关键在于找到尖锐头端并尝试将其移动。一旦尖锐头端被游离出来，就可以抓住并取出异物。夹持尖锐物体的柄或钝部可能会导致尖锐部分嵌入气管支气管黏膜中。

21.9 病例分享

一名既往健康的 34 岁男性因在胸部 X 线检查中偶然发现放射学异物（图 21.4 A）而从当地医疗机构

急诊转入。

患者诉 3 周前接受拔牙，过程顺利，但术后很快出现干咳，持续 3 周。拔牙术后的第 2 天，患者开始咳嗽，一直持续至此处就诊。因考虑到存在异物吸入的可能，患者被转诊过来准备接受可弯曲支气管镜下异物取出术。

异物移除术在设备齐全的支气管镜室内进行，术前给予静脉注射咪达唑仑和吗啡的中度镇静和利多卡因局部麻醉。支气管镜操作包括了全面的气道评估，从健侧开始。在仔细检查后，确定异物在右下肺叶，

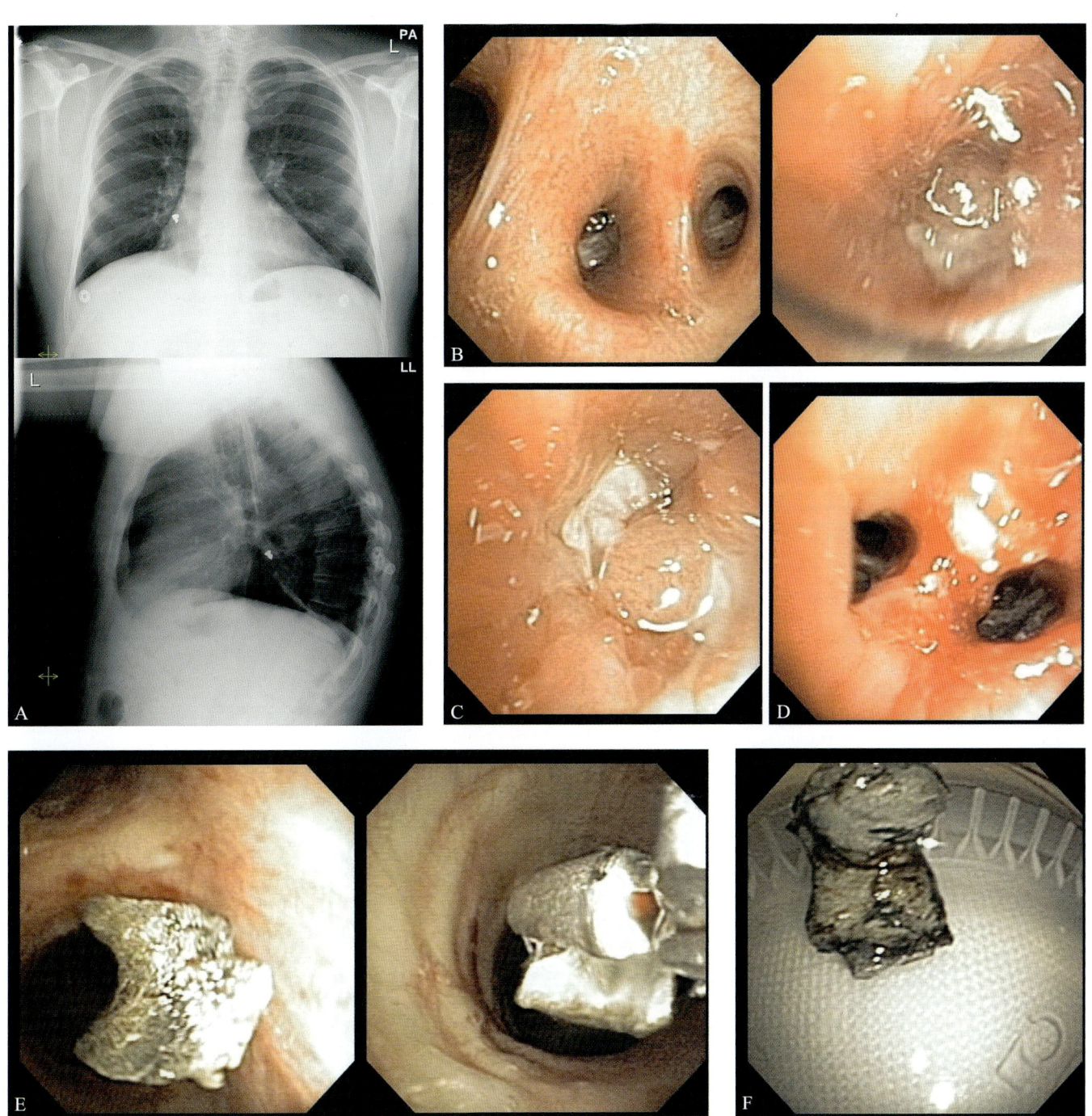

图 21.4　典型病例

A. 后前位和侧位胸片显示放射性异物位于右肺下叶后基底部；B. 支气管镜观察到右下叶后基底段气道区域有肉芽组织阻塞；C. 支气管镜下观察到右下叶后基底段阻塞，周围有脓液溢出；D. 清除肉芽组织后暴露出异物；E. 在 Fogarty 球囊的帮助下，异物被拉向近端，随后被活检钳夹住；F. 确认异物为牙齿充填物。

但由于肉芽组织的存在，无法看清异物（图 21.4 B）。在用 4 号 Fogarty 球囊探查了该区域后，发现肉芽组织周围的管腔存在一个小腔隙。用活检钳清理肉芽组织后，引流出被包裹于异物周围的脓性物质（图 21.4 C）。在 Fogarty 球囊的拖拽下，金属异物被暴露出来（图 21.4 D）。最后，用活检钳夹住了这枚形状不规则的异物并取出（图 21.4 E）。确认异物是一块牙齿填充物（图 21.4 F）。

在成功移除异物后，对病变所在区域再次进行了支气管镜探查，确认所有化脓物质均已被吸除，梗阻得到了解决。患者当天出院回家。

参考文献

1 Du Rand, I.A., Blaikley, J., Booton, R. et al. (2013). British Thoracic Society guideline for diagnostic flexible bronchoscopy in adults: accredited by NICE. *Thorax* 68 (Suppl 1): i1–i44.

2 Dikensoy, O., Usalan, C., and Filiz, A. (2002). Foreign body aspiration: clinical utility of flexible bronchoscopy. *Postgrad. Med. J.* 78: 399–403.

3 Salih, A.M., Alfaki, M., and Alam-Elhuda, D.M. (2016). Airway foreign bodies: a critical review for a common pediatric emergency. *World J. Emerg. Med.* 7: 5–12.

4 Lin, L., Lv, L., Wang, Y. et al. (2014). The clinical features of foreign body aspiration into the lower airway in geriatric patients. *Clin. Interv. Aging* 9: 1613–1618.

5 Feinberg, M.J., Knebl, J., Tully, J., and Segall, L. (1990). Aspiration and the elderly. *Dysphagia* 5: 61–71.

6 Martinot, A., Closset, M., Marquette, C.H. et al. (1997). Indications for flexible versus rigid bronchoscopy in children with suspected foreign-body aspiration. *Am. J. Respir. Crit. Care Med.* 155: 1676–1679.

7 Swanson, K.L., Prakash, U.B., Midthun, D.E. et al. (2002). Flexible bronchoscopic management of airway foreign bodies in children. *Chest* 121: 1695–1700.

8 Roberts, C.A. and Carr, M.M. (2018). Morbidity and mortality in children undergoing bronchoscopy for foreign body removal. *Laryngoscope* 128: 1226–1229.

9 Tenenbaum, T., Kahler, G., Janke, C. et al. (2017). Management of foreign body removal in children by flexible bronchoscopy. *J. Bronchol. Interv. Pulmonol.* 24: 21–28.

10 Injury Facts (2017). National Safety Council. https://injuryfacts.nsc.org/

11 Mittleman, R.E. and Wetli, C.V. (1982). The fatal cafe coronary. Foreign-body airway obstruction. *JAMA* 247: 1285–1288.

12 Fang, Y.F., Hsieh, M.H., Chung, F.T. et al. (2015). Flexible bronchoscopy with multiple modalities for foreign body removal in adults. *PLoS One* 10: e0118993.

13 al-Majed, S.A., Ashour, M., al-Mobeireek, A.F. et al. (1997). Overlooked inhaled foreign bodies: late sequelae and the likelihood of recovery. *Respir. Med.* 91: 293–296.

14 Baharloo, F., Veyckemans, F., Francis, C. et al. (1999). Tracheobronchial foreign bodies: presentation and management in children and adults. *Chest* 115: 1357–1362.

15 McGuirt, W.F., Holmes, K.D., Feehs, R., and Browne, J.D. (1988). Tracheobronchial foreign bodies. *Laryngoscope* 98: 615–618.

16 Mantor, P.C., Tuggle, D.W., and Tunell, W.P. (1989). An appropriate negative bronchoscopy rate in suspected foreign body aspiration. *Am. J. Surg.* 158: 622–624.

17 Hoeve, L.J., Rombout, J., and Pot, D.J. (1993). Foreign body aspiration in children. The diagnostic value of signs, symptoms and pre-operative examination. *Clin. Otolaryngol. Allied Sci.* 18: 55–57.

18 Wiseman, N.E. (1984). The diagnosis of foreign body aspiration in childhood. *J. Pediatr. Surg.* 19: 531–535.

19 Banerjee, A., Rao, K.S., Khanna, S.K. et al. (1988). Laryngo-tracheo-bronchial foreign bodies in children. *J. Laryngol. Otol.* 102: 1029–1032.

20 Pasaoglu, I., Dogan, R., Demircin, M. et al. (1991). Bronchoscopic removal of foreign bodies in children: retrospective analysis of 822 cases. *Thorac. Cardiovasc. Surg.* 39: 95–98.

21 Cleveland, R.H. (1979). Symmetry of bronchial angles in children. *Radiology* 133: 89–93.

22 Steen, K.H. and Zimmermann, T. (1990). Tracheobronchial aspiration of foreign bodies in children: a study of 94 cases. *Laryngoscope* 100: 525–530.

23 Ramchandani, R., Dewan, R.K., and Ramchandani, S. (2016). Incidental intraoperative diagnosis of retained foreign body lung misdiagnosed as pulmonary tuberculosis. *Lung India* 33: 444–446.

24 Heimlich, H.J. (1975). A life-saving maneuver to prevent food-choking. *JAMA* 234: 398–401.

25 Task Forces of the American Heart Association (2005). American Heart Association guidelines for cardiopulmonary resuscitation and emergency cardiovascular care. *Circulation* 112: IV1–IV203.

26 Daniilidis, J., Symeonidis, B., Triaridis, K., and Kouloulas, A. (1977). Foreign body in the airways: a review of 90 cases. *Arch. Otolaryngol.* 103: 570–573.

27 Abdulmajid, O.A., Ebeid, A.M., Motaweh, M.M., and Kleibo, I.S. (1976). Aspirated foreign bodies in the tracheobronchial tree: report of 250 cases. *Thorax* 31: 635–640.

28 Elhassani, N.B. (1988). Tracheobronchial foreign bodies in the Middle East. A Baghdad study. *J. Thorac. Cardiovasc. Surg.* 96: 621–625.

29 Mahmoud, M., Imam, S., Patel, H., and King, M. (2012). Foreign body aspiration of a dental bridge in the left main stem bronchus. *Case Rep. Med.* 2012: 798163.

30 Yapici, D., Atici, S., Birbicer, H., and Oral, U. (2008). Manufacturing defect in an endotracheal tube connector: risk of foreign body aspiration. *J. Anesth.* 22: 333–334.

31 Schembri, J., Cortis, K., Mallia Azzopardi, C., and Montefort, S. (2013). Aspiration of a speaking valve. *BMJ Case Rep.* 2013.

32 Kupeli, E., Khemasuwan, D., Lee, P., and Mehta, A.C. (2013). "Pills" and the air passages. *Chest* 144: 651–660.

33 Santos Costa, A. and Afonso, A. (2008). Endobronchial Helix

pomatia. A very rare foreign-body aspiration. *Rev. Port. Pneumol.* 14: 415–419.

34 Parvez, Y. and Kandath, M.A. (2016). Accidental aspiration of head scarf pin in left bronchus piercing the lung parenchyma: a rare case in a child. *Lung India* 33: 424–426.

35 Gencer, M., Ceylan, E., and Koksal, N. (2007). Extraction of pins from the airway with flexible bronchoscopy. *Respiration* 74: 674–679.

36 Al-Ali, M.A., Khassawneh, B., and Alzoubi, F. (2007). Utility of fiberoptic bronchoscopy for retrieval of aspirated headscarf pins. *Respiration* 74: 309–313.

37 Svedstrom, E., Puhakka, H., and Kero, P. (1989). How accurate is chest radiography in the diagnosis of tracheobronchial foreign bodies in children? *Pediatr. Radiol.* 19: 520–522.

38 Burton, E.M., Riggs, W. Jr., Kaufman, R.A., and Houston, C.S. (1989). Pneumomediastinum caused by foreign body aspiration in children. *Pediatr. Radiol.* 20: 45–47.

39 Esclamado, R.M. and Richardson, M.A. (1987). Laryngotracheal foreign bodies in children. A comparison with bronchial foreign bodies. *Am. J. Dis. Child.* 141: 259–262.

40 Shepard, J.A. (1995). The bronchi: an imaging perspective. *J. Thorac. Imaging* 10: 236–254.

41 Cevizci, N., Dokucu, A.I., Baskin, D. et al. (2008). Virtual bronchoscopy as a dynamic modality in the diagnosis and treatment of suspected foreign body aspiration. *Eur. J. Pediatr. Surg.* 18: 398–401.

42 Imaizumi, H., Kaneko, M., Nara, S. et al. (1994). Definitive diagnosis and location of peanuts in the airways using magnetic resonance imaging techniques. *Ann. Emerg. Med.* 23: 1379–1382.

43 Kitanaka, S., Mikami, I., Tokumaru, A., and O'Uchi, T. (1992). Diagnosis of peanut inhalation by MRI. *Pediatr. Radiol.* 22: 300–301.

44 O'Uchi, T., Tokumaru, A., Mikami, I. et al. (1992). Value of MR imaging in detecting a peanut causing bronchial obstruction. *Am. J. Roentgenol.* 159: 481–482.

45 Mu, L., He, P., and Sun, D. (1991). The causes and complications of late diagnosis of foreign body aspiration in children. Report of 210 cases. *Arch. Otolaryngol. Head Neck Surg.* 117: 876–879.

46 Falase, B., Sanusi, M., Majekodunmi, A. et al. (2013). Preliminary experience in the management of tracheobronchial foreign bodies in Lagos, Nigeria. *Pan Afr. Med. J.* 15: 31.

47 Atmaca, S., Unal, R., Sesen, T. et al. (2009). Laryngeal foreign body mistreated as recurrent laryngitis and croup for one year. *Turk. J. Pediatr.* 51: 65–66.

48 Barben, J., Berkowitz, R.G., Kemp, A., and Massie, J. (2000). Bronchial granuloma – where's the foreign body? *Int. J. Pediatr. Otorhinolaryngol.* 53: 215–219.

49 Saliba, J., Mijovic, T., Daniel, S. et al. (2012). Asthma: the great imitator in foreign body aspiration? *J. Otolaryngol. Head Neck Surg.* 41: 200–206.

50 Dong, Y.C., Zhou, G.W., Bai, C. et al. (2012). Removal of tracheobronchial foreign bodies in adults using a flexible bronchoscope: experience with 200 cases in China. *Intern. Med.* 51: 2515–2519.

51 Oka, M., Fukuda, M., Takatani, H. et al. (1996). Chronic bronchial foreign body mimicking peripheral lung tumor. *Intern. Med.* 35: 219–221.

52 Matsuse, H., Shimoda, T., Kawano, T. et al. (2001). Airway foreign body with clinical features mimicking bronchial asthma. *Respiration* 68: 103–105.

53 Kosloske, A.M. (1982). Bronchoscopic extraction of aspirated foreign bodies in children. *Am. J. Dis. Child.* 136: 924–927.

54 Kosloske, A.M. (1980). Tracheobronchial foreign bodies in children: back to the bronchoscope and a balloon. *Pediatrics* 66: 321–323.

55 Law, D. and Kosloske, A.M. (1976). Management of tracheobronchial foreign bodies in children: a reevaluation of postural drainage and bronchoscopy. *Pediatrics* 58: 362–367.

56 Bose, P. and El Mikatti, N. (1981). Foreign bodies in the respiratory tract. A review of forty-one cases. *Ann. R. Coll. Surg. Engl.* 63: 129–131.

57 Cotton, E.K., Abrams, G., Vanhoutte, J., and Burrington, J. (1973). Removal of aspirated foreign bodies by inhalation and postural drainage. A survey of 24 cases. *Clin. Pediatr.* 12: 270–276.

58 Panchabhai, T.S. and Mehta, A.C. (2015). Historical perspectives of bronchoscopy. Connecting the dots. *Ann. Am. Thorac. Soc.* 12: 631–641.

59 Jackson, C. and Jackson, C.L. (1936). Diseases of the Air and Food Passages of Foreign-Body Origin. Philadelphia: Saunders.

60 Limper, A.H. and Prakash, U.B. (1990). Tracheobronchial foreign bodies in adults. *Ann. Intern. Med.* 112: 604–609.

61 Hsu, W., Sheen, T., Lin, C. et al. (2000). Clinical experiences of removing foreign bodies in the airway and esophagus with a rigid endoscope: a series of 3217 cases from 1970 to 1996. *Otolaryngol. Head Neck Surg.* 122: 450–454.

62 Faro, A., Wood, R.E., Schechter, M.S. et al. (2015). Official American Thoracic Society technical standards: flexible airway endoscopy in children. *Am. J. Respir. Crit. Care Med.* 191: 1066–1080.

63 Debeljak, A., Sorli, J., Music, E., and Kecelj, P. (1999). Bronchoscopic removal of foreign bodies in adults: experience with 62 patients from 1974–1998. *Eur. Respir. J.* 14: 792–795.

64 Heinz, G.J. 3rd, Richardson, R.H., and Zavala, D.C. (1978). Endobronchial foreign body removal using the bronchofiberscope. *Ann. Otol. Rhinol. Laryngol.* 87: 50–52.

65 Mehta, A.C. and Grimm, M. (1988). Breakage of Nd-YAG laser sapphire contact probe inside the endobronchial tree. *Chest* 93: 1119.

66 Fieselmann, J.F., Zavala, D.C., and Keim, L.W. (1977). Removal of foreign bodies (two teeth) by fiberoptic bronchoscopy. *Chest* 72: 241–243.

67 Klayton, R.J., Donlan, C.J., O'Neil, T.J., and Foreman, D.R. (1975). Letter: Foreign body removal via fiberoptic bronchoscopy. *JAMA* 234: 806.

68 Lee, M., Fernandez, N.A., Berger, H.W., and Givre, H. (1982). Wire basket removal of a tack via flexible fiberoptic bronchoscopy. *Chest* 82: 515.

69 Rohde, F.C., Celis, M.E., and Fernandez, S. (1977). The removal of an endobronchial foreign body with the fiberoptic

70 Hiller, C., Lerner, S., Varnum, R. et al. (1977). Foreign body removal with the flexible fiberoptic bronchoscope. *Endoscopy* 9: 216–222.

71 Cunanan, O.S. (1978). The flexible fiberoptic bronchoscope in foreign body removal. Experience in 300 cases. *Chest* 73: 725–726.

72 Clark, P.T., Williams, T.J., Teichtahl, H. et al. (1989). Removal of proximal and peripheral endobronchial foreign bodies with the flexible fibreoptic bronchoscope. *Anaesth. Intensive Care* 17: 205–208.

73 Nunez, H., Perez Rodriguez, E., Alvarado, C. et al. (1989). Foreign body aspirate extraction. *Chest* 96: 698.

74 Lan, R.S., Lee, C.H., Chiang, Y.C., and Wang, W.J. (1989). Use of fiberoptic bronchoscopy to retrieve bronchial foreign bodies in adults. *Am. Rev. Respir. Dis.* 140: 1734–1737.

75 Chen, C.H., Lai, C.L., Tsai, T.T. et al. (1997). Foreign body aspiration into the lower airway in Chinese adults. *Chest* 112: 129–133.

76 Moura e Sa, J., Oliveira, A., Caiado, A. et al. (2006). Tracheobronchial foreign bodies in adults – experience of the Bronchology Unit of Centro Hospitalar deVila Nova de Gaia. *Rev. Port. Pneumol.* 12: 31–43.

77 Nussbaum, E. (1983). Flexible fiberoptic bronchoscopy and laryngoscopy in infants and children. *Laryngoscope* 93: 1073–1075.

78 Bolliger, C.T. and Mathur, P.N. (2000). Interventional Bronchoscopy. Basel: Karger.

79 Gibson, W.S. Jr. and Vrabec, D.P. (2000). Encounters with challenging bronchial foreign bodies: impromptu adaptation of technique. *Ann. Otol. Rhinol. Laryngol.* 109: 86–88.

80 Downey, R.J., Libutti, S.K., Gorenstein, L., and Mercer, S. (1995). Airway management during retrieval of the very large aspirated foreign body: a method for the flexible bronchoscope. *Anesth. Analg.* 81: 186–187.

81 Verea-Hernando, H., Garcia-Quijada, R.C., and Ruiz de Galarreta, A.A. (1990). Extraction of foreign bodies with fiberoptic bronchoscopy in mechanically ventilated patients. *Am. Rev. Respir. Dis.* 142: 258.

82 Hirai, T., Yamanaka, A., Fujimoto, T. et al. (1999). Bronchoscopic removal of bronchial foreign bodies through the laryngeal mask airway in pediatric patients. *Jpn. J. Thorac. Cardiovasc. Surg.* 47: 190–192.

83 McGrath, G., Das-Gupta, M., and Clarke, G. (2001). Bronchoscopy via continuous positive airway pressure for patients with respiratory failure. *Chest* 119: 670–671.

84 Kim, J.H., Jeong, G.M., Park, K.H. et al. (2015). Large endobronchial hamartoma successfully resected by snare through flexible bronchoscopy. *Ann. Thorac. Surg.* 100: 1107–1109.

85 Yun, S.C., Na, M.J., Choi, E. et al. (2013). Successful removal of endobronchial lipoma by flexible bronchoscopy using electrosurgical snare. *Tuberc. Respir. Dis.* 74: 82–85.

86 Saito, H., Saka, H., Sakai, S., and Shimokata, K. (1989). Removal of broken fragment of biopsy forceps with magnetic extractor. *Chest* 95: 700–701.

87 Mayr, J., Dittrich, S., and Triebl, K. (1997). A new method for removal of metallic-ferromagnetic foreign bodies from the tracheobronchial tree. *Pediatr. Surg. Int.* 12: 461–462.

88 Zhang, L., Yin, Y., Zhang, J., and Zhang, H. (2016). Removal of foreign bodies in children's airways using flexible bronchoscopic CO_2 cryotherapy. *Pediatr. Pulmonol.* 51: 943–949.

89 Lee, H., Leem, C.S., Lee, J.H. et al. (2014). Successful removal of endobronchial blood clots using bronchoscopic cryotherapy at bedside in the intensive care unit. *Tuberc. Respir. Dis.* 77: 193–196.

90 Rubio, E., Gupta, P., Ie, S., and Boyd, M. (2013). Cryoextraction: a novel approach to remove aspirated chewing gum. *Ann. Thorac. Med.* 8: 58–59.

91 Mehta, A.C. and Dweik, R.A. (1996). Nasal versus oral insertion of the flexible bronchoscope: pro-nasal insertion. *J. Bronchol. Interv. Pulmonol.* 3: 224–228.

92 Mehta, A.C. and Dasgupta, A. (1997). Bronchoscopic approach to tracheobronchial foreign bodies in adults pro-flexible bronchoscopy. *J. Bronchol. Interv. Pulmonol.* 4: 173–178.

93 Boelcskei, P.L., Wagner, M., and Lessnau, K.K. (1995). Laser-assisted removal of a foreign body in the bronchial system of an infant. *Lasers Surg. Med.* 17: 375–377.

94 Rees, J.R. (1985). Massive hemoptysis associated with foreign body removal. *Chest* 88: 475–476.

95 Hayashi, A.H., Gillis, D.A., Bethune, D. et al. (1990). Management of foreign-body bronchial obstruction using endoscopic laser therapy. *J. Pediatr. Surg.* 25: 1174–1176.

第 22 章

支气管镜在咯血中的应用

Guo-wu Zhou[1,2], Hai-dong Huang[1,3,4], Chong Bai[1], and Sunit R. Patel[5]

[1] Respiratory and Critical Care Medicine, Changhai Hospital,
Second Military Hospital, Shanghai, China
[2] Respiratory and Critical Care Medicine, China-Japan Friendship Hospital, Beijing, China
[3] Interventional Pulmonology Center of SMMU Respiratory and Critical Care Medicine,
Changhai Hospital, Second Military Medical University (SMMU), Shanghai, China
[4] International Training Center for Interventional Pulmonology,
Henry Ford Hospital, Shanghai, China
[5] Medical Group, Trulock, CA, USA

（译者：周国武　译者单位：中日友好医院）

咯血是指将声门以下出血咳出的过程[1]。它是临床常见的症状[2]。6.8%肺科门诊患者[3]和11%肺科住院患者因咯血[4]就诊，38%普胸外科手术患者[5]及15%的肺科门诊患者存在咯血[6]。咯血的诊断是一项挑战，因为多种心肺疾病和血液系统疾病均可导致咯血[7-11]。引起咯血最常见的病因是慢性支气管炎、支气管扩张症、支气管肺癌和结核[4,7,8,12-15]。然而多年来，由于引起咯血的疾病谱一直在变化，导致了咯血的诊断面临困境[4,7,16,17]。

评估咯血患者时应关注以下4个方面：①能否排除肺癌；②明确潜在病变是否可治；③定位出血部位以便需要进一步的介入治疗[6]；④如果出血持续存在或再发大咯血，需决定何时进行何种治疗。鉴于此，支气管镜技术特别是可弯曲支气管镜已经成为诊断、定位出血点和治疗咯血的核心手段[18]。事实上，咯血是支气管镜检查最常见的指征之一，其病例数在一些大的医疗中心占10%~30%[7,15,19,20]。例如，1989年美国胸科医师协会（ACCP）对871名支气管镜医师进行的调查发现，81.1%的受访者报告咯血是支气管镜检查最常见的五大原因之一。

在此背景下，本章回顾了咯血的定义、病理生理机制、鉴别诊断以及系统的诊断路径，并将重点阐述支气管镜在咯血诊疗中的作用。

22.1　大咯血与非大咯血的定义

咯血可表现为从痰中带血至大咯血导致窒息和休克等。因为对于咯血的整体管理是基于其严重程度，所以多数学者将咯血分为大咯血（存在潜在致命风险）和非大咯血[1,11,22,23]。虽然目前关于非大咯血没有明确的定义，但一般是指少量到中等量咯血，界定为痰中带血和24 h内咯血量小于30 mL[1,23,24]。较大量的咯血一般是指咯血量比大咯血小，但是比血痰要多[11]。

表22.1总结了一些关于大咯血的定义。这些定义均从咯血量（如24 h咯血600 mL）和咯血引起的严重并发症（如咯血引起的窒息）两方面来进行描述[2,25-31]。文献报道大咯血的标准从24 h内咯血100~1 000 mL。一般24 h内咯血小于100 mL都认为

是非大咯血[26,27]。大咯血最宽松的定义由 Amirana[25]、Bobbrowitz[26]等提出。他们将大咯血的标准制定为 1 天内至少 1 次 100 mL 或以上的咯血。Crocco 等[28]提出将大咯血的标准定为 48 h 内咯血 600 mL 以上，而 Corey 和 Hla[29]则将大咯血的标准定为 24 h 内咯血量至少 1 000 mL。

表 22.1　大咯血的定义

根据容量定义
≥100 mL/24 h [25,26]
>600 mL/48 h [27]
较大量咯血（≥200 mL/24 h）对大咯血（≥1 000 mL/24 h）[28]
根据咯血后果定义
出现大量误吸
危及生命的气道阻塞、低血压和贫血
根据咯血量和速度定义
咯血量≥1 000 mL 或速度≥150 mL/h
广为接受的概念
24 h 咯血量≥600 mL

引自：Stoller[2]。

其他一些学者则使用临床严重程度代替咯血量来定义大咯血。气道的解剖无效腔多数为 100~200 mL，大咯血带来的风险主要是咯出的血液阻塞了气道，从而导致危及生命的气道阻塞、低血压、血气交换障碍以及血液流失。最后，Holsclaw 等[27,30]提出了一种具备操作性的大咯血定义，即符合以下 3 条：①咯血导致死亡或需要住院救治；②咯血导致失血引起的临床表现或实验室异常；③咯血导致需要进行输血或输血浆。

Garzon 等[27,31]提出大咯血不仅仅是通过窒息（因气道被阻塞）危及生命，同时也会因为大量失血导致低血压，此时失血量>1 000 mL 或失血速度≥150 mL/h。虽然目前广为接受的大咯血的定义是 24 h 咯血量至少超过 600 mL，但在临床实践中，精确计算咯血量比较困难[2]。同时，在临床中，咯血的频率和咯血量一样的重要[37,39]。Crocco 等[28]通过对 67 例 48 h 内咯血量超过 600 mL 的患者进行观察，发现排除治疗因素，患者死亡率和咯血速度相关。特别是 4 h 内咯血量达到 600 mL 的患者，其死亡率为 71%；4~6 h 咯血量达到 600 mL 的患者，其死亡率为 45%；而 16~48 h 内咯血量为 600 mL 的患者，其死亡率约为 5%。

22.2　咯血的病因

有时尽管做了很多工作，甚至包括可弯曲支气管镜检查，仍不能明确咯血的病因。这类咯血被称为特发性咯血、原发性咯血或隐源性咯血，占咯血患者的 2%~18%[4,8-10,13,15,38]。特发性咯血的典型表现是只有咯血而甚少或无其他呼吸系统症状，且胸片和支气管镜检查未见异常，支气管肺泡灌洗液也无感染或恶性肿瘤的证据[7,40]。幸运的是，特发性咯血一般 6 个月内会停止[40]。此外，上消化道出血（呕血），也称假性咯血，表现类似真性咯血（当血液被吸入肺内时），它是由于血液经口腔或鼻咽腔回流到喉后壁，激惹咳嗽反射所致。利福平服药过量的患者也可表现为红色痰液。

随着疾病发病率的变化（如新发支气管扩张的降低）和诊断技术的进步（如自 20 世纪 70 年代以来可弯曲支气管镜的应用），咯血的常见病因谱也在发生相应变化。研究发现，在 20 世纪 40~50 年代，最常见的咯血原因是结核、支气管扩张及支气管肺癌[5,12-15]。然而，研究发现，如今咯血最常见的原因是支气管炎，而结核和支气管扩张导致的咯血在逐渐减少[16,17]。

只有少数患者表现为大咯血（咯血住院患者 4.8%~6.7% 发生大咯血）[4,29]，且大咯血的病因谱较窄。引起大咯血最常见的原因是支气管扩张、结核（活动性或非活动性）、支气管肺癌、肺脓肿及足分枝菌病等[2,28,31,33,34,47-49]。与导致普通咯血的病因不同（咯血的病因中，结核和支气管扩张所占比重已经逐渐降低）[16,17]，大咯血的病因在过去 30 年中，未发生明显的变化。

22.3　咯血的病理生理机制

肺出血的来源包括低压的肺动脉循环系统（正常肺动脉收缩压为 15~20 mmHg，舒张压为 5~10 mmHg）、支气管动脉循环系统（其起源于主动脉，压强等同于体循环压），以及支气管静脉（通过全身静脉系统进入右心）[2]。支气管动脉是气道（从主气管到终末细支气管）和肺支撑结构（如胸膜、肺内淋巴组织、大的肺血管及神经）的主要供血血管[11,50]。

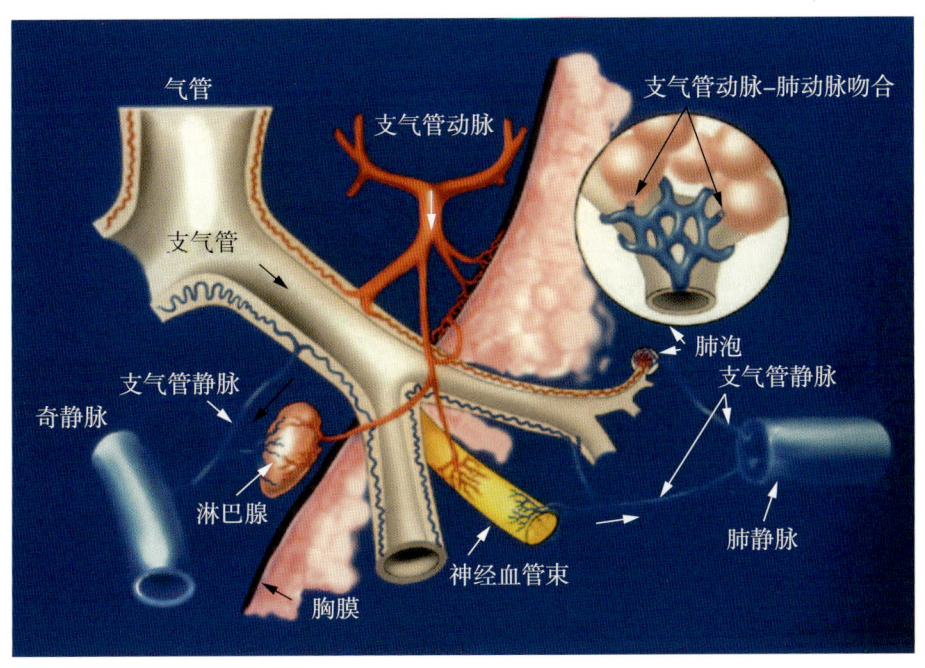

图 22.1 肺血供系统示意图

血流灌注到肺内支气管和支撑结构后回流至右心，而肺内血管引流至肺静脉并汇入左心。来源：经 Deffebach 等许可转载。[45]

肺动脉主要向肺实质包括呼吸性细支气管供血[11,50]。

如图 22.1 所示，支气管循环和肺循环是相连的，滋养近端气道的支气管动脉血流入支气管静脉并最终汇入右心，而灌注肺内支气管和肺组织的支气管动脉则通过支气管肺循环吻合引流至肺静脉并汇入左心[2,51]。尸检报告显示，位于支气管动脉和肺静脉分支之间的吻合负责正常的肺内右向左的分流，这可能是大咯血的主要来源[51]。动脉血管造影结果显示，在活动性咯血的患者（92%的患者）中，出血点位于支气管循环系统[51]。动脉造影显示支气管动脉扩张、膨大侧支循环形成，或可见与局部出血部位相符的活动性出血[51]。另外，肺循环也有可能是咯血的来源。例如，由于 Swan-Ganz 动脉导管置入所造成的肺动脉破裂、继发于胶原血管疾病的肺动脉瘤以及肺动脉血管炎等[27]。

22.4 咯血的诊断流程

所有的咯血均需经仔细评估后探明病因及出血部位。支气管镜检查有助于同时达成上述目标。

22.4.1 支气管镜术前常规评估

支气管镜术前常规评估的目的主要包括两方面，一方面通过临床特征初步判断可能的咯血原因和部位，以指导制定支气管镜检查的策略；另一方面，通过术前常规检查，排除可能存在的手术禁忌证。

如前所述，咯血的病因纷繁复杂，需要通过详细的病史、体格检查、实验室检查以及影像学检查进行细致的鉴别诊断。需要注意的是，超过 30%的患者胸片并无异常[11]，需要做进一步检查[10]。一些可能引起咯血但是胸片阴性的疾病包括：支气管炎、支气管扩张、支气管结石、局部感染、血管瘤、梗死形成、主动脉支气管瘘以及一些尚未导致支气管闭塞的支气管腔内病变[27,66]。

如果明确了出血来源于肺，则需尽快明确出血部位，尤其是针对反复咯血或者大咯血的患者，只有明确了出血部位，才能够选择最佳的治疗方式[2]。明确出血部位也有利于选择下一步的诊断技术，如灌洗和活检。综合使用各种手段定位出血点的总体成功率达 75%~93%[38,68]。即便无法到达特定肺叶水平，95%的病例也可明确出血侧[69]。Pursel 和 Lindskog 对 105 例咯血患者进行统计分类，比较了不同定位策略的准确率[4]，发现有 10%的患者进行了自我评估，但准确率最低，错误率达到了 30%；临床体格检查等准确定位了 43%的出血来源，错误率为 2%；胸部影像学准确识别了 60%患者的出血部位，错误率为 0%；支气管镜检查的准确率最高（86%），但是只有20%的患者接受了支气管镜检查。

鉴于支气管镜检查已广泛地作为定位咯血（无论是否大咯血）[11,49]部位的首选方式，为了制定一条完美的诊断路径我们必须深入了解支气管镜的作用。

22.4.2 支气管镜检查的适应证

咯血和影像学确诊的肺实质浸润影（如肿块影、渗出、空洞、肺不张等）已公认是支气管镜检查的适应证。对于这类患者而言，支气管镜检查的诊断率约为80%[20,70-76]，其中癌症占了1/3[70]。

对于胸片正常或者影像学改变不局限的咯血患者来说，是否行支气管镜检查存在争议。当患者存在以下临床表现时（特别是怀疑为肺癌时），支气管镜检查的阳性率会提高，包括年龄>40岁、出血持续时间超过1周、痰血量>30 mL、吸烟量>40包/年以及男性患者[69-71,77,78]。

如患者无上述临床特征，是否需行支气管镜检查尚且存争议。虽然有些研究建议应在痰细胞学阴性以及耳鼻喉镜检查后再行支气管镜检查[70-72,77-79]，但其他研究则推荐对所有咯血患者都进行支气管镜检查，因为有4%~22%的咯血患者胸片正常，或者不存在局限性影像学改变[20,73,80-82]。例如，Poe等对196位患者进行支气管镜检查，结果发现6%患者为支气管肺癌，另外有17%的患者存在其他病变[78]。O'Neil发现119位支气管镜受检患者中，5%为恶性肿瘤[70]。Lee等在一项回顾性研究中对478位咯血但胸片无异常的患者进行了支气管镜检查，其中2.1%的患者诊断为恶性肿瘤，支气管镜检查的阳性率为4.2%[63]。Lederle等对106位40岁以上、咯血但是胸片无异常或者无局部浸润影的患者进行了支气管镜检查，发现其中4.7%的患者为支气管肺癌[64]。

尽管不常见，但40岁以下的年轻患者中存在支气管源性肿瘤，对于这类患者也应考虑行支气管镜检查。例如，Snider报道在955例患者中，有5%诊断为支气管肺癌的患者均在45岁以下[52]。类似的，Cortese等报道，5.5%的影像学诊断肺癌的患者年龄<50岁[65]。基于这些研究，笔者认为，除非咯血原因已明，否则所有的咯血患者都应该行支气管镜检查。

虽说所有明显或新发咯血患者都有进行支气管镜检查的指征，但有些临床情况也可能不需要。包括：慢性支气管炎患者偶发的轻微痰中带血，尤其是急性气管支气管炎发作期[11,18]；急性下呼吸道感染的患者[11]；最近已经通过支气管镜检查明确了出血部位的患者[11]；患者有心脏和肺血管的疾病，如充血性心力衰竭以及肺血栓栓塞症[11]。尽管支气管镜检查的适应证很宽泛，实施支气管镜检查的决定应个体化，需根据可能的病因区别对待。

22.4.3 支气管镜检查的时机

是尽早（急性出血48 h内）还是推迟进行支气管镜检查，目前尚有争议。表22.2展示了3项早期对比延迟行支气管镜检查的研究[4,20,66,3]。3项研究的结果都显示早期行支气管镜检查可以增加定位出血点的成功率。然而，仔细分析支气管镜检查的诊断价值，发现尽管早期检查较延迟检查能更好地观察到活动性出血和出血部位（分别为34%和11%），但是支气管镜检查的时机并不能改变病因判断和患者整体治疗方案[20]。尽管存在这些争议，我们还是建议尽早地行支气管镜检查来明确出血部位，因为其随时可能发展为大咯血，并且尽早行支气管镜检查也能减少陈旧性的血块因为咳嗽或重力影响而重新分布的概率[49]。

表22.2 比较对咯血患者早期和延迟行支气管镜检查的相关文献总结

研究	数量	支气管镜	延迟	尽早
Pursel, 1961[4]	105	硬质	52	86
Smiddy, 1973[66]	71（active）	可弯曲	NS	93
Gong, 1981[20]	129	可弯曲	11	34
Bobrowitz, 1983[26]	25	可弯曲	NS	86
Rath, 1973[73]	31	可弯曲	NS	68
Corey, 1987[28]	59	NS	NS	39
Saumench, 1989[85]	36	可弯曲	50	91

表头"定位出血部位诊断率（%）"横跨"支气管镜"、"延迟"、"尽早"三列。

NS，未说明。摘自：Stoller JK. 大咯血的诊断和处理：综述。Respir Care 1992；32：564-581.

22.4.4 设备的选择

可弯曲支气管镜适用于非大咯血的患者，因其仅需局麻，在门诊和床旁即可开展。大多数患者的耐受性好，可以清晰地看到亚肺段，包括上叶支气管[7,49,54]。

对于大咯血的患者，使用硬质支气管镜还是可弯曲支气管镜存在争议，目前研究也尚无定论。目前来看，选择取决于操作者的经验。外科医生偏向于使用硬质支气管镜，而内科医生则偏向于可弯曲支气管镜。硬质支气管镜最大的优点是吸引能力强，腔道大，可送入填塞止血材料、进行灌洗，且能持续掌控气道[6]。

然而，硬质支气管镜视野受限，操作需在手术室全麻下进行。Neff总结道，在急诊大咯血的患者中，硬质支气管镜较可弯曲支气管镜看起来更有优势。其实重要的是经验丰富的内、外科医生的密切交流，而选择哪种支气管镜并不那么重要[67]。

对近期有大咯血的患者行可弯曲支气管镜检查时，需使用大内径的经口气管插管进行气道管理，气管镜可经此进入[37]。如果气管镜镜头被血液糊住需要清理时，气管插管也可以保证气管镜可以快速地进出[37,68]。除了气道管理，还可经气管插管送入大孔径的吸引导管去吸引血块[69]。可弯曲支气管镜下可对每个亚段支气管进行冲洗，并抵近观察有无新鲜出血[37]。

1998年，ACCP[69]开展了一项有关大咯血气道急症处理的调研，共有230位医师参加，其中79%倾向经气管插管使用可弯曲支气管镜，较之10年前的48%明显增加[69]。如果选择可弯曲支气管镜，推荐使用大工作通道的支气管镜（2.6~3.0 mm的通道，最新的治疗型支气管镜吸引通道甚至已达3.2 mm）[32]。如果出血速度超出了可弯曲支气管镜的吸引能力，可经硬质支气管镜置入可弯曲支气管镜，这样既安全（如气道管理、吸引能力等）又操作灵活[36,70]。这个操作也可应用在气管支气管腔内肿瘤的激光治疗上[18,71,72]。

如检查过程中需持续机械通气，不管是硬质支气管镜还是可弯曲支气管镜，都可以使用高频喷射通气。其开放式系统既可以保证通气，又可以同时进行支气管镜检查、吸引以及定位。

22.4.5　可弯曲支气管镜进镜路径

如果明确出血部位位于声门下，那么从鼻腔或者口腔进入气道都可以。但如对出血来源还存疑，则应对上气道开展评估。Selecky指出支气管镜经口进入时对鼻咽后壁有一个独特的视角，操作者需要将镜头朝头端弯曲180°来查看后鼻道和后鼻甲[7]。如果怀疑上气道有出血且经鼻进镜，那么双侧鼻道都需要进行评估。

22.4.6　支气管镜检查发现

虽然支气管镜检查是最好的诊断咯血和确认出血部位的方法，但是它并不一定能够精确地找到出血点。例如，Smiddy和Elliot[68]对71例咯血患者进行可弯曲支气管镜检查，仅46.5%的患者找出了出血点。38%的病例能将出血部位定位至段支气管，8.45%明确为多点出血，还有7.0%的患者未找到出血部位。为了提高支气管镜检查的阳性率，应尽可能将支气管镜送至其能到达的最远端，最好可以到达亚段支气管[18]。有时候，选用小外径的支气管镜或者小儿支气管镜可以提高诊断率，因为可以到达更远的支气管树[71]。在上文中也讨论过[37]，在段支气管水平以无菌生理盐水灌洗也有助于明确出血的来源。支气管镜检查时，需要对黏膜和可见的血管特别注意，因为显而易见的血管、支气管炎性改变以及微小的黏膜改变都是有价值的发现[18]。

在1988年ACCP对于咯血的调查中[32]，要求临床医生对支气管镜镜下表现及其对临床诊断的意义进行打分，虽然特异性的诊断（如肺癌）比非特异性的结果更有用，但是超过80%的人认为支气管镜检查下非特异性的发现（如支气管炎性改变、正常气道、局部的或者弥漫性的气管支气管内出血）都对临床诊断有作用。

根据潜在的疾病不同，所有的不正常表现都需要活检、刷检或者进行灌洗以留取足够的标本进行检验[7]，但是需要注意的是，对于富含血供，尤其是怀疑支气管黏膜血管畸形的病灶，行活检时应慎重，且均需完善胸部增强CT检查或支气管动脉造影，以评估局部血供情况。Katoh等[73]对比了7位咯血的患者的支气管镜下表现和支气管动脉造影结果。结果发现，病变均位于第2到第5级支气管，表现为隆起性或肿块性病灶。5位患者经支气管镜检查发现了隆起性病灶。这5位患者中，有1位患者经动脉造影术后确认为动脉瘤，另外4位患者的隆起性病变经支气管动脉造影提示为血管丛聚。另外2位患者的支气管肿块性病灶，经动脉造影提示1例为血管阻塞伴局部扩张，另1例为血管丛聚。支气管动脉栓塞术后这些病灶均缩小或消失。然而，有研究报道，某些支气管动脉病灶在支气管镜下类似肿瘤，如果行活检术，会造成后果严重的出血[74,75]。

Dieulafoy病是一种以黏膜下动脉扭曲发育不良为特点的血管畸形病[76-78]。虽然这种畸形更常见于胃黏膜，但是也有报道Dieulafoy病有可见于支气管黏膜。需对此提高警惕，因其破裂可能造成反复大咯血。支气管镜检查如果镜下发现直径数毫米的隆起性病变，且其表面黏膜正常时，需要怀疑 Dieulafoy 病（避免活检术）。出血灶常被血液或血块所包绕。气道 Dieulafoy 病也偶有报道。近期一项研究报道了 81 例隐源性咯血的患者，其中有 9 例患者最终诊断为 Dieulafoy 病，其中 5 例最终行外科手术治疗才控制住咯血[77]。

22.5　支气管镜在咯血治疗中的作用

随着支气管镜下局部治疗技术的发展，支气管镜在咯血中的应用有了很大的改变[79]。这些技术被用来治疗大咯血或者危及生命的咯血，也能和外科治疗结合使用。作为辅助措施，支气管镜下治疗能为稳定患者病情赢得时间，从而完善必要的诊断，以决定是采取栓塞还是外科治疗。支气管镜下治疗技术包括肺隔离和气道管理技术、支气管内球囊或支气管镜下直接填塞、冰生理盐水冲洗、激光治疗、电凝止血、近距离放疗、使用血管收缩剂和促凝血剂等。

22.5.1　肺隔离和气道管理

能否稳定得住咯血患者的气道情况，取决于医生是否有能力进行气管插管，保护健侧肺，隔离患侧肺，填塞出血部位，或者应用各种内镜技术或药物干预的方法成功止血。下文将介绍几种可以达此目的的技术。

如在寻找出血灶的过程中发现存在活动性出血，可单独使用硬质支气管镜或经大内径的气管插管置入可弯曲支气管镜的办法来保持气道畅通。可弯曲支气管镜也可用来辅助进行气管插管、更换气管插管。如果担心存在上气道水肿或陷闭，还可以在支气管镜引导下拔除气管插管[80]。对于气道管理来说，5 mm 外径的纤维支气管镜最为适用。在成人中要使用这个型号的支气管镜，则气管插管的内径至少需 8 mm[80]。这种外径的支气管镜即使是留置在气管内，气管内剩余空间仍能容下一根 7 mm 内径的气管插管。不推荐在气管插管内使用 6 mm 外径的纤维支气管镜，除非是出血已控制且支气管镜仅用来引导气管插管。

22.5.2　双腔气管插管

大咯血抢救时，必须防止健侧肺被血液阻塞[81-86]，一个办法就是在支气管镜引导下置入双腔气管插管[81-82]。可用的双腔气管插管包括 Carlen 插管[81]（1949 年发明，现被内径更小的插管逐渐替代）、Robertahaw 插管[84]（包括左侧和右侧两种型号）、一次性聚乙烯材料制成的 Robertshaw 套管（包括 Mallinckrodt 气管插管、Rusch 气管插管及 Sheridan 气管插管）[81]。最新的一些双腔气管插管在其呼吸机接口上还有隔膜，这样能维持支气管镜检查时机械通气的压力避免漏气[81]。目前的双腔插管有 5 种型号：28F、35F、37F、39F 和 41F。型号的选择依患者而定。一般倾向于选择能通过声门的最大径的气管插管，这样既不会太过深入至左主支气管，又能保证气密性。小号的插管需要更高的支气管内截断压力，这样可能在隆突周围形成过大的气管插管气囊而导致气道阻塞[81]。一般成年男性患者可以选用 41F 插管，女性患者选用 39F 插管[85]。

可弯曲支气管镜在双腔插管中发挥两方面作用，一个是协助困难气道的插管，另一方面是确认导管的位置正确。由于双腔导管的内径较小，治疗用的支气管镜一般难以通过。如果需要通过支气管镜进行插管，则须将双腔导管的近端缩短至 7 cm 以给支气管镜预留充足的空间[86]。如果患者使用了小于 39F 的双腔导管[81-82]，则推荐使用儿科支气管镜，因为最细的成人支气管镜的外径也达 4.9 mm，难以通过双腔导管[81]。

Dellinger[80] 介绍了可弯曲支气管镜引导下双腔导管的插入方法。首先，在支气管镜或直视喉镜引导下完成插管，插管进入气管后立即将气管插管的气囊充气，开始实施机械通气。然后将支气管镜经气管插管插入并引导插管的支气管段向下推送至主支气管腔内。例如，对左侧支类型的双腔管，就将支气管镜推送至左主支气管腔内。一般都选用左侧支类型的双腔管，因为右侧球囊难以达到很好的密封效果。右侧距离隆突近，右主支气管分支出现早，这都使得右侧支类型的双腔管放置困难，且难以保证气密性。支气管镜固定于左主支气管腔内后，沿镜身下推双腔管使其左侧支进入左主支气管腔内（图 22.2）。然后将支气管镜退至插管气管支腔内。在镜下确认双腔插管的左侧支进入左主支气管后，将插管左侧支上的气囊充盈至合适位置。正确的双腔插管位置应该是轻易就能看到支气管侧支的蓝色气囊应位于隆突附近，气囊没有疝出，双腔管道没有太过深入主支气管的远端[79]。

22.5.3　支气管镜下球囊填塞

另一种能经支气管镜放置的导管是支气管腔内填塞球囊，其可用于未插管患者控制威胁生命的咯

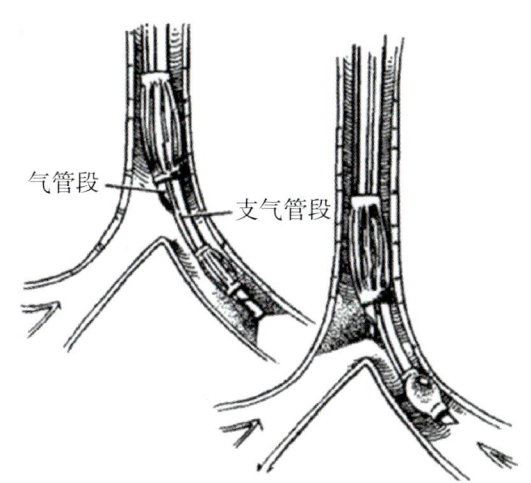

图 22.2 支气管镜引导下双腔导管置入术（左侧型）

可以参考 Dellinger 的书来了解详细的操作步骤[80]。

血[87-91]。球囊填塞就是通过纤维支气管镜或者硬质支气管镜置入 Fogarty 取栓球囊（段支气管使用 4F，左主支气管可以用到 14F）[2]，充气后阻塞出血的气道，然后再退出支气管镜（图 22.3）。留置 24~48 h 后，将球囊放气后移除。还有一种方法就是沿可弯曲支气管镜外围置入 Fogarty 球囊[92]达到压迫止血的目的[126]。

1974 年，Hiebert[84]报道了 1 例活动性咯血的病例，硬质支气管镜下无法保持视野。迫不得已，他们在右主支气管置入了 Fogarty 球囊，充盈后成功止血，并因此挽救了患者的生命。在这之后，相继有成功应用这项技术的报道[88-91]。Saw 等[89]报道了 10 例应用球囊填塞成功控制急性出血，且在之后 9 个月的随访中没有患者因为咯血死亡或再发咯血（没有外科手术）。Swersky 等[91]成功使用球囊填塞控制了 4 名患者的急性出血，虽然之后有 3 名患者出现再次出血。目前这些研究中都没有报道支气管内球囊填塞止血的并发症。

Valipour 等[93]报道在 57 名咯血患者中，经可弯曲支气管置入氧化纤维素网填塞来治疗咯血，有 56 例患者得以控制。

总的来说，虽然报道的病例并不多，但是普遍认为支气管内球囊填塞止血可以达到止血的作用且没有副作用，故该技术得到了广泛应用[2]。球囊填塞能快速保护健侧肺，维持患者生命体征平稳，确保患者的下一步有效止血治疗的实施[37]。

22.5.4 选择性支气管插管

若只能将出血部位定位至某侧肺而非特定肺叶，Garzon 和 Gourin[94-95]推荐使用选择性支气管插管或

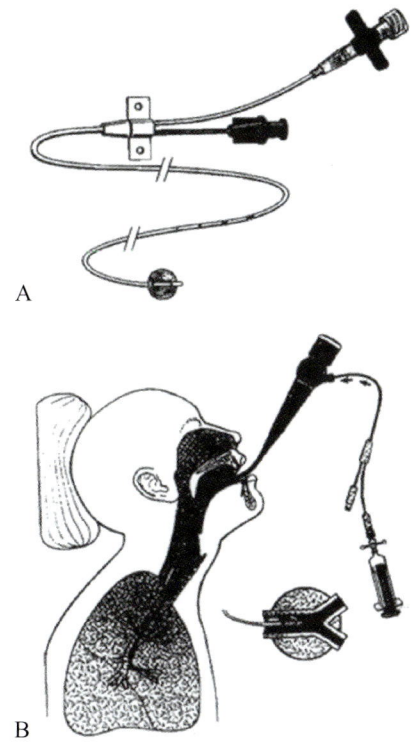

图 22.3 Fogarty 取栓球囊及应用

A. Fogarty 取栓球囊充气状态下；B. Fogarty 取栓球囊通过可弯曲支气管镜工作通道插入，到达病灶后充盈球囊完成填塞止血。

者球囊导管填塞止血技术。当右侧肺出血时，可以在支气管镜引导下将气管插管推进至左主支气管内，这样既能进行单肺通气，又能防止血液从右肺淹入左肺（图 22.4 A）。

由于解剖结构的不对称，右主支气管内单侧插管有阻塞右上支气管的风险，因其开口紧邻隆突[37]。因此，左侧出血的处理方式有所不同。可以将 Fogarty 球囊填塞左主支气管，然后将气管插管末端留置在气管内维持右肺单侧通气（图 22.4 B）。在 Garzon 和 Gourin[94]报道了 25 名选择性支气管插管的患者，对其中的 18 例咯血患者予以单侧支气管插管或球囊导管封堵。术后胸片示仅 3 例患者对侧肺淹入血液，仅 1 例死亡（死于呼吸衰竭和肾衰竭）。选择性支气管内插管让外科手术和血管栓塞术得以安全进行[79]。如果有药物治疗的适应证，可以继续支持治疗[79]。支气管内插管技术在维持对健侧肺通气的同时，还能允许向出血部位灌注冰生理盐水。这在处理支气管血管瘘时也是作为首选方式加以考虑[79]。

另一种隔离出血侧肺的技术是置入一根带自膨胀气囊的气管导管。这种导管一般在胸外科中或胸腔

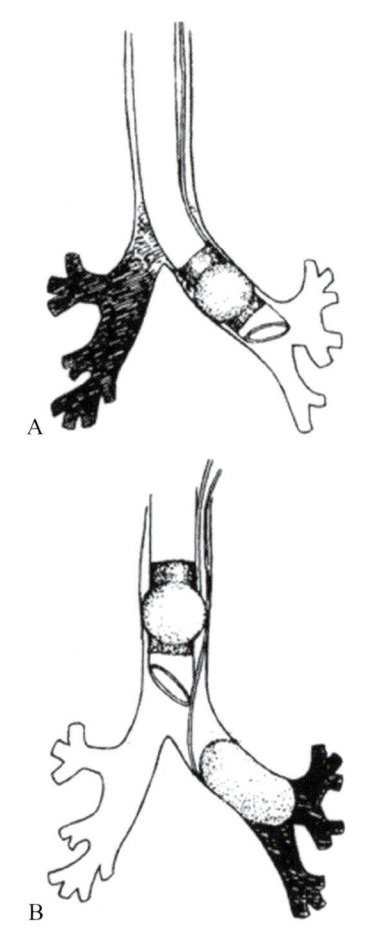

图 22.4　气管插管与支气管出血处理
A. 右肺出血时，将气管插管送入左主支气管，维持左肺通气，同时防止右肺的血进入左肺；B. 左肺出血时，先在左主支气管侧放入一个 Fogarty 球囊压迫填塞，气管插管末端在气管下段，维持右肺的通气[95]。

镜时单肺通气或者萎陷肺时使用。可经气管插管盲插或在支气管镜引导下送入目标主支气管。它在隔离出血肺的同时还能吸除血液[27]。

22.5.5　支气管镜直接填塞

如果在支气管镜检查的过程中大量出血，可在直视下将可弯曲支气管镜直接推入出血的段或亚段支气管，类似一个堵塞的楔子[37,96]。这是一种暂时的止血方法，可以让血液形成血凝块，同时防止血液流入其他正常的区域。如果硬质支气管镜检查时发生大气道出血，硬质的器械也可用来直接填塞出血部位，还可在维持气道通畅的同时，使用硬质镜侧壁直接压迫出血部位止血[18]。

22.5.6　局部使用缩血管药和促凝药

经支气管镜往气道内注入肾上腺素溶液（1∶20 000）可以起到局部血管收缩的作用，在减少血液流速的同时也可以促进末梢血管形成血栓，从而达到止血的目的[18,97,97]。局部使用肾上腺素对血管瘤活检后的出血或者严重的黏膜出血也有止血作用[80,97]。采用球囊填塞止血后，推荐常规性往支气管腔内滴注肾上腺素[91]。例如，Poe 等在一项对 4 273 例患者的回顾性研究中发现，有 2.8% 的患者在活检之后出现出血，局部使用肾上腺素有很好的止血作用[99]。

但局部使用肾上腺素在大咯血治疗中的作用尚不确定。

血管加压素是另一种可以用来治疗咯血的缩血管药。Worth 等[100]比较了气管内滴入或静脉使用血管加压素在治疗肺出血中的疗效差别。11 例患者经静脉使用了 1 mg 血管加压素治疗，而 16 例患者在出血部位滴注了同等剂量的血管加压素。结果发现支气管腔内应用一样有效，且不影响血流动力学。Ramon 等[101]也报道在 20 例重症咯血患者中紧急使用肠外特利加压素，14 例患者得以成功控制。最后，有研究报道在 3 例轻、中度咯血患者的保守治疗中，使用雾化血管加压素成功控制住了咯血[102]。

经支气管镜注入促凝剂也可以起到止血的作用，已报道过的止血药包括 Bosmin[103]、蛇毒凝血酶[104]、凝血酶[105]、纤维蛋白原凝血酶[106,107]、纤维蛋白原前体[85]。Tsukamoto 等[106]在一项研究中，对 19 位患者使用了凝血酶（5~10 mL，1 000 U/mL 溶液），并且对疗效进行了记录，14 例（74%）基本有效（2 周内未再次咯血），1 例部分有效（治疗后在 24 h 到 2 周内再次出现咯血），4 例（21%）没有起到止血作用。另外有 14 例接受纤维蛋白原凝血酶（5~10 mL 2% 纤维蛋白原溶液）治疗的患者中，11 例（79%）基本有效，3 例（21%）部分有效。

Bense[108]报道局部使用的促凝剂都含有纤维蛋白前体细胞（如纤维蛋白原、纤连蛋白、XII 因子、抑肽酶等），加入无水氯化钙和凝血酶之后就会被激活。使用这一方法，Bense 将一个外径 2 mm 的四通道的导管沿可弯曲支气管镜插入出血的支气管，两种主要成分及纤维蛋白胶混合并加热至 37℃，经这个四通道注射器中的两条通道各自同时注入支气管腔内。运用这个技术，Bense 安全控制了这 4 名其他治疗无效患者的咯血[108]。

尽管人们对使用促凝剂治疗大咯血也很有热情，但目前缺乏对照性研究，鉴于研究有限，读者们可对此保留意见。更深的担心在于，大咯血时持续不断的出血可能会在血凝块形成之前就把这些纤维蛋白胶冲走[18]。

22.5.7　支气管镜下冷生理盐水灌洗

冷生理盐水灌洗在上消化道出血治疗中的疗效确切，该方法也在大咯血的止血中有所应用。例如，Conlan和Hurwitz[109]对12例大咯血患者通过硬质支气管镜分次注入50 mL的冰生理盐水（4℃），达到了止血的效果。总共需要的盐水量约为500 mL（300~750 mL）。该疗法止血的机制可能是低温引起血管收缩，减小出血速度，促成末梢血管内血栓形成。

22.5.8　支气管镜下激光治疗、电凝止血及其他相关介入技术

在之前的章节中讨论过，通过可弯曲支气管镜或硬质支气管镜进行Nd:YAG激光疗法，可以治疗由于气道肿瘤所导致的咯血。同样，内镜下氩等离子电凝术，一种非接触性电凝术，也可以在肺部肿瘤引起的咯血中达到止血的效果[110]。Morrice等对60例支气管腔内病灶引起的咯血或气道阻塞进行氩等离子电凝术治疗，结果在治疗后平均97天的随访中发现咯血均得到了良好的控制[97]。

电凝也可以作为支气管镜下治疗咯血的方法之一。Gerasin和Shafirovsky[110]在可弯曲支气管镜下使用电圈套对14例气管支气管肿瘤患者进行电凝治疗，9例良性的气道肿瘤都被成功切除，另外5例恶性气道肿瘤患者有3例成功地进行了气道廓清。其中有1例患者因甲状腺癌气道转移而导致出血，通过电凝成功止血。相较于激光治疗而言，电凝止血费用低、设备可及性高、电圈套切除肿瘤速度更快，且可用于含软骨或骨性成分等激光不敏感肿瘤等的切除。但是，对于肿瘤新生物基底部太大、气道被完全阻塞或者段支气管内的肿瘤，电凝治疗的应用受限[111]。

在电凝治疗过程中，需要警惕以下两点：①避免电凝头直接接触支气管镜的尖端，因为支气管镜并非绝缘体；②闭合圈套器时避免电流过大或用力过度，以免快速切割时伤及血管而加重出血。一些新型支气管镜改良了绝缘技术，使用新型单电极和双电极探头，使其在良恶性气道肿瘤的治疗中，较之激光而言更加便宜和安全[111]。

其他的支气管镜介入手段，包括冷冻治疗和光动力学疗法，由于它们在气道起效的延迟性，在咯血的治疗中应用有限。

22.5.9　硅胶塞支气管封堵治疗大咯血

一项新的支气管镜介入技术，即经可弯曲支气管镜暂时性放置硅胶塞填塞，可以在支气管动脉栓塞术前、术中防止气道内血液四溢[112]。支气管动脉栓塞术后可以取出硅胶塞。这项经济且简单的技术仅使用活检钳来放置硅胶塞。但在广泛推广前还需积累更多的经验。

总之，虽然有多种支气管镜下治疗咯血的介入技术，但要做出首选推荐，尚缺乏对照性研究证据。对于非大咯血的患者，我们的经验是局部喷洒肾上腺素，然后使用支气管球囊填塞。对大咯血的患者，急救措施包括静脉使用血管加压素、患侧卧位，在实施支气管动脉栓塞或外科手术之前，可对患者行选择性支气管插管以维持生命体征平稳。

22.6　支气管镜操作相关大咯血

随着呼吸内镜诊疗技术的发展，接受内镜诊疗的人数日趋增多，与此同时，支气管镜操作相关的并发症也日益增加，其中出血是支气管镜诊疗操作最常见的并发症，约占所有并发症的40%[113]。根据病变的类型及接受的内镜操作不同，其发生率为0.5%~5.3%。虽然大多数出血是可控的，但仍时有致命性的大出血发生，这也是最令支气管镜检查医师沮丧和棘手的难题。

多项研究将"支气管镜操作相关大出血"定为支气管镜诊断或治疗性操作所引起的下呼吸道单次出血量>100 mL。由此所致的患者死亡是最为严重的意外不良事件之一。它不仅极大消耗医疗资源，而且会严重影响支气管镜检查医生制定医疗决策。

22.6.1　流行病学及病因

Zhou等[121]对33家三级医院做了一项多中心回顾性队列研究，结果显示，2001—2013年共520 343例接受可弯曲支气管镜诊疗的患者中，发生支气管镜诊疗操作相关大出血194例，发生率为0.037%。原发病主要包括恶性肿瘤（74/194，38.1%）、肺结核（34/194，17.5%）、慢性炎症（23/194，11.9%）、肉芽肿性疾病（17/194，8.8%）、曲霉病（6/194，3.1%）、良性肿瘤（5/194，2.6%）、血管畸形（4/194，2.1%）、

间质性肺病（4/194，2.1%）、栓塞（3/194，1.5%）及其他疾病（24/194，12.4%，包括 11 例病因不明）。这一结果与 Carr[117] 和 Cordasco[114] 的研究一致，他们的结果显示，原发性肺癌和肺结核是支气管镜操作相关大出血的主要病因。而 Zhou[121] 的研究显示导致大出血的诊疗操作包括经支气管活检（0.065%）、刷检（0.007%）、支气管肺泡灌洗术（0.004%）、球囊扩张（0.043%）、热消融（0.106%）及支架植入（0.055%）。

总体而言，支气管镜操作相关大咯血的发生率很低。肿瘤性疾病是支气管镜操作相关大咯血的主要病因，而治疗性操作大咯血的发生率明显高于诊断性操作。

22.6.2 治疗

支气管镜操作相关大咯血的治疗原则与前述普通大咯血的救治是一致的，即迅速提高氧浓度、保持重要脏器的氧供、肺隔离和气道控制、维持气道开放，尽快给予止血措施如局部灌注止血药物、全身静脉使用止血药、机械性压迫填塞、电凝或激光止血、支气管动脉栓塞手术和手术等。但由于支气管镜操作相关大出血具有一定的不可预测性和突发性，因此，其救治也有一些特殊性。首先，面对突如其来的大出血，术者应尽量地保持沉着、镇定，保持内镜负压吸引状态，尽量吸除健肺积血，同时指挥其他医护人员有序配合，尽快实施救治措施。其次，对于局麻或者静脉适度镇静的患者，由于没有人工气道进行肺隔离和气道保护，气道极易被血凝块阻塞引起窒息，而此时最快的办法是调整患者体位至患侧卧位，这可有效防止患者肺内的积血淹入健侧肺，同时可使已经残留于健侧肺内的积血通过咳嗽排出体外，这对于改善患者通气、改善氧合具有极其重要的意义（图 22.5）。再者，对于没有人工气道保护的患者，盲目地退出支气管镜可能因为大量出血而丧失再次进镜或气管插管的视野，这也是支气管镜操作相关大出血的主要救治难点。为此，黄海东和柯明耀等发明了一种带导丝引导通道的气管插管（图 22.6），一旦出现大出血，先将金属导丝经支气管镜工作通道插入气道内，然后退镜，再沿金属导丝迅速插入加长型气管插管，从而建立人工气道，随后再次进镜采取进一步的救治措施止血（图 22.7）。

22.6.3 预后

Zhou 等[121] 的研究结果显示，194 例支气管镜操作相关大出血患者中死亡 21 例（死亡率为 0.004%，致死率为 10.8%）；其原发病依次为肿瘤（9 例）、慢性炎症（2 例）、肉芽肿性疾病（2 例）、气管淀粉样变（1 例）、曲霉病（1 例）、血管畸形（1 例）以及无明确病因者（5 例）。导致死亡的支气管镜操作依次为经支气管活检 12 例（死亡率为 0.007%，致死率为 10.1%）、

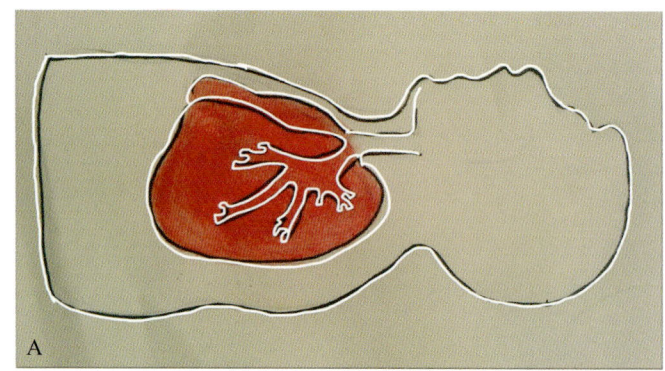

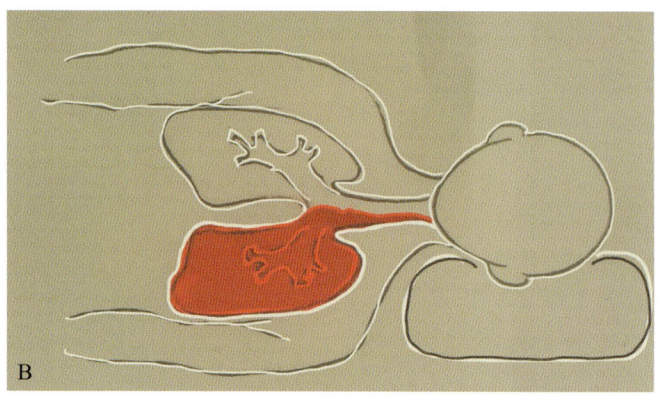

图 22.5 不同体位对支气管镜诊疗操作相关大咯血的气道血液和通气的影响

A. 当患者处于仰卧位时，大量的血液容易淹没到肺的两侧，导致气道阻塞迅速发生；B. 将患者迅速翻转为患侧卧位后，该体位使得对侧健康肺位于患侧肺上方，气道中的血液不容易淹没，这为建立人工气道争取了时间。

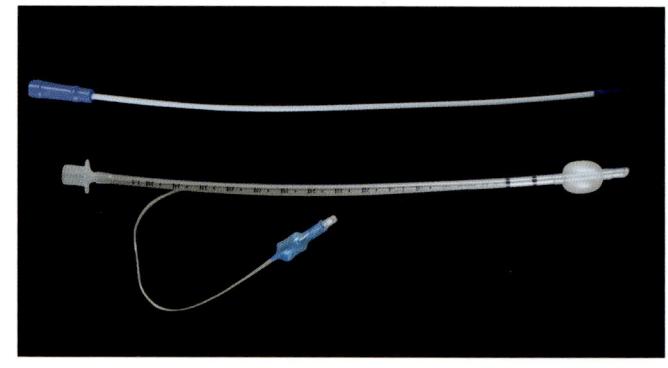

图 22.6 用于支气管镜诊疗操作相关大咯血的一种特殊设计的加长型气管插管

热消融术（4例）(0.022%，21.1%）、球囊扩张（2例）（0.017%，40%）、刷检（1例）(0.0004%，6.7%）、腔内冷冻（1例）(0.007%，14.3%）等。总体而言，支气管镜操作相关大咯血的死亡率很低。

Zhou的研究提示可弯曲支气管镜检查诱发的大咯血是一种威胁生命的并发症。总体致死率为10.8%，而治疗性操作致死率甚至达14.3%~40%。但仍然低于原发病所致大咯血的死亡率。文献报道，后者的致死率高达50%~80%，且死亡多发生在发病后1 h内[28,29,122]。究其原因，可能是大咯血发生的地点不同所致，支气管镜操作相关大咯血均发生于医院内，这意味着在大咯血出现后可以尽快开展急诊多学科抢救[123,124]。尽管如此，年龄65岁以上，气管内出血，出血量超过500 mL以及继发休克提示预后不良。然而，多因素分析显示，急诊手术可能是一项独立保护因素。咯血的复发率低，随访1个月后约3.1%。

22.6.4 预防

充分的术前风险评估是预防支气管镜操作相关大咯血的重要措施，评估内容包括病史、查体、实验室

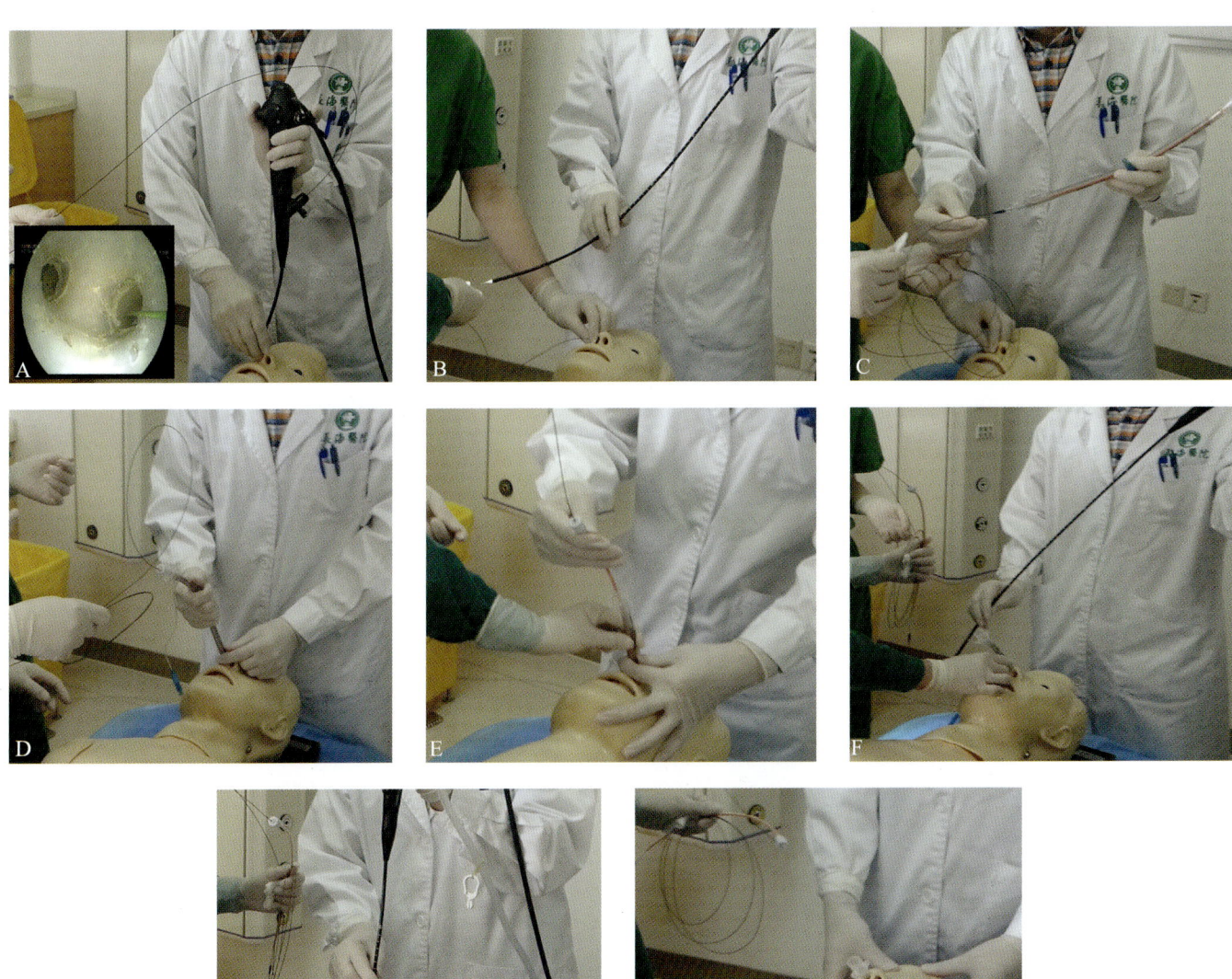

图 22.7　支气管镜引导快速插管治疗大咯血

模型上演示发生支气管镜诊疗操作相关大咯血时，经支气管镜引导下通过导丝迅速插入加长型气管插管。

及影像学检查结果。胸部增强CT有助于鉴别是血管发育不良还是恶性肿瘤中丰富的血管。应急计划、抢救用药及设备、有经验的支气管镜操作者、外科手术支援都非常必要。此外，针对如何有效救治支气管镜检查诱发的大咯血的标准化培训也非常重要。

22.6.5 病例分享

一位25岁男性患者，因"反复发热3个月，面色苍白1周，双下肢出血点2天"收入医院。经外周血检查及骨髓穿刺活检，他被诊断为"急性髓细胞白血病"。遂予化疗，化疗后出现发热、白细胞降低，并逐渐出现咳嗽、咳痰，伴痰中带血。胸部CT提示双肺散在片状高密度阴影，以右下肺明显，考虑真菌感染可能。多次痰培养提示烟曲霉。先后以两性霉素及伏立康唑抗真菌治疗。复查胸部CT提示双肺片状影好转，右中下肺实变影较前好转（图22.8 A）。为进一步明确病因，行支气管镜检查，术中发生致命性大咯血窒息及心跳骤停，经患侧卧位，静脉应用垂体后叶素，迅速建立左主支气管插管后机械通气，积极抗休克等治疗后，自主心率在90 min后恢复，生命体征趋于平稳，后行急诊胸外科手术治疗后转危为安。

术后病理示支气管镜下标本含坏死的支气管结构。HE染色见支气管黏膜彻底坏死，透明软骨变性、坏死，坏死组织中可见大量曲霉菌丝及孢子（图22.8 H）。切除的右中下肺组织内见积血（图22.8 I）。右中间段支气管周围组织大量坏死和曲霉侵犯，最终诊断为侵袭性支气管曲霉病。

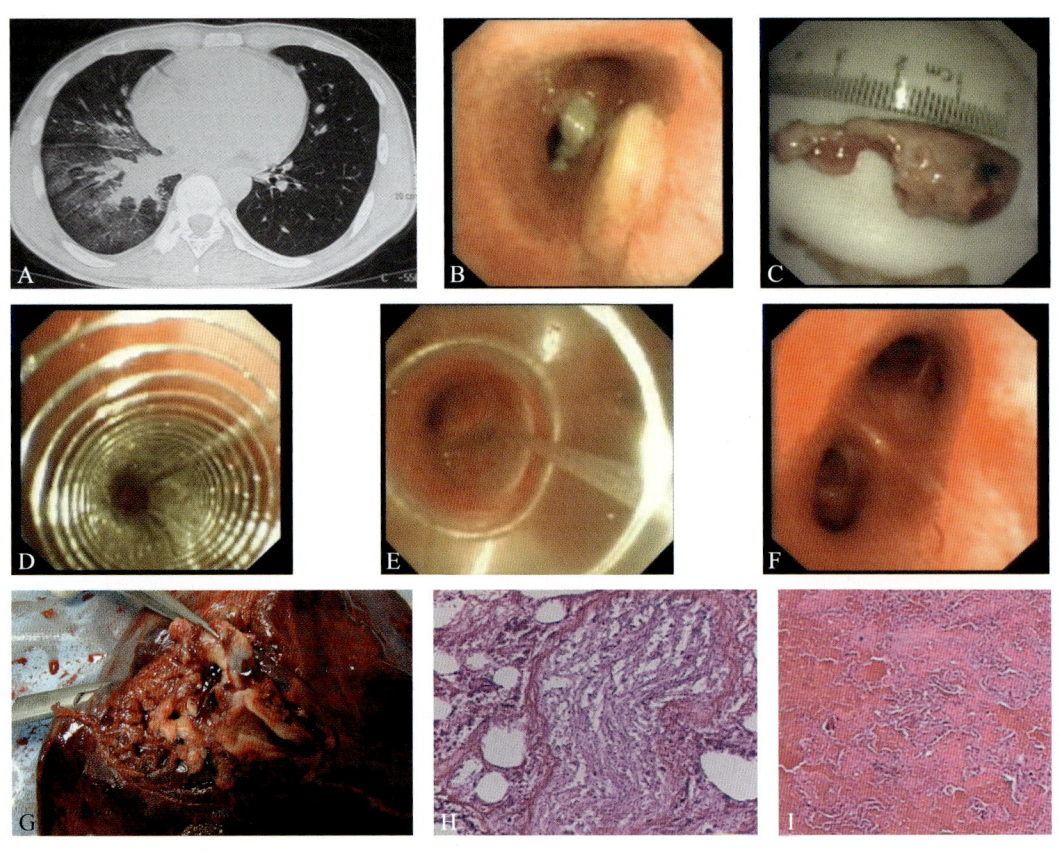

图22.8 典型病例

A. 胸部CT显示右下肺部出现斑片状浸润，右下叶支气管腔完全阻塞；B. 支气管镜检查显示气管支气管黏膜充血，并有大量坏死组织附着在右主支气管和中间支气管黏膜上，中间支气管的开口被坏死组织完全堵塞；C. 进行了冷冻冻切以去除坏死组织，坏死物质以约3.5 cm×1.5 cm×1.2 cm的条状物被冻切取出。随后发生了致命性大咯血；D. 在清除口腔和鼻腔中大量血块后，通过间接喉镜引导进入气道腔道，成功行气管插管；E. 支气管镜成功插入气管插管的腔道，并通过支气管镜引导将气管插管的远端放置在左主支气管内；F. 在气管插管气囊充气后，左主支气管被有效封闭，右侧大量出血无法进入左主支气管和远端气道；G. 急诊开胸手术取出的右中下肺组织。我们可以看到远端中间支气管和右下叶支气管及其周边大血管已被曲霉完全侵蚀；H. 术后病理检查（HE×100）显示支气管镜下标本为坏死组织。HE染色显示支气管黏膜完全坏死，透明软骨退变和坏死，并在坏死组织中观察到大量曲霉菌丝和孢子；I. 切除标本显示右中叶和下叶肺泡组织内为血液完全填塞。

参考文献

1. Marini, J. (1987). Hemoptysis. In: *Respiratory Medicine for the House Officer*, 2e, 223-225. Baltimore: Williams and Wilkins.
2. Stoller, J.K. (1992). Diagnosis and management of massive hemoptysis: a review. *Respir. Care* 32: 564 581.
3. Chaves, A.D. (1951). Hemoptysis in chest clinic patients. *Am. Rev. Tuberc.* 63: 144-201.
4. Pursel, S.E. and Lindskog, G.E. (1961). Hemoptysis: a clinical evaluation of 105 patients examined consecutively on a thoracic surgical service. *Am. Rev. Respir. Dis.* 84: 329-336.
5. Abbott, O.A. (1948). The clinical significance of pulmonary hemorrhage: a study of 1316 patients with chest disease. *Dis. Chest* 14: 824-842.
6. Johnston, R.N., Lockhart, W., Ritchie, R.T., and Smith, D.M. (1960). Hemoptysis. *Br. Med. J.* 1: 592-595.
7. Selecky, P.A. (1978). Evaluation of hemoptysis through the bronchoscope. *Chest* 73: 741-745.
8. Lyons, H.A. (1976). Differential diagnosis of hemoptysis and its treatment. *ATS News*: 26-30.
9. Barrett, R.J. and Tuttle, W.M. (1960). A study of essential hemoptysis. *J. Thorac. Cardiovasc. Surg.* 40: 468-474.
10. Wolfe, J.D. and Simmons, D.H. (1977). Hemoptysis: diagnosis and management. *West. J. Med.* 127: 383-390.
11. Irwin, R.S. and Curley, F.J. (1991). Hemoptysis. In: *Intensive Care Medicine*, 2e (eds. J.M. Rippe, R.S. Irwin, J.S. Alpert, et al.), 513-524. Boston: Little, Brown.
12. Jackson, C.R. and Diamond, S. (1942). Hemorrhage from the trachea, bronchi, and lungs of non-tuberculosis origin. *Am. Rev. Tuberc.* 46: 126-138.
13. Souders, C.R. and Smith, A.T. (1952). The clinical significance of hemoptysis. *N. Engl. J. Med.* 247: 790-793.
14. Heller, R. (1946). The significance of hemoptysis. *Tubercule* 26: 70-74.
15. Moersch, H.J. (1952). Clinical significance of hemoptysis. *JAMA* 148: 1461-1465.
16. Johnston, H. and Reisz, G. (1989). Changing spectrum of hemoptysis: underlying causes in 148 patients undergoing diagnostic flexible bronchoscopy. *Arch. Intern. Med.* 149: 1666-1668.
17. Santiago, S., Tobias, J., and William, A.J. (1991). A reappraisal of the causes of hemoptysis. *Arch. Intern. Med.* 151: 2449-2451.
18. Prakash, U.B.S. (1993). Bronchoscopy. In: *Pulmonary and Critical Care Medicine*, vol. 1 (eds. R.C. Bone, D.R. Dantzker, R.D. George, et al.), 1-18. St Louis: Mosby-Year Book.
19. Kahn, M.P., Whitcomb, M.E., and Snider, G.L. (1976). Flexible fiberoptic bronchoscopy. *Am. J. Med.* 61: 151-155.
20. Gong, H. and Salvatierra, C. (1981). Clinical efficacy of early and delayed fiberoptic bronchoscopy in patients with hemoptysis. *Am. Rev. Respir. Dis.* 124: 221-225.
21. Prakash, U.B.S., Offord, K.P., and Stubbs, S.E. (1991). Bronchoscopy in North America: the ACCP survey. *Chest* 100: 1668-1675.
22. Howard, W., Rosario, E.J., and Calhoon, S.L. (1985). Hemoptysis: causes and practical management approach. *Postgrad. Med.* 77: 53-57.
23. Karlinsky, J.B., Lau, J., and Goldstein, R.H. (1991). Hemoptysis. In: *Decision Making in Pulmonary Medicine*, 10-11. Philadelphia: B.C. Decker.
24. Clausen, J.L. (1991). Hemoptysis. In: *Manual of Clinical Problems in Pulmonary Medicine* (eds. R.A. Nordew and K.M. Moser), 67-71. Boston: Little, Brown.
25. Amirana, M., Prater, R., Tirschwell, P. et al. (1968). An aggressive surgical approach to significant hemoptysis in patients with pulmonary tuberculosis. *Am. Rev. Respir. Dis.* 97: 187-192.
26. Bobrowitz, F.D., Ramkrishna, S., and Shim, Y.S. (1983). Comparison of medical vs. surgical treatment of major hemoptysis. *Arch. Intern. Med.* 143: 1343-1346.
27. Comforti, J. (2006). Management of massive hemoptysis. In: *Thoracic Endoscopy: Advances in Interventional Pulmonology*, vol. 23 (eds. M.J. Simoff, D.H. Sterman and A. Ernst), 330-343. Ames: Blackwell Futura.
28. Crocco, J.A., Rooneyn, J.J., Fankushen, D.S. et al. (1968). Massive hemoptysis. *Arch. Intern. Med.* 121: 495-498.
29. Corey, R. and Hla, K.M. (1987). Major and massive hemoptysis: reassessment of conservative management. *Am. J. Med. Sci.* 294: 301-309.
30. Holsclaw, D.S., Grand, R.J., and Shuachman, H. (1970). Massive hemoptysis in cystic fbrosis. *J. Pediatr.* 76: 829-838.
31. Garzon, A.A., Cerruti, M.M., and Golding, M.E. (1982). Exsanguinating hemoptysis. *Thorac. Cardiovasc. Surg.* 84: 829-833.
32. Haponik, E.P. and Chin, R. (1990). Hemoptysis: clinician's perspective. *Chest* 97: 469-475.
33. Gourin, A. and Garzon, A.A. (1974). Operative treatment of massive hemoptysis. *Ann. Thorac. Surg.* 18: 52-60.
34. Conlan, A.A., Hurwitz, S.S., Krige, L. et al. (1983). Massive hemoptysis: a review of 123 cases. *J. Thorac. Cardiovasc. Surg.* 85: 120-124.
35. Bone, R.C. (1982). Massive hemoptysis. In: *Pulmonary Emergencies* (ed. S. Sahn), 225-236. New York: Churchill Livingstone.
36. Rogers, R.M. (1976). The management of massive hemoptysis in a patient with pulmonary tuberculosis. *Chest* 70: 519-526.
37. Winter, S.M. and Ingbar, D.H. (1988). Massive hemoptysis: pathogenesis and management. *J. Intensive Care Med.* 3: 171-188.
38. Ozgul, M.A., Turna, A., Yildiz, A. et al. (2006). Risk factors and recurrence patterns in 203 patients with hemoptysis. *Tuberk. Toraks* 54: 243-248.
39. Wedzicha, J.A. and Pearson, M.C. (1990). Management of massive hemoptysis. *Respir. Med.* 84: 9-12.
40. Adelman, M., Haponik, E.P., Bleecker, E.R., and Britt, E.J. (1985). Cryptogenic hemoptysis. *Ann. Intern. Med.* 102: 829-834.
41. Uflacker, R., Kaemmerer, A., Picon, P.D. et al. (1985). Bronchial artery embolization in the management of hemoptysis: technical aspects and long-term results. *Radiology* 157: 637-644.

42 McCollum, W.B., Mattox, K.L., Guinn, G.A., and Beall, A.C. (1975). Immediate operative treatment for massive hemoptysis. *Chest* 67: 152–155.

43 Yang, C.T. and Berger, H.W. (1978). Conservative management of life threatening hemoptysis. *Mt Sinai J. Med.* 45: 329–333.

44 Remy, J., Arnaud, A., Pardou, H. et al. (1977). Treatment of hemoptysis by embolization of bronchial arteries. *Radiology* 122: 33–39.

45 Deffebach, M.E., Charau, N.B., and Lakshminarayan, S. (1987). State of the art: the bronchial circulation – small but a vital attribute of the lung. *Am. Rev. Respir. Dis.* 135: 463–481.

46 Strickland, B. (1986). Investigating hemoptysis. *Br. J. Hosp. Med.* 35: 246–251.

47 Smiddy, J.R. and Elliot, R.C. (1973). The evaluation of hemoptysis with fiberoptic bronchoscopy. *Chest* 64: 158–162.

48 Shamji, P.M., Vallieres, E., Todd, E.R., and Sach, H.J. (1991). Massive or life-threatening hemoptysis. *Chest* 100: 78S.

49 Ingbar, D. (1989). A systematic workup for hemoptysis. *Contemp. Intern. Med.* Aug: 60–70.

50 O'Neil, K.M. and Lazarus, A.A. (1991). Hemoptysis: indications for bronchoscopy. *Arch. Intern. Med.* 151: 171–174.

51 Weaver, L.J., Solliday, N., and Cugell, D.W. (1979). Selection of patients for fiberoptic bronchoscopy. *Chest* 76: 7–10.

52 Snider, G.L. (1979). When not to use the bronchoscope for hemoptysis. *Chest* 76: 1–2.

53 Zavala, D.C. (1975). Diagnostic fiberoptic bronchoscopy. *Chest* 68: 12–19.

54 Mitchell, D.M., Emerson, C.J., Collyer, J., and Collins, J.V. (1980). Fiberoptic bronchoscopy ten years on. *Br. Med. J.* 281: 360–363.

55 Rath, G.S., Schaff, J.T., and Snider, G.L. (1973). Flexible fiberoptic bronchoscopy: techniques and review of 100 bronchoscopies. *Chest* 63: 689–693.

56 Peters, J., McClung, H., and Teague, R. (1984). Evaluation of hemoptysis in patients with a normal chest roentgenogram. *West. J. Med.* 141: 624–626.

57 Jackson, C.V., Savage, P.J., and Quinn, D.L. (1985). Role of fiberoptic bronchoscopy in patients with hemoptysis and a normal chest roentgenogram. *Chest* 87: 142–144.

58 Poe, R.H., Israel, R.H., Marin, M.G. et al. (1988). Utility of fiberoptic bronchoscopy in patients with hemoptysis and a non-localizing chest roentgenogram. *Chest* 92: 70–75.

59 Heimer, D., Bar-Ziv, J., and Scharf, S.M. (1985). Fiberoptic bronchoscopy in patients with hemoptysis and non-localizing chest roentgenographs. *Arch. Intern. Med.* 145: 1427–1428.

60 Kallenbach, J., Song, E., and Zwi, S. (1981). Hemoptysis with no radiologic evidence of tumors: the value of early bronchoscopy. *S. Afr. Med. J.* 59: 556–558.

61 Richardson, R.H., Zavala, D.C., Mukerjee, P.K., and Bedell, G.N. (1974). The use of fiberoptic bronchoscopy and brush biopsy in the diagnosis of suspected pulmonary malignancy. *Am. Rev. Respir. Dis.* 109: 63–66.

62 Heaton, R.W. (1987). Should patients with hemoptysis and normal chest x-ray be bronchoscoped? *Postgrad. Med. J.* 63: 947–949.

63 Lee, C.J., Lee, C.H., Lan, R.S. et al. (1989). The role of fiberoptic bronchoscopy in patients with hemoptysis and a normal chest roentgenogram. *Changgeng Yi Xue Za Zhi* 12: 136–140.

64 Lederle, F.A., Nichol, K.L., and Parenti, C.M. (1989). Bronchoscopy to evaluate hemoptysis in older men with nonsuspicious chest roentgenograms. *Chest* 10: 43–47.

65 Cortese, D.A., Parvolero, P.C., Bergstrach, E.J. et al. (1983). Roentgenographically occult lung can a ten-year experience. *J. Thorac. Cardiovasc. Surg.* 86: 373–380.

66 Saumench, J., Escarrabil, J., Padro, I. et al. (1989). Value of fiberoptic bronchoscopy and angiography for diagnosis of the bleeding site in hemoptysis. *Ann. Thorac. Surg.* 48: 272–274.

67 Neff, J.A. (1977). Hemoptysis. *West. J. Med.* 127: 411–412.

68 Imgrund, S.P., Goldberg, S.K., Walkenstein, M.D. et al. (1985). Clinical diagnosis of massive hemoptysis using the fiberoptic bronchoscope. *Crit. Care Med.* 13: 438–443.

69 Haponik, E.F., Fein, A., and Chin, R. (2000). Managing life-threatening hemoptysis: has anything really changed? *Chest* 118: 1431–1435.

70 Newton, R.W. and Forest, A.R.W. (1975). Rifmpicin overdosage -"the red man syndrome.". *South. Med. J.* 20: 55–57.

71 George, P.J.M., Garrett, C.P.O., Nixon, C. et al. (1987). Laser treatment for tracheobronchial tumors: local or general anesthesia? *Thorax* 42: 656–660.

72 Prakash, U.B.S. (1985). The use of the pediatric fiberoptic bronchoscope in adults. *Am. Rev. Respir. Dis.* 132: 715–717.

73 Katoh, O., Yamada, H., Hiura, K. et al. (1987). Bronchoscopic and angiographic comparison of bronchial arterial lesions in patients with hemoptysis. *Chest* 91: 486–489.

74 Takeuchi, Y., Namikawa, S., Kusagawa, M. et al. (1985). Bronchofiberscopic findings of bronchial artery lesions: a report of two cases. *J. Jpn. Soc. Bronchol.* 7: 71–76.

75 Flick, M.K., Wasson, K., Dunn, L.J., and Block, A.J. (1975). Fatal pulmonary hemorrhage after transbronchial lung biopsy through the fiber optic bronchoscope. *Am. Rev. Respir. Dis.* 111: 853–856.

76 Kuzucu, A., Gurses, I., Soysal, O. et al. (2005). Dieulafoy's disease: a cause of massive hemoptysis that is probably under diagnosed. *Ann. Thorac. Surg.* 80: 1126–1128.

77 Savale, L., Parrot, A., Khalil, A. et al. (2007). Cryptogenic hemoptysis: from a benign to a life-threatening pathogenic vascular condition. *Am. J. Respir. Crit. Care* 175: 1181–1185.

78 Loschhorn, C., Nierhoff, N., Mayer, R. et al. (2006). Dieulafoy's disease of the lung: a potential disaster for the bronchoscopist. *Respiration* 73: 562–565.

79 Conlan, A.A. (1985). Massive hemoptysis: diagnostic and therapeutic implications. *Surg. Annu.* 17: 337–355.

80 Dellinger, R.P. (1990). Fiberoptic bronchoscopy in adult airway management. *Crit. Care Med.* 18: 882–887.

81 Strange, C. (1991). Double-lumen endotracheal tubes. *Clin. Chest Med.* 12: 497–506.

82 Shivaram, U., Finch, P., and Nowak, P. (1987). Plastic endobronchial tubes in the management of life-threatening hemoptysis. *Chest* 92: 1108–1110.

83 Bjork, V.O. and Carlens, E. (1951). The prevention of spread during pulmonary resection by the use of a double-lumen

catheter. *J. Thorac. Surg.* 20: 151–154.

84 Robertshaw, F.L. (1962). Low resistance double-lumen endobronchial tubes. *Br. J. Anaesth.* 34: 576–579.

85 Brodsky, J.B. (1990). Isolation of the lungs. *Probl. Anesth.* 4: 264–269.

86 Shulman, M.S., Brodsky, J.B., and Levesque, P.R. (1987). Fiberoptic bronchoscopy for tracheal and endobronchial intubation with a doublelumen tube. *Can. J. Anaesth.* 34: 172–175.

87 Hiebert, C.A. (1974). Balloon catheter control of life-threatening hemoptysis. *Chest* 66: 308–309.

88 Gottlieb, L.S. and Hillberg, R. (1975). Endobronchial tamponade therapy for intractable hemoptysis. *Chest* 67: 482–483.

89 Saw, E.C., Gottlieb, L.S., Yokoyama, T., and Lee, B.C. (1976). Flexible fiberoptic bronchoscopy and endobronchial hemoptysis. *Chest* 70: 589–591.

90 Faloney, J.P. and Balchum, O.J. (1978). Repeated massive hemoptysis: successful control using multiple balloon-tipped catheters for endobronchial tamponade. *Chest* 74: 683–685.

91 Swersky, R.B., Chang, J.B., Wisoff, B.G., and Gorvoy, J. (1979). Endobronchial balloon tamponade of hemoptysis in patients with cystic fibrosis. *Ann. Thorac. Surg.* 27: 262–264.

92 Thompson, A.B., Teschler, H., and Rennard, S. (1992). Pathogenesis, evaluation and therapy for massive hemoptysis. *Clin. Chest Med.* 13: 69–82.

93 Valipour, A., Kreuzer, A., Koller, H. et al. (2005). Bronchoscopy-guided topical hemostatic tamponade therapy for the management of life-threatening hemoptysis. *Chest* 127: 2118.

94 Garzon, A.A. and Gourin, A. (1978). Surgical management of massive hemoptysis: a ten-year experience. *Ann. Surg.* 187: 267–271.

95 Gourin, A. and Garzon, A.A. (1975). Control of hemorrhage in emergency pulmonary resection for massive hemoptysis. *Chest* 68: 120–121.

96 Israel, R.H. and Poe, R.H. (1987). Hemoptysis. *Clin. Chest Med.* 8: 197–205.

97 Morice, R.C., Ece, T., Ece, F., and Keus, L. (2001). Endobronchial argon plasma coagulation for treatment of hemoptysis and neoplastic airway obstruction. *Chest* 19: 781–787.

98 Zavala, D.C. (1976). Pulmonary hemorrhage in fiberoptic transbronchial biopsy. *Chest* 70: 584–588.

99 Poe, C.A. and Pacht, E.R. (1995). Complications of fiberoptic bronchoscopy at a university hospital. *Chest* 107: 430–432.

100 Worth, H., Breuer, H.W.M., Charchut, S. et al. (1987). Endobronchial versus intravenous application of Glypressin for the therapy and prevention of lung bleeding during bronchoscopy. *Am. Rev. Respir. Dis.* 135: A108.

101 Ramon, P.H., Wallaert, B., Devollez, M. et al. (1989). Traitement des hemoptysis graves par la terlipressine. *Rev. Mal. Respir.* 6: 365–368.

102 Anovar, D., Schaad, N., and Mazzocato, C. (2005). Aerosolized vasopressin is a safe and effective treatment for mild to moderate recurrent hemoptysis in palliative care patients. (letter). *J. Pain Symptom Manag.* 29: 427–429.

103 Kaneko, M., Ono, R., Yoneyama, T., and Ikada, S. (1980). A case of aortitis syndrome with massive hemorrhage following a transbronchial biopsy. *J. Jpn. Soc. Bronchol.* 3: 73–80.

104 Nakano, S. (1986). Use of Reptilase with an endoscope against bronchial hemorrhage. *Chin. Rep.* 20: 229–235.

105 Kinoshita, M., Shiraki, R., Wagai, F. et al. (1982). Thrombin instillation therapy through the fiberoptic bronchoscope in cases of hemoptysis. *Jpn. J. Thorac. Dis.* 20: 251–254.

106 Tsukamoto, T., Sasaki, H., and Nakamura, H. (1989). Treatment of hemoptysis patients by thrombin and fibrinogen-thrombin infusion therapy using a fiber optic bronchoscope. *Chest* 96: 473–476.

107 Takagi, O., Kohda, Y., Yamazaki, K. et al. (1983). Effect on bronchial bleeding by local infusion of fibrinogen and thrombin solution. *J. Jpn. Soc. Bronchol.* 5: 455–464.

108 Bense, L. (1990). Intrabronchial selective coagulative treatment of hemoptysis. *Chest* 97: 990–996.

109 Conlan, A.A. and Hurwitz, S.S. (1980). Management of massive hemoptysis with the rigid bronchoscope and cold saline lavage. *Thorax* 35: 901–904.

110 Gerasin, V.A. and Shafrovsky, B.B. (1988). Endobronchial electrosurgery. *Chest* 93: 270–274.

111 Jantz, M. and Silvestvi, G. (2006). Fire and ice: laser bronchoscopy, electrocautery and cryotherapy. In: *Thoracic Endoscopy: Advances in Interventional Pulmonology*, vol. 8 (eds. M.J. Simoff, D.M. Sterman and A. Ernst), 134–154. Ames: Blackwell Futura.

112 Dutau, H., Palot, A., Han, A. et al. (2006). Endobronchial embolization with a silicon spigot as a temporary treatment for massive hemoptysis. A new bronchoscopic approach of the disease. *Respiration* 73: 830–832.

113 Asano, F., Aoe, M., Ohsaki, Y. et al. (2012). Deaths and complications associated with respiratory endoscopy: a survey by the Japan Society for Respiratory Endoscopy in 2010. *Respirology* 17: 478–485.

114 Cordasco, E.M. Jr., Mehta, A.C., and Ahmad, M. (1991). Bronchoscopically induced bleeding. A summary of nine years' Cleveland clinic experience and review of the literature. *Chest* 100: 1141–1147.

115 Bjørtuft, O., Brosstad, F., and Boe, J. (1998). Bronchoscopy with transbronchial biopsies: measurement of bleeding volume and evaluation of the predictive value of coagulation tests. *Eur. Respir. J.* 12: 1025–1027.

116 Chinsky, K. (2005). Bleeding risk and bronchoscopy: in search of the evidence in evidence-based medicine. *Chest* 127: 1875–1877.

117 Carr, I.M., Koegelenberg, C.F., von Groote-Bidlingmaier, F. et al. (2012). Blood loss during flexible bronchoscopy: a prospective observational study. *Respiration* 84: 312–318.

118 Tukey, M.H. and Wiener, R.S. (2012). Population-based estimates of transbronchial lung biopsy utilization and complications. *Respir. Med.* 106: 1559–1565.

119 Smyth, C.M. and Stead, R.J. (2002). Survey of flexible fibreoptic bronchoscopy in the United Kingdom. *Eur. Respir. J.*

19: 458–463.
120 Suratt, P.M., Smiddy, J.F., and Gruber, B. (1976). Deaths and complications associated with fiberoptic bronchoscopy. *Chest* 69: 747–751.
121 Zhou, G.W., Zhang, W., Dong, Y.C. et al. (2016). Flexible bronchoscopy-induced massive bleeding: a 12-year multicenter retrospective cohort study. *Respirology* 21 (5): 927–931.
122 Hirshberg, B., Biran, I., Glazer, M., and Kramer, M.R. (1997). Hemoptysis: etiology, evaluation, and outcome in a tertiary referral hospital. *Chest* 112: 440–444.
123 Sakr, L. and Dutau, H. (2010). Massive hemoptysis: an update on the role of bronchoscopy in diagnosis and management. *Respiration* 80: 38–58.
124 Valipour, A., Kreuzer, A., Koller, H. et al. (2005). Bronchoscopy-guided topical hemostatic tamponade therapy for the management of life-threatening hemoptysis. *Chest* 127: 2113–2118.

第 23 章

气道支架

Septimiu D. Murgu[1], Jonathan S. Kurman[2], J. Francis Turner, Jr.[3,4], Atul C. Mehta[5], and Ko-Pen Wang[6]

[1] Department of Medicine, Section of Pulmonary and Critical Care, University of Chicago, Chicago, IL, USA

[2] Division of Pulmonary and Critical Care, Department of Medicine, Medical College of Wisconsin, Milwaukee, WI, USA

[3] Division of Pulmonary and Critical Care Medicine, University of Tennessee Graduate School of Medicine, Knoxville, TN, USA

[4] National Supercomputing Institute, University of Nevada, Las Vegas, NV, USA

[5] Lerner College of Medicine, Buoncore Family Endowed Chair in Lung Transplantation, Department of Pulmonary Medicine, Respiratory Institute, Cleveland Clinic, Cleveland, OH, USA

[6] Division of Pulmonary and Critical Care Medicine, Johns Hopkins Bayview Medical Center, Johns Hopkins University School of Medicine, Baltimore, MD, USA

（译者：陈 愉 王绮霞 徐逸铧 温梓键 译者单位：广州医科大学附属第一医院）

23.1 引言

自本书 2012 年第 3 版出版以来，本领域又已发表 500 多篇关于支架设计、生理学、应用和潜在并发症的文章。许多关于支架使用的基本原则仍然没有显著变化，本章对此进行了回顾。然而，关于支架在良、恶性疾病中的应用指征以及不同材料支架在气管支气管树内的相互作用和并发症一直存在争议，对此我们也将予以回顾，并介绍我们自己这些年的临床经验。

希波克拉底首次提出了将芦苇插入气管以帮助窒息患者的想法。现代支气管镜医生在气管支气管树内放置支架的技术成功实现了希波克拉底的设想。然而，大约在希波克拉底之后过了 2 000 年，英国牙医查尔斯·R. 斯坦特制造了牙科模型和夹板，能为移植物或吻合物提供支持，他的名字（Stent）因此成了希波克拉底数世纪前提出的想法的代名词[1]。自 19 世纪 70 年代起，已经有文献报道通过放置气道假体以帮助窒息患者减轻痛苦并改善呼吸[2-6]。

随着支架技术的发展，我们用于帮助呼吸窘迫患者的材料也在不断改进。早期由橡胶或银等金属制成的支架已经被硅酮、金属合金以及由聚合物和金属合金组成的复合支架所取代（图 23.1）。Montgomery 在 1965 年开创性地使用了橡胶-硅酮管。当时他描述了使用一个带侧支的中空管，经气切口置入来治疗声门下狭窄的方法[8]。1990 年，Jean-Francois Dumon 回顾了他开发专用支气管内支架治疗主气道外压狭窄的经验[9]。在这项开创性工作中，他概述了他首次使用改进的 Montgomery T 管，并随后研制了一种基于硅酮模具制作的气管支气管假体。其他研究人员尝试在 Dumon 的原始设计基础上进行改进，随后陆续开发了

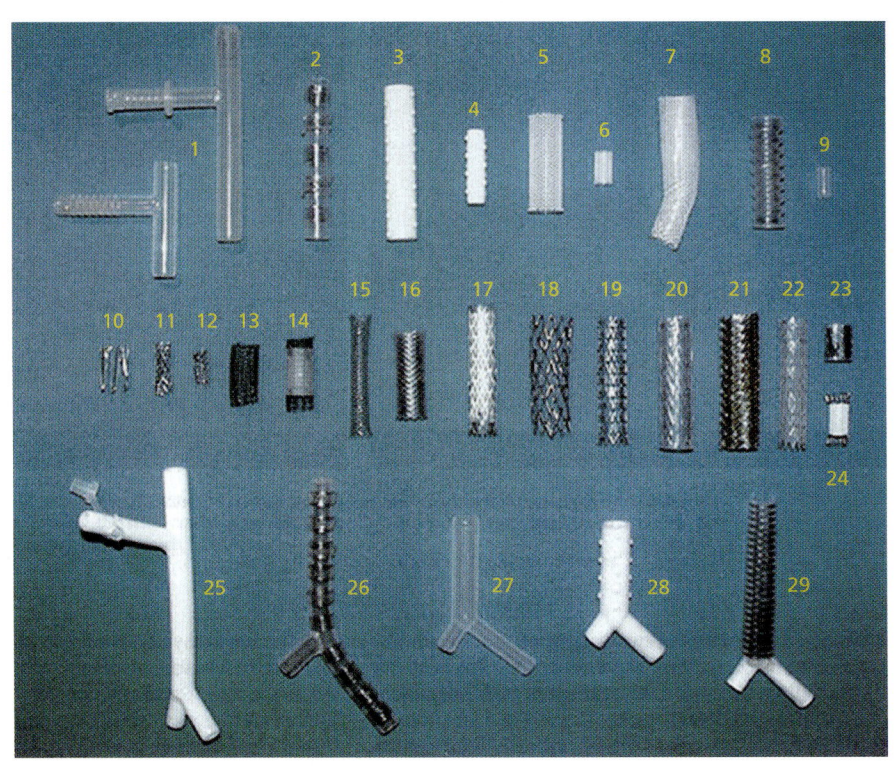

图 23.1　气道支架

1. Montgomery T 管；2. Orlowski 气管支架；3. Dumon 气管支架；4. Dumon 支气管支架；5. Polyflex 气管支架；6. Polyflex 支气管支架；7. Polyflex 残端支架；8. Noppen 气管支架；9. Hood 支气管支架；10. Gianturco 支架；11. Palmaz 支架；12. Strecker 钽支架；13. 非覆膜的 Ultraflex 支架；14. 覆膜 Ultraflex 支架；15. 非覆膜 Wallstent 支架；16. 覆膜 Wallstent 支架；17~24. 支架原型；25. Westaby T-Y 支架；26. Orlowski "Y" 形支架；27. Hood "Y" 形支架；28. Dumon "Y" 形支架；29. Rusch 动态支架。资料来源：经来自 Freitag 的 John Wiley & Sons 许可转载[7]。

由橡胶硅酮、金属合金或由先前使用的材料组成的复合支架。

23.2　工程与材料

气道是弹性结构，受到呼吸过程中产生的跨壁压的影响[10]。在过去的 30 年里，气道支架已被证明可以改善特定的中央气道阻塞（central airway obstruction，CAO）患者的症状，但它们确实也是气道中的异物，因此容易发生可预见的不良事件。随着气管支气管支架的发展，人们对气道和假体材料之间相互作用的重要性及其固有特性有了更深入的了解。了解中央气道解剖结构和流体力学对于正确选择气道支架至关重要。

如前文所述，正常成人气管长 10~14 cm，直到分叉进入左右主支气管。气管由 18~22 个 "C" 形软骨环支撑，软骨环由后部膜状部分连接。气管直径平均为 25 mm，左右主支气管直径平均为 16 mm，右主支气管长约 2 cm，左主支气管长约 5 cm。除了气管支气管树的个体解剖差异和跨壁压的影响外，还需要考虑到气管支气管黏液纤毛运输的作用[11]。黏膜纤毛清除功能的异常与多种疾病有关，咳嗽一种是帮助清除气管支气管树分泌物和异物的机制[12]。随着支架需要留置的时间越来越长，以及解剖和生理特征之间复杂的相互作用，要求我们在支架工程和材料使用方面取得进展。因此，当今支架的开发正是基于对特定技术和生物力学的深入理解[13]。

1）稳定气道。任何气管支气管支架的设计首先需要能够对抗施加在气道上的跨壁压，同时还能解除其放置所针对的外源性或内源性狭窄，以保持气道的通畅性[13,14]。

2）生物相容性。选择的材料应无刺激性，目标是容易插入和可能重建黏膜纤毛活动梯度。

3）易于插入和放置。支架应具有抗迁移性，能够适应病变气管支气管树的不规则形状，并具有不同的长度和直径。插入后应能调整和移除。

4）整合治疗性药物或材料。支架的设计最终应允许个体化整合能持续治疗恶性肿瘤的化疗药物或放射性材料、抗纤维化药物（用于潜在治疗良性气管狭窄）或促纤维化药物（用于潜在治疗气管支气管软化）。

从上述清单中可以迅速推断出，理想的支架尚未开发出来。目前，介入性肺病学的奥妙在于根据个体患者的适应证、禁忌证、特殊气道解剖结构以及支气管镜操作者的技能和经验，选择支架材料、尺寸和置入方式。

23.3 生物力学特性

在确定特定情况下最佳支架类型时，需要考虑许多生物力学特性。临床指征和狭窄部位特定的气道形态也是关键因素。笔者认为，对每个患者选择支架时，都应考虑以下因素。

23.3.1 可回收性

支架的放置可能是暂时的，也可能由于并发症而需要移除。放射治疗或全身治疗后，恶性 CAO 的程度可能会降低。在这种情况下，可能需要取出支架以防止移位，或取出已经移位的支架[15]。良性 CAO 的患者在支架移除后可能不会出现狭窄复发。支架诱导的肉芽组织增生、支架断裂、新生上皮化将部分覆膜或非覆膜支架完全包埋在气道壁内，这些因素将使得支架的移除变得复杂。因此，开展气道支架的支气管镜医师必须采用安全、有效的技术来移除支架。

23.3.2 扩张径向力

这一因素在现用的气道支架中因设计不同而有所差异。一项研究表明，硅酮支架具有比自膨式金属支架（self-expanding metallic stents, SEMS）更大的径向力[16]。因此，当气道受压严重且气道直径较大时，倾向于选择硅酮支架。了解每种类型支架的特性将使操作者能够根据扩张狭窄所需的压力选择最佳支架。这种压力可以通过在腔内应用带压力传感器的球囊来测量。该方法将允许个性化的、基于生理学的方法来选择气道支架。然而，目前支气管镜检查者尚无法获得这些参数。

23.3.3 抗变形能力

这种特性指的是支架抵抗成角的能力，当遇到弯曲或扭曲的气道时，这一能力尤为重要[16]。抗成角阻力将决定支架是否既贴合气道形态，又能保持其通畅性。这种挑战最常见于左主支气管，因为左主支气管是一条弯曲、锥形的气道，可能会因隆突下大肿瘤的外源性压迫而变形，还可见于右上叶缺失，需要从气管隆突向中间支气管远端插入支架时（锥形气道）。在这种情况下，SEMS 可能比硅酮支架更好，因为它具有更好的抗成角性。这一观点得到了一项研究的支持，该研究发现，带凸点的硅酮支架最常用于气管和右主干支气管，而部分覆膜的 SEMS（Ultraflex®，Boston Scientific，Natick，MA）在左主支气管中最常用[16]。

23.3.4 亲水性

支架内壁上有一层亲水涂层，用于防止黏液积聚。制造商没有公开每种支架类型的具体材料。这种特性和支架其他一些特性可能会造成黏液堵塞的风险。虽然硅酮和完全覆膜/部分覆膜的 SEMS 都会产生黏液潴留，但在我们看来，与硅酮支架相关的黏液往往更厚且"像胶水一样"，清除起来更具挑战性。

23.3.5 形态

支架形态（即形状）取决于气道狭窄的位置。例如，Montgomery T 管需通过气管造口术置入，而直筒形支架则用于开放气管和主支气管（在较新的型号中，甚至是肺叶支气管）。Y 形支架可置于主隆突或偶尔至副隆突。在某些情况下需要定制支架，可以在现场制作或向制造商订购。

23.3.6 尺寸

支架应将气道通畅性恢复到正常气道直径的至少 50%，以完全改善气流动力学。过大尺寸的支架可能会导致无法成功展开（即支架不会展开），或压力过大阻碍黏膜供血。黏膜缺血是肉芽组织形成的危险因素。对于直筒形硅酮支架，一项研究表明，支架与气道直径的比率达到 90% 时是肉芽组织形成的阈值[17]。另一方面，支架与气道直径比越小，移位率越高[18]。一篇文章报道，当比率为 0.9~1 时，移位率为 5%，但当比率<0.8 时，移位率增加到 15%。如果支架的整个周长都与气道壁接触，那么其扩张力的分布区域很大。如果支架只接触气道壁的一小部分，那么该区域的压力将明显更高，因为所有的扩张力将集中在那个有限的区域。这将导致黏膜血流明显

受损，从而导致组织缺血、损伤和肉芽组织形成。这种情况可见于在气管造口术后三角形狭窄处放置圆柱形支架。SEMS 的金属丝在接触组织的地方也可能限制黏膜血流。扩张后，选择比扩张支气管镜或球囊大 1~2 mm 的支架。可用计算机断层扫描（computed tomography，CT）的测量设备确定最佳支架尺寸。选择支架尺寸的理想方法是测量堵塞毛细血管所需的压力，然后在移位风险（尺寸过小）、黏膜缺血和肉芽组织形成风险（尺寸太大）之间进行权衡。

23.3.7 长度

气道狭窄类型相似时，长的狭窄较之简单狭窄（<1 cm），其狭窄段的总压强降低幅度仅轻度升高[19]。因此，从流体力学的角度来看，狭窄段长度和支架的长度都不是影响气流限制和症状的重要因素。然而，为了防止移位并适当缓解气道狭窄，支架的长度应超过狭窄的长度。支架应向近端和远端延伸超过狭窄区域 0.5~1.0 cm（即比狭窄总共长 1~2 cm，在有瘘道的情况下甚至更长）。狭窄段或瘘道的长度和精确位置是决定气道手术可行性和类型的关键因素（如气管袖状切除术、喉气管切除术等）。

23.3.8 疲劳性

疲劳寿命被定义为在正常通气周期中，特别是在用力呼气和咳嗽期间，由于反复压迫而导致支架疲软和断裂所需的时间。这种特性与良性 CAO，尤其是气管支气管软化的病例特别相关。因为考虑到良性疾病患者的寿命更长，这些支架往往可以放置更长的时间。支架的结构完整性更有可能随着时间的推移而受损，因为它将承受更多的压缩循环。支架断裂是一种罕见的并发症，主要与金属支架置入有关，可能导致气道壁穿孔或咯血，这可能是致命的。美国食品药品监督管理局（FDA）警告称，只有在探索了替代治疗方案（如手术和硅酮支架置入）后，才能在良性气道疾病患者中使用金属气管支架[20]。虽然新型金属支架有不同的设计，许多支架是在 2005 年 FDA 警告后上市的，但在推荐新型金属支架用于良性疾病的常规治疗之前，需要进行良好设计的可行性和安全性研究。考虑到所有上述生物力学特性将可以降低支架置入后并发症的风险。目前，制造商将这些特性视为专有信息，因此支气管镜医生无法获得。公司可能会考虑在未来向医生提供这些信息，以提高气道支架置入的安全性。

23.4 生理学原理

23.4.1 气管狭窄

在气道狭窄中，呼吸困难取决于呼吸做功，而呼吸做功与沿狭窄段的压降大小直接相关。这种压降不仅取决于狭窄程度（即半径），还取决于狭窄处的流速，这是气道狭窄程度相似的患者症状不同的原因。这是因为流速取决于活动水平。因此，在确定气道支架置入是否合理时，必须评估功能状态。功能状态和呼吸困难量表实际上可能比静态肺功能测量更适用，后者与喉气管狭窄的呼吸困难量值相关性较弱[21]。在一个分类系统中，50% 和 70% 的阈值分别用于定义中度和重度狭窄[22]。

生理学原理如图 23.2 中所述。正常的声门口径面积约相当于正常气管直径的 50%。因此，从流体力学的角度来看，50% 或更低的气管狭窄甚至可能没有临床意义或不需要治疗。基于该值，支架必须达到正常气道直径的至少 50% 的通畅性。通常在 75%、85% 和 90% 的狭窄度观察到压力的显著降低。在这些阈值下，呼吸功会增加[19]。狭窄环的范围和形态也会影响压力沿狭窄段的下降，但较气道狭窄程度的影响要小。例如，同样程度的气道狭窄，气管造口术后的三角形狭窄就比环形狭窄的症状轻。

23.4.2 呼气性中央气道塌陷

有临床意义的中央气道塌陷（exhalatory central airway collapse，ECAC）是如何形成的尚不清楚。目前也缺乏非侵入性手段来预测支架置入后的反应。当患者无法清除分泌物、反复发生肺炎或呼吸衰竭时，无论潜在病因如何，都需要进行气道支架置入。从生理学的角度看，问题的关键在于支架置入是否能改善呼气气流。了解气道生理学有助于理解 ECAC 状态下的气流动力学。

在给定的肺容量下，当呼气流速逐渐变小时，会在胸腔内气道中形成等压点（equal pressure point，EPP），支气管壁内、外压力相等[23]。EPP 和口腔之间的气道在用力呼气期间会受到压缩，甚至在特定情况下，潮汐呼气期间也可能受到压缩。这个被压缩区域或减小的管腔内径被称为限流段（flow-limiting segment，FLS）或"检查点"。随着呼气期间肺容量的减少和胸膜腔压力的增加，EPP 向下游移动，导致

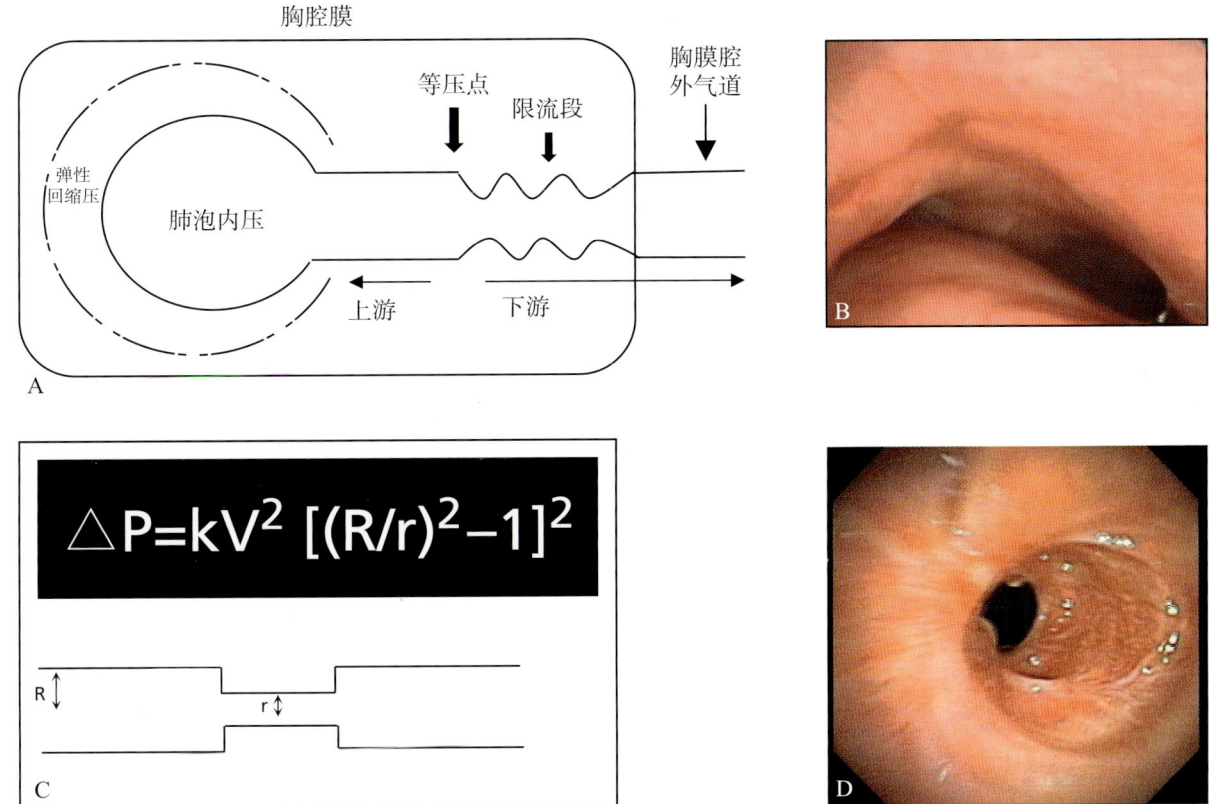

图 23.2 流量限制理论和梗阻生理学

A. 肺泡内压（Palv）使呼气时空气流动，大约相当于肺的弹性回缩压（Pst）和胸膜腔内压的总和。在用力呼气时，等压点（EPP）处的管腔内压力与胸膜腔内压相等。其上、下游跨壁压力分别为正、负。在一定肺容积下，来自 EPP 上游的驱动压力等于 Pst，而由于管腔内压力小于胸膜腔压力，下游气道被压缩。这个压迫区域是一个限流段或"阻塞点"。B. 在病态肥胖患者中，限制引起的 Pst 降低加上胸膜腔内压增加导致过度的动态气道塌陷（EDAC）。C. 对于气管狭窄，症状取决于沿狭窄段的压力降低程度。这是由阻碍程度（r）和流速（V）决定的。D. 对于固定阻塞，如结核后复杂气管狭窄，当狭窄程度为正常气管直径的 50% 时，应考虑置入支架，因为这时管径大约是正常声门的大小。鉴于其不断变化的严重程度，此建议不适用于动态狭窄。

FLS 延长。这会增加气道阻力，防止呼气流速进一步增加。当气流流速固定时，EPP 也将停止移动。在高肺容量（总肺活量）下，EPP 和 FLS 位于气管。然而，随着肺容量的减少，FLS 将向外围移动，但仍处于中央气道中[24]。由于人体中 FLS 通常位于叶支气管，尽管在 CT 扫描或支气管镜检查中可观察到主支气管或气管塌陷，但不应导致口腔和 FLS 之间的任何压降。因此，流速不应受到影响（图 23.2）。

基于这一分析，生理学家建议在发现呼气性气管或主支气管塌陷时，应到肺的更远端气道中寻找气流阻塞的迹象[25]。ECAC 可能只是外周气道阻塞或胸膜腔压力增加的表现。事实上，这可能是由于病态肥胖引起的，这会导致静息状态下胸膜腔压力增加，可能会导致气流受限。支架仍然可以通过改善分泌物引流或减少气流湍流来改善一些气管支气管软化或过度动态气道塌陷（excessive dynamic airway collapse，EDAC）患者的功能状态。其原理类似于采用氦氧混合气提高中重度慢性阻塞性肺病（chronic obstructive pulmonary disease，COPD）患者的运动能力，尽管这些患者的阻塞点位于小气道[26]。

23.5 适应证

支架置入适用于各种良性和恶性疾病。事实上，30% 的肺癌患者在诊断时会出现中央气道异常（其中一些是真正的阻塞性病变）[27]。在置入任何支架之前，应仔细考虑，导致患者气道狭窄的病因有无可能通过外科手术治愈[28]。此外，对于特定的病变，使用减瘤策略或辅以激光/电凝术扩张可能就足够了。

一旦确定无法手术根治，可以考虑支架置入，其适应证主要包括以下的良性或恶性疾病（表 23.1）。

表 23.1 支架作为大气道阻塞的姑息性治疗手段

	紧急	支气管腔内	激光/支架
新生物		黏膜下层	支架
		外压型	支架
	可选用	支气管内	
		外生型	激光,冷冻,PDT,电凝
气管狭窄		黏膜下层	XRT,近距离放疗,支架
		外压型	XRT,支架
		瘢痕狭窄	激光,支架,扩张
		非瘢痕狭窄	支架
		炎症后	系统的治疗,支架
气管支气管软化			支架

PDT,光动力治疗;XRT,放射治疗。资料来源:经 Metha,Dasgupta[33] 许可转载。

(1)良性梗阻

1)声门下狭窄[29-32]:
  a. 感染后;
  b. 气管插管后;
  c. 声门下和喉部囊肿或网眼;
  d. 气管环;
  e. 声门下血管瘤;
  f. 膜性蹼状网眼;
  g. 气管软化症;
  h. 第一气管环闭合;
  i. 创伤;
  j. 系统性疾病(如干燥综合征等结缔组织病)。

2)气管支气管的良性疾病:
  a. 创伤后;
  b. 感染后;
  c. 系统性疾病;
  d. 肺移植后;
  e. 气管支气管软化;
  f. 良性肿瘤;
  g. 来自主动脉瘤的外压;
  h. 躯体畸形导致的气管变形;
  i. 食管支架引起的大气道梗阻;
  j. 先天性气管食管瘘。

(2)恶性肿瘤

1)外压;
2)由黏膜下疾病引起的内在梗阻;
3)气管支气管食管瘘[33]。

气道支架置入的适应证因梗阻机制不同而有所差别,如外压、管腔内梗阻和混合性梗阻等。其他适应证包括残端瘘、食管气道瘘(esophago-respiratory fistulas,ERF)和 ECAC。

无论支架置入的梗阻机制如何,CAO 患者的肺功能在置入后都会得到改善。前瞻性研究表明,支气管镜对恶性 CAO 的干预与 6 min 步行试验、肺活量测定和呼吸困难的改善相关[34]。支气管镜下治疗可以快速缓解梗阻,提高生活质量,并充当全身治疗起效之前的过渡手段[35-37]。通过保持气道通畅,支架还可以预防阻塞性肺炎,协助拔管及启动全身治疗,进而改善生存。与历史对照组相比,PS 评分中度的患者最能生存获益,因此在恶性 CAO 并发症发生之前,及时进行气道支架置入可能会改善生存[38]。一项针对初治和终末期肺癌患者的研究表明,支架置入后的中位生存时间分别为 5.6 个月和 1.6 个月,1 年生存率分别为 25%和 5.1%[39]。

23.5.1 支架置入治疗气道外压

良性或恶性纵隔或实质性肺疾病、甲状腺肥大或巨大淋巴结可引起有症状的外压性气道压迫。对于不适于手术的外压患者,当症状严重且其他治疗方法显效较慢时(即由纵隔肿块引起的气管严重压迫,伴有呼吸困难),支架可能是唯一选择。极少情况下,无法手术矫正的血管异常,如主动脉瘤和双主动脉弓,可能也需行气道支架置入。

23.5.2 管腔内阻塞(狭窄环或外生性)

如果使用腔内疗法去除梗阻的管腔内成分后,残余狭窄仍超过 50%,则应考虑支架。这一原则通常适用于恶性梗阻[40]。良性管腔内梗阻可能是特发性、创伤性的,或与多种疾病有关,包括肉芽肿伴多血管炎、淀粉样变性、结节病、溃疡性结肠炎或结核病。支架仅适用于特定的病例(如无法手术和扩张失败的患者)。复发性呼吸道乳头状瘤病(recurrent respiratory papillomatosis,RRP)是一种良性 CAO,如果其他医疗手段无法保持气道通畅,可能需要支架置入。病例报告表明,使用硅酮支架可充分控制 RRP 继发的 CAO[41]。特发性气管狭窄、气管插管后和气管造口术后狭窄的支架置入应仅在非手术候选者中考虑。与其他形式的 CAO 一样,这些患者在考虑使用支架之前必须有大于 50% 的狭窄并出现症状。复杂的狭窄,即长度>1 cm 的狭窄,通常伴有软骨炎,所以仅仅扩张通常是无效的[42]。在这些情况下，硅酮支架是首选[42,43]。在一项针对复杂狭窄患者的研究中，只有20%的患者适合外科治疗；80%的患者使用硅酮支架治疗，成功率为70%[18]。对于复杂狭窄，如支架放置约12个月或更长时间后再移除，支气管镜治疗的成功率将会提高[44]。单纯狭窄，即范围<1 cm，无软化的狭窄，单用支气管镜治疗（激光或电凝辅助机械扩张）的成功率更高。据报道，气管插管至治疗的潜伏期可以独立预测支气管镜干预的成功率，这可能是因为存在发展为复杂狭窄的风险[45,46]。白光支气管镜检查可能难以评估气道壁支架的完整性，这可能解释了为什么一些患者会因复杂狭窄而进行反复扩张。基于球囊的径向探头支气管内超声可用于检测潜在的软骨缺损[47]。硅酮T管，也称为Montgomery T管，可用于喉气管狭窄的良性病例，这些患者既不适合手术，也不适合置入直筒形气道支架[42]。在良性疾病中，尤其是上气道/声门下区域，SEMS与重大并发症有关，如可能应尽量避免使用[20]。

23.5.3 混合性阻塞

混合性外源性和管腔内阻塞通常由恶性病变引起，这是需放置支架的最常见的阻塞形式[48]。支架放置的适应证不变，但由于需要多种操作，这些患者可能需要结合使用多种镜下治疗技术（即去除腔内部分、扩张和放置支架）。

23.5.4 残端瘘

使用支架来覆盖肺叶切除术或肺切除术后的大型残端瘘是支架置入的少见适应证[49]。治疗策略取决于潜在的病因、瘘管的大小、持续时间和患者的健康状况。支气管镜治疗通常适用于无法手术或需要推迟手术的患者[50]。对于需要机械通气的患者来说，手术修复是一个糟糕的选择，因为作用在修复后残端的持续气压伤使得手术的失败率很高[50]。一般来说，在这种情况下，必须使用大尺寸支架，以便尽可能紧密地密封残端瘘，避免吸入性肺炎，并在需要机械通气支持的情况下允许单肺通气。

23.5.5 食管呼吸道瘘（ERF）

大多数ERF见于食管切除术后、气管插管后或恶性肿瘤中。良性ERF在支架放置后可能不会改善，甚至瘘口进一步增大。因此，只有在手术矫正不可行的情况下才应考虑支架置入[51]。大多数恶性ERF放置支架的目的是缓解症状，提高生活质量[52]。恶性ERF的缓解通常需置入食管支架、气道支架或两者同时置入[52]。一种专用于瘘道的支架，即DJ袖扣形假体，是专门为恶性ERF设计的，其尺寸可以调整以适应瘘道[53,54]。研究表明，硅酮"Y"形支架可以改善恶性ERF症状，减少感染，并提高生活质量。较早的研究表明，这些患者平均存活时间仅约2个月[55]。如果不进行治疗，存活时间可能仅几天[54]。最近的一项研究发现，平均总生存期为236.6天[52]。气道支架、食管支架和气道-食管联合支架的平均生存时间分别为219.1、262.8和252.9天[52]。

原则上讲，任何良性ERF都应考虑外科修复。SEMS和硅酮支架偶可用于无法手术的患者。覆膜SEMS似可作为首选，这是因为其和气道壁的接触更紧密，从而可更持久的闭合瘘道。对于良性ERF，支架应仅看作能耐受外科手术治疗前的一种临时措施[56-58]。对于恶性ERF，食管支架是优选的，除非同时存在气道阻塞。值得注意的是，食管支架置入后，气道阻塞可能会加重。有时，首先进行气道支架置入，只有在影像学检查提示仍有残留瘘的情况下才放置食管支架。

23.5.6 呼气性中央气道塌陷

气道支架置入已被用于改善ECAC患者的咳嗽、分泌物和生活质量[59,60]。在这种情况下是否置入支架需考虑到以下两点：①对异常狭窄的标准化定义和阈值尚不明晰；②这种狭窄是否是导致气流限制的真正原因[61]。研究表明，在短期内（10~14天），ECAC患者使用硅酮支架来稳定气道可以改善症状、生活质量和功能状态。然而，在一项研究中，支架相关并发症的发生率接近10%[59]。在另一项主要针对气管支气管软化症患者的研究中，83%的患者在置入后29天内至少出现1种并发症[60]。由于ECAC的动态性质，支架与气道壁之间的接触点不断变化，导致摩擦和黏膜刺激，可能更频繁地出现黏液栓、支架移位和肉芽组织形成。虽然并不致命，但这些并发症需要频繁的支气管镜介入治疗[60]。

ECAC中过度的气道狭窄会导致湍流，从而增加气道阻力。因此，需要更大的跨肺压来维持呼气气流。这会增加呼吸做功，并可能导致呼吸困难。无创气道正压通气可以作为气动支架，通过保持气道通畅来降低肺阻力。这可以促进分泌物排出并改善呼气流量。有限的证据表明，在接受支架置入的ECAC患者中，生活质量和功能状况得到改善，但通过 FEV_1 测量，肺功能并未显示出与支架置入或膜性气管成形术相一致的改善[59]。这也引起了疑惑，从生理角度看，在该类型疾病中支架置入是否合适。只有使用支气管镜假手术作为对照的随机研究才能澄清在该综合征中支架置入的合理性。

23.6 禁忌证

气管支气管树支架置入术的绝对和相对禁忌证与以下因素有关。

23.6.1 患者病情

气管支气管支架术的绝对禁忌证很少。能够进行手术重建并治愈的潜在良性或恶性疾病，是置入人工假体的绝对禁忌证。事实上，SEMS 不应用于需要手术切除的潜在候选者[62]。那些行动不便和预计只能存活很短时间的患者应该避免进一步干预，考虑进行姑息治疗。然而，这并不排除在重病患者中使用支架以及联合多模式治疗的可能性。在 Colt 和 Harrell 的一项回顾性综述中，1994—1996 年，32 名需要机械通气的患者接受了联合模式治疗[63]。在这 32 名患者中，15 人接受了支架置入术（9 例恶性疾病和 6 例良性疾病）。在这项研究中，通过支架置入和包括硬质支气管镜在内的联合治疗，52.6% 的患者能够立即停用机械通气。在随访中，只有 5 名患者发生支架移位或肉芽组织形成，均为良性气道疾病和高位气管病变。

其他研究支持了采用气管支气管支架术治疗恶性气道阻塞和终末期疾病患者的理念[64-67]。Monnier 的研究中指出，对 40 名无法手术的气管支气管癌患者，临床及内镜下改善了术后 1 天、30 天和 90 天对呼吸困难指数，平均 Karnofsky 表现指数也从 40 提高到 70[65]。Vonk-Noordegraaf 等随后于 2001 年发表的一项研究中，评估了 14 名因中央气道阻塞即将窒息的患者置入支架的姑息效果[66]。尽管这是个小型研究，但其目的是评估在临终护理的边缘临床情况下姑息治疗的界限。总体而言，该研究中患者的平均生存期为 11 周，14 名患者中有 12 人存活出院。Vonk-Noordegraaf 的研究值得注意，是因为它包括了患者的初诊全科医生的评估，以回顾性判断姑息干预的最终效果。结论是尽管患者面临即将窒息的困境，但通过支架的置入，大多数患者在全科医生的照料下，能够在家中（80%）去世，而这些医生最终负责患者在家中的临终护理。因此，可以得出结论，在 58% 即将窒息的癌症患者中放置支架是值得的。Murgu 等最近的研究进一步证明，患有非小细胞肺癌和呼吸衰竭的患者进行支架置入是有必要的，因为它能够减轻护理负担并启动全身治疗[68]。

相对禁忌证更多地取决于患者的病情和阻塞程度。那些不能耐受中度镇静或全身麻醉的患者，目前的支架置入技术存在相对禁忌证。对于恶性气道梗阻，这些患者接受介入性支气管镜检查时，全身麻醉可能更安全[69]。事实上，在这项注册研究中，中度镇静、紧急性支气管镜检查的需求、ASA 评分＞3、低功能状态和再次支气管镜检查是 30 天发病率和死亡率以及资源利用风险增加的独立危险因素。

23.6.2 阻塞的程度和持续时间

在评估支架置入的可能性时，必须在置入前评估阻塞的程度和影响。为了成功置入支架，在尝试置入支架之前，必须确定气道管腔具有扩张潜力。这取决于支气管镜医生是否能够通过支气管镜或探头将阻塞远端打开。CAO 的分类系统表明气道狭窄可以通过结构或动态特征、狭窄程度（管腔阻塞的百分比）、病灶与气管或主支气管的位置关系来描述[70]（表 23.2 至表 23.4、图 23.3）。当前的狭窄分级体系主要是围绕喉气管狭窄尤其是声门下狭窄，对其回顾后笔者提出了上述表格中的建议[71-76]。

表 23.2 狭窄分类

狭窄	类型	特点
结构性	1	外生型 / 内生型
	2	外压的
	3	变形
	4	瘢痕 / 狭窄
动力性或功能性	1	软骨受损 / 软化
	2	膜部活动度增大（软膜）

资料来源：经 John Wiley & Sons、Freitag 等许可转载[70]。

表 23.3 气道狭窄的程度

级数	程度（%）
0	没有狭窄
1	25#
2	26~50#

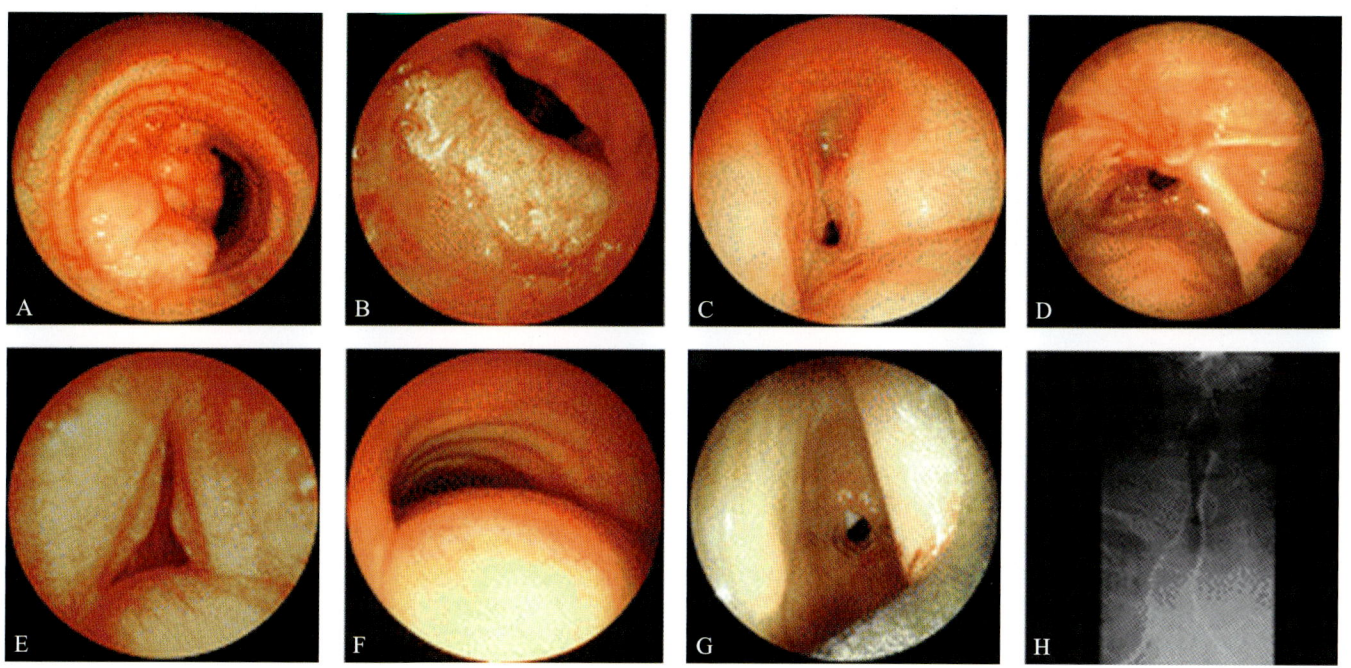

图 23.3 不同类型气道狭窄的临床实例

A. 腔内肿瘤或肉芽肿；B. 变形或扭曲；C. 外压性狭窄；D. 瘢痕狭窄；E. 剑鞘形气管；F. 膜部松弛；G. 急剧变窄（网眼狭窄）；H. 锥形变窄（沙漏狭窄）。资料来源：经来自 Freitag 等的 John Wiley & Sons 许可转载[70]。

（续表）

级数	程度（%）
3	51~75#
4	76~90#
5	91~完全闭塞

#横截面积减小。资料来源：经 John Wiley & Sons、Freitag 等许可转载[70]。

表 23.4 根据位置进行的狭窄分类

分级	位置
I	气管的上 1/3
II	气管的中间 1/3
III	气管的下 1/3
IV	右主支气管
V	左主支气管

资料来源：经 John Wiley & Sons、Freitag 等许可转载[70]。

在尝试置入支架之前，应该已经识别出气道管腔，并经球囊扩张或切除多余组织。如果无法确定可用的气道管腔，或者扩张程度不允许放置支架，则应放弃这种尝试[77]。还应认识到，在尝试打开管腔和放置支架之前，应评估新开通的气道通向的肺的状态。如果阻塞腔远端的肺组织已经萎缩，则再膨胀的可能性较小[78,79]。如果目标管腔通向的部位在影像上提示存在肺脓肿或肿瘤，则应重新考虑开通管腔的效果，或做好引流肺脓肿的准备。大气道（肺叶或主干）持续闭塞时，相应肺血管并发血栓闭塞的概率相对较高。在这种情况下，支气管再通可能没有任何功能益处，甚至会通过增加死腔通气而恶化气体交换[80]。因此，通气/灌注比和仔细评估增强胸部CT扫描可能有助于支气管镜干预的决策过程。

23.6.3 阻塞位置

虽然没有绝对的位置禁忌，但声门下因距离声带太近，放置支架可能更具挑战性。鉴于此，我们不推荐在声门下间隙置入支架，因其耐受性差（如咳嗽、误吸等）和移位率高。理想情况下，声门下间隙不应使用支架，因为导致狭窄的最初损伤通常是由人工气道引起的。然而，有时也使用支架来支撑移植物和皮瓣，这对支撑重建喉气管骨架、防止瘢痕形成具有重要作用[81,82]。

此外，各种支架均有过尝试。Colt 等描述了支气管镜下放置声门下支架，经皮外固定的技术[83]。英国的 Morris 报道了 Montgomery T 管在治疗声门下狭窄中的应用[84]。此外，Miyazawa 在声门下区域使用了

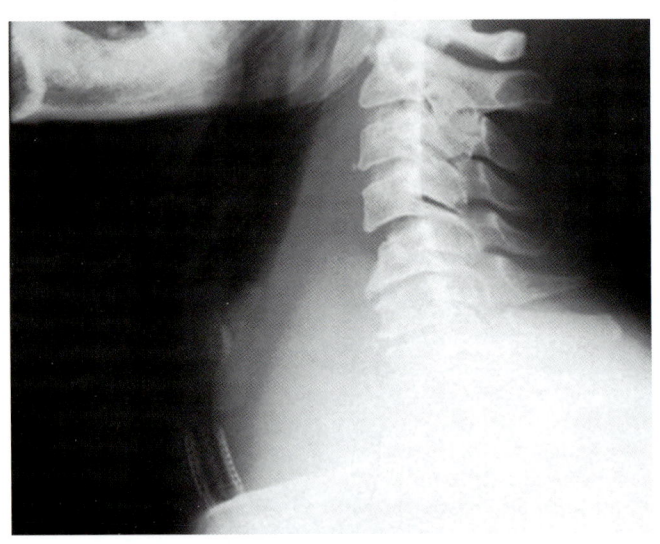

图 23.4 声门下梗阻患者放置镍钛合金（Ultraflex）支架后的侧位胸片

资料来源：经来自 Freitag 等的 John Wiley & Sons 许可转载[70]。

一些新的混合支架（图 23.4）[85]。

气管支气管树的其余部分（肺叶和段支气管）的阻塞通常可以使用支架（尤其是新型号的支架）。然而，需要对患者的潜在益处或风险进行严格评估，对叶支气管支架的有效性进行批判性判断。ACQUIRE 注册研究表明，阻塞越远（肺叶及以上），患者症状越轻（PS 评分<2），支气管镜干预的益处就越小[69]。基于这些数据，目前尚不清楚叶支气管支架是否能改善恶性 CAO 患者的预后。尽管如此，一项小型回顾性研究评估了 14 例同时患有恶性和良性叶支气管狭窄的患者，结果显示小型 SEMS 叶支气管支架可立即缓解 92% 的患者的呼吸困难，并在良性病变患者中产生持久性肺功能测试（pulmonary function test，PFT）和临床症状的改善[86]。如此看来，即使是段支气管支架（平均每位患者 4 次手术）也可以改善影像学和临床结果[87]。这需要更多的研究来证实这些发现。

23.6.4 可调用的人员和设备

所需的设备取决于阻塞的类型、要放置的支架以及可能的并发症。在尝试放置支架之前，应确定合适的设备和人员。团队必须意识到，即使是计划中的常规 SEMS 置入也可能有严重的并发症，需要立即或随后使用重新定位器械，如活检钳、球囊、硬质支气管镜和硬质活检钳。

无论使用何种类型的支架，我们建议由受过支架放置和移除培训的团队进行支架放置。该团队应该熟悉潜在的不良反应，并能对潜在的严重并发症（如气道阻塞）作出快速反应，正如我们之前对于支气管镜下激光术所推荐的那样[78]。尽管 SEMS 允许在中度镇静下放置，但气道阻塞的程度，特别是在中央气道，可能需要更深的镇静，采用全身麻醉和肌松。因此，团队必须有一位了解复杂气道并能和介入肺脏病医师共同管理气道的麻醉医师。靶控全静脉麻醉（target-controlled total intravenous anesthesia，TIVA）可能是首选，特别是在使用开放系统（硬质支气管镜下支架置入术）时[88]。通常采用多种麻醉技术的组合。这些可能包括静脉镇静药和阿片类药物以及吸入麻醉药物。这些与各种人工气道和通气方式结合使用，包括喉罩通气（laryngeal mask airway，LMA），硬质支气管镜通气，自主呼吸和喷射通气。

23.7 支架类型和放置要求

由于不同患者的病情需要不同，阻塞和狭窄的类型不同，人员和专业经验知识及设备存在不同，所以目前不存在理想的支架，最重要的原则仍然是"不同的病情-不同的支架"。因此，支架的类型、放置技术和所需人员可能会根据患者的具体情况而有所调整。下面描述不同的放置方法和支架类型，目的是讲述不同类型支架的适应证和局限性，并非是针对个别患者情况的指导。这需要在初始的支气管镜评估和治疗时根据具体情况确定。

23.7.1 橡胶支架和硅酮支架

23.7.1.1 Montgomery T 管

在 1965 年，一种 T 管被引入用于治疗声门下狭窄。虽然早期的 T 管是由丙烯酸制成的，但后来被硅橡胶所取代。Montgomery T 管可用于治疗高至声带水平的狭窄，需在气管切开术下实施。在气管切开时及之后，通过现有的气管造口置入支架。先把 T 管的远端支穿过切开口置入气管，然后用钳子夹住 T 管，将 T 管的近端支拉入适当的位置并在内镜下调整位置（图 23.5）。

暴露在外的 T 管颈部支可保持开放以便于进行抽吸及通气（图 23.6）。如果不存在更近端的声门阻塞且患者可以发声，那么就可将 T 管颈部支封堵。这种情况需要有正常的声带和口咽部才能说话。由于固定的 T 管颈部支通过气管切开口，因此 T 管不易发生移位。干燥的分泌物以及反复出现的切开口感染或肉芽组织

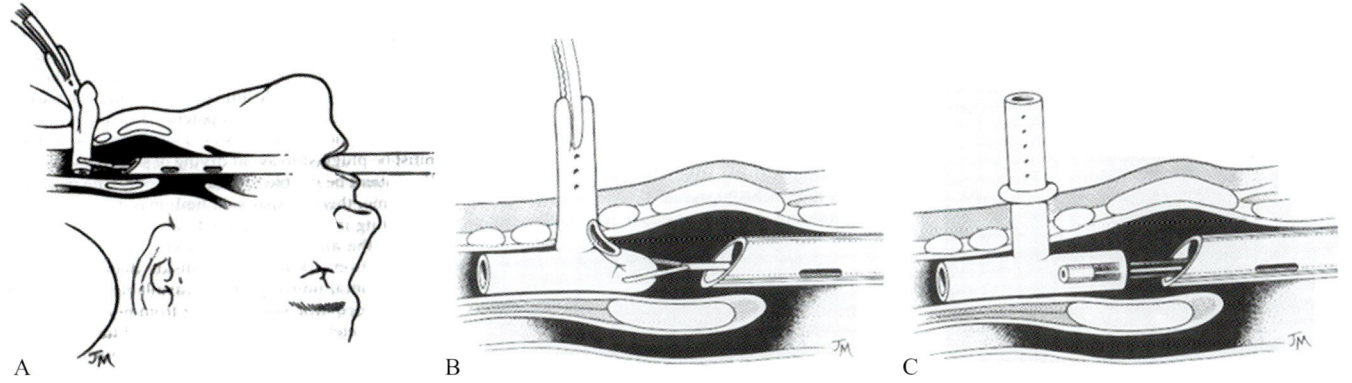

图 23.5　Montgomery T 管

A. 通过气管切开口置入 Montgomery T 管，运用 Kelly 钳和硬质异物钳将 T 管远端支向下推；B. 一旦 T 管远端支位置放置正确，使用硬质支气管镜异物钳向上拉 T 管近端支，同时将硬质支气管镜牢固地固定在声门下间隙内；C. 一旦近端支展开，将硬质支气管镜轻轻后撤，以评估近端支与声带之间的距离。资料来源：经 John Wiley & Sons 公司许可转载[89]。

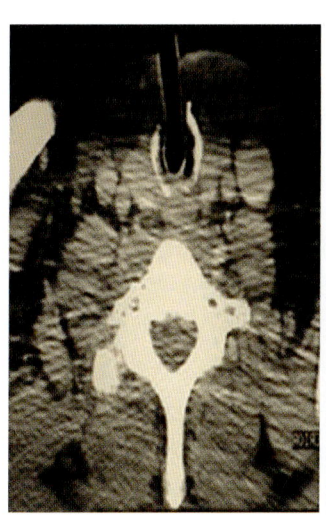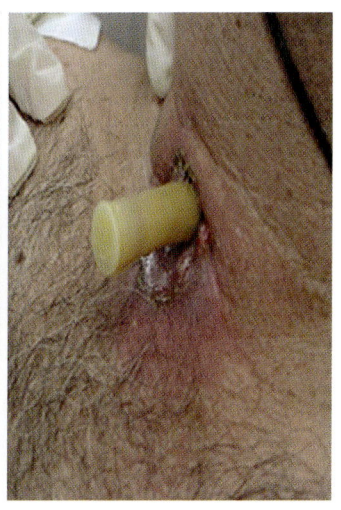

图 23.6　颈部 CT 显示 Montgomery T 管的颈部支

患者 T 管颈部支有肉芽组织形成和蜂窝组织炎。资料来源：经 John Wiley & Sons 公司许可转载。

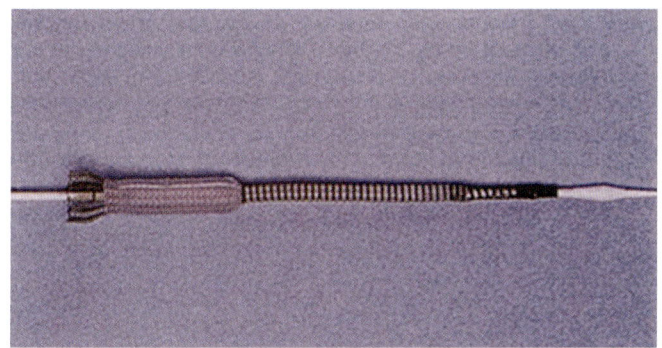

图 23.7　Ultraflex 支架部分约束在推送器上

通过拉动推送器近端的释放绳来进一步释放支架，然后拔出塑料输送导管。资料来源：经 John Wiley & Sons 公司许可转载。

可能造成管腔阻塞（图 23.6）。尤其是当 T 管的近端分支紧靠声带和声门开口时，声带功能可能因而受损。

23.7.1.2　Hood 支架

Hood 支架[图 23.1（9）]是一种带有突缘的防移位的硅酮管。这些分叉硅酮支架的气管直径为 14 mm，需要使用硬质支气管镜才能置入。

23.7.1.3　Dumon 支架

1990 年推出的 Dumon 支架[图 23.1（3,4,28）]（法国阿巴约内的诺瓦泰克公司生产）可能是世界上使用最频繁的硅酮支架。它们都设计了用于防止迁移的外部硅酮螺柱，并且有不同的长度和直径。Dumon 支架的"Y"形支架也适用于气管和支气管性阻塞。Dumon 支架用途广泛，通过气道壁和硅酮螺柱之间的接触压力固定在位。支架的放置通常需要使用硬质支气管镜和专用的 Dumon 支架释放装置。不过，也可使用其他技术，包括带霍普金斯光源镜或不同直径的硬质支气管镜。在没有硬质支气管镜的情况下，也可使用气管插管进行放置。作者并不推荐这些替代技术，因为这些技术发生术中并发症方面的安全性不确切。

Dumon 支架的并发症相对较少，Dumon 在 1987—1994 年放置了共 1 574 个支架，值得注意的是移位发生率为 9.5%，分泌物阻塞的发生率为 3.6%。此外，对于硅酮支架的较大规模的研究提示，分泌物潴留的并发症在 3%～4% 之间，肉芽组织的形成在 6%～20% 之间，移位发生率高达 17%。最近的研究表明，在恶性 CAO 患者中，与 SEMS 相比，Dumon 直形硅酮支架的移位率更高。这些发现很耐人寻味，因为硅酮支架的径向扩张力远高于 SEMS。由于 Dumon 支架需要使用硬质支气管镜，因而有可能导致 Dumon 支架尺寸过小。自从 Montgomery T 管和 Dumon 硅酮支架的开发以来，为了防止移位等并发症发生，其设计上发生了变化。Reynders-NoppenTyron 带螺纹气管支架与标准 Dumon 支架进行了比较［图 23.1（8）］。对 46 名需要放置 50 个支架的气管狭窄患者进行研究，并将其与标准的 Dumon 支架进行配对，便于支架置入和随访。在良性气管狭窄的患者中，螺纹组与传统的 Dumon 支架相比，移位率显著减少（24% 比 5%）。

23.7.2 金属及合金支架

在气管支气管树中置入金属支架已有数十年历史。坎菲尔德和诺顿植入了一根银管来治疗气道狭窄，Harkins 随之利用铬钴合金制成支架，这些都普及了金属支架在治疗气管和支气管狭窄中的使用。由合金制成的金属支架可以根据基本成分、生物力学性能或其置入、展开的技术或并发症来区分。下面概述了需要球囊扩张或自膨胀的金属支架。金属和合金支架使用得越来越多，因为它们可以通过导丝或可弯曲支气管镜进行放置，这与需硬质支气管镜递送的支架有所区别。这些支架其中的一些，在商业上已无法应用于气道，但由于其历史价值，本章仍将对其进行讨论。

23.7.2.1 球囊辅助膨胀金属和合金支架

23.7.2.1.1 Strecker 支架

Strecker 支架（波士顿科学公司）［图 23.1（12）］是一种钽丝网状管，源于血管假体。支架在透视下放置，当定位到狭窄处时，通过球囊充气展开。这种支架的并发症包括肉芽组织的形成和肿瘤向支架内生长。

23.7.2.1.2 Palmaz Stent

Palmaz Stent（强生公司，沃伦，新泽西州）［图 23.1（11）］是一种由导管递送和透视下定位的钢丝支架。Palmaz 钢支架需要球囊扩张来完成释放且支架更僵硬。一旦因呼吸压力改变而变形，如剧烈咳嗽，它无法重新膨胀到原来的直径，可能造成气道阻塞。

23.7.2.2 自膨胀金属和合金支架

最近，由导管递送的自膨式金属或合金支架已经被开发出来，其递送系统简单，应用广泛。

23.7.2.2.1 Gianturco 支架

Gianturco 支架（库克公司，比耶韦尔斯科夫，丹麦）［图 23.1（10）］是一个连续的不锈钢环，末端有金属钩，在放置时具有自膨胀的能力。支架的存在的问题包括肿瘤向内生长和穿孔。金属钩使得这种特殊的支架很难被调整或移除。

23.7.2.2.2 Wallstent™

Wallstent 支架（波士顿科技公司）［图 23.1（15,16）］由钴基合金长丝编织而成，对于一些型号，该支架经导丝和置入装置或可弯曲支气管镜的工作通道来递送。该支架已用于良性和恶性狭窄。覆膜 Wallstent 结合了 Wallstent 的原始设计，带有钴基合金细丝和聚亚安酯覆膜。其被设计成经导丝递送，具备自膨胀能力。钴合金的聚亚安酯覆膜不会降低支架的灵活性或放置性能。开发这种聚氨酯覆盖物是为了防止肉芽组织向内生长。置入时也存在类似的并发症，此外，如果覆膜 Wallstent 发生移位，则存在引起气管或支气管闭塞的可能性。Wallstent 不再被批准用于气道，但一些术者仍对那些市场上用于胃肠道产品进行"标签使用"。

23.7.2.2.3 镍钛合金支架

钛和镍合金（镍钛合金）支架（波士顿科学公司）［图 23.1（13,14）］的结合具有形状记忆特性，允许在放置时自膨胀，也可以通过插入导丝和透视来递送（图 23.7、图 23.8）。镍钛支架在置入人体后会自膨胀到预定的直径，并迅速嵌到周围的上皮中，在 3~4 个月的时间里会被纤毛黏膜覆盖。置入气道初期可通过异物钳钳夹支架上缘的调整线，使支架局部塌陷而调整支

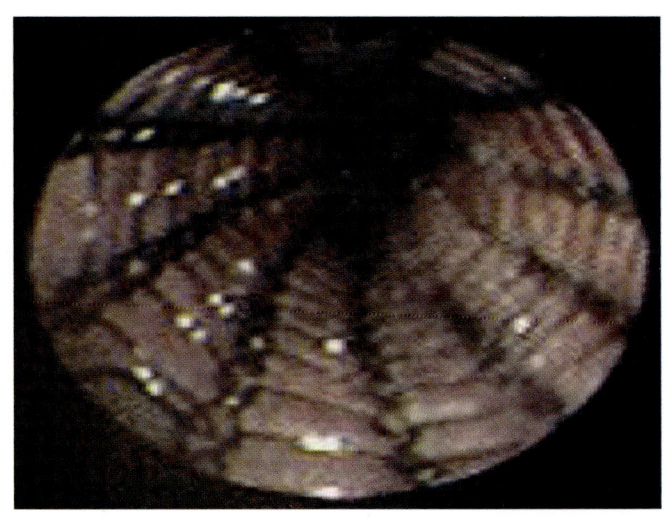

图 23.8 完全复张的 Ultraflex 支架

该支架被放置在声门下间隙，如图 23.3 H 胸片所示。资料来源：经 John Wiley & Sons 公司许可转载。

架,但一旦支架完全嵌入气管支气管壁后,这种操作就会变得十分困难。事实上,在 SEMS 移除过程中多数并发症见于非覆膜 SEMS 和长期支架置入的患者。

23.7.3. 复合型支架

复合型支架是将聚合物和金属或合金技术结合在一起的支架。

23.7.3.1 Ultraflex 支架

Ultraflex 支架(微创,波士顿科学公司)由钽丝制成,也有聚亚安酯覆膜的型号。覆膜的目的与其他覆膜支架一致,即试图防止肿瘤向内生长(图 23.9、图 23.10)。Ultraflex 支架可在可弯曲支气管镜下经导丝引导放置。网眼末端仍可能形成肉芽组织或肿瘤内生。这种肿瘤向内生长很可能是部分覆膜支架相较全覆膜支架移位率低的原因。对恶性 CAO 的研究表明,这些支架的并发症发生率低,可有效地用于具有明显不对称和不规则气道结构的复杂恶性 CAO。

23.7.3.2 Polyflex™ 支架

Polyflex 支架(波士顿科学公司,马萨诸塞州纳蒂克)是一种硅酮和聚酯纤维构成的复合型支架。它的强度来自将聚酯纤维交织入硅酮覆盖物中。Polyflex 支架需在硬质支气管镜或悬吊式喉镜下插入及放置。一项研究表明,在良性气道疾病中,使用 Polyflex 支架的并发症发生率高,并发症包括需要紧急支气管镜处理的移位和黏液堵塞。

23.7.3.3 Aero® 气管支气管支架

Aero® 气管支气管支架(MERIT 医疗系统,南约旦,犹他州)是一款完全覆膜 SEMS。金属网由激光切割的镍钛而成,上覆聚安酯。这种支架的设计带有防移位鳍片,意在嵌入到气道黏膜中。其完全覆膜的设计使其更容易回收。这种支架仍然会发生移位,其发生率可能高于部分覆膜或非覆膜 SEMS。一项病例系列报道,对肺移植受体患者放置了 6 个支架,有 5 个支架移位(83%),6 个黏液堵塞(100%),所有患者(100%)吻合口复发狭窄[109]。对于恶性疾病,这些支架显示可以改善症状和肺功能,相关并发症发生率为 33%,其中移位是最常见的(14%)[69]。这些支架的尺寸较小,可置入叶支气管中。

23.7.3.4 Dynamic™ (Freitag) 支架

Dynamic 支架(波士顿科学公司)是一种"Y"形硅酮支架,在前面和侧面的硅酮支架中嵌入了不锈钢钢丝,以模拟"C"形气管软骨环。因此,支架后方膜部是有弹性的,可模仿呼吸过程中气管膜部的运动。通过削剪气管或支气管侧支到预定长度,可调整支架的整体长度(图 23.11)。经喉镜看到声带后,可使用硬质钳子递送器械来放置支架。我们也能联合使用

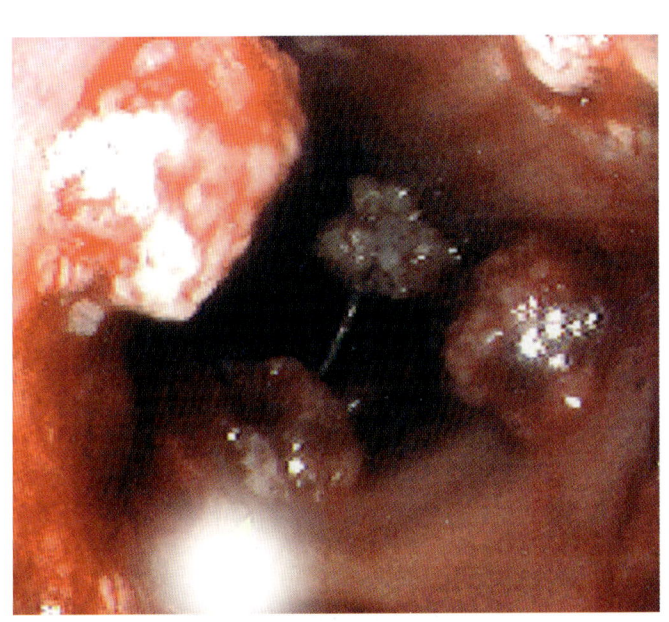

图 23.9 气管内多发息肉样转移瘤,伴内源性和外源性阻塞
资料来源:大卫·布里基博士提供。

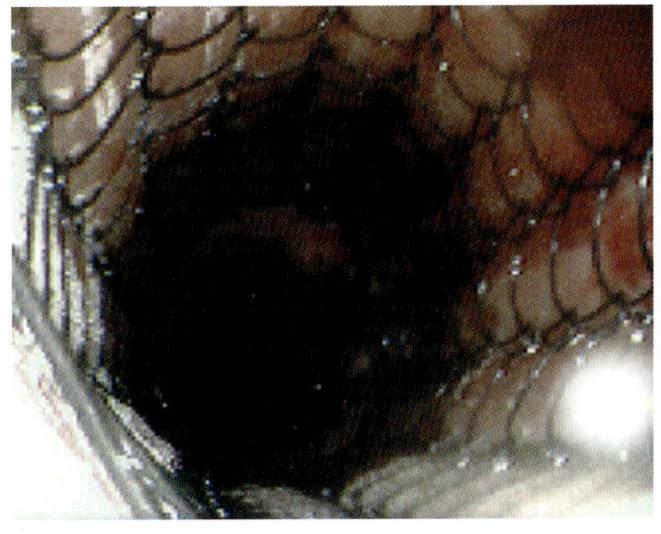

图 23.10 Ultraflex 支架
在氩等离子体凝固治疗后,放置了一个覆膜 Ultraflex 支架。资料来源:大卫·布里基博士提供。经 John Wiley & Sons 公司许可转载。

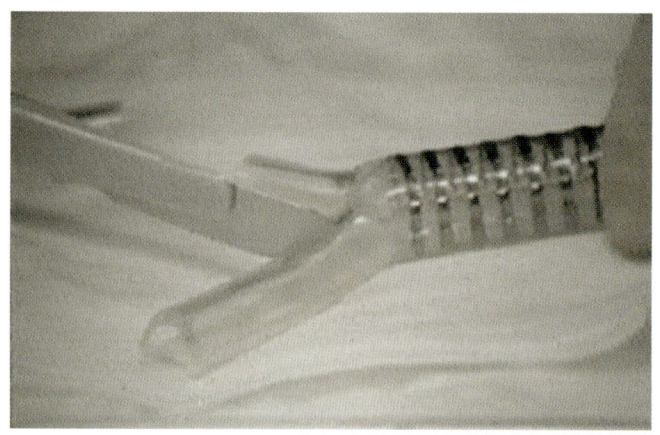

图 23.11 左主支气管支被截短的 Dynamic 支架
资料来源：经 John Wiley & Sons 许可转载。

霍普金斯窥镜和硬镜鳄鱼钳来完成抓持、观察和置入 Dynamic 支架（图 23.12、图 23.13）。还可以使用可视喉镜和硬质支气管镜来放置。

这些支架通常用于隆突肿瘤或严重的气管支气管软化症。值得注意的是，文献表明，在恶性 CAO 患者中，"Y" 形支架的置入与直筒形支架相比死亡率更高。在新月形气管支气管软化症患者中，已有该支架断裂的报道。

硅酮支架和复合支架的开发不仅可以保持气道的通畅，也可封闭在气管支气管壁上形成的瘘管。图 23.14 显示一位出现咳嗽和呼吸急促，进食后加重的患者，吞下钡餐后，显示在气管支气管树中出现钡剂。图 23.15 显示该患者的支气管镜下所见，气管和左侧

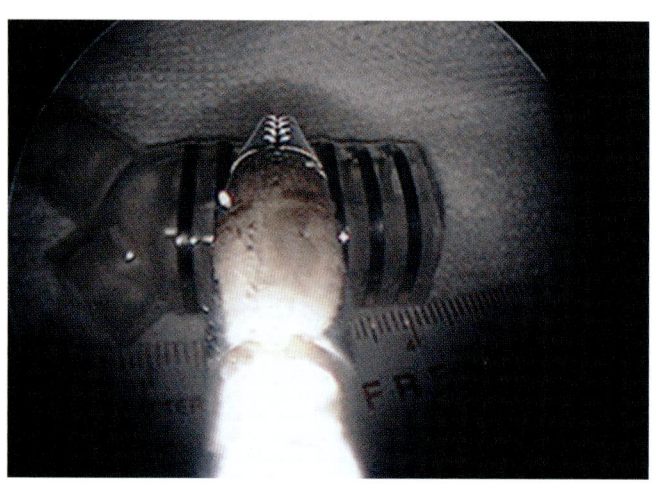

图 23.12 硬质活检钳夹住 Dynamic 支架
资料来源：经 John Wiley & Sons 许可转载。

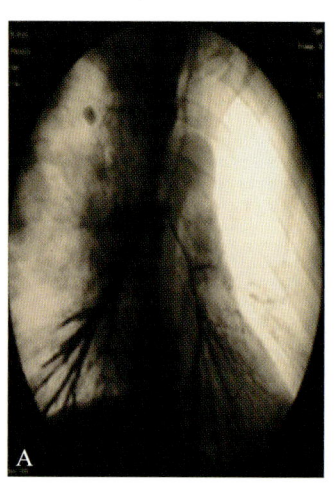

图 23.14 钡餐造影
咳嗽和进食后气促加重的患者吞钡后的后前位（A）和侧位片（B）显示了气管支气管树中的钡影。资料来源：经 John Wiley & Sons 许可转载。

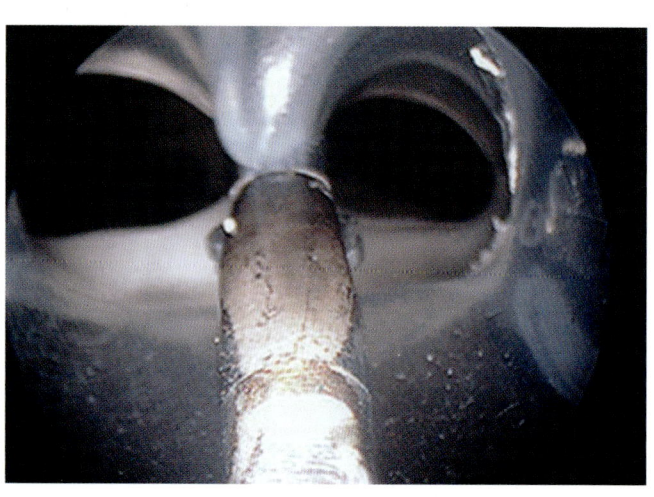

图 23.13 硬质钳在 Dynamic 支架内并夹住支架
该视角是通过霍普金斯 0° 硬镜视频光源镜所观察的。资料来源：经 John Wiley & Sons 许可转载。

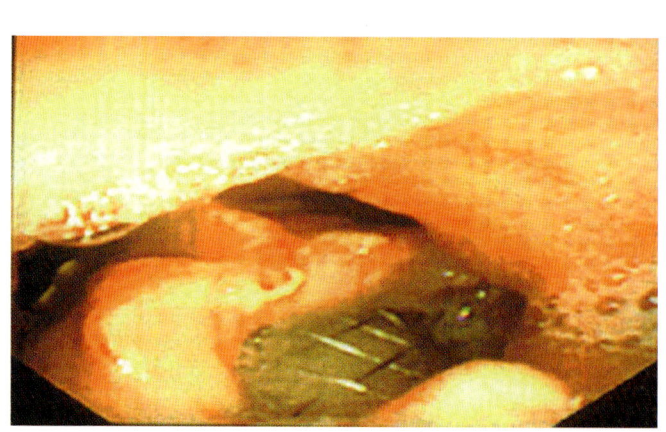

图 23.15 镜下所示
支气管镜检查显示气管和左侧主支气管食管瘘，可见先前置入的食道支架。资料来源：经 John Wiley & Sons 许可转载。

主支气管食管瘘。图中所示的支架之前曾被放置在食管内。图 23.16 显示了一个 Dynamic 支架，封堵了气管和左主支气管瘘。

23.8 新型金属支架

自 2005 年 FDA 发出警告以来，已经推出了几种型号的金属支架。因此，与这一警告相关的几个问题可能不适用于这些新的气道假体。然而，在推荐常规使用这些新器械之前，必须有可重复和可靠的证据。这些呼吸道支架大多采用混合式设计，可以自行膨胀或球囊辅助扩张。它们的设计和被发表的刊物摘要见表 23.5。

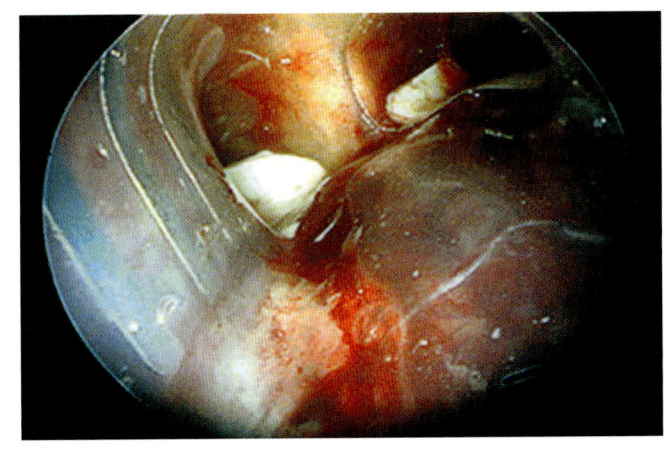

图 23.16 Dynamic 支架封堵气管食管瘘

置入 Dynamic 支架，封闭气管和左侧主支气管瘘。资料来源：经 John Wiley & Sons 许可转载。

表 23.5 新型金属支架的设计和数据

支架名称/生产商	支架设计	临床数据
Bonastent EndoChoice, Inc.（美国乔治亚州阿尔法利塔）	覆盖一层硅酮膜的镍钛合金交叉线支架	·小样本研究，无早期并发症（30 天内）[112]
MICRO-TECH（中国南京公司）	全覆膜 SEMS：镍钛网内部被硅酮膜完全覆盖"Y"形支架也适用	·基于病例系列的证据[113]；一项研究在 16 例 CAO 患者中置入 21 个支架，支架置入术平均持续时间为 282 天，肉芽组织（35%），移位（30%）和痰潴留（15%），55% 的支架因为各种并发症不得不被移除
Aerstent and ECO-Y 支架，（Leufen，德国）	全覆膜 SEMS	·一项研究的中位随访时间为 44 天，未出现移位或断裂[114] ·有 86% 出现黏液潴留而无黏液栓，轻度肉芽组织形成占 31.7%，硅酮涂层脱落率为 9%，聚氨酯涂层穿孔率在 4%
	覆膜金属"Y"形支架	·对"Y"形支架的研究有限（无长期随访）[115,116] ·用于恶性 CAO、TEF ·最常见的并发症是黏液堵塞 ·一项研究纳入了 43 例良恶性 CAO 患者[117]，随访了 18 例患者，44.4% 的患者对支架耐受，11.1% 需要进一步支架置入，33.3% 有分泌物增多、咳嗽、呼吸困难或肉芽组织形成等并发症
Silmet Novatech（La Coitat，法国）	全覆膜以聚酯纤维的镍钛金属支架 锥形、直线形等定制型号	·几个大型病例系列研究（$n>30$ 例）[118,119] ·技术性成功率 >90%，肿瘤向内生长/肉芽组织 10%~32%，移位 7%~8%，支架破裂 5%，可弯曲支气管镜检查无法清除分泌物 7% ·在一项研究中，由于并发症，50% 的支架在中位时间为 77 天内被移除
COMVI（韩国泰雄医疗）	采用聚四氟乙烯膜的全覆膜 SEMS 镍钛丝结构	·经验有限[119]；在一项 30 例患者的研究中，支架放置成功率为 100%，但组织增生、支架移位和 LUL 支气管阻塞分别发生在 36.7%、13.3% 和 3.3% 的患者中，所有支架均在 2 个月和 6 个月时成功取出，平均随访时间为 24 个月
iCAST（美国新罕布什尔州哈德逊）	球囊扩张释放 不锈钢框架覆以聚四氟乙烯 可以通过 2.8 mm 支气管镜 专为叶支气管设计	·在一项 38 例患者的研究中，因支气管狭窄放置了 120 个支架[87]，18.5% 的患者放置了 >1 个支架，每个患者平均经历了 4 次操作，平均支架移除时间为 85 天，常见的并发症包括移位（10%）、肉芽组织增生（5%）、放置困难（2%）、支架置入后立即移位（2%）、黏液阻塞（1%）和肿瘤阻塞（1%） ·另一项对 18 例置入 21 个支架的患者的研究显示，MRC 呼吸困难评分有所改善[120]，移位（9.5%）、肉芽组织增生（9.5%）和黏液阻塞（4.8%）

CAO，中央气道阻塞；LUL，左上肺叶；MRC，英国医学研究委员会；SEMS，自膨式覆膜金属支架；TEF，气管食管瘘。

23.9 支架相关不良事件

支架置入术引起的并发症在一定程度上是可预测和可预防的，与下列因素有关：支架的选择、置入和放置的技术、移位、阻塞和感染、支架故障和穿孔。

表 23.6 列出了一些最常见的不良事件及其相关发病率。

表 23.6 支架并发症及发病率

并发症	发病率
肉芽组织增生	使用金属支架为 9%~67%[121] 使用硅酮支架为 6%~15%
支架破裂	仅有病例报告
下呼吸道感染及黏液阻塞	36%~39%[48]
移位	5%~15%，取决于支架-气道直径[17]

23.9.1 支架选择相关并发症：覆膜与非覆膜

如前所述，理想的支架尚未开发，因此必须采用"不同病情，不同支架"的原则。如果选择的支架在长度、直径上不匹配，那么患者的气道梗阻或许只能部分缓解，甚至面临更大的支架移位的风险。此外，如果在内生性肿瘤和瘘的地方使用非覆膜支架，则可能分别出现反复的阻塞或分泌物潴留。在纤毛功能保持方面，覆膜与非覆膜的支架相比，硅酮支架和混合支架会破坏黏膜纤毛活动梯的正常运输，导致分泌物积聚。这种黏液的堆积和后续支架的焦痂样痰栓可导致阻塞，故需要使用生理盐水雾化来预防。

对非覆膜金属支架与黏膜的相互作用的考虑也时有提及，因为这些 SEMS 对下方黏膜和浅表肿瘤会施加持久的径向力。由于上皮化，支架也可能嵌入黏膜，使移除变得困难或不安全。支架与组织的相互作用需要进一步研究。在 Hauck 的一份报告中，评估了支架置入前和置入 1 周后的支气管内组织学改变。在平均 122 天的随访时间内，作者报道的再狭窄事件极少。在他们为期 1 周的随访研究中，支架对邻近肿瘤组织施加的压力导致完整肿瘤细胞数量减少，在取样区域识别到更多的坏死或非肿瘤细胞。这很可能是由于剪切力导致浅表肿瘤区域细胞活力下降，从而有助于维持支架通畅。

23.9.2 置入和放置期间的并发症

尽管硅酮支架很容易用硬镜进行放置和操作，但有时也需要调整，必要时需用球囊或硬镜扩张。然而，当使用自膨胀式金属支架或复合支架时，很难甚至无法进行调整。因此，需要更加小心地选择合适的尺寸，以确保能恰当地放置。图 23.17 展示了一个需要被移除的金属支架。在内镜下，可以看到活检钳扯松了一根单独的支架丝。虽然该金属支架被成功取出，但该操作花费了更多的时间，因为它难以轻易地整体取出。此外，放置一个尺寸不合适的支架可能导致肉芽组织增生和支架置入后再狭窄。在 Kim 等的一项前瞻性研究中，对 38 例良性气道狭窄的患者放置了镍钛合金支架。文章作者认为，尺寸过小的支架导致金属支架与气道壁的过度摩擦，相反，过大的支架导致过大的径向压力，从而损害黏膜微循环；两种情况都可能导致肉芽组织过度增生。

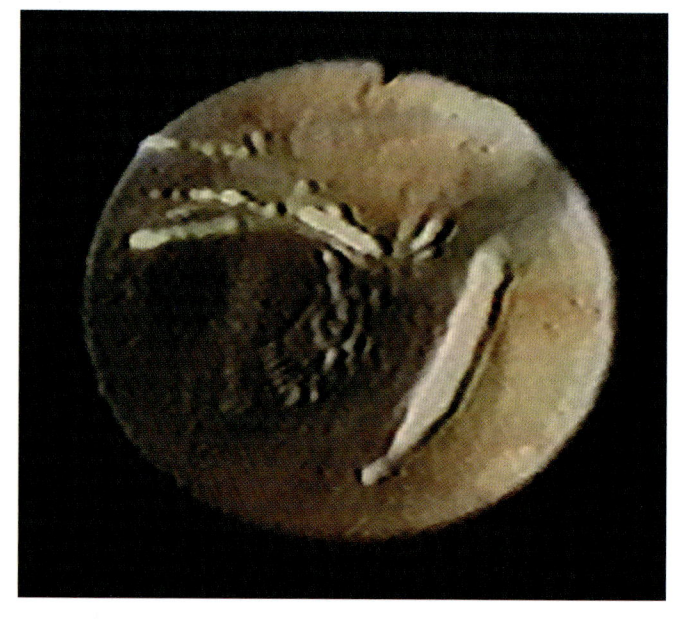

图 23.17 需要移除的金属支架
资料来源：经 John Wiley & Sons 许可转载。

23.9.3 移位

当肿瘤产生的外力通过联合治疗得到缓解后，支架可能会发生移位。在良性气道狭窄中，如气管软化症，报道中支架移位的发生率高达 20%。支架移位在良性气道狭窄中尤为明显，如结核后气道狭窄和

ECAC 分别有 51% 和 10% 的移位发生率。一项有关混合硅酮支架（Polyflex）应用在良性气管支气管疾病患者中的研究指出，由于总并发症的发生率高（75%），特别是 69%（16 例中的 11 例）的患者发生移位，作者所在的机构放弃使用该支架。当患者接受全身治疗（如免疫、放疗、靶向或化疗等）后，支架可能出现移位，因为局部病灶反应会导致支架松动而有移位的可能。有证据表明，支架移位在良性气道疾病（由于长期支架置入扩张气道）和硅酮支架置入术后中更常见，尽管后者可能是由于尺寸问题。

23.9.4 支架堵塞和感染

随着正常黏膜纤毛活动的中断和分泌物的干燥，支架可能会出现堵塞。可能会出现支架内菌群定植和分泌物潴留，导致反复咳嗽和黏液产生。留置气道支架的患者中，下呼吸道感染的发生率为 36%~39%，并伴有显著的发病率和死亡率。吸烟、无效咳嗽、左侧支架、硅酮支架和支架置入术后化疗是支架相关呼吸道感染的危险因素。生理盐水雾化可能有助于防止分泌物的积聚，但不建议常规使用抗生素，除非怀疑感染。

所有类型的支架都可能出现肿瘤过度生长或肉芽组织增生。肉芽组织增生和肿瘤过度生长可能出现在非覆膜金属支架任何部位，也可能出现在混合支架非覆膜的末端（图 23.18）。在 Thornton 等的一项回顾性研究中，分析了 40 例因良性气管支气管疾病置入支架的患者，11 例患者中有 10 例通过 CT 发现需要再次内镜治疗来改善支架通畅性[127]。这些良性疾病置入的支架通畅率在第 1 年是 60%，随后逐渐降低，46% 的支架在 6.8 年内保持通畅。由于缺乏活检资料证实，很难从已发表的文献中区分肿瘤内向性生长或肉芽组织增生的发生率。然而，当发生阻塞时，肉芽组织增生或肿瘤过度生长在大约 25% 的患者中可能有临床意义。肉芽组织增生在瘢痕体质和慢性呼吸道感染的患者中更常见。有报道近 50% 良性气道疾病接受 SEMS 置入的患者出现肉芽组织增生。

23.9.5 支架破裂和穿孔

气管支气管树是可移动的，处在波幅较大的压力变化环境中。在反复运动的情况下，支架的材料可能发生断裂，导致支架失去完整性。这是由于金属疲劳所致。此外，支架的反复移位，特别是边缘锋利的支架，可能导致穿孔。一名接受支架和辅助治疗后因穿

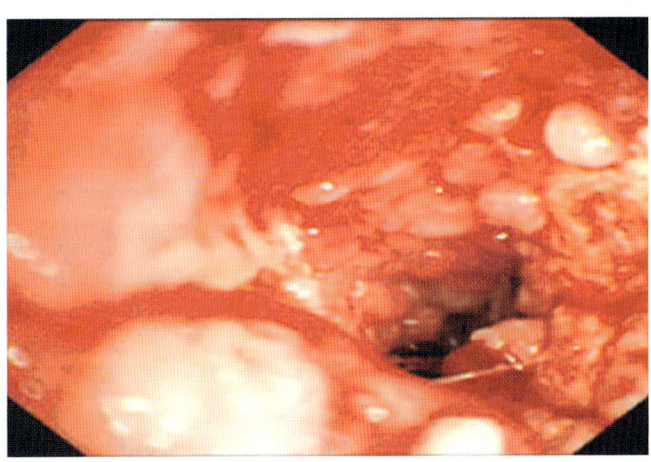

图 23.18 气管支架被肿瘤压迫和覆盖

可以看到支架的近端和中段的一些金属丝。资料来源：经 John Wiley & Sons 许可转载。

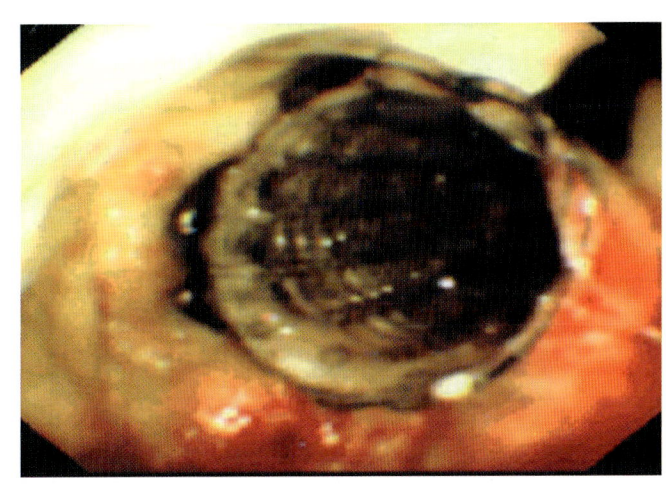

图 23.19 金属支架从气管空洞瘘里突出

资料来源：经 John Wiley & Sons 许可转载。

孔转来笔者单位就诊（图 23.19）。由于气管旁非小细胞癌引起内源性和外源性阻塞，患者接受了金属支架置入。后续的化疗和放疗导致肿瘤肿块空洞化，形成气管瘘，继而支架移位纵隔瘘道中。

如上所述，一些支架，特别是 Gianturco 和 Palmaz 支架的使用，由于穿孔和断裂的报道而变得复杂。随后的研究表明，支架失效最常与黏液阻塞、肉芽组织增生导致再狭窄、支架断裂、移位和穿孔有关[129,130]。

23.10 移除支架的考虑

支架移除的指征包括支架感染、黏液或肉芽组织

堵塞、支架断裂、支架移位、需要重新修复瘘管以及恶性肿瘤的治疗后反应[105,130]。

硅酮或全覆膜的复合支架可通过可弯曲或硬质支气管镜取出，这通常没有难度。而移除 SEMS 则可能具有挑战性，这取决于支架的类型和放置的时间。早期的 SEMS 类型，以 Gianturco 支架为例，因锋利的金属突出点导致穿孔而备受质疑。随着时间的推移，这些锋利的突出和上皮化，让支架嵌入黏膜中，使得移除支架变得困难。因此，移除 SEMS 可能需要使用硬质支气管镜的前端铲切或用异物钳钳夹取出，这是个非常耗时的操作。新款的 SEMS，如镍钛合金覆膜支架，末端设计得更圆润。其中 Ultraflex 支架在近端有一根调整线，操作者可以钳夹调整线后取出支架。

由于移除困难，SEMS 在良性疾病中的应用受到了广泛关注，以至于 FDA 发布了关于在良性疾病中使用 SEMS 的警告[131]。Noppen 等描述了移除此类支架的方法，通过抓住调整丝线，推进硬性支气管镜，直到支架近端进入硬镜内，然后用异物钳钳夹旋转将支架拔出[130]。支架近端或远端上皮组织的过度生长可能会增加支架移除的难度。由于 4~6 周后支架上皮化，Rampey 等描述了在特定病例中联合内镜和开放入路移除 SEMS 的方法[132]。

支架移除后的潜在并发症包括以下几种[133]：
1）支架断裂；
2）支架无法完整移除（气道失用）；
3）气道穿孔伴纵隔气肿/气胸；
4）气道出血；
5）喉部外伤、水肿、痉挛；
6）支架碎片残留；
7）再阻塞；
8）麻醉相关问题（取决于合并症），包括呼吸衰竭；
9）死亡。

在一项研究中，每位患者平均需接受 2.6 次手术以移除支架和处理与支架相关的并发症。大多数支架移除的适应证都是在良性 CAO 患者中报道的，支架移除时的并发症多见于非覆膜的 SEMS 和长期支架置入的患者[105,134]。

由于支架移除可能会带来严重的并发症，我们建议通过详细评估气道解剖、血管结构与气管壁的关系以及支架的状况（如断裂、嵌入等）以进行全面的术前计划。当考虑移除内嵌的支架时，有必要进行增强胸部 CT 检查，以评估毗邻大血管结构的情况。

23.11　未来的方向

最近，生物可吸收和 3D 打印气道支架的出现对传统的气道支架及置入模式提出了挑战。随着支持这两种类型支架使用的数据的积累，最终它们可能取代传统的气道支架。生物可吸收支架由惰性材料制成，可在置入后一段时间内被吸收降解，因而无须移除[135,136]。作为一种临时置入的措施，支架可以留置原处，额外的移除及其相关的风险和花费就无必要了。这些支架可能包被或浸渍药物，从而能将药物靶向输送到气道的特定位置。

市售的支架几乎不能完美贴合气道，特别是当气道因病变而扭曲时。这种差异导致气道壁和支架之间的接触点产生不同水平的张力。3D 打印的出现使得针对特定患者定制优化支架成为可能[137-140]。根据影像学和支气管镜数据，可以打印出与患者解剖结构完美贴合的支架，以施加最佳水平的张力，从而最大限度地减少与气道支架相关的常见并发症。气道对 3D 打印支架的生理和症状反应，以及支架本身的长期耐久性和安全性仍有待确定。

23.12　进一步的思考

支架置入用于多种良性疾病中，包括瘢痕性狭窄、插管后损伤和感染。有时，在不幸吸入化学物导致的气管狭窄也需要置入支架治疗。例如，Wang 等报道了 1 例患者由于掉进 35% 盐酸的大桶里激烈挣扎大量吸入盐酸，导致气管支气管多节段狭窄，需要置入多个支架（图 23.20）[141]。

良性疾病使用支架治疗还见诸肺移植患者。来自美国克利夫兰的 Mehta 的团队，回顾性分析了 112 例 SEMS，发现其中 11 例用于治疗肺移植术后气道并发症，21 例用于治疗其他良性病变[142]。肺移植患者的中位随访时间为 329 天，其他气道受损患者的中位随访时间为 336 天。后续为了预防肉芽组织增生或改善气道通畅性，27.3% 的肺移植患者和 47.6% 的其他良性气道疾病的患者需要进一步干预。没有出现黏液堵塞、慢性咳嗽、瘘管形成或致死性咯血的病例。他们的结论是，对于那些不适合手术的 CAO 患者，SEMS 是一种可接受的治疗方式。

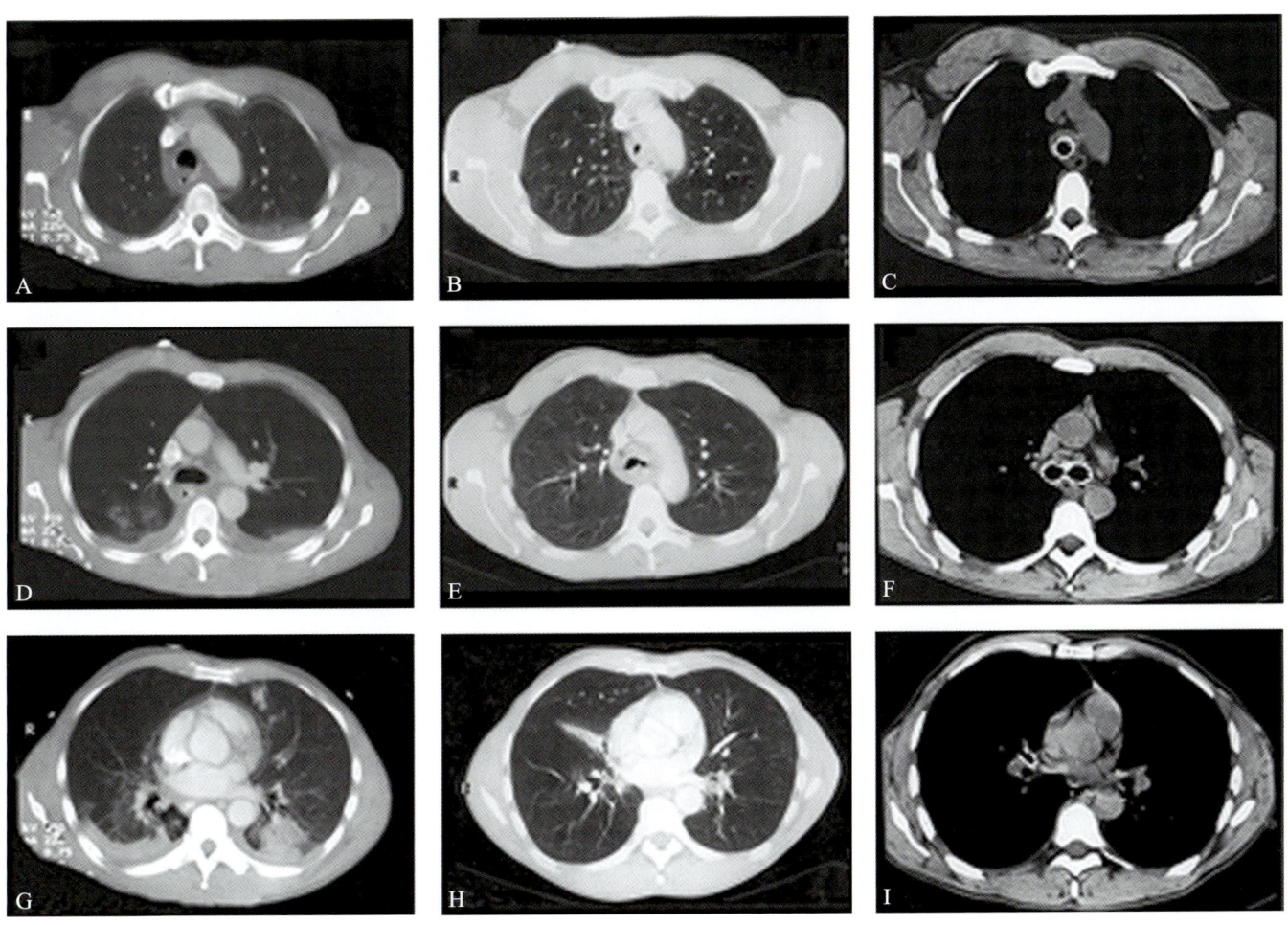

图 23.20 事故后气管支气管 CT 图像随时间的变化与支架置入效果
A、D、G. 事故发生后的即时 CT 图像；B、E、H. 事故发生后 2 个月的 CT 图像；C、F、I. 置入多个支架后的 CT 图像；在远端气管（A~C）、主隆突（D~F）和右侧支气管中/下叶（G~I）的水平上拍摄代表性图像。值得注意的是，事故发生后肺炎立即主要出现在下肺叶（G），随后消退（H、I）。与初次表现相比（分别为 A、D），气管（B）和隆突处可见明显的气道狭窄（E）。通过支架置入矫正了这些狭窄，如 C、F 所示。来源：经来自 Rubin 等的 John Wiley & Sons 许可转载[141]。

来自德国汉诺威的 Gottlieb 等随后进行的一项回顾性研究，详细介绍了 SEMS 在肺移植患者中的应用。这些研究者们回顾了 1998 年 1 月至 2008 年 2 月间 111 例肺移植病例。患者由于出现有症状的气道阻塞，狭窄直径 <5 mm，或者吻合口广泛开裂[143]而置入 SEMS。80% 的患者支架置入后的临床症状缓解，短期并发症（30 天）包括黏液阻塞（7 例）和移位（2 例）。中位随访时间为 777 天后，65 例患者中有 52 例（80%）出现晚期并发症，包括再狭窄、细菌定植、支架断裂、咯血和肺不张。1 名患者死于致命性的咯血，尸检显示移植肺有侵袭性曲霉感染，支架处没有出血。研究者得出结论，再狭窄率为 52%，高于其他研究（良性和恶性疾病为 10%~47%），这可能是因为较长的随访时间和主要使用了非覆膜支架。

这些研究者和其他团队报道了较高的气道细菌定植率，在本研究中为 77%，Burns 等的研究为 56%，两者都为 SEMS 置入后的肺移植患者[144]。相比之下，Noppen 等报道了未移植患者置入硅酮支架后的细菌定植率为 80%[145]。有趣的是，在 Burns 等的报告中，尽管细菌气道定植情况如上所述，但在支架放置后长达 1 年的时间里，实际上肺部感染的发生率有所降低，这可能是由于气道通畅和肺功能改善的缘故。

与长时间放置金属支架相比，Zhou 等的中国经验值得关注。他们在由炎症病因（如结核）引起的良性气管支气管狭窄高发人群中短期放置金属支架[146]，40 名患者中放置了 49 个支架，放置中位时间 18 天内没有出现重大并发症。支架置入前气道直径为 3.3~4.2 mm，置入后中位数提升到 7.4 mm。随访 3 年余，FEV_1 和 6 min 步行测试显著改善，提示短期支架置入可能对一些良性气道疾病患者有益。

23.13 支架置入术后随访

尽管存在上述潜在的不良事件，气管支气管支架通常有良好的耐受性，并且可以轻松留置多年。Matsuo 和 Colt 指出，硅酮支架置入后不需要进行常规支气管镜检查，但如果出现新症状，则应再次进行支气管镜检查[147]。然而，最新的数据表明，在未经选择的有气道支架[金属、硅酮（直筒形、"Y"形、"T"形管）和复合支架]留置的患者中，随访支气管镜检查可以发现支架并发症，并且进一步治疗[148]。在这项研究中，134 名患者放置了 147 个支架，其中 10 个患者置入了多枚支架。94 例患者在置入后平均 41.2 天内进行了支气管镜随访。尽管随访支气管镜检查时的患者的症状与支架并发症无关，但 2/3 的患者在随访支气管镜检查时发现了支架相关并发症。在本研究中，与其他支架相比，复合型支架更容易移位或被分泌物阻塞。

气道形态特征和支架远端的气道动力学对评估支架是否失效具有价值。因此，胸部 CT 可以补充信息[149]。在一项研究中，除了支架起始处肉芽组织增生所致的中度狭窄（20%），CT 显示了支气管镜检查发现的其他所有明显异常[150]。这些研究的作者建议在支架置入后进行支气管镜检查。随访支气管镜检查的频率必须根据后续治疗个体化，如全身化疗、免疫治疗或放射治疗[151,152]。

23.14 结论

尽管关于气道支架的综述和文献总是讨论"理想的支架"，但它尚未开发出来。通常涉及的参考因素包括材料、覆膜与非覆膜的形式、生物相容性和亲水性。从生物力学的角度来看，支架应该具有相对较大的径向力，以维持气道通畅并防止移位。然而，如果径向力过大，则会引起黏膜缺血和肉芽组织增生。较低的轴向力会使支架更好地适应扭曲的气道形态。轴向力较大时，支架不能很好地适应气道的轮廓。而且，支架若不能很好地适应局部气道解剖结构，随后可能会出现移位。

目前在导丝辅助下通过可弯曲支气管镜置入支架的技术并不适用于所有情况，在置入或取出支架时可能需要使用硬质支气管镜。关于生物可降解支架的更多研究，以及可以输送化疗或放疗药物的材料，都是我们积极研究的主题。由于理想的支架并不存在，我们要回归根据症状、阻塞类型和位置个体化支架置入的基本原则。支气管镜介入医师和他们的团队应有相应的工具来操作和快速移除支架，保护气道。因此，支气管镜介入团队不仅应接受支架置入方面的培训，还应接受其他介入性支气管镜手术方面的培训，如高频电灼、冷冻治疗和激光治疗，以便在支架置入或移除期间处理肿瘤、肉芽组织或气道出血形成的阻塞。展望未来，对支架生物力学的更深入理解、生物相容性材料的开发以及基于患者个体解剖结构的定制气道支架可能会减少支架相关不良事件的发生率。

参考文献

1 (1989). *Taber's Cyclopedic Medical Dictionary*. Philadelphia: Davis.
2 Trendelenburg, F. (1872). Beatrice zoo den Operationen an den Luftwegen. *Lange Becks Arch Chir* 13: 335.
3 Bond, C.J. Note on the treatment of tracheal stenosis by a new T-shaped tracheostomy tube. *Lancet* 1891 (i): 539–540.
4 Burnings, W. and Albrecht, W. (1915). *Directed Endoskopie der Loftund Speisewege*, 134–138. Stuttgart: Eke.
5 Canfield, N. and Norton, N. (1949). Bony stenosis of the larynx. *Ann. Otol. Rhinol. Laryngol.* 58 (2): 559–565.
6 Harkins, W.B. (1952). An endobronchial metallic prosthesis in the treatment of stenosis of the Trachea. *Ann. Otol. Rhinol. Laryngol.* 61: 663–675.
7 Freitag, L. (2000). Tracheobronchial stents. In: *Interventional Bronchoscopy* (eds. C.T. Bolliger and P.N. Mathur), 176. Basel: Karger.
8 Montgomery, W.W. (1965). T-tube tracheal stent. *Arch. Otolaryngol.* 82: 320–321.
9 Dumon, J.F. (1990). A dedicated tracheobronchial stent. *Chest* 97: 328–332.
10 Rotate, J.R. and Shardonofsky, F.R. (2000). Respiratory system mechanics. In: *Textbook of Respiratory Medicine*, 3e (eds. J.F. Murray and J.A. Navel), 91–117. Philadelphia: W.B. Saunders.
11 Yeates, D.B., Bess Eris, G.J., and Wong, L.B. (1997). Physiochemical properties of mucus and its propulsion. In: *The Lung: Scientific Foundations* (eds. R.G. Crystal, J.B. West, E.R. Weibel, et al.), 487–503. Philadelphia: Lippincott-Raven.
12 Yates, D.B. and Mortensen, J. (2000). Deposition and clearance. In: *Textbook of Respiratory Medicine*, 3e (eds. J.F. Murray and J.A. Navel), 349–379. Philadelphia: W.B. Saunders.
13 Freitag, L. (1998). Tracheobronchial stents. In: *Pulmonary Endoscopy and Biopsy Techniques*. European Respiratory Monograph (ed. J. Strausz), 79–105. Sheffield: European Respiratory Society Journals.

14 Freitag, L., Eicker, K., Donavan, T.J. et al. (1995). Mechanical properties of airway stents. *J. Bronchol.* 2: 270–278.

15 Witt, C., Dinges, S., Schmidt, B. et al. (1997). Temporary tracheobronchial stenting in malignant stenoses. *Eur. J. Cancer* 33: 204–208.

16 Chajed, P.N., Somandin, S., Baty, F. et al. (2010). Therapeutic bronchoscopy for malignant airway stenoses: choice of modality and survival. *J. Cancer Res. Ther.* 6: 204–209.

17 Hu, H.-C., Liu, Y.-H., Wu, Y.-C. et al. (2011). Granulation tissue formation following Dumon airway stenting: the influence of stent diameter. *Thorac. Cardiovasc. Surg.* 59: 163–168.

18 Galluccio, G., Lucantoni, G., Battistoni, P. et al. (2009). Interventional endoscopy in the management of benign tracheal stenoses: definitive treatment at long-term follow-up. *Eur. J. Cardiothorac. Surg.* 35: 429–433.

19 Brouns, M., Jayaraju, S.T., Lacor, C. et al. (2007). Tracheal stenosis: a flow dynamics study. *J. Appl. Physiol.* 102: 1178–1184.

20 Schultz, D. (2005). FDA Public Health Notification: Complications from Metallic Tracheal Stents in Patients with Benign Airway Disorders. www.jsre.org/info/0801_fda.pdf.

21 Nouraei, S.A.R., Nouraei, S.M., Randhawa, P.S. et al. (2008). Sensitivity and responsiveness of the Medical Research Council dyspnoea scale to the presence and treatment of adult laryngotracheal stenosis. *Clin. Otolaryngol.* 33: 575–580.

22 Myer, C.M., O'Connor, D.M., and Cotton, R.T. (1994). Proposed grading system for subglottic stenosis based on endotracheal tube sizes. *Ann. Otol. Rhinol. Laryngol.* 103: 319–323.

23 Mead, J., Turner, J.M., Macklem, P.T. et al. (1967). Significance of the relationship between lung recoil and maximum expiratory flow. *J. Appl. Physiol.* 22: 95–108.

24 Smaldone, G.C. and Smith, P.L. (1985). Location of flow-limiting segments via airway catheters near residual volume in humans. *J. Appl. Physiol.* 59: 502–508.

25 Baram, D. and Smaldone, G. (2006). Tracheal collapse versus tracheobronchomalacia: normal function versus disease. *Am. J. Respir. Crit. Care Med.* 174: 724–725.

26 Hogg, J.C., Macklem, P.T., and Thurlbeck, W.M. (1968). Site and nature of airway obstruction in chronic obstructive lung disease. *N. Engl. J. Med.* 278: 1355–1360.

27 Dutau, H., Toutblanc, B., Lamb, C. et al. (2004). Use of the Dumon Y-stent in the management of malignant disease involving the carina. A retrospective review of 86 patients. *Chest* 126: 951–958.

28 Grillo, H.C. and Mathisen, D.J. (1988). Surgical management of tracheal strictures. *Surg. Clin. North Am.* 68: 511–524.

29 Siegal, P.D. and Katz, J. (1996). Respiratory complications of gastroesophgeal reflux disease. *Prim. Care* 23: 433–441.

30 Cohen, L.F. (2000). Stridor and upper airway obstruction in children. *Pediatr. Rev.* 21: 4–5.

31 Sano, H., Kita, Y., Nowata, Y. et al. (1999). Case of recurrent subglottic stenosis later followed by the development of Wegener's granulomatosis. *Nihon Naika Gakka Zasshi* 88: 2469–2470.

32 Freidman, E.M., Healy, G.B., and McGill, T.J. (1983). Carbon dioxide laser management of subglottic and tracheal stenosis. *Otolaryngol. Clin. North Am.* 16: 871.

33 Mehta, A.C. and Dasgupta, A. (1999). Airway stents. *Clin. Chest Med.* 20: 139–151.

34 Oviatt, P.L., Stather, D.R., Michaud, G. et al. (2011). Exercise capacity, lung function, and quality of life after interventional bronchoscopy. *J. Thorac. Oncol.* 6: 38–42.

35 Stanopoulos, I.T., Beamis, J.F., Martinez, F.J. et al. (1993). Laser bronchoscopy in respiratory failure from malignant airway obstruction. *Crit. Care Med.* 21: 386–391.

36 Lo, C.P., Hsu, A.A., and Eng, P. (2000). Endobronchial stenting in patients requiring mechanical ventilation for major airway obstruction. *Ann. Acad. Med. Singap.* 29: 66–70.

37 Jeon, K., Kim, H., Yu, C.-M. et al. (2006). Rigid bronchoscopic intervention in patients with respiratory failure caused by malignant central airway obstruction. *J. Thorac. Oncol.* 1: 319–323.

38 Razi, S.S., Lebovics, R.S., Schwartz, G. et al. (2010). Timely airway stenting improves survival in patients with malignant central airway obstruction. *Ann. Thorac. Surg.* 90: 1088–1093.

39 Furukawa, K., Ishida, J., Yamaguchi, G. et al. (2010). The role of airway stent placement in the management of tracheobronchial stenosis caused by inoperable advanced lung cancer. *Surg. Today* 40: 315–320.

40 Bolliger, C.T. (1996). Introduction to different approaches to intrabronchial treatment. *Monaldi Arch. Chest Dis.* 51: 316–324.

41 Bondaryev, A., Makris, D., Breen, D.P. et al. (2009). Airway stenting for severe endobronchial papillomatosis. *Respiration* 77: 455–458.

42 Brichet, A., Verkindre, C., Dupont, J. et al. (1999). Multidisciplinary approach to management of postintubation tracheal stenoses. *Eur. Respir. J.* 13: 888–893.

43 Patelli, M. and Gasparini, S. (2007). Post-intubation tracheal stenoses: what is the curative yield of the interventional pulmonology procedures? *Monaldi Arch. Chest Dis.* 67: 71–72.

44 Cavaliere, S., Bezzi, M., Toninelli, C. et al. (2007). Management of post-intubation tracheal stenoses using the endoscopic approach. *Monaldi Arch. Chest Dis.* 67: 73–80.

45 Nouraei, S.A.R., Ghufoor, K., Patel, A. et al. (2007). Outcome of endoscopic treatment of adult postintubation tracheal stenosis. *Laryngoscope* 117: 1073–1079.

46 Cooper, J.D. and Grillo, H.C. (1969). The evolution of tracheal injury due to ventilatory assistance through cuffed tubes: a pathologic study. *Ann. Surg.* 169: 334–348.

47 Murgu, S.D., Colt, H.G., Mukai, D. et al. (2010). Multimodal imaging guidance for laser ablation in tracheal stenosis. *Laryngoscope* 120: 1840–1846.

48 Ost, D.E., Shah, A.M., Lei, X. et al. (2012). Respiratory infections increase the risk of granulation tissue formation following airway stenting in patients with malignant airway obstruction. *Chest* 141: 1473–1481.

49 Deschamps, C., Bernard, A., Nichols, F.C. III et al. (2001). Empyema and bronchopleural fistula after pneumonectomy: factors affecting incidence. *Ann. Thorac. Surg.* 72: 243–248.

50 Lois, M. and Noppen, M. (2005). Bronchopleural fistulas. *Chest*

128: 3955–3965.

51 Shen, K.R. (2017). Management of acquired nonmalignant tracheoesophageal fistula: surgical pearls. *J. Thorac. Cardiovasc. Surg.* 154: e123.

52 Herth, F.J.F., Peter, S., Baty, F. et al. (2010). Combined airway and oesophageal stenting in malignant airway-oesophageal fistulas: a prospective study. *Eur. Respir. J.* 36: 1370–1374.

53 Rodriguez, A.N. and Diaz-Jimenez, J.P. (2010). Malignant respiratory-digestive fistulas. *Curr. Opin. Pulm. Med.* 16: 329–333.

54 Diaz-Jimenez, J.P. (2005). New cufflink-shaped silicon prosthesis for the palliation of malignant tracheobronchial-esophageal fistula. *J. Bronchol.* 12: 207–209.

55 Dumon, J.-F. and Dumon, M.C. (2000). Dumon-Novatech Y-stents. *J. Bronchol.* 7: 26–32.

56 Boyd, M. and Rubio, E. (2012). The utility of stenting in the treatment of airway gastric fistula after esophagectomy for esophageal cancer. *J. Bronchology* 19: 232–236.

57 Sahebazamani, M., Rubio, E., and Boyd, M. (2012). Airway gastric fistula after esophagectomy for esophageal cancer. *Ann. Thorac. Surg.* 93: 988–990.

58 Yasuda, T., Sugimura, K., Yamasaki, M. et al. (2012). Ten cases of gastro-tracheobronchial fistula: a serious complication after esophagectomy and reconstruction using posterior mediastinal gastric tube. *Dis. Esophagus* 25: 687–693.

59 Ernst, A., Majid, A., Feller-Kopman, D. et al. (2007). Airway stabilization with silicone stents for treating adult tracheobronchomalacia: a prospective observational study. *Chest* 132: 609–616.

60 Murgu, S.D. and Colt, H.G. (2007). Complications of silicone stent insertion in patients with expiratory central airway collapse. *Ann. Thorac. Surg.* 84: 1870–1877.

61 Murgu, S.D. and Colt, H.G. (2007). Description of a multidimensional classification system for patients with expiratory central airway collapse. *Respirology* 12: 543–550.

62 Gaissert, H.A., Grillo, H.C., Wright, C.D. et al. (2003). Complication of benign tracheobronchial strictures by self-expanding metal stents. *J. Thorac. Cardiovasc. Surg.* 126: 744–747.

63 Colt, H.G. and Harell, J.H. (1997). Therapeutic rigid bronchoscopy allows level of care changes in patients with acute respiratory failure from central airways obstruction. *Chest* 112: 202–206.

64 Sutedja, G., Schrage, F., van Kralingen, K. et al. (1995). Stent placement is justifiable in end stage patients with malignant airway tumor. *Respiration* 62: 148–150.

65 Monnier, P., Muddy, A., Stanzel, F. et al. (1996). The use of the covered Wallstent for the palliative treatment of inoperable tracheabronchial cancers: a prospective, multicenter study. *Chest* 110: 1161–1168.

66 Vonk-Noordegraaf, A., Postmus, P.E., and Sutedja, T.G. (2001). Tracheobronchial stenting in the terminal care of cancer patients with central airways obstruction. *Chest* 120: 1811–1814.

67 Chawla, M. and Finley, D. (2009). Outcomes after airway stenting: how do we know it is the right move? *Am. J. Respir. Crit. Care Med.* 179: A6161.

68 Murgu, S., Langer, S., and Colt, H. (2012). Bronchoscopic intervention obviates the need for continued mechanical ventilation in patients with airway obstruction and respiratory failure from inoperable non-small-cell lung cancer. *Respiration* 84: 55–61.

69 Ost, D.E., Ernst, A., Grosu, H.B. et al. (2015). Complications following therapeutic bronchoscopy for malignant central airway obstruction: results of the AQuIRE registry. *Chest* 148: 450–471.

70 Freitag, L., Ernst, A., Unger, M. et al. (2007). A proposed classification system of central airway stenosis. *Eur. Respir. J.* 30: 7–12.

71 Cotton, R.T. (1984). Pediatric laryngotracheal stenosis. *J. Pediatr. Surg.* 19: 699–704.

72 Grundfast, K.M., Morris, M.S., and Bentley, C. (1987). Subglottic stenosis: retrospective analysis and proposal for standard reporting system. *Ann. Otol. Rhinol. Laryngol.* 96: 101–105.

73 McCaffrey, T.V. (1992). Classification of laryngotracheal stenosis. *Laryngoscope* 102: 1335–1340.

74 Grillo, H.C., Mark, E.J., Mathisen, D.J. et al. (1993). Idiopathic laryngotracheal stenosis and its management. *Ann. Thorac. Surg.* 56: 80–87.

75 Anand, V.K., Alomar, G., and Warren, E.T. (1992). Surgical considerations in tracheal stenosis. *Laryngoscope* 102: 237–243.

76 Myer, C.M., O'Connor, D.M., and Cotton, R.T. (1994). Proposed grading system for subglottic stenosis based on endotracheal tube sizes. *Ann. Otol. Rhinol. Laryngol.* 103: 319–323.

77 Hauck, R.W., Lembeck, R.M., Emslander, H.P. et al. (1997). Implantation of Accuflex and Strecker stents in malignant bronchial stenosis by flexible bronchoscopy. *Chest* 112: 134–144.

78 Turner, J.F. and Wang, K.P. (1999). Endobronchial laser therapy. *Clin. Chest Med.* 20: 107–122.

79 Mehta, A.C., Lee, F.Y.W., and DeBoer, G.E. (1995). Flexible bronchoscopy and the use of lasers. In: *Flexible Bronchoscopy* (eds. K.P. Wang and A.C. Mehta), 247–274. Cambridge: Blackwell Science.

80 Macha, H.N., Becker, K.O., and Kemmer, H.P. (1994). Pattern of failure and survival in endobronchial laser resection. A matched pair study. *Chest* 105: 1668–1672.

81 Cotton, R.T. (2000). Management of subglottic stenosis. *Otolaryngol. Clin. North Am.* 33: 111–130.

82 Simpson, G.T., Strong, M.S., Healy, G.B. et al. (1982). Predictive factors of success or failure in the endoscopic management of laryngeal and tracheal stenosis. *Ann. Otol. Rhinol. Laryngol.* 91: 384–388.

83 Colt, H.G., Harrell, J., Newman, T.R. et al. (1984). External fixation of subglottic tracheal stents. *Chest* 105: 1653.

84 Morris, D.P., Malik, T., and Rothera, M.P. (2001). Combined 'trachea-stent': a useful option in the treatment of complex case of subglottic stenosis. *J. Laryngol. Otol.* 115: 430–433.

85 Miyazawa, T., Yamakito, M., Ikeda, S. et al. (2000). Implantation of Ultraflex nitinol stents in malignant tracheobronchial stenoses. *Chest* 118: 959–965.

86 Fruchter, O., Abed El Raouf, B., Rosengarten, D. et al. (2017). Long-term outcome of short metallic stents for lobar airway stenosis. *J. Bronchol.* 24: 211–215.

87 Sethi, S., Gildea, T.R., Almeida, F.A. et al. (2018). Clinical success stenting distal bronchi for "lobar salvage" in bronchial stenosis. *J. Bronchol.* 25: 9–16.

88 Conacher, I.D. (2003). Anesthesia and tracheobronchial stenting for central airway obstruction in adults. *Br. J. Anaesth.* 90: 367–374.

89 Colt, H.G. (1999). Silicone airway stents. In: *Interventional Pulmonology* (eds. J.B. Beamis and P.N. Mathur), 100. New York: McGraw-Hill.

90 Acuff Tea, E., Mack, M.J., and Ryan, W.H. (1994). Simplified placement of silicone tracheal Y-stent. *Ann. Thorac. Surg.* 57: 496–497.

91 Nomori, H., Horio, H., and Suemasu, K. (1999). Dumon stent placement via endotracheal tube. *Chest* 115: 582–583.

92 Strausz, J. (1997). Management of postintubation tracheal stenosis with stent implantation. *J. Bronchology* 4: 294–296.

93 Becker, H.D. (1995). Stenting the central airways. *J. Bronchol.* 2: 98–106.

94 Dumon, J.F., Cavaliere, S., Diaz-Jimenez, J.P. et al. (1996). Seven-year experience with the Dumon prosthesis. *J. Bronchol.* 3: 6–10.

95 Colt, H.G. and Dumon, J.F. (1993). Tracheobronchial stents: indications and applications. *Lung Cancer* 9: 301–306.

96 Bolliger, C.T., Probst, R., Tschopp, K. et al. (1993). Silicone stents and the management of inoperable tracheobronchial stenosis: indications and limitations. *Chest* 104: 1653–1659.

97 Sonett, J.R., Keenan, R.J., Ferson, P.F. et al. (1995). Endobronchial management of benign malignant and lung tranplantation airway stenosis. *Ann. Thorac. Surg.* 59: 1417–1422.

98 Martinez-Ballarin, J.I., Diaz-Jimenez, J.P., Castro, M.J. et al. (1996). Silicone stents in the management of benign tracheobronchial stenosis: tolerance and early results in 63 patients. *Chest* 109: 626–629.

99 Noppen, M., Meysman, M., Claes, I. et al. (1999). Screw-thread vs. Dumon endoprosthesis in the management of tracheal stenosis. *Chest* 115: 532–535.

100 Strecker, E.P., Liermann, D., Barth, K.H. et al. (1990). Expandable tubular stents for treatment of arterial occlusive diseases: experimental and clinical results. *Radiology* 175: 87–102.

101 Palmaz, J. (1988). Balloon expandable intravascular stent. *Am. J. Roentgenol.* 150: 1263–1269.

102 Bolliger, C.T., Heitz, M., Hauser, R. et al. (1996). An airway Wallstent for the treatment of tracheobronchial malignancies. *Thorax* 51: 1127–1129.

103 Bolliger, C.T., Arnoux, A., Oeggerli, M.B. et al. (1995). Covered Wallstent insertion in a patient with conical tracheobronchial stenosis. *J. Bronchol.* 2: 215–218.

104 Buehler, W.F., Gilfrich, J.V., and Wiley, R.C. (1963). Effect of low-temperature phase changes of the mechanical properties of alloys near composition TiNi. *J.Appl. Phys.* 34: 1475–1477.

105 Lunn, W., Feller-Kopman, D., Wahidi, M. et al. (2005). Endoscopic removal of metallic airway stents. *Chest* 127: 2106–2112.

106 Madden, B.P., Park, J.E.S., and Sheth, A. (2004). Medium-term follow-up after deployment of ultraflex expandable metallic stents to manage endobronchial pathology. *Ann. Thorac. Surg.* 78: 1898–1902.

107 Breitenbücher, A., Chhajed, P.N., Brutsche, M.H. et al. (2008). Long-term follow-up and survival after Ultraflex stent insertion in the management of complex malignant airway stenoses. *Respiration* 75: 443–449.

108 Gildea, T.R., Murthy, S.C., Sahoo, D. et al. (2006). Performance of a self-expanding silicone stent in palliation of benign airway conditions. *Chest* 130: 1419–1423.

109 Tan, J.H., Fidelman, N., Durack, J.C. et al. (2010). Management of recurrent airway strictures in lung transplant recipients using AERO covered stents. *J. Vasc. Interv. Radiol.* 21: 1900–1904.

110 Yarmus, L., Gilbert, C., Akulian, J. et al. (2012). Novel use of the GlideScope for rigid bronchoscopic placement of a dynamic (Y) stent. *Ann. Thorac. Surg.* 94: 308–310.

111 Popilevsky, F., Al-Ajam, M.R., Ly, V. et al. (2012). Dynamic Y stent fractures in crescentic tracheobronchomalacia. *J. Bronchol.* 19: 206–210.

112 Holden, V.K., Alape, D., Chee, A.C. et al. (2018). Safety and efficacy of a new fully covered self-expandable metallic airway stent. *Am. J. Respir. Crit. Care Med* 197: A7315.

113 Dahlqvist, C., Ocak, S., Gourdin, M. et al. (2018). Fully covered metallic stents for the treatment of benign airway stenosis. *Can. Respir. J.*: 1–7.

114 Rosell, A., Carnevali, L., Cubero, N. et al. (2015). Two-year experience with the use of fully covered self- expandable metal stents. *Eur. Respir. J.* 46: PA4875.

115 Özdemir, C., Sökücü, S.N., Karasulu, L. et al. (2016). Placement of self-expandable bifurcated metallic stents without use of fluoroscopic and guidewire guidance to palliate central airway lesions. *Multidiscip. Respir. Med.* 11: 15.

116 Madan, K., Dhooria, S., Sehgal, I.S. et al. (2016). A multicenter experience with the placement of self- expanding metallic tracheobronchial Y stents. *J. Bronchol.* 23: 29–38.

117 Gompelmann, D., Eberhardt, R., Schuhmann, M. et al. (2013). Self-expanding Y stents in the treatment of central airway stenosis: a retrospective analysis. *Ther. Adv. Respir. Dis.* 7: 255–263.

118 Marchese, R., Poidomani, G., Paglino, G. et al. (2015). Fully covered self-expandable metal stent in tracheobronchial disorders: clinical experience. *Respiration* 89: 49–56.

119 Fortin, M., Lacasse, Y., Elharrar, X. et al. (2017). Safety and efficacy of a fully covered self-expandable metallic stent in benign airway stenosis. *Respiration* 93: 430–435.

120 Majid, A., Kheir, F., Chung, J. et al. (2017). Covered balloon-expanding stents in airway stenosis. *J. Bronchology* 24: 174–177.

121 Dalupang, J.J., Shanks, T.G., and Colt, H.G. (2001). Nd-YAG laser damage to metal and silicone endobronchial

121. stents: delineation of margins of safety using an in vitro experimental model. *Chest* 120: 934–940.
122. Hauck, R.W., Barbur, M., and Lembeck, R. (2002). Cellular composition of stent-penetrating tissue. *Chest* 122: 1615–1621.
123. Kim, J.H., Shin, J.H., Song, H.-Y. et al. (2007). Benign tracheobronchial strictures: long-term results and factors affecting airway patency after temporary stent placement. *Am. J. Roentgenol.* 188: 1033–1038.
124. Orlowski, T.M. (1987). Palliative intubation of the tracheobronchial tree. *J. Thorac. Cardiovasc. Surg.* 94: 343–348.
125. Monnier, P., Mudry, A., Stanzel, F. et al. (1996). The use of covered Wallstent for the palliative treatment of inoperable tracheobronchial cancers. A prospective multicenter study. *Chest* 110: 1161–1168.
126. Kim, Y.J., Yu, C.M., Choi, J.C. et al. (2006). Use of silicone stents for the management of post-tuberculosis tracheobronchial stenosis. *Eur. Respir. J.* 28: 1029–1035.
127. Thornton, R.H., Gordon, R.L., Kerlan, R.K. et al. (2006). Outcomes of tracheobronchial stent placement for benign disease. *Radiology* 240: 273–282.
128. Chung, F.-T., Lin, S.-M., Chou, C.-L. et al. (2010). Factors leading to obstructive granulation tissue formation after Ultraflex stenting in benign tracheal narrowing. *Thorac. Cardiovasc. Surg.* 58: 102–107.
129. Chin, C.S., Little, V., Yun, J. et al. (2008). Airways stents. *Ann. Thorac. Surg.* 85: S792–S796.
130. Noppen, M., Stratakos, G., d'Haese, J. et al. (2005). Removal of covered self-expandable metallic airway stents in benign disorders: indications, techniques, and outcomes. *Chest* 127: 482–487.
131. Lund, M.E. and Force, S. (2007). Airway stenting for patients with benign airway disease and the Food and Drug Administration advisory. A call for restraint. *Chest* 132: 1107–1108.
132. Rampey, A.M., Silvestri, G.A., and Gillespie, M.B. (2007). Combined endoscopic and open approach to the removal of expandable metallic tracheal stent. *Arch. Otolaryngol. Head Neck Surg.* 133: 37–41.
133. Doyle, D.J., Abdelmalak, B., Machuzak, M. et al. (2009). Anesthesia and airway management for removing pulmonary self-expanding metallic stents. *J. Clin. Anesth.* 21: 529–532.
134. Bolliger, C. (1997). Airway stents. *Semin. Respir. Crit. Care Med.* 18: 563–570.
135. Dutau, H., Musani, A.I., Laroumagne, S. et al. (2015). Biodegradable airway stents – bench to bedside: a comprehensive review. *Respiration* 90: 512–521.
136. Freitag, L., Gördes, M., Zarogoulidis, P. et al. (2017). Towards individualized tracheobronchial stents: technical, practical and legal considerations. *Respiration* 94: 442–456.
137. Cheng, G.Z., San Jose Estepar, R., Folch, E. et al. (2016). Three-dimensional printing and 3D slicer: powerful tools in understanding and treating structural lung disease. *Chest* 149: 1136–1142.
138. Cheng, G.Z., Folch, E., Brik, R. et al. (2015). Three-dimensional modeled T-tube design and insertion in a patient with tracheal dehiscence. *Chest* 148: e106–e108.
139. Young, B.P., Machuzak, M.S., and Gildea, T. (2017). Initial clinical experience using 3D printing and patient-specific airway stents: compassionate use of 3D printed patient-specific airway stents. *Am. J. Respir. Crit Care Med.* 195: A1711.
140. Gildea, T.R., Young, B.P., and Machuzak, M.S. (2018). Application of 3D printing for patient-specific silicone stents: 1-year follow-up on 2 patients. *Respiration* 96: 488–494.
141. Rubin, A.E., Wang, K.P., and Liu, M.C. (2003). Tracheobronchial stenosis from acid aspiration presenting as asthma. *Chest* 123: 643–646.
142. Saad, C.P., Murthy, S., and Krizmanaich, G. (2003). Self-expandable metallic airway stents and flexible bronchoscopy: long-term outcomes analysis. *Chest* 124: 1993–1999.
143. Gottlieb, J., Fuehner, T., and Dierich, M. (2009). Are metallic stents really safe? A long-term analysis in lung transplant recipients. *Eur. Respir. J.* 34: 1417–1422.
144. Burns, K.E.A., Orons, P.D., and Dauber, J.H. (2002). Endobronchial metallic stent placement for airway complications after lung transplantation: longitudinal results. *Ann. Thorac. Surg.* 74: 1934–1941.
145. Noppen, M., Peirard, D., and Meysman, M. (1999). Bacterial colonization of central airways after stenting. *Am. J. Respir. Crit. Care Med.* 160: 672–677.
146. Shou, G.W., Huang, H.D., Sun, Q.Y. et al. (2015). Temporary placement of metallic stent could lead to benefits for benign tracheobronchial stenosis. *J. Thorac. Dis.* 7 (S4): S398–S404.
147. Matsuo, T. and Colt, H.G. (2000). Evidence against routine scheduling of surveillance bronchoscopy after stent insertion. *Chest* 118: 1455–1459.
148. Lee, H.J., Labaki, W., Yu, D.H. et al. (2017). Airway stent complications: the role of follow-up bronchoscopy as a surveillance method. *J. Thorac. Dis.* 9: 4651–4659.
149. Lehman, J.D., Gordon, R.L., Kerlan, R.K. et al. (1998). Expandable metallic stents in benign tracheobronchial obstruction. *J. Thorac. Imaging* 13: 105–115.
150. Ferretti, G.R., Kocier, M., Calaque, O. et al. (2003). Follow-up after stent insertion in the tracheobronchial tree: role of helical computed tomography in comparison with fiberoptic bronchoscopy. *Eur. Radiol.* 13: 1172–1178.
151. Burt, M., Diehl, W., Martini, N. et al. (1991). Malignant esophagorespiratory fistula: management options and survival. *Ann. Thorac. Surg.* 52: 1222–1228.
152. Menna, C., Poggi, C., Ibrahim, M. et al. (2017). Coated expandable metal stents are effective irrespective of airway pathology. *J. Thorac. Dis.* 9: 4574–4583.

第 24 章

球囊扩张支气管成形术

Ben Bevill[1], Luca Paoletti[2], and Nicholas J. Pastis Jr.[2]
[1] Division of Pulmonary and Critical Care Medicine,
University of Tennessee Graduate School of Medicine, Knoxville, TN, USA
[2] Division of Pulmonary and Critical Care Medicine,
Medical University of South Carolina, Charleston, SC, USA

（译者：朱　莹　译者单位：解放军总医院）

24.1　引言

气管支气管狭窄可表现为多种形式，包括恶性狭窄和非恶性狭窄。轻度狭窄所导致的气道阻塞基本不会引起任何临床症状，而重度气道阻塞可能会导致呼吸困难、反复感染甚至危及生命。一般而言，只有在气道达到重度狭窄的程度时，患者才会出现临床症状。例如，气管直径为 8 mm 时，患者可能会在活动时感到气短，而在气管直径为 5 mm 时，其在静息条件下就会出现呼吸困难[1]。多种外科手段可用于治疗气道狭窄，包括气管造口术、切除术和狭窄段切除后再吻合术，或采用气管/支气管成形术等方法进行气道重建[2]。而微创手术，如支气管镜下治疗，由于其风险小、获益快，成了临床医师常用的一线治疗手段。气道扩张治疗就是其中一种，可采用球囊和探条（硬质）扩张器进行气道扩张，也可在硬质支气管镜和气管导管下完成气道扩张。

血管成形术导管最先被应用于球囊支气管成形术。20 世纪 80 年代，Groff 和 Allen 首次报道了使用血管成形球囊扩张 1 例气管插管后支气管狭窄的婴幼儿[3]。Cohen 等同样使用球囊支气管成形术扩张 1 例婴幼儿的先天性气管狭窄[4]。自此之后，设计用于球囊支气管成形术的相关体系逐渐得以发展，其与可弯曲支气管镜相结合使用成为主流。本章将着重介绍这一技术。

24.2　适应证

一般气道狭窄程度超过 50% 的患者，可出现临床症状，并需要进行干预。基于流体力学原理，气道狭窄程度<50% 的患者出现临床症状的可能性较小。典型症状包括喘息、呼吸困难、喘鸣、反复感染、分泌物黏稠排出困难和明显的呼吸衰竭[5]。气管支气管狭窄的恶性和非恶性病因详见表 24.1。

表 24.1　中央气道梗阻病因

恶性疾病	非恶性疾病
腔内肿瘤生长或气道外部压迫（原发性）	医源性
支气管癌	气管插管后
腺样囊性癌	气道支架相关阻塞
黏液表皮样癌	外科吻合术
类癌	感染性
	结核病
腔内肿瘤生长或气道外部压迫（转移性）	乳头状瘤病
	会厌炎
肾细胞癌	先天性
乳腺癌	完整（"O"形）气管环
甲状腺癌	吊带狭窄（环吊综合征）
结肠癌	膜状狭窄

(续表)

恶性疾病	非恶性疾病
肉瘤	血管异常
黑色素瘤	**自身免疫/炎症性**
邻近结构的肿瘤	肉芽肿性多血管炎（韦格纳肉芽肿）
喉癌	复发性多软骨炎
食管癌	纤维化纵隔炎
胸腺瘤	结节性硬化症
甲状腺癌	淀粉样变性
生殖细胞瘤	**其他**
淋巴瘤	错构瘤
	甲状腺肿
	气管软化/支气管软化
	黏液栓
	血栓

来源：McArdle 等[6]。

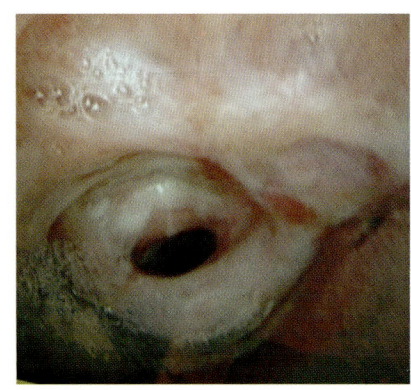

图 24.1　硬质支气管镜下良性膜状气管狭窄

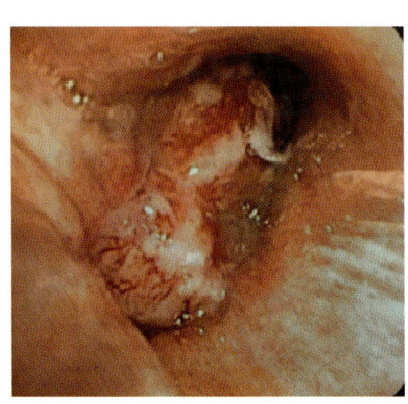

图 24.2　左肺门肿块导致左上叶和左下叶恶性（腔内和腔外混合型）气道狭窄

临床上，我们可以通过病史采集、体格检查、肺功能流量容积曲线、计算机断层扫描（computed tomography，CT）、磁共振成像（magnetic resonance imaging，MRI）和/或支气管镜检查等手段相结合诊断症状性气道狭窄（图 24.1、图 24.2）。由于阻塞程度和位置不同，体格检查的结果在气道狭窄中会有较大差异。气道远端狭窄可在受累区域闻及局限性哮鸣音或呼吸音消失，而近端狭窄可在上气道闻及哮鸣音。但对有些气道狭窄，体格检查却可能是正常的。流量容积曲线在这方面极其有价值，固定性上气道阻塞的经典表现为吸气相和呼气相均出现平台样改变，但在可变性胸内段气道阻塞中，仅在呼气相出现平台样改变。

气管插管和气管切开术导致的气道狭窄，其发病率介于 10%~22% 之间，但只有 1%~2% 的气道狭窄患者会出现症状或严重的后遗症。气管插管后的气道狭窄是由于气囊压超过毛细血管灌注压（正常为 22~32 mmHg），从而阻断血流，使气道内易于形成纤维母细胞和瘢痕[7]。大容量、低压 ETT 球囊的出现已经大大减少了气管插管后气道狭窄的发病率。而气管切开术后的气道狭窄主要是由于切口处伤口的异常愈合，伴有过多的肉芽组织形成所致[8]。

Feretti 等得出结论，只有纤维化所致的狭窄患者可以从球囊支气管成形术的一线治疗中获益。研究还认为，球囊扩张术对于局部支气管软化症并不起作用[9]。此外，其他研究已经证实，当气道内炎症反应活化时，单用球囊支气管成形术难以给患者带来获益，还需要进一步联合治疗，包括冷冻、电凝、激光治疗，甚至是支架置入[10,11]。已有研究发现，在气道周围软骨和气道结构被某些潜在病因破坏后，仅靠球囊支气管成形术并不能有效重建气道的通畅性[11]。

支气管狭窄是肺移植后最常见的气道并发症，发病率介于 1%~32% 之间[12]。随着外科介入手段的进步，支气管吻合口狭窄的发病率已经逐步下降。例如，望远镜式（套叠式）吻合术的狭窄发病率较高（34%），而端-端吻合术的狭窄发病率较低（5%），后者是现在首选的外科治疗手段[13]。肺移植后吻合处支气管狭窄使用球囊扩张术治疗在短期内已被证实是成功的[14]。目前普遍认为吻合口处发生坏死和形成肉芽肿通常都是短暂的。如果能在这一段时间内进行治疗，基本不会再次出现气道狭窄[15,16]。

24.3　技术

明确气道狭窄的病因对于制订治疗计划至关重要。

非恶性狭窄（图 24.1）通过使用球囊支气管成形术即可获益，而恶性病因导致的狭窄（图 24.2）在使用球囊扩张术后仍可能面临复发，并需要进一步治疗，甚至支架置入。同其他支气管镜操作一样，开展球囊支气管成形术需要仔细的术前评估，包括病史采集、体格检查、明确合并症以及利用已有的影像学资料确定狭窄段长度、周围正常结构和对侧气道的直径以及远端气道的通畅性。值得一提的是，在进行手术之前，要充分考虑手术适应证、禁忌证以及术者经验。Colt 和 Murgu 描述了一种支气管镜介入治疗的"四步"实用方法，其中包括初步评估、操作策略、操作技能和结果以及长期管理计划[17]。

可弯曲支气管镜通常需要中度镇静后经口或在有麻醉监护下经喉罩完成插入。如果支气管镜能够进入鼻腔，也可经鼻插入支气管镜进行球囊扩张，但并不常用。进行球囊扩张时，一般要避免气管内插管，因其不利于对上气道包括声门下部位的观察。根据术者经验和气道狭窄的严重程度，也可使用硬质支气管镜。特别是在症状严重或高度怀疑气道重度狭窄的患者中，首选硬质支气管镜（配备完整管径）（图 24.1）。

支气管镜对气道进行全面检查时，需重点关注狭窄段的直径和长度，这对选择球囊尺寸至关重要。可在支气管镜直视下进行气道内测量，也可通过透视下使用金属标识对可见病变末端做标记测量。

通过支气管镜工作通道或由带有软硅胶端的导丝直视引导下，将球囊送入狭窄段及远端气道。一般使用工作孔径为 2.8 mm 的可弯曲支气管镜可以通过球囊，如果使用工作孔径为 2.0 mm 的支气管镜，则需要在带有软硅胶端导丝引导下进行球囊扩张术，以减少操作过程中发生气胸的风险。操作中应用改良 Seldinger 技术，沿着导丝将球囊送入狭窄段后进行充填扩张，该过程可在支气管镜直视下或透视引导下进行。理想的球囊长度应能超过狭窄段两端至少 0.5 cm，以保证球囊稳固且不易移位。如果球囊过于靠近狭窄近端或远端，则球囊容易脱落并滑出。因此，操作前确定气道狭窄段长度是确保球囊放置最佳位置的唯一方法，这一操作最好在支气管镜直视及放射透视辅助下进行。

膜状或瘢痕病变在使用球囊进行支气管成形术之前需要介入手段进行干预（图 24.3），包括电凝术（electrocautery，EC）、氩等离子体凝固术（argon plasma coagulation，APC）、二氧化碳（carbon dioxide，CO_2）激光、Nd:YAG 和 Nd:YAP 激光等，这些介入方法各有优缺点。比如，电凝刀需要直接接触组织，其精确度不如激光，但止血效果良好。APC 无须接触组织，止血效果佳，但对组织的穿透深度较浅。CO_2 激光也是一种非接触技术，精确度佳但同样穿透深度浅，适合精细切割网状狭窄，但止血效果差。Nd:YAG 激光也是一种非接触手段，有较深的穿透性，止血效果良好，但容易损伤邻近组织[18]。同 Nd:YAG 激光，Nd:YAP 激光也属于非接触技术，但由于两种激光的物理特性不同，其治疗效果也不同。Nd:YAP 激光波长更长，光凝固性更好，但气化和切割能力较低[19]。网状狭窄可使用激光或其他热疗法进行径向切割（图 24.3 B），以充分释放并延展病变组织，提高球囊扩张的成功率[20]。

丝裂霉素 C 局部应用于气道狭窄处可降低再狭窄发生率并延长至下一次手术的时间间隔。回顾性研究报道丝裂霉素 C 的局部应用成功率高达 75%~93%[21]，可改善球囊扩张后的短期再狭窄[22]。但丝裂霉素 C 的疗效目前仍不十分确定，因其对狭窄复发率的报道没有显著差异[23,24]。此外，有报道黏膜下注射糖皮质激素治疗声门下狭窄，但由于病变类型不同而疗效各异，这一方法并未被广泛接受[25]。

在球囊扩张操作中，可在支气管镜下直接观察气道直径的改善（图 24.3）。研究表明，有些病变行 1 次

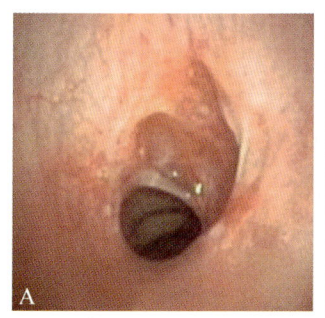 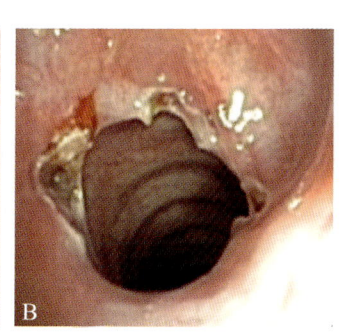 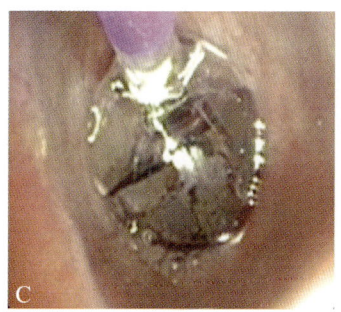 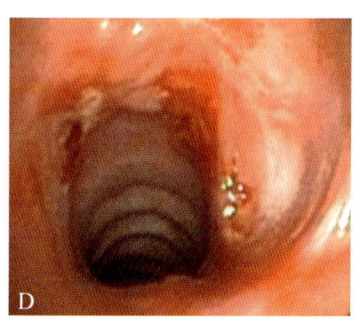

图 24.3　球囊扩张支气管成形术步骤
A. 严重膜状气道狭窄；B. 使用电刀径向切割；C. 填充加压时正确放置球囊；D. 球囊扩张后，气管狭窄有所改善。

球囊扩张术即可成功[10]，而有些则需要多次扩张甚至需要配合其他介入治疗技术[11]。

退出球囊操作前，务必确保气道内没有发生明显的并发症，且已达到预期扩张效果。

专为支气管镜下使用的球囊，其主要材质为硅胶且适应高填充压力。不同的填充压力可使球囊扩张到3种不同的直径来逐步扩张气道而无须更换球囊。这种球囊均配有带三通管的特殊高压注射器进行适当的填充加压。球囊和填充加压系统示例见图24.4和图24.5。球囊内通常注入生理盐水或稀释的水溶性造影剂，以减少球囊意外破裂时对肺部造成损伤。水溶性造影剂则更有助于在放射透视下观察，一般球囊扩张注入生理盐水即可。

扩张时间取决于狭窄段位置。越靠近中央气道（如气管），扩张时间越短，通常至少扩张30 s。越远端部位的病变（如主支气管和亚段），扩张时间越长，至少60~90 s，具体取决于患者耐受性。

球囊支气管成形术操作尚无最佳镇静方案。近端气道狭窄（如气管）通常需要深度镇静甚至肌松以确保操作安全。建议在麻醉师协助下进行，一方面更安全，另一方面更能确保疗效[26]。然而，尚未有随机临床试验对此进行研究。

24.4　其他扩张方法

如上文所述，球囊支气管成形术辅助治疗包括EC、APC、激光和冷冻治疗。可以单用硬质支气管镜来扩张狭窄气道以及铲除长入中心气道的病变组织（图24.2）。球囊支气管成形术可直接通过硬质支气管镜进行，有无可弯曲支气管镜均可。

支架置入（参见第23章）可与球囊支气管成形术相结合，在首次扩张或首次扩张复发后均可使用。此时球囊的主要功能是为支架置入做准备，一是扩张气道，二为测量气道大小。恶性气道阻塞是置入自膨胀金属支架或硅酮支架的适应证，通常作为姑息疗法。但可膨胀金属支架通常禁用于非恶性狭窄，特殊情况下可以使用硅酮支架。在气管造口术后气管狭窄的患者亚组中，初始球囊扩张失败后，短期支架置入可有效缓解症状[27]。

24.5　并发症

球囊扩张支气管成形术的并发症很少见[9-11]。主

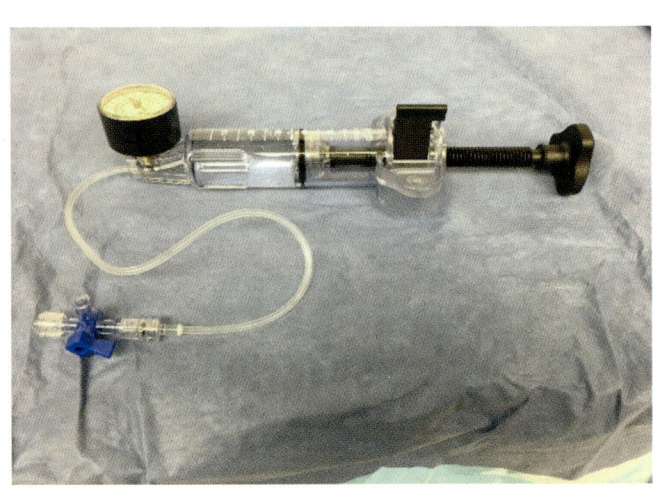

图24.4　高压注射器
波士顿科学，马塞诸塞州，美国。

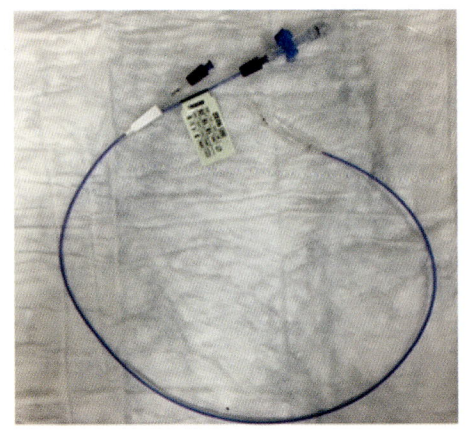
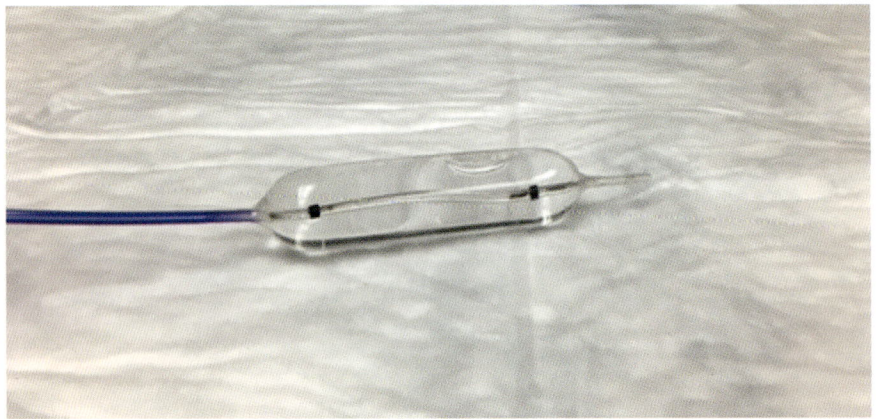

图24.5　一次性肺部球囊扩张器
波士顿科学，马塞诸塞州，美国。

要是可弯曲支气管镜操作常见的并发症，包括气胸、出血、呼吸衰竭、感染、肺不张以及对周围结构（包括声带）的损伤[18]；以及球囊扩张特有的并发症包括气管支气管撕裂或破裂、纵隔气肿、纵隔炎及死亡[14]。球囊扩张过程中发生气管支气管撕裂的发生率据报道可高达51.6%[28]。但大部分气道撕裂为表浅性，可在1个月内自愈，没有临床意义。较深的气道撕裂也可在短时间内通过保守治疗愈合，无进展为透壁撕裂或破裂的报道。球囊扩张特有的其他并发症很少见，在文献中也很少被报道。

24.6　疗效

据文献报道，球囊扩张的成功率差异较大，介于40%~90%之间。Feretti等[9]报道了36例球囊扩张病例，近期疗效为68%，远期疗效为56%。Sheski和Mathur等[10]发现71%（共14例）的非恶性气管支气管狭窄患者经过一次治疗即可获得成功。Hautmann等[29]在一项纳入126例大部分为恶性气道狭窄患者的临床研究中发现，79%的患者经过治疗即可改善狭窄程度；52%的患者可获得长于7天的长期改善。需要多次进行支气管镜检查评估再狭窄发生率。随访时间从数周到数月不等。根据患者的狭窄类型及其症状的严重程度确定球囊扩张的次数。

患者的狭窄类型决定了使用何种治疗方法。球囊扩张术对非恶性狭窄的疗效更好，这是因为气道内纤维化成分更多而炎症反应更少，而恶性狭窄则需要与其他介入技术配合治疗，如支架置入、激光治疗或电凝术[11]。

在非恶性病变中，特别是气管插管后的气管狭窄，最佳治疗是由胸外科或耳鼻喉科医师行气管切除。切除长度取决于狭窄长度。Grillo等[30]报告了503名气管插管后气道狭窄患者，其气管切除长度为1~7.5 cm不等。大多数切除长度为2~4 cm。球囊扩张一般用于初始治疗，但如果无效，适合手术的患者行外科修复治疗是最佳的方案。

24.7　结论

球囊扩张是一种安全的治疗方法。操作者通过适当培训，可以有效治疗多种原因导致的气管支气管狭窄。可以单独应用或联合其他介入治疗技术，进行多次操作以缓解症状。建议多学科联合，与外科医生密切合作确保最佳治疗方案。

参考文献

1. Al-Bazzaz, F., Grillo, H., and Kazemi, H. (1975). Response to exercise in upper airway obstruction. *Am. Rev. Respir. Dis.* 111 (5): 631-640.
2. Greenhill, S. and Kovitz, K. (2012). Balloon bronchoplasty. In: *Flexible Bronchoscopy*, 3e (eds. K. Wang, A. Mehta and F. Turner), 294-300. Ames: Wiley-Blackwell.
3. Groff, D. and Allen, J. (1985). Gruentzig balloon catheter dilation for acquired bronchial stenosis in an infant. *Ann. Thorac. Surg.* 39 (4): 379-381.
4. Cohen, M., Weber, T., and Rao, C. (1984). Balloon dilatation of tracheal and bronchial stenosis. *Am. J. Roentgenol.* 142 (3): 477-478.
5. Brouns, M., Jayaraju, S., Lacor, C. et al. (2007). Tracheal stenosis: a flow dynamics study. *J. Appl. Physiol.* 102 (3): 1178-1184.
6. McArdle, J., Gildea, T., and Mehta, A. (2005). Balloon bronchoplasty: its indications, benefits, and complications. *J. Bronchol.* 12 (2): 123-127.
7. Seegobin, R.D. and van Hasselt, G.L. (1984). Endotracheal cuff pressure and tracheal mucosal blood flow: endoscopic study of effects of four large volume cuffs. *Br. Med. J. (Clin. Res. Ed.)* 288 (6422): 965-968.
8. Zias, N., Chroneou, A., Tabba, M. et al. (2008). Post tracheostomy and post intubation tracheal stenosis: report of 31 cases and review of the literature. *BMC Pulm. Med.* 8: 18.
9. Feretti, G., Jouvan, F., Thony, F. et al. (1995). Benign noninflammatory bronchial stenosis: treatment with balloon dilation. *Radiology* 196 (3): 831-834.
10. Sheski, F. and Mathur, P. (1998). Long-term results of fiberoptic bronchoscopic balloon dilation in the management of benign tracheobronchial stenosis. *Chest* 114 (3): 796-800.
11. Shitrit, D., Kuchuk, M., Zismanov, V. et al. (2010). Bronchoscopic dilatation of tracheobronchial stenosis: long-term follow-up. *Eur. J. Cardiothorac. Surg.* 38 (2): 198-202.
12. Frye, L. and Machuzak, M. (2017). Airway complications after lung transplantation. *Clin. Chest Med.* 38 (4): 693-706.
13. Garfein, E.S., Ginsberg, M., Gorenstein, L. et al. (2001). Superiority of end-to-end versus telescoped bronchial anastomosis in single lung transplantation for pulmonary emphysema. *J. Thorac. Cardiovasc. Surg.* 121 (1): 149-154.
14. Keller, C. and Frost, A. (1992). FIberoptic bronchoplasty: description of a simple adjunct technique for the management of bronchial stenosis following lung transplantation. *Chest* 102 (4): 995-998.
15. Mahajan, A.K., Folch, E., Khandhar, S. et al. (2017). The diagnosis and management of airway complications following lung transplantation. *Chest* 152: 627-638.
16. Chhajed, P., Malouf, M., Tamm, M. et al. (2001). Interventional bronchoscopy for the management of airway

complications following lung transplantation. *Chest* 120 (6): 1894-1899.

17 Colt, H. and Murgu, S. (2012). *Bronchoscopy and Central Airway Disorders: A Patient-Centered Approach*. St Louis: Elsevier.

18 Hsia, D. and Musani, A. (2011). Interventional pulmonology. *Med. Clin. NorthAm.* 95 (6): 1095-1114.

19 Lee, H.J., Malhotra, R., Grossman, C. et al. (2011). Initial report of neodymium:yttrium aluminum-perovskite (Nd: YAP) laser use during bronchoscopy. *J. Bronchol. Interv. Pulmonol.* 18 (3): 229-232.

20 Brichet, A., Verkindre, C., Dupont, J. et al. (1999). Multidisciplinary approach to management of postintubation tracheal stenoses. *Eur. Respir. J.* 13 (4): 888-893.

21 Ubell, M.L., Ettema, S., Toohill, R. et al. (2006). Mitomycin-c application in airway stenosis surgery: analysis of safety and costs. *Otolaryngol. Head Neck Surg.* 134 (3): 403-406.

22 Simpson, B. and James, J. (2006). The efficacy of mitomycin-c in the treatment of laryngotracheal stenosis. *Laryngoscope* 116 (10): 1923-1925.

23 Valdez, T.A. and Shapshay, S.M. (2002). Idiopathic subglottic stenosis revisited. *Ann. Otol. Rhinol. Laryngol.* 111 (8): 690-695.

24 Smith, M.E. and Elstad, M. (2009). Mitomycin C and the endoscopic treatment of laryngotracheal stenosis: are two applications better than one? *Laryngoscope* 119 (2): 272-283.

25 Wierzbicka, M., Tokarski, M., Puszczewicz, M. et al. (2016). The efficacy of submucosal corticosteroid injection and dilatation in subglottic stenosis of different aetiology. *J. Laryngol. Otol.* 130 (7): 674-679.

26 Kern, M., Kerner, T., and Tank, S. (2017). Sedation for advanced procedures in the bronchoscopy suite: proceduralist or anesthesiologist? *Curr. Opin. Anaesthesiol.* 30 (4): 490-495.

27 Park, J.H., Kim, J., Song, H. et al. (2014). Management of benign tracheal strictures caused by tracheostomy. *Cardiovasc. Intervent. Radiol.* 37 (3): 743-749.

28 Kim, J.H., Shin, J., Song, H. et al. (2007). Tracheobronchial laceration after balloon dilation for benign strictures: incidence and clinical significance. *Chest* 131 (4): 1114-1117.

29 Hautmann, H., Gamarra, F., Pfeifer, K. et al. (2001). Fiberoptic bronchoscopic balloon dilatation in malignant tracheobronchial disease: indications and results. *Chest* (1): 43-49.

30 Grillo, H.C., Donahue, D., Mathisen, D. et al. (1995). Postintubation tracheal stenosis. Treatment and results. *J. Thorac. Cardiovasc. Surg.* 109 (3): 486-492; discussion 492-493.

第 25 章

硬质支气管镜技术

J. Francis Turner, Jr.[1,2] and Ko-Pen Wang[3]
[1] Division of Pulmonary and Critical Care Medicine,
University of Tennessee Graduate School of Medicine, Knoxville, TN, USA
[2] National Supercomputing Institute, University of Nevada, Las Vegas, NV, USA
[3] Division of Pulmonary and Critical Care Medicine, Johns Hopkins Bayview Medical Center,
Johns Hopkins University School of Medicine, Baltimore, MD, USA

（译者：林 欢 黄海东 译者单位：海军军医大学第一附属医院）

25.1 引言

Gustav Killian 被称为"支气管镜之父"，虽然 Rosenheim 和 Mikulicz 之前也曾用过食管镜探查气道，但首次采用硬质内镜探查气管并进行治疗性操作的是 Killian[1]（图 25.1）。1897 年 3 月 30 日，Killian 采用硬镜从一个德国农夫的右主支气管腔内成功取出了一块猪骨头，从而开创了硬镜操作的先河[2]。在美国，支气管镜的操作始于 Chevalier Jackson，他改良了当时的食管镜，并发明了硬质支气管镜，之后的 H. H. Hopkins 发明了"霍普金斯"可视光源镜，从而改善了硬质支气管镜的视野清晰度[3]。1970 年，随着池田茂人发明的可弯曲支气管镜应用于临床，硬质支气管镜的时代不再辉煌[4,5]。因此，美国以及其他地方的新一代支气管镜医师在其成长中缺少对硬质支气管镜技术的认识以及对硬质支气管镜操作技艺的体会。硬质支气管镜使用率下降十分显著，大约 92% 的支气管镜操作者在临床实践中从未使用过硬质支气管镜[6]。

但在某些情况下，硬质支气管镜较可弯曲支气管镜更有优势。硬质支气管镜大的工作通道更容易处理，如大咯血、取异物和支架置入等情况，同时气道安全也可保障[7,8]。虽然目前激光治疗常通过可弯曲支气管镜下进行，但相比可弯曲支气管镜橡胶的外皮，硬质

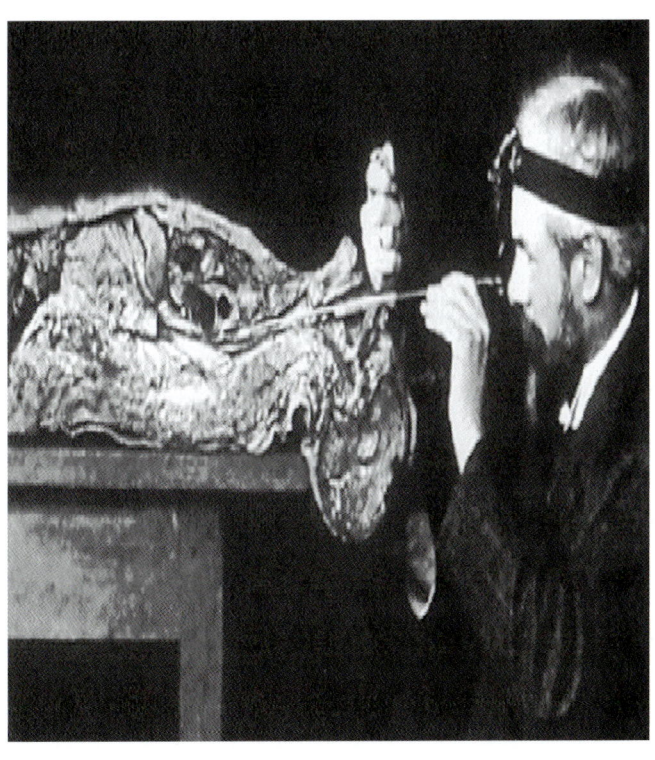

图 25.1 Gustov Killian 医生在尸体上操作硬质支气管镜
来源：Heinrich Becker 医生提供。

支气管镜金属镜身结构更有助于降低气道着火的风险[9]。此外，硬质支气管镜可用来直接铲除腔内阻塞性病灶，缩短操作时间，提高操作效率。使用硬质支气管镜操作时可以同时进行机械通气，较适合处理重度气管支气管狭窄的患者。

Clot 和 Harell 回顾性分析了急诊硬镜在重症 ICU 急性呼吸衰竭患者中的应用[10]，19 例中央型气道狭窄患者接受了急诊治疗性硬质支气管镜操作，52.6% 术后无须机械通气。7 例患者术后成功拔除气管插管，71.4% 患者术后降低了护理等级，62.5%（20/32）术后可立即降低护理等级。硬质支气管镜操作下，可以采用较大的配件获得更多更大的活检组织。最后，硬质支气管镜在处理操作中并发症方面优势明显，可以确保气道通畅和控制出血。

相比可弯曲支气管而言，硬质支气管镜对于远端气道的应用有限且大多数患者需全麻。此外，硬质支气管镜不适用于颈椎不稳定、严重的颈项强直或颞颌关节活动受限的患者[9]。

25.2 设备

硬质支气管镜设备的设计立足于解决通气且型号相对统一，根据患者为成年或儿童可选择不同型号金属管，硬质支气管镜内径可达 14~16 mm，硬质支气管镜镜长约 30 cm，成人通气型硬质支气管镜镜长约 40 cm（图 25.2）[11]。

不同的硬质支气管镜生产商都参照 Jean-Francois Dumon 设计的硬质支气管镜并在此基础上做修改，Jean-Francois Dumon 有以他的名字命名的硬质支气管镜品牌，较新的型号包括 Dumon-Harrell 通用硬质支气管镜（Bryon Corp，沃本，马萨诸塞州）。

虽然硬质支气管镜插入部远端管道内仅采用了一个微小的棒状发光装置照明，但内置于硬质支气管镜插入部管道内的霍普金斯可视光源镜可以提供足够的硬质支气管镜视野。图 25.3 为不锈钢材质的硬质支气管镜金属管（Storz 样品，Karl Storz 内镜，卡尔佛城，加利福尼亚州）、霍普金斯镜、硬质支气管镜活检钳和吸引导管（从硬质支气管镜机械通气接口斜行插入，在硬质支气管镜远端亮光下缘穿出）。硬质支气管镜的远端可以提供 0°、30° 和 90° 的视角。图 25.4 为硬质支气管镜附属配件，用于活检和介入操作。霍普金斯可视光源镜可以通过硬质支气管镜管道，配合不同型

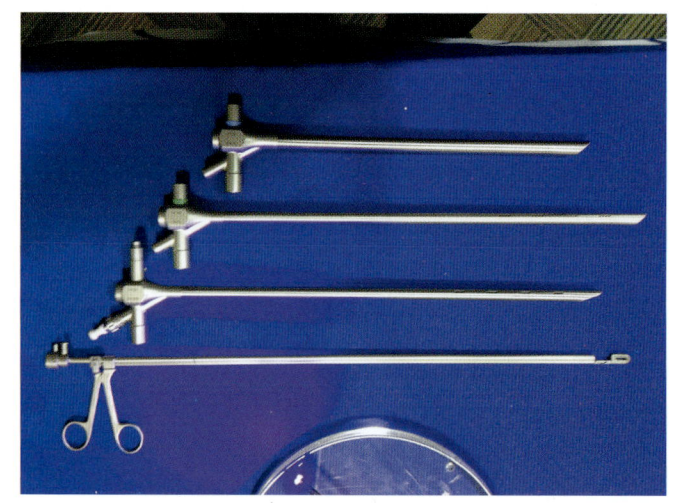

图 25.2 硬质支气管镜

自上而下，分别是硬质气管镜镜管、两种尺寸的硬质支气管镜镜管、霍普金斯硬质"花生钳"。

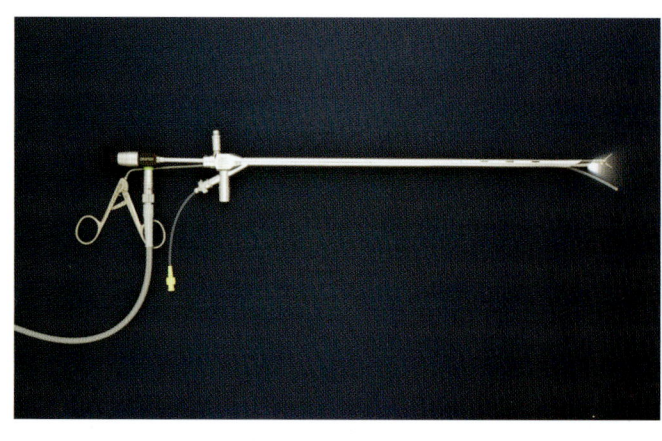

图 25.3 插入了霍普金斯可视光源镜、硬质支气管镜活检钳和专用软式吸引管的可进行机械通气的硬质支气管镜

图片来源：Turner 等。经 Wolters Kluwer Health, Inc. 许可复制。

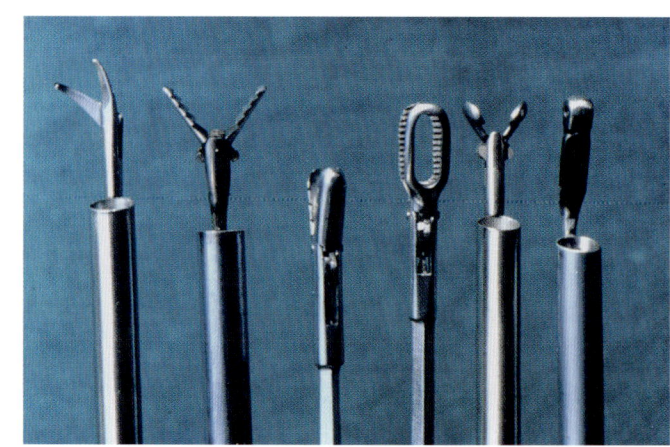

图 25.4 硬质支气管镜配件

图片来源：Turner 等。经 Wolters Kluwer Health, Inc. 许可复制。

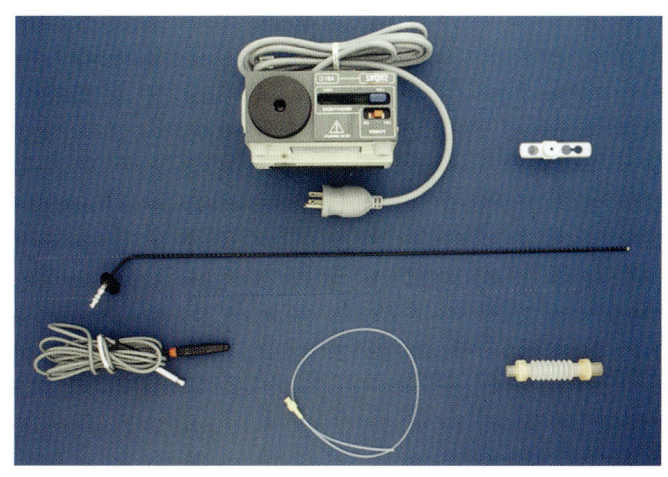

图 25.5　硬质支气管镜配件

顺时针方向：便携式光源，"FLUVOG"转换接口（接在硬质支气管镜近端开口位置），硬质支气管镜用电凝探头和接线，硬质支气管镜用吸引管和呼吸机转换接口。图片来源：Turner 等。经 Wolters Kluwer Health, Inc. 许可复制。

号活检钳一起对腔内病灶开展诊治。硬质支气管镜插入部近端配有含透明玻璃的小帽，可以套在硬质支气管镜插入近端的通道上封堵镜体，避免机械通气时气体外泄。一些玻璃小帽上有一个很小的"钥匙孔"，是硬质支气管镜配件的插入通道。图 25.5 中物品分别为（顺时针方向）：图片正上方为便携式光源，可以用来套在硬质支气管镜近端的 FLUVOG 帽，硬质支气管镜用高频电凝配件和仪器线，硬质支气管镜用吸引导管和螺纹通气接口。FLUVOG 接口可以滑动，是一种三合一的多功能接口，如果选择玻璃镜片接口，不仅可以封闭镜体避免漏气，还便于观察气道内的情况。选择有小孔的玻璃接口，则可以可视下通过小孔置入硬质支气管镜配件进行操作。选择没有镜片的大通道接口则可以置入多种硬质支气管镜配件和设备（如活检钳、可弯曲支气管镜）开展综合腔内介入诊疗。

25.3　适应证和禁忌证

25.3.1　适应证

目前常将硬质支气管镜和可弯曲支气管镜联合使用，这样可以充分发挥两者的优势。然而，在一些情境下硬质支气管镜效果更佳。

因硬质支气管镜具备较大的工作通道和大型号的钳子，所以通过硬质支气管镜可以获取更大的组织标本。虽然对于上叶病灶，因硬质支气管镜无法弯曲，故单纯硬质支气管镜操作活检取病理组织非常困难，但一旦硬质支气管镜结合可弯曲支气管镜，对于上叶病灶开展活检就非常容易了，可以取到更多的病理组织。其他的适应证还包括以下几个方面。

25.3.1.1　气道异物取出

如硬质支气管镜最初应用，成人或儿童气道异物的移除是硬质支气管镜的重要适应证之一[13-16]。异物是通过硬质支气管镜镜管取出的，故气管、喉部肌肉和声门得以保护，避免异物损伤。如果异物直径过大，则用钳子抓住异物并将其拉到硬质支气管镜的远端，后将硬质支气管镜与异物一同取出（视频 25.1）。

视频 25.1　智障成人患者，因吸入硬币就诊。通过硬质支气管镜和可弯曲支气管镜联合操作，从右中间段支气管取出硬币。

25.3.1.2　大咯血

大咯血会迅速导致患者通气困难和氧饱和度下降。此时，应用硬质支气管镜能更好地控制气道，改善通气。硬质支气管镜的工作通道可以允许使用较大内径的吸引导管吸出血液，钳夹纱布填塞出血部位或支气管分支[17,18]。1980 年，Conlan 等报道了 12 例通过硬质支气管镜使用冰生理盐水灌洗治疗大咯血的病例，这些患者 24 h 内咯血量超过 600 mL[19]。操作者使用硬质支气管镜将活动性出血的支气管隔离，用 4℃生理盐水进行灌洗，量 50~750 mL（平均 500 mL）。所有患者均止血成功，但有 2 例患者再次接受了生理盐水灌洗治疗。

25.3.1.3　中央气道阻塞

采用硬质支气管镜可以直接对腔内肿瘤实施机械性铲切，这项技术在过去已被使用于声门下狭窄的扩张治疗（图 25.6、图 25.7）。

25.3.1.4　热消融术

由于气道内没有易于燃烧的气管插管，硬质支气管镜下实施热消融治疗（如激光、氩等离子凝固术和高频电治疗）更加安全，激光治疗过程中产生的烟气等物质更容易在硬质支气管镜下排出体外（图 25.8，视频 25.2）。

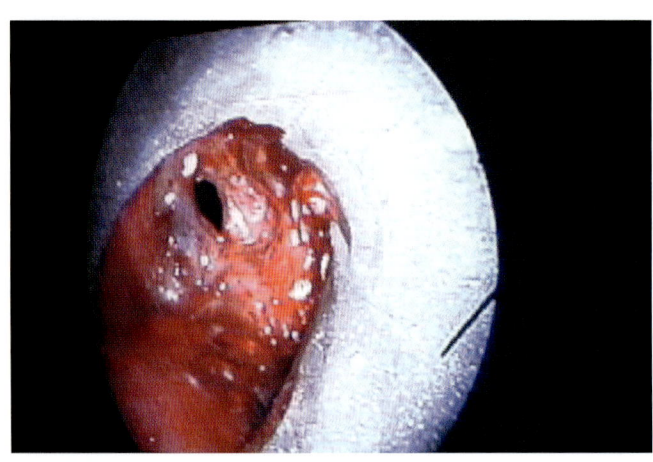

图 25.6　硬镜的远端位于声门下狭窄区域的正上方

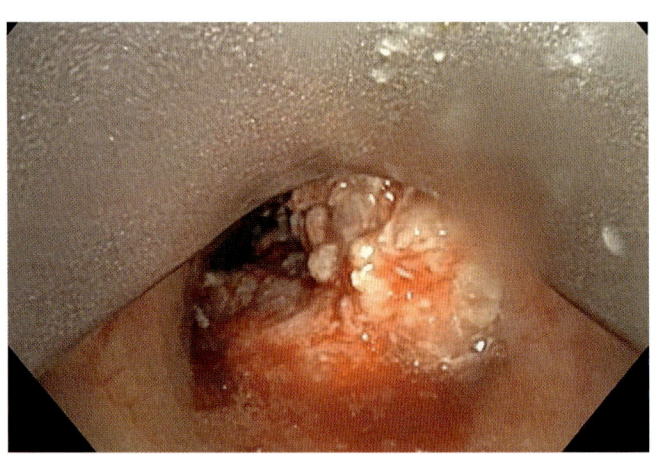

图 25.7　硬质支气管镜下铲切术

一位 56 岁的白人男性患者，气管阻塞超过 80%，侵犯长度 5 cm，活检显示为鳞状细胞癌，硬质支气管镜下"铲切"造成气管阻塞的肿瘤。

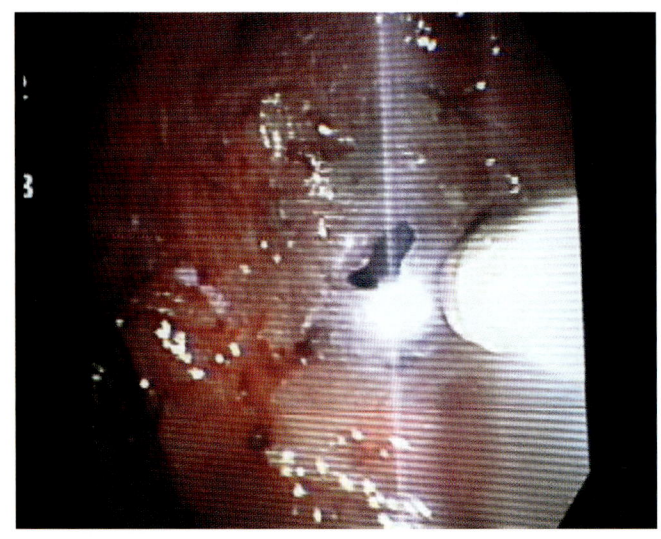

图 25.8　声门下气管狭窄区域的硬镜下激光消融术

视频 25.2　70 岁白人男性患者，右肺上叶支气管腔内息肉样肿物阻塞，采用钕：钇铝石榴石（Nd:YAG）激光消融治疗，右主支气管及右中间段支气管恢复通畅。

25.3.1.5　支架的置入和取出

目前还没有适用于各种类型气道狭窄的理想支架，选择支架仍然依据"不同需求，不同支架"的原则。支架的类型、支架释放的技术和所需的医疗团队取决于患者的实际状况。硬质支气管镜依旧用于硅酮和金属支架的置放和取出（视频 25.3）。

（1）　　　　（2）

视频 25.3　28 岁非裔美国男性，诊断为转移性骨肉瘤（左肺转移），肿瘤完全阻塞左主支气管并向上生长延伸至气管腔内。在硬质支气管镜下联合应用氩等离子体凝固术（APC）消融瘤体后，硬质支气管镜下肿瘤铲除术成功解除气道梗阻，随后于气管至右主支气管置入覆膜支架，术后患者气道恢复通畅，自主呼吸功能恢复良好。

25.3.2　禁忌证

25.3.2.1　缺乏训练有素的人员

目前大多数支气管镜操作者都热衷于使用可弯曲支气管镜，所以能够操作硬质支气管镜的训练有素的人员明显减少。一支训练有素的团队应包括支气管镜操作者、麻醉医师、呼吸治疗师和护理团队（图 25.9）。

25.3.2.2　颈椎不稳定

对于颈椎不稳定或因颈部先天畸形、关节炎或机械性融合术导致的颈椎固定患者，硬质支气管镜插入非常困难或无法完成。

25.3.2.3　循环系统不稳定或非气道阻塞所致的低氧血症

合并心肌缺血、血流动力学不稳定或其他一些全麻高风险患者，硬质支气管镜操作期间出现并发症的风险会增加。如果患者低氧血症或呼吸机依赖是气道阻塞导致的，硬质支气管镜操作仍是适应证。

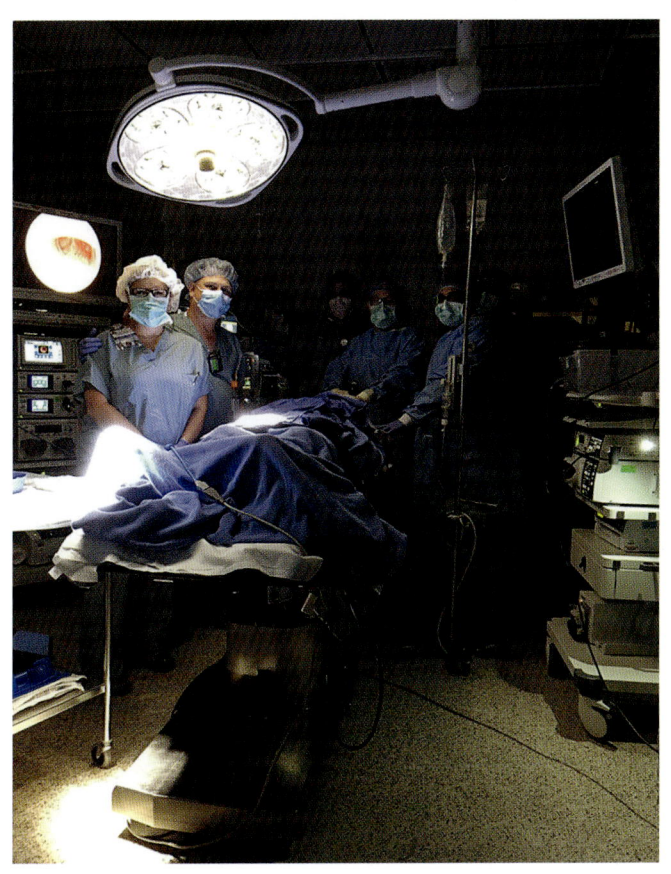

图 25.9　田纳西大学医学中心的支气管镜诊疗团队

25.4　麻醉

支气管镜操作的麻醉已在第 5 章进行阐述，然而，此处特别提出硬质支气管镜操作中的麻醉。虽然硬质支气管镜可以在适度镇静、局部麻醉和自主呼吸的情况下进行，但这会增加低氧血症的风险，现在这种方式已基本上被放弃[9,11]。目前硬质支气管镜操作通常在全麻下进行。机械通气方式由支气管镜操作者、麻醉医师的操作经验和相关的硬件设备决定。当给患者注射麻醉诱导剂后，硬质支气管镜插入气管。进入气管后，硬质支气管镜近端侧面端口需连接机械通气管路，管路另一端可连接简易呼吸器（Ambu bag）、麻醉机或喷射通气呼吸机。喷射通气可以采用手动喷气阀（50 psi 流速，吸入氧浓度为 100%）或高频喷射呼吸机。通常采用吸入药物或静脉药物，或者两者联合开展全麻硬质支气管镜操作[20]。我们更喜欢使用全身静脉麻醉，尤其是在使用硬质支气管镜操作的时候。因为麻醉气体可能会在操作过程中泄露到周围环境中，这可能会影响整个支气管镜团队。当采用简易呼吸器（Ambu bag）、麻醉机通气时，须谨防气体从鼻腔、口腔和硬质支气管镜近端泄漏出来，检查室需保持足够的通气。下面简要介绍间歇喷射通气和填塞鼻腔和口腔的方法[21]。笔者个人比较喜欢采用喷射通气机开展硬质支气管镜操作，这样硬质支气管镜近端可以保持开放，允许可弯曲支气管镜和其他器械有足够大的空间进入。大多数介入呼吸病专业医师熟悉喷射通气机，喷射通气机通过文丘里原理实现通气，麻醉师需随时监测氧饱和度。在某些使用高喷射通气（high-frequency jet ventilation，HFJV）进行硬质支气管镜检查时，可进行呼气末二氧化碳分压监测。与经皮监测相比，这种方法也被认为是准确的[22]。在行治疗性硬质支气管镜操作时尤其要注意吸入氧浓度，硬质支气管镜下开展激光等热治疗，高浓度氧有导致气道着火的可能[13]。

目前，还有一些其他通过联合应用一些辅助外部设备进行通气和氧气交换的方法。Natalini 等阐述了在硬质支气管镜操作中应用间歇负压通气和外部高频振荡通气，或应用同步体外膜肺氧合（extracorporeal membrane oxygenation，ECMO）[24-27]。

25.5　操作方法

患者肌松后，调整患者头部位置处于颈部后仰位，让口腔、口咽到声门呈一条直线。右手握持硬质支气管镜的近端调整硬质支气管镜插入端，使硬质支气管镜远端唇样突出的金属末端位于前方位置。若采用硬质支气管镜内置入霍普金斯光源视频镜（图 25.3）引导下完成硬质支气管镜插入，在插入前必须旋转校正视频图像位置，使电视视频图像和硬质支气管镜插入部末端图像方向一致（即硬质支气管镜远端唇样突出的金属末端位于 12 点钟的位置）（图 25.10）。右手虎口将霍普金斯光源视频镜与硬质支气管镜镜身固定，使其插入时稳定不滑动，光源视频镜的插入末端必须位于硬质支气管镜插入部唇样突起金属管末端的内部，这样有利于插入过程。保持患者头部位于"嗅探"位置，确认硬质支气管镜插入部唇样突起调整至 12 点位置，左手示指、中指、无名指和小指探入患者口腔，用以在整个插入过程中固定患者的头部。左手大拇指和示指辅助硬质支气管镜插入口咽部。示指用以保护下牙槽和下唇避免和硬质支气管镜直接接触，大拇指保护上牙槽和上唇。

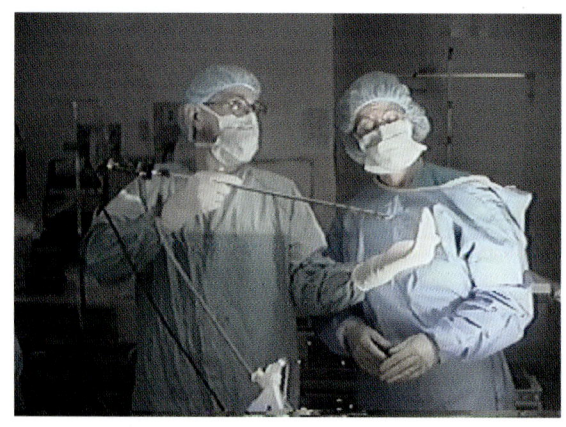

图 25.10　硬质支气管镜操作方法

右手持硬质支气管镜近端部分，调整硬质支气管镜远端使硬质支气管镜插入部远端唇样突起金属部分位于前位，然后调整视频图像位置，确保镜下所见图像位置和实际硬质支气管镜金属末端位置一致。

　　硬质支气管镜首先置于与口腔呈 90°垂直角度进入（图 25.11）。硬质支气管镜沿着左手拇指、示指扩展的通道进入直至看到悬雍垂，一旦硬质支气管镜插入末端到达悬雍垂，此时以左手拇指为支点使硬质支气管镜长轴逐渐向下趋于水平位向前推进。左手示指在保护下唇和下牙槽的同时引导硬质支气管镜向前推进。操作者不能让硬质支气管镜推进过程中接触上牙槽和嘴唇，以免导致唇部创伤和牙齿断裂。

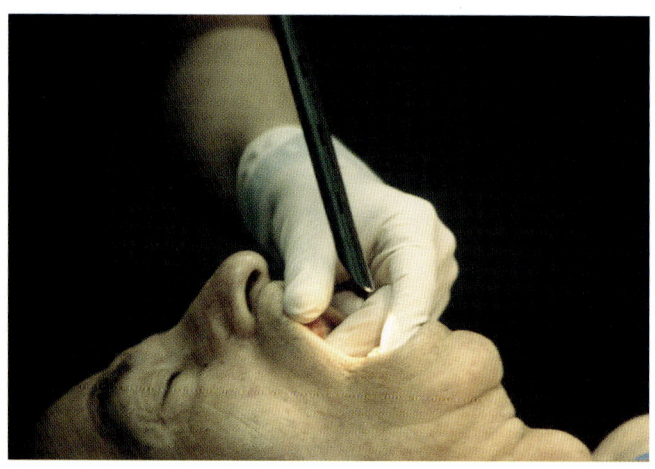

图 25.11　硬质支气管镜进镜角度

硬质支气管镜插入端与张开的口腔呈 90°方向垂直进入。图片来源：Turner 等[12]。经 Wolters Kluwer Health, Inc. 许可复制。

　　操作硬质支气管镜沿中线位置向前推进直至看到会厌，采用类似用喉镜插管的操作，将硬质支气管镜插入端唇样金属末端挑起会厌（图 25.12），从其下方通过并旋转 90°，这样硬质支气管镜插入端较容易通过声门而不损伤声带，通过声门时需非常谨慎且动作轻柔，可微微旋转并小心地推开两侧声带进入。当患者声门开放至最大但所选的硬质支气管镜仍然太粗通过困难时，可考虑换用小一个型号的硬质支气管镜重新插入，当硬质支气管镜插入部唇样金属突起通过声门后，将硬质支气管镜旋转使唇样金属突起置于 6 点钟位置，这样使硬质支气管镜可以暂时固定在口咽部（图 25.13），另外使用硬质支气管镜过程中注意用纱布或橡皮牙垫保护患者的牙齿和牙龈。

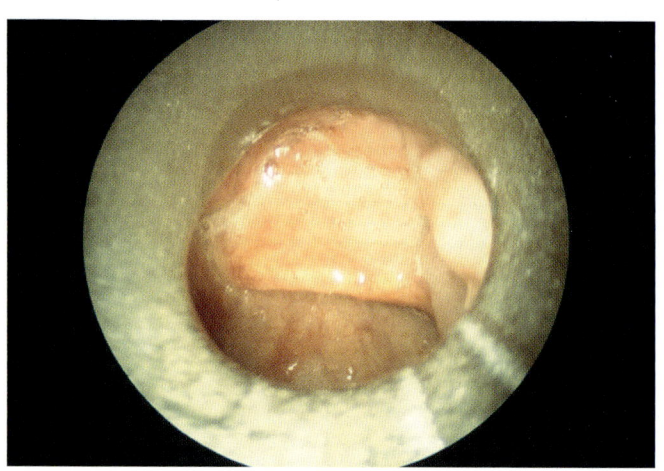

图 25.12　硬质支气管镜进境

硬质支气管镜插入端缓缓向前推进直至探查发现会厌软骨。图片来源：Turner 等[12]。经 Wolters Kluwer Health, Inc. 许可复制。

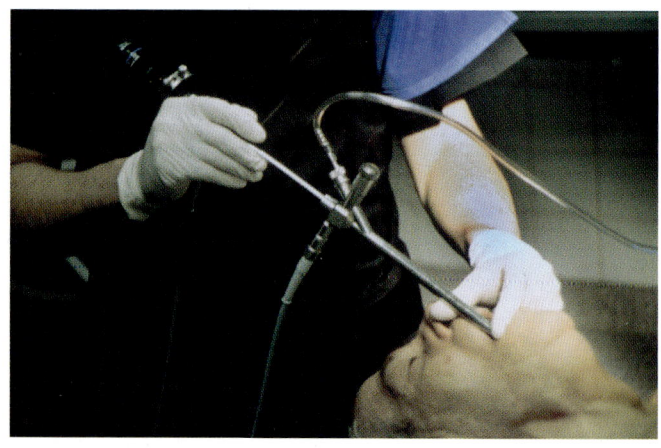

图 25.13　硬质支气管镜近端部分镜管置于口咽部

操作者正用霍普金斯光源视频镜插入硬质支气管镜管腔内实施气道探查。图片来源：Turner 等[12]。经 Wolters Kluwer Health, Inc. 许可复制。

还有一些其他方法也可以将硬质支气管镜插入气管，具体方法的选择取决于器械的可及性及困难气道的具体情况。

1）操作者可以不使用视频光源镜，通过硬质支气管镜直接肉眼观察口腔和声门插入声门下区域，其间可使用棱镜附件实现远端照明，利于插入。

2）操作者可将可弯曲支气管镜置入硬质支气管镜管腔内，将可弯曲支气管镜的插入端固定于硬质支气管镜的末端，像使用霍普金斯光源视频镜一样插入。

3）操作者也可采用喉镜或可视喉镜，如 GlideScope 可视喉镜暴露声门，像气管插管一样将硬质支气管镜直接插入声门下气管区域（图 25.14、图 25.15）。

4）操作者先给患者完成气管插管后，然后将硬质支气管镜经口插入，沿着气管插管直至看见声门口，此时缓慢的撤出气管插管，再将硬质支气管镜向前推进完成插入声门（图 25.16，视频 25.4）。

采用霍普金斯可视光源镜引导完成硬质支气管镜插入时，必须让霍普金斯远端不超过硬质支气管镜插入部唇样金属末端，这样做可避免硬质支气管镜插入过程中唇样金属末端所致的意外气道损伤。如果不采用霍普金斯可视光源镜引导，则必须保持硬质支气管镜插入部的唇样金属末端插入过程中始终在可视范围内。

硬质支气管镜通过声门进入气管后，将硬质支气管镜缓缓向前推进并仔细探查气管内结构，推进过程中如遇阻力不可强行推进。到达气道隆突后可轻轻转动患者头部使硬质支气管镜进入左右主支气管进一步探查远端气道。向左转动患者头部便于硬质支气管镜插入右主支气管，反之亦然，向右转动患者头部便于硬质支气管镜插入左主支气管。一般情况下，通过硬质支气管镜可探查至上下叶段支气管开口层面的水平。采用 0° 视角的可视镜可探查右中叶和下叶亚段开口，对于右上叶，除非采用 90° 视角镜头探查，否则硬质支气管镜无法观察到所有亚段支气管，上述大角度的叶段腔内活检操作，可借助可弯曲支气管镜完成。硬质支气管镜探查左侧固有上叶、左舌叶和右上叶的情况基本一致。在常规完成气道评估检查后，就可以在硬质支气管镜下完成其他气道介入治疗操作。

硬质支气管镜操作完成后，需插入硬质支气管镜专用软式吸引管将硬质支气管镜内的分泌物持续吸引干净。如果操作者使用霍普金斯可视光源镜插入硬质支气管镜内，其远端需不超过硬质支气管镜插入部唇样金属末端，避免硬质支气管镜插入过程中唇样金属

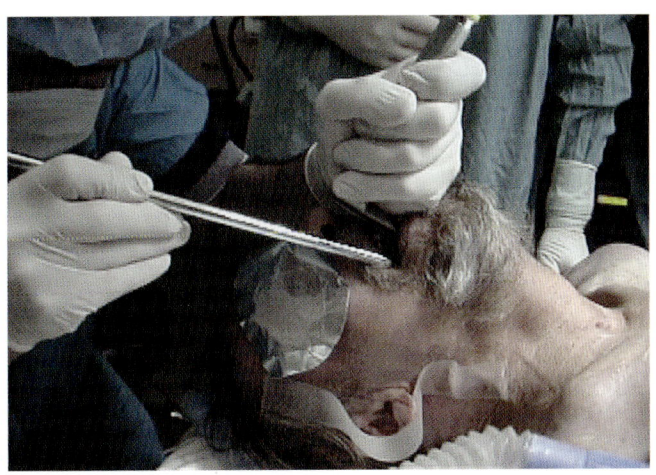

图 25.14　喉镜辅助下暴露声门后完成硬质支气管镜的插入

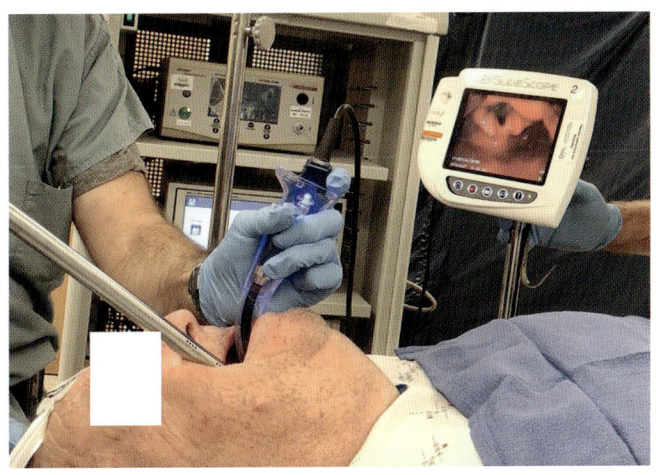

图 25.15　使用可视喉镜 GlideScope 直视下完成硬质支气管镜的插入

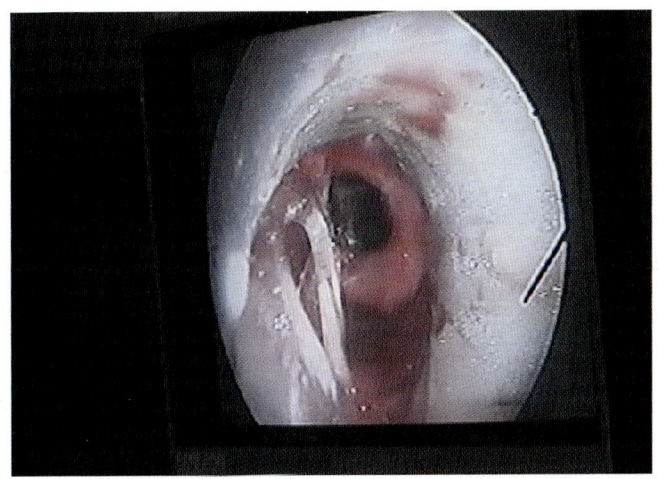

图 25.16　硬质支气管镜插入过程

硬质支气管镜经口沿着气管插管进入，然后慢慢拔出气管插管，同时将硬质支气管镜插入端在两侧声带之间向前推动完成插入。

末端所致的意外气道损伤。操作者一边持续吸引，一边将硬质支气管镜顺畅地无明显阻力地退出气道。

（1）　　　　（2）

视频 25.4　吸入性损伤患者（术前已行气管插管）

（1）硬质支气管镜沿气管导管插入；（2）在霍普金斯光源镜直视引导下，将硬质支气管镜插入到声门下区域，同步撤出气管导管。

25.6　并发症

并发症往往与肺部基础疾病有关，硬质支气管镜操作往往会导致以下并发症：

1）低氧血症：因肺部基础疾病所致，因硬质支气管镜在气道内致无法插管；

2）血流动力学不稳定；

3）气管和食管穿孔：因硬质支气管镜及相关器械强行进入或推进方向错误所致的上气道、气管和食管穿孔；

4）牙齿损伤；

5）声带水肿。

硬质支气管镜插入时切忌过快或用蛮力推进，这样做易导致插入方向错误而意外进入梨状窦，损伤食管或误伤声门。硬质支气管镜插入时过度匆忙而准备不足易导致插入方向错误和声带脱位，尤其在既往有头颈部外科手术病史的患者，操作硬质支气管镜时需非常小心且保持镜下视野清晰。不管采用哪种硬质支气管镜插入方式，操作者都必须认识到在此过程中患者需无自主呼吸，如果插入过程不顺利或插入耗时过长，此时操作者应该及时给予患者机械通气。完善的术前计划非常重要，术前硬质支气管镜操作医师和麻醉医师应充分交流，共同解决硬质支气管镜建立后的气道通气问题和应对可能的对气道"失去控制的"情况。同时，各种不同直径和型号的硬质支气管镜、气管插管、喉罩都需备齐，紧急环甲膜穿刺包和气管切开包也应该作为硬质支气管镜操作的必需备件。

25.7　培训目标

总之，并非所有支气管镜操作医生都必须掌握硬质支气管镜，目前大部分的支气管镜相关操作都可以在可弯曲支气管镜下高效开展。但如上所述，有些情况下硬质支气管镜还起着至关重要的作用。目前硬质支气管镜的操作数量在全美支气管镜操作总数上仅占一小部分，故建议全美主要的几个接受转诊患者的大型医疗中心，每个中心至少拥有1名既精通硬质支气管镜也能用可弯曲支气管镜的介入呼吸病专家。

这并非意味着会使用硬质支气管镜的医师，其能力就比其他支气管镜操作医师强，内镜医师获得一些临床经验后，其水平的提高取决于进一步的培训和个人领悟的能力。所有的内镜操作者都应该知道，任何一项内镜操作技术，首先必须通过一定数量的练习才能掌握，然后确保一定数量的操作才能维持这种技能。Kvale 在1990年提出建议，医师完成支气管镜下激光治疗至少操作25例/年才能被认为具备了操作激光的能力[28]。美国胸科医师协会制定的支气管镜操作指南中指出，接受内镜规范化培训的医师必须在指导老师带教下完成50例次的可弯曲支气管镜诊断性操作才能被认为具备了独立解决支气管镜操作中发生的意外和并发症的能力[29,30]。对于硬质支气管镜培训而言，参与学习的医师需首先在模型上练习，然后在指导老师带教下至少完成50例次硬质支气管镜操作，才能开始独立操作硬质支气管镜。

25.8　结论

在 Killian 发明硬质支气管镜100年后的今天，硬质支气管镜技术仍然是一种非常有价值的技术。硬质支气管镜的大直径的管腔具备了操作的同时，还可进行控制通气的优点，这点是小工作通道的可弯曲支气管镜所无法做到的。对于介入呼吸病医师而言，应该继续开展培训并精通这项技术，以应对临床工作的需求。

参考文献

1　Zollner, F. (1965). Gustav Killian: father of bronchoscopy. *Arch. Otolaryngol.* 82: 656-659.

2　Von Eiken, C. (1904). The clinical application of the method of direct examination of the respiratory passes and upper alimentary tract. *Arch Laryngol. Rhinol.*: 15.

3　Prakash, U.B.S. (1994). Introduction. In: *Bronchoscopy* (ed. U.B.S. Prakash). New York: Raven Press.

4　Panchabhai, T.S. and Mehta, A.C. (2015). Historical perspectives of bronchoscopy. *Ann. Am. Thorac. Soc.* 12 (5): 631-641.

5. Miyazawa, T. (2000). History of the flexible bronchoscope. In: *Progress in Respiration Research, Vol. 30: Interventional Bronchoscopy* (eds. C.T. Bollieger and P.N. Mathur), 16–21 Basel: Karger.
6. Prakash, U.B.S., Offord, K.P., and Stubbs, S.E. (1991). Bronchoscopy in North America: the ACCP survey. *Chest* 100: 1668–1675.
7. Wedzicha, J.A. and Pearson, M.C. (1990). Management of massive hemoptysis. *Respir. Med.* 84: 9–12.
8. Freitag, L. (1995). Flexible versus rigid bronchoscopic placement of tracheobronchial prosthesis (stents). Pro rigid bronchoscopy. *J. Bronchol.* 2: 248–251.
9. Ayers, M.L. and Beamis, J.F. (2001). Rigid bronchoscopy in the twenty-first century. *Clin. Chest Med.* 22 (2): 355–364.
10. Colt, H.G. and Harrell, J.H. (1997). Therapeutic rigid bronchoscopy allows level of care changes in patients with acute respiratory failure from central airway obstruction. *Chest* 112: 202–206.
11. Yarmus, L. and Batra, H. (2018). Indications and complications of rigid bronchoscopy. *Expert Rev. Respir. Med.* 12 (6): 509–520.
12. Turner, J.F., Ernst, A., and Becker, H.D. (2000). "How I do it"; rigid bronchoscopy. *J. Bronchol.* 7: 172.
13. Beamis, J. (1999). Rigid bronchoscopy. In: *Interventional Pulmonology* (eds. J.F. Beamis and P.N. Mathur), 17–28. New York: McGraw-Hill.
14. Kollofrath, O. (1897). Entfernung eines Knochenstucks aus dem rechten Bronchus auf anturlichem Wege und Anwendung der directed Laryngoscopie. *Munch. Med. Wochenschr.* 38: 1038–1039.
15. Folch, E. and Mehta, A.C. (2008). Airway interventions in the tracheobronchial tree. *Semin. Respir. Crit. Care Med.* 29 (4): 441–452.
16. Oki, M., Saka, H., and Hori, K. (2017). Airway stenting in patients requiring intubation due to malignancy airway stenosis: a 10-year experience. *J. Thorac. Dis.* 9 (9): 3154–3160.
17. Valipour, A., Kreuzer, A., Koller, H. et al. (2005). Bronchoscopy-guided topical hemostatic tamponade therapy for the management of life-threatening hemoptysis. *Chest* 127 (6): 2113–2118.
18. Reisz, G. (2005). Topical haemostatic tamponade: another tool in the treatment of massive hemoptysis. *Chest* 127 (6): 1888–1889.
19. Conlan, A.A. and Hurwitz, S.S. (1980). Management of massive haemoptysis with the rigid bronchoscope and cold saline lavage. *Thorax* 35: 901–904.
20. Pathak, V., Welsby, I., Mahmoood, K. et al. (2014). Ventilation and anesthetic approaches for rigid bronchoscopy. *Ann. Am. Thorac. Soc.* 11: 628–634.
21. Ginsberg, R.J. (1995). Rigid bronchoscopy. In: *Textbook of Bronchoscopy* (eds. S.H. Feinsilver and A.M. Fein), 486–493 Baltimore: Williams & Wilkins.
22. Simon, M., Bottschall, R., Gugel, M. et al. (2003). Comparison of transcutaneous and endtidal CO_2-monitoring for rigid bronchoscopy during high-frequency jet ventilation. *Acta Anaesthesiol. Scand.* 47: 861–867.
23. Turner, J.F. and Wang, K.P. (1999). Endobronchial laser therapy. *Clin. Chest Med.* 20: 107.
24. Natalini, G., Cavaliere, S., Seramondi, V. et al. (2000). Negative pressure ventilation vs. external high-frequency oscillation during rigid bronchoscopy. *Chest* 118: 18–23.
25. Natalini, G., Vitacca, M., Cavaliere, S. et al. (1998). Negative pressure ventilation vs. spontaneous assisted ventilation during rigid bronchoscopy. *Acta Anaesthesiol. Scand.* 42: 1063–1069.
26. Natalini, G., Vitacca, M., Cavaliere, S. et al. (1997). Use of Hayek oscillator during rigid bronchoscopy under general anesthesia [abstract]. *Br. J. Anaesth.* 78 (Suppl 1): 23.
27. Dunkman, W.J., Nicoara, A., Schroder, J. et al. (2017). Elective venovenous extracorporeal membrane oxygenation for resection of endotracheal tumor: a case report. *AA Case Rep.* 9 (4): 97–100.
28. Kvale, P. (1990). Training in laser bronchoscopy and proposal for credentialing. *Chest* 97: 983–989.
29. American College of Chest Physicians, Section of Bronchoscopy (1982). Guidelines for competency and training in fiberoptic bronchoscopy. *Chest* 81: 739.
30. Ernst, A., Silvestri, G., and Johnstone, D. (2003). Interventional pulmonary procedures: guidelines from the American College of Chest Physicians. *Chest* 123 (5): 1693–1717.

第 26 章

儿科可弯曲支气管镜

Xicheng Liu[1], Chen Meng[2], Jing Ma[2], and Shunying Zhao[1]
[1] Department of Interventional Pulmonology, Beijing Children's Hospital,
Capital University of Medicine, Beijing, China
[2] Department of Interventional Pulmonology,
Qilu Children's Hospital of Shandong University, Jinan, China
（译者：马　静　译者单位：山东大学附属儿童医院）

26.1　引言

近10年来，支气管镜介入技术迅速发展。儿科可弯曲支气管镜在临床诊疗中的重要作用日益彰显[1-3]。儿科医生开创性地将热消融技术（如高频电、氩气等离子凝固术、激光等），冷冻、球囊扩张治疗术，支架置入术等应用于气道阻塞性疾病及气道重建。在防污染采样毛刷、经支气管镜肺活检术（transbronchial lung biopsy，TBLB）、经支气管镜针吸活检术（transbronchial needle aspiration，TBNA）及内科胸腔镜方面进行了大量探索性临床应用研究。适用于儿童的气道支架、球囊的开发，以及肺内局部用药的研究等也在进行中。新介入技术的应用，无论在儿科呼吸系统感染、变态反应、间质性肺疾病等的诊治，还是在气道肿瘤、结核、外伤、外压以及先天发育异常导致的气道狭窄的诊治方面都获得了革命性的进展。

26.2　操作注意事项

26.2.1　可弯曲支气管镜的选择

选择合适外径的可弯曲支气管镜非常重要。现有不同型号的可弯曲支气管镜以满足不同年龄的儿童患者，包括新生儿。儿童常用的可弯曲支气管镜外径为2.8~4.0 mm，吸引/工作通道直径为1.2~2.2 mm。此外"超细"支气管镜（外径2.2 mm）虽不具有吸引/工作通道，但在评价早产儿和低体重新生儿的远端小气道方面发挥了重要作用。较大直径的支气管镜（≥4.9 mm）适用于学龄儿童和青少年患者。有不同型号的活检钳可适配于2~2.2 mm以及1.2 mm工作通道。

支气管镜的选择取决于检查的目的和患儿气道的大小。儿童的气道直径可以通过以下计算公式来估计：

气道直径（mm）= 4 + 年龄（岁）/4

因支气管镜会部分占用管腔空间，如果经气管插管（endotracheal tube，ETT）实施支气管镜检查，支气管镜外径的选择尤为重要[2]。支气管镜进入气管插管后阻塞的面积比例可以从以下公式计算：

$[1-(支气管镜半径^2/ETT半径^2)] \times 100\%$

由此可知，将2.8 mm支气管镜插入4.0 mm的气管插管将导致57%的管腔直径被阻塞。为保证术中有足够的通气，气管插管的外径至少要比支气管镜外径粗1 mm。如果超过50%的管腔通气受阻或者患儿本身已存在明显的气体交换障碍，检查过程中往往需要实施辅助通气。

儿童出生时气管内径为4.0~5.0 mm，并随年龄增长。根据不同年龄选用合适型号的支气管镜是成功、安全地进行检查的前提。直径<3.0 mm 的支气管镜可用于各年龄组，直径 4.0~4.9 mm 的支气管镜适用于 1 岁以上各年龄组。1.2 mm 的工作通道的支气管镜下可进行吸引、给氧、灌洗、活检、刷检、球囊扩张和激光等诊疗操作，而 2.0 mm 的工作通道下还可以进行电凝、冷冻、金属支架置入、TBNA 和 TBLB 等各种操作。

26.2.2 术前准备

术前准备区域应设计成能尽量减轻可弯曲支气管镜检查给患儿带来的焦虑。可采取转移注意力、提前开放静脉通路等减少痛苦的措施。对于烦躁及不合作的儿童可酌情使用镇静剂或抗焦虑药，如口服咪达唑仑。

确保患者佩戴印有身份标识的腕带，并至少有一条有效的静脉通道。

26.2.2.1 术前评估

由于镇静、麻醉剂对呼吸系统、心血管系统都有不同程度的抑制作用，加之原有的呼吸系统疾病，患儿在支气管镜检查时可能出现呼吸抑制、低氧血症、喉、气管支气管痉挛，血压下降，心律失常等。因此，有必要选择最佳的手术时间和麻醉方式，并在手术前评估耐受性，制定应急预案。

26.2.2.2 签署知情同意书

无论局部或全身麻醉，医生必须告知患者的监护人（或对于年龄较大的儿童本人）支气管镜检查的目的、其他替代方案以及手术期间和手术后可能出现的并发症。监护人必须签署知情同意书。对于全身麻醉，麻醉医师必须明确麻醉药过敏史，监护人必须签署麻醉知情同意书。

术前的一段时间对父母和孩子来说都很煎熬，一方面对支气管镜操作本身感到焦虑，也担心支气管镜可能会发现潜在不能接受的疾病。此外，孩子们经常因为饥饿和陌生的环境而变得烦躁和焦虑，尤其 3 岁以上的幼儿，应进行心理护理，尽可能消除其紧张和焦虑，并获得其配合。

26.2.2.3 术前检查

常规术前检查包括血常规、凝血功能、乙肝及丙肝血清学检查、人类免疫缺陷病毒（HIV）、梅毒螺旋体抗体、胸部 X 线或胸部 CT、心电图等。部分患儿需要术前检查血型、肝肾功能、肺功能、超声等。

26.2.2.4 术前禁食

根据食物在胃内排空的时间长短，确定不同的禁食时间。包括：轻饮料 2 h；母乳 4 h；牛奶、配方奶、淀粉类固体食物 6 h；脂肪类固体食物 8 h。婴儿及新生儿因糖原储备少，禁食 2 h 后可在病房内静脉输注含糖液体，以防止发生低血糖和脱水。

26.2.2.5 介入设备及电脑工作站准备

必备的常规药物及急救设施如下：

1）常规药物：37℃生理盐水、2% 利多卡因、润滑剂等；

2）急救药物：4℃生理盐水、肾上腺素、支气管舒张剂、止血药物（如血凝酶、垂体后叶素等）、糖皮质激素（静脉及雾化用）、利尿剂等；

3）急救设备：氧源、吸引器、复苏气囊、不同型号气管插管、脉氧监护仪、除颤仪等。建议配备麻醉机或呼吸机；

4）不同型号的支气管镜；

5）常规器械：灌洗液留置瓶、鼻导管、活检钳等；

6）专用设备和器械：激光工作站、冷冻工作站、电工作站、不同型号的球囊与支架等；

7）电脑工作站处于正常工作状态。

26.3 支气管镜检查

26.3.1 镇静与麻醉

给儿童镇静富有挑战性。选择合适的麻醉入路是成功的关键。有几个因素需要考虑，包括：在手术过程中儿童的安全性；术前、术中和术后患儿的舒适度；防止儿童和家长出现过度焦虑；达到适当的镇静以完成手术。可弯曲支气管镜的镇静通常是通过局部应用利多卡因联合静脉镇静药或吸入麻醉剂来实现的。镇静的深度和镇静剂的选择由支气管镜操作的目的决定。气道动力学特性可因深度镇静或全身麻醉引起的肌肉张力和呼吸的变化而改变。

26.3.1.1 联合使用局部利多卡因和镇静，边麻醉边进镜法

刘玺诚[5]最早采用边麻醉边进镜的方法，即用局部利多卡因喷在黏膜表面麻醉，随后对该方法进行了改进和完善。先雾化吸入 2% 利多卡因，入手术室后给予咪达唑仑 0.1~0.3 mg/kg，总剂量<10 mg，中等

剂量 0.03 mg/kg 的阿托品可预防幼儿出现迷走神经相关性心动过缓，减少腺体分泌。

当支气管镜进入声门、喉部、气管、左右主支气管时，局部喷洒 1%~2% 利多卡因 1~2 mL（6 个月以下婴儿 1%）；必要时可重复喷洒，总药量不超过 7 mg/kg[6]。1：10 000 肾上腺素可与利多卡因合用，收缩黏膜血管，防止肿胀出血，并可舒张支气管平滑肌，增强心肌收缩力，抗过敏。

医生在患儿镇静后开始支气管镜检查。如果患儿有明显的肢体运动或咳嗽，因个体差异对镇静剂反应较差，则可使用异丙酚 0.5~1 mg/kg，必要时可重复使用，常规剂量使用非常安全[7]。

26.3.1.2　全身麻醉

根据通气方式的不同又分为静脉复合全麻、气管插管全麻、喉罩通气全麻和高频通气全麻。一般由麻醉医师执行，合理选择镇静药、镇痛药，必要时使用肌松药以达到适当的麻醉深度，使患儿能够平稳地耐受手术并保持生命体征的稳定。最常用的是喉罩通气全麻，适用于喉部及以下部位的支气管镜诊疗操作，对于气管狭窄，尤其是上段狭窄的患儿，喉罩通气可能是目前唯一能有效控制气道的方法。

26.3.1.3　喉罩

喉罩比面罩、鼻导管能够更好地进行气道的管理[8]。在行支气管镜检查过程中，喉罩能够帮助气体交换异常的患儿进行通气。喉罩的置入和维持较面罩需更深的镇静及麻醉。然而，深度麻醉可降低喉罩置入时喉痉挛及支气管痉挛的风险。不同年龄组，甚至新生儿都有适配型号的喉罩（表 26.1）。如果使用一次性喉罩，则可在放置前将孔径处的栅栏移除，以方便支气管镜的插入。

表 26.1　喉罩型号

喉罩型号	儿童体重（kg）
1	<5
1.5	5~10
2	10~20
2.5	20~30
3	30~50
4	50~70

引用自 http://www.lmana.com。

喉罩的缺点包括置入时可能会使上气道的解剖结构发生扭曲。喉罩的栅栏覆盖于会厌的上方，会部分阻塞支气管镜的通道。另外，喉罩置入时所需的麻醉深度可能会改变气道的动力学和声带的运动。

26.3.1.4　全麻下气管插管

全麻下气管插管主要适用于较大儿童长时间的气管远端与支气管内的诊疗操作。在不需要评估上气道或者在检查过程中存在明显风险的患儿，经气管插管能够方便地到达下气道进行肺泡灌洗和其他诊断操作。还可以借此研究气道正压对下气道的动力学的影响。使用气管插管的主要缺点是看不见上气道和近端气道。此外，气管插管及麻醉深度往往会掩盖气道动力学异常。

26.3.1.5　高频通气

全麻高频通气适用于时间较短的支气管镜检查及诊疗操作。因此，在无呼吸支持下给患儿行支气管镜操作时，应该通过鼻咽导管（流量每分钟 0.5~2 L）或面罩（流量每分钟 2~4 L），或必要时经工作通道（流量每分钟 0.5~1 L）给氧，后者需监控胸内压并间歇给氧。

吸入性麻醉药应用于全身麻醉的诱导，适用于一部分人，尤其对一些不需要评估气道动力学改变的患者。吸入性麻醉药常在放置喉罩或气管插管以及静脉穿刺前给药。

26.3.2　监护

术中常规监测项目包括：心电图、呼吸、无创血压和血氧饱和度、呼气末二氧化碳。理想的血氧饱和度应达到 95% 以上，如出现血氧饱和度 <90%、心率减慢、心律失常等情况，应暂停操作并对症治疗。视患儿恢复情况决定是否继续进行操作。支气管镜操作结束后，继续心电监护直至患儿意识完全恢复。必要时给予吸氧、雾化吸入等治疗，密切观察患儿，预防术后并发症。

26.4　支气管镜检查

术前医生、护士和麻醉医师共同核对患儿身份。患儿多采取仰卧位，肩部略垫高。支气管镜经鼻孔轻柔送入，注意观察鼻腔、咽部有无异常（经口腔进入者观察口腔、舌）、扁桃体、会厌及声门时，观察会厌有无塌陷、声带运动是否良好及对称；进入气管后观察形态、黏膜色泽、软骨环的清晰度、隆突、主支气管。一般先查健侧再查患侧，病灶不明确时先查右侧后查左侧。发现病变可吸引留取分泌物、毛刷涂片、钳夹活检及留取灌洗液。

检查过程中注意观察各叶、段支气管黏膜外观，有无充血、水肿、坏死及溃疡；有无出血及分泌物；管腔及开口是否通畅、有无变形；是否有狭窄、异物及新生物等。

检查时尽量保持视野位于气管、支气管腔中央，避免触碰管壁。刺激管壁引起咳嗽、支气管痉挛及损伤黏膜。操作要熟练、准确、快捷，尽量缩短手术时间。

26.5 儿童肺脏疾病的诊断及治疗

26.5.1 支气管镜下诊断

26.5.1.1 气管支气管管壁异常

黏膜改变（如充血、水肿、粗糙不平、肥厚、萎缩、环形皱褶、纵形皱襞、溃疡、坏死、瘢痕、结节等）、肉芽、肿瘤、瘘管、憩室、血管扩张或迂曲、黏液腺孔扩大、色素沉着、钙化物质、支气管残端、气管支气管膜部增宽、完全性气管环、囊性变等。

26.5.1.2 气管支气管管腔异常

阻塞、狭窄、扩张、闭锁、气管和支气管异常分支。

26.5.1.3 气管支气管管腔内异常物质

1）分泌物：浆液性、黏液性、脓性及血性、牛奶样；
2）出血：鲜血或陈旧性血凝块；
3）异物：外源性和内源性；
4）干酪样物。

26.5.1.4 动力学改变

1）声带麻痹：双侧或单侧；
2）隆突活动消失；
3）气管运动紊乱，如完全性气管软骨环、气管骨化症等；
4）支气管痉挛；

5）软化：气管、支气管在呼气相时管腔内陷，管腔直径缩窄不足 1/2 为轻度，1/2～3/4 为中度，3/4 以上管腔缩窄近闭合为重度。可原发或继发于血管、心脏、肿物等的压迫。

26.5.2 诊断方法

26.5.2.1 刷检

支气管镜进入气管、支气管及肺段后刷检涂片、染色及培养，主要用于细胞学及病原学检测。

26.5.2.2 活检

26.5.2.2.1 细胞学、组织活检

1）毛刷活检。
2）活检钳活检：黏膜活检及 TBLB，可以借助电子导航、电磁导航、环形超声、超声支气管镜（endobronchial ultrasound，EBUS）等技术提高活检阳性率。
3）TBNA、EBUS-TBNA：取气管、支气管周围淋巴结，提高诊断的阳性率。
4）支气管镜下冷冻活检：分冷冻黏膜活检和冷冻肺活检。

26.5.2.2.2 支气管肺泡灌洗活检

支气管肺泡灌洗技术在成人和儿童是相似的（见第 14 章）。支气管镜的先端部楔入段或亚段支气管，注入定量的生理盐水，然后吸引回收完成灌洗。最佳灌洗量尚不清楚[9]。通常，采用生理盐水 1 mL/kg 分次灌洗，最大量为 5 mL/kg。然而，研究表明，根据儿童的年龄调整生理盐水灌洗的总量可能是更恰当的方法[10]。通常情况下，灌入的生理盐水中近 30%～60% 被回收。在随后的灌洗中，回收的液体量将逐渐增加。儿童肺泡灌洗液的细胞成分正常值如下[9,11]：细胞成分正常值（比值）为淋巴细胞<15%，粒细胞<3%，嗜酸性粒细胞<0.5%，巨噬细胞 80%～95%。肺泡灌洗液的细胞组分在肺部疾病状态下会出现变化[12,13]。很多研究都通过支气管肺泡灌洗术来检测炎症介质[14,15]。治疗性的灌洗可以通过清除阻塞的气道黏稠分泌物治疗肺不张，也可用于治疗肺泡蛋白沉积症[16]。

26.5.2.3 快速现场评估

在呼吸系统疾病的诊治中，快速现场评估（raid on-site evaluation，ROSE）是一种伴随于诊断性介入操作的快速细胞学判读技术[17]。它能判读细胞形态、分类、计数、构成比、排列、相互关系、背景、细胞中的异物以及病原体。可协助呼吸系统感染性疾病和

肿瘤性疾病的快速现场初步诊断。

26.5.3 支气管镜下治疗技术

26.5.3.1 基本治疗技术

26.5.3.1.1 支气管肺泡灌洗术

是通过支气管镜通道向支气管肺段内注入37℃生理盐水或药物，并随即抽吸清除呼吸道和/或肺泡中滞留的物质，用以缓解气道阻塞，改善呼吸功能，控制感染的治疗方法。支气管肺泡灌洗术分为支气管肺段灌洗术和全肺灌洗。支气管肺段灌洗术主要用于肺部感染性疾病、肺不张、支气管扩张症、迁延性细菌性支气管炎、过敏性肺泡炎、少量咯血或痰中带血等的治疗。全肺灌洗术主要用于肺泡蛋白沉着症等疾病的治疗。

26.5.3.1.2 局部注药、给药术

喷洒及注射药物用于止血、稀释分泌物、抗感染等。

26.5.3.1.3 毛刷刷取术

刷除分泌物、拖拽内生性异物等以清理气道。

26.5.3.1.4 钳取术

应用与内镜工作通道相匹配的钳子钳除气道管腔内、外源性异物、增生组织及坏死物等。异物网篮多用于活检钳难以取出的异物。

26.5.3.2 高级介入治疗技术

26.5.3.2.1 球囊扩张术

用于气道狭窄的治疗，协助特殊异物的取出。

26.5.3.2.2 消融术

1）热消融术：包括激光、氩等离子体凝固术以及电凝、电切等，主要应用于气道腔内肉芽、肿块、占位、囊肿等增生性病变的消融[18-21]。电凝、电切术尤其适用于体积较大病变，电圈套器适用于带蒂增生物的切割治疗。氩等离子体凝固术对弥漫性、浅表性增生病变更为适用，在浅表性气道出血的治疗中有优势。激光光纤纤细，可通过1.2 mm的工作通道，可精准治疗喉部、声门及亚段支气管病变。

2）冷冻消融术：包括冻融和冻切技术。冻融术可应用于气道内良、恶性肿瘤和良、恶性气道狭窄的治疗，可抑制肉芽增生[22-23]，冻切技术可应用于肺活检、清理气道内血栓或支气管塑型物。

26.5.3.2.3 支架置入术

适用于气管、支气管软化及气道软骨薄弱处的支撑；气管支气管狭窄的气道重建；气管食管瘘的姑息治疗。儿童气道支架种类包含金属非覆膜支架、覆膜金属支架、硅酮支架等；形状上可为直筒形、"T"形、"L"形及"Y"形[24-29]。支架的选择应综合考虑气道病变的部位、类型、患儿病情、内镜中心的设备及操作人员技术能力等因素。

26.5.3.2.4 其他

协助困难气管插管、胃管置入术。

26.6 儿科支气管镜检查的适应证、禁忌证

26.6.1 适应证

儿童支气管镜检查最常见的适应证为排除解剖学异常或异物吸入。能得到何种诊断信息取决于进行支气管镜检查的目的。

1）喉鸣；
2）反复或持续性喘息；
3）局限性喘鸣；
4）不明原因的慢性咳嗽；
5）反复呼吸道感染；
6）可疑异物吸入；
7）咯血；
8）呼吸机脱机困难；
9）影像学异常：
　　a. 气管、支气管肺发育不良和/或畸形；
　　b. 肺不张；
　　c. 肺气肿；
　　d. 肺部结节性病变；
　　e. 肺部弥漫性病变；
　　f. 纵隔气肿；
　　g. 气道、纵隔占位；
　　h. 血管、淋巴管、食管发育异常；
　　i. 胸膜腔病变需鉴别诊断者。
10）肺部感染性疾病的病原学诊断及治疗；
11）胸部外伤、怀疑有气管支气管裂伤或断裂者；
12）需经支气管镜行各种介入治疗者；
13）心胸外科围手术期患儿的气道评估和管理；
14）引导气管插管、胃管置入；
15）其他：如不明原因的生长发育迟缓、睡眠障碍等需鉴别诊断者。

26.6.2 禁忌证

儿科支气管镜术没有绝对禁忌证，禁忌证取决于术者的技术水平和必要的设备条件。其相对禁忌证为：

1）严重心肺功能不全者；

2）严重心律失常，如心房、心室颤动及扑动，Ⅲ度及以上房室传导阻滞者；

3）高热患者：持续高热而又亟需行支气管镜术者，可将其体温降至38.5℃以下再行手术，以防高热惊厥；

4）活动性大咯血者：严重的出血性疾病、凝血功能严重障碍、严重的肺动脉高压以及可能诱发大咯血者等；

5）严重营养不良、身体状况明显衰弱者。

26.7 鉴别诊断

26.7.1 喉鸣

喉软化症（图26.1）是迄今为止导致婴幼儿喉鸣最常见的病因[30]，喉鸣也可见于其他功能性病变，如声带麻痹（图26.2）。声门上或声门下区的结构异常同样可能导致喘鸣，包括声门上囊肿（图26.3）和声门下狭窄（图26.4）。某些病变如喉裂需要硬质支气管镜

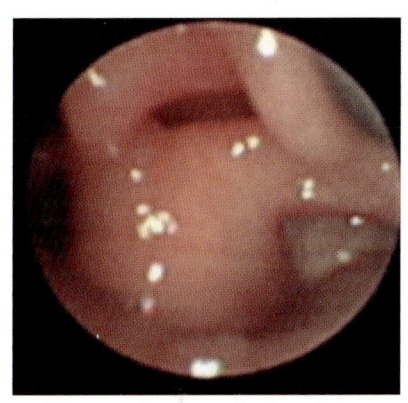

图26.1 喉软化症（5月龄男孩），临床症状为喘鸣

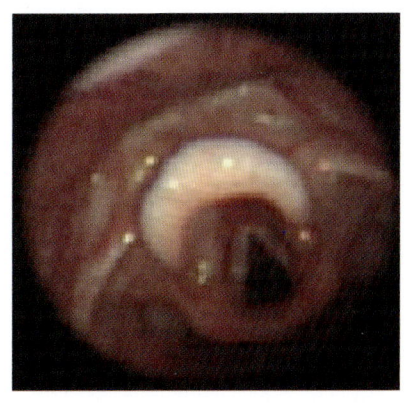

图26.2 声带麻痹（2月龄女孩），临床症状为喘鸣

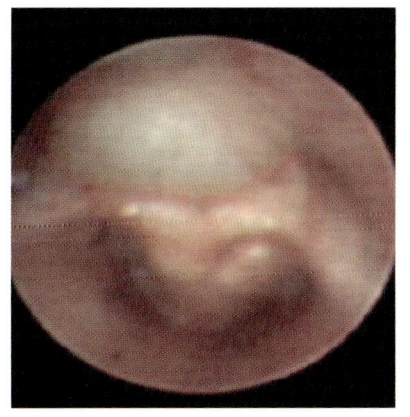

图26.3 声门上区囊肿（3月龄男孩）

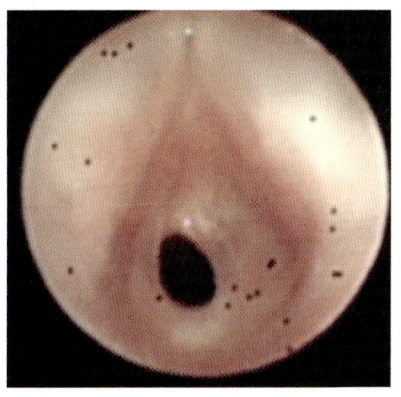

图26.4 气管插管后，声门下狭窄（6月龄女孩）

检查来显示[31]。

26.7.2 持续性喘息

Wood[32]在1 000例回顾分析中发现，喘息的患儿其中70%支气管镜检查可见相关异常。

在评估持续或反复喘息患儿时，支气管镜检查结合其他资料如CT、透视或胃食管反流（gastroesophageal reflux，GER）检测可提高检出率[33]。有多种气道解剖异常可表现为持续喘息。气道动力学的改变，如支气管软化症在呼气相气流通过受限（图26.5），可通过支气管镜检查诊断。其他原发病变如完全性气管环相对少见（图26.6）。因囊肿、血管瘤（图26.7）等占位导致的气道阻塞，也可表现为喘息或持续肺不张。气道内肿瘤在儿童非常罕见，支气管镜可明确诊断（图26.8）。伴有搏动感的气道外压提示血管环的存在。先天性心脏病的患儿，常因异常的血管结构或心脏增大致气道明显软化、压迫症状。

异物吸入也可导致持续喘息，有时可通过体格检

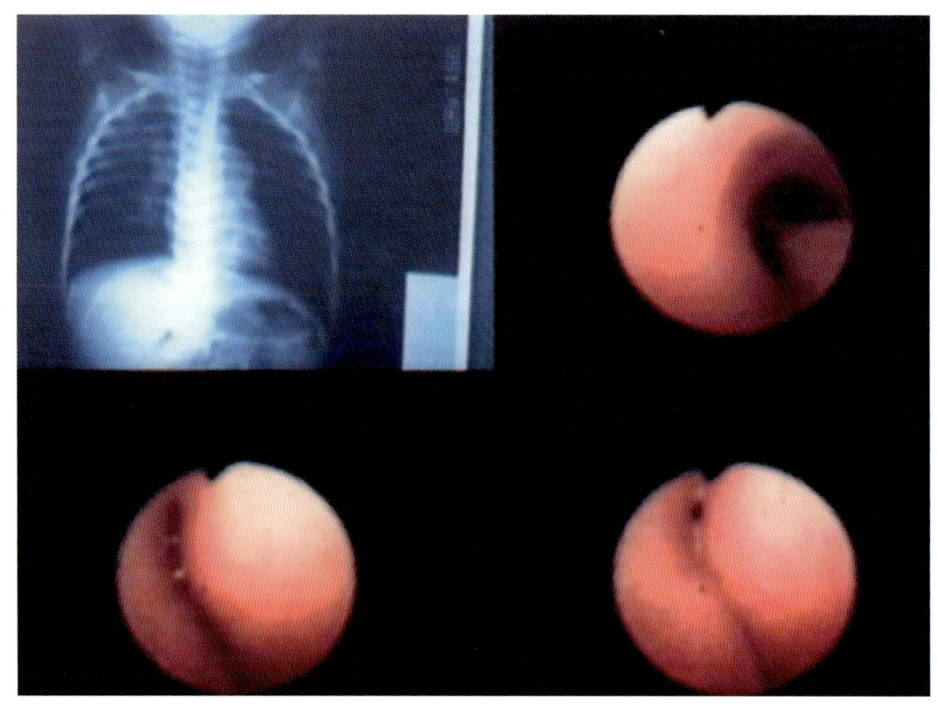

图 26.5　支气管软化症（5 月龄男孩），临床表现为喘息

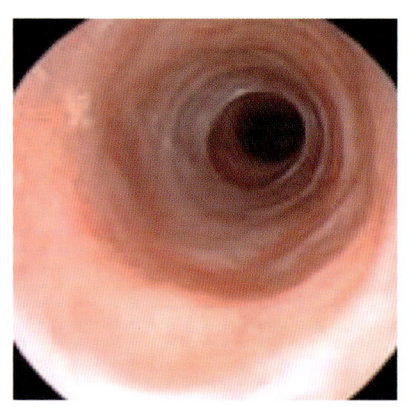

图 26.6　完全性气管环（13 月龄男孩），临床表现为持续性喘息

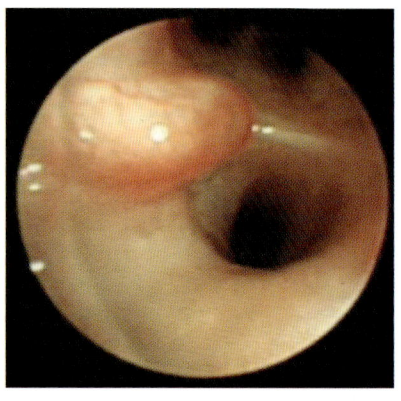

图 26.7　声门下血管瘤（12 岁男孩慢性咳嗽伴咯血 2 年）

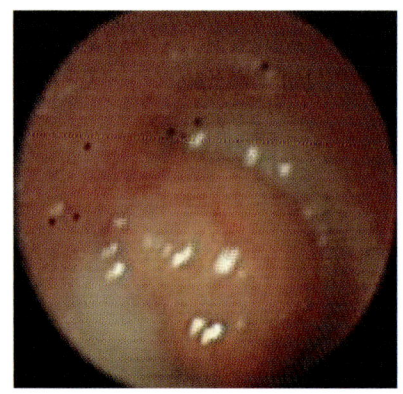

图 26.8　右主支气管肿瘤（4 岁男孩反复咳嗽、肺炎）

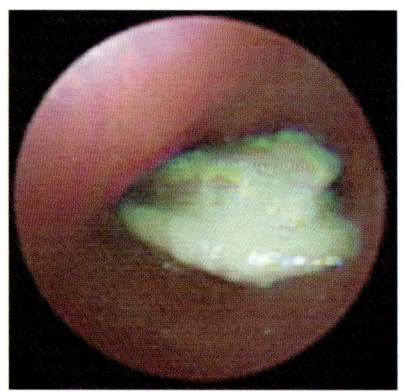

图 26.9　肺下叶亚段支气管内的花生碎块（1.5 岁男孩，反复咳嗽、肺炎）

查定位,但也有些查体阴性。图 26.9 显示吸入的花生残块诱发的炎症反应。异物取出术通常在硬质支气管镜下完成,但在儿童,也有应用可弯曲支气管镜成功取出异物的经验报道[34]。如果异物的可能性小,先行可弯曲支气管镜检查是一种有效的鉴别方法[35]。

吞咽功能失调相关的慢性吸入是引起婴幼儿喘息的一种常见病因,这往往会导致下气道黏膜水肿。上气道红斑和水肿提示胃食管反流症的存在,但慢性吸入的确诊不能仅通过支气管镜检查。

在肺泡灌洗液中找到富含脂质的巨噬细胞(lipid-laden macrophages,LLM)往往提示存在慢性吸入。但很多证据表明 LLM 并不是特异表现[36-38]。在肺泡灌洗液中找到 LLM 必须与患儿的吞咽功能评估、GER 程度及肺部疾病的严重程度相结合。停止经口喂养后观察婴幼儿的反应往往是诊断慢性吸入的最佳方法。支气管镜检查可鉴别气管食管瘘引起的慢性吸入。

26.7.3 慢性咳嗽

支气管镜检查常用于儿童慢性咳嗽的病因学诊断。Wood[32] 发现在慢性咳嗽的患儿中,55% 存在有诊断意义的异常。Saito 等[39] 发现,在 5~26 月龄慢性咳嗽的 19 例患儿中,有 12 例(63%)存在下气道畸形。病毒和细菌是常被检出的病原。在大多数"湿性咳嗽"的患儿中,慢性支气管炎为常见的病因之一[40]。在婴幼儿组,与喘息相类似,慢性吸入同样为咳嗽的常见原因。

26.7.4 肺不张

肺不张最常见的原因是气道内黏液栓堵塞[32,41],因此,治疗性灌洗、清除分泌物为治疗肺不张的有效疗法。其他的常见病因还有异物、气道狭窄、支气管软化和气道外压[41]。

26.7.5 肺炎及可疑感染

因为儿童咳痰困难,支气管镜在诊断感染病原方面起到重要的作用,包括正常及免疫功能低下的儿童。例如,在骨髓移植后合并肺炎的患儿中,支气管肺泡灌洗液微生物检出率为 29%~52%[42]。

在经验性应用广谱抗感染药物之前进行支气管镜检查,可增加病原检出率。应用可弯曲支气管镜可为呼吸机相关性肺炎提供治疗建议,这是经气管导管吸引无法比及的[43]。

支气管内感染如结核,通过支气管镜很容易被识别(图 26.10)。微生物如肺部铜绿假单胞菌等引起的肺部感染对囊性肺纤维化的患者有显著影响。这类患儿通常采用口咽分泌物培养来监测病原体,然而,这些培养可能无法提供一个完整的下气道微生物病原信息[44-46]。因此,一些囊性纤维化中心应用支气管镜进行诊断和定期随访[45]。然而,常规进行支气管镜检查的价值尚存在争议[47]。

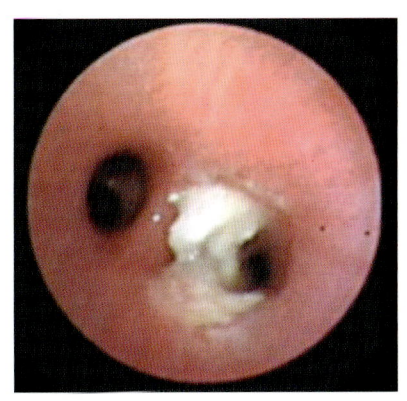

图 26.10 支气管结核(1 岁男孩,肺门淋巴结肿大)

26.8 气道管理

在手术室、ICU 中可使用可弯曲支气管镜辅助困难气道的气管插管。美国胸科协会推荐对气管切开的患者每 6~12 月常规进行气管检查"评估潜在的气道病理情况,监测和治疗并发症,评估套管的尺寸和位置"[48]。气道支架在幼儿中的应用存在争议。但对经正确筛选的患儿,应用可弯曲支气管镜放置支架可成功治疗重度气道阻塞[49]。

26.9 支气管镜检查常见并发症及处理

1)支气管镜操作者的技术及经验不足。
2)术前未充分评估患儿病情。
3)支气管镜的型号选择与患者不匹配。
4)麻醉镇静方法选择不恰当。
5)应用不恰当的供氧方式,如低流量、高流量、高频或辅助通气。
6)感染防控不足。

7）未建立有效的静脉通道[50]。

26.9.1　药物过敏

支气管镜诊疗围手术期用药有可能引起变态反应。症状包括皮疹、皮肤瘙痒、胸闷、脉搏微弱、面色苍白、血压降低甚至过敏性休克。

处理：轻者停止用药后变态反应可逐渐好转，重者加用抗过敏药物，有喉头水肿、过敏性休克时就地抢救。对心跳呼吸骤停者，立即行人工心肺复苏。

预防：术前应询问患儿药物过敏史，对有药物过敏史者，应高度重视，做好过敏的应急预案。既往有相关药物过敏者，应避免使用。

26.9.2　缺氧或血氧饱和度下降、窒息

轻度患者口唇轻度发绀，外周血氧饱和度轻度降低；严重的患者表现为面部发绀，外周血氧饱和度明显降低。

处理：积极查找并解除引起低氧的原因，必要时撤出支气管镜，提高氧流量，加压吸氧。待末梢血氧饱和度恢复正常再继续进行支气管镜操作。

预防：管控导致支气管镜检查并发症常见原因，可降低该类并发症的发生率。

26.9.3　心律失常

轻者出现心动过速或过缓；严重者术中、术后可出现明显的心律失常，甚至心脏骤停。

处理：轻者停止支气管镜诊疗可以自行缓解；严重者需行人工心肺复苏。

预防：支气管镜检查时应动作轻柔。

26.9.4　喉痉挛或支气管痉挛

喉痉挛时咽喉部肌肉、真假声带发生痉挛性收缩，使声门和呼吸道部分或完全紧闭与梗阻，导致患儿呼吸困难，血氧饱和度进行性下降，迅速发绀，稍有贻误可危及生命，需紧急处理。支气管痉挛时，呼吸困难，双肺出现广泛的哮鸣音，正压通气时气道阻力急剧增高，潮气量减少，血氧饱和度下降，呼气末二氧化碳升高，严重时可窒息死亡[51]。

喉痉挛的处理：立即祛除喉痉挛的可能诱因，如声门和会厌附近的分泌物等；用100%氧气进行正压通气；应用静脉或吸入麻醉药加深麻醉。上述处理无效时，可应用短效肌肉松弛药或进行气管插管来改善氧合。

支气管痉挛的处理：停止支气管镜操作、100%氧气吸入、加深麻醉、气管内应用糖皮质受体激动剂及糖皮质激素，必要时气管插管呼吸机辅助通气。

预防：对于有气道痉挛的高风险患儿，术前给予β_2受体激动剂及糖皮质激素雾化吸入；术中充分的表面麻醉；及时清除呼吸道分泌物和血液；避免浅麻醉下行口腔、咽喉和气道内操作。

26.9.5　出血

轻度受支气管镜操作影响的患者气道少量出血；严重患者可出现大咯血[52]。

处理：少量出血无须治疗，凝血功能正常的患者可自行止血。局部出血用生理盐水、1∶10 000肾上腺素或凝血酶治疗。大出血时，应局部静脉使用止血药物和垂体后叶素，并立即将患者置于侧卧位。如有必要，应气管插管以保持气道畅通。应防止鼻咽出血流回喉咙。使用局部止血药物和纱布止血。气道局部出血用生理盐水、1∶10 000肾上腺素或凝血酶治疗。大出血时，应局部静脉使用止血药物和垂体后叶素，并立即将患者置于侧卧位。当下呼吸道出血时，应将支气管镜置于出血部位吸出患侧的血液。如有必要，可将球囊导管置于患侧，通过局部压迫、数字减影血管造影（digital subtraction angiography，DSA）栓塞或紧急开胸或急诊肺叶切除术止血。

预防：经鼻道进行支气管镜检查可引起黏膜出血。对于易导致气道出血的疾病，需与患儿家长沟通并制定计划，如血液制品的可及性、在手术室进行支气管镜操作以及能随时行胸外科手术。

26.9.6　感染和发热

感染和发热是常见并发症，约15%的患者可发生感染和发热，特别是那些有大量分泌物、呼吸道病原体位于下呼吸道的患者和免疫功能低下的患者。这可能与细胞因子的释放或局部病原体的播散有关。依据发热的原因进行相应的处理。

预防：严格执行消毒流程、加强防护管理是减少感染发生的根本措施。操作人员在操作前要洗手，佩戴无菌手套。清除上呼吸道分泌物，用75%乙醇棉签擦拭鼻腔。在支气管镜进入下呼吸道前不要吸痰，以免上呼吸道的病原体移入下呼吸道。常规支气管镜检查不需要灌洗。围手术期抗感染治疗是非常必要的，特别是对于免疫功能异常、内分泌异常、遗传代谢性疾病的患儿。支气管结核患者应在手术前2周内接受

26.9.7 气胸、纵隔或皮下气肿

少量气胸、纵隔或皮下气肿可自行吸收。当大量气胸、纵隔或皮下气肿导致呼吸困难时，应进行紧急通气。

处理：气胸一般选择锁骨中线第二肋间或气肿最明显处穿刺排气，纵隔、皮下气肿可选择气管前筋膜或气肿最明显处切开或穿刺针抽吸排气。张力性气胸需进行持续闭式引流，必要时持续负压引流。如在支气管镜术前即存在明显漏气，应先引流再行支气管镜。

预防：选择与患者的气道相匹配型号的支气管镜。选择合理的给氧方式。支气管镜操作避免粗暴。支气管镜的介入治疗技术需要培训。

参考文献

1. Bronchoscopy Collaboration Subgroup of Respiratory Group and Pediatric Section of Chinese Medical Association (2009). Guideline of pediatric bronchoscopy (2009 version). *Chin. J. Pediatr.* 47 (10): 740–744.
2. Expert Group of Pediatric Respiratory Endoscopy, Talent Exchange Service Center of National Health Commission, Endoscopy Committee et al. (2018). Guideline of pediatric flexible bronchoscopy in China (2018 version). *Chin. J. Appl. Clin. Pediatr.* 33 (13): 983–989.
3. Expert Group of Pediatric Respiratory Endoscopy, Talent Exchange Service Center of National Health Commission, Endoscopy Committee et al. (2018). Expert consensus on respiratory interventional diagnosis and treatment of airway foreign bodies in children in China. *Chin. J. Appl. Clin. Pediatr.* 33 (18): 1392–1402.
4. Balfour-Lynn, I.M. and Harcourt, J. (2010). Bronchoscopic equipment. In: *Pediatric Bronchoscopy*, vol. 38 (eds. K.N. Priftis, M.B. Anthracopoulos, A.C. Koumbourlis and R.E. Wood), 12–21. Basel: Karger.
5. Liu, X.C., Jiang, Q.B., Gao, H. et al. (1994). Application of local surface anesthesai in diagnostic and treatment of pediatric fiberoptic bronchoscopy. *Chin. J. Pediatr.* (1): 38.
6. Amitai, Y., Zylber-Katz, E., Avital, A. et al. (1990). Serum lidocaine concentrations in children during bronchoscopy with topical anesthesia. *Chest* 98: 1370–1373.
7. Hasan, R.A. and Reddy, R. (2009). Sedation with propofol for flexible bronchoscopy in children. *Pediatr. Pulmonol.* 44: 373–378.
8. Naguib, M.L., Streetman, D.S., Clifton, S. et al. (2005). Use of laryngeal mask airway in flexible bronchoscopy in infants and children. *Pediatr. Pulmonol.* 39: 56–63.
9. de Blic, J., Midulla, F., Barbato, A. et al. (2000). Bronchoalveolar lavage in children. ERS task force on bronchoalveolar lavage in children. *Eur. Respir. J.* 15: 217–231.
10. Ratjen, F. and Bruch, J. (1996). Adjustment of bronchoalveolar lavage volume to body weight in children. *Pediatr. Pulmonol.* 21: 184–188.
11. Brennan, S., Gangell, C., Wainwright, C. et al. (2008). Disease surveillance using bronchoalveolar lavage. *Paediatr. Respir. Rev.* 9: 151–159.
12. Najafi, N., Demanet, C., Dab, I. et al. (2003). Differential cytology of bronchoalveolar lavage fluid in asthmatic children. *Pediatr. Pulmonol.* 35: 302–308.
13. Ratjen, F., Costabel, U., Griese, M. et al. (2003). Bronchoalveolar lavage fluid findings in children with hypersensitivity pneumonitis. *Eur. Respir. J.* 21: 144–148.
14. Khan, T.Z., Wagener, J.S., Bost, T. et al. (1995). Early pulmonary inflammation in infants with cystic fibrosis. *Am. J. Respir. Crit. Care Med.* 151: 1075–1082.
15. Kim, C.K., Kim, S.W., Kim, Y.K. et al. (2005). Bronchoalveolar lavage eosinophil cationic protein and interleukin-8 levels in acute asthma and acute bronchiolitis. *Clin. Exp. Allergy* 35: 591–597.
16. Mahut, B., Delacourt, C., Scheinmann, P. et al. (1996). Pulmonary alveolar proteinosis: experience with eight pediatric cases and a review. *Pediatrics* 97: 117–122.
17. National Health and Planning Commission Cross-Strait Medical and Health Exchange Association Respiratory Disease Committee, Respiratory Endoscopy Specialized Committee of Tuberculosis Society of Chinese Medical Association, Endoscopy Specialized Committee of Pediatric Society of Chinese Medical Doctor Association et al. (2017). Clinical guidelines for rapid field evaluation of diagnostic interventional pulmonary diseases. *Tianjin Med. J.* 45 (4): 441–448.
18. Liu, X., Ma, J., Zhao, F.M. et al. (2013). Application of electric coagulation treatment via bronchoscopy in the management of congenital vallecular cyst in children. *Chin. J. Pediatr.* 51 (11): 846–849.
19. Wang, H., Zhang, N., Tao, M. et al. (2012). Application of interventional bronchoscopic therapy in eight pediatric patients with malignantairway tumors. *Tumori* 98 (5): 581–587.
20. Xu, X., Zhu, B., Shi, M.Q. et al. (2015). Study on tracheal intubation related severe subglottic stenosis under laryngeal mask by using holmium laser combined with argon plasma coagulation and cryotherapy through bronchoscopy. *Chin. J. Appl. Clin. Pediatr.* 30 (19): 1479–1482.
21. Wang, Y.J., Shi, Y.S., Wang, Z.T. et al. (2016). Clinical characteristics of severe infant laryngomalacia diagnosed by flexible bronchoscopy and the curative effect of laser therapy. *Chin. J. Appl. Clin. Pediatr.* 31 (16): 1242–1244.
22. Ni, C.Y., Liu, X., Ma, J. et al. (2012). Effect of bronchoscopic cryosurgery in twenty-two children with lower airway stenosis. *Zhonghua ErKe Za Zhi* 50 (1): 45–49.
23. Xu, X., Liu, X., Zhu, B. et al. (2014). Argon plasma coagulation combined CO_2 freezing through the flexible bronchoscope for treatment of airway granulation proliferation in children. *Zhonghua ErKe Za Zhi* 52 (5): 368–372.
24. Zhang, Z., Ma, J., Liu, S. et al. (2017). Fully-covered metallic stenting in an infant with tracheoesophageal fistula due to button battery ingestion. *Int. J. Pediatr. Otorhinolaryngol.* 95: 80–83.

25 Ding, H. and Liu, X.C. (2015). Airway stents in children. *Chin. J. Appl. Clin. Pediatr.* 30 (16): 1204–1206.
26 Meng, C., Ma, J., Zhang, Z.X. et al. (2015). Transbronchoscopic application of vascular balloon expandable metal stents in treating an infant with bridging bronchus combined with stenosis deformity. *Chin. J. Appl. Clin. Pediatr.* 30 (16): 1260–1261.
27 Meng, C., Li, C.X., Liu, X. et al. (2015). Two cases of post-intubation tracheal stenosis treated successfully with a Montgomery T-tube. *Chin. Appl. Clin. Pediatr.* 30 (16): 1258–1259.
28 Meng, F.Z., Wang, L.N., Zhang, L. et al. (2015). The clinical treatment of tracheoesophageal fistula by coated stent in trachea. *Chin. J. Appl. Clin. Pediatr.* 30 (16): 1206–1208.
29 Xu, X., Ding, H., Li, D.D. et al. (2011). Balloon dilatation and expandable metallic stent placement bronchoscopically for two children with tracheal stenosis. *Chin. J. Evid. Based Pediatr.* 6 (4): 250–254.
30 Zoumalan, R., Maddalozzo, J., and Holinger, L.D. (2007). Etiology of stridor in infants. *Ann. Otol. Rhinol. Laryngol.* 116: 329–334.
31 Wood, R.E. (2008). Evaluation of the upper airway in children. *Curr. Opin. Pediatr.* 20: 266–271.
32 Wood, R.E. (1985). The diagnostic effectiveness of the flexible bronchoscope in children. *Pediatr. Pulmonol.* 1: 188–192.
33 Saglani, S., Nicholson, A.G., Scallan, M. et al. (2006). Investigation of young children with severe recurrent wheeze: any clinical benefit? *Eur. Respir. J.* 27: 29–35.
34 Ramirez-Figueroa, J.L., Gochicoa-Rangel, L.G., Ramirez-San Juan, D.H. et al. (2005). Foreign body removal by flexible fiberoptic bronchoscopy in infants and children. *Pediatr. Pulmonol.* 40: 392–397.
35 Righini, C.A., Morel, N., Karkas, A. et al. (2007). What is the diagnostic value of flexible bronchoscopy in the initial investigation of children with suspected foreign body aspiration? *Int. J. Pediatr. Otorhinolaryngol.* 71: 1383–1390.
36 Chang, A.B., Cox, N.C., Purcell, J. et al. (2005). Airway cellularity, lipid laden macrophages and microbiology of gastric juice and airways in children with reflux oesophagitis. *Respir. Res.* 6: 72.
37 Ding, Y., Simpson, P.M., Schellhase, D.E. et al. (2002). Limited reliability of lipid-laden macrophage index restricts its use as a test for pulmonary aspiration: comparison with a simple semiquantitative assay. *Pediatr. Dev. Pathol.* 5: 551–558.
38 Rosen, R., Fritz, J., Nurko, A. et al. (2008). Lipid-laden macrophage index is not an indicator of gastroesophageal reflux-related respiratory disease in children. *Pediatrics* 121: e879–e884.
39 Saito, J., Harris, W.T., Gelfond, J. et al. (2006). Physiologic, bronchoscopic, and bronchoalveolar lavage fluid findings in young children with recurrent wheeze and cough. *Pediatr. Pulmonol.* 41: 709–719.
40 Marchant, J.M., Masters, I.B., Taylor, S.M. et al. (2006). Evaluation and outcome of young children with chronic cough. *Chest* 129: 1132–1141.
41 Wood, R.E. (1984). Spelunking in the pediatric airways: explorations with the flexible fiberoptic bronchoscope. *Pediatr. Clin. North Am.* 31: 785–799.
42 Collaco, J.M., Gower, W.A., and Mogayzel, P.J. Jr. (2007). Pulmonary dysfunction in pediatric hematopoietic stem cell transplant patients: overview, diagnostic considerations, and infectious complications. *Pediatr. Blood Cancer* 49: 117–126.
43 Bar-Zohar, D. and Sivan, Y. (2004). The yield of flexible fiberoptic bronchoscopy in pediatric intensive care patients. *Chest* 126: 1353–1359.
44 Rosenfeld, M., Emerson, J., Accurso, F. et al. (1999). Diagnostic accuracy of oropharyngeal cultures in infants and young children with cystic fibrosis. *Pediatr. Pulmonol.* 28: 321–328.
45 Hilliard, T.N., Sukhani, S., Francis, J. et al. (2007). Bronchoscopy following diagnosis with cystic fibrosis. *Arch. Dis. Child.* 92: 898–899.
46 Armstrong, D.S., Grimwood, K., Carlin, J.B. et al. (1996). Bronchoalveolar lavage or oropharyngeal cultures to identify lower respiratory pathogens in infants with cystic fibrosis. *Pediatr. Pulmonol.* 21: 267–275.
47 Wainwright, C.E., Vidmar, S., Armstrong, D.S. et al. (2011). Effect of bronchoalveolar lavage-directed therapy on *Pseudomonas aeruginosa* infection and structural lung injury in children with cystic fibrosis: a randomized trial. *JAMA* 306: 163–171.
48 Sherman, J.M., Davis, S., Albamonte-Petrick, S. et al. (2000). Care of the child with a chronic tracheostomy. *Am. J. Respir. Crit. Care Med.* 161: 297–308.
49 Nicolai, T. (2008). Airway stents in children. *Pediatr. Pulmonol.* 43: 330–344.
50 Pérez-Frías, J., Moreno Galdó, A., Pérez Ruiz, E. et al. (2011). Pediatric bronchoscopy guidelines. *Arch. Bronconeumol.* 47 (7): 350–360.
51 Shen, K.L., Deng, L., Li, Y.Z. et al. (2018). Consensus on the use of inhalation of glucocorticoid with nebulizer in pediatric patients (2018 revised). *J. Clin. Pediatr.* 36 (2): 95–107.
52 Respiratory Society of Chinese Medical Association (2016). Expert consensus on prevention and treatment of major bleeding related to diagnosis and treatment of bronchoscopy. *Chin. J. Tuberc. Respir. Dis.* 39 (8): 588–591.

第 27 章

可弯曲支气管镜在重症监护室中的应用

Ali Sadoughi[1] and Alexander Chen[2]
[1] Division of Pulmonary and Critical Care,
Albert Einstein College of Medicine/Montefiore Medical Center, New York, USA
[2] Division of Pulmonary and Critical Care, Washington University School of Medicine, St Louis, MO, USA

（译者：秦　浩　王　俊　译者单位：海军军医大学第一附属医院）

27.1 引言

池田茂人在 20 世纪 60 年代后期开发的可弯曲支气管镜大大拓宽了支气管镜的潜在应用范围。如今，越来越多不同的器械得以开发，并被应用于可弯曲支气管镜的诊断与治疗中。由于可弯曲支气管镜在重症监护室（intensive care unit，ICU）的重要应用及其在患者诊治中的显著效果，已成为重症医师不可或缺的工具。

危重患者的定义是因一个或多个脏器遭受病理性损伤，导致机体功能严重受损的患者。这些患者需要经过专业人员予以密切监测和观察，以处理疾病和可能发生的严重并发症。

呼吸功能损害可能是首发的病理过程，也可能随着其他疾病的进展而发生。ICU 患者病情危重的特质意味着他们不适合转出重症监护病房。因此，具备在严密监测条件下在床边开展诊断和治疗性支气管镜操作的能力是有很大优势的。

27.2 可弯曲支气管镜

在可弯曲支气管镜发明之前，硬质支气管镜被用于上呼吸道检查。尽管硬质支气管镜仍有其实用性，也被推荐用于处理一些临床状况，但也存在局限性，包括需要全身麻醉、无法检查中央气道以外的支气管和无法在临床上广泛推广。相反，可弯曲支气管镜操作可以在床边、中度镇静下进行且广大重症监护人员都能用得上。

27.3 适应证

ICU 支气管镜操作的适应证非常广泛，可大致分为气道管理、诊断或治疗。表 27.1 总结了一些较常见的适应证。

表 27.1 ICU 内支气管镜操作主要适应证

气道管理
直视下引导气管插管
气道内插管定位
诊断性操作
气道检查
收集下呼吸道标本
治疗性操作
误吸
解除气道梗阻
气道异物取出
引导经皮扩张气管切开术
气道支架置入
咯血

关于 ICU 支气管镜操作的适应证，已有大量的综述和研究发表[1-6]。虽然不同机构和重症监护环境（即外科、内科）的适应证有所不同，但诊断性和治疗性支气管镜操作的比例总体上是平衡的，有些操作既用于诊断，也用于治疗。

27.4 设备

在任何情况下进行支气管镜操作都需要包括医师、护士、技术人员和呼吸治疗师在内的医务人员参与。在危重患者中，这些工作人员必须能够处理诸如进行性呼吸衰竭、血流动力学不稳定、气胸和可能继发于潜在疾病的大出血等并发症[7]。后文将进一步讨论支气管镜操作的潜在并发症和对机械通气的影响。

当在 ICU 内进行支气管镜操作时，必须对患者进行连续监测[8]。如果患者需要机械通气，应连续监测氧饱和度、呼气末二氧化碳水平、血压和心率，并监测所有呼吸机参数。

27.5 镇静与麻醉

大多数 ICU 患者都有镇静的医嘱，特别是那些机械通气的患者。这些患者的镇静通常由一种短效苯二氮䓬类药物和一种阿片类药物组成。支气管镜操作时可以使用这种镇静镇痛方案，这将产生术中遗忘的效果，同时达到镇痛的作用。另外，异丙酚作为一种镇静剂，因其快速起效和短半衰期的药理特性目前被广泛使用于支气管镜镇静方案中。

气管插管患者经支气管镜向气道内注入 2.5~5 mL 1% 利多卡因行表面麻醉。在非插管患者中，可通过雾化器雾化利多卡因局部麻醉喉部和口咽。局部喷洒利多卡因或将利多卡因浸透的纱布敷在鼻黏膜上，可达到鼻腔麻醉的效果。

27.6 机械通气患者的支气管镜操作

机械通气患者可以安全地接受支气管镜操作，但必须注意以下事项[9]：首先是可弯曲支气管镜对气管插管内吸气和呼气气流的影响。在没有气管插管的情况下，支气管镜约占成人气管横截面的 10%。外径为 5.7 mm 的支气管镜占据 8 mm 气管插管 51% 的横截面，导致气流阻力显著增加[10]。表 27.2 显示，气管插管内支气管镜的存在对其他几个因素也有显著影响[11]。

表 27.2 经气管插管实施支气管镜操作时对不同呼吸生理参数的影响

呼吸力学参数	影响
气管内压	增加
气道压	增加
功能残气量（FRC）	增加
第 1 秒内用力呼气容积（FEV_1）	减少
呼气末正压	增加
重吸入潮气量	减少

在支气管镜操作期间，通常采用两种通气策略：① 在维持 CO_2 基线稳定的基础上使用定容通气；② 允许潮气量（tidal volume，VT）降低并限制峰值的定压通气。由于支气管镜操作时呼气流量受限，前一种策略有过度充气的风险。Greenstein 等在限制 VT 的情况下研究了 16 名气管插管受试者在支气管镜操作期间的呼气末肺容积（end-expiratory lung volume，EELV）。任何受试者的 EELV 均未出现显著性增加。EELV 的下降与负压吸引动作同步。限制峰压通气保护了受试者免受过度通气的影响，随之而来的是可耐受的 VT 降低和高碳酸血症[12]。

为了降低风险，如果使用容量控制通气模式（volume-controlled ventilation，VCV），建议在接受标准诊断性支气管镜操作时，通过内径≥8 mm 的气管插管进行。首选外径 4.9 mm 的支气管镜，但外径 5.2 mm 的支气管镜也可以接受。对机械通气患者进行支气管镜操作的其他建议包括在插入支气管镜前以纯氧进行预氧合，降低呼气末正压（positive end-expiratory pressure，PEEP）或将其调为 0，降低吸气流速以抵消气管插管内支气管镜引起的气道高压。

27.7 并发症

即使在危重症患者中，支气管镜操作通常也耐受良好[13]。对在 ICU 中进行的 1 000 多例支气管镜操作的回顾分析显示，没有因支气管镜操作引起的死亡。可弯曲支气管镜在机械通气患者中应用的安全性也经过了专门评估。尽管在一篇综述中提到支气管肺泡灌洗（bronchoalveolar lavage，BAL）没有导致需要提前终止操作的并发症，但BAL确实与肺泡-动脉氧梯度的增加有关。

一过性低氧血症通常发生在支气管镜操作期间，特别是在存在呼吸衰竭基础的危重患者中，并且通常在操作后恢复到基线水平[15]。在支气管镜操作期间保持FiO_2为100%并避免不必要的吸痰可能有助于降低低氧血症的发生和严重程度，但操作中应随时准备好退出支气管镜并在必要时使用Ambu袋（Ambu Bag）手动给患者通气。或者，如果需要的话也可以直接通过支气管镜的吸引通道给患者供氧。

经鼻高流量氧疗已成为低氧血症患者无创呼吸支持的一种技术。经鼻高流量氧疗的疗效可以通过以下几种机制来解释：通过冲刷上气道死腔、降低吸气时鼻咽腔阻力、产生一定水平的气道正压效应来缓解呼吸窘迫症状和改善氧合[16]。一项前瞻性、多中心研究对30例ICU内急性呼吸衰竭（acute respiratory failure，ARF）重症患者进行了支气管镜操作，结果表明接受经鼻高流量氧疗支持的患者完成了所有BAL操作。对需经鼻支气管镜操作的低氧性急性呼吸衰竭患者，经鼻高流量氧疗可能是一种有效的、耐受性良好的呼吸支持手段[17]。

支气管镜操作对心血管系统有多方面影响，这些影响在危重疾病的情况下可能会放大。3%~11%的接受支气管镜操作患者可出现心律失常，但心脏骤停非常罕见。其他异常，如心率、血压和心输出量升高，可能是交感神经活动激增所致。患有潜在心血管疾病，特别是冠状动脉疾病的患者发生心脏并发症的可能性增加。因此，建议持续监测心率、血压、血氧饱和度和心电遥测（如果有的话）。

支气管镜操作不易并发出血，除非患者有凝血功能障碍且未纠正。考虑到尿毒症患者血小板功能障碍，可以提前使用去氨加压素进行预防。血小板减少症在骨髓移植患者中很常见，在支气管镜操作之前可以给予额外的血小板输注，即使在这种情况下，在进行BAL时也很少出现无法控制的出血[18-24]。

27.8 气道管理

27.8.1 困难气道

困难气道是ICU内气管插管的挑战。患者可能存在颈部活动受限或上呼吸道病变导致标准喉镜视野不佳[25]。在以下情况下，建议采用可弯曲支气管镜引导插管：① 清醒插管，以防止血流动力学或神经系统功能障碍；② 当其他步骤失败时，支气管镜引导插管可作为一种抢救方式。观察性研究结果表明，纤支镜引导插管（气管插管通过支气管镜进入气管）在87%~100%困难气道患者中取得了成功[26]。

27.8.2 双腔气管插管放置

双腔气管插管的适应证较为局限，主要用于择期胸外科手术。其在ICU的适应证仅限于气道大咯血，以及由于肺出血后双肺顺应性不同或其他原因导致需要差异性设置每侧肺的机械通气参数的临床情况。双腔气管插管的正确放置需要可弯曲支气管镜检查确认。长管的末端通常固定在左主支气管，而短管的末端则固定在气管内[27-32]。

27.8.3 气管插管堵塞

由于气管插管部分或完全阻塞，吸入和呼出时肺内的空气流动可能受到限制，这可能是由于插管内过多的黏液或气管的机械形变。此时可导致明显的临床表现：气道峰压骤升、低吸气流速、手动通气阻力增高。在这些情况下，可使用可弯曲支气管镜操作并通过气道内吸引解除堵塞。

27.8.4 气管插管定位与更换

正确的气管插管位置是危重患者机械通气管理的重要组成部分。有研究报道，高达15%的机械通气患者的气管插管位置放置不正确[33,34]。而可弯曲支气管镜检查提供了一种快速、直接的最佳方法。有几个因素可能导致气管插管的意外移动，如患者翻身。尽管胸片可以提示放置不当，但为了确保气道得到适当保护，镜下直视观察是必要的。

纤维支气管镜也使得更换气管插管变得简单。将新的气管插管套到支气管镜上，然后沿旧的气管插管一起推送到声门，在直视下缓慢取出旧气管插管。当旧的气管插管被移除时，将支气管镜推过声带，新的气管插管通过支气管镜送入气管。这种续贯更换气管插管的方法全程可视，从而降低了插入食管或无法找到气管的可能性。

27.9 诊断性支气管镜操作

27.9.1 支气管肺泡灌洗（BAL）

院内感染是医院获得性肺炎死亡的主要原因。呼吸机相关性肺炎（ventilator-associated pneumonia，VAP）指在插管 48 h 后机械通气患者发生的肺炎。大量研究表明，与那些接受药物敏感的抗生素治疗的 VAP 患者相比，早期抗菌药物治疗不充分的患者死亡率更高[35-45]。因此，有必要早期明确病原生物体。BAL 是一种微创的收集下呼吸道标本的方法，可用于指导危重患者的抗菌治疗。

在一项针对 130 例患者的研究中，BAL 的结果导致近 60% 的病例改变治疗方案或停止抗菌治疗[46]。调整抗菌方案的最常见指征是分离培养出耐药革兰氏阴性菌或耐甲氧西林金黄色葡萄球菌，并需要额外使用抗生素。

27.9.1.1 机械通气患者的 BAL 操作技术

对接受机械通气的危重患者采集呼吸道标本应遵循标准化的 BAL 流程。表 27.3 列出了机械通气患者行 BAL 所需的材料。其应包括连接支气管镜和气管插管的适配转接头、2 个无菌标本容器和生理盐水。

表 27.3 机械通气患者行 BAL 时物品准备

支气管镜插入适配转接头
2 个无菌标本容器
生理盐水
咬口
60 mL 注射器
2 个四通接头
管路

使患者处于仰卧位，首先给予充分镇静，通常以苯二氮䓬类药物联合阿片类药物，或使用异丙酚。在患者口中放置咬口以保护支气管镜，在气管插管和呼吸机管道之间放置用于支气管镜的三通转换接头。可通过气管插管注入 2.5~5 mL 1% 利多卡因进行腔内局部麻醉，支气管镜经三通转接头进入目标段支气管。

一旦支气管镜进入叶段或亚段支气管内，通过支气管镜的吸引通道注入 50 mL 生理盐水，然后进行回收，将吸出的液体收集在无菌标本容器中。初始 50 mL 生理盐水的灌注后吸引的液体作为支气管洗涤液应被丢弃。用另外 50 mL 生理盐水重复该过程，回收的灌洗液作为送检的支气管肺泡灌洗液。可以再注入 50 mL，直到支气管肺泡灌洗液量足以进行所需的检测（即病原微生物学、细胞学）。

BAL 会降低机械通气患者的动脉血氧饱和度，但在手术后 12~15 h 内其值似乎会恢复到基线水平。一项研究表明，150 mL 和 40 mL 的 BAL 灌注量在降低氧合方面没有显著差异[47]。图 27.1 列出了笔者医院进行 BAL 操作时连接到支气管镜的配件。

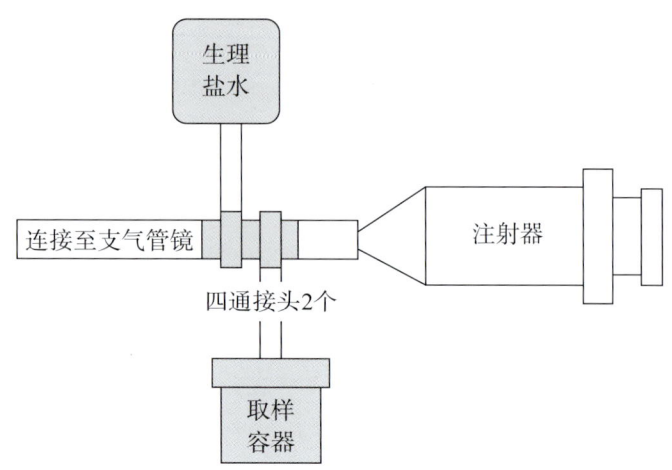

图 27.1 进行 BAL 时配件示意图

27.9.1.2 疑诊 VAP 患者 BAL 的时机

如果要进行 BAL，应在怀疑 VAP 后尽早进行，且不能因操作而延误使用恰当的广谱抗菌药物。数项研究表明，在支气管肺泡灌洗液培养结果回报后再将抗菌药物调整至充分覆盖，其死亡率与继续接受不充分抗菌药物覆盖的患者相似[46,48]。图 27.2 概述了 VAP 患者 BAL 的建议流程。

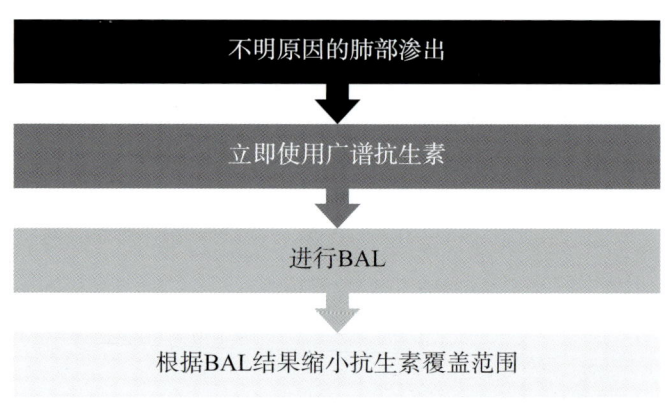

图 27.2 机械通气患者怀疑 VAP 进行 BAL 的流程图

27.9.1.3 肺组织活检

在机械通气的危重患者中常出现病因不明的肺部

阴影。虽然 BAL 提供了一种侵入性较小的下呼吸道标本取样方法，但当 BAL 结果不确定时，可能需要肺组织活检来做出特定诊断。开胸肺活检是一种成熟的获得肺组织的方法，但需要将患者转运到手术室，进行插管开胸的外科手术，所有这些都可能增加发病率和死亡率[49,50]。机械通气患者的经支气管镜肺活检术（transbronchial lung biopsy，TBLB）随后被用于不需要开胸活检的病例。以前，机械通气被认为是经支气管活检的一个相对禁忌证，但也有一些研究表明，在这类患者群体中，机械通气下可以安全成功地进行经支气管肺活检[51,52]。

一项分析报告称，60% 机械通气患者经支气管活检获得的组织检查改变了医疗决策，而肺移植后机械通气患者的这一数字明显较低[53]。医疗决策的变化包括开始或停止使用抗菌药物，开始或停止使用皮质类固醇，或在诊断为淋巴瘤后停止治疗。

机械通气患者 TBLB 后气胸的发生率一直存在争议[54]。一项对非呼吸机依赖患者在择期插管和机械通气下进行 TBLB 的回顾性研究显示，机械通气组和非机械通气组的并发症发生率无显著差异。选择性正压机械通气对非呼吸机依赖患者的 TBLB 是安全的，不会增加并发症的风险[55]。透视下操作已被证明可降低经支气管活检的气胸风险[54]。因此，如条件允许应予使用。

27.10 治疗性支气管镜操作

27.10.1 中央气道阻塞

中央气道阻塞（central airway obstruction，CAO）是患者发病和死亡的重要原因。危重患者的气道阻塞可由多种恶性和非恶性病因引起，解剖学上可分为固定或动态狭窄。非恶性原因包括先前插管或气管切开术后瘢痕狭窄、异物梗阻、气管支气管软化和过度动态气道塌陷。气道损伤时的支气管镜操作适应证还包括外伤性气道损伤、吸入烟雾或腐蚀性物质造成气道损伤[56,57]。

支气管来源的肿瘤是导致大气道阻塞的主要原因，但确切的发病率和流行病学尚不清楚。20%~30% 的支气管肿瘤患者会因 CAO 而出现并发症，包括肺不张、反复发生阻塞性肺炎、呼吸困难和呼吸衰竭[58]。评估阻塞气道远端的通畅性是很重要的，它能预测支气管镜下扩张或支气管内支架置入成功的概率。

可弯曲支气管镜操作可直接测量阻塞程度，并可在需要时协助组织病理诊断。如果没有腔内病变，超声引导下经支气管针吸活检（endobronchial ultrasound-assisted transbronchial needle aspiration,, EBUS-TBNA）可以用于诊断，也可以在需要时为肺癌患者获取活检组织开展分子学检测。

可弯曲支气管镜下可开展多种介入手术，如冷冻治疗、氩等离子体凝固术（argon plasma coagulation，APC）和热消融，以解除支气管内阻塞病变。

27.10.2 气道支架

一些研究已经证实了放置气道支架对中央气道疾病继发呼吸衰竭患者的疗效[58]。一些报道称，在气管或主支气管内放置金属支架后，多达 50% 的危重患者成功脱离机械通气。气道支架置入可在床边通过可弯曲支气管镜进行，可直接在支气管镜下观察或在透视下辅助[59,60]。图 27.3 显示了金属支架置入治疗气道外源性压迫后气道直径的改善。

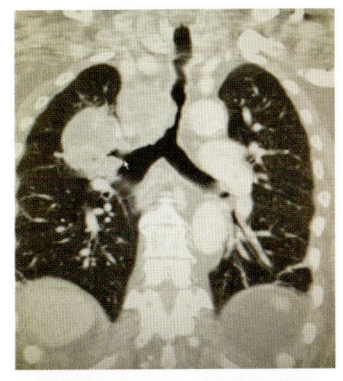
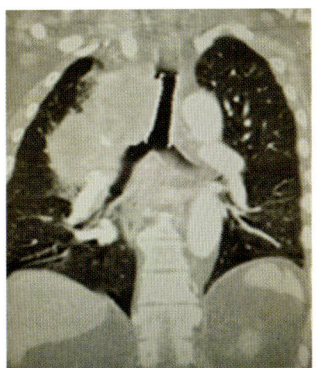
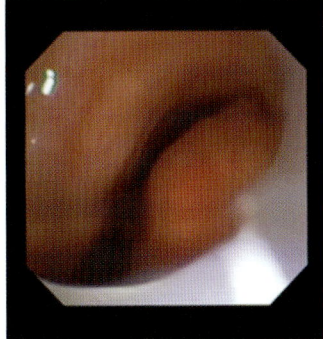
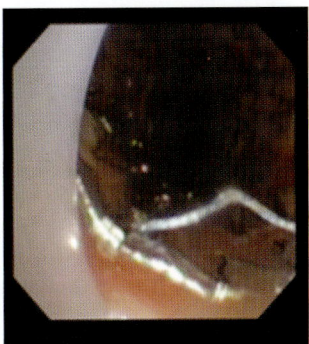

图 27.3　气道外源性压迫致气道狭窄患者的治疗
可弯曲支气管镜下球囊扩张和金属支架置入后气管直径改善。干预后，患者脱离机械通气。

27.10.3 气道异物取出

可弯曲支气管镜下可以通过使用网篮、异物钳和冷冻等器械移除异物。较大或尖锐的物体可能需要硬质支气管镜下取出[61,62]。

27.10.4 肺移植术后气道并发症管理

肺移植术后气道并发症虽不常见，但仍与死亡率和发病率升高有关。解剖学上，气道并发症可分为狭窄、肉芽组织、感染、坏死、畸形、撕裂和瘘管形成。不同类型的气道并发症采用不同的治疗方式，包括球囊扩张支气管成形术、冷冻疗法、电凝、APC、激光、机械清理、支架置入[硅酮支架或自膨胀金属支架（self-expanding metallic stents，SEMS）]。可弯曲支气管镜检查通常是早期诊断的第一步。一旦发生并发症通常需要反复镜下介入治疗。治疗后吻合口并发症患者与无并发症患者的早期死亡率相当[63]。

27.10.5 误吸

肺不张常见于机械通气危重患者。传统上，治疗由黏液堵塞引起的肺不张的重点一直是物理疗法、体位引流和气道内吸引分泌物。可弯曲支气管镜常用于误吸患者的气道内吸引，这是其在ICU中最常见的应用[64,65]。根据笔者经验，使用大外径治疗性支气管镜可以高效地吸除大量气道分泌物，操作时应当考虑气管插管或气管切开套管的直径和呼吸的气流流速，可直接通过支气管镜注入气道黏液溶解剂以促进分泌物吸除（但很少需要这样做）。

黏稠、干结的分泌物可能形成堵塞，阻塞中央气道甚至气管插管管腔从而导致严重的低氧血症。在这种情况下，即使大外径支气管镜也可能无法成功清除。通过可弯曲支气管镜进行冷冻治疗对于缓解由液体成分（如黏液或血块）引起的气道阻塞非常有帮助。在这个过程中，冷冻治疗探头通过支气管镜推进到梗阻物中，冷冻气体就会使梗阻物在探针周围收缩并黏附，然后将支气管镜带着冷冻治疗探头和梗阻物一起通过气管插管整体移除。这种方法对于清除大的黏液栓和血块是有用的，并且有显著的临床效果。

支气管镜下治疗肺不张时，把支气管镜嵌塞到目标气道，将支气管镜连接到Ambu袋，经工作通道将空气吹入目标肺段[65]。通过这种方法，可改善影像学和氧合，但考虑到医源性气胸的可能性，必须谨慎使用。

27.10.6 经皮扩张气管造口术

经皮扩张气管造口术（percutaneous dilational tracheostomy，PDT）已成为重症监护室重症患者进行气管切开术的一种广泛方法，主要是因为它可以在床边进行，从而避免了需要转运可能不稳定的患者。使用可弯曲支气管镜直视下操作提高了该手术的安全性，现已被广泛推荐[66]。

27.10.7 大咯血

对危重患者来说，大咯血可能是一种危及生命的并发症。气道保护至关重要，可弯曲支气管镜检查可以根据需要辅助定位气管插管或放置封堵球囊。在某些情况下，也可用硬质支气管镜操作辅助[67-70]。

27.10.8 持续性漏气

支气管胸膜瘘和肺泡胸膜瘘是主支气管、叶支气管或节段支气管或肺实质与胸膜腔之间形成交通。持续的漏气是患者死亡的重要原因。由于患肺的愈合能力差，治疗颇具有挑战性。在漏气无法解决时，可以考虑支气管镜下治疗。当手术等常规干预措施存在禁忌或效果不理想时，可对孤立的持续性漏气的部位放置支气管内单向活瓣[71-74]。

27.11 结论

可弯曲支气管镜是现代重症监护室医师不可缺少的工具，它使得医师能在床边进行一系列诊断和治疗操作。有了适当的设备和人员，这些操作就可以安全地开展，并对危重患者的临床进程产生重大影响。

参考文献

1 Raoof, S., Mehrishi, S., and Prakash, U.B. (2001). Role of bronchoscopy in modern medical intensive care unit. *Clin. Chest Med.* 22: 241–261.

2 Olopade, C.O. and Prakash, U.B. (1989). Bronchoscopy in the critical care unit. *Mayo Clin. Proc.* 64: 1255–1263.

3 Jolliet, P.H. and Chevrolet, J.C. (1992). Bronchoscopy in the intensive care unit. *Intensive Care Med.* 18: 160–169.

4 Turner, J.S., Willcox, P.A., Hayhurst, M.D., and Potgieter, P.D. (1994). Fiberoptic bronchoscopy in the intensive care unit – a prospective study of 147 procedures in 107 patients. *Crit. Care Med.* 22: 259–264.

5 Labbé, A., Meyer, F., and Albertini, M. (2004). Bronchoscopy in intensive care units. *Paediatr. Respir. Rev.* 5 (SupplA): S15–S19.

6 Bone, R.C., McElwee, N.E., Eubanks, D.H., and Gluck, E.H. (1993). Analysis of indications for intensive care unit admission. Clinical efficacy assessment project: American

College of Physicians. *Chest* 104: 1806–1811.
7. Krell, W.S. (1988). Pulmonary diagnostic procedures in the critically ill. *Crit. Care Clin.* 4: 393–407.
8. Dunagan, D.P., Burke, H.L., Aquino, S.L. et al. (1998). Fiberoptic bronchoscopy in coronary care unit patients: indications, safety, and clinical implications. *Chest* 114: 1660–1667.
9. Anzueto, A., Levine, S.M., and Jenkinson, S.G. (1992). The technique of fiberoptic bronchoscopy: diagnostic and therapeutic uses in intubated, ventilated patients. *J. Crit. Illn.* 7: 1657–1664.
10. Lindholm, C.E., Ollman, J.S., Millen, E.G., and Grenvik, A. (1978). Cardiorespiratory effects of flexible fiberoptic bronchoscopy in critically ill patients. *Chest* 74: 362–368.
11. Matsushima, Y., Jones, R., King, E. et al. (1984). Alterations in pulmonary mechanics and gas exchange during routine fiberoptic bronchoscopy. *Chest* 86: 184–188.
12. Greenstein, Y.Y., Shakespeare, E., Doelken, P. et al. (2017). Defining a ventilation strategy for flexible bronchoscopy on mechanically ventilated patients in the medical intensive care unit. *J. Bronchol. Interv. Pulmonol.* 24: 206–210.
13. Jin, F., Mu, D., Chu, D. et al. (2008). Severe complications of bronchoscopy. *Respiration* 76: 429–433.
14. Hertz, M.I., Woodward, M.E., Gross, C.R. et al. (1991). Safety of bronchoalveolar lavage in the critically ill, mechanically ventilated patient. *Crit. Care Med.* 19: 1526–1532.
15. Albertini, R.E., Harrell, J.H., Kurihara, N., and Moser, K.M. (1974). Arterial hypoxemia induced by fiberoptic bronchoscopy. *JAMA* 230: 1666–1667.
16. Ricard, J.D. (2012). High flow nasal oxygen in acute respiratory failure. *Minerva Anestesiol.* 78: 836–841.
17. La Combe, B., Messika, J., Labbe, V. et al. (2016). High-flow nasal oxygen for bronchoalveolar lavage in acute respiratory failure patients. *Eur. Respir. J.* 47: 1283–1286.
18. Dunagan, D.P., Baker, A.M., Hurd, D.D., and Haponik, E.F. (1997). Bronchoscopic evaluation of pulmonary infiltrates following bone marrow transplantation. *Chest* 111: 135–141.
19. Azoulay, E., Mokart, D., Rabbat, A. et al. (2008). Diagnostic bronchoscopy in hematology and oncology patients with acute respiratory failure: prospective multicenter data. *Crit. Care Med.* 36: 100–107.
20. Kim, Y.H., Suh, G.Y., Kim, M.H. et al. (2008). Safety and usefulness of bronchoscopy in ventilator-dependent patients with severe thrombocytopenia. *Anaesth. Intensive Care* 36: 411–417.
21. Rabbat, A., Chaoui, D., Lefebvre, A. et al. (2008). Is BAL useful in patients with acute myeloid leukemia admitted in ICU for severe respiratory complications? *Leukemia* 22: 1361–1367.
22. Gruson, D., Hilbert, G., Valentino, R. et al. (2000). Utility of fiberoptic bronchoscopy in neutropenic patients admitted to the intensive care unit with pulmonary infiltrates. *Crit. Care Med.* 28: 2224–2230.
23. White, P., Bonacum, J.T., and Miller, C.B. (1997). Utility of fiberoptic bronchoscopy in bone marrow transplant patients. *Bone Marrow Transplant.* 20: 681–687.
24. Kim, Y.H., Suh, G.Y., Kim, M.H. et al. (2008). Safety and usefulness of bronchoscopy in ventilator-dependent patients with severe thrombocytopenia. *Anaesth. Intensive Care* 36: 411–417.
25. Elizondo, E., Navarro, F., Pérez-Romo, A. et al. (2007). Endotracheal intubation with flexible fiberoptic bronchoscopy in patients with abnormal anatomic conditions of the head and neck. *Ear Nose Throat J.* 86: 682–684.
26. Apfelbaum, J.L., Hagberg, C.A., Caplan, R.A. et al. (2013). Practice guidelines for management of the difficult airway: an updated report by the American Society of Anesthesiologists Task Force on Management of the Difficult Airway. *Anesthesiology* 118: 251–270.
27. Cahill, B.C. and Ingbar, D.H. (1994). Massive hemoptysis. Assessment and management. *Clin. Chest Med.* 15: 147–167.
28. Karmy-Jones, R., Cuschieri, J., and Vallières, E. (2001). Role of bronchoscopy in massive hemoptysis. *Chest Surg. Clin. North Am.* 11: 873–906.
29. Valipour, A., Kreuzer, A., Koller, H. et al. (2005). Bronchoscopy-guided topical hemostatic tamponade therapy for the management of life-threatening hemoptysis. *Chest* 127: 2113–2118.
30. Fartoukh, M., Parrot, A., and Khalil, A. (2008). Aetiology, diagnosis and management of infective causes of severe haemoptysis in intensive care units. *Curr. Opin. Pulm. Med.* 14: 195–202.
31. Ong, T.H. and Eng, P. (2003). Massive hemoptysis requiring intensive care. *Intensive Care Med.* 29: 317–320.
32. Shigemura, N., Wan, I.Y., Yu, S.C. et al. (2009). Multidisciplinary management of life-threatening massive hemoptysis: a 10-year experience. *Ann. Thorac. Surg.* 87: 849–853.
33. Weiss, Y.G. and Deutschman, C.S. (2000). The role of fiberoptic bronchoscopy in airway management of the critically ill patient. *Crit. Care Clin.* 16: 445–451.
34. Schmidt, U., Hess, D., Kwo, J. et al. (2008). Tracheostomy tube malposition in patients admitted to a respiratory acute care unit following prolonged ventilation. *Chest* 134: 288–294.
35. Pereira Gomes, J.C., Pedreira, W.L. Jr., Araújo, E.M. et al. (2000). Impact of BAL in the management of pneumonia with treatment failure: positivity of BAL culture under antibiotic therapy. *Chest* 118: 1739–1746.
36. Fagon, J.Y., Chastre, J., Wolff, M. et al. (2000). Invasive and noninvasive strategies for management of suspected ventilator-associated pneumonia. A randomized trial. *Ann. Intern. Med.* 132: 621–630.
37. Hayon, J., Figliolini, C., Combes, A. et al. (2002). Role of serial routine microbiologic culture results in the initial management of ventilator-associated pneumonia. *Am. J. Respir. Crit. Care Med.* 165: 41–46.
38. Canadian Critical Care Trials Group (2006). A randomized trial of diagnostic techniques for ventilator-associated pneumonia. *N. Engl. J. Med.* 355: 2619–2630.
39. Heyland, D.K., Cook, D.J., Marshall, J. et al. (1999). The clinical utility of invasive diagnostic techniques in the setting of ventilator-associated pneumonia. Canadian Critical Care Trials Group. *Chest* 115: 1076–1084.
40. Luna, C.M., Vujacich, P., Niederman, M.S. et al. (1997).

Impact of BAL data on the therapy and outcome of ventilator-associated pneumonia. *Chest* 111: 676–685.

41 Timsit, J.F., Cheval, C., Gachot, B. et al. (2001). Usefulness of a strategy based on bronchoscopy with direct examination of bronchoalveolar lavage fluid in the initial antibiotic therapy of suspected ventilator-associated pneumonia. *Intensive Care Med.* 27: 640–647.

42 Fagon, J.Y., Chastre, J., and Rouby, J.J. (2007). Is bronchoalveolar lavage with quantitative cultures a useful tool for diagnosing ventilator-associated pneumonia? *Crit. Care* 11: 123.

43 Shorr, A.F., Sherner, J.H., Jackson, W.L., and Kollef, M.H. (2005). Invasive approaches to the diagnosis of ventilator-associated pneumonia: a meta-analysis. *Crit. Care Med.* 33: 46–53.

44 Bonten, M.J., Bergmans, D.C., Stobberingh, E.E. et al. (1997). Implementation of bronchoscopic techniques in the diagnosis of ventilator-associated pneumonia to reduce antibiotic use. *Am. J. Respir. Crit. Care Med.* 156: 1820–1824.

45 Mentec, H., May-Michelangeli, L., Rabbat, A. et al. (2004). Blind and bronchoscopic sampling methods in suspected ventilator-associated pneumonia. A multicentre prospective study. *Intensive Care Med.* 30: 1319–1326.

46 Kollef, M.H. and Ward, S. (1998). The influence of mini-BAL cultures on patient outcomes: implications for the antibiotic management of ventilator-associated pneumonia. *Chest* 113: 412–420.

47 Bauer, T.T., Torres, A., Ewig, S. et al. (2001). Effects of bronchoalveolar lavage volume on arterial oxygenation in mechanically ventilated patients with pneumonia. *Intensive Care Med.* 27: 384–393.

48 Joffe, A.R., Muscedere, J., Marshall, J.C. et al. (2008). The safety of targeted antibiotic therapy for ventilator-associated pneumonia: a multicenter observational study. *J. Crit. Care* 23: 82–90.

49 Papazian, L. and Gainnier, M. (2003). Indications of BAL, lung biopsy, or both in mechanically ventilated patients with unexplained infiltrations. *Eur. Respir. J.* 21: 383–384.

50 Baumann, H.J., Kluge, S., Balke, L. et al. (2008). Yield and safety of bedside open lung biopsy in mechanically ventilated patients with acute lung injury or acute respiratory distress syndrome. *Surgery* 143: 426–433.

51 Papin, T.A., Grum, C.M., and Weg, J.G. (1986). Transbronchial biopsy during mechanical ventilation. *Chest* 89: 168–170.

52 Ghamande, S., Rafanan, A., Dweik, R. et al. (2002). Role of transbronchial needle aspiration in patients receiving mechanical ventilation. *Chest* 122: 985–989.

53 O'Brien, J.D., Ettinger, N.A., Dhevlin, D., and Kollef, M.H. (1997). Safety and yield of transbronchial biopsy in mechanically ventilated patients. *Crit. Care Med.* 25: 440–446.

54 White, C.S., Templeton, P.A., and Hasday, J.D. (1997). CT-assisted transbronchial needle aspiration: usefulness of CT fluoroscopy. *Am. J. Roentgenol.* 169: 393–394.

55 Asai, M., Samayoa, A.X., Hodge, C. et al. (2017). Elective intubation and positive pressure ventilation for transbronchial lung biopsy. *J. Surg. Res.* 219: 296–301.

56 Dissanaike, S., Shalhub, S., and Jurkovich, G.J. (2008). The evaluation of pneumomediastinum in blunt trauma patients. *J. Trauma* 65: 1340–1345.

57 Johnson, S.B. (2008). Tracheobronchial injury. *Semin. Thorac. Cardiovasc. Surg.* 20: 52–57.

58 Ernst, A., Feller-Kopman, D., Becker, H.D. et al. (2004). Central airway obstruction. *Am. J. Respir. Crit. Care Med.* 169: 1278–1297.

59 Chhajed, P.N., Baty, F., Pless, M. et al. (2006). Outcome of treated advanced non-small cell lung cancer with and without central airway obstruction. *Chest* 130: 1803–1807.

60 Lin, S.M., Lin, T.Y., Chou, C.L. et al. (2008). Metallic stent and flexible bronchoscopy without fluoroscopy for acute respiratory failure. *Eur. Respir. J.* 31: 1019–1023.

61 Folch, E. and Mehta, A.C. (2008). Airway interventions in the tracheobronchial tree. *Semin. Respir. Crit. Care Med.* 29: 441–452.

62 Colt, H.G. and Harrell, J.H. (1997). Therapeutic rigid bronchoscopy allows level of care changes in patients with acute respiratory failure from central airways obstruction. *Chest* 112: 202–206.

63 Machuzak, M., Santacrus, J.F., Gildea, T. et al. (2015). Airway complications after lung transplantation. *Thorac. Surg. Clin.* 25: 55–75.

64 Kreider, M.E. and Lipson, D.A. (2003). Bronchoscopy for atelectasis in the ICU: a case report and review of the literature. *Chest* 124: 344–350.

65 Tsao, T.C., Tsai, Y.H., Lan, R.S. et al. (1990). Treatment for collapsed lung in critically ill patients. *Chest* 97: 435–438.

66 Yuca, K., Kati, I., Tekin, M. et al. (2008). Fibre-optic bronchoscopy-assisted percutaneous dilational tracheostomy by guidewire dilating forceps in intensive care unit patients. *J. Otolaryngol. Head Neck Surg.* 37: 76–80.

67 Sakr, L. and Dutau, H. (2010). Massive hemoptysis: an update on the role of bronchoscopy in diagnosis and management. *Respiration* 80: 38–58.

68 Hetzel, M.R. and Smith, S.G. (1991). Endoscopic palliation of tracheobronchial malignancies. *Thorax* 46: 325–333.

69 Morice, R.C., Ece, T., Ece, F. et al. (2001). Endobronchial argon plasma coagulation for treatment of hemoptysis and neoplastic airway obstruction. *Chest* 119: 781–787.

70 Homasson, J.P. (1997). Endobronchial electrocautery. *Semin. Respir. Crit. Care* 18: 535–543.

71 Travaline, J.M., McKenna, R.J. Jr., de Giacomo, T. et al. (2009). Treatment of persistent pulmonary air leaks using endobronchial valves. *Chest* 136: 355–360.

72 Kovitz, K.L. and French, K.D. (2013). Endobronchial valve placement and balloon occlusion for persistent air leak: procedure overview and new current procedural terminology codes for 2013. *Chest* 144: 661–665.

73 Gillespie, C.T., Sterman, D.H., Cerfolio, R.J. et al. (2011). Endobronchial valve treatment for prolonged air leaks of the lung: a case series. *Ann. Thorac. Surg.* 91: 270–273.

74 Hance, J.M., Martin, J.T., and Mullett, T.W. (2015). Endobronchial valves in the treatment of persistent air leaks. *Ann. Thorac. Surg.* 100: 1780–1786.

第 28 章

支气管热成形术治疗哮喘

Ara A. Chrissian[1], Samir Makani[2], and Michael J. Simoff[2]
[1] Pulmonary and Critical Care, Loma Linda University, Loma Linda, CA, USA
[2] Division of Pulmonary and Critical Care Medicine, Henry Ford Hospital, Detroit, MI, USA
（译者：陈 巍　译者单位：上海交通大学医学院附属瑞金医院）

28.1　引言

哮喘是一种广泛分布的慢性肺部疾病，全球超过3亿人受其影响。在美国，因医疗支出和停工停学，哮喘所造成的花费每年估计超过560亿美元[1]。这一经济负担主要由少数重症哮喘患者承担，这些患者因频繁地急性加重，导致急诊就诊和住院。因此，人们花费了大量的精力开发新的创新性疗法来管理严重哮喘患者。这些包括针对靶向白三烯信号通路、抑制炎症细胞激活和各种抗细胞因子的药物。然而，由于该病的复杂性、受影响人群的异质性以及经济和现实情况的限制，这些疗法的有效性仍然不一致。

支气管热成形术（bronchial thermoplasty，BT）是一种新型的支气管镜介入技术，旨在将热能传递到气道壁。其目的是减少平滑肌数量，从而减少在哮喘急性加重时的多种病理效应。基于临床前数据展示的前景，数项人体研究也得以展开，并证实了安全性可接受及多项一致的临床获益。因此，2010年美国食品药物监督管理局（FDA）批准BT用于未完全控制的成年重度哮喘患者。累积的长期数据显示，最初的临床获益持续存在。随访研究还在持续进行着，以期更精确地识别最有可能对BT疗法反应良好的患者。

28.2　病理生理基础

哮喘是一种复杂的炎症性疾病，由多种机制介导。它的特点是分化的T辅助细胞响应来自下呼吸道上皮的刺激，释放各种细胞因子，招募白细胞到气道壁周围并激活。这进一步触发了多种炎症介质的产生和释放，导致了某些临床表型。慢性哮喘的特点是持续的气道炎症导致气道重塑，可见于各种管径的大、小气道。其确切的机制尚不清楚，但这是一个热门的研究方向[2]。气道重塑的特征包括上皮增厚、黏液腺肥大、细胞外基质（extracellular matrix，ECM）沉积增加、血管活化、气道平滑肌（airway smooth muscle，ASM）增生和肥大。最后一点似乎在持续重度哮喘中发挥了重要作用。

ASM延续至呼吸性细支气管水平的整个气道。尽管它被认为具有保护功能，有助于优化通气，其蠕动能为呼吸道各种动作提供支撑，但它在呼吸道中的确切作用仍存在争议。无论它在正常状态下的重要性如何，它都参与形成了严重的慢性疾病。变形和肥大的ASM不仅侵占气道管腔，而且肌肉缩短和收缩力增强，从而增加了气道阻力[3]。此外，ASM是炎症细胞和细胞因子介质的重要来源和储藏库，其表面含有乙酰胆碱反应性毒蕈碱受体[4-7]。因此，ASM很可能是一个炎性支气管收缩、黏液产生和ECM沉积的关键效应物。

ASM 的变化与重度哮喘表型之间的关联性已有广泛研究。哮喘患者的尸检标本上已观察到 ASM 的肥大和增生[8]。此外，已证明 ASM 量和气道重塑的程度与哮喘的严重程度相关，甚至可以在临床前期预测儿童中的哮喘发病[9-13]。因此，ASM 对重度哮喘明显的机械和生理影响使其成为一个合理的干预靶点。

体外和动物研究表明，皮质类固醇和 β 气体激动剂能通过多种机制调节 ASM。β 气体激动剂可促进气管平滑肌松弛，皮质类固醇可导致培养的平滑肌细胞的细胞周期停滞和收缩蛋白表达降低[14-16]。皮质类固醇也被证明可以防止小鼠肌成纤维细胞的积累和气道重塑，并减少甚至逆转气道重塑[17,18]。然而，尽管还有少量重度哮喘患者对现有的药物治疗反应不佳，但对其机制仍不完全明了，也尚未在人体中得到充分的研究。

28.3　支气管热成形术概述和临床证据

BT 是首次尝试以 ASM 为靶标，通过非药物性、内镜操作性的干预措施来减轻哮喘症状的内镜治疗方法。该干预措施是通过支气管镜下的射频消融术（radiofrequency ablation，RFA）来完成的，RFA 利用电极使组织产生交流电，交流电的离子活动会产生摩擦热，从而导致细胞损伤来达到减少支气管平滑肌。RFA 已安全有效地应用于多种临床场景，如癌症和心脏传导异常的治疗[19,20]。BT 遵循类似的原理，将能量传递到支气管。通过支气管镜，将射频导管插入各级呼吸道，并将能量系统地作用于气道壁（图 28.1）。能量的应用会导致 ASM 的变性、肌动蛋白-肌凝蛋白网络的破坏，并最终导致平滑肌量的减少[21-23]。

BT 通过消融 ASM 治疗哮喘的初步数据来源于犬模型。Danek 等发现，使用四电极篮状 BT 导管将热能传递到气道壁可减少 ASM 量，并导致气道对乙酰胆碱的反应性降低[24]。每只犬的肺被分为 4 个区域（对照组和 3 个治疗区域），并在每个区域给予了不同温度（55℃、65℃ 和 75℃）的消融。总共检查了 300 个单独的气道部位。在 55℃ 区域，气道高反应性（airway hyperresponsiveness，AHR）与对照组相比无显著差异，而在 75℃ 区域，AHR 在所有时间点均有显著差异。组织学上，所有治疗组在术后 1 周就发现了 ASM 的变化（图 28.2）。这种情况在随后 3 年的随访中一直存在（当时发现成熟的胶原蛋白已经取代了 ASM），并且在 75℃ 组中最为显著。在一项单独的研究中，

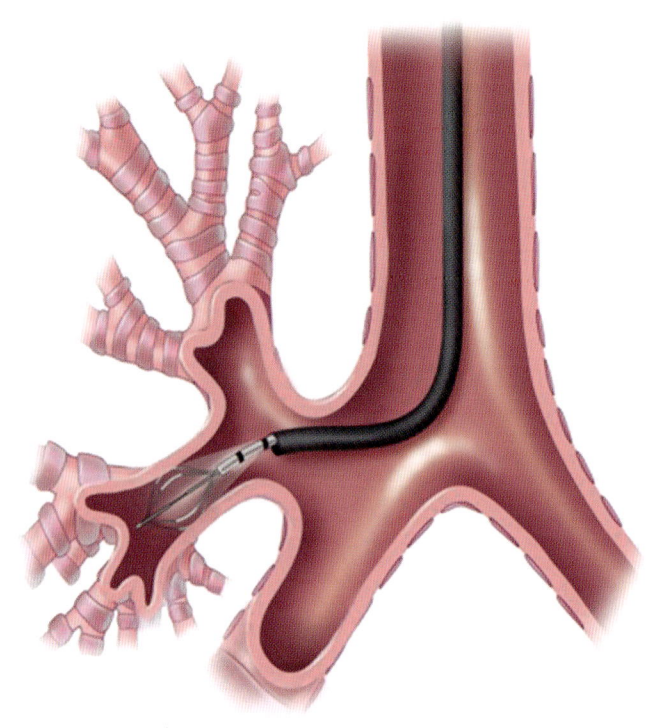

图 28.1　支气管热成形术
使用可弯曲支气管镜引入的专用导管将射频能量输送到气道壁。资料来源：图片由波士顿科学公司提供。©2018 波士顿科学公司或其附属公司。

Brown 等发现，与未经治疗的气道相比，经 BT 治疗的犬的气道在基线时具有较低的支气管运动张力，并且在不同的气道压力下更容易扩张[25,26]。这些研究结果共同为人体可行性和安全性试验奠定了基石。

第一项人体 BT 研究在 8 名计划切除肺叶的无哮喘病史的肺癌患者中进行[27]。前 2 名受试者接受 55℃ 治疗，随后 6 名接受 65℃ 治疗。被切除的肺组织学标本显示 ASM 减少。经 65℃ 治疗的标本总体上比 55℃ 治疗的标本变化更明显。患者对 BT 的耐受性良好，均按计划接受手术。

Cox 等首次对哮喘患者开展了 BT 的前瞻性分析，他们评估了 16 例稳定的轻中度哮喘和使用支气管扩张剂后第 1 秒用力呼气量（forced expiratory volume in first second，FEV_1）值正常的患者[28]。除 1 名患者因复发感染而无法完成第 3 次治疗外，所有受试者均安全地进行了治疗。研究人员发现，BT 术后即时常见不良事件包括咳嗽、喘息和呼吸困难等，但可在 1 周内缓解。在治疗后的前 12 周内没有急诊就诊或住院记录，受试者反馈无症状天数增多。通过乙酰胆碱激发试验，在 12 周时 AHR 有所改善，效果持续了 2 年。

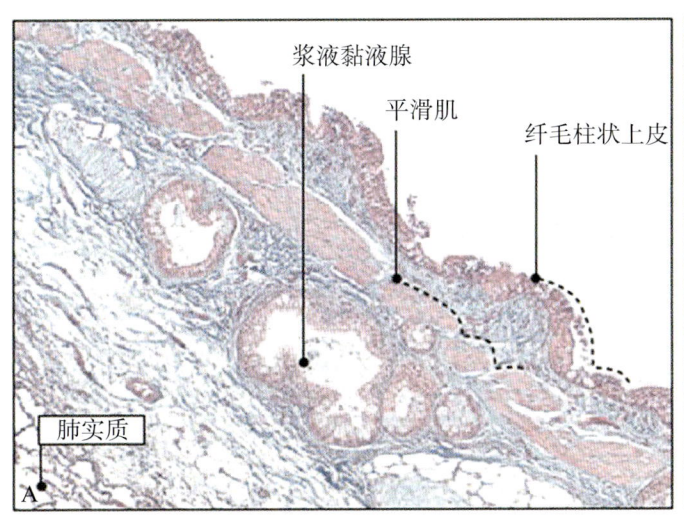 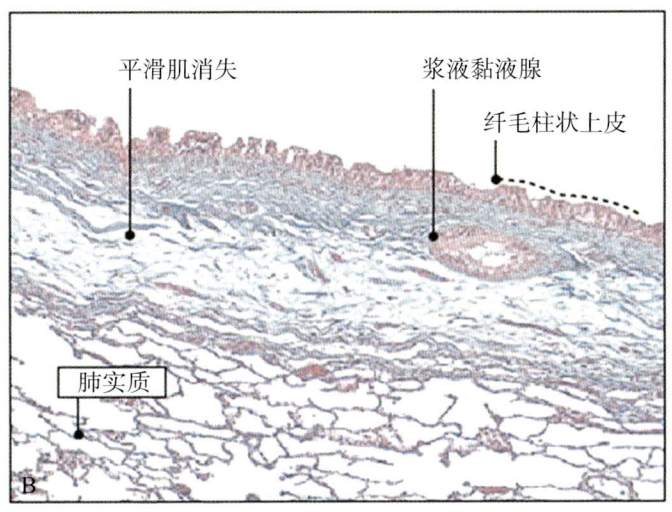

图 28.2 支气管热成形术（BT）术前、术后变化

A. 未经治疗的对照组气道壁；B. BT 术后的组织学标本，显示平滑肌减少。资料来源：图片由波士顿科学公司提供。©2018 波士顿科学公司或其附属公司，保留所有权利。

这些研究为随机对照研究奠定了基础，研究汇总见表 28.1。

第一个是哮喘干预研究，试验招募了 112 名符合全球哮喘倡议（GINA）定义的中度至重度哮喘患者[29]。支气管扩张剂前的 FEV_1 预测值在 60%~85% 之间。在停用长效 β 激动剂（long-acting B-agonist, LABA）2 周后出现哮喘加重的患者才纳入研究。受试者被随机分配到 LABA+ 吸入性皮质类固醇（inhaled corticosteroid，ICS）基础上，联合或不联合 BT 治疗。主要研究结果：与基线相比，BT 组的轻度急性加重率（定义为呼气峰流速较基线下降 20%，急救吸入器的使用增加，或夜间憋醒）在治疗后 3 个月和 12 个月的随访时降低，在 6 个月时无差异。哮喘生活质量问卷（AQLQ）和哮喘控制问卷（ACQ）在所有随访点的评分，与对照组相比，BT 治疗的受试者在哮喘相关生活质量方面有所改善。在治疗后的所有随访时间内，两组之间的 FEV_1 值、AHR 或急性加重率的变化没有差异。

重度哮喘研究试验是第一项评估重度持续性哮喘患者的 BT 研究[30]。32 名 $FEV_1 \geq 50\%$ 预测值、AHR 或可逆性支气管收缩，以及尽管接受了高剂量 ICS 和 LABA 治疗但症状仍持续存在的受试者被随机分配接受 BT 治疗或继续先前的治疗。BT 组和对照组的基线平均支气管扩张剂前 FEV_1 分别为预测值的 63% 和 66%。从治疗后 16 周开始，受试者在 1 年内停止口服激素或 ICS 的治疗。主要结果是比较不良事件的数量。在治疗期间，不良事件在 BT 组中更常见，但仅 10% 被归类为严重。BT 组中有 4 名患者（27%）需要住院 6 次，所有住院均与呼吸事件相关，而对照组中无住院。治疗后的随访期间，两组的不良事件和住院率相

表 28.1 评价入支气管热成形术的前瞻性、随机对照试验总结

研究	设计	关键纳入标准	主要研究结果，与对照组比较
AIR	RCT 多中心 112 名受试者	中度或重度持续性哮喘，稳定 6 周，FEV_1 60%~85% 预测值，LABA 停药后 AHR 加重	在 BT 后 3 个月和 12 个月的轻度急性加重率降低，6 个月时无差异
RISA	RCT 多中心 32 例受试者	重度持续性哮喘，高剂量 ICS 和 LABA，$FEV_1 \geq 50\%$ 预测值，AHR	治疗期间不良事件更多（10% 重度），治疗后也发生了类似的不良事件
AIR-2	双盲、假手术对照多中心 297 名受试者	重度持续性哮喘，高剂量 ICS 和 LABA，AQLQ ≤ 6.25，$FEV_1 \geq 60\%$ 预测值，AHR	AQLQ 评分较基线水平提高，持续平均超过 1 年

AHR，气道高反应性；AIR，哮喘干预研究[29]；AIR-2，哮喘干预研究-2[31]；AQLQ，哮喘生活质量问卷；ICS，吸入性皮质类固醇；RCT，随机对照试验；RISA，严重哮喘研究[30]。

似。研究者还注意到，在 22 周的随访中，接受 BT 治疗的受试者的支气管扩张剂前 FEV_1 值较高，AQLQ 和 ACQ 评分改善，急救药物使用减少。

对 AIR 和 RISA 试验的主要质疑在于它们的非盲设计，这引起了人们对未评估的安慰剂效应的顾虑，并由此质疑 BT 的真实疗效。哮喘干预研究-2（AIR-2）试验解决了这一问题，该试验设置了一个假手术对照组[31]，以 2∶1 的方式将 297 例重度、未控制哮喘患者随机分为 BT 治疗组和假手术组。表 28.2 汇总了纳入和排除标准。BT 组 190 名受试者和对照组 98 名受试者至少接受了一次支气管镜术。对照组（假手术组）支气管镜术流程与 BT（治疗）组相似。这包括将 RF 导管进入到气道中、扩展电极阵列以及激活假 RF 控制器。除了没有射频能量输送，所产生的听觉和视觉感知与有源射频控制器无法区分。目的是使每次支气管镜术的持续时间和假激活的数量与激活的治疗程序相匹配。虽然未对支气管镜治疗组采取盲法，但所有随访评估的访视均由盲法医护团队进行。预设的主要结果是 AQLQ 评分相较于基线值的变化（6 个月、9 个月、12 个月随访时间点的平均值）。

研究发现，两组的 AQLQ 评分均有所改善，接受 BT 治疗的受试者增加了 1.35 ± 1.0 个单位，而接受假 BT 治疗的受试者增加了 1.16 ± 1.23 个单位。BT 组中达到 0.5 AQLQ 单位的最小重要差异（MID）的受试者比例较高（79% 比 64%，后验概率为 99.6%）。在治疗后的随访期（最后一次 BT 治疗后的 6～52 周），接受 BT 治疗的受试者急性加重、急诊就诊、住院频次均减少。由于哮喘症状平稳，他们停工停学的天数也更少。

BT 组和假手术组的 ACQ 评分和总症状评分、晨起呼气峰流速以及急救药物使用率均有所改善，但组间差异无统计学意义。两组中支气管扩张剂使用前和使用后的 FEV_1 值均无变化。

与 AIR 和 RISA 试验相似，AIR-2 中接受 BT 治疗的受试者在治疗期间发生的不良事件多于对照组。其中绝大多数被归类为轻度或中度，包括气道刺激、上呼吸道感染或哮喘急性加重（如喘息、胸部不适、咳嗽等）的典型症状。如之前的临床试验所示，这些不良事件大多在支气管镜术后 1 周内消退。BT 组中有 16 名受试者（8.4%）因呼吸系统症状需住院 19 次，而假手术组中有 2 名受试者（2.0%）。BT 组 19 例住院病例中有 10 例发生在手术当天。

AIR-2 研究已经过仔细分析，医学界对其优点进行了讨论。AIR-2 研究队列的哮喘严重程度受到了质疑。总体上只有 2.8% 的受试者（BT 组中为 3.7%）在口服皮质类固醇，平均剂量约为 6 mg/天。此外，作为研究设计的一部分，前 1 年内发生 3 次以上的下呼吸道感染、3 次哮喘相关皮疹或 4 次口服类固醇的患者被排除在外。然而，根据研究期间美国胸科协会的标准，86% 的 AIR-2 研究 BT 队列符合重度、未控制哮喘的定义。其他关注点围绕着在假手术组中观察到的安慰剂效应以及评估哮喘相关生活质量的主要外部测量方法。批评者指出，两组之间的绝对平均 AQLQ 变化（0.19 个单位）缺乏统计学和临床意义上的差异。然而，AIR-2 研究人员得出结论，虽然观察到安慰剂效应，但根据对 AQLQ 有意义改善的受试者比例（0.5 个单位）的分析，治疗效果更好。该方法不是比较组

表 28.2 AIR-2 研究的主要纳入和排除标准

纳入标准	排除标准
18～65 岁成人	危及生命的哮喘
过去 4 周内至少有 2 天哮喘症状	慢性鼻窦疾病
高剂量 ICS（每天 1 000 µg 倍氯米松或同等药物）	肺气肿
高剂量 LABA（沙美特罗每天 100 µg 或同等）	使用免疫抑制剂、β 阻断剂和抗凝剂
口服皮质类固醇剂量每天 10 mg	前 1 年 3 次以上的哮喘相关住院治疗
基线 AQLQ 评分为 ≤6.25	前 1 年 3 次以上的下呼吸道感染
基线支气管扩张剂前 $FEV_1 \geq 60\%$	前 1 年 4 次以上口服皮质类固醇治疗哮喘
AHR（乙酰甲胆碱 $PC_{20} < 8$ mg/mL）	基线支气管扩张剂后 $FEV_1 < 65\%$
戒烟至少 1 年，且吸烟史 10 年以下	
入组前病情稳定 4 周	

AHR，气道高反应性；AIR-2，哮喘干预研究-2[31]；AQLQ，哮喘生存质量问卷；ICS，吸入性皮质类固醇；PC_{20}，激发浓度导致 FEV_1 下降至少 20%。

间的汇总值差异，而是评估受试者间的变化，因此遵循 AQLQ 评分的验证[32,33]。

基于 AIR-2 及之前研究的一致结果，FDA 于 2010 年批准 BT 用于使用 ICS 和 LABA 治疗后仍未完全控制的重度持续性哮喘成人患者。从那时起，GINA 和英国胸科协会还增加了 BT 作为治疗哮喘第 5 级患者的辅助治疗推荐方案。然而，截至 2013 年版，国际 ERS/ATS 指南对重度哮喘患者的治疗仅在机构审查委员会批准的注册或临床研究背景下对成年患者进行 BT[34]。读者可以通过多篇评论对 BT 争议进行更详细的分析[35-40]。

28.4 患者筛选

选择合适的患者开展 BT 治疗至关重要。最重要的初始步骤是确认哮喘诊断的准确性，并排除疑似哮喘的临床表现，或者类似哮喘症状加重的其他疾病。通过仔细的病史和体格检查以及常规的实验室和胸部影像学检查，可排除这些潜在的原发性疾病，如慢性鼻窦疾病、声带功能障碍、胃食管反流、肺气肿、过敏性支气管肺曲霉病、支气管扩张、结节病、气管支气管狭窄或软化等。对于所有准备进行 BT 治疗的患者，建议进行全血细胞计数及分类计数、代谢全套、基线肺功能检测（包括一氧化碳弥散能力和流量容积环的测定）以及胸部 CT。还可针对其他疑似诊断进行额外检查（表 28.3）。

表 28.3 疑似或加重哮喘的疾病建议检查项目

疑似致病的情况	建议进一步检查的项目
肺气肿	全套 PFT、HRCT、α1-抗胰蛋白酶水平
弥漫性肺实质病变	全套 PFT、HRCT、相关血清学检查、超声心动图
慢性鼻窦疾病	鼻窦 CT、过敏原检测
声带功能异常	喉镜
胃食管反流或误吸	食管 pH 测定，吞咽功能评估
支气管扩张	HRCT、免疫蛋白水平、痰培养、皮肤和血清过敏原检测、汗液氯化物测定
结节病	胸部 CT、支气管镜下纵隔淋巴结和肺组织活检
气管支气管狭窄或软化	流量容积环、动态 CT、支气管镜
充血性心力衰竭	血清 BNP、超声心动图

HRCT，高分辨率计算机断层扫描；BNP，脑钠肽；PFT，肺功能检查。

一旦确诊为重度哮喘，并且排除或控制对症状有显著影响的其他疾病后，应严格评估患者对哮喘药物治疗的依从性。如果依从性差，医护人员应适当教育患者，根据需要调整药物种类或给药技术，并安排重新评估。随后，医护人员应使用专用的检查表审查 BT 的候选资格。患者筛选通常应遵循 AIR-2 研究的纳入和排除标准（表 28.2）。患者应至少需要第 5 级哮喘治疗（高剂量 ICS 和 LABA）。一旦确定患者为合适的 BT 目标治疗人群，应讨论合理的预期，包括短期和长期风险和获益。2018 年，该手术的医疗保险覆盖范围在美国各地仍存在较大差异，应对此进行审核。应排除患者是否存在支气管镜手术的常见禁忌证（如不稳定型心肺疾病、严重凝血障碍等）。

对病情控制较差或有更严重的临床特征从而不符合 AIR-2 纳入标准的哮喘患者，是否进行 BT 治疗，目前仍存在争议。这些包括支气管扩张剂前 FEV_1 值低于预测值 60% 的患者、口服高剂量皮质类固醇和/或近期频繁加重住院的患者。RISA 研究是唯一一项纳入 FEV_1 阈值以下患者的随机、对照研究，但也是受试者最少的一项研究（15 名患者接受 BT 治疗）。最近一项由 8 名患者组成的小型病例系列研究表明，对于严重气流阻塞（FEV_1 平均 52% 预测值，其中 5 名受试者被归类为非常严重）的受试者，可以安全地进行 BT[41]。

正在进行的 FDA 批准后的评估重度持续性哮喘行 BT 的临床研究（PAS-2）纳入标准与 AIR-2 研究相比，纳入了在 BT 前一年中年龄更大、更肥胖、接受更高剂量皮质类固醇治疗以及哮喘急性加重和住院频率更高的患者[42]。这可能更符合"真实世界"的重度哮喘人群。此项前瞻性、观察性研究中对前 190 名受试者的中期分析显示，在 3 年随访时，BT 治疗后每年的急性加重、急诊就诊和住院人数均减少，与 AIR-2 的结果一致。然而，该队列总体上没有出现严重的气流阻塞（基线平均支气管扩张剂前 FEV_1 为预测值的 80%，与 AIR-2 研究 BT 组类似）。此外，未报告 BT 后 AQLQ 评分，与 AIR-2 研究一样，未将对照组纳入长期分析。因此，在获得更可靠的数据确定 BT 治疗控制不佳且伴有严重气流阻塞的哮喘患者的安全性和有效性之前，应仅在个案基础上考虑对这些患者进行 BT 治疗，并应在有经验的中心进行。

28.5 操作流程

BT 应由有经验的支气管镜医师开展。完整治疗需要3次支气管镜手术，每次间隔2~3周。例如，第1疗程治疗右下叶，第2疗程治疗左下叶，最后治疗双上叶。由于担心右肺中叶支气管容易陷闭，因此未予以治疗。每次手术前，患者必须处于临床稳定期，在前2周内无皮疹、感染或增加使用吸入剂。为了最大限度地减少围手术期的呼吸相关不良事件，从支气管镜手术前3天开始，给患者为期5天的50 mg泼尼松口服预防性治疗。手术当天，应检查FEV_1，并观察其是否在其基线值的10%以内，且指脉血氧饱和度应大于90%。

支气管镜下BT治疗的现场准备应符合机构标准，并熟悉BT操作，标准治疗持续时间为30~60 min。BT的支气管镜下治疗可在中度镇静、无气道辅助设备或深度镇静/全身麻醉下进行。要求使用诊断性支气管镜，其最小工作通道直径为2.0 mm，以便通过RF导管。不鼓励使用较大外径的治疗性支气管镜，较细的支气管镜可进入较小的气道并进行更完整的治疗。患者应在手术前接受短效β激动剂治疗，有研究者建议给予止涎药（如格隆溴铵0.2~0.4 mg静脉注射或肌肉注射），尽量减少分泌物并优化视野[43]。正确使用表面麻醉，如支气管镜术前雾化吸入利多卡因和手术过程中随时向气道黏膜喷洒利多卡因溶液，以尽量减少咳嗽。根据支气管镜术中热能量输送的推荐意见，供氧应保持在$FiO_2<40\%$，以防止理论上的气道着火。

每次支气管镜术均从完整的气道检查开始。在第2或第3疗程中，应对先前治疗过的区域进行仔细检查。支气管镜医师应注意观察有无气道持续性炎症、黏液生成过多、新的狭窄或其他病变。如果有发现上述情况，特别是如果有临床意义或同时存在，应考虑推迟预定的BT治疗。如无上述情况，需仔细检查治疗目标肺叶，并制订系统的治疗计划。建议所有直径>3 mm的可见气道都应实施BT治疗，治疗可从远端气道开始，逐步移动至近端肺段支气管，最后治疗叶支气管。每个部位应治疗一次。

2018年，采用Alai支气管热成形术系统（Boston Scientific，Natick，MA）来开展BT。能量由一次性Alair射频导管输送，导管远端装有一个四臂阵列，并通过一个可压下的驱动器连接到手柄上，该驱动器控制阵列的展开和收缩（图28.3）。导管被设计成适宜进入直径在3~10 mm之间的气道且能与气道壁接触。导管的近端连接到Alair控制器，控制器又连接到脚踏开关，当踩下脚踏开关一次时，触发的热能通过导管输送（最大120焦耳）。此"激活"将持续10 s，除非再次踩下脚踏开关，而这将提前终止射频传输。控制器监测功率和阻抗，确保一致的射频能量输送，并将气道壁调节加热至65℃。为了形成电回路，在患者（通常为背部或大腿）上放置一个返回电极，并在手术前连接至控制器。

具体操作时，确定目标气道后，通过工作通道将导管插入气道。导管远端不应超出内镜视野范围，导管不应扭转或弯曲。然后将阵列展开，并检查是否贴合良好，确保阵列所有4个臂与气道壁接触（图28.4）。然后，支气管镜医师踩下脚踏开关一次，以输

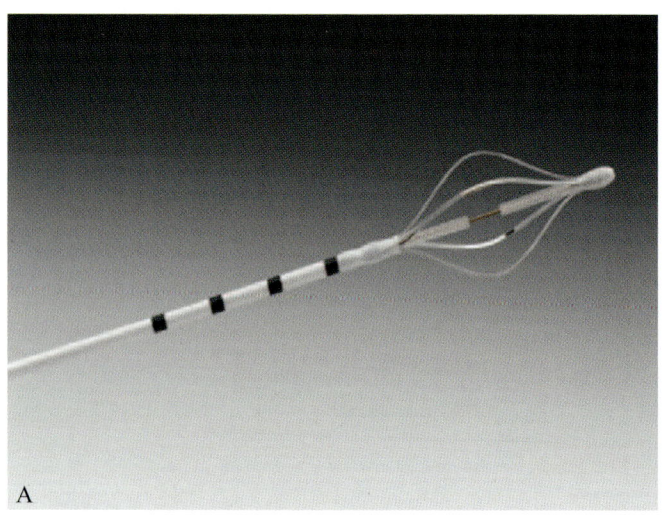
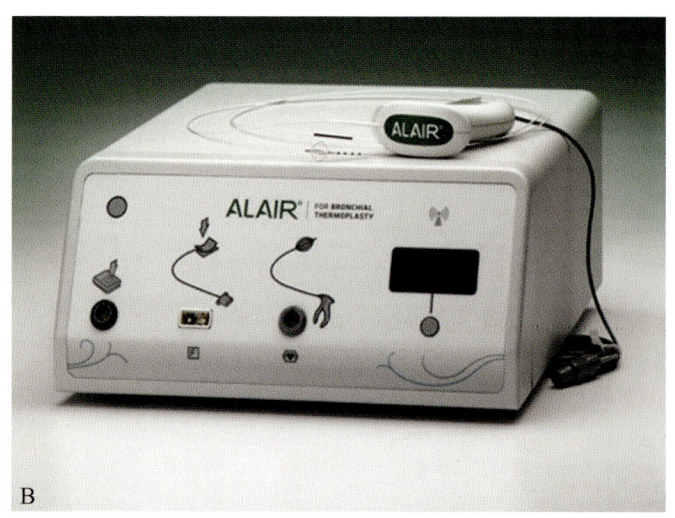

图28.3　一次性Alair射频导管

A. 射频导管远端装有一个四臂阵列，可以使用带有可调节的驱动器手柄来展开和折叠阵列；B. 可调节的驱动器又连接到Alair控制器单元。2018波士顿科学公司或其附属公司保留所有权利。

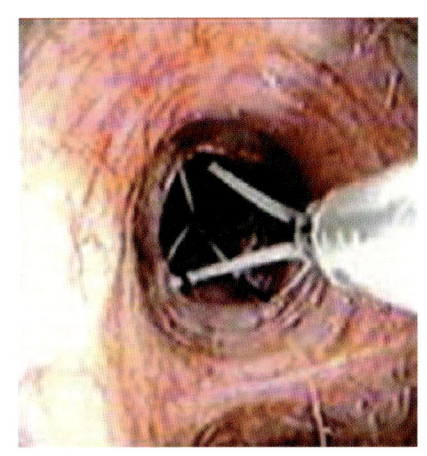

图 28.4 电极阵列 4 个臂与气道壁接触

导管被激活前，电极阵列的 4 个臂均应与气道壁接触。2018 波士顿科学公司或其附属公司保留所有权利。

送射频能量，该能量由控制器发出听觉提示信号，重复 10 s，直到激活完成。此时，释放驱动器以使阵列回纳，并将导管在气道中移动 5~10 mm 的距离，确保治疗区域无重叠（图 28.5）。然后在新位置重复激活，如此循环。电极篮 4 根电线中的 1 根有反馈回路，其中包含接地。如果在任何激活过程中，此导线失去了与气道壁的充分接触，控制器则会发出具有不同音调的听觉信号，以提醒术者修改阵列位置，并且终止激活。

助手应在专用的纸质气道树图谱上记录所有接受治疗的气道，以尽量减少遗漏并确保最大程度的治疗。一旦靶肺叶的所有气道都接受了射频能量治疗，该疗程即完成。每次支气管镜操作预期激活数为 80~120 次。

BT 治疗后，应根据常规的医疗指南指导患者康复。由于大多数患者会在 BT 治疗后即刻表现出哮喘症状加重（AIR-2 研究中为 85%），因此建议术后密切监测数小时。术后住院标准包括持续或重度咳嗽、呼吸困难、低氧血症、血流动力学不稳定、咯血（4 h 恢复期内＞50 mL）或非预期的感觉异常。应仔细指导出院的患者自我关注这些体征和症状的发生、发展，并尽早通知相关医疗照护人员或急诊就诊。建议在第 1 天、第 2 天和第 7 天进行电话随访，并在下一次 BT 治疗前进行临床访视。

28.6　长期疗效和未来研究方向

BT 研究中观察到的组织学和临床效应似乎都持续了至少数年。RISA 和 AIR-2 研究对各自的 BT 队列进行了治疗后 5 年的随访[44,45]。结果发现在长期随访期间，BT 治疗后第 1 年观察到的急性加重率、急诊就诊率和住院率的下降基本保持不变。此外，肺功能的几项指标保持稳定，在高分辨率 CT 上未发现新的结构异常。在随机研究中，只有 AIR 研究对对照组受试者

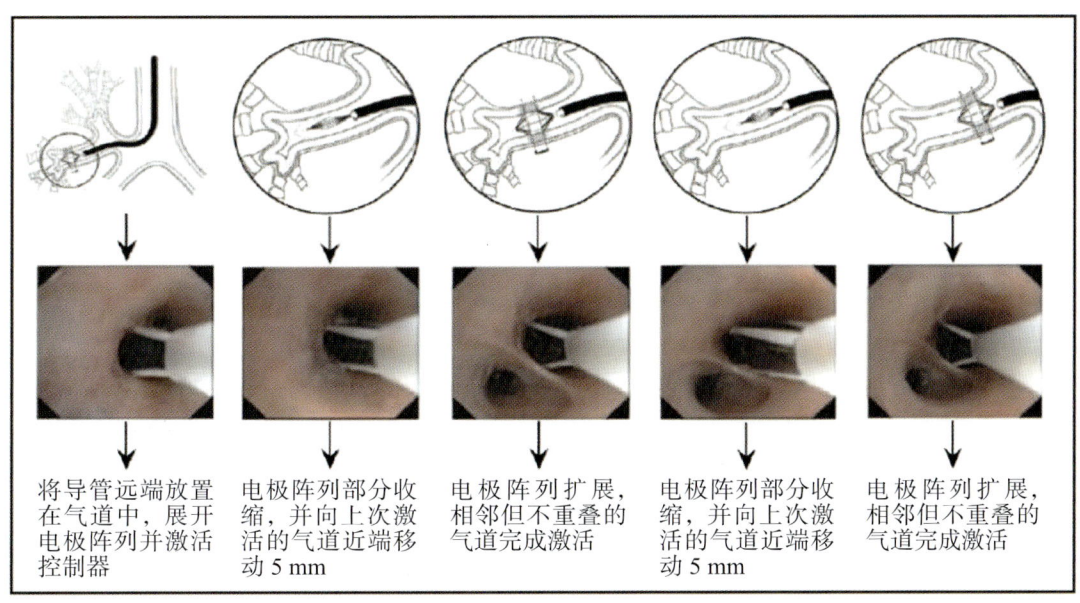

图 28.5　支气管热成形术期间进行连续激活的建议操作顺序

波士顿科学公司或其附属公司保留所有权利。

进行了长期随访，与 BT 队列相比，24 名对照组受试者接受了总计 3 年的研究后评估[46]。在第 2 年和第 3 年，与接受 BT 治疗的队列相比，对照组中的 AHR 更严重。两组的呼吸系统不良事件、急诊就诊和住院率均保持在较低水平且稳定。

最近的几个对 BT 治疗期间和术后 ASM 变化的研究发现，ASM 量减少和 I 型胶原沉积的结果相一致。在治疗后即刻和长期随访期间，这些变化与 BT 治疗后临床结果的改善相关[23,47-49]。

尽管有越来越多的证据支持 BT 对 ASM 的影响，但其背后确切机制仍不完全清楚，需要进一步评估。最近的一项研究发现，BT 相关 ASM 降低的同时伴有上皮下基底膜、上皮神经内分泌细胞以及黏膜下 ASM 相关神经的变化[49]。分析 ASM 内炎性细胞（如中性粒细胞、嗜酸性粒细胞和肥大细胞）数量和功能与 BT 相关变化的研究很少且相互矛盾[23,49,50]。此外，BT 相关作用对气道上皮、ECM 和血管网络的影响程度和意义尚未明确。

BT 对气道的影响范围也尚不清楚。最近的一份报告指出，约 1/3 的患者在 BT 治疗后，未治疗肺叶即刻出现急性放射影像异常[51]。有趣的是，Pretolani 等在重度哮喘患者未治疗的右肺中叶发现 ASM 减少和其他组织学变化（对照部位：与来自同一个体，经 BT 治疗的气道进行比较）[22]。这些发现表明热效应扩展到了直接治疗区以外。使用肺泡一氧化氮测定，Van Veen 等证明了哮喘严重程度与外周气道受累之间的相关性[52]。Dolhnikoff 等发现，致死性哮喘会造成小气道外壁发生显著的重塑[53]。这些研究和其他研究表明，外周气道树在严重疾病中可能发挥更大的作用[8]。总之，这些发现不仅突出了 BT 可能获益的复杂病理生理机制，而且对当前方法的适度性提示了疑问：过于激进、不够或恰到好处？新型支气管镜和引导技术能使支气管镜医师到达比 AIR-2 研究更远的气道。如果未来的研究支持这种方法，结合其他新兴技术，这可以扩大治疗领域和更精确地输送能量。

其他的研究也有助于确定最佳的 BT 目标治疗人群。非特异性（非 Th2 型）哮喘患者可能更适合 BT，因为他们往往有更频繁的住院和耐药性[34,54-56]。然而，BT 临床研究尚未特别关注这些表型。另一个值得关注的领域是使用 HRCT、磁共振成像（magnetic resonance imaging，MRI）和光学相干断层扫描（optical coherence tomography，OCT）等成像模式来帮助识别更有可能受益于 BT 的患者[57-60]。OCT 是一种基于光的高分辨率成像技术，已被证明可预测组织学结果，可能具有广阔的应用前景。其特点允许对单个气道壁层进行准确和可重复的体内评估，因此可能有助于更精确地识别 BT 目标治疗人群、实时定位靶气道和监测治疗反应。

最后，分子表型和生物标志物的揭示有助于区分应答者和非应答者，这将为个性化哮喘治疗提供重要的临床辅助手段。分析这些问题的大型注册和随机研究正在进行中。

28.7 结论

BT 是一种治疗重度持续性哮喘的新型非药物内镜治疗方法。支气管镜操作中向支气管壁施加射频能量以减少气道平滑肌量，可改善哮喘患者相关的生活质量，降低急性加重率，减少急诊就诊和住院次数。总体而言，这是一个耐受良好的手术，很少发生严重的不良事件。治疗后，临床效应可至少持续数年。正在进行的研究可能会加深对其病理生理学作用机制的理解，并有助于进一步定义和明确最有可能受益的患者。

参考文献

1. Nunes, C., Pereira, A.M., and Morais-Almeida, M. (2017). Asthma costs and social impact. *Asthma Res. Pract.* 3: 1.
2. Doeing, D.C. and Solway, J. (2013). Airway smooth muscle in the pathophysiology and treatment of asthma. *J. Appl. Physiol.* 114: 834–843.
3. Ma, X., Cheng, Z., Kong, H. et al. (2002). Changes in biophysical and biochemical properties of single bronchial smooth muscle cells from asthmatic subjects. *Am. J. Physiol. Lung Cell. Mol. Physiol.* 283: L1181–L1189.
4. Brightling, C.E., Bradding, P., Symon, F.A. et al. (2002). Mast-cell infiltration of airway smooth muscle in asthma. *N. Engl. J. Med.* 346: 1699–1705.
5. Hirst, S.J. (2003). Regulation of airway smooth muscle cell immunomodulatory function: role in asthma. *Respir. Physiol. Neurobiol.* 137: 309–326.
6. Damera, G., Tliba, O., and Panettieri, R.A. (2009). Airway smooth muscle as an immunomodulatory cell. *Pulm. Pharmacol. Ther.* 22: 353–359.
7. Koziol-White, C.J. and Panettieri, R.A. (2011). Airway smooth muscle and immunomodulation in acute exacerbations of airway disease. *Immunol. Rev.* 242: 178–185.
8. James, A.L., Elliot, J.G., Jones, R.L. et al. (2012). Airway smooth muscle hypertrophy and hyperplasia in asthma. *Am. J. Respir. Crit. Care Med.* 185: 1058–1064.
9. Carroll, N., Elliot, J., Morton, A., and James, A. (1993). The structure of large and small airways in nonfatal and fatal

asthma. *Am. Rev. Respir. Dis.* 147: 405–410.
10 Benayoun, L., Druilhe, A., Dombret, M.C. et al. (2003). Airway structural alterations selectively associated with severe asthma. *Am. J. Respir. Crit. Care Med.* 167: 1360–1368.
11 James, A.L., Bai,T.R., Mauad,T. et al. (2009). Airway smooth muscle thickness in asthma is related to severity but not duration of asthma. *Eur. Respir. J.* 34: 1040–1045.
12 Gordon, I.O., Husain, A.N., Charbeneau, J. et al. (2013). Endobronchial biopsy: a guide for asthma therapy selection in the era of bronchial thermoplasty. *J. Asthma* 50: 634–641.
13 O'Reilly, R., Ullmann, N., Irving, S. et al. (2013). Increased airway smooth muscle in preschool wheezers who have asthma at school age. *J. Allergy Clin. Immunol.* 131: 1024–1032.
14 Fernandes, D., Guida, E., Koutsoubos,V. et al. (1999). Glucocorticoids inhibit proliferation, cyclin D1 expression, and retinoblastoma protein phosphorylation, but not activity of the extracellular-regulated kinases in human cultured airway smooth muscle. *Am. J. Respir. Cell Mol. Biol.* 21: 77–88.
15 Fernandes, D.J., Mitchell, R.W., Lakser, O. et al. (2003). Do inflammatory mediators influence the contribution of airway smooth muscle contraction to airway hyperresponsiveness in asthma? *J.Appl. Physiol.* 95: 844–853.
16 Ammit, A.J. and Panettieri, R.A. (2003). Airway smooth muscle cell hyperplasia: a therapeutic target in airway remodeling in asthma? *Prog. Cell Cycle Res.* 5: 49–57.
17 Miller, M., Cho, J.Y., McElwain, K. et al. (2006). Corticosteroids prevent myofibroblast accumulation and airway remodeling in mice. *Am. J. Physiol. Lung Cell. Mol. Physiol.* 290: L162–L169.
18 Bullone, M., Vargas, A., Elce,Y. et al. (2017). Fluticasone/salmeterol reduces remodelling and neutrophilic inflammation in severe equine asthma. *Sci. Rep.* 7: 8843.
19 Fernando, H.C., de Hoyos, A., Landreneau, R.J. et al. (2005). Radiofrequency ablation for the treatment of non-small cell lung cancer in marginal surgical candidates. *J. Thorac. Cardiovasc. Surg.* 129: 639–644.
20 Benussi, S., Nascimbene, S., Calori, G. et al. (2005). Surgical ablation of atrial fibrillation with a novel bipolar radiofrequency device. *J. Thorac. Cardiovasc. Surg.* 130: 491–497.
21 Dyrda, P., Tazzeo, T., DoHarris, L. et al. (2011). Acute response of airway muscle to extreme temperature includes disruption of actin-myosin interaction. *Am. J. Respir. Cell Mol. Biol.* 44: 213–221.
22 Pretolani, M., Dombret, M.C., Thabut, G. et al. (2014). Reduction of airway smooth muscle mass by bronchial thermoplasty in patients with severe asthma. *Am. J. Respir. Crit. Care Med.* 190: 1452–1454.
23 Denner, D.R., Doeing, D.C., Hogarth, D.K. et al. (2015). Airway inflammation after bronchial thermoplasty for severe asthma. *Ann. Am. Thorac. Soc.* 12: 1302–1309.
24 Danek, C.J., Lombard, C.M., Dungworth, D.L. et al. (2004). Reduction in airway hyperresponsiveness to methacholine by the application of RF energy in dogs. *J. Appl. Physiol.* 97: 1946–1953.
25 Brown, R.H., Wizeman,W., Danek, C., and Mitzner, W. (2005). Effect of bronchial thermoplasty on airway distensibility. *Eur. Respir. J.* 26: 277–282.
26 Brown, R.H., Wizeman,W., Danek, C., and Mitzner, W. (2005). In vivo evaluation of the effectiveness of bronchial thermoplasty with computed tomography. *J. Appl. Physiol.* 98: 1603–1606.
27 Miller, J.D., Cox, G., Vincic, L. et al. (2005). A prospective feasibility study of bronchial thermoplasty in the human airway. *Chest* 127: 1999–2006.
28 Cox, G., Miller, J.D., McWilliams, A. et al. (2006). Bronchial thermoplasty for asthma. *Am. J. Respir. Crit. Care Med.* 173: 965–969.
29 Cox, G., Thomson, N.C., Rubin, A.S. et al. (2007). Asthma control during the year after bronchial thermoplasty. *N. Engl. J. Med.* 356: 1327–1337.
30 Pavord,I.D., Cox, G., Thomson,N.C. et al. (2007). Safety and efficacy of bronchial thermoplastyin symptomatic, severe asthma. *Am. J. Respir. Crit. CareMed.* 176: 1185–1191.
31 Castro, M., Rubin, A.S., Laviolette, M. et al. (2010). Effectiveness and safety of bronchial thermoplasty in the treatment of severe asthma: a multicenter, randomized, double-blind, sham-controlled clinical trial. *Am. J. Respir. Crit. Care Med.* 181: 116–124.
32 Juniper, E.F., Guyatt, G.H., Willan, A., and Griffith, L.E. (1994). Determining a minimal important change in a disease-specific quality of life questionnaire. *J. Clin. Epidemiol.* 47: 81–87.
33 Sheshadri, A., McKenzie, M., and Castro, M. (2014). Critical review of bronchial thermoplasty: where should it fit into asthma therapy? *Curr. Allergy Asthma Rep.* 14: 470.
34 Chung, K.F., Wenzel, S.E., Brozek, J.L. et al. (2014). International ERS/ATS guidelines on definition, evaluation and treatment of severe asthma. *Eur. Respir. J.* 43: 343–373.
35 Bel, E.H. (2010). Bronchial thermoplasty: has the promise been met? *Am. J. Respir. Crit. Care Med.* 181: 101–102.
36 Michaud, G. and Ernst, A. (2011). Counterpoint: efficacy of bronchial thermoplasty for patients with severe asthma. Is there sufficient evidence? Not yet. *Chest* 140: 576–577.
37 Shifren, A., Chen, A., and Castro, M. (2011). Point: efficacy of bronchial thermoplasty for patients with severe asthma. Is there sufficient evidence? Yes. *Chest* 140: 573–575.
38 Iyer,V.N. and Lim,K.G. (2014). Bronchial thermoplasty: reappraising the evidence (or lack thereof). *Chest* 146: 17–21.
39 Castro, M., Cox, G., Wechsler, M.E., and Niven, R.M. (2015). Bronchial thermoplasty: ready for prime time – the evidence is there! *Chest* 147: e73–e74.
40 Laxmanan, B., Egressy, K., Murgu, S.D. et al. (2016). Advances in bronchial thermoplasty. *Chest* 150: 694–704.
41 Doeing, D.C., Mahajan, A.K., White, S.R. et al. (2013). Safety and feasibility of bronchial thermoplasty in asthma patients with very severe fixed airflow obstruction: a case series. *J. Asthma* 50: 215–218.
42 Chupp, G., Laviolette, M., Cohn, L. et al. (2017). Long-term outcomes of bronchial thermoplasty in subjects with severe asthma: a comparison of 3-year follow-up results from two prospective multicentre studies. *Eur. Respir. J.* 50.
43 Sheshadri, A., Castro, M., and Chen, A. (2013). Bronchial

44 Pavord, I.D., Thomson, N.C., Niven, R.M. et al. (2013). Safety of bronchial thermoplasty in patients with severe refractory asthma. *Ann. Allergy Asthma Immunol.* 111: 402–407.

45 Wechsler, M.E., Laviolette, M., Rubin, A.S. et al. (2013). Bronchial thermoplasty: long-term safety and effectiveness in patients with severe persistent asthma. *J. Allergy Clin. Immunol.* 132: 1295–1302.

46 Thomson, N.C., Rubin, A.S., Niven, R.M. et al. (2011). Long-term (5 year) safety of bronchial thermoplasty: Asthma Intervention Research (AIR) trial. *BMC Pulm. Med.* 11: 8.

47 Chakir, J., Haj-Salem, I., Gras, D. et al. (2015). Effects of bronchial thermoplasty on airway smooth muscle and collagen deposition in asthma. *Ann. Am. Thorac. Soc.* 12: 1612–1618.

48 Salem, I.H., Boulet, L.P., Biardel, S. et al. (2016). Long-term effects of bronchial thermoplasty on airway smooth muscle and reticular basement membrane thickness in severe asthma. *Ann. Am. Thorac. Soc.* 13: 1426–1428.

49 Pretolani, M., Bergqvist, A., Thabut, G. et al. (2017). Effectiveness of bronchial thermoplasty in patients with severe refractory asthma: clinical and histopathologic correlations. *J. Allergy Clin. Immunol.* 139: 1176–1185.

50 d'Hooghe, J.N.S., ten Hacken, N.H.T., Weersink, E.J.M. et al. (2018). Emerging understanding of the mechanism of action of bronchial thermoplasty in asthma. *Pharmacol. Ther.* 181: 101–107.

51 d'Hooghe, J.N.S., van den Berk, I.A.H., Annema, J.T., and Bonta, P.I. (2017). Acute radiological abnormalities after bronchial thermoplasty: a prospective cohort trial. *Respiration* 94: 258–262.

52 van Veen, I.H., Sterk, P.J., Schot, R. et al. (2006). Alveolar nitric oxide versus measures of peripheral airway dysfunction in severe asthma. *Eur. Respir. J.* 27: 951–956.

53 Dolhnikoff, M., da Silva, L.F., de Araujo, B.B. et al. (2009). The outer wall of small airways is a major site of remodeling in fatal asthma. *J. Allergy Clin. Immunol.* 123: 1090–1097.

54 Woodruff, P.G., Modrek, B., Choy, D.F. et al. (2009). T-helper type 2-driven inflammation defines major subphenotypes of asthma. *Am. J. Respir. Crit. Care Med.* 180: 388–395.

55 Moore, W.C., Meyers, D.A., Wenzel, S.E. et al. (2010). Identification of asthma phenotypes using cluster analysis in the Severe Asthma Research Program. *Am. J. Respir. Crit. Care Med.* 181: 315–323.

56 Wenzel, S. (2012). Severe asthma: from characteristics to phenotypes to endotypes. *Clin. Exp. Allergy* 42: 650–658.

57 Hou, R., Le, T., Murgu, S.D. et al. (2011). Recent advances in optical coherence tomography for the diagnoses of lung disorders. *Expert Rev. Respir. Med.* 5: 711–724.

58 Castro, M., Fain, S.B., Hoffman, E.A. et al. (2011). Lung imaging in asthmatic patients: the picture is clearer. *J. Allergy Clin. Immunol.* 128: 467–478.

59 Trivedi, A., Hall, C., Hoffman, E.A. et al. (2017). Using imaging as a biomarker for asthma. *J. Allergy Clin. Immunol.* 139: 1–10.

60 d'Hooghe, J.N.S., Goorsenberg, A.W.M., de Bruin, D.M. et al. (2017). Optical coherence tomography for identification and quantification of human airway wall layers. *PLoS One* 12: e0184145.

第 29 章

肺气肿的内镜下治疗

Stefano Gasparini[1,2] and Martina Bonifazi[1,2]
[1] Department of Biomedical Sciences and Public Health,
Università Politecnica delle Marche, Ancona, Italy
[2] Pulmonary Diseases Unit, Department of Internal Medicine,
Azienda Ospedaliero-Universitaria 'Ospedali Riuniti', Ancona, Italy

（译者：郑　宇　译者单位：上海交通大学医学院附属仁济医院）

29.1　引言

慢性阻塞性肺疾病（chronic obstructive pulmonary disease，COPD）是一种在有害颗粒和气体的作用下，以持续性气流受限伴气道和肺慢性炎症为特征的常见呼吸系统疾病[1]。尽管近年来对其发病机制的研究、治疗和管理方面取得了许多进展，但COPD仍然是全球发病和死亡最常见的原因之一，造成相应的社会和经济负担，并且这种情况在未来几十年仍将进一步加剧。由于危险因素（如吸烟、室外/室内空气污染）日趋普遍和全球人口老龄化[1]，按照目前的流行病学趋势，到2020年COPD将成为全球第三大死亡原因。根据联合国《2015年世界人口展望（修订版）》，到2100年，预计60岁以上的人口总数将增加1倍以上，而80岁以上的人口数将增加7倍以上[2]。由于寿命延长使得在危险因素下暴露的时间增加，同时老龄本身也是COPD发病和发展的危险因素，因此年龄结构的巨大变化在COPD流行病学和疾病负担中扮演了重要角色。

COPD当前的治疗策略包括戒烟、接种流感和肺炎球菌疫苗、肺康复、氧疗和药物治疗[1]。支气管扩张剂治疗虽然不能改善长期的肺功能下降，但被强烈推荐用于缓解症状、减少急性加重、改善运动能力和生活质量[1]。然而，在最新的GOLD报告中强调COPD是一种包含不同表型的疾病，治疗策略应当个性化，根据患者的具体特征量身定制[1]。由于缺乏减少过度充气的有效手段，晚期肺气肿患者在现有药物的治疗中获益有限。

肺过度充气是指在潮气末（自主）呼气结束时肺和气道内气体量的异常增加[3]。重度肺气肿患者的肺泡结构被破坏，周围结缔组织消失，肺的弹性回缩力下降，以及缺乏肺泡支撑所导致的小气道过度塌陷。这些呼吸力学的改变，加上气道的内在炎症，导致显著的呼气气流受限和进行性空气潴留，从而转为肺功能评估时的残气量（residual volume，RV）增加。在这种情况下，呼吸系统的静态/弹性平衡点上移到更大的容积位，其最主要的后果是呼气时的胸内正压以及通气负荷增加[3]。当呼吸急促时，呼气时间缩短，上述的恶性循环进一步加剧。此外，肺容积的增大使得膈肌缩短变平，肌长度–肌张力呈负性关系，收缩力降低。与此同时，整个胸廓的改变在力学上不利于吸气肌工作，降低了其产生压力的能力。

总而言之，在肺气肿患者呼吸困难和活动耐量下降的病理生理过程中，肺过度充气是关键原因，并且导致预后不佳[4,5]。

这种病理生理机制为靶向治疗的研发——肺减

容术提供了理论依据。该手术（外科或内镜下）目的是通过去除肺实质受损最严重的区域来减少过度充气，从而改善剩余组织的呼吸功能，减少呼吸做功。

尽管外科肺减容（surgical lung volume reduction，LVRS）在20世纪50年代就开始首次尝试，但直到2003年[6]，随着美国国家肺气肿治疗试验（NETT）结果公布[7]，该手术才被证实可显著改善肺气肿患者的临床症状和肺功能。在NETT研究中，共有1 218名受试者随机接受LVRS（n=608）或最佳医疗照护（n=610），与对照组相比，LVRS组患者活动耐量总体得到改善（长达24个月）。另一方面，因为在术后90天内观察到死亡率为7.9%，并且高达1/3的患者因出现并发症并在术后1个月仍在接受住院治疗[6]，使得人们对其安全性和成本效益存在顾虑。而亚组分析显示，以上叶为主的肺气肿以及经康复治疗后仍运动能力低下的患者与对照组相比死亡率更低（分别为2.9%和3.3%），随访5年中生存获益证实了这点。

LVRS是一种适用于非均质型上叶肺气肿患者的治疗选择[1]。然而，与LVRS相关的死亡率和成本效益存疑，使得人们反思如何选择创伤更小的替代方法实现LVR，如内镜技术［生物性肺减容（biological lung volume reduction，BLVR）][8]。

过去15年来，取得同样临床获益的同时降低风险和成本的这一宗旨在介入肺脏病领域一直深入人心，并已成功研发了多种不同的技术。根据其潜在的作用机制和可逆性，可将其主要分为两类：可逆性封堵装置和不可逆性非封堵装置（表29.1）。第一类以单向活瓣为代表，主要是将过度充气最明显的肺叶闭塞和不张。非封堵性装置是通过诱导不可逆的肺实质反应来达到去除目标肺叶的目的，包括线圈和硬化剂，如密封剂和热蒸汽消融[8]。活瓣、线圈和热蒸汽消融已在欧洲获批上市[9]。

表29.1 支气管镜肺减容技术（按照作用机制和可逆性划分）

可逆的封堵装置	不可逆的非封堵装置
单向活瓣	线圈
EBV	密封剂
IBV	热蒸汽消融

EBV、IBV，支气管内单向活瓣。

29.2 单向活瓣

单向活瓣是在BLVR领域研究最广泛的装置，迄今为止接受治疗的患者数量最多。目前有两种单向活瓣可供使用：EBV：endobronchial valves（Zephyr®，Pulmonx公司，加利福尼亚州，美国）和IBV：intrabronchial valves（奥林巴斯公司，华盛顿州，美国）。虽然略有不同，但两者均可阻止气体被吸入，而在呼气时允许空气和分泌物排出，减少过度充气。

EBV有不同的尺寸，由覆盖有硅胶的镍钛合金网制成，内有双层硅胶膜，在呼气时打开，吸气时关闭（图29.1 A）。IBV有4种不同尺寸，为伞形装置，由覆盖有聚氨酯膜的镍钛合金网制成，通过5个钩状锚钉固定在支气管壁上（图29.1 B）。[8]

EBV用于治疗肺气肿的首个大型随机试验VENT研究，纳入了美国的31个中心共321例患者[10]和欧洲的23个中心共171例患者[11]，结果显示：与接受最佳药物治疗的对照组受试者相比，尽管治疗组的肺功能、运动耐量和生活质量的改善幅度不大，但具有统计学意义。治疗组总体的获益可能没有临床意义，但之后的亚组分析显示非均质型肺气肿（美国队列）和叶间裂完整的患者效果更佳[12]。随后所有的大型临床试验也证实了完整的叶间裂，即不存在叶间侧支通气（interlobar collateral ventilation，CV），是手术成功的预测因素[13-16]，成为置入活瓣治疗的必要条件。肺叶之间存在侧支通气确实会抵消活瓣效果，因此，对这一特征的准确判断是筛选患者的关键。活瓣治疗的成功取决于是否能达到肺叶的完全封堵从而导致肺不张。而封堵不完全时，气体可通过活瓣与支气管壁间的缝隙进入而造成漏气[8]。VENT研究中首次确认了达到完全肺不张的重要性，尽管这会使气胸发生的风险升高。此后Eberhardt等也相继证实，单侧的完全封堵疗效优于双侧的不完全封堵[17]。

15年来，EBV治疗的大量经验明确显示基线肺形态学特征（完整的叶间裂和非均质型肺气肿）和手术效果方面（手术后达到完全性肺不张）(图29.2)对于治疗结局至关重要。因此，强烈建议术前对患者进行仔细筛选并予以娴熟的手术技术保障。

通过高分辨率计算机断层扫描（high-resolution computed tomography，HRCT）对叶间裂的完整性进行分析已开展数年，并且成为术前常规的准备工作。

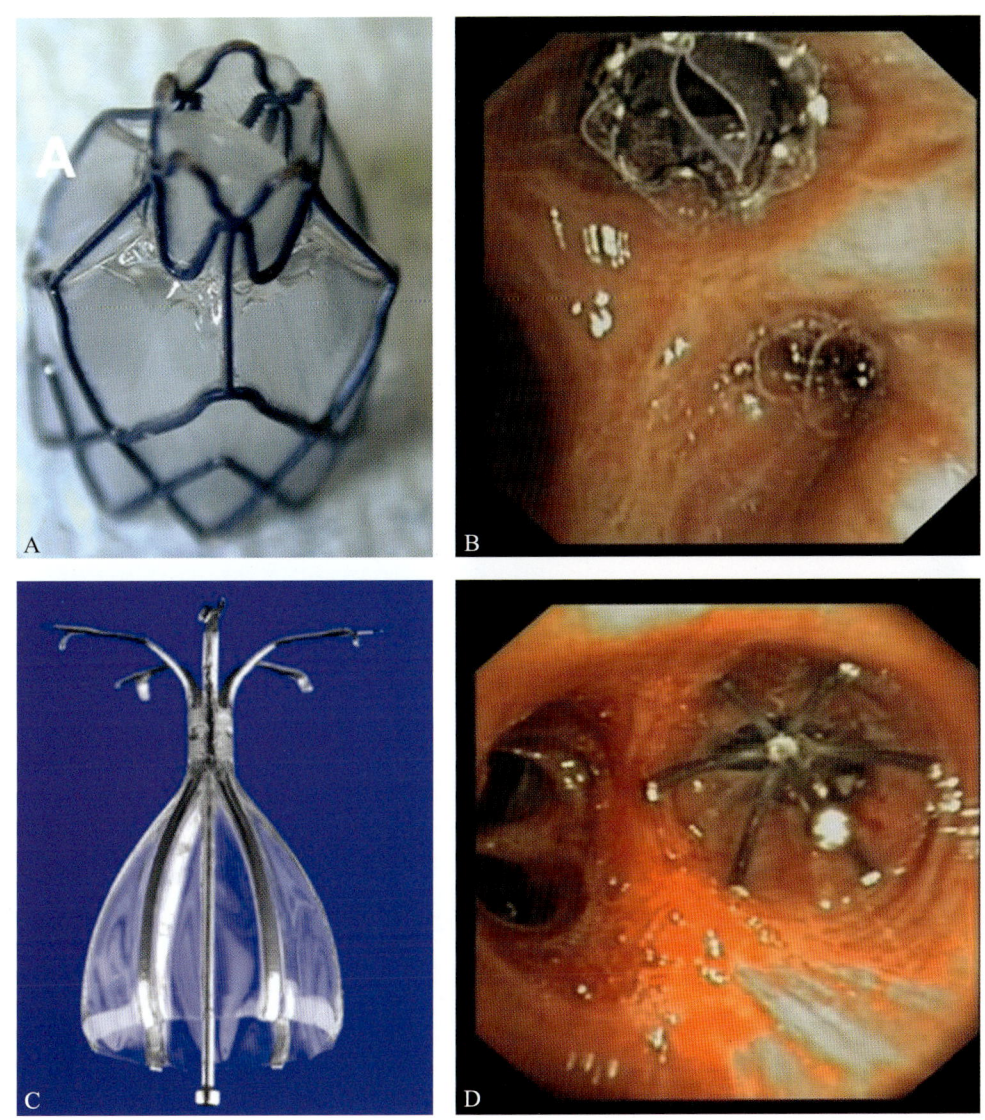

图 29.1　支气管内单向活瓣
A、B. Zephyr® 支气管内单向活瓣（EBV）；C、D. 支气管内单向活瓣（IBV）。

然而，这种评估的主观性使其在某些情况下不太可靠，并且严重依赖于操作人员的经验，目前已开发了其他的方法来客观评估叶间裂的完整性和是否存在 CV，如 Chartis 系统和定量 CT。

Chartis 系统（Pulmonx 公司）可在支气管镜下采用一根连接外部控制台的球囊导管直接测量靶区肺叶是否存在 CV[18]。进入目标支气管后导管球囊充气阻塞空气进入，同时允许远端肺组织呼出气体。如呼气流量持续存在即表明 CV 的存在，而流量逐渐下降到零则表明 CV 不存在。在 BeLieVer-HIfi 研究中，使用 Chartis 进行患者筛选显著改善了疗效[14]，在后续的研究[13,15,16,19]中只对叶间裂完整和 Chartis 测量阴性的患者进行治疗，治疗结果均显示成功。

通过回顾性分析 HRCT 和 Chartis 系统对患者预后的预测价值，发现两种方法都能准确预测活瓣治疗的效果，HRCT 可准确预测叶间裂完整度在 90% 以上的患者的预后。换言之，当患者被经验丰富的操作人员通过薄层 HRCT 评估为叶间裂完整度在 90% 以上时，可认为患者适合接受活瓣置入而无须进一步评估，因为 Chartis 系统在这种情况下较 HRCT 没有明显优势。相比之下，对于叶间裂完整度在 75%~90% 之间的病例则情况较为复杂，建议增加 Chartis 系统评估，因为它可以优化患者的选择。最后，HRCT 显示叶间裂完整度低于 75% 的患者，达到肺不张的阴性预测值为

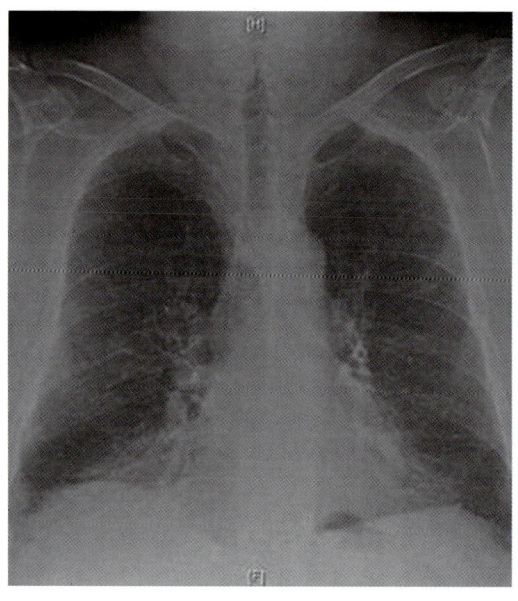 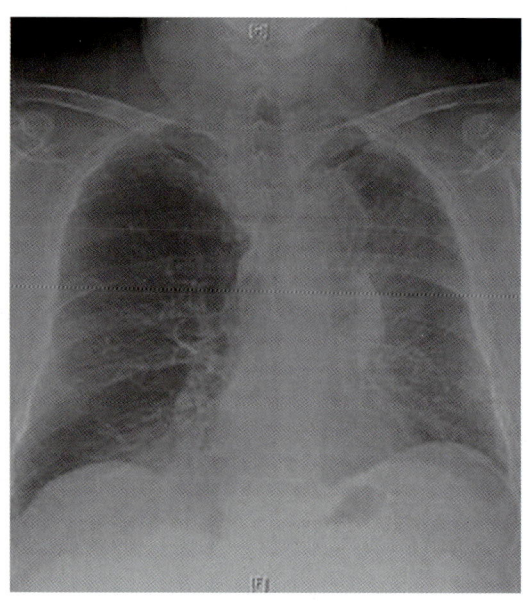

图 29.2　活瓣置入后影像学可见左肺下叶不张和膈肌抬高

100%，因此，在这种情况不适合 EBV 治疗，Chartis 系统评估也没有意义[20]。

但考虑到人为因素对于 HRCT 视觉评估上的局限性，最近数家公司开发了计算机半自动化程序，以减少观察者之间的差异，最大程度减少人为的不准确性。定量 CT（quantitative CT，QCT）是其中一种很有应用前景的工具，可以提供叶间裂完整性、组织密度和血管容积的定量测量。现已有回顾性研究分析了它与 Chartis 系统联合预测 EBV 治疗效果。研究发现，Chartis 系统仅对叶间裂完整度为 80%~95% 的患者提供了额外的价值[21]。在另一项研究中，将 QCT 与 Chartis 系统进行回顾性比较[22]。首先，作者在 34 个基线变量中确定了主要的 QCT 预测因子（结局定义为 3 个月时目标肺叶体积减少>350 mL），这些变量包括叶间裂完整度、低衰减区和小血管的血管容积百分比。使用这些预测因子的 QCT 准确度与 Chartis 相当（78.8% 比 75.8%），进一步证实了其在患者筛选中的前景。因此，在最新的专家共识推荐，如有条件的情况下内镜下肺减容应当术前使用 QCT 进行分析评估[20]。

IMPACT 研究评估了在不存在 CV 且均质型肺气肿患者中 EBV 治疗的价值，仅仅纳入了这一特定人群。在这项前瞻性多中心研究中，83 名患者被随机分组到 EBV 联合标准治疗组或单纯标准治疗组，主要终点是 FEV_1 的百分比变化。治疗 3 个月的结果显示 FEV_1、生活质量和运动耐量显著改善，6 个月时有 87.6% 的患者至少仍然能达到其中一个研究终点[15]。

最终，在德国进行的一项前瞻性、观察性多中心临床研究——LIVE 研究中，评价了 Chartis 系统用于日常筛选肺气肿患者并置入 EBV 治疗的长期疗效。总体来看，其治疗耐受性良好，6 个月时的数据显示大多数肺功能参数持续显著改善[19]。

尽管活瓣置入总体上是安全的，但也可能会出现并发症，应引起注意。最常见的不良事件是气胸，发生率高达 25%，其次是 COPD 加重、肺炎、咯血、瓣膜移位和肉芽增生。80% 以上气胸需要置入胸腔引流管，中位发病时间为 2 天。因此，建议常规住院 48~72 h 进行密切监测。在少数病例中，气胸发生在出院后，患者应当有意识到这种风险，以便在症状出现时尽快寻医。该并发症并不会对这些患者的临床结果产生负面影响，因为这是肺容量迅速减少的一种表现，也说明由于精确的筛选使得治疗更加成功[13]。此外，保持卧床休息 48 h 和镇咳治疗可以降低气胸的风险[23]。

自首次发表以来的近十几年，数项随机对照研究和一项真实世界研究提供的许多证据证明，对于以上叶或下叶为主的，不存在 CV 的非均质型肺气肿患者采用单向活瓣治疗，能够持续显著改善肺功能、运动耐量和生活质量。而目前 EBV 对于均质型肺气肿患者的疗效方面的数据仍然有限，可以在登记备案情况下予以考虑。

IBV 治疗的有效性和安全性仅在一项随机对照研究中进行了评估，即在中国进行的 REACH 研究，其在 2016 年伦敦 ERS 大会上发表。大约 100 例非均质型肺气肿（55%上叶，45%下叶）且不存在 CV 的患者随机接受 IBV 置入或最佳药物治疗，主要结果是靶肺叶体积缩小和 FEV_1 的改善。与对照组相比，在治疗 6 个月时观察到两个研究终点均有显著改善。急性加重和气胸是常见的不良事件，分别发生 12 例和 5 例[24]。然而，这项研究尚未发表。虽然研究结果应该与 EBV 相似，但目前该装置的临床数据太过有限，不能直接套用。

29.3 线圈

线圈生物学肺减容术（biological LVR with coils，BLVRC）是指采用线圈（PneumRx 公司，加利福尼亚州，美国）进行肺减容。这种创新疗法旨在恢复肺组织张力并减少肺气肿最严重区域的肺实质过度充气。线圈采用形状记忆镍钛合金装置，以拉直的状态通过可弯曲支气管镜递送到气道，随后在展开时恢复为原始的双圆环形状，达到使受损最严重的肺实质收缩的目的[8]。线圈可在中度镇静或全身麻醉下，使用特定的推送装置通过 X 线透视引导置入。有多种尺寸可供选择，平均每个肺叶需要 10~12 个线圈才能达到足够的疗效。通常双侧上、下肺叶均需治疗，分两个阶段进行（一侧和对侧手术之间间隔 1~4 个月）（图29.3）。尽管线圈可在展开后立即取出，但总的来说还是一种不可逆的治疗方式[12]。

2010 年，Herth 等首次报道了关于应用线圈进行肺减容的初步试验，证明了该治疗方法的可行性和安全性，此后，又有 6 项临床试验进一步评估了其在重度肺气肿患者中的作用[26-31]。无论是否存在 CV，患者的肺容量、运动能力和生活质量均显著改善。尤其是在REVOLENS 研究中，线圈组的 18 例患者（36%）较标准治疗组的 9 例患者（18%）在治疗 6 个月时 6 min 步行试验至少增加 54 m，组间差异为 18%，然而由于短期成本较高，成本-效益比被质疑[27]。

关于线圈技术的进一步的探究来自最新的 RCT 研究——RENEW 研究，这也是迄今为止已发表的最大规模的相关研究。该研究纳入了 315 例重度肺气肿（不均质型和均质型）和重度过度充气（前 170 名患者 RV 占预测值＞225%，后续降至 170%）患者，并在 21 个北美和 5 个欧洲的中心展开。主要研究终点是基线与治疗 12 个月时 6 min 步行试验的绝对值变化（最小临床意义差值，25 m）。治疗组患者的中位变化值为 10.3 m，组间差值为 14.6 m（$P=0.02$）。线圈组中 40.0% 的患者和对照组中 26.9% 的患者出现了 25 m 以上的改善，具有临床意义。治疗组的主要并发症（如需收住院的肺炎和其他潜在危及生命或致死性事件）显著高于对照组，发生率分别为 34.8% 和 19.1%。由于运动耐量的中位变化值不一定具有临床意义，而严重的并发症发生率却明显升高，故该手术风险和获益值得深思。然而，亚组分析（根据肺过度充气和肺气肿的类型将患者分为 4 个亚组）显示不均质型肺气肿亚组和 RV＞225% 预计值的患者治疗效果较好[20]。

这些结果证实了需根据肺气肿的特征和分布正确选择目标肺叶。在技术上，BLVRC 可行的首要条件是在 HRCT 观察到足够的肺实质密度，因为该装置要获得最佳疗效需要有一定的组织量保证，如果肺叶损伤太多或存在巨大肺大疱则不适合应用。换言之，理想的靶肺叶应该是受损严重且过度充气的肺叶，但同时，

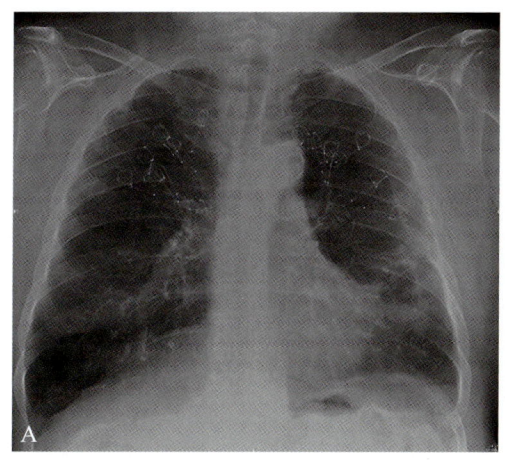 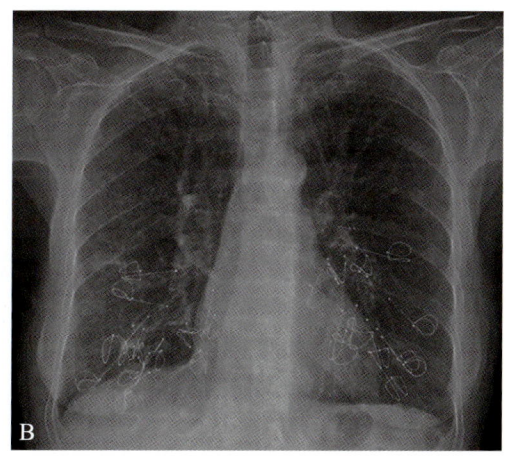

图 29.3 双侧线圈（A. 双肺上叶；B. 双肺下叶）置入后的影像学表现

应该具有足够的健康肺实质，便于线圈发挥效果。

与 BLVRC 相关的最常见并发症包括肺炎、气胸和 COPD 加重。超过 1/3 的肺炎病例为线圈相关的非感染性异常阴影，可能是线圈刺激局部气道导致的炎症反应。尽管这样的情况似乎与良好的疗效有一定关系，但仍需将其视为术后并发症并密切监测。另外术后出血也有报道，而肺不张不常见。因此，无论是胸片或 CT 出现线圈近端的肺部实变应当考虑有肺部并发症的可能。

在最近一项对 86 例患者进行的单中心真实世界回顾性分析中，有 4 例患者因并发症死亡，并且术后得到初步改善的各项肺功能参数，在术后 1 年时基本回到术前状态，这引起了对 BLVRC 技术的长期风险和效益的质疑。

总体而言，基于现有数据，BLVRC 适用于叶间裂不完整、非均质型肺气肿和可能存在重度过度充气（RV＞预计值的 225%）的患者。这项技术在均质型肺气肿患者中的价值已在一项初步研究（n=10）中进行了探讨[30]，同样多项 RCT 的亚组分析[26]中也提示该技术对于均质型肺气肿患者可能有所获益。但是，由于数据有限，需进行相关 RCT 研究后再考虑是否用于均质型肺气肿患者的治疗。

29.4 硬化剂

29.4.1 密封剂

密封剂作用于肺泡水平，主要是诱导肺实质炎性反应，从而导致气道阻塞引起肺不张以及严重受损肺叶的重塑，与叶间裂的完整性无关。第一代生物制剂在一项大型多中心 II 期剂量试验进行了测试，该研究纳入了 50 例非均质型上叶肺气肿患者，结果显示可改善肺功能且安全性可接受。随后两项非盲试验和一项多中心随机试验（ASPIRE）采用合成聚合物泡沫密封剂（Aeris Therapeutics 医疗公司，马塞诸塞州，美国）替代生物制品，但由于缺乏经费而提前终止。然而，由于其在疗效方面的初步数据令人鼓舞，目前正在对该技术进行 RCT 研究，以期通过缓慢增加剂量及支气管镜多次注入增进疗效（NCT 02877479）[20]。

29.4.2 热蒸汽消融

经支气管镜热蒸汽消融（bronchoscopic thermal vapor ablation，BTVA）（InterVapor®，Uptake Medical 公司，华盛顿州，美国）使用高温水蒸气诱导局部炎症反应，促进纤维化和瘢痕形成，从而导致靶肺叶体积减小。该技术的主要优点是其可选择性，因为它可以在肺段水平而不是肺叶水平进行减容，BTVA 可精确定位病变严重和过度充气的肺段，同时保留健康肺段（图 29.4）。从技术上讲，BTVA 是一种相对简单的操作，包括将导管引入目标支气管，通过导管末端膨胀球囊隔离目标肺段，最后输送加热的水蒸气。术前根据肺组织的密度和容积使用专用软件选择目标气道和计算蒸汽剂量。

最初纳入 11 例患者的初步研究显示肺功能改善有限且安全性存疑（7 例严重不良事件），但后来的两项研究证实，无论是否存在叶间侧支通气，非均质型上

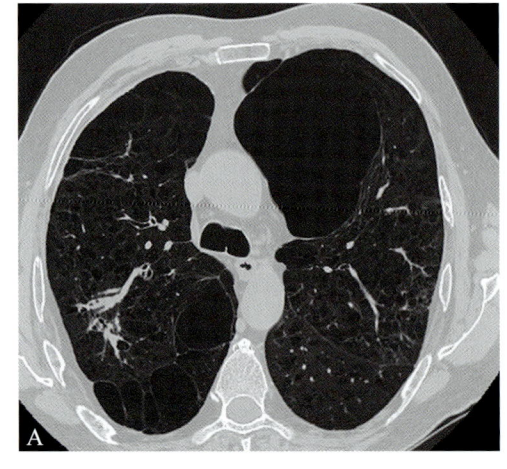
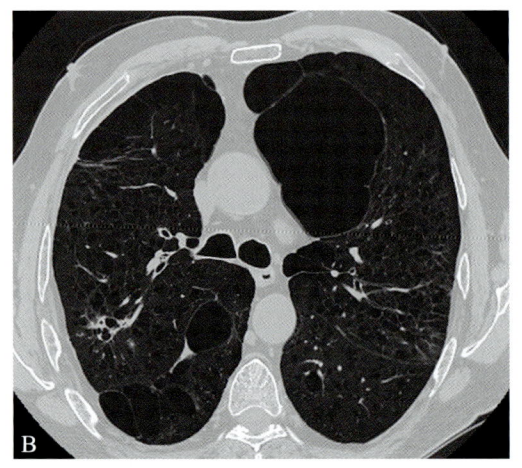

图 29.4 经支气管镜热蒸汽消融术（BVTA）后影像学

A、B. 胸部 CT 显示，BTVA 术后 1 个月，右上肺叶支气管出现节段性纤维化。

叶肺气肿患者的肺功能改善明显。STEP-UP研究是第一项BTVA相关的RCT研究，选择性地只针对受损更严重的上叶部分，同时保留健康的肺段。主要终点为治疗组（$n=45$）和对照组（$n=24$）FEV_1和SGRQ评分[32]。该手术首先在一侧上叶的1个肺段进行，90天后在另一侧上叶的1~2个肺段进行。治疗6个月的结果显示，无论是否存在CV、FEV_1和SGRQ评分的改善均有临床和统计学意义，并且安全性可接受，观察到的唯一的不良事件是25%的患者出现COPD加重。13%的患者在BTVA治疗后的3个月出现炎症反应，如肺部炎症或肺部感染，并伴有不同的症状，如咳嗽、发热、呼吸困难、咯血和炎症标志物升高[33]。为减少炎症反应的风险，所有患者需预防性给予抗生素2周。治疗12个月的数据显示FEV_1和SGRQ评分持续改善，未发生后期并发症[34]。

因此，无论CV是否存在，BTVA可能是对于上叶为主的肺气肿患者的一种有效的治疗选择。其在下叶为主或均质型肺气肿患者的安全性、可行性和有效性，目前正在进行前瞻性研究。

29.5 患者的筛选和治疗原则

29.5.1 临床功能评估

患有严重COPD伴弥漫性肺气肿的患者，尽管已戒烟、接受药物治疗和进行肺康复后但仍有症状时，应评估是否选择BLVR。另一个必要标准是存在明显的肺过度充气，其定义为体积描记法测量肺总量（total capacity，TLC）>100%和RV>175%。其他标准包括FEV_1占预计值的15%~45%，吸入空气时PaO_2>45 mmHg，6 min步行测试>140 m，没有明显的高碳酸血症。禁忌证包括未戒烟、α_1抗胰蛋白酶缺乏、感染活动期、严重肺动脉高压、心脏疾病未稳定以及手术前7天内不能暂停抗血小板或抗凝治疗[4]。BLVR治疗没有绝对禁忌证，除非它们可能严重影响患者的短期预后，因此术前应仔细评估各项合并症。

尽管一些学者建议治疗年龄在40~75岁之间，但目前对于年龄上限未达成共识。由于研究人群的年龄很少超过70岁，故老年患者的数据非常有限。然而仅凭年龄就将老年患者排除在BLVR的适应证之外是不合适的，应根据总体状态来指导患者的选择，如肺气肿的严重度和合并症情况。不适合手术或肺部受损过于严重的患者不太可能从BLVR中获益。

29.5.2 放射学评估

放射学评估建议使用非增强CT，并要求薄层（0.6~1.25 mm）扫描。评估患者是否存在相对或绝对的禁忌证是放射科医师的首要任务，如疑似癌症、间质纤维化、支气管扩张、严重的气管支气管软化或其他可能影响手术预后和风险-获益的异常情况。随后，肺气肿形态学的评估对选择何种BLVR的方法起到至关重要的作用。特别是需要对叶间裂的完整性和肺气肿的分布范围（非均质型/均质型）进行详细的评估，以选择合适的目标肺叶以及治疗方法。

如前所述，当叶间裂完整度百分比低于或高于特定阈值时，叶间裂完整度的定性、半定量和定量评估均能提供较高的预测价值（阳性或阴性）。而在不太明确的情况下，应当结合如Chartis系统等其他措施来进一步评估。

多年来，肺气肿范围和严重程度的术前评估一直基于半定量HRCT视觉评分（0~5分，其中5分表示损伤最严重的区域），但这种方法受观察者间的差异性影响很大。使用"密度掩膜"（density mask）法可以对肺气肿的评估更加客观、更具重复性。该方法是通过预设的CT阈值用以区分正常衰减区域和低衰减区域（low attenuation areas，LAA）。CT衰减值的测量使用亨氏单位（Hounsfield units，HU）。肺气肿应用密度值低于设定阈值的区域占肺的百分比（LAA%）来表示，在吸气末扫描时为-950 HU或-910 HU。后一个阈值适用于厚层（>3 mm）CT扫描。在1 mm的非增强CT扫描时通常采用-950 HU作为阈值。目前已经开发了许多专用的自动化程序（如QCT）来优化肺气肿的测量。这些程序可计算肺总量、左右肺容积、平均肺密度、低衰减区百分比（LAA%）、叶间裂完整度和肺气肿的区域分布。同侧肺叶不均质通常定义为各肺叶之间LAA的百分比差异，阈值为-950 HU时为LAA%>15%，阈值为-910 HU时为>25%。

然而，肺气肿定量评估的预测价值尚未确定，因为测量值可能受到与患者相关手术因素（如年龄、吸气深度等）以及解剖结构异常（如病变和浸润）的影响。此外，目前还没有数据可用于验证线圈治疗的特定LAA%阈值。

在选择目标肺叶时需要考虑的另一个特征是局部肺灌注。越来越多的证据表明肺气肿破坏程度与肺毛细血管血容量之间存在密切关系。与单纯CT相比，

CT联合肺灌注显像在评估非均质型肺气肿方面更具优势。因此，在基线时进行肺叶灌注的评估能为非均质型肺气肿的评估提供有用信息。此外，有数据表明BLVRC使治疗区域相邻的未放置线圈区域的血流灌注显著增加，同样情况也出现在同侧肺叶未进行治疗的区域。另外6 min步行距离增加与灌注增加之间也存在明显的相关性（$P=0.0027$，$R^2=0.3850$）。这就提示BLVR可能起到改善通气/灌注关系的作用。

灌注显像对于活瓣肺减容手术的预测作用也已被研究，结果显示在非目标肺叶较高的血流灌注与6 min步行试验的改善直接相关（$P=0.014$），而各肺叶间较高的不均质性是FEV_1增加的预测因子。因此，在一些中心，灌注显像已被列入目标肺叶的筛选程序，尽管仍需要前瞻性研究进一步确定其预测价值。

29.5.3 BLVR治疗原则

非均质型肺气肿且不存在CV的患者应首先考虑使用活瓣治疗，因为该方法已进行了广泛的研究，证据明确，效果确切。另外，使用活瓣治疗是可逆的，如疗效不佳或出现并发症，患者可以转为其他方法治疗。对于非均质型肺气肿并且存在CV的患者应评估是否使用BLVRC或BTVA治疗。对于肺组织密度（目前还无密度测量的阈值）足够的患者，当存在明显的过度充气（$RV>225\%$）时，BLVRC应该是治疗首选。其余的情况（肺组织密度不足且没有明显的过度充气的患者）则可以考虑BTVA，尤其是存在肺叶内的异质性情况时，因为BTVA能够选择性的诱导肺段硬化（图29.5）。

对于均质型肺气肿，有证据表明活瓣减容的治疗效果有限，线圈的治疗尚存争议，而BTVA治疗没有证据。总体而言，对于均质型肺气肿可以采用相同的治疗路径，但仅限于RCT研究或注册研究。此外，对于存在CV且没有足够肺组织量来使用线圈的情况，目前还没有任何可选的治疗方式。

29.6 结论

由于COPD患病率逐渐升高，目前COPD已经成为全球公共卫生的重要问题，并且在未来几十年发病情况仍将成倍增加。目前突出的问题是肺气肿患者疾病负担日益增加，标准治疗只能起到辅助作用。这使得人们对BLVR技术越来越关注，并且已经研发了数种内窥镜微创手术方式，成为介入呼吸病领域最令人

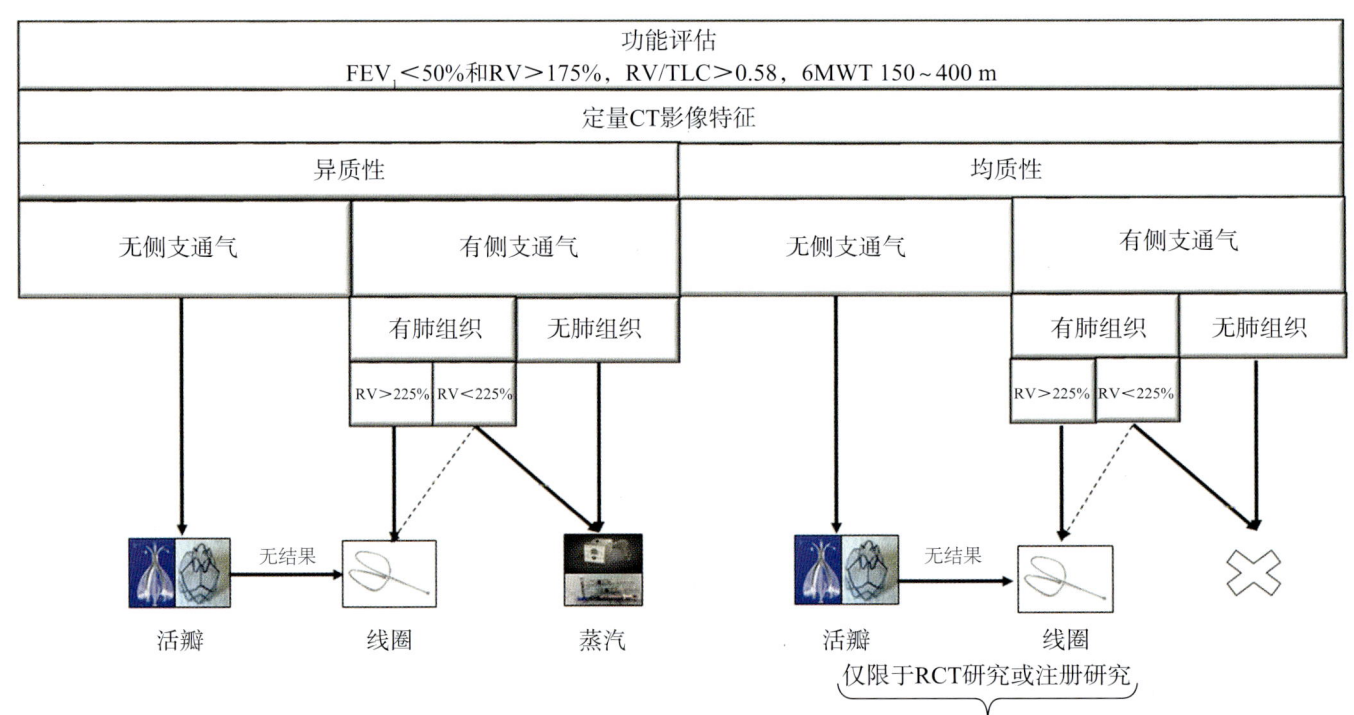

图29.5 经支气管肺减容（BLVR）推荐的治疗流程图

FEV_1，第1秒用力呼气量；RV，残气量；TLC，肺总量；6MWT，6 min步行试验；RCT，随机对照试验。

激动的技术创新之一。尽管这些手术总体上显示出令人鼓舞的结果，但是必须仔细筛选患者，包括全面评价肺气肿的形态、合并症和预期寿命，以降低风险和得到更多获益。此外，这些技术需要进一步的前瞻性研究来更好地探索其应用价值。因此，患者需在有经验的中心接受治疗并登记备案。

参考文献

1. Global Initiative for Chronic Obstructive Lung Disease (GOLD). Global Strategy for the Diagnosis M, and Prevention of Chronic Obstructive Pulmonary Disease. https://goldcopd.org/wp-content/uploads/2017/11/GOLD-2018-v6.0-FINAL-revised-20-Nov_WMS.pdf
2. United Nations Department of Economic and Social Affairs Population Division. World population prospects: the 2015 revision. www.un.org/en/development/desa/publications/world-population-prospects-2015-revision.html
3. Rossi, A., Aisanov, Z., Avdeev, S. et al. (2015). Mechanisms, assessment and therapeutic implications of lung hyperinflation in COPD. *Respir. Med.* 109: 785–802.
4. Van Geffen, W.H., Kerstjens, H.A.M., and Slebos, D.J. (2017). Emerging bronchoscopic treatments for chronic obstructive pulmonary disease. *Pharmacol. Ther.* 179: 96–101.
5. Moore, A.J., Soler, R.S., Cetti, E.J. et al. (2010). Sniff nasal inspiratory pressure versus IC/TLC ratio as predictors of mortality in COPD. *Respir. Med.* 104: 1319–1325.
6. Brantigan, O.C. and Mueller, E. (1957). Surgical treatment of pulmonary emphysema. *Am. Surg.* 23: 789–804.
7. Fishman, A., Martinez, F., Naunheim, K. et al. (2003). A randomized trial comparing lung-volume-reduction surgery with medical therapy for severe emphysema. *N. Engl. J. Med.* 348: 2059–2073.
8. Gasparini, S., Zuccatosta, L., Bonifazi, M. et al. (2012). Bronchoscopic treatment of emphysema: state of the art. *Respiration* 84: 250–263.
9. Gompelmann, D., Eberhardt, R., and Herth, F. (2014). Endoscopic volume reduction in COPD – a critical review. *Dtsch. Arztebl. Int.* 111: 827–833.
10. Sciurba, F.C., Ernst, A., Herth, F.J. et al. (2010). A randomized study of endobronchial valves for advanced emphysema. *N. Engl. J. Med.* 363: 1233–1244.
11. Herth, F.J., Noppen, M., Valipour, A. et al. (2012). Efficacy predictors of lung volume reduction with Zephyr valves in a European cohort. *Eur. Respir. J.* 39: 1334–1342.
12. Koegelenberg, C.F., Slebos, D.J., Shah, P.L. et al. (2015). Time for the global rollout of endoscopic lung volume reduction. *Respiration* 90: 430–440.
13. Klooster, K., ten Hacken, N.H., Hartman, J.E. et al. (2015). Endobronchial valves for emphysema without interlobar collateral ventilation. *N. Engl. J. Med.* 373: 2325–2335.
14. Zoumot, Z., Davey, C., Jordan, S. et al. (2015). A randomised controlled study of BronchoscopicLung Volume Reduction with endobronchial valves for patients with Heterogeneous emphysema and Intact interlobar Fissures: the BeLieVeR-HIFi study. www.ncbi.nlm.nih.gov/pubmed/26378336
15. Valipour, A., Slebos, D.J., Herth, F. et al. (2016). Endobronchial valve therapy in patients with homogeneous emphysema. Results from the IMPACT study. *Am. J. Respir. Crit. Care Med.* 194: 1073–1082.
16. Kemp, S.V., Slebos, D.J., Kirk, A. et al. (2017). A multicenter randomized controlled trial of Zephyr endobronchial valve treatment in heterogeneous emphysema (TRANSFORM). *Am. J. Respir. Crit. Care Med.* 196: 1535–1543.
17. Eberhardt, R., Gompelmann, D., Schuhmann, M. et al. (2012). Complete unilateral vs partial bilateral endoscopic lung volume reduction in patients with bilateral lung emphysema. *Chest* 142: 900–908.
18. Herth, F.J., Eberhardt, R., Gompelmann, D. et al. (2013). Radiological and clinical outcomes of using Chartis to plan endobronchial valve treatment. *Eur. Respir. J.* 41: 302–308.
19. Skowasch, D., Fertl, A., Schwick, B. et al. (2016). A long-term follow-up investigation of endobronchial valves in emphysema (the LIVE study): study protocol and six-month interim analysis results of a prospective five-year observational study. *Respiration* 92: 118–126.
20. Herth, F.J.F., Slebos, D.J., Criner, G.J. et al. (2017). Endoscopic lung volume reduction: an expert panel recommendation – update 2017. *Respiration* 94: 380–388.
21. Koster, T.D., van Rikxoort, E.M., Huebner, R.H. et al. (2016). Predicting lung volume reduction after endobronchial valve therapy is maximized using a combination of diagnostic tools. *Respiration* 92: 150–157.
22. Schuhmann, M., Raffy, P., Yin, Y. et al. (2015). Computed tomography predictors of response to endobronchial valve lung reduction treatment. Comparison with Chartis. *Am. J. Respir. Crit. Care Med.* 191: 767–774.
23. Herzog, D., Poellinger, A., Doellinger, F. et al. (2015). Modifying post-operative medical care after EBV implant may reduce pneumothorax incidence. *PLoS One* 10: e0128097.
24. Li, S.W.G., Wang, C., Jin, F. et al. (2016). The REACH study, a randomized controlled trial assessing the safety and effectiveness of the Spiration Valve System endobronchial therapy for severe emphysema. *Eur. Respir. J.* 48: OA3013.
25. Herth, F.J., Eberhard, R., Gompelmann, D. et al. (2010). Bronchoscopic lung volume reduction with a dedicated coil: a clinical pilot study. *Ther. Adv. Respir. Dis.* 4: 225–231.
26. Deslee, G., Klooster, K., Hetzel, M. et al. (2014). Lung volume reduction coil treatment for patients with severe emphysema: a European multicentre trial. *Thorax* 69: 980–986.
27. Deslee, G., Mal, H., Dutau, H. et al. (2016). Lung volume reduction coil treatment vs usual care in patients with severe emphysema: the REVOLENS randomized clinical trial. *JAMA* 315: 175–184.
28. Shah, P.L., Zoumot, Z., Singh, S. et al. (2013). Endobronchial coils for the treatment of severe emphysema with hyperinflation (RESET): a randomised controlled trial. *Lancet Respir. Med.* 1: 233–240.
29. Slebos, D.J., Klooster, K., Ernst, A. et al. (2012). Bronchoscopic lung volume reduction coil treatment of patients with severe heterogeneous emphysema. *Chest* 142: 574–582.

30 Klooster, K., ten Hacken, N.H., Franz, I. et al. (2014). Lung volume reduction coil treatment in chronic obstructive pulmonary disease patients with homogeneous emphysema: a prospective feasibility trial. *Respiration* 88: 116–125.

31 Sciurba, F.C., Criner, G.J., Strange, C. et al. (2016). Effect of endobronchial coils vs usual care on exercise tolerance in patients with severe emphysema: the RENEW randomized clinical trial. *JAMA* 315: 2178–2189.

32 Herth, F.J., Valipour, A., Shah, P.L. et al. (2016). Segmental volume reduction using thermal vapour ablation in patients with severe emphysema: 6-month results of the multicentre, parallel-group, open-label, randomised controlled STEP-UP trial. *Lancet Respir. Med.* 4: 185–193.

33 Gompelmann, D., Sarmand, N., and Herth, F.J. (2017). Interventional pulmonology in chronic obstructive pulmonary disease. *Curr. Opin. Pulm. Med.* 23: 261–268.

34 Shah, P.L., Gompelmann, D., Valipour, A. et al. (2016). Thermal vapour ablation to reduce segmental volume in patients with severe emphysema: STEP-UP 12 month results. *Lancet Respir. Med.* 4: e44–e45.

第 30 章

支气管胸膜瘘的内镜管理

Ming-yao Ke[1], Hai-dong Huang[2,3,4], and J. Francis Turner, Jr.[5,6]

[1] Department of the Respiratory Centre,
Second Affiliated Hospital of XiaMen Medical College, Xiamen, Fujian, China

[2] Respiratory and Critical Care Medicine, Second Military Medical University, Shanghai, China

[3] Interventional Pulmonology Center of SMMU Respiratory and Critical Care Medicine,
Changhai Hospital, Second Military Medical University (SMMU), Shanghai, China

[4] International Training Center for Interventional Pulmonology,
Henry Ford Hospital, Shanghai, China

[5] Division of Pulmonary and Critical Care Medicine,
University of Tennessee Graduate School of Medicine, Knoxville, TN, USA

[6] National Supercomputing Institute, University of Nevada, Las Vegas, NV, USA

（译者：柯明耀　曾俊莉　译者单位：厦门医学院附属第二医院）

支气管胸膜瘘（bronchopleural fistula，BPF）是指支气管树与胸膜腔之间相互交通形成瘘管。尽管该病较为少见，但处理极为棘手，死亡率高[1]。传统治疗手段主要包括内科保守治疗和外科手术治疗。BPF多见于肺切除术后，这些患者往往因一般情况差而无法耐受再次手术治疗。而且，BPF的瘘口通常难以通过内科保守治疗自行闭合。因此，BPF一直是复杂的难治性胸部疾病，也是困扰胸科医生的一大难题。近年来，随着呼吸介入技术的快速发展，尤其是内镜下诊疗技术的进步，内镜下介入已被证实可为BPF提供有效的治疗选择[2]。本章将重点介绍支气管镜下介入治疗在BPF中的应用。

30.1　病因和发病率

BPF可源于多种疾病及诊疗操作，最常见的病因是肺切除术后并发症，其次还可见于肺部坏死合并感染、持续性自发性气胸、肺结核，以及医源性损伤如肺活检、胸腔闭式引流、胸腔穿刺术、肺部肿瘤的放化疗等[1,3]。

目前缺乏BPF的大型流行病学数据，文献报道的术后BPF的发生率为0.5%~20%[4]。肺解剖性切除后支气管残端裂开仍是术后BPF的主要原因。导致术后BPF的非手术相关危险因素包括：支气管残端肿瘤复发、术前放疗、合并感染（尤其是真菌感染）、术后长期机械通气、成人呼吸窘迫综合征、慢性阻塞性肺疾病、营养不良、低蛋白血症、激素的使用、糖尿病以及术后长期住院等[4-6]。Vester等[7]对2 234名行不同肺切除术式的患者分析后发现，行肺段切除者BPF发生率为0.3%，单个肺叶切除者BPF发生率为0.82%，双肺叶切除者的BPF发生率为0.93%，而全肺切除者BPF的发生率高达4.5%。还有研究结果也显示，接受右肺全切和右下叶切除手术者BPF的发生率最高[4,8]。此外，瘘口形成的手术相关危险因素还包括：手术切缘肿瘤残留、支气管残端过长、缝合张力过大、气管或支气管旁组织切除过多等[1]。

30.2 临床表现与诊断

30.2.1 临床表现

BPF的临床表现多样、轻重不一，按病程大致可分为急性、亚急性和慢性三大类。术后BPF则可以根据术后发现瘘的时间分为早期BPF（术后1周内）、中期BPF（术后7~30天）及晚期BPF（术后30天后）[9]。BPF较为典型的临床表现为突发的呼吸困难、低血压、皮下气肿、咳出脓性分泌物，查体发现气管、纵隔偏移或胸腔引流后引流管瓶内可见持续漏气。亚急性临床表现则更为隐匿，常表现为刺激性咳嗽、发热伴咯血痰或脓痰。而慢性BPF或非外科所致BPF，其临床表现则与感染进程相关[3]。一旦出现发热、频繁咳嗽、胸片显示新出现或增加的气液平面，需警惕BPF的可能[1]。

30.2.2 诊断

BPF诊断常通过病史及临床表现即可明确，尤其是胸腔闭式引流患者，持续存在漏气，则高度怀疑存在BPF。目前已有多种技术设备可用于BPF的诊断，包括影像技术和气管镜技术两大类。

影像技术主要指胸部X线平片和胸部CT检查。提示BPF的影像特征包括：① 胸腔内气腔增大；② 新发气液平面；③ 已存在的气液平面改变；④ 未经胸腔导管引流者气液平面下降超过2 cm[10]。胸部CT相较于X线平片可更为准确地显示上述改变，而且通过薄层CT扫描有可能发现支气管残端与胸膜腔交通的瘘口。

支气管镜作为胸肺疾病的重要检查方法，可用于瘘的诊断和定位[11]。多数病例可经支气管镜确定瘘口位置、大小、形态，甚至可以通过瘘口观察到胸腔内的情况。除了直接观察到瘘口之外，气管镜还可通过镜下冲洗发现持续气泡产生而间接提示瘘口的存在。对于气管镜下难以直接清晰显示瘘口的患者，对可疑部位行支气管造影可帮助诊断。而对于已行胸腔闭式引流者，还可通过气管镜下向可疑支气管段内注射美蓝的方法，观察胸腔引流液的颜色来辅助诊断[1,3]。此外，还可通过气管镜下球囊扩张封堵可疑支气管，观察胸腔引流气体是否消失或减少辅助诊断。

随着科技进步，一些新的技术也可用于BPF的诊断和定位，包括通气闪烁显像[12]、体积渲染成像[13]、虚拟支气管镜[14]，以及计算机断层支气管造影[15]等。

30.3 传统治疗方法

BPF的最佳治疗方法尚缺乏共识。传统治疗方法包括内科保守治疗和外科手术治疗。

内科保守治疗是基础，适用于所有患者。建立通畅的胸腔引流是治疗BPF最重要的治疗措施之一，其他内科保守治疗还包括使用抗生素、营养支持以及必要时机械通气等。胸腔闭式引流可通过引流胸腔内脓液和积气，促进感染控制以及受压肺的复张。因此，一旦确诊BPF则应行胸腔置管引流[16]，而且嘱患者尽量取患侧卧位以免胸腔内渗出物流向健侧；如合并脓胸，更应立即行胸腔引流防止吸入性肺炎，并同时给予静脉广谱抗生素治疗及胸腔局部灌洗[17]。反复胸腔灌洗可以有效控制感染，促进瘘口闭合。据报道，小瘘口有可能通过内科保守治疗达到完全愈合[16,18]。

外科手术治疗是BPF的传统根治方法。外科开胸手术方式包括：长期开窗引流、直接缝合支气管残端并用血供良好的自体组织加固、带蒂大网膜/肌瓣移植术、经胸骨支气管残端闭合术、胸廓成形术[19]。随着微创外科的发展，电视胸腔镜也开始应用于BPF[20]，尤其是早期BPF的治疗。已有报道在胸腔镜下用带血管蒂的皮瓣缝合封闭支气管残端瘘成功治疗BPF的病例[21,22]。据文献报道，外科方法封闭BPF的成功率可高达80%~95%[23]。尽管如此，BPF患者往往因体质差而无法接受外科手术治疗。因此，实际上可进行外科手术患者的数量是很有限的。详细讨论外科手术方式的选择及其适应证并非本章重点，不做过多展开。

30.4 气管镜下介入治疗

对于大多数BPF（尤其是术后BPF），单纯内科保守治疗瘘口闭合率很低，而外科手术治疗对于大部分患者而言又无法耐受。随着介入治疗技术的发展，经支气管镜介入诊疗BPF的模式正逐渐受到认可。气管镜检查甚至可发现直径<5 mm的小瘘口[1]；气管镜下治疗BPF具有创伤小、并发症少、可重复操作、患者耐受性好、花费少、操作相对简单等诸多优点。以下我们将介绍几种气管镜下治疗BPF的主要方法。

30.4.1 硝酸银

1984 年，Hoier-Madsen 等[24]首次尝试使用硝酸银治疗 BPF。他们通过硬质支气管镜下应用硝酸银的方法成功治愈了 10 名 BPF 患者。应用硝酸银可引起局部组织灼伤和炎症反应，随后瘘周黏膜进入正常修复愈合和瘢痕形成的阶段，促进瘘口闭合。该方法适用于位于中央气道的小瘘口。然而，自此 25 年内再无该方法应用于 BPF 治疗的报道。直至 2009 年，Stratakos 等[25]再次报道了在可弯曲支气管镜下使用支气管刷在<5 mm 的瘘口周围反复涂抹硝酸银成功治疗 BPF 的病例。此外，Boudaya 等[18]也同样通过镜下使用硝酸银成功闭合 BPF 的瘘口。

30.4.2 乙醇

可弯曲支气管镜下直接将无水乙醇注射到瘘周黏膜下层可快速诱导组织脱水，并通过可再生的方式促进瘢痕形成[26]。理想情况下，无水乙醇应注射到皮下组织层与下方的肌肉层之间，但在临床实践中这一目标很难实现。而且快速地将无水乙醇注射到组织内可能会引起组织毒性，导致组织坏死。因此，使用无水乙醇进行治疗时需非常谨慎，应缓慢、少量注射。根据现有的报道，黏膜下注射 0.1 mL 的无水乙醇似乎是安全有效的剂量[26,27]。但是，值得注意的是，该方法只适用于直径<5 mm 的小瘘口，尤其是那些直径<3 mm 的瘘口。目前未报道无水乙醇注射治疗相关的并发症[1,26]。

30.4.3 聚多卡醇

聚多卡醇是一种局麻剂，最初作为硬化疗法用于蜘蛛痣和静脉曲张的治疗。直至 1988 年，Varoli 等[9]率先报道了聚多卡醇在 35 例术后 BPF 中的应用。该研究中，镜下注射聚多卡醇成功闭合 66%（23/35）的瘘口，包括直径长达 10 mm 的大瘘口。随后，Kanno 等[28]也报道了应用聚多卡醇和环氧丙烷作为硬化疗法治疗 BPF 的成功病例。该文章中指出硬化治疗不仅操作简单，而且还可有效治疗 BPF。此外，还有报道气管镜下注射聚多卡醇的相关化合物乙醇胺亦可使 80%（12/15）胸腔内持续漏气患者的漏气问题得到解决[29]。

30.4.4 石炭酸

石炭酸，又称苯酚，是一种具有甜味的无色液体，用于制备树脂、防腐剂、杀菌剂和药物，还可用于消毒手术器械。苯酚可与黏膜组织产生强烈反应，纯苯酚可在 60 秒内完全腐蚀黏膜。当苯酚与黏膜表面接触时，组织会迅速变性，刺激黏膜炎症渗出和组织增生，最终导致瘘口闭合。Wang 等[30]首次报道了气管镜下注射苯酚在 BPF 中的应用。如果初次应用苯酚后仍然存在漏气，可重复给予苯酚治疗。治疗时间的长短不一，治愈率最高可达 100%，并且尚无治疗相关并发症的报道。但是，目前的应用经验少，还需要进行更多的研究来确认其疗效和安全性。

30.4.5 纤维蛋白胶

瘘口小的 BPF，还可通过纤维支气管镜下注射纤维蛋白密封剂来进行诊断和治疗。该方法已被成功地应用于小瘘口的 BPF 患者及多发术后支气管残端瘘的患者[11,31-34]。纤维蛋白胶是一种双组分生物黏合剂，其作用模拟了凝血的最后阶段，即纤维蛋白原（以冷冻沉淀形式存在）在凝血因子XIII、凝血酶和钙的作用下聚合形成纤维蛋白凝块的过程，这些蛋白最终逐渐通过纤溶作用吸收。需要注意的是，这两种纤维蛋白组分应分别直接注入瘘口处并使它们在预定的位置混合，因为二者混合后几秒内就会形成凝块。具体的操作是通过气管镜将导管放置在瘘口附近，首先注射 1 mL 浓缩纤维蛋白原，紧接着注射 1 mL 外用凝血酶（1 000 IU/mL），二者混合后形成的纤维凝块将封堵瘘口。一般认为纤维蛋白胶最终可被重吸收，从而防止产生异物反应[35]。此外，纤维蛋白胶还可与氧化再生纤维素贴片[33]和海绵状小牛腿骨片[36]等材料联合应用于 BPF 瘘口的封堵。

30.4.6 氰基丙烯酸酯胶

氰基丙烯酸酯胶和纤维蛋白胶同样都属于最为常见的密封剂化合物。它们先是作为塞子堵塞瘘口，而后诱导局部炎症反应导致纤维化和黏膜增生从而使瘘口永久闭合[37,38]。通过支气管镜将导管沿工作通道放置在瘘口附近；随后将氰基丙烯酸酯胶通过导管注入瘘口，该胶水在与体液或组织接触时聚合为固体材料，并可与创伤表面形成紧密连接，从而堵塞瘘口。若单次操作无法完全密封瘘口，则可以重复上述过程。据现有资料，氰基丙烯酸酯胶的最佳注射剂量为 0.5~1 mL[39]。

30.4.7 激光

可弯曲支气管镜下能量消融技术已被应用于 BPF 的治疗。其原理是诱导周围组织产生炎症反应。将 Nd:YAG 激光束瞄准瘘口周围的支气管黏膜，然后通过非聚焦的YAG激光束在瘘口周围造成表浅的糜烂和出血,继而凝固[40]。Nd:YAG激光适用于直径2 mm以内的小瘘口的治疗。Kiriyama等报道了运用Nd:YAG激光(功率5~20 W,持续0.5 s)治疗8名BPF患者的经验,其中4名患者的瘘口成功愈合[41]。然而,这项技术尚未被广泛地应用于BPF的治疗,其疗效和安全性还需进一步的研究探索。

30.4.8　线圈

目前,线圈已被单独或与其他密封剂联合用于治疗BPF[42-44]。Ponn等报道了在5名患者中使用Gianturco血管闭塞线圈完全或显著地控制了漏气,并且未发生治疗相关的并发症[45]。此外,线圈联合氰基丙烯酸酯胶治疗BPF同样也取得了成功。在该组合模式下,线圈充当了氰基丙烯酸酯胶支撑,从而更有效达到治疗BPF的目的[43,44]。

30.4.9　支气管内活瓣

支气管内活瓣(endobronchial valves,EBV)最初是为了替代外科肺减容而设计的用于气管镜下肺减容的材料。EBV可用于治疗BPF的理论基础是其可阻止气流进入瘘口,从而为瘘口闭合创造条件。Feller-Kopman等[46]首次报道使用EBV成功治疗BPF和脓胸的病例。随后,其他研究结果也发现,EBV可安全、有效地治疗BPF[47-49]。近期的一项单中心回顾性研究分析了EBV治疗75例BPF患者的临床价值。这些患者共放置了195个EBV[平均每位患者放置2.6个(范围1~8个)EBV],漏气治愈的中位时间为16天(范围2~56天)[49]。

30.4.10　Amplatzer封堵器

Amplatzer封堵器(Amplatzer device,AD)作为经导管治疗先天性心脏缺损的医疗器械而为大家所熟知。它是由镍钛合金编织而成、具有自膨性能的双盘网状结构(图30.1)。现被发现亦可用于BPF的治疗,最常用于BPF的类型是Amplatzer房间隔封堵器和Amplatzer导管封堵器Ⅱ(AGA Medical公司,明尼苏达州,美国)。Amplatzer房间隔封堵器的双盘之间有一个直径为4~40 mm的中央腰部,而双盘的远端和近端的直径分别比中央腰部的直径大14 mm和10 mm,以在周边形成5~7 mm的锚定边缘。网片内部的聚酯纤维织物有助于缺损的封堵和组织的生长。腰部放置在缺损内部,而双盘则固定在缺损两侧。Amplatzer导管封堵器Ⅱ装置的结构大体与房间隔封堵器相似,但中央腰部直径为3~6 mm,长度范围为4~6 mm,网片内部没有布料。盘片比中央腰围大6 mm。由于设备尺寸可选择范围大,

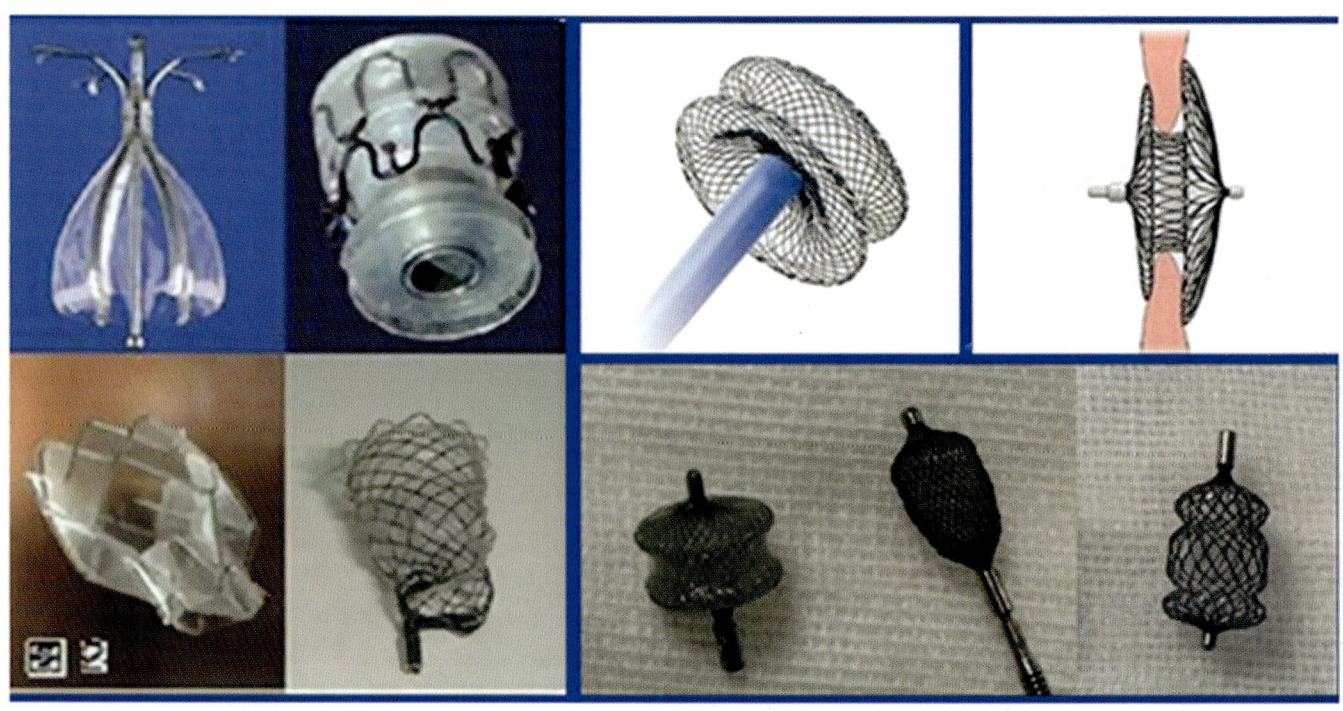

图30.1　临床中常用的各种封堵器

故可根据不同病变的直径和长度进行适当匹配。

经支气管镜下 Amplatzer 封堵器治疗 BPF 主要适用于位于主支气管的大瘘口，尤其适于那些因瘘口过大而无法通过弹簧圈、生物胶等闭合的 BPF。Butera 等[50]最先将 AD 应用于 BPF 的治疗。随后其他团队也相继报道了应用 AD 有效治疗 BPF 的成功病例[51-54]。Fruchter 等[53]对 31 名 BPF 患者进行气管镜下 AD 置入封堵瘘口，其中 30 名患者瘘口成功闭合，AD 放置 6 个月后复查气管镜发现 AD 的表面被肉芽组织覆盖，瘘口封堵良好，而且随访期间未出现严重并发症。然而需特别注意的一点是，AD 有移位脱落入胸腔的风险，并且一旦脱落则无法再利用，这就限制了其临床应用。

2018 年 5 月，笔者单位收治了 1 名右中叶切除联合右上叶病灶切除的 BPF 伴脓胸患者。胸部 CT 显示右侧胸腔和胸壁间的瘘口（图 30.2 A）。气管镜检查探及 2 个瘘口，较大者位于右中叶支气管（直径约 12 mm），较小者位于右上叶支气管（直径约 2 mm）。由于右中叶瘘口位于中央气道且瘘口直径过大，难以通过传统的方式有效治疗。因此，我们选择 AD 对较大瘘口进行封堵（图 30.2 B），并裁剪合适大小的硅胶条封堵右上叶小瘘口（图 30.2 C）。经气管镜下封堵治疗后，该患者的咳嗽明显缓解，液气胸明显改善。复查支气管镜示 AD 被肉芽组织覆盖，瘘口封堵良好。

30.4.11 硅胶塞

使用一种支气管内硅胶塞（endobronchial Watanabe spi-got，EWS）封堵支气管可有效治疗持续性 BPF[55-58]。EWS 由 Watanabe 等开发，他们发现通过 EWS 堵塞靶支气管后可有效减少管腔漏气[59]。EWS 由硅胶制成并有 3 种规格可供选择（小号 5 mm、中号 6 mm 以及大号 7 mm）。EWS 主要适用于封堵亚段支气管[59]。使用 EWS 进行支气管内封堵的主要并发症是 EWS 移位。如果 EWS 发生移位，可在气管镜下重复操作放回目标位置。目前尚缺乏 EWS 置入后的长期随访数据。EWS 已在日本获批难治性气胸的适应证，但截至目前 EWS 仍未获得 FDA 的应用批准。

30.4.12 支架

气道支架置入是中央气道阻塞的主要治疗手段。如今，已有少量个案和病例系列报告报道，气道支架可用于 BPF 的治疗。支架置入的目的是尽可能地贴合气道隔绝瘘口，从而防止误吸和肺炎。用于 BPF 的支架主要分两大类，分别是金属支架和硅酮支架（图 30.3）。

众所周知，金属支架会诱发组织炎症反应并刺激肉芽组织增生。这一刺激作用可能对瘘口的闭合有利。而金属支架有多种类型，特性各异。选择合适的支架需要考虑到病变类型、病灶位置、支架的物理特性以及支架潜在的短期和长期并发症。最近，Han 等[60]的一项大型系列研究报道了覆膜金属支架个体化应用于 148 例 BPF 的治疗。研究结果发现，96.6%（143/148）的患者漏气现象得到有效解决。而其余 5 例患者尝试重新置入支架后获得满意的封堵效果。这项大样本的研究表明，金属支架置入为 BPF 提供了一种可行且有效的治疗方式。另一项纳入 7 名大瘘口术后 BPF 患者的回顾性研究发现，硬镜下置入全覆膜自膨胀金属支架的即刻瘘口封堵成功率可达 100%[61]。该研究同时还提供了增加成功率的建议：① 术前测量支架需覆盖的范围，以便定制支架的中心正好置于瘘口处；② 支架直径应比瘘口周围气道直径大 10%~20%。典型病例图片参见图 30.4。

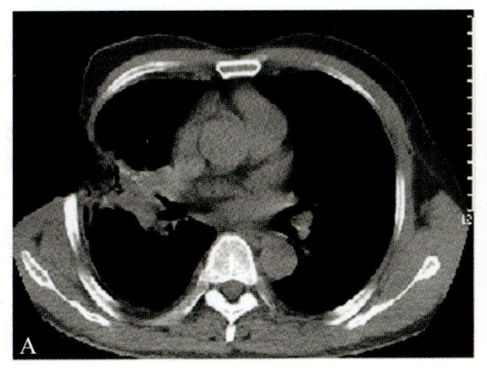
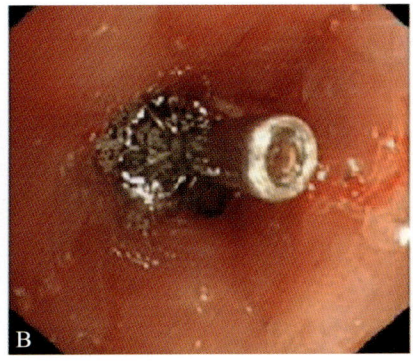
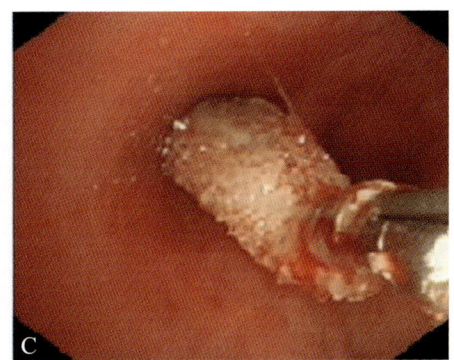

图 30.2 应用 Amplatzer® 封堵器（AD）和硅胶条治疗支气管胸膜瘘（BPF）的典型病例
A. 胸部 CT 显示右侧胸腔与胸壁间的瘘口；B. AD 用于封堵位于右肺中叶的大瘘口；C. 根据瘘口大小修剪的硅胶条用于封堵右上叶的小瘘口。

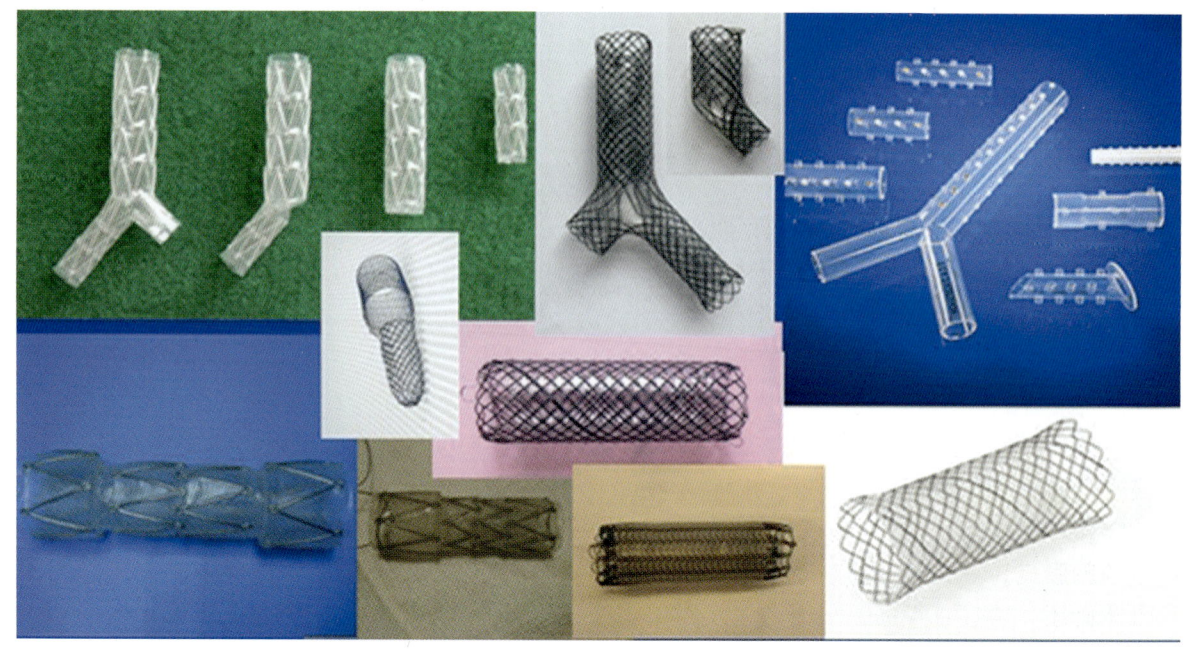

图 30.3　临床中应用于治疗支气管胸膜瘘（BPF）的金属和硅酮支架

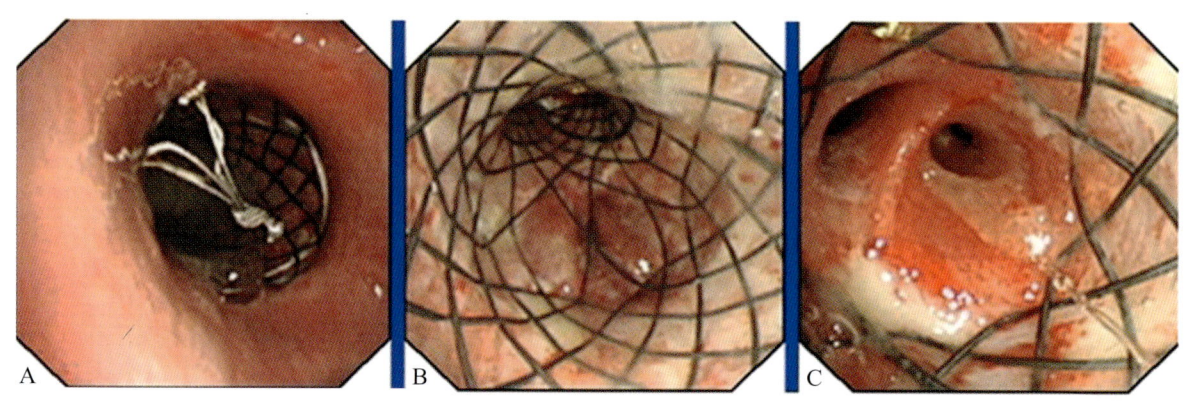

图 30.4　金属覆膜支架用于治疗支气管胸膜瘘（BPF）的典型病例

硬质支气管镜下放置硅酮支架也被用于治疗术后 BPF。2005 年，Tsukada 等首次采用改良 Dumon 硅酮支架成功治疗 1 例术后 BPF 的患者[62]。此外，Ferraroli 等[63]同样使用改良的 Dumon "Y" 形硅酮支架治疗 1 名右主支气管残端瘘（2 mm）的患者。该改良支架的右侧支被来自支架自身的硅胶材料所封闭[63]。

支架置入与其他所有治疗方式一样，也存在缺点。支架在气道内作为异物，不仅会刺激黏膜分泌增加，而且支架覆盖影响了气道内纤毛活动，继而导致分泌物难以排出。尽管气道支架材料和放置技术在不断的改良和进步，气道支架置入引起的相关问题如胸部不适感、痰液潴留、肉芽组织增生等，仍难以完全避免[60,64]。

在临床工作中，我们会遇到非常复杂的病例。以本中心收治的 1 名患者为例：该患者 20 年前因空洞型肺结核行右上叶切除术，8 年前又因右肺曲霉感染再次行右肺切除术，具体术式不详。第 2 次术后，患者反复出现液气胸，提示存在 BPF。该患者在外院进行多次气管镜下氩气等离子凝固治疗，以刺激肉芽组织的增生，但疗效不佳。故该患者于 2018 年 4 月至笔者单位就诊，支气管镜检查发现右上叶支气管残端瘘，根据瘘口情况放置了 1 枚 "Y" 形硅酮支架（Y16-13-13，右上叶支用尼龙网缝合密闭形成封堵器）封堵瘘口。然而硅酮支架封堵效果并不理想。于是我们取出了原 Dumon 支架并用 2 块合适大小的明胶海绵填塞右上叶瘘口（图 30.5 A）；再对硅酮支架进行加工裁剪，在 "Y" 形 Dumon 支架的右中间支和右主支分别套接一个直径 15 mm 和 18 mm 的支架环（图 30.5 B、C），以扩大支架外径使其与气道贴合紧密，增强封堵效果。治疗后，胸腔内漏气明显减少并最终消失，而且患者症状得到明显缓解。胸部 CT 显示瘘口被支架完全覆盖（图 30.5 D）。该患者病史长且复杂，单一治疗手段难以达到满意的效果。在这种情况下，我们应该根据患者个体情况，联合应用多种治疗手段，使得治疗效益最大化。

30.4.13 自体血

已有系列病例报告可通过胸腔引流管内注射自体血形成胸膜固定从而有效控制胸腔的持续漏气[65]。该方法的成功有赖于血液凝固所带来的即时封堵效果以及随之产生的胸膜炎症反应。除了通过胸腔内注射的方式外，自体血还可通过可弯曲支气管镜下注射达到封堵的效果。首先通过可弯曲支气管镜和活检钳，先涂抹几层止血药，然后通过改良的 Fogarty 球囊导管在瘘口位置注射自体血，漏气可即刻停止[66]。倘若漏气持续存在，可重复该过程。有作者指出，每个病例应用的自体血总量不应超过 25 mL[67]。

30.5 结论

综上，我们虽然介绍了诸多治疗 BPF 的方法，但并不存在任何情况下均适用的最佳方式。多数学者认为，瘘口的大小是决定治疗方式的关键因素。通过查阅文献，我们发现气管镜下注射硬化剂、注射纤维胶的方式更适用于直径＜5 mm 的小瘘口的治疗，尤适于那些直径＜3 mm 者。而 AD 和支架置入则可在直径＞5 mm 的较大瘘口中发挥良好的封堵效果。除瘘口的大小之外，瘘口的位置、感染的控制情况以及伴发病等都是影响治疗成功率的重要因素。最后，无证据支持某种化合物或联合方式优于另一种。因此，需根据具体情况进行个体化的选择。此外，治疗方式的选择还有赖于操作者对该方法的熟练程度及治疗经验。

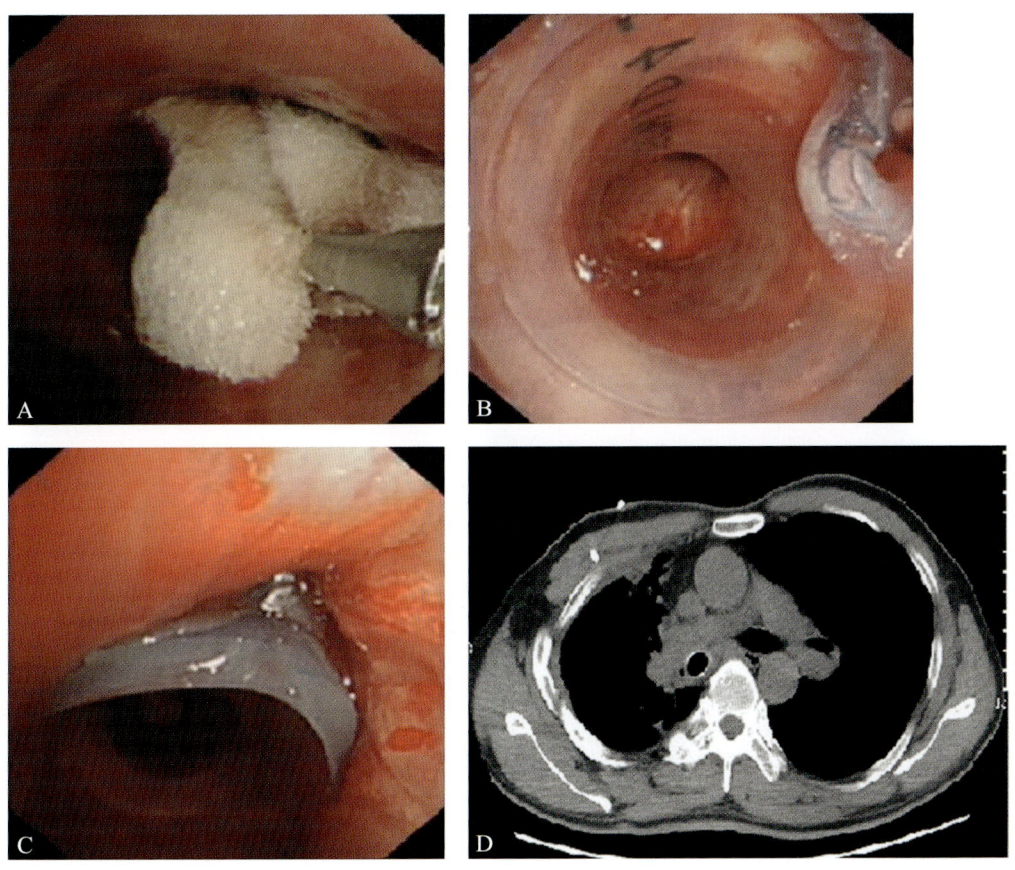

图 30.5 改良 Dumon 硅酮支架联合明胶海绵封堵难治性支气管胸膜瘘（BPF）
A. 明胶海绵用于填塞封堵瘘口；B. 原硅酮支架右中间支套接外径 15 mm 的硅酮支架环；C. 原硅酮支架的右主支套接外径 18 mm 的硅酮支架环；D. 治疗后胸部 CT 影像显示瘘口被改良硅酮支架完全覆盖。

参考文献

1. Lois, M. and Noppen, M. (2005). Bronchopleural fistulas: an overview of the problem with special focus on endoscopic management. *Chest* 128: 3955–3965.
2. Keshishyan, S., Revelo, A.E., and Epelbaum, O. (2017). Bronchoscopic management of prolonged air leak. *J. Thorac. Dis.* 9: S1034–S1046.
3. Sarkar, P., Chandak, T., Shah, R., and Talwar, A. (2010). Diagnosis and management bronchopleural fistula. *Indian J. Chest Dis. Allied Sci.* 52: 97–104.
4. Cerfolio, R.J. (2001). The incidence, etiology, and prevention of postresectional bronchopleural fistula. *Semin. Thorac. Cardiovasc. Surg.* 13: 3–7.
5. Panagopoulos, N.D., Apostolakis, E., Koletsis, E. et al. (2009). Low incidence of bronchopleural fistula after pneumonectomy for lung cancer. *Interact. Cardiovasc. Thorac. Surg.* 9: 571–575.
6. Algar, F.J., Alvarez, A., Aranda, J.L. et al. (2001). Prediction of early bronchopleural fistula after pneumonectomy: a multivariate analysis. *Ann. Thorac. Surg.* 72: 1662–1667.
7. Vester, S.R., Faber, L.P., Kittle, C.F. et al. (1991). Bronchopleural fistula after stapled closure of bronchus. *Ann. Thorac. Surg.* 52: 1253–1257, 1257–1258.
8. Darling, G.E., Abdurahman, A., Yi, Q.L. et al. (2005). Risk of a right pneumonectomy: role of bronchopleural fistula. *Ann. Thorac. Surg.* 79: 433–437.
9. Varoli, F., Roviaro, G., Grignani, F. et al. (1998). Endoscopic treatment of bronchopleural fistulas. *Ann. Thorac. Surg.* 65: 807–809.
10. Kim, E.A., Lee, K.S., Shim, Y.M. et al. (2002). Radiographic and CT findings in complications following pulmonary resection. *Radiographics* 22: 67–86.
11. York, E.L., Lewall, D.B., Hirji, M. et al. (1990). Endoscopic diagnosis and treatment of postoperative bronchopleural fistula. *Chest* 97: 1390–1392.
12. Carp, L., de Bondt, P., van Schil, P., and Blockx, P. (1999). Ventilation scintigraphy for the detection of bronchopleural fistulae. *Eur. J. Nucl. Med.* 26: 1379–1380.
13. Lawler, L.P. and Fishman, E.K. (2001). Multi-detector row CT of thoracic disease with emphasis on 3D volume rendering and CT angiography. *Radiographics* 21: 1257–1273.
14. De Wever, W., Vandecaveye, V., Lanciotti, S., and Verschakelen, J.A. (2004). Multidetector CT-generated virtual bronchoscopy: an illustrated review of the potential clinical indications. *Eur. Respir. J.* 23: 776–782.
15. Sarkar, P., Patel, N., Chusid, J. et al. (2010). The role of computed tomography bronchography in the management of bronchopleural fistulas. *J. Thorac. Imaging* 25: W10–W13.
16. Cooper, W.A. and Miller, J.J. (2001). Management of bronchopleural fistula after lobectomy. *Semin. Thorac. Cardiovasc. Surg.* 13: 8–12.
17. Davies, H.E., Davies, R.J., and Davies, C.W. (2010). Management of pleural infection in adults: British Thoracic Society Pleural Disease Guideline 2010. *Thorax* 65 (Suppl 2): i41–i53.
18. Boudaya, M.S., Smadhi, H., Zribi, H. et al. (2013). Conservative management of postoperative bronchopleural fistulas. *J. Thorac. Cardiovasc. Surg.* 146: 575–579.
19. Wang, D.L., Cheng, G.Y., Sun, K.L. et al. (2008). Treatment and prevention of bronchus-pleural fistula after pneumonectomy for lung cancer. *Zhonghua WaiKe Za Zhi* 46: 193–195.
20. Karfis, E.A. and Kakadellis, J. (2009). Video-thoracoscopic management of a postpneumonectomy bronchopleural fistula. *Gen. Thorac. Cardiovasc. Surg.* 57: 675–677.
21. Baldwin, J.C. and Mark, J.B. (1985). Treatment of bronchopleural fistula after pneumonectomy. *J. Thorac. Cardiovasc. Surg.* 90: 813–817.
22. Deschamps, C., Allen, M.S., Miller, D.L. et al. (2001). Management of postpneumonectomy empyema and bronchopleural fistula. *Semin. Thorac. Cardiovasc. Surg.* 13: 13–19.
23. Stamatis, G., Freitag, L., Wencker, M., and Greschuchna, D. (1994). Omentopexy and muscle transposition: two alternative methods in the treatment of pleural empyema and mediastinitis. *Thorac. Cardiovasc. Surg.* 42: 225–232.
24. Hoier-Madsen, K., Schulze, S., Moller, P.V., and Halkier, E. (1984). Management of bronchopleural fistula following pneumonectomy. *Scand. J. Thorac. Cardiovasc. Surg.* 18: 263–266.
25. Stratakos, G., Zuccatosta, L., Porfyridis, I. et al. (2009). Silver nitrate through flexible bronchoscope in the treatment of bronchopleural fistulae. *J. Thorac. Cardiovasc. Surg.* 138: 603–607.
26. Takaoka, K., Inoue, S., and Ohira, S. (2002). Central bronchopleural fistulas closed by bronchoscopic injection of absolute ethanol. *Chest* 122: 374–378.
27. Fujisawa, T., Hongo, H., Yamaguchi, Y. et al. (1986). Intratumoral ethanol injection for malignant tracheobronchial lesions: a new bronchofiberscopic procedure. *Endoscopy* 18: 188–191.
28. Kanno, R., Suzuki, H., Fujiu, K. et al. (2002). Endoscopic closure of bronchopleural fistula after pneumonectomy by submucosal injection of polidocanol. *Jpn. J. Thorac. Cardiovasc. Surg.* 50: 30–33.
29. Lim, A.L., Kim, C.H., Hwang, Y.I. et al. (2012). Bronchoscopic ethanolamine injection therapy in patients with persistent air leak from chest tube drainage. *Tuberc. Respir. Dis.* 72: 441–447.
30. Wang, Z., Yu, H.B., Luo, Q., and Liu, Y.Y. (2015). Treatment of bronchopleural fistula with carbolic acid instilled through bronchofiberscope in post-pulmonectomy patients. *J. Cardiothorac. Surg.* 10: 120.
31. Glover, W., Chavis, T.V., Daniel, T.M. et al. (1987). Fibrin glue application through the flexible fiberoptic bronchoscope: closure of bronchopleural fistulas. *J. Thorac. Cardiovasc. Surg.* 93: 470–472.
32. Shrestha, P., Safdar, S.A., Jawad, S.A. et al. (2014). Successful closure of a bronchopleural fistula by intrapleural administration of fibrin sealant: a case report with review of literature. *NorthAm. J. Med. Sci.* 6: 487–490.
33. Fiorelli, A., Frongillo, E., and Santini, M. (2015).

Bronchopleural fistula closed with cellulose patch and fibrin glue. *Asian Cardiovasc. Thorac. Ann.* 23: 880–883.

34 Goussard, P., Gie, R.P., Kling, S. et al. (2008). Fibrin glue closure of persistent bronchopleural fistula following pneumonectomy for post-tuberculosis bronchiectasis. *Pediatr. Pulmonol.* 43: 721–725.

35 McCarthy, P.M., Trastek, V.F., Bell, D.G. et al. (1988). The effectiveness of fibrin glue sealant for reducing experimental pulmonary air leak. *Ann. Thorac. Surg.* 45: 203–205.

36 Hollaus, P.H., Lax, F., Janakiev, D. et al. (1998). Endoscopic treatment of postoperative bronchopleural fistula: experience with 45 cases. *Ann. Thorac. Surg.* 66: 923–927.

37 Scappaticci, E., Ardissone, F., Ruffini, E. et al. (1994). Postoperative bronchopleural fistula: endoscopic closure in 12 patients. *Ann. Thorac. Surg.* 57: 119–122.

38 York, J.A. (2013). Treating bronchopleural fistulae percutaneously with N-butyl cyanoacrylate glue. *J. Vasc. Interv. Radiol.* 24: 1581–1583.

39 Chang, C.C., Hsu, H.H., Kuo, S.W., and Lee, Y.C. (2007). Bronchoscopic gluing for post-lung-transplant bronchopleural fistula. *Eur. J. Cardiothorac. Surg.* 31: 328–330.

40 Wang, K.P., Schaeffer, L., Heitmiller, R., and Baker, R. (1993). NdYAG laser closure of a bronchopleural fistula. *Monaldi Arch. Chest Dis.* 48: 301–303.

41 Kiriyama, M., Fujii, Y., Yamakawa, Y. et al. (2002). Endobronchial neodymium: yttrium-aluminum garnet laser for noninvasive closure of small proximal bronchopleural fistula after lung resection. *Ann. Thorac. Surg.* 73: 945–948, 948–949.

42 Uchida, T., Wada, M., Sakamoto, J., and Arai, Y. (1999). Treatment for empyema with bronchopleural fistulas using endobronchial occlusion coils: report of a case. *Surg. Today* 29: 186–189.

43 Clemson, L.A., Walser, E., Gill, A. et al. (2006). Transthoracic closure of a postpneumonectomy bronchopleural fistula with coils and cyanoacrylate. *Ann. Thorac. Surg.* 82: 1924–1926.

44 Hirata, T., Ogawa, E., Takenaka, K. et al. (2002). Endobronchial closure of postoperative bronchopleural fistula using vascular occluding coils and n-butyl-2-cyanoacrylate. *Ann. Thorac. Surg.* 74: 2174–2176.

45 Ponn, R.B., d'Agostino, R.S., Stern, H., and Westcott, J.L. (1993). Treatment of peripheral bronchopleural fistulas with endobronchial occlusion coils. *Ann. Thorac. Surg.* 56: 1343–1347.

46 Feller-Kopman, D., Bechara, R., Garland, R. et al. (2006). Use of a removable endobronchial valve for the treatment of bronchopleural fistula. *Chest* 130: 273–275.

47 Alexander, E.S., Healey, T.T., Martin, D.W., and Dupuy, D.E. (2012). Use of endobronchial valves for the treatment of bronchopleural fistulas after thermal ablation of lung neoplasms. *J. Vasc. Interv. Radiol.* 23: 1236–1240.

48 Akil, A., Reichelt, J., Freermann, S. et al. (2018). Application of intrabronchial valves in high risk patients with bronchopleural fistula: an alternative therapeutic option. *Zentralbl. Chir.* 143: 296–300.

49 Gilbert, C.R., Casal, R.F., Lee, H.J. et al. (2016). Use of one-way intrabronchial valves in air leak management after tube thoracostomy drainage. *Ann. Thorac. Surg.* 101: 1891–1896.

50 Butera, G., Chessa, M., and Carminati, M. (2007). Percutaneous closure of ventricular septal defects. *Cardiol. Young* 17: 243–253.

51 Gulkarov, I., Paul, S., Altorki, N.K., and Lee, P.C. (2009). Use of Amplatzer device for endobronchial closure of bronchopleural fistulas. *Interact. Cardiovasc. Thorac. Surg.* 9: 901–902.

52 Fruchter, O., Kramer, M.R., Dagan, T. et al. (2011). Endobronchial closure of bronchopleural fistulae using amplatzer devices: our experience and literature review. *Chest* 139: 682–687.

53 Fruchter, O., El, R.B., Abdel-Rahman, N. et al. (2014). Efficacy of bronchoscopic closure of a bronchopleural fistula with amplatzer devices: long-term follow-up. *Respiration* 87: 227–233.

54 Klotz, L.V., Gesierich, W., Schott-Hildebrand, S. et al. (2015). Endobronchial closure of bronchopleural fistula using Amplatzer device. *J. Thorac. Dis.* 7: 1478–1482.

55 Kaneda, H., Minami, K., Nakano, T. et al. (2015). Efficacy and long-term clinical outcome of bronchial occlusion with endobronchial Watanabe spigots for persistent air leaks. *Respir. Invest.* 53: 30–36.

56 Morikawa, S., Okamura, T., Minezawa, T. et al. (2016). A simple method of bronchial occlusion with silicone spigots (Endobronchial Watanabe Spigot; EWS (R)) using a curette. *Ther. Adv. Respir. Dis.* 10: 518–524.

57 Kostopanagiotou, K., George, R.S., Kefaloyannis, E., and Papagiannopoulos, K. (2015). Novel technique in managing bronchobiliary fistula in adults: endobronchial embolization using silicone spigots in 2 cases. *Ann. Thorac. Med.* 10: 67–68.

58 Uchida, S., Igaki, H., Izumo, T., and Tachimori, Y. (2017). Effective treatment of empyema with bronchopleural fistula after esophagectomy by endobronchial embolization using endobronchial Watanabe Spigots. *Int. J. Surg. Case Rep.* 33: 1–3.

59 Adachi, T., Oki, M., and Saka, H. (2016). Management considerations for the treatment of idiopathic massive hemoptysis with endobronchial occlusion combined with bronchial artery embolization. *Intern. Med.* 55: 173–177.

60 Han, X., Yin, M., Li, L. et al. (2018). Customized airway stenting for bronchopleural fistula after pulmonary resection by interventional technique: single-center study of 148 consecutive patients. *Surg. Endosc.* 32: 4116–4124.

61 Dutau, H., Breen, D.P., Gomez, C. et al. (2011). The integrated place of tracheobronchial stents in the multidisciplinary management of large post-pneumonectomy fistulas: our experience using a novel customised conical self-expandable metallic stent. *Eur. J. Cardiothorac. Surg.* 39: 185–189.

62 Tsukada, H. and Osada, H. (2005). Use of a modified Dumon stent for postoperative bronchopleural fistula. *Ann. Thorac. Surg.* 80: 1928–1930.

63 Ferraroli, G.M., Testori, A., Cioffi, U. et al. (2006). Healing of bronchopleural fistula using a modified Dumon stent: a case report. *J. Cardiothorac. Surg.* 1: 16.

64 Cao, M., Zhu, Q., Wang, W. et al. (2016). Clinical application of fully covered self-expandable metal stents in the treatment of

bronchial fistula. *Thorac. Cardiovasc. Surg.* 64: 533–539.

65 Manley, K., Coonar, A., Wells, F., and Scarci, M. (2012). Blood patch for persistent air leak: a review of the current literature. *Curr. Opin. Pulm. Med.* 18: 333–338.

66 Wiaterek, G., Lee, H., Malhotra, R., and Shepherd, W. (2013). Bronchoscopic blood patch for treatment of persistent alveolar-pleural fistula. *J. Bronchol. Interv. Pulmonol.* 20: 171–174.

67 Mizumori, Y., Nakahara, Y., Kawamura, T. et al. (2016). Intrabronchial infusion of autologous blood plus thrombin for intractable pneumothorax after bronchial occlusion using silicon spigots: a case series of 9 patients with emphysema. *J. Bronchol. Interv. Pulmonol.* 23: 199–203.

第 31 章

良性气道狭窄和气管支气管软化症的临床诊疗

Qiang Li[1] and Yang Xia[2]
[1] Department of Respiratory and Critical Care Medicine, Shanghai East Hospital,
Tongji University School of Medicine, Shanghai, China
[2] Division of Pulmonary and Critical Care Medicine,
Second Affiliated Hospital of Zhejiang University School of Medicine, Hangzhou, China
（译者：夏　旸　周凌霄　陈　婷　译者单位：浙江大学医学院附属第二医院）

成人和儿童的气管支气管狭窄均有多种临床表现，其病因多样，治疗选择也有所不同。气管支气管狭窄的症状差异较大，表现为轻微或无呼吸困难、反复感染甚至危及生命的气道阻塞。良性气道狭窄（benign airway stenosis，BAS）既往主要通过手术治疗，但随着支气管镜技术的快速创新、应用范围不断扩大、新技术和新器械的开发都推进了气管支气管狭窄或阻塞的治疗方式的革新。根据狭窄的类型、位置、程度和长度不同，球囊扩张、冷冻治疗、热消融和支架置入术都已被用于良性气管支气管狭窄的治疗。

31.1　流行病学和病因

BAS 的病因各不相同，最常见的原因是医源性狭窄、炎症、感染、动态塌陷和气道良性肿瘤（表 31.1）[1]。

表 31.1　良性气道狭窄（BAS）的病因

特发性事件
气管内插管
气管切开术
肺移植

（续表）

感染
结核病
曲霉菌
克雷伯氏鼻疽杆菌
白喉棒状杆菌
梅毒螺旋体
炎症
肉芽肿性多血管炎
复发性多软骨炎
结节病
淀粉样变性
炎症性肠病
气道良性肿瘤
错构瘤
多形性腺瘤
软骨瘤
纤维瘤
鳞状细胞乳头状瘤
血管瘤
动态塌陷
软膜症
气管软化症

在北美和欧洲，BAS 最常见的病因是气管插管、气管切开和肺移植[2,3]。然而，在中国的病因却不尽

相同,最主要的病因是支气管结核,占患者总数的 64.3%,而气管插管或气管切开约占 15%[4]。

31.1.1 医源性病因

由医源性事件引起的气道狭窄在全球范围内受到越来越多的关注。在北美和欧洲,造成气道大范围狭窄的最常见原因是医源性气道狭窄,包括气管切开、气管插管和胸外科手术(如肺移植)[2,5]。气管狭窄最常涉及的两个部位是气管切开部位和气管插管气囊接触的气管壁[5]。这些病变通常是在患者出现拔管困难时才被发现。

插管后气道狭窄由 MacEwen 于 1880 年首次报道[6]。数据显示,多达 1/3 的危重患者在经皮扩张气管造口术(percutaneous dilational tracheostomy,PDT)后

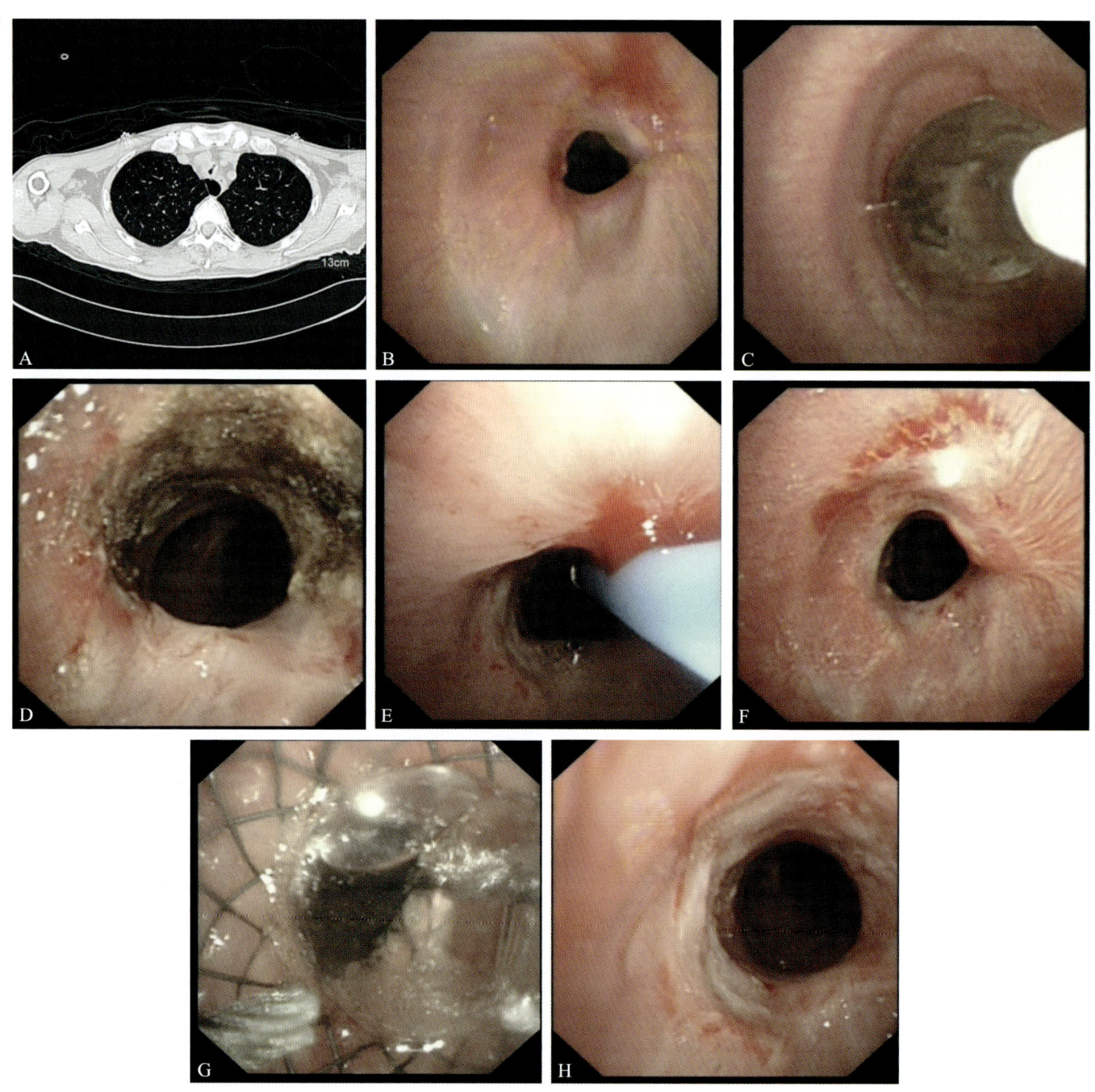

图 31.1　经皮气管切开术导致的气管狭窄
A、B. 胸部 CT 和支气管镜图片示 2 型气管狭窄(bT2L2D4L1.5);C~E. 采用激光切除、球囊扩张和冷冻疗法进行气管扩张;F. 狭窄段很快再次阻塞;G. 置入气管覆膜金属支架 1 个月后;H. 支架移除后气管狭窄段维持通畅。

出现气道狭窄（图 31.1）[7]。迄今为止，气管切开术后和插管术后气道狭窄的发生率仍为 10%~22%，无症状比例较高，严重狭窄的比例较低[8]。气管插管后狭窄一般是由于气囊过度充气导致气管壁受压引起缺血，而气管造口术后狭窄则是由于伤口愈合异常伴有肉芽组织形成过度所致。

气道狭窄是肺移植最常见的并发症，发生率为 5%~15%[5,9,10]。曲霉菌或假单胞菌感染、年龄＜45 岁、气道坏死、长时间气管插管和免疫抑制与气道狭窄相关[5,9,11]。

此外，近年来因不恰当的介入操作手术而导致气道狭窄的发生率也在增加，值得支气管镜医师注意。

31.1.2 感染

在中国某些地方和印度等结核病流行地区，支气管结核是导致 BAS 的主要原因（图 31.2）[12,13]。10%~37% 的肺结核累及气道，90% 的支气管结核患者会出现气道狭窄[5]。气道狭窄可由增生性改变和炎性水肿引起，有时也可由邻近的淋巴结肿大引起。

结核病以外的微生物也会引起良性气管狭窄（benign tracheal stenosis，BTS）。真菌，尤其是曲霉菌会引起气管支气管炎，继而导致气道狭窄。鼻硬结克雷伯菌、白喉棒状杆菌和梅毒螺旋体感染也会引起气道硬结，形成肿块、结节和纤维化，最终导致气道狭窄[1]。值得注意的是，气道狭窄通常发生在愈合期，而不是感染的急性期。

31.1.3 炎症

导致气道狭窄的全身性炎症疾病包括肉芽肿性血管炎（又称韦格纳肉芽肿）、复发性多软骨炎、结节病、淀粉样变性、炎症性肠病和其他全身性胶原血管病[1]。

31.1.4 气管良性肿瘤

气管良性肿瘤都可能导致气道阻塞，如错构瘤、多形性腺瘤、软骨瘤、纤维瘤、鳞状细胞乳头状瘤和血管瘤。甲状腺肿大或甲状腺肿瘤也会造成气道狭窄。

31.1.5 呼气性中央气道塌陷

呼气性中央气道塌陷（exhalatory central airway collapse，ECAC）是指呼气时中央气道的狭窄，主要包括两种病理生理类型：过度动态气道塌陷（excessive dynamic airway collapse，EDAC）和气管支气管软化（tracheobronchomalacia，TBM）（表 31.2）。

表 31.2 气管支气管软化的原因

局限性气管软化	弥漫性气管软化
局限性复发性多软骨炎	严重性复发性多软骨炎
肺结核	食管闭锁
慢性阻塞性肺病	气管食管瘘
慢性支气管炎	气管支气管肥大（Monuier-Kuhn 综合征）
肥胖	
甲状腺肿大	

过度动态气道塌陷的特征是呼气时气道膜部向内鼓起，气道管腔横截面变窄。TBM 是由于纵向弹性纤维减少和/或萎缩以及软骨完整性受损导致的气道壁薄弱。大多数 TBM 病例发生在胸腔内，但也有胸腔外 TBM 的报道[14]。由于对气道塌陷程度的定义不同，TBM 的发病率也不同。最近的证据表明，无症状的健康人也可表现出 TBM[15,16]。因此，诊断标准应加以验证，看是否能将真正的 TBM 和生理范围内的动态气道塌陷区分开来。

TBM 有多种分类方式。从镜下大体形态上看，侧壁塌陷狭窄的 TBM 被称为"剑鞘型"或"裂隙型"，而前后壁塌陷狭窄的 TBM 被称为"新月型"或"鞘状"，第 3 种类型被称为"环状狭窄"，其特征是前两种类型的结合[14]。另一种分类系统将 TBM 分为先天型和后天型[17]。先天性气管软化很少见；而创伤、外科手术、慢性刺激、炎症、机械性改变和恶性肿瘤是后天型气管软化的主要原因。

根据我们的经验，我们建议将 TBM 分为局限性和弥漫性。局限性 TBM 通常发生在局限性复发性多软骨炎、结核、慢性阻塞性肺病和肥胖的患者身上。弥漫性 TBM 由整个气管支气管树的破坏或缺损引起。弥漫性气管支气管软化症常见病因是严重的复发性多软骨炎和先天性软化，常见于食管闭锁和气管食管瘘。另一种罕见的病因是气管支气管巨大症，又称 Mounier-Kuhn 综合征，表现为气道弥漫性扩张和软化。这些患者的特点是反复呼吸道感染和肺炎[18]。

31.2 表现

气管支气管狭窄的表现可无症状或症状轻微，也可出现呼吸困难、感染，甚至危及生命。这主要取决于病变所在区域和狭窄程度。患者最常见的主诉是呼吸困难，其次是肺炎和呼吸衰竭，其中呼吸窘迫只占

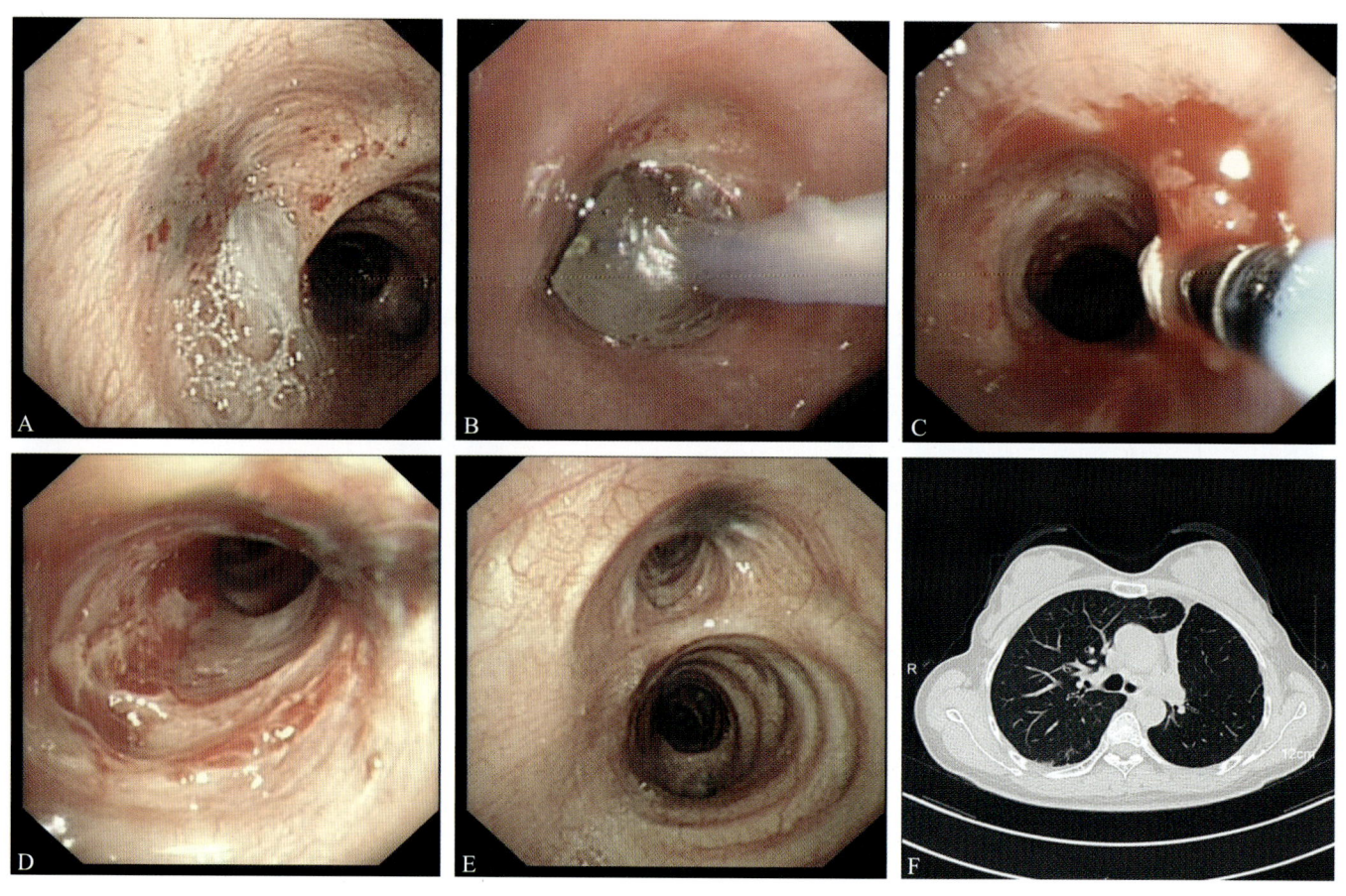

图 31.2　肺结核继发右主支气管阻塞（bT2L4D5L2）
A. 右主支气管严重阻塞，黏液堵塞；B、C. 于右主支气管行反复球囊扩张和冷冻治疗；D. 治疗后的右主支气管。E、F. 最后一次干预 6 个月后，支气管镜检查和胸部 CT 显示右主支气管通畅。

一小部分[9]。如果狭窄位于中央气道，患者可能会出现胸闷、呼吸困难，甚至呼吸窘迫；当狭窄位于支气管时，症状表现为由于局部引流不畅引起的反复感染。

31.3　诊断及评估

良性气管支气管狭窄的诊断根据以下因素确定。

31.3.1　症状

如上所述，不同区域和不同程度的狭窄对应的临床表现各异。体格检查时，可出现吸气性或双相性哮鸣音。此外，还可发现三凹征和发绀。

31.3.2　影像学检查

胸片是评估气道狭窄的经典工具，但诊断敏感性有限。计算机断层扫描（computed tomography，CT）是一种高效、无创的气道狭窄识别方法，可提高诊断率。多平面重组的灵敏度为 86%~89%，特异性为 100%[19]。目前，三维 CT 扫描的层面比传统 CT 扫描更薄，可精确重建气道内外解剖结构，利于定制支架[20]。这种重建技术也被称为虚拟导航支气管镜，有助于更准确地评估病变的长度和程度。此外，吸气和呼气双相 CT 扫描在动态气道狭窄的诊断中也起着举足轻重的作用。呼气相气道面积比吸气相减少 >50% 即为动态气道狭窄[21]。然而，将 50% 作为阈值仍存在争议。对怀疑 TBM 的患者，需要去注意他们的年龄和性别，这对用力呼气时的气道塌陷有很大影响。

31.3.3　肺功能检查

肺功能检查广泛应用于气道狭窄的评估。肺容积和流速容积曲线的测量可为评估气道狭窄提供重要信息。有趣的是，呼气峰流速（peak expiratory flow rate，PEFR）和最大通气量（maximal voluntary ventilation，

MVV）比第 1 秒用力呼气量（forced expiratory volume in first second，FEV$_1$）对气道狭窄更敏感。通常情况下，呼气流速的达峰时间延迟或峰值下降，以及最大通气量受损都支持气道狭窄的诊断[1]。对于流速容积曲线，FEV$_1$ 的下降可能提示诊断，但呼吸环的形状提供了更直接的证据[9]。在固定气道阻塞的病例中，曲线的吸气和呼气相均变平，而在气管上 1/3 的动态塌陷中，仅吸气相变平[1]。肺功能检查对 TBM 的诊断价值非常有限。ECAC 不会导致气流受限。相当多的中、重度 TBM 患者（21%）可显示正常的流速容积曲线[22]。不过，我们仍建议对这类患者进行常规肺功能检查，以排除阻塞性气道疾病等合并症。

31.3.4 支气管镜检查

支气管镜检查被认为是诊断气道塌陷和狭窄的"金标准"，能全面地获得相关信息，包括气道塌陷和狭窄的位置、形状、长度和严重程度。此外，还可根据需要进行直接活检或针吸活检。此外，支气管腔内超声检查有助于评估气道力学完整性，这是制定治疗策略的决定性参数。

31.4 分类

气道狭窄有多种分类方法。Cotton 等主要研究喉-气管狭窄，最先提出根据狭窄的横截面积将其分为 4 个等级[23]。McCaffrey 根据狭窄部位升级了喉-气管狭窄的分期概念：① 1 期：在声门下或气管，长度<1 cm；② 2 期：在声门下，长度>1 cm；③ 3 期：在声门下和气管上部；④ 4 期：在声门，声带固定和麻痹[24]。Myer 等[23]对气管狭窄程度进行了分类：Ⅰ级（≤50%）；Ⅱ级（51%~70%）；Ⅲ级（>70%）；Ⅳ级（完全阻塞）。

目前的共识是，一个成熟的分类系统可以准确、全面、简明地概括气管支气管狭窄的情况，并方便支气管镜医生进行治疗判断。因此，我们对 Freitag 以前的分类系统进行了修改，提出了"TLDL"系统，指的是类型（type）、位置（location）、程度（degree）和长度（length），这与肺癌采用的 TNM 分期系统类似。

31.4.1 狭窄类型

BAS 可根据结构支持的完整性分为 3 种类型（表 31.3、图 31.3）。CT 和/或超声可用于评估力学完整性。类型 1 指力学完整性完好的狭窄，2 型指力学完整性轻度受损的狭窄，3 型指力学完整性重度损伤的狭窄（表 31.3）。

表 31.3 狭窄类型

类型	狭窄
1	力学完整性完好
2	力学完整性部分受损
3	力学完整性严重受损

31.4.2 狭窄位置

狭窄的位置与手术风险直接相关。我们定义了中央气道内的 5 个位置（表 31.4）。

1）位置 1：声门下区，距离真声带远端<2 cm，高危；
2）位置 2：气管区，距离真声带远端>2 cm，中危；
3）位置 3：隆突区，中-高危；
4）位置 4：左/右主支气管，低-中危；
5）位置 5：双侧主支气管，中-高危。

表 31.4 气道狭窄的位置

位置	风险
1 声门下区	高
2 气管区	中
3 隆突区	中-高
4 左/右主支气管	低-中
5 双侧主支气管	中-高

31.4.3 狭窄程度

狭窄程度可用于任何部位[25]。具体来说，0 表示无明显的狭窄，1、2、3 和 4 分别表示横截面积减少 25%、50%、75% 和 90%；5 表示完全阻塞（表 31.5）。

表 31.5 气道狭窄的程度

分级	程度（%）
0	无狭窄
1	<25

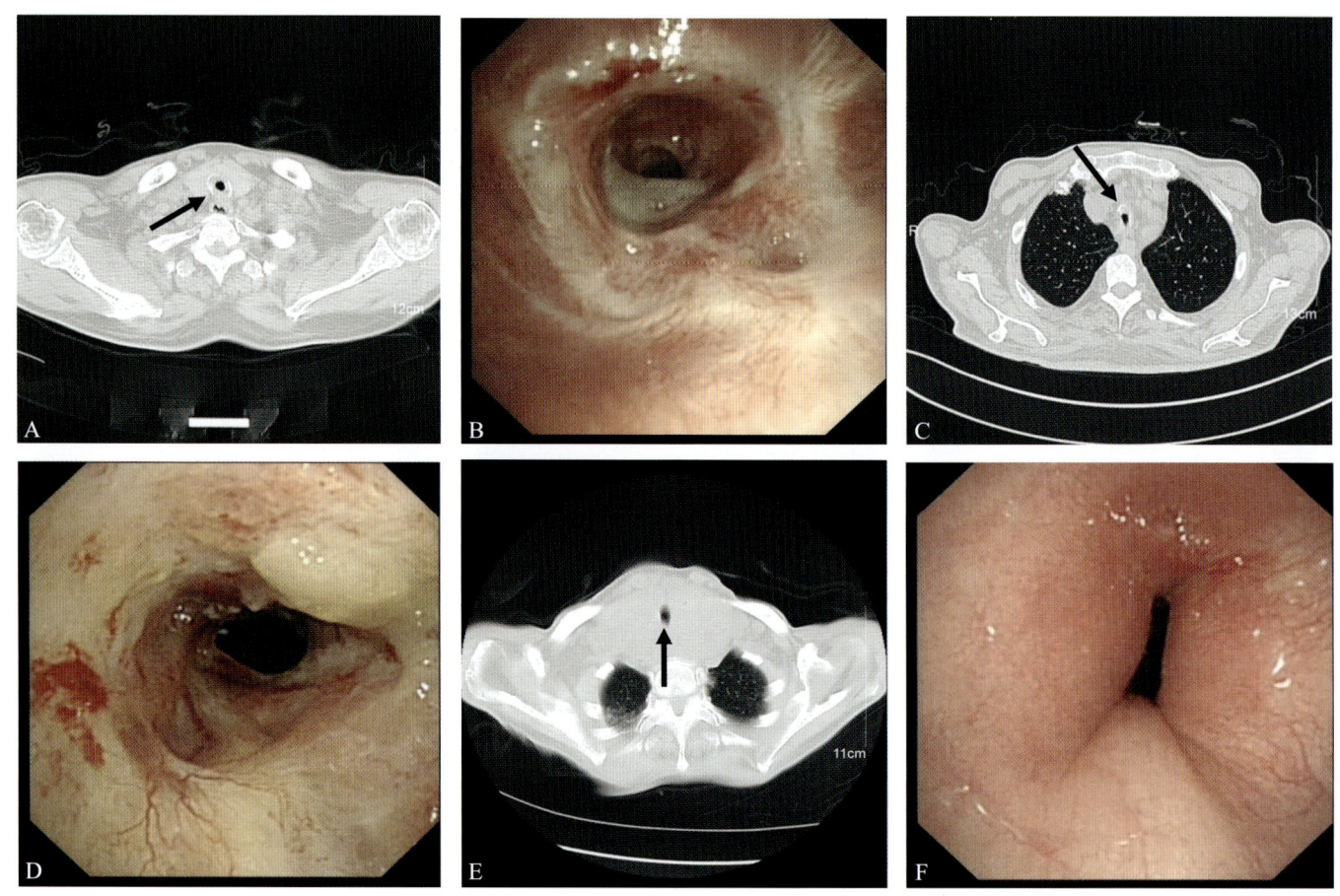

图 31.3 支气管镜和 CT 显示的良性气道狭窄（BAS）形态类型

A、B. 力学完整性完好的气管狭窄（箭头示）；C、D. 力学完整性部分受损的气道狭窄（箭头示）；E、F. 力学完整性严重受损的狭窄。

（续表）

分级	程度（%）
2	26~50
3	51~75
4	76~90
5	91~100

31.4.4 狭窄长度

我们建议记录绝对值来描述狭窄长度。值得注意的是，如果狭窄长度>5 cm，则不适合外科手术。此外，还应考虑到狭窄处与周围正常气道交界是逐渐过渡还是突然形成的。

总之，我们将狭窄的类型、位置、程度和长度等信息整合在一起。同时，如果数据是通过支气管镜收集的，我们在 TLDL 前使用"b"。同样，如果数据来自 CT、MRI 或虚拟支气管镜，我们在前面使用"r"。

例如，标注为 bT1L2D4L3 的狭窄表示经支气管镜证实的长度 3 cm、狭窄程度 76%~90% 且结构支撑完好的距声带 2 cm 以上的气管狭窄。

31.4.5 Cotton-Meyer 系统

对于声门下气道狭窄，一般采用 Cotton-Meyer 系统（表 31.6）[23]。不过，该系统只能反映狭窄的程度，而我们的 TLDL 系统能提供更广泛的信息。

表 31.6 Cotton-Meyer 分级系统

分级	阻塞比例（%）
Ⅰ级	0~50
Ⅱ级	51~70
Ⅲ级	71~99
Ⅳ级	无法探及管腔

31.5 治疗

BAS 的治疗原则是通过最小的侵入性方法重新开通气道，以带给患者最小风险和最大的受益。具体的治疗方案取决于病因、TLDL 分级，以及患者的年龄和健康状况。一般来说，结构支撑是否完整对治疗策略的选择起着核心作用。对于 T1 型（力学完整性完好的狭窄），建议采用球囊扩张、冷冻疗法和硬质支气管镜/扩张器，必要时还可采用电针刀松解术。除非情况紧急，否则很少置入支架。同样，对于 T2 型（力学完整性轻度受损的狭窄），也会常规使用扩张、冷冻治疗和电刀松解。与 T1 型不同，支架置入术是 T2 型的替代方案。对于 T3 型（力学完整性受损的狭窄），单一的球囊扩张和冷冻疗法只有短暂的效果。包括硅酮和金属在内的支架置入术是首选方法。

31.5.1 球囊扩张

球囊扩张是目前广泛应用于 BAS 的治疗技术。1991 年，Nakamura 等首次报道了使用可弯曲支气管镜进行球囊扩张治疗 BAS[26,27]。研究人员发现，固定狭窄（T1 和 T2）患者对球囊扩张的反应较好，而软骨损伤（T3）患者的反应相对较差[1,28]。

一般来说，球囊扩张术是一种安全、简便、有效的介入治疗，可用于治疗多种病因引起的气道狭窄。它可以单独使用，也可以作为其他手术的辅助手段，必要时还可以重复多次。在手术过程中，大多数患者需要深度镇静或全身麻醉。在局部麻醉或中度镇静的情况下，中心气道的扩张时间不能超过 1 min。球囊扩张的关键因素是球囊的大小和长度，这取决于狭窄段的直径和长度（D 和 L 参数）以及治疗后的预期直径。理想情况下，球囊的长度应超过狭窄段约 1 cm。球囊直径的判断标准是充气后的直径比治疗后的预期直径大 2~3 mm。气管镜下直视非常重要，可以及时监视扩张过程和发现可能的并发症。通常建议逐步扩张，以避免气道撕裂。使用连接到压力计的注射器将球囊充气并保持在设计压力下。每次扩张大约持续 1 min，根据扩张的难易程度可重复多次。

球囊扩张可以处理复杂的狭窄（图 31.4）。当遇到瘢痕挛缩时，建议将电刀松解术和随后的球囊扩张术结合起来，作为标准化的治疗方法。有的管腔内肿瘤局部组织质脆，或出现坏死，血管成形球囊导管（如 Fogarty 球囊）等顺应性好的球囊将是更好的选择[1]。对于张力大的狭窄区域，应考虑使用硬质球囊，如可控径向扩张球囊[1]。

球囊扩张术鲜有并发症的报道。它可能会出现气管支气管破裂、气胸、气道阻塞、出血、黏液堵塞和呼吸功能不全。

31.5.2 热消融治疗

热消融治疗，包括激光治疗、电烧灼和氩等离子体凝固术（argon plasma coagulation，APC），广泛应用于治疗性支气管镜操作，以清除肿瘤、控制出血、去除肉芽组织，以及治疗其他导致气道狭窄的良性疾病。选择合适的工具和合理的治疗方案极为重要。否则，不恰当的治疗，尤其是热消融本身，可能会对气道造成不可逆的损伤，最终导致气道狭窄恶化。

31.5.2.1 激光

激光切除术是治疗气管支气管阻塞的一种安全、有效的工具，可迅速缓解症状。最常用的激光类型有 Nd:YAG、钬激光和二氧化碳激光。Nd:YAG 具有凝固特性，可穿透 10 mm，比二氧化碳激光更深，而二氧化碳激光的切割更精确。因此，二氧化碳激光和钬激光更适合用于 L1 型患者，而 Nd:YAG 则更适合用于其他位置的气管狭窄。激光治疗适用于 T1 型和 T2 型狭窄的患者，特别是气管插管和气管切开造成的狭窄、与感染有关的炎性肉芽组织、手术引起的吻合口肉芽、吻合处肉芽肿、良性或低度恶性肿瘤、支气管结石以及胶原血管疾病。

激光治疗的并发症一般不严重，但一旦出现就可能是致命的。术中的严重并发症包括气管内起火、大出血、气管食管瘘、体循环空气栓塞、气胸和纵隔气肿。

31.5.2.2 电烧灼和氩等离子体凝固术（APC）

电烧灼和 APC 治疗 BAS 的适应证相对有限，如 T1、T2 型患者的腔内病变。重要的是，过度使用电烧灼和 APC 治疗可能会对结缔组织和软骨造成损伤。因此，在靠近病灶底部进行剥离时，最好避免使用电烧灼或 APC。相比之下，电刀松解术后再用球囊扩张被认为是治疗瘢痕挛缩的首选方法。

电烧灼和 APC 的并发症与激光相似，经验丰富的操作者可大大降低风险。

31.5.3 冷冻疗法

冷冻疗法是一项极其重要的技术。呼吸道由对低

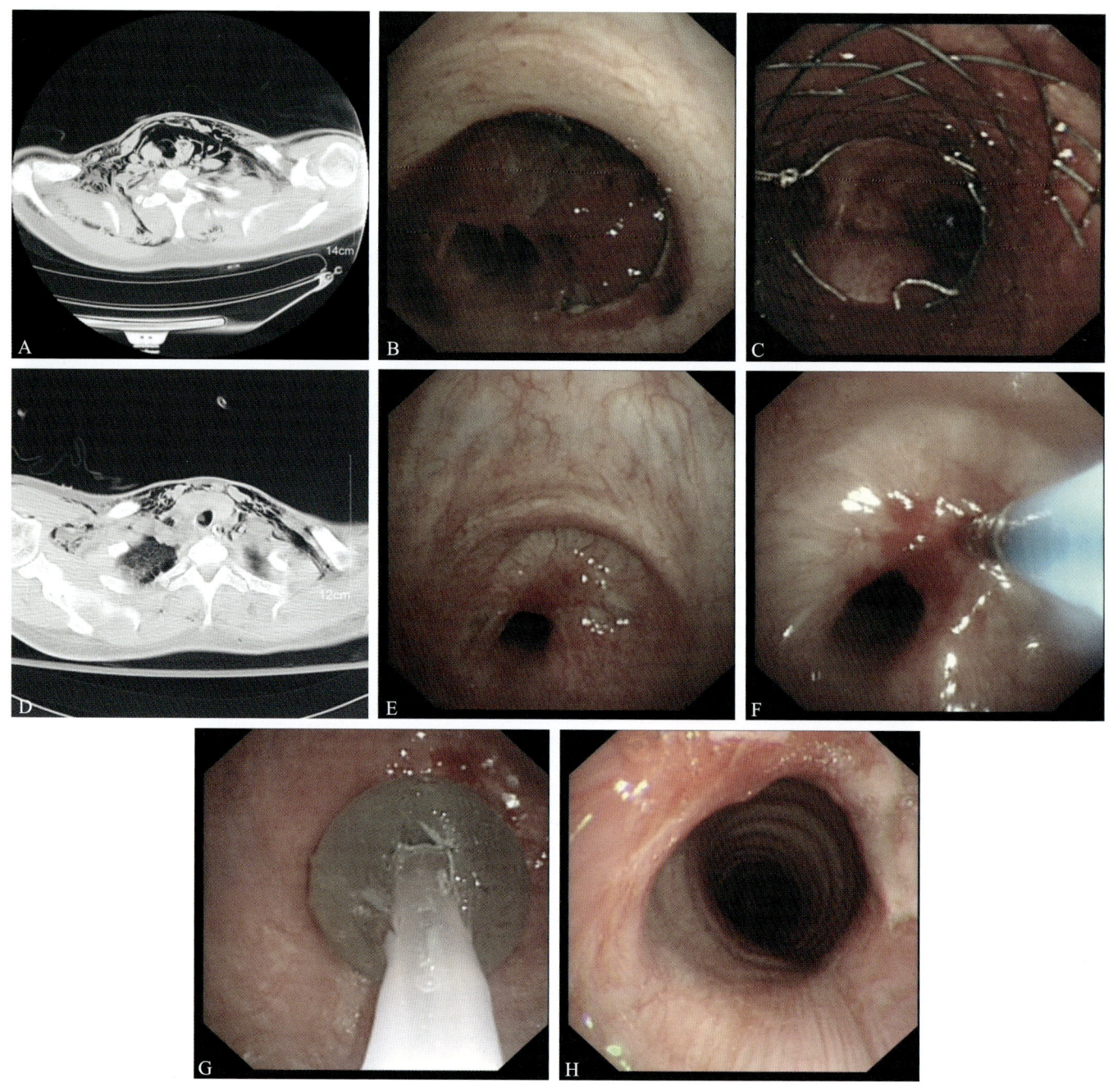

图 31.4　车祸导致气管破裂（bT3L1D4L2.5）

A. 气管破裂导致皮下气肿和纵隔气肿；B. 颈部气管被纵隔结缔组织阻塞；C、D. 置入全覆膜镍钛金属合金支架，症状迅速缓解；E. 狭窄得到缓解；F~H. 实施球囊扩张和冷冻疗法。

温敏感的组织（包括黏膜和肉芽组织）以及对低温不敏感的组织（如脂肪、软骨、纤维和结缔组织）组成。因此，冷冻疗法可完全破坏黏膜和黏膜下腺体，却同时维持结缔组织和软骨框架的完整性。

因此，冷冻疗法是 T1 型和 T2 型患者的首选方法（图 31.5）。通常来说，在球囊扩张后，我们会开始冷冻治疗。用冷冻探头直接接触狭窄段，每次 1 min，每个点可重复 3 次冻融循环。组织被冷冻到 −40~−30℃后，镜下可以观察到相应的组织破坏。

目前冷冻治疗主要有两种：接触式和喷雾式。接触式冷冻治疗通过低温和恢复至人体温度的交替形成冻融循环。喷雾冷冻疗法使用液氮作为基础冷冻剂，就像激光疗法一样，能量转移过程中温度降低达到冷冻治疗的目的。

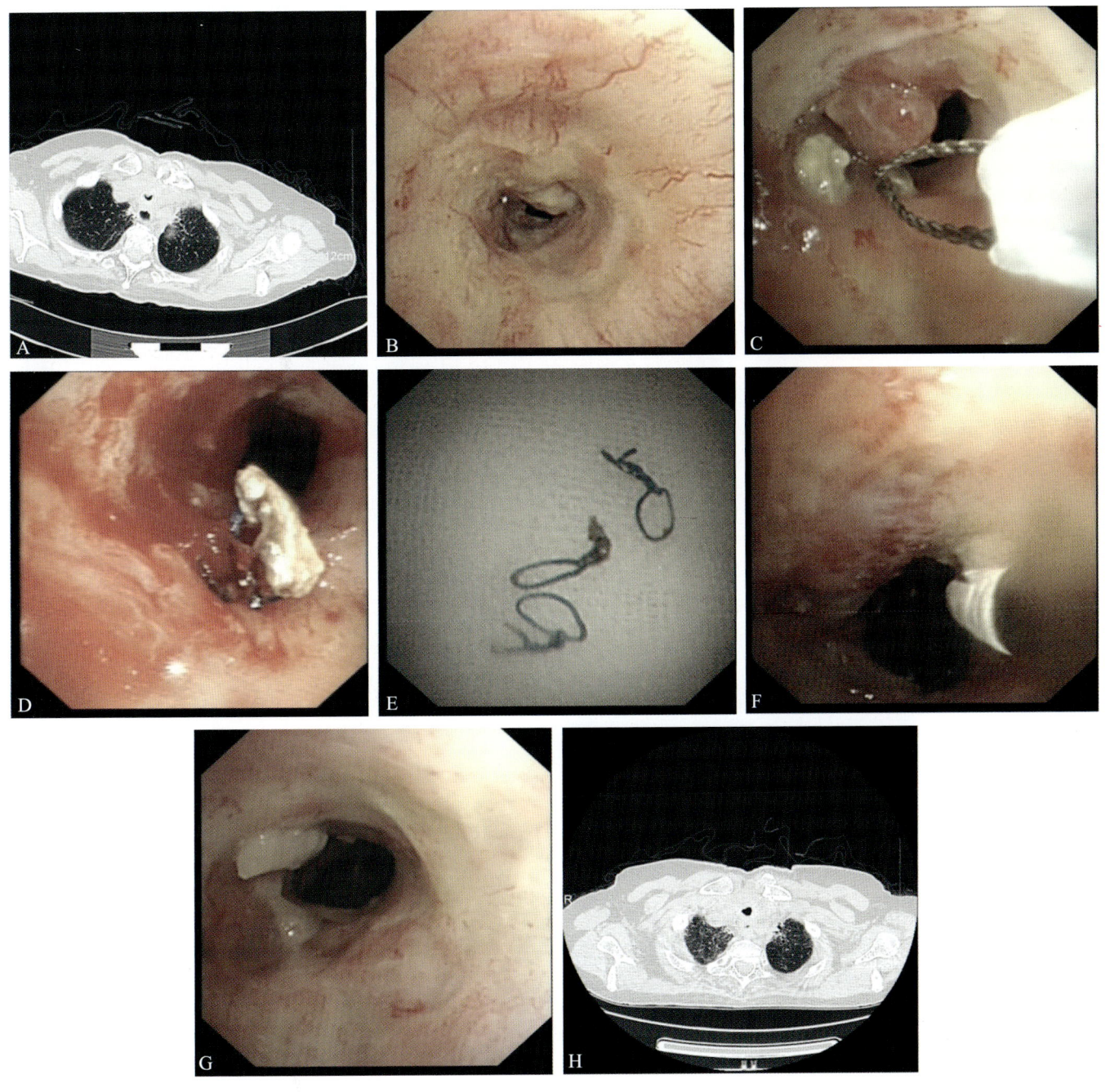

图 31.5 外科左胸锁关节脓肿（bT1L2D5L2）术后

A、B. 胸部 CT 和支气管镜视图显示 1 型气管狭窄；C、D. 用电圈套器切除肉芽组织后，露出手术缝合线；E、F. 钳除缝线，并用冷冻治疗基底部；G、H. 3 个月后随访时气管通畅。

与球囊扩张类似，冷冻疗法安全、易于操作、价格低廉且并发症少。

31.5.4 支架

近几十年来，支架技术已发展成为治疗 BAS 的一项重要技术。气道是受呼吸影响的弹性结构，因此在治疗 BAS 时应考虑到气道的固有特性以及支架的材料和工程学。

在上文中，我们指出了热消融、球囊扩张和冷冻治疗对 BAS 的价值，尤其是对 T1 或 T2 型患者。然而，对于 T3 型患者，这 3 种方法或许只能作为辅助。如果没有可通过手术治愈的病变，且球囊扩张只能暂时缓解狭窄，则需要置入支架[29]。在评估支架置入的可能性时，必须事先进行仔细的 TLDL 评估。

31.5.4.1 硅酮支架

硅酮支架是治疗 BAS 最常用的气道植入物。现代硅酮支架从 Montgomery "T" 管改良而来，由 Dumon 于 1990 年首次推出。硅酮支架的置入比较简单，需要在全身麻醉下通过硬质支气管镜，使用专用的推送器置入。与金属支架相比，硅酮支架的突出优点是肉芽形成的概率较低，且易于取出。此外，硅酮支架可以重复放置，是 BAS 的理想选择。

以 Dumon 支架为例，硅酮支架具有多种设计，可用于不同情况：L1（声门下区）和 L2（气管）可使用不同厚度的气管支架（TD/TF 支架）；L4（左/右主支气管）使用支气管支架（BD 支架）；用于 L3（隆突）和 L5（双侧第二隆突）可使用分叉支架（"Y"形支架）、L1、L2 和 L4 可以选用气管–支气管支架（ST 支架）、L4 可选用隆突–支气管支架（CB 支架），以及用于右 L4 加中间支气管的 Oki 支架（由名古屋医疗中心的 Masahide Oki 发明）。目前，大多数型号的 Dumon 支架都可以定制，并且可以制作成不透射线/透射线的。

然而，硅酮支架移位和分泌物潴留是一个重要问题[30]。据报道，总体移位率为 9.5%，分泌物阻塞率为 3.6%。气管软化患者的移位率可能会增加到 20%，最终导致治疗失败[28,31-33]。为了解决这些问题，支架外突起硅胶钉突和支架袖口样设计来固定支架不移位。目前已开发出一些特殊设计，如沙漏形支架（Dumon ST 支架）和近端带有固定帽的 I 形支架（Dumon CB 支架）。此外，还有研究概述了各种经皮在 L1 腔内固定硅酮支架（Dumon TD/TF 支架）的方法[34,35]。对于分泌物阻塞，雾化生理盐水加湿有助于防止分泌物积聚；但除非怀疑感染，不建议立即使用抗生素。使用硅酮支架的患者也可能出现肉芽组织；据报道，肉芽形成率在 6%~20% 之间[32,36]。

硅酮支架置入的目的可以是治愈性也可以是姑息性。Martinez-Ballarin 等的研究进行了 486（±260）天的随访，他们发现 43% 的患者在疾病根治后可以取出支架；而如果只是为了缓解病情，硅酮支架也可以永久放置[37]。目前还没有明确的硅酮支架移除时机。过早取出支架可能会导致气管再狭窄，而过晚取出支架可能会引起与支架相关的并发症。研究发现，再狭窄率与支架放置时间呈负相关。支架放置超过 14 个月的结核后的患者无一例出现再狭窄[38]。在笔者单位，支架放置时长由力学完整性的恢复情况决定。例如，对于支持组织完全破坏的 T3 型患者，将每 6 个月进行一次 HRCT 进行支气管树重建，如果出现钙化影，表明支撑结构正在重建，因此这可能是取出支架的合适时机。通常，这一过程将持续至少 8 个月，但需要进一步研究来确定。

Montgomery "T" 管是一种特殊形式的硅酮支架，用于气管切开后的 L1 患者。它于 1891 年问世，1965 年由蒙哥马利改良成稍柔软的硅酮材料装置[39]。由于其独特的设计，它具有多项优点[40]：

1）双重通气通道保证了双重安全。即使近声门端被黏液或肉芽堵塞，T 支（即外支）仍可开放，用于抽吸和通气；

2）由于 T 支通过气管切开部位固定，因此不太可能发生移位；

3）由于保留了发音功能，患者的生活质量得到了显著提高；

4）由于 Montgomery "T" 管不存在移位问题，因此我们倾向于选择比气管切口小的尺寸，以便减少肉芽组织；

5）Montgomery "T" 管也有缺点。放置过程比较复杂，需要在气管切开部位使用硬质支气管镜和钳子；可能会影响声带功能，尤其是当 "T" 管近端与声带、声门相邻时。

31.5.4.2 金属支架

金属支架和硅酮支架有诸多不同，因此适用于不同的情况。金属支架由网状金属丝制成，通常可自行膨胀，具有良好的重塑能力，可适应各种狭窄情况。由于金属支架可以通过导丝和压缩输送系统经由可弯曲支气管镜置入，因此其应用越来越广泛。最近，Jiang 等[41]对导引器进行了改进，直接通过支气管镜工作通道插入释放系统，然后在实时可视的情况下展开支架。然而，金属支架易刺激肉芽肿形成，且难以移动，这些弊病限制了金属裸支架的使用，因此主要用于恶性的气道狭窄[42,43]。与金属裸支架相比，聚氨酯覆膜金属支架是良性病变的一种选择（图 31.6）。不同公司生产的覆膜支架有完全覆盖型和部分覆盖型。覆膜支架对肿瘤生长的抵抗力比金属裸支架更强，且易于移除，但也更容易移位。金属支架有多种形状可供选择，如用于常规用途的 I 形、用于 L3（隆突）和 L5（双侧第二隆突）的 "Y" 形、用于 L2（气管）和 L4（左/右主支气管）的带角度的 "J" 形。为了克服移位问题，我们最近设计了一种新的沙漏形全覆膜金属支架，可用于 L1（声门下区）、L2 和 L4 患者（图 31.7）。

如前所述，在植入硅酮支架之前，应先进行球囊

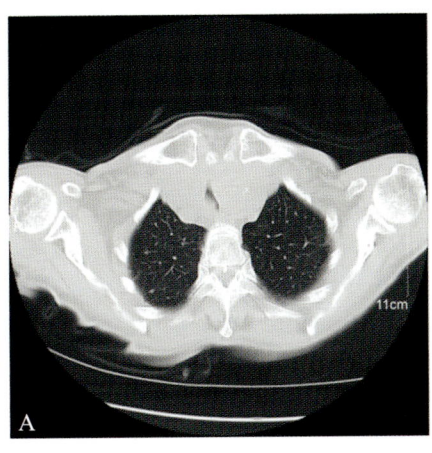
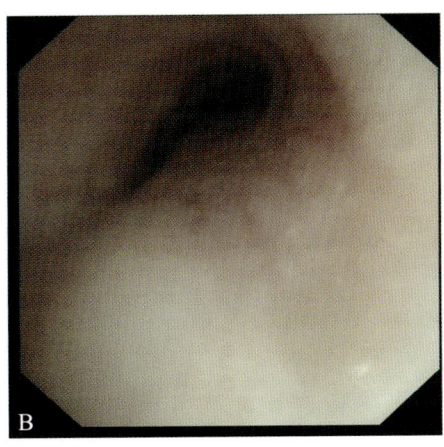
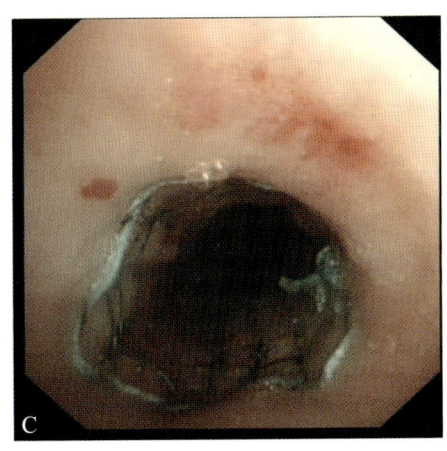

图 31.6 甲状腺肿大引起的 3 类上气道狭窄（bT3L2D5L3）
A. 胸部 CT 显示气管被胸内甲状腺肿压迫；B. 支气管镜下可见外压性狭窄；C. 使用镍钛合金（Ultraflex™）支架治疗阻塞。

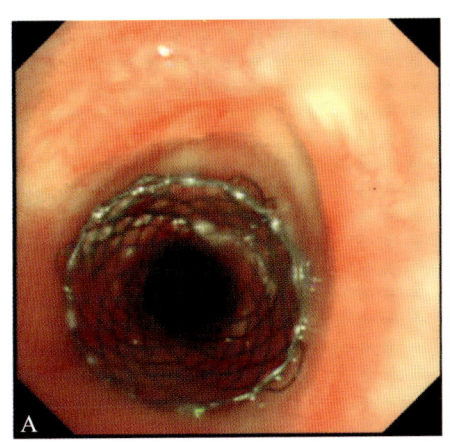
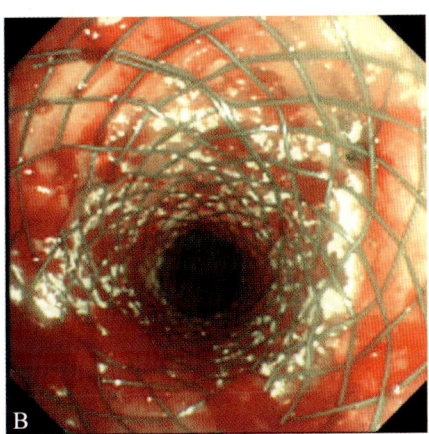
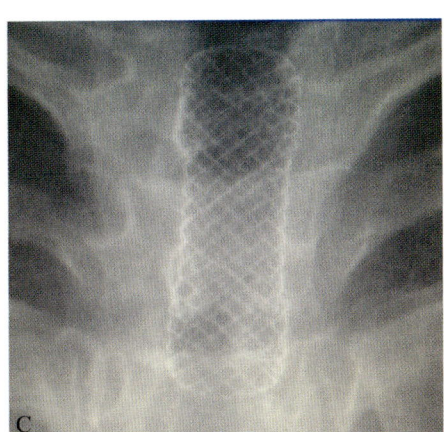
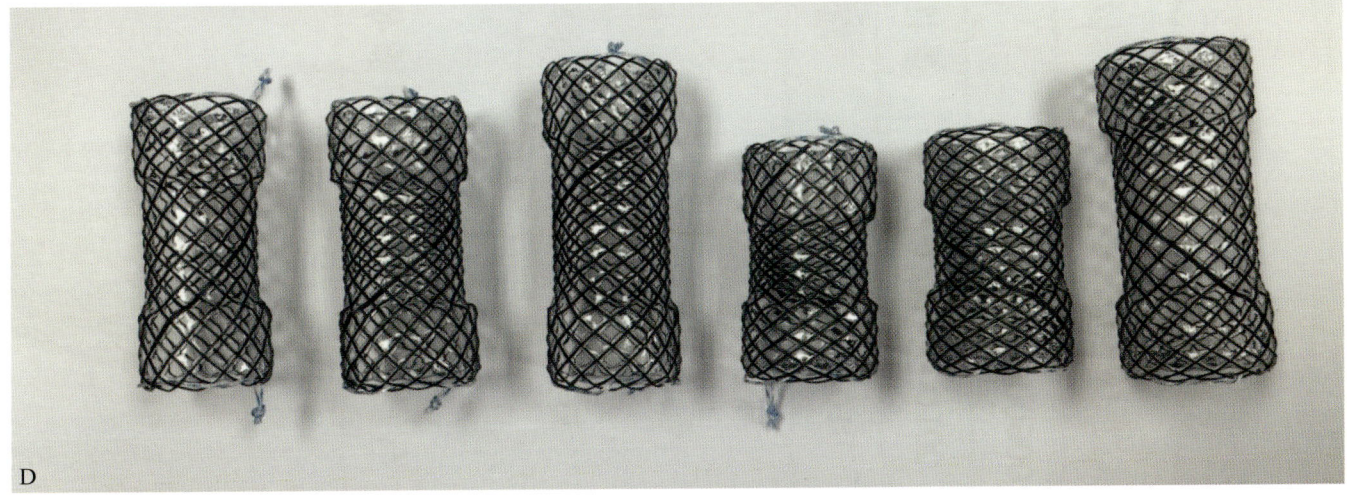

图 31.7 沙漏形全覆膜金属支架
A~C. 沙漏形金属支架置入治疗 L1 狭窄（bT3L1D4L1）；D. 全覆膜沙漏形金属支架。

扩张或清理气道，以确保支架的正确置入。此外，我们还尝试了"暂时性支架置入"的概念。简而言之，我们将一个自膨胀金属支架进行短期置入，通常 1~2 周，让支架在狭窄部位产生持续的扩张力。在这种情况下，我们得以减少反复球囊扩张的次数。另外，与球囊扩张产生的瞬时暴力扩张相比，金属支架的扩张力更温和也更持久。为了便于移除这种暂时支架，我们在支架的两端都加装了调整线，这使取支架操作更加简便。此外，置入暂时支架的材料和手术费也比多次球囊扩张术更便宜。总之，对于 BAS 难治性病例，暂时支架置入术是一种安全、可靠、经济的策略。

31.5.4.3 其他支架

复合支架兼具金属和硅酮支架的特点。Freitag 动力支架是一种主要用于 L2 和 L3 患者的复合支架，但其插入和放置的器械比较特殊，需经专门培训。其他类型的复合支架，包括 Orlowski 支架和 Nova 支架等的数据还需进一步的临床统计。工业新进展使得临床医师能够尝试使用 3D 打印的支架治疗 BAS。一些来自动物模型和人体的试验性研究都获得了令人鼓舞的数据[44,45]。药物洗脱支架也被应用于恶性和良性气道狭窄。据观察，丝裂霉素 C 和西罗莫司可通过减少肉芽肿组织的形成来帮助支架的成功置入[46]。最近，包括吉非替尼微球在内的抗癌药物被载入聚氨酯结构作为药物洗脱支架涂层[47]。此外，支架表面处理也是一个重要方向，如化学物质（如氯己定）、金属离子（如银离子）和抗生素（如米诺环素、利福平）涂层都可用于控制感染[48]。一些研究人员对可降解材料进行了研究，旨在发明可按预定方式降解的支架。

尽管前景乐观，但在投入商业应用之前，以上理想的支架仍有相当多的工艺和法律限制需要攻克。

31.5.5 病灶内注射药物

再狭窄是 BAS 的主要问题，其中成纤维母细胞发挥重要作用。已开展了一些减少再狭窄的治疗方法，包括局部注射类固醇、曲尼司特、紫杉醇和丝裂霉素 C[49]。一项针对成人喉气管狭窄患者的前瞻性、随机、对照研究发现，丝裂霉素 C 可延缓但不能完全阻止伤口愈合反应[49]。另一项在中国进行的临床试验发现，采用曲安奈德局部注射联合传统介入技术治疗的患者，其再狭窄间期更长，气道狭窄率更低，呼吸困难评分更低[50]。

31.5.6 手术治疗

开放性手术治疗，如环状软骨前切开术、喉气管重建术、环状软骨气管重建术、气管切除并残端吻合术、滑动气管成形术、袖状切除术和支气管成形术仍是高度狭窄（D4 和 D5）的一线治疗方式。当狭窄累及喉部时，切除吻合术应延伸至声门下，治疗方案也因狭窄部位及长度、气管受累长度以及对声门开放度和声带活动度的细致评估来综合决定。

（1）手术指征 手术指征包括：

1）气管插管后狭窄；

2）气管切开术后狭窄；

3）创伤后狭窄；

4）继发性气管肿瘤；

5）气管食管瘘和气管内隐匿的瘘口。

（2）预后

然而，对于以下患者，药物治疗或内镜介入治疗会带来更好的预后：

1）炎症和非环形梗阻的患者，如肉芽肿和部分纤维瘢痕狭窄；

2）气管支架置入的患者[51]；

3）伴有"O"形环和气管软化的长距离先天性气管狭窄患者；

4）严重慢性阻塞性肺病、糖尿病和缺血性心血管疾病患者[52]。

（3）并发症

手术并发症包括：

1）吻合口感染和炎症；

2）肺炎；

3）吻合口瘘；

4）吻合口开裂；

5）再狭窄；

6）气管软化；

7）喉部受累时出现喉功能障碍；

8）出血。

（4）其他

再狭窄的原因包括[53]术后水肿、吻合口张力过大以及吻合口感染和炎症。吻合口感染和炎症是造成吻合口再狭窄和瘘的主要原因，需要术后对气道进行精心护理。重复手术、切除时间过长、扩大切除范围至喉部是出现手术并发症的常见危险因素[54]。

31.5.7 呼气性中央气道塌陷（ECAC）的治疗

其他良性气道狭窄的治疗原则也适用于 ECAC。由于 ECAC 是由于气道膜部向腔内膨出，而 TBM 是由于气道壁（包括弹性纤维和软骨完整性）薄弱所致，因此 ECAC 和 TBM 都属于 T3 狭窄。所以支架置入是重要的治疗方法。为 ECAC 置入支架后，70% 的患者短期内生活质量和功能状态得到改善，90% 的患者呼吸困难得到改善。然而，在支架植入或膜部气管成形术后，肺功能似乎并无改善[55]。重要的是，我们要注意常见的支架相关并发症。对于严重、弥漫性和有症状的病例来说，硅酮支架是首选。硅酮支架的形状和大小取决于 L 因素（长度和位置）。此外，TBM 患者也可从自膨胀金属支架的短期扩张中获益[56]，这完全符合我们的"暂时性支架置入"理论。为 TBM 患者置入支架的一个问题是气流受限的病理生理部位。我们将支架置入呼气时出现塌陷最明显的区域，这会使气流受限的部位向更远端移动[16]，但还需要进一步的研究来帮助预测哪些患者能从中获益。

为 TBM 置入支架的一个目的是缓解症状，另一个目的是为外科干预做好准备。气管支气管成形术是稳定胸内气管（包括主支气管和右中间支气管）支气管壁的最广泛应用的外科治疗。软化的气管支气管在手术治疗稳定后，可显著改善呼吸相关的生活质量、呼吸困难指数和活动耐量[56]。气道正压通气可作为气管支架置入的替代选择。持续气道正压通气可改善症状、减少分泌物。维持气道通畅所需的压力可通过间歇正压通气辅助支气管镜检查来确定[57]。

参考文献

1. Puchalski, J. and Musani, A.I. (2013). Tracheobronchial stenosis: causes and advances in management. *Clin. Chest Med.* 34: 557–567.
2. Grillo, H.C. and Donahue, D.M. (1996). Post intubation tracheal stenosis. *Semin. Thorac. Cardiovasc. Surg.* 8: 370–380.
3. Wain, J.C. Jr. (2009). Postintubation tracheal stenosis. *Semin. Thorac. Cardiovasc. Surg.* 21: 284–289.
4. Li, Y.Q., Li, Q., Bai, C. et al. (2008). Causes of benign central airway stenoses and the efficacy of interventional treatments through flexible bronchoscopy. *Zhonghua Jie HeHeHuXi Za Zhi* 31: 364–368.
5. Grenier, P.A., Beigelman-Aubry, C., and Brillet, P.Y. (2010). Nonneoplastic tracheal and bronchial stenoses. *Thorac. Surg. Clin.* 20: 47–64.
6. Macewen, W. (1880). Clinical observations on the introduction of tracheal tubes by the mouth, instead of performing tracheotomy or Laryngotomy. *Br. Med. J.* 2: 163–165.
7. Norwood, S., Vallina, V.L., Short, K. et al. (2000). Incidence of tracheal stenosis and other late complications after percutaneous tracheostomy. *Ann. Surg.* 232: 233–241.
8. Zias, N., Chroneou, A., Tabba, M.K. et al. (2008). Post tracheostomy and post intubation tracheal stenosis: report of 31 cases and review of the literature. *BMC Pulm. Med.* 8: 18.
9. Thistlethwaite, P.A., Yung, G., Kemp, A. et al. (2008). Airway stenoses after lung transplantation: incidence, management, and outcome. *J. Thorac. Cardiovasc. Surg.* 136: 1569–1575.
10. Alvarez, A., Algar, J., Santos, F. et al. (2001). Airway complications after lung transplantation: a review of 151 anastomoses. *Eur. J. Cardiothorac. Surg.* 19: 381–387.
11. Herrera, J.M., McNeil, K.D., Higgins, R.S. et al. (2001). Airway complications after lung transplantation: treatment and long-term outcome. *Ann. Thorac. Surg.* 71: 989–993.
12. Ryu, Y.J., Kim, H., Yu, C.M. et al. (2006). Use of silicone stents for the management of post-tuberculosis tracheobronchial stenosis. *Eur. Respir. J.* 28: 1029–1035.
13. Kashyap, S., Mohapatra, P.R., and Saini, V. (2003). Endobronchial tuberculosis. *Indian J. Chest Dis. Allied Sci.* 45: 247–256.
14. Carden, K.A., Boiselle, P.M., Waltz, D.A. et al. (2005). Tracheomalacia and tracheobronchomalacia in children and adults: an in-depth review. *Chest* 127: 984–1005.
15. Boiselle, P.M., O'Donnell, C.R., Bankier, A.A. et al. (2009). Tracheal collapsibility in healthy volunteers during forced expiration: assessment with multidetector CT. *Radiology* 252: 255–262.
16. Litmanovich, D., O'Donnell, C.R., Bankier, A.A. et al. (2010). Bronchial collapsibility at forced expiration in healthy volunteers: assessment with multidetector CT. *Radiology* 257: 560–567.
17. Feist, J.H., Johnson, T.H., and Wilson, R.J. (1975). Acquired tracheomalacia: etiology and differential diagnosis. *Chest* 68: 340–345.
18. Wright, C.D. (2003). Tracheomalacia. *Chest Surg. Clin. North Am.* 13: 349–357.
19. Morshed, K., Trojanowska, A., Szymanski, M. et al. (2011). Evaluation of tracheal stenosis: comparison between computed tomography virtual tracheobronchoscopy with multiplanar reformatting, flexible tracheofiberoscopy and intra-operative findings. *Eur. Arch. Otorhinolaryngol.* 268: 591–597.
20. Zwierzak, I., Cosentino, D., Narracott, A.J. et al. (2014). Measurement of in vitro and in vivo stent geometry and deformation by means of 3D imaging and stereo-photogrammetry. *Int. J. Artif. Organs* 37: 918–927.
21. Lee, K.S., Ernst, A., Trentham, D.E. et al. (2006). Relapsing polychondritis: prevalence of expiratory CT airway abnormalities. *Radiology* 240: 565–573.
22. Majid, A., Sosa, A.F., Ernst, A. et al. (2013). Pulmonary function and flow-volume loop patterns in patients with tracheobronchomalacia. *Respir. Care* 58: 1521–1526.
23. Myer, C.M. 3rd, O'Connor, D.M., and Cotton, R.T. (1994). Proposed grading system for subglottic stenosis based on endotracheal tube sizes. *Ann. Otol. Rhinol. Laryngol.* 103: 319–323.
24. McCaffrey, T.V. (1992). Classification of laryngotracheal stenosis. *Laryngoscope* 102: 1335–1340.
25. Freitag, L., Ernst, A., Unger, M. et al. (2007). A proposed classification system of central airway stenosis. *Eur. Respir. J.* 30: 7–12.
26. Nakamura, K., Terada, N., Ohi, M. et al. (1991). Tuberculous bronchial stenosis: treatment with balloon bronchoplasty. *Am. J. Roentgenol.* 157: 1187–1188.
27. Sheski, F.D. and Mathur, P.N. (1998). Long-term results of fiberoptic bronchoscopic balloon dilation in the management of benign tracheobronchial stenosis. *Chest* 114: 796–800.

28 Strausz, J. (1997). Management of postintubation tracheal stenosis with stent implantation. *J. Bronchol. Interv. Pulmonol.* 4: 294–296.

29 Freitag, L. and Darwiche, K. (2014). Endoscopic treatment of tracheal stenosis. *Thorac. Surg. Clin.* 24: 27–40.

30 Kim, H. (1998). Stenting therapy for stenosing airway disease. *Respirology* 3: 221–228.

31 Dumon, J.F. (1990). A dedicated tracheobronchial stent. *Chest* 97: 328–332.

32 Dumon, J.-F., Cavaliere, S., Diaz-Jimenez, J.P. et al. (1996). Seven-year experience with the Dumon prosthesis. *J. Bronchol. Interv. Pulmonol.* 3: 6–10.

33 Becker, H.D. (1995). Stenting of the central airways. *J. Bronchol. Interv. Pulmonol.* 2: 98–106.

34 Musani, A.I., Jensen, K., Mitchell, J.D. et al. (2012). Novel use of a percutaneous endoscopic gastrostomy tube fastener for securing silicone tracheal stents in patients with benign proximal airway obstruction. *J. Bronchol. Interv. Pulmonol.* 19: 121–125.

35 Miwa, K., Takamori, S., Hayashi, A. et al. (2004). Fixation of silicone stents in the subglottic trachea: preventing stent migration using a fixation apparatus. *Ann. Thorac. Surg.* 78: 2188–2190.

36 Lee, P., Kupeli, E., and Mehta, A.C. (2010). Airway stents. *Clin. Chest Med.* 31: 141–150.

37 Martinez-Ballarin, J.I., Diaz-Jimenez, J.P., Castro, M.J. et al. (1996). Silicone stents in the management of benign tracheobronchial stenoses. Tolerance and early results in 63 patients. *Chest* 109: 626–629.

38 Eom, J.S., Kim, H., Park, H.Y. et al. (2013). Timing of silicone stent removal in patients with post-tuberculosis bronchial stenosis. *Ann. Thorac. Med.* 8: 218–223.

39 Montgomery, W.W. (1965). T-tube tracheal stent. *Arch. Otolaryngol.* 82: 320–321.

40 Carretta, A., Casiraghi, M., Melloni, G. et al. (2009). Montgomery T-tube placement in the treatment of benign tracheal lesions. *Eur. J. Cardiothorac. Surg.* 36: 352–356; discussion 356.

41 Jiang, J., Mao, J., Huang, J. (2016). A pilot study of a new Chinese nitinol alloy airway stent deployed system through bronchoscope. Presented at the 19th World Association for Bronchology and Interventional Pulmonology, Italy, p. 358.

42 Gaissert, H.A., Grillo, H.C., Wright, C.D. et al. (2003). Complication of benign tracheobronchial strictures by self-expanding metal stents. *J. Thorac. Cardiovasc. Surg.* 126: 744–747.

43 Madden, B.P., Loke, T.K., and Sheth, A.C. (2006). Do expandable metallic airway stents have a role in the management of patients with benign tracheobronchial disease? *Ann. Thorac. Surg.* 82: 274–278.

44 Kaye, R., Goldstein, T., Aronowitz, D. et al. (2017). Ex vivo tracheomalacia model with 3D-printed external tracheal splint. *Laryngoscope* 127: 950–955.

45 Cheng, G.Z., San Jose Estepar, R., Folch, E. et al. (2016). Three-dimensional printing and 3D slicer: powerful tools in understanding and treating structural lung disease. *Chest* 149: 1136–1142.

46 Freitag, L., Gordes, M., Zarogoulidis, P. et al. (2017). Towards individualized tracheobronchial stents: technical, practical and legal considerations. *Respiration* 94: 442–456.

47 Chen, W., Clauser, J., Thiebes, A.L. et al. (2017). Gefitinib/gefitinib microspheres loaded polyurethane constructs as drug-eluting stent coating. *Eur. J. Pharm. Sci.* 103: 94–103.

48 Schuurmans, M.M., Palheiros Marques, M., Freitag, L. et al. (2015). Biofilm formation in a permanent tracheal stent implanted for twenty-five years. *Respiration* 90: 327–328.

49 Smith, M.E. and Elstad, M. (2009). Mitomycin C and the endoscopic treatment of laryngotracheal stenosis: are two applications better than one? *Laryngoscope* 119: 272–283.

50 Chen, Y., Wu, H.Y., and Li, S.Y. (2012). Intralesional triamcinolone acetonide injection combined with conventional interventional modalities for the management of recalcitrant benign central airway stenosis: preliminary experience. *Zhonghua Jie HeHeHuXiZa Zhi* 35: 415–418.

51 Nashef, S.A., Dromer, C., Velly, J.F. et al. (1992). Expanding wire stents in benign tracheobronchial disease: indications and complications. *Ann. Thorac. Surg.* 54: 937–940.

52 Rea, F., Callegaro, D., Loy, M. et al. (2002). Benign tracheal and laryngotracheal stenosis: surgical treatment and results. *Eur. J. Cardiothorac. Surg.* 22: 352–356.

53 Pearson, F.G. and Andrews, M.J. (1971). Detection and management of tracheal stenosis following cuffed tube tracheostomy. *Ann. Thorac. Surg.* 12: 359–374.

54 Stoelben, E., Koryllos, A., Beckers, F. et al. (2014). Benign stenosis of the trachea. *Thorac. Surg. Clin.* 24: 59–65.

55 Ernst, A., Majid, A., Feller-Kopman, D. et al. (2007). Airway stabilization with silicone stents for treating adult tracheobronchomalacia: a prospective observational study. *Chest* 132: 609–616.

56 Buitrago, D.H., Wilson, J.L., Parikh, M. et al. (2017). Current concepts in severe adult tracheobronchomalacia: evaluation and treatment. *J. Thorac. Dis.* 9: E57–E66.

57 Murgu, S.D., Egressy, K., Laxmanan, B. et al. (2016). Central airway obstruction: benign strictures, tracheobronchomalacia, and malignancy-related obstruction. *Chest* 150: 426–441.

附 录

本书配套视频资源汇总

- 本书英文版配套视频资料网址：http://www.wiley.com/go/wang4e

本书英文版视频资料密码：patients

- 本书中文版配套视频资料网址：https://mp.zhizhuma.com/c/36l/121544JOB31.q

本书中文版视频资料总二维码